Clinicopathological Correlation of Oral Diseases

Wanninayake M Tilakaratne • Thomas George Kallarakkal
Editors

Clinicopathological Correlation of Oral Diseases

Springer

Editors
Wanninayake M Tilakaratne
Department of Oral and Maxillofacial Clinical Sciences
Faculty of Dentistry
Universiti Malaya
Kuala Lumpur, Malaysia

Thomas George Kallarakkal
Department of Oral and Maxillofacial Clinical Sciences
Faculty of Dentistry
Universiti Malaya
Kuala Lumpur, Malaysia

ISBN 978-3-031-24407-0   ISBN 978-3-031-24408-7 (eBook)
https://doi.org/10.1007/978-3-031-24408-7

This Springer imprint is published by the registered company Springer Nature Switzerland AG
The registered company address is: Gewerbestrasse 11, 6330 Cham, Switzerland

Foreword

This comprehensive textbook consisting of 66 chapters is an excellent reference source on oral diseases written by invited experts in the field. The book concisely addresses a range of topics comprehensively covering the curriculum in Oral Medicine, Oral Pathology, Oral Surgery and also includes the broader aspects of Cariology and Periodontology.

This book is unique in its coverage in a number of aspects. Each chapter starts with a guide to history taking based on a patient's complaint to explore the symptomatology of a large range of oral disorders. The reasoning behind the selection of key questions during history taking is explained to the reader, and based on the responses each chapter presents a differential diagnosis that leads to appropriate special investigations. Based on the findings the reader is taken through steps in decision making and is directed to a final diagnosis. This is followed by a comprehensive clinicopathological description of the disorder and the basic clinical management helpful to the clinician. For the practicing Oral Medicine and Oral Surgery specialists and trainees, additional information is included on staging of the disease, an update on the current opinion, and steps in surgical management. This book, in my opinion, will change the way how the readers will approach history taking in their clinical practice.

In the recent decade there has been some tremendous advances in our understanding of the biology and genetics of oral diseases. The molecular biology sections presented in some chapters in this textbook summarise the important achievements made on this rapidly expanding topic. These scientific advances are presented in a clear and understandable way that the reader would find it easy to grasp rather than having to grapple through journals or very extensive published literature.

I found the overall presentation of the book very pleasing. The individual chapters are presented in a reader friendly manner. The core information is presented in an easily accessible format that is ideally suited to student understanding and to help in revision when preparing for examinations. Each chapter is well illustrated with photographs, to convey to the reader clinical presentations and the intricate details from pathological processes to surgical techniques.

The contributors are well-known teachers in dental schools mostly from South and Southeast Asia, and this book has drawn them together in a unique collaboration to provide an all-encompassing review of the current state of knowledge on oral diseases. The textbook is edited by an eminent globally recognised academic in the field of Oral and Maxillofacial Pathology and Medicine together with another experienced academic colleague. Professor Wanninayake M Tilakaratne, former Dean of the Faculty of Dental Sciences, University of Peradeniya and currently Professor and Senior Consultant in Oral Pathology Faculty of Dentistry Universiti Malaya, is a world-renowned Professor who has contributed to teaching Oral Pathology in several universities including Queen Mary University and Guy's and St Thomas Hospitals in the United Kingdom. His in-depth knowledge from his widely published research in Oral Pathology and Medicine has indeed helped to raise the didactic standard of this textbook. Co-editor Associate Professor Thomas George Kallarakkal is a dedicated teacher and a researcher at the Universiti Malaya with years of experience in Oral Pathology and Medicine. He has recently contributed to the WHO book on Head and Neck Tumours. His areas of interest include verrucopapillary oral lesions, epithelial dysplasia, testing for HPV, and developing large databases for image analysis of high-risk oral lesions.

The book will appeal to a wide variety of readers including undergraduate students in dentistry, general dentists, and primary care practitioners. I would also especially recommend this book to higher trainees who are seeking specialisation in Oral Medicine, Oral Pathology, Maxillofacial Surgery, and other branches of dentistry.

With very best wishes!

Saman Warnakulasuriya
Emeritus Professor of Oral Medicine and Experimental Pathology,
King's College London, London, UK
WHO Collaborating Centre for Oral Cancer,
London, UK

20 March 2023

Preface

Clinicopathological Correlation of Oral Diseases is a book aimed at undergraduates, early-stage postgraduates, and practitioners. This book differs from most conventional clinical textbooks at present in many aspects. Clinicopathological correlation is the most widely accepted concept in teaching clinical students on how to arrive at a rational and accurate diagnosis.

The book discusses case-based scenarios, which help in case-based learning and clinical reasoning. Every chapter consists of a detailed approach to the definitive diagnosis of a given disease starting from history taking, clinical examination, and investigations. A detailed account is included in each chapter as a justification for differential diagnosis and necessary investigations. Moreover, a well-designed format of asking questions in order to gather information about a patient's history and examination findings has been proposed in each chapter. A detailed and up-to-date account on each specific disease is described after the section featuring a case-based scenario in every chapter. Salient features of the disease are embedded in a table for easy reference and understanding. One of the unique features in the book is the inclusion of a diagnostic and management algorithm, which imparts a broader knowledge to the reader on related entities to a particular disease and the ways in which they can be differentiated from each other. Finally, a self-assessment exercise is included, covering all major aspects of the disease.

We as editors hope that the novel approach we have tried to introduce will help the readership to improve diagnostic skills in oral and maxillofacial diseases. We would like to extend our gratitude to all contributors for accepting our invitation with generosity. Special thanks are due to Dr. Goh Yet Ching and Dr. Nur Fauziani Binti Zainul Abidin for the help extended in providing histopathological pictures. In addition, we would like to thank all our friends and family members for their help and constructive comments.

This book is planned to be published as part of the Golden Jubilee celebrations of the Faculty of Dentistry, Universiti Malaya, Kuala Lumpur, Malaysia.

Wanninayake M Tilakaratne
Kuala Lumpur, Malaysia

Thomas George Kallarakkal
Kuala Lumpur, Malaysia

Contents

XVIII Orofacial Syndromes

XIX Forensic Odontology

Contributors

Nur Fauziani Zainul Abidin, BDS, MClinDent Department of Oral and Maxillofacial Clinical Sciences, Faculty of Dentistry, Universiti Malaya, Kuala Lumpur, Malaysia

Ajith Manjula Attygalla, BDS, MS, FDSRCS Department of Oral and Maxillofacial Surgery, Faculty of Dental Sciences, University of Peradeniya, Peradeniya, Sri Lanka

Dhanushka Leuke Bandara, BDS, MD Department of Oral Medicine and Periodontology, Faculty of Dental Sciences, University of Peradeniya, Peradeniya, Sri Lanka

Siew Wui Chan, DDS, MClinDent Department of Oral and Maxillofacial Clinical Sciences, Faculty of Dentistry, Universiti Malaya, Kuala Lumpur, Malaysia

Manil Fonseka, BDS, MS (Resto), LDSRCS Department of Restorative Dentistry, Faculty of Dental Sciences, University of Peradeniya, Peradeniya, Sri Lanka

Yet Ching Goh, BDS, MClinDent Department of Oral and Maxillofacial Clinical Sciences, Faculty of Dentistry, Universiti Malaya, Kuala Lumpur, Malaysia

Firdaus Hariri, BDS, MBBS, MDS (OMFS) Department of Oral and Maxillofacial Clinical Sciences, Faculty of Dentistry, Universiti Malaya, Kuala Lumpur, Malaysia

Muhammad Kamil Hassan, BDS, MSc, FFDRCSI Department of Oral and Maxillofacial Clinical Sciences, Faculty of Dentistry, Universiti Malaya, Kuala Lumpur, Malaysia

Pilana Vithanage Kalani Shihanika Hettiarachchi, BDS, MD (OMFS) Department of Oral Medicine and Periodontology, Faculty of Dental Sciences, University of Peradeniya, Kandy, Sri Lanka

Siti Mazlipah Ismail, BDS, FDSRCS Department of Oral and Maxillofacial Clinical Sciences, Faculty of Dentistry, Universiti Malaya, Kuala Lumpur, Malaysia

Oral Cancer Research and Coordinating Centre, Faculty of Dentistry, Universiti Malaya, Kuala Lumpur, Malaysia

Ruwan Jayasinghe, BDS, MS, FDS RCPS Department of Oral Medicine and Periodontology, Faculty of Dental Sciences, University of Peradeniya, Peradeniya, Sri Lanka

Nadeena S. S. Jayasuriya, BDS, MS (OMFS) Department of Oral and Maxillofacial Surgery, Faculty of Dental Sciences, University of Peradeniya, Kandy, Sri Lanka

Jacob John, BDS, MDS (Prosthodontics) Department of Restorative Dentistry, Faculty of Dentistry, Universiti Malaya, Kuala Lumpur, Malaysia

Kathreena Kadir, BDS, MClinDent (OMFS) Department of Oral and Maxillofacial Clinical Sciences, Faculty of Dentistry, Universiti Malaya, Kuala Lumpur, Malaysia

Thomas George Kallarakkal, BDS, MDS Department of Oral and Maxillofacial Clinical Sciences, Faculty of Dentistry, Universiti Malaya, Kuala Lumpur, Malaysia

Daniel Lim, BDS, MClinDent (OMFS) Department of Oral and Maxillofacial Clinical Sciences, Faculty of Dentistry, Universiti Malaya, Kuala Lumpur, Malaysia

Phrabhakaran Nambiar, BDS, BSc Dent, MSc Dent, FF OMP Department of Oral and Maxillofacial Clinical Sciences, Faculty of Dentistry, Universiti Malaya, Kuala Lumpur, Malaysia

MAHSA University, Bandar Saujana Putra, Selangor, Malaysia

Wei Cheong Ngeow, BDS, FFDRCS, FDSRCS, MDSc, PhD Department of Oral and Maxillofacial Clinical Sciences, Faculty of Dentistry, Universiti Malaya, Kuala Lumpur, Malaysia

P. L. Ranganayaki Devi S. Palaniappan, BDS, MFDS RCSEd, MClinDent Department of Restorative Dentistry, Faculty of Dentistry, Universiti Malaya, Kuala Lumpur, Malaysia

Prasangi Madubhashini Peiris, BDS Department of Oral Medicine and Periodontology, Faculty of Dental Sciences, University of Peradeniya, Peradeniya, Sri Lanka

Rabi'ah Al-Adawiyah Rahmat, BDS, GDipForOdont, PhD Department of Oral and Maxillofacial Clinical Sciences, Faculty of Dentistry, Universiti Malaya, Kuala Lumpur, Malaysia

Jasmin Raja, MMed, MBBS Rheumatology unit, Faculty of Medicine, Universiti Malaya, Kuala Lumpur, Malaysia

Anand Ramanathan, BDS, MDS Department of Oral and Maxillofacial Clinical Sciences, Faculty of Dentistry, Universiti Malaya, Kuala Lumpur, Malaysia

Oral Cancer Research and Coordinating Center, Faculty of Dentistry, Universiti Malaya, Kuala Lumpur, Malaysia

Zakiah Mat Ripen, BDS, MClinDent (OMFS) Department of Oral and Maxillofacial Clinical Sciences, Faculty of Dentistry, Universiti Malaya, Kuala Lumpur, Malaysia

Karthick Sekar, BDS, MDS, MFDSRCS, FICD Department of Oral and Maxillofacial Clinical Sciences, Faculty of Dentistry, Universiti Malaya, Kuala Lumpur, Malaysia

Benedict Seo, BDS, DClinDent, PhD Department of Oral Diagnostic and Surgical Sciences, Faculty of Dentistry, University of Otago, Dunedin, New Zealand

P. Shanmuhasuntharam, BDS, FDSRCS Department of Oral and Maxillofacial Clinical Sciences, Faculty of Dentistry, Universiti Malaya, Kuala Lumpur, Malaysia

Harsha Lal De Silva, BDS, MS, FFDRCS, DClinDent Department of Oral Diagnostic and Surgical Sciences, Faculty of Dentistry, University of Otago, Dunedin, New Zealand

Dunedin Hospital, Southern District Health Board, Otago, New Zealand

B. S. M. S. Siriwardena, BDS, MPhil, MD, PhD, FRCPath Department of Oral Pathology, Faculty of Dental Sciences, University of Peradeniya, Peradeniya, Sri Lanka

Chuey Chuan Tan, BDS, MClinDent (OMFS) Department of Oral and Maxillofacial Clinical Sciences, Faculty of Dentistry, Universiti Malaya, Kuala Lumpur, Malaysia

Aruni Tilakaratne, BDS, PhD Department of Oral Medicine and Periodontology, Faculty of Dental Sciences, University of Peradeniya, Peradeniya, Sri Lanka

Department of Restorative Dentistry, Faculty of Dentistry, Universiti Malaya, Kuala Lumpur, Malaysia

Wanninayake M Tilakaratne, BDS, MS, FDSRCS, FRCPath, PhD Department of Oral and Maxillofacial Clinical Sciences, Faculty of Dentistry, Universiti Malaya, Kuala Lumpur, Malaysia

Parakrama Wijekoon, BDS, MS Department of Oral and Maxillofacial Surgery, Faculty of Dental Sciences, University of Peradeniya, Peradeniya, Sri Lanka

Zuraiza Mohamad Zaini, BDS, MDSc, MRACDS, PhD Department of Oral and Maxillofacial Clinical Sciences, Faculty of Dentistry, Universiti Malaya, Kuala Lumpur, Malaysia

Oral Cancer Research and Coordinating Center, Faculty of Dentistry, Universiti Malaya, Kuala Lumpur, Malaysia

Nurul Izyan Zainuddin, BDS, DClinDent Department of Oral and Maxillofacial Clinical Sciences, Faculty of Dentistry Universiti Malaya, Kuala Lumpur, Malaysia

Introduction

Contents

Guide to Diagnose Oral Lesions: Principles of Clinicopathological Approach

Thomas George Kallarakkal and Wanninayake M Tilakaratne

Contents

W. M Tilakaratne, T. G. Kallarakkal (eds.), *Clinicopathological Correlation of Oral Diseases*,
https://doi.org/10.1007/978-3-031-24408-7_1

Learning Goals

1. Devise the correct way of compiling the history with appropriate questions.
2. Deduce appropriate procedures in clinical examination.
3. Justify the relevant investigations required to arrive at the diagnosis.
4. Comprehend the importance of clinicopathological correlation in arriving at the correct diagnosis.

A clinician when encountering a patient with oral and maxillofacial disease is faced with vast amount of information pertaining to the patient's chief complaint, personal and medical history. The formulation of a provisional diagnosis or a differential diagnosis is one of the most critical and intellectually challenging aspects of medical reasoning. The clinician must be able to judiciously compare the probabilities of various diseases that could have caused the patient's signs and symptoms using his/her vast knowledge of oral health and disease.

Clinicopathological correlation is a thought process that combines clinical information and findings from microscopic examination of biopsy specimens together with findings from other investigations. It helps to confirm clinical suspicions and provide more information in uncertain clinical cases. Many a time, histopathological examination may not suffice to arrive at a definitive diagnosis but requires correlation with the patient's chief complaint, pertinent clinical examination findings and findings from other relevant ancillary tests such as imaging studies, haematological, serological and biochemical investigations. In this perspective, a better understanding of the disease, its definitive diagnosis and most importantly, proper and correct management of the patient is not compromised.

Diagnosis is the process of identifying a disease process from its signs and symptoms and other relevant investigations. It requires acquisition of data about the patient and their presenting complaint through observation, hearing, touching and sometimes smelling. In the present age, patients have access to a wide variety of sources of information on health care. This may be used by them for self-diagnosis or to demand a specific treatment. The clinician must be able to allay their concerns and initiate optimal scientific and evidence-based treatment. A correct diagnosis facilitates appropriate and effective treatment as well as prognostication. The diagnostic process comprises three main components:

1. History taking: A thorough history taking usually provides the diagnosis in 80% of the cases.
2. Physical examination.
3. Investigations which may be essential to validate the history and examination findings.

1.1 History Taking

The initial contact with the patient is crucial in establishing good communication between the patient and the clinician. The clinician should be courteous and professional in his approach and should ensure that the patient is the focus of attention. History taking needs to be designed to suit the individual patient. Patients may differ from one another with some being articulate while the others may be nervous or confused. It is very essential to build a good rapport with the patients to elicit useful information. This can be initiated by posing open-ended questions (those questions which do not suggest an answer) to the patient that allows them to open-up and speak at length, thereby helping them to gain some confidence. The clinician should be careful to avoid unwanted use of medical jargon and leading questions (those questions which suggest the answer) that may compel the patients to agree with the clinician. Questions seeking relevant social or psychological history and information on embarrassing medical conditions can be delayed until the patient has gained enough confidence to reveal everything unconditionally to the clinician. The patient should be encouraged to tell their story in their own words, and when required, methodical questioning should be employed to elicit more information. The clinician will be able to assess the psychological status and the patient's expectation from the consultation and the treatment during the history taking. It is important to gauge demographic information such as age, gender and ethnicity of the patient. Certain disease states such as degenerative joint diseases involving the temporomandibular joint tend to occur more commonly in the elderly while mucocutaneous disorders such as lichen planus have a predilection for female patients.

The history of the presenting complaint which is recorded in the patient's own words should describe the state of health before the occurrence of the present complaint, the duration of the symptoms, any aggravating or relieving factors and any change in the course of the symptoms over the period of time. Any previous treatment that the patient has had should be detailed. A lack of response to a specific treatment in the past may prompt the diagnosis to be revisited. The patient's medical history will help to understand whether the patient's presenting complaint is an oral manifestation of an underlying systemic disease. Similarly, adequate knowledge regarding the patient's medical history is crucial as it may influence the patient's dental or surgical treatment. A detailed dental history provides comprehensive information on the dental treatment that the patient has had previously. Inappropriate dental treatments in the past such as an ill-fitting denture or a faulty restoration with high bite may result in pain. A lack of timely dental intervention in the past could have aggravated a carious process eventually resulting in pulpal inflammation or necrosis with resultant severe pulpal pain. A comprehensive subjective review of systems (ROS) (◘ Table 1.1) will help gather information on diseases affecting the different body systems which could either affect the dental treatment or may be a clue to the presenting oral manifestations.

Questions pertaining to the family history will uncover any hereditary disorders such as haemophilia or amelogenesis imperfecta that have a recessive pattern of inheritance. Details of the patient's social history will reveal whether the patient has a partner or a family and the extent of support that can be anticipated as it will influence the implementation of a treatment regimen. Information on patient's habits and sexual history is relevant to the diagnosis of specific oral mucosal lesions.

◘ **Table 1.1** Subjective symptoms associated with different body systems

Body systems/ organs	Symptoms
General	Fever, weight loss
Eyes	Changes in vision, photophobia, blurring of vision
Ears	Hearing changes, tinnitus, vertigo
Psychiatric disorders	Changes in mood or sleep pattern, emotional disturbances, anxiety, depression
Skin	Rashes, pruritus, vesicles, bullae
Nervous system	Sensory changes, seizures, unilateral or bilateral weakness, changes in coordination and memory
Respiratory system	Cough, dyspnea, wheezing, chest pain
Cardiovascular system	Chest pain, dyspnea, orthopnea, oedema
Gastrointestinal system	Changes in appetite, constipation, diarrhea, bloating, melena, abdominal pain, hematemesis
Genitourinary system	Changes in urinary frequency or urgency, dysuria, hematuria, nocturia, incontinence
Endocrine system	Skin or mucosal pigmentations, polyuria, polydipsia, polyphagia, temperature intolerance
Musculoskeletal system	Muscle and joint pain, deformities, joint swellings, spasms, changes in range of motion
Circulatory system	Easy bruising, epistaxis, spontaneous gingival bleeding, increased bleeding after trauma
Lymphatic system	Swollen and enlarged lymph nodes

1.2 Clinical Examination

A thorough history and clinical examination will facilitate the clinician to make a provisional diagnosis or a differential diagnosis. The clinician should be able to determine if the patient has any physical difficulties such as abnormal gait, or learning disability as soon as the patient enters the clinic and is greeted by the clinician. Other disabilities such as blindness, deafness, speech or language disorders as well as the patient's mood and general well-being will also be evident. A general examination includes recording of the patient's body weight and vital signs. The vital signs include:

1. Conscious state: An alteration in the conscious state may be a reflection of a head injury or drug abuse.
2. Temperature: The normal body temperature is 36.6 °C (oral). An adult with an oral temperature above 37.8 °C is pyrexic. The fever may be caused due to an underlying infection (bacteria/viral), inflammatory conditions (rheumatoid arthritis) and malignancy besides other causes.
3. Pulse: The normal reference range for pulse rate is 60–80 beats/min in an adult and is elevated due to exercise, anxiety, fever, cardiac disorders and hyperthyroidism among many other factors. Any change in the rhythm, character and the volume of the pulse should be brought to the attention of a medical physician.
4. Blood pressure: The normal systolic/diastolic blood pressure is 120/80 mm of Hg. The blood pressure may be elevated in health conditions such as cardiovascular disease, kidney disease, adrenal disorders and thyroid disease. Several factors including stress, obesity, smoking, excess intake of alcohol, increased salt in the diet, old age and family history can contribute to an elevated blood pressure.
5. Respiration: A reference range of 12–20 breaths/min is considered a normal respiratory rate in an adult. Tachypnea may be caused to several pathological states including asthma, chronic obstructive pulmonary disease (COPD), heart failure and anaemia.

Extra oral examination of the face and the neck can determine whether the patient has anaemia (pallor of the skin and palpebral conjunctiva), jaundice (yellowish sclera), thyroid disease (exophthalmos) and lymphadenopathy. Swellings due to inflammatory or neoplastic disorders and malar rash indicative of lupus erythematosus will be easily apparent. The parotid and submandibular salivary glands and the lymph nodes in the neck should be palpated. Lymphadenopathy is a common manifestation of infection or a lymphoreticular malignancy. The character (site, size, shape, consistency and tenderness) of the enlarged lymph nodes should be recorded. Evaluation of the temporomandibular joint (TMJ) involves examination for any facial asymmetry indicative of masseteric hypertrophy suggestive of bruxism, mandibular opening and closing paths (straight/corrected deviation/uncorrected deviation), range of mandibular movements (open movements/lateral excursions/protrusive movements), joint noises (click/crepitus) during opening and closing and joint locking. The TMJ and the muscles of mastication should be palpated. The pain induced in the joint and the muscles due to palpation is a classical clinical test to determine if the induced pain replicates the patient's chief complaint of pain if any. Maxillary sinuses should be palpated for tenderness over the maxillary antrum to exclude any sinus infections. The cranial nerves particularly the trigeminal nerve and the facial nerve that guide the facial movement and sensation from the face should be examined for defective function (◘ Table 1.2).

◘ Table 1.2 Signs indicative of defective function of the cranial nerves

Cranial nerve	Signs indicative of defective function
I. Olfactory	Impaired sense of smell for common odours
II. Optic	Visual acuity determined using a hand-held eye chart or a Snellen chart is impaired Visual fields determined by confrontation using the examiner's finger or coloured pen are impaired Pupil responses are impaired
III. Oculomotor	Diplopia (double vision) Strabismus (eye looks down and laterally) Ptosis (drooping of eyelid) Pupil dilated Pupillary reactions: Direct reflex (constriction that occurs when the pupil is exposed to light) is impaired Indirect reflex/consensual reflex (simultaneous constriction of the opposite pupil that occurs when the pupil is exposed to light) is impaired
IV. Trochlear	Diplopia (double vision) Strabismus (eye looks down and laterally) Patients with defective trochlear nerve function will have normal pupillary reactions and not have ptosis contrary to patients with defective oculomotor nerve function
V. Trigeminal	Reduced sensation over the face Impaired corneal reflex Impaired taste sensation Reduced motor power of masticatory muscles Weakness on opening of jaw
VI. Abducens	Diplopia (double vision) Strabismus (eye looks down and laterally) Lateral eye movements impaired to the affected side
VII. Facial	Flattening of the nasolabial groove Impaired motor power of facial muscles (inability to smile, blow-out cheeks, show the teeth) Impaired corneal reflex Impaired taste perception
VIII. Vestibulocochlear	Impaired hearing Impaired balance Nystagmus (an involuntary rhythmic side-to-side, up and down or circular motion of the eyes) Tinnitus
IX. Glossopharyngeal	Reduced gag reflex Deviation of the uvula Reduced taste sensation Voice may have a nasal tone
X. Vagus	Reduced gag reflex Voice may be impaired
XI. Accessory	Impaired motor power of trapezius and sternocleidomastoid muscle
XII. Hypoglossal	Impaired motor power of the tongue Abnormal speech Ipsilateral deviation on protrusion

The muscles of facial expression are innervated by the facial nerve. A lower motor neuron lesion involving the facial nerve results in Bell's palsy characterized by paresis/paralysis of all the ipsilateral muscles. Bell's palsy and stroke are the most common causes of abrupt onset of unilateral facial weakness. The clinical presentation of patients with orofacial pain (OFP) is usually complex and may be driven by many factors. The patients may be well or may have significant comorbidities that may be psychological or related to other medical problems. A clinician consulting a patient with OFP should have excellent communication skills as the pain is invisible, and a diagnosis is based upon what the patients communicate with the clinician. A thorough pain history (▫ Table 1.3) is a cornerstone in establishing a diagnosis in patients with OFP.

Examination of the lips is useful to assess cyanosis which is seen in cardiac or respiratory disease. Angular chelitis is observed very commonly in oral candidiasis, iron or vitamin deficiency disorders. Intraoral examination should be performed only with a good light source, mouth mirrors and compressed air for drying the teeth. If the patient is wearing any removable prostheses or appliances, it should be removed first to ensure that all the areas are thoroughly visualized. The fit, function and the relationship of the prosthesis to any lesion if present should be assessed. Evidence of oral dryness as observed by sticking of the mouth mirror to the oral mucosa, absence of normal saliva pooling in the floor of the mouth, presence of lipstick stains on the anterior teeth and food residues on the teeth suggest reduced secretory function of the salivary glands. The soft tissues of the mouth should be examined first in a systematic manner to include all the areas. The floor of the mouth, soft palate and tonsillar areas are high-risk sites for oral squamous cell carcinoma and should not be missed during the examination. The tongue should be held in a piece of gauze and extended from side to side to enable better visualization of the lateral tongue and posterior floor of the mouth. Suspicious areas should be palpated to check for the presence of any induration. The opening of the salivary ducts and the patency of the ducts should be assessed by checking the flow of saliva through the ducts. Dental examination should encompass the status of the periodontal health, caries and restorative state of all the teeth present in the mouth. Teeth vitality must be checked if they are symptomatic and if they are located in the region of jaw swellings or radiolucent jaw lesions.

▫ Table 1.3 SOCRATES—mnemonic for pain assessment

Site—Where is the pain? Or the maximal site of the pain.
Onset—When did the pain start, and was it sudden or gradual? (State whether it is progressive or regressive.)
Character—What is the pain like? An ache? Stabbing?
Radiation—Does the pain radiate anywhere?
Associations–Any other signs or symptoms associated with the pain?
Time course—Does the pain follow any pattern?
Exacerbating/Relieving factors—Does anything change the pain?
Severity—How bad is the pain?

Lumps and swellings are relatively common in the mouth. They may be developmental, inflammatory, traumatic or neoplastic in origin. They may also be caused due to drugs, hormonal imbalances or may be a manifestation of specific disorders such as fibro-osseous lesions. The important features to be assessed when making a provisional diagnosis of a swelling are summarized in ▫ Table 1.4.

Oral ulcers may arise as a result of local or systemic factors and are generally very painful. They can be broadly classified into acute and chronic ulcers. Acute oral ulcers have an abrupt onset and persist for a short duration. The more common acute oral ulcers include traumatic ulcers, recurrent aphthous stomatitis and ulcers due to viral infections. It is generally agreed that an ulcer which persists for more than 2 weeks is a chronic ulcer. Examples of chronic ulcers are drug-induced ulcers, ulcers due to altered immunity as seen in pemphigus vulgaris, mucous membrane pemphigoid and erosive oral lichen planus. A persistent ulcer that shows no evidence of healing could be highly suspicious of a mucosal malignancy such as squamous cell carcinoma. Vital information that is essential when making a diagnosis of an oral ulcer is whether the ulcers are a) acute or chronic, b) primary or recurrent and c) single or multiple. Features that need to be assessed during examination of an ulcer are summarized in ▫ Table 1.5.

The diagnosis and the optimal treatment plan may be deduced from the history and examination findings. Very often, there are various possible diagnoses which should be recorded in their order of probability based on their prevalence and likelihood of causing the signs and symptoms. The types of diagnosis include:

Clinical diagnosis: made from the history and examination.

Provisional diagnosis: an initial diagnosis from which further investigations need to be planned.

Differential diagnosis: the process of making a diagnosis by considering the similarities and differences between similar conditions.

Table 1.4 Important features to be assessed in reviewing a swelling

Feature
Duration—Reactive lesions such as mucoceles and swellings due to infections arise rapidly within a few days. Benign tumours grow slowly and may be present for many years, while malignant tumours grow rapidly within a period of months
Alteration in size—A mucocele may increase and decrease in size over time, while benign and malignant neoplasms usually do not decrease in size
Position—The anatomical position and the proximity to adjacent structures should be recorded Midline lesions —are usually developmental in origin (e.g. torus palatinius) Bilateral lesions —are usually benign (e.g. dialysis) Unilateral lesions—tend to be neoplastic in nature
Size: The size should always be measured and recorded
Shape—Some swellings have a characteristic shape. A parotid swelling usually fills the space between the posterior border of the mandible and the mastoid process
Colour—The colour of the lesion reflects the content of the swelling. A haemagioma may appear purple or red due to the vascularity of the lesion. A naevus or a melanoma usually appears brown or black due to the presence of the melanin pigment in the lesion
Temperature—Inflammatory swellings such as abscesses are warm to touch
Tenderness—Inflammatory swellings are tender
Mobility—Neoplastic swellings tend to be fixed to the underlying structures or the overlying skin or mucosa
Consistency—They may be soft and fluctuant, firm or stony hard in consistency. Fluctuant swellings contain fluid, while stony hard or indurated swellings are highly suggestive of a malignancy or a lesion with hard tissue formation
Surface texture—The surface characteristics should be recorded. Papillomas have a warty or papillary surface. Malignant neoplasms tend to have a nodular or verrucous surface and may show surface ulceration
Margins—Malignant swellings have ill-defined margins, while benign swellings have clearly defined margins
Number—Multiple swellings are suggestive of an infective or developmental origin. Specific syndromes may have multiple similar swellings

Table 1.5 Important features to be assessed during the examination of an ulcer

Inspection findings:
Site
Size (Extent)
Tender/painful
Margin (Shape)—Regular/irregular
Edge: Sloping (healing ulcer)/punched out (trophic ulcer)/undermined (tuberculous ulcer)/rolled-out (basal cell carcinoma)/everted (squamous cell carcinoma)
Floor—Healthy/granulation tissue (healing ulcer)/slough (necrotic tissue—non-healing ulcer)
Discharge—Serous/serosanguinous/purulent
Palpation findings:
Margin/edge
Base—Marked induration at the base of the ulcer is a characteristic feature of squamous cell carcinoma

1.3 Investigations

Investigations are intended to determine specific answers regarding a probable diagnosis. They should not be employed as a routine procedure. Prior to ordering the investigations, the clinician should explain to the patient: a) the nature of the investigation, b) the potential benefits and possible adverse effects associated with the investigation and c) the implications of not carrying out the investigation. A witnessed and informed consent should be obtained for all invasive procedures. Strict infection control protocols should be in place prior to the procedure as all body fluids are considered potentially infectious. Certain lesions such as a pyogenic granuloma, which manifests as a gingival overgrowth, will need only a biopsy and histopathological examination to determine the diagnosis. There are other disease conditions such as Paget disease of bone which will require a corroboration of imaging, serological and histopathological investigations to determine the definitive diagnosis.

1.4 Imaging

Imaging techniques most commonly employed in the head and neck region are plain radiography, computerized tomography (CT), cone beam computerized tomography (CBCT), magnetic resonance imaging (MRI) and ultrasound. The clinician ordering the imaging investigation should be able to justify the need for the investigation due to the cumulative effect of radiation hazard. A formal radiologist's report should always be requested when the radiographic features appear unusual or beyond the comprehension of a clinician. The imaging modality and their specific applications are detailed in ◘ Table 1.6.

◘ **Table 1.6** Imaging modalities and their specific applications

Imaging modality	Applications
Intraoral radiography	
Periapical radiograph	• To demonstrate any pathology in the tooth (dental caries), periapical region (such as a granuloma and cyst), periodontium and adjacent bone
Bitewing radiograph	• To reveal any approximal caries and for reviewing the alveolar bone crest
Occlusal radiograph	• To review the facial and lingual bony cortices and adjacent areas such as floor of the mouth and palate
Extraoral radiography	
Dental panoramic tomography	• Valuable for a general full mouth survey including review of the antra and the temporomandibular joint • The radiation dose is significantly lower than a full mouth survey using intraoral periapical films
Sialography	• To assess patients with hyposalivation and salivary gland swelling • To detect salivary gland ductal obstruction • To detect developmental salivary gland disorders such as aplasia
Salivary scintigraphy	• To diagnose patients with salivary gland disorders such as Sjogren syndrome, salivary gland neoplasms, ductal obstruction and aplasia
Arthrography	• To assess patients with suspected internal derangements of the temporomandibular joint
Angiography	• To diagnose vascular anomalies and tumours • To assist in surgical procedures (microvascular surgery or embolization)
Computed axial tomography (CAT/CT)	• To visualize head and neck areas inaccessible to conventional radiographs • To clearly visualize hard tissue lesions • To determine tumour spread • To exclude intracranial or cranial base pathologies • To plan surgery and implant placement
Cone beam CT (CBCT)	• Similar to CT for imaging of jaws and related structures, but the scanning time and radiation dosage are significantly lower than a conventional CT.
Positron emission tomography (PET)	• To detect second primary tumours and metastasis. This is facilitated by mapping tissue metabolic activity based either on blood flow or glucose utilization.
Magnetic resonance imaging (MRI)	• To visualize soft tissues and lesions • To detect bone invasion • To review the temporomandibular joints
Ultrasound scanning (US)	• To review soft tissues including subcutaneous tissues, tendons, muscles, vessels and internal organs such lymph nodes and salivary glands

1.5 Histopathology

Biopsy and histopathological examination are critical for a definitive diagnosis of diseases of the mucosa, soft tissue and bone. Biopsy involves the removal and examination of a part (incisional biopsy) or whole of the lesion (excisional biopsy). An ideal incisional biopsy should be of sufficient size (10 mm × 5 mm × 4 mm) to provide enough information about the lesion and should include the lesional and peri-lesional tissue. For ulcerated lesions, much of the relevant information is obtained from the peri-lesional tissue as the lesion is often entirely denuded off the epithelium. Care should be taken in handling the soft tissues to avoid any crush artefacts that may be caused due to inadvertent squeezing of the tissues. The tissues for histopathological examination should be immediately fixed preferably in tenfold volume of buffered formalin or other fixatives at room temperature. Indications for a biopsy are summarized in ◘ Table 1.7.

Fine needle aspiration (FNA) biopsy is a process where a 21-gauge needle is inserted into the lesion and the aspirated cells are smeared on a slide. FNA biopsy does not always provide a definitive diagnosis but provides reliable information to differentiate benign from malignant neoplasms, determine the need for further investigations or initiate treatment. It is usually indicated for lymph node swellings, parotid gland tumours and deep-seated swellings. There are relatively less complications related to the procedure as the small-size needle does not cause any damage to the vital structures of the head and neck. However, the interpretation of the FNA biopsy requires thorough experience.

◘ Table 1.7 Indications for biopsy

Persistent soft or hard tissue lesions that do not respond to treatment
Persistent soft or hard tissue lesions of uncertain origin
Lesions that cause extreme concern to the patient such as a persistent lump or a red/white/pigmented lesion that is increasing in size
Lesions suspicious of a malignancy
Oral potentially malignant disorders such as leukoplakia, erythroplakia and lichen planus
To confirm the clinical diagnosis of conditions such as Sjogren syndrome
Non-healing ulcers and extraction sockets

1.6 Exfoliative Cytology

This is a process that involves the examination of cells scraped from the surface of a lesion. The process is relatively easy and is primarily useful for detecting candidal hyphae, virally damaged cells and acantholytic cells from vesiculobullous diseases such as pemphigus. A major disadvantage of exfoliative cytology is that it samples only the surface cells, while the deeper tissues cannot be assessed and hence, unreliable for diagnosing epithelial dysplasia or cancer.

1.7 Brush Biopsy

This technique utilizes a stiff-bristle brush to collect cells from the surface and the deeper layers by scraping. It is a non-invasive procedure that is relatively painless. The cells obtained are smeared on to a microscopic slide and are screened either manually or using an image analyser to identify the abnormal cells.

1.8 Molecular Tests

Molecular diagnostics are extremely useful for identification of genetic abnormalities and for rapid identification of bacteria and viruses. Malignant neoplasms which harbour characteristic genetic alterations can be detected by cytogenetics, polymerase chain reaction (PCR) or fluorescence in situ hybridization (FISH). The diagnosis of lymphomas is greatly aided with the use of molecular techniques which is otherwise difficult with conventional histopathology and immunohistochemistry (IHC). Specimens for immunofluorescence should not be fixed in formalin but should be sent to the laboratory for freezing or snap frozen on solid carbon dioxide or liquid nitrogen and sent to the laboratory within an hour. Vesiculobullous disorders such as pemphigus and mucous membrane pemphigoid are diagnosed by a direct immunofluorescence (DIF) test. It detects the presence of immune deposits (autoantibodies and/or complement) in the tissues. A fluorescein stain which fluoresces apple green under ultraviolet light is utilized for the DIF test. Indirect immunofluorescence test which detects the immune deposits (circulating autoantibodies and/or complement) in the serum is also utilized for the diagnosis and management of autoimmune disorders.

1.9 Haematological, Serological and Biochemical Investigations

Many systemic diseases have oral manifestations. Anaemias are associated with recurrent aphthous stomatitis and glossodynia or painful tongue. Leukaemias and multiple myelomas may primarily manifest as gingival enlargement and mobility of adjacent teeth. Appropriate haematological investigations can detect these specific disease states. These investigations are also essential to establish a definitive diagnosis in patients presenting with a variety of oral conditions and should be requested only when it is clinically indicated (Table 1.8).

The request form for the investigations should always include sufficient clinical details to allow the haematologist or the clinical expert to ensure that the appropriate test has been ordered and also to allow for the proper interpretation of results. A full blood count/picture useful to detect anaemias and leukaemias utilizes whole blood and should be collected in tubes containing EDTA. Assays to detect antibodies useful for detection of infections and autoimmune disorders and biochemical substances such as enzymes utilize serum obtained by collection of whole blood without anticoagulant. Table 1.9 summarizes the various commonly employed blood tests useful in the diagnosis of systemic diseases with oral manifestations.

Table 1.8 Common oral conditions that require a blood test to arrive at a definitive diagnosis

- Recurrent aphthous stomatitis
- Persistent sore and or dry mouth
- Oral lesions unusually resistant to treatment
- Persistent orofacial candidosis
- Abnormal taste sensation
- Oral signs and symptoms of anaemia, leukaemia and other systemic diseases

Table 1.9 Commonly used blood tests useful in the diagnosis of oral conditions

Test	Main uses
Full blood picture/complete blood count includes erythrocyte number, size and haemoglobin indices and differential white cell count	Anaemias and the effects of iron and vitamin B_{12} deficiency associated with common oral disorders, leukaemias
Blood film	Leukaemias, anaemias, infectious mononucleosis
Erythrocyte sedimentation rate (ESR)	Raised in systemic inflammatory and autoimmune disorders Particularly useful in the diagnosis of giant cell arteritis and granulomatosis with polyangitis
Serum iron and total iron-binding capacity	Iron deficiency associated with common oral disorders
Serum ferritin	Iron deficiency associated with common oral disorders
Red cell folate level	Folic acid deficiency associated with recurrent aphthous stomatitis and recurrent oral candidiasis
Vitamin B_{12} level	Vitamin B_{12} deficiency associated with recurrent aphthous stomatitis and recurrent oral candidiasis
Autoantibodies (rheumatoid factor, antinuclear factor, DNA-binding antibodies, SS-A, SS-B)	Raised in autoimmune disorders
Viral antibody titres (Herpes simplex, varicella zoster, mumps virus)	A rising titre of specific antibody indicates infection by a virus
Complement component levels	Systemic lupus erythematosus (SLE)
Serum angiotensin converting enzyme	Sarcoidosis
Serum calcium, phosphate and parathormone levels	Paget disease and hyperparathyroidism
Serum alkaline phosphatase	Paget disease and hyperparathyroidism
C-Reactive protein (CRP)	Acute and chronic infections including periodontal disease

1.10 Urinalysis

Urinalysis performed with dipsticks is used to detect the presence of blood, glucose, proteins, ketones, bilirubin and urobilinogen in the urine (Table 1.10).

A culture and sensitivity (C&S) test is the most useful microbiological investigation in the context of pus-producing bone and soft tissue oral infections to determine the causative microorganisms and their sensitivity to antibiotics. Empirical treatment is usually initiated for osteomyelitis, cellulitis, acute parotitis, systemic mycoses and other severe infections which is refined further based on the results of the C&S test. There are no other microbiological tests that can offer specific diagnostic value in oral infections. Direct gram-stained smears can diagnose oral candidiasis while haematoxylin and eosin (H & E) stained smears can show altered epithelial cells characteristic of viral infections without the need for additional microbiological tests to detect the causative organisms.

Table 1.10 Significance of findings from urinalysis

Condition	Significance
Glycosuria	Suggests diabetes mellitus
Ketonuria	May indicate diabetic ketoacidosis or starving
Bilirubin or urobilinogen	May indicate hepatobiliary disorders
Proteinuria	Suggestive of renal, urinary tract or cardiac disease
Haematuria	Indicative of renal or urinary tract disease

1.10.1 Skin Patch Test

Oral contact allergies (OCAs) arise as a result of exposure of the oral mucosa to dental materials, food and oral hygiene products. Flavouring agents and preservatives contained in food and oral hygiene products often serve as etiologic agents for OCA. The signs and symptoms of OCA are varied and comprise erythema, oedema, desquamation, vesicle formation and ulceration, leukoplakia-like lesions and lichenoid reactions. A skin patch test helps to determine the specific substances that cause allergic inflammation of a patient's skin. The allergens used for the test include dental materials as well as other additional allergens. Skin testing is preferred to mucosal testing owing to its higher sensitivity and specificity. In addition to mucosal testing, the concentration of the allergen should be 5–12 times higher in the oral mucosa compared to the skin resulting in more adverse events.

Once a definitive diagnosis has been established based on the history, clinical examination findings and investigations, the clinician should be able to effectively communicate the findings of the assessment to the patient or his/her representative. It is the responsibility of the clinician to ensure that the information regarding the disease is clearly understood by the patient or his/her representative. The clinician should follow ethical principles and professional responsibility to refer the patient to another health care professional if deemed necessary in the best interests of the patient.

1.11 Diagnostic Pathway

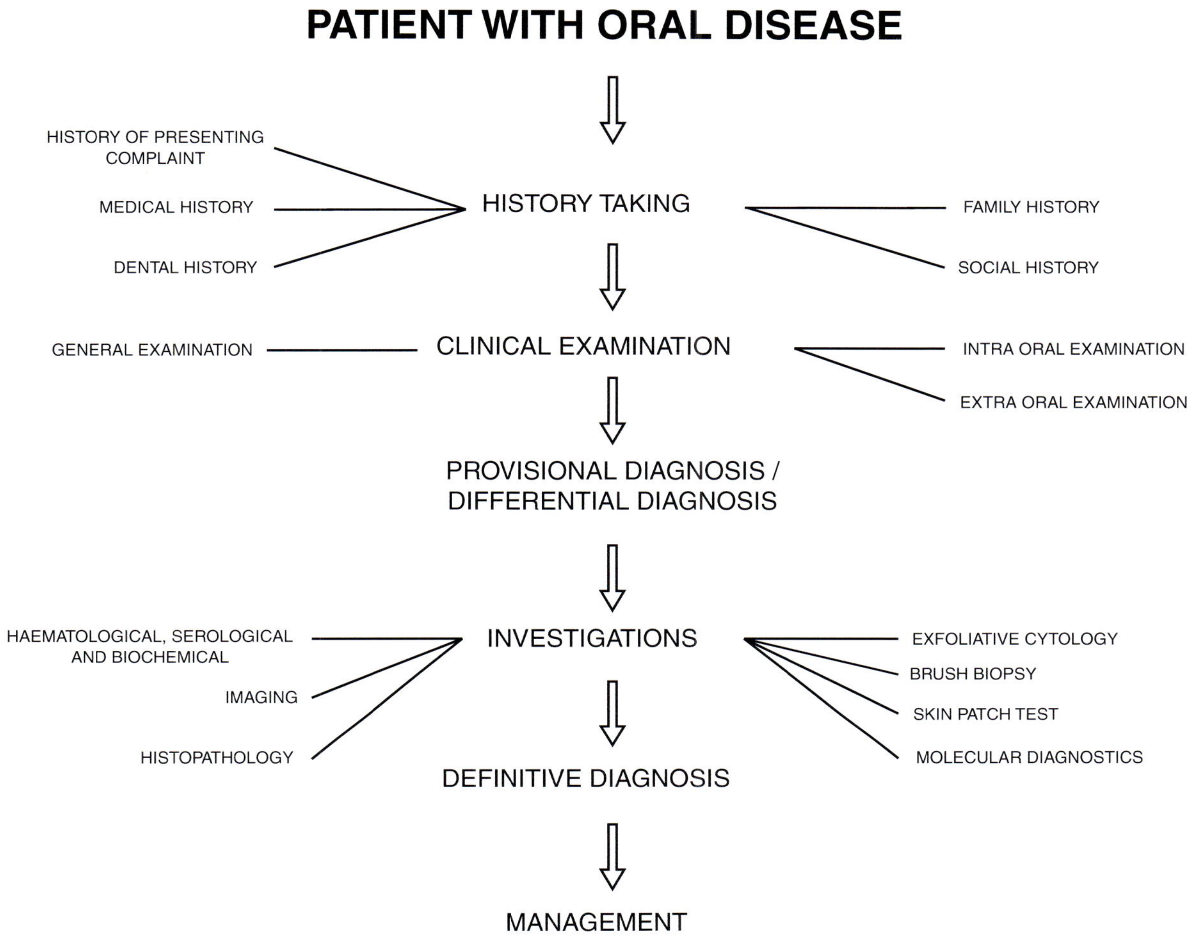

Summary

A clinical diagnostic process starts with medical history and physical examination where the clinician uses his professional and communication skills. Formulating a provisional diagnosis and differential diagnosis follows next. Appropriate investigations help to establish a definitive diagnosis. Establishing a definitive diagnosis is crucial for the optimal management and prognosis of the patient. Once a diagnosis has been established, the clinician should be able to effectively communicate the findings of the assessment to the patient or his/her representative. It is the responsibility of the clinician to ensure that the information regarding the disease is clearly understood by the patient or his/her representative. The clinician should follow ethical principles and professional responsibility in managing the patient or refer the patient to another health care professional if deemed necessary in the best interests of the patient.

Further Reading

1. Scully C. Oral and maxillofacial medicine: the basis of diagnosis and treatment. Elsevier Health Sciences; 2012.
2. Glick M. Burket's oral medicine. PMPH USA; 2015.
3. Cawson RA, Odell EW. Cawson's essentials of oral pathology and oral medicine e-book. Elsevier Health Sciences; 2017.
4. Dios PD, Scully C, de Almeida OP, Bagán JV, Taylor AM. Oral medicine and pathology at a glance. John Wiley & Sons; 2016.
5. Bruch JM, Treister NS. Clinical oral medicine and pathology. Humana Press; 2010. p. 66–8.
6. Ongole R. Text book of oral medicine, oral diagnosis and oral radiology. Elsevier India; 2009.

Pulp and Periodontal Diseases

Contents

Pain in an Upper Back Tooth: Pulpitis

Manil Fonseka

Contents

W. M Tilakaratne, T. G. Kallarakkal (eds.), *Clinicopathological Correlation of Oral Diseases*,
https://doi.org/10.1007/978-3-031-24408-7_2

Learning Goals

1. Understand the different presentations of a toothache
2. Understand the differential diagnosis of toothache based on its clinical presentation
3. Select the most appropriate treatment option for the management of pulpitis
4. Appreciate the indications of different treatment modalities in the management of pulpitis

2.1 Main Complaint

A 50-year-old patient complains of pain in relation to one of his upper left posterior teeth for a duration of 3 days.

2.2 History of Complaint

Question: When does the pain occur?

The pain is more pronounced when consuming hot/cold or sweet food or beverages. Occasionally, there is a sudden onset of pain without any reason.

Question: How long does the pain last?

The pain lasts for a long duration. It sometimes lasts for a few minutes to about an hour or 2 h.

Question: What is the nature of the pain?

It is a dull aching-type pain.

2.3 Additional Complaints

Question: Have you noticed any other problems?

There is retention of food between the upper right posterior teeth after a meal. Occasionally, I use a toothpick to remove the food debris. I also feel there is a cavity in relation to the upper right posterior teeth between the left premolars.

Question: Does the pain disturb your sleep?

I woke up the previous night with pain. I sat up and rinsed my mouth and took an analgesic. The pain settled down in about an hour.

Question: Did you notice anything unusual in the teeth prior to this episode of pain?

I had noticed a slight discoloration of one of my teeth on the upper right posterior region. The tooth had initially been slightly sensitive to hot and cold stimulation but was not unbearable. I had felt a bad taste in this region. I had noted these changes for about 2–3 months.

Question: Tell me about your meal habits?

I snack on biscuits and fruit drinks on a regular basis. These are consumed in between main meals. I consume three cups of milk tea with two teaspoons of sugar. I also have a habit of eating a bar of chocolate after lunch.

Question: How do you clean your teeth?

I brush twice a day using a herbal toothpaste. The night-time brushing session is missed frequently. I occasionally use a saltwater rinse.

Question: Are you suffering from any other medical problems such as heart disease, high blood pressure, diabetes, bleeding disorders or respiratory diseases? If yes, what kind of medications have you been taking until now?

I don't have any other medical problem. However, I feel that my mouth is quite dry, and I also have difficulty in swallowing. I sip water while eating to help in the swallowing.

Question: Have you undergone any surgery?

I have not undergone any surgery in the past.

Question: Have you undergone any dental treatment?

I have about six restorations done for decayed teeth. Two lower teeth had been extracted due to decay at the age of 12 years. Many of my milk teeth were also decayed and restored during my childhood.

Question: What is your occupation?

I am a proprietor of a grocery shop.

Question: Do you have any habits?

I do not have any betel-chewing habits. I am a non-smoker. I occasionally consume alcohol.

2

2.4 With the Findings from History, What Is Your Differential Diagnosis?

1. Irreversible pulpitis
2. Reversible pulpitis
3. Cracked tooth/cracked cusp
4. Abfraction/abrasion
5. Gingival recession
6. Maxillary sinusitis

2.5 How Do You Justify Your Differential Diagnosis After History Taking?

1. The history of pain is suggestive of irreversible pulpitis considering the onset of pain with or without stimulation, the relatively longer duration of pain and the nature of pain. Pain at night that disturbs the patient's sleep supports this diagnosis as well.
2. Pain on hot, cold and sweet stimulation may suggest reversible pulpitis. However, the duration, spontaneous occurrence of pain and the pain that disturbs the patient's sleep are not clear features of reversible pulpitis.
3. With a cracked tooth or a cusp, the patient could end up with spontaneous pain or pain especially with biting. The pain will be very sharp in nature. With a chronic cracked tooth, irreversible pulpitis could develop leading to a similar clinical presentation.
4. Abfraction and abrasion are common conditions affecting this age group where the cervical enamel, dentine and cementum are lost due to wear. Pain on stimulation and extreme sensitivity on stimulation could be a manifestation.
5. Gingival recession leads to exposure of radicular dentine which again could present as a tooth or teeth exhibiting similar symptoms. Complications of chronic periodontitis could lead to extreme recession.
6. Maxillary sinusitis could occasionally present as a dull ache in relation to the teeth whose roots are in close proximity to the maxillary sinus. The pain could be aggravated by various stimuli. Tilting the head forward may aggravate the discomfort.

2.6 Findings of Examination

The upper left second premolar (25) shows cavitation especially on the distal surface. Discoloration of the tooth is also noticeable (◘ Fig. 2.1). Examination and flossing of the proximal embrasures show food debris. A blast of air or water from a three-way syringe triggers the episode of pain. There is no tenderness of the tooth on percussion. The gingiva around the distal surface of the tooth appeared inflamed due to the long-term accumulation of food debris or due to improper hygiene measures due to the pain. The particular tooth did not show any wear facets, evidence of cracks and gingival recession. Electrical pulp testing or pulp sensibility testing was carried out which revealed a positive response.

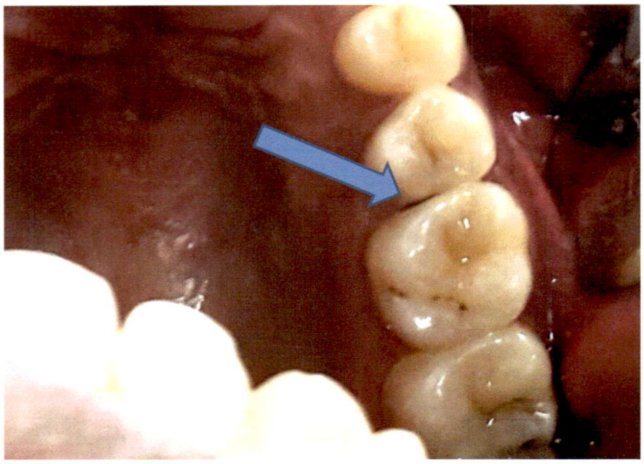

◘ **Fig. 2.1** Discoloration of the distal surface and food impaction are early signs of proximal caries on 25

2.7 What Other Relevant Features You Look for with the Findings You Have so Far?

Examination of the other teeth as well may show evidence of caries (decay). Trans-illumination of the teeth would show a darkened area of the caries-affected tooth or teeth. A general examination of the oral cavity should be carried out to assess the caries state of the patient. This includes the state and number of other restored and decayed teeth, any failing restorations, state of oral hygiene, any evidence of abscesses, gingival swellings, sinus tract openings, tenderness of the gingiva and mobility of teeth.

2.8 What Is Your Clinical Differential Diagnosis?

1. Irreversible pulpitis
2. Reversible pulpitis

2.9 How Would You Exclude Other Conditions and Justify the Inclusion of the Diseases That You Have Mentioned in the Differential Diagnosis to Arrive at a Working Diagnosis?

2.9.1 Cracked Tooth

This is common in the older age groups due to the progressive brittleness of teeth due to reduction in the moisture content of the tooth as a result of a reduced vasculature. On the other hand, the progressive deposition of secondary dentine also contributes to this. Heavily restored teeth and endodontically treated teeth are also prone to this condition. The pain mostly occurs on biting due to the opening of the cracked area due to occlusal forces. More remarkably, the pain is more intense on releasing of the bite as the herniated pulpal contents are being compressed due to the recoil of the opened crack. There could be tenderness localized on one cusp or area of the tooth if the cusp is involved. There will not be any evidence of caries. The crack may be visible or be observed on trans-illumination. Food packing which is generally associated with a cavitated tooth is not a feature of a cracked tooth. The pain is generally short-lasting. The patient may not bite on this side due to intense pain, and as a result, occlusal calculi may be noted due to lack of function (Fig. 2.2).

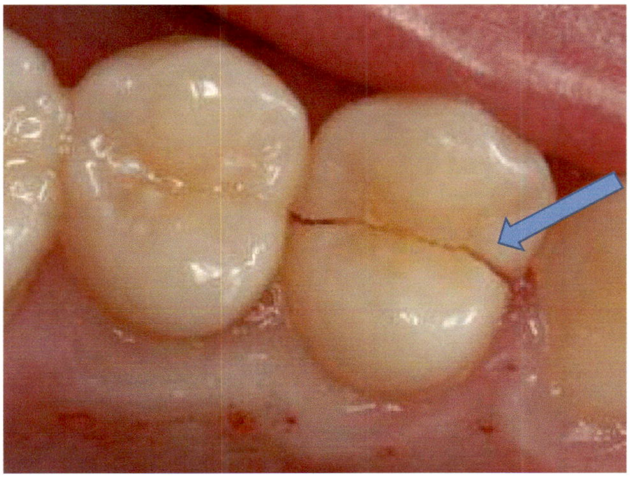

Fig. 2.2 Cracked upper right first premolar showing a visible crack may commonly give a similar complaint as described in this patient

2.9.2 Abfractions/Abrasions

The characteristic feature of this condition is that there will be wear facets mainly on the buccal cervical region of the tooth/teeth. Abfractions classically present as "V"-shaped defects on the cervical region of the teeth. The pain is mainly on stimulation and is short-lasting. The patient may avoid consuming hot or cold beverages due to the intense sensitivity or pain.

2.9.3 Gingival Recession

This condition presents as gross loss of gingiva covering the roots of teeth. The yellowish root dentine would be clearly visible on examination. The condition mainly presents as sensitivity on hot or cold stimulation. Underlying periodontal diseases may be noted on examination with deep pocketing, mobility and bone loss.

2.9.4 Maxillary Sinusitis

In this condition, there would not be any apparent cavitation, food stagnation or discoloration of teeth. The primary complaint would be a dull pain more pronounced on biting. Tilting the head would aggravate the condition. The patient may present with a history of allergic sinusitis or may be recovering from a common cold.

The above conditions can be excluded as associated features were not obvious in this patient.

2.10 What Is the Most Likely Diagnosis?

Irreversible pulpitis

2.11 How Would You Investigate This Patent?

1. Radiography—Periapical radiographs or dental-panoramic tomography
2. Electric pulp sensibility testing

2.12 What Are the Findings of Radiography and the Importance of Radiography in the Assessment of the Teeth Prior to Treatment?

A periapical radiograph obtained using a paralleling technique is mandatory in the assessment of teeth with pulpitis. Though it will not lead to a definitive diagnosis, it would help in assessment of the extent of caries (◘ Fig. 2.3). In addition, any changes in the periapical region such as loss of the lamina dura or development of periapical radiolucencies are suggestive of periapical pathology. The state of the alveolar process and bone loss suggestive of periodontal diseases may determine the prognosis of the tooth and help in deciding the treatment modality and the management plan for this tooth. If the patient has multiple teeth which require assessment, a dental-panoramic tomogram could be obtained which would help in assessment of not only the tooth in question but also the general state of the entire dentition in terms of caries, periodontal diseases and even traumatic injuries. The periapical radiograph of 25 shows a large carious lesion on the distal aspect with no periapical changes.

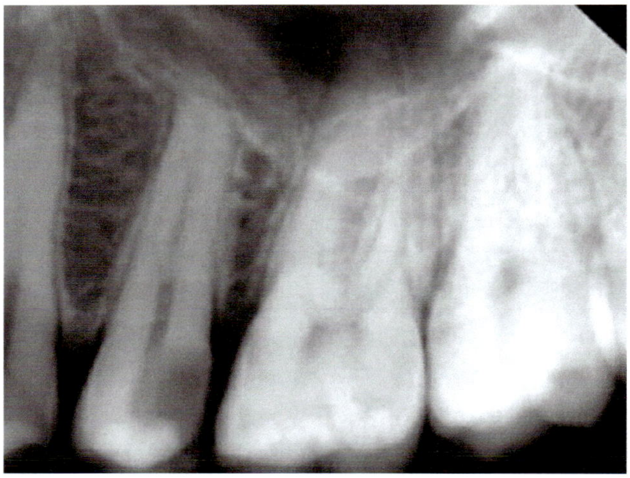

◘ **Fig. 2.3** Periapical radiograph showing caries extending in the distal proximal region of 25

2.12.1 Interpretation of Electric Pulp Tester Results

Electric pulp testing or pulp sensibility testing could be carried out which may reveal a hyper-responsive tooth. However, this may not be required if the patient provides a clear and coherent history coupled with examination and radiographic findings.

2.13 What Is the Definitive Diagnosis?

Considering the history and clinical findings, the condition should be irreversible pulpitis. Based on the ICDAS (International Caries Detection and Assessment System) classification, a score of 4 was given for the extent of caries (◘ Table 2.1).

◘ **Table 2.1** ICDAS classification system for caries

Score	Description
0	No or slight change in enamel translucency after prolonged air drying (5S)
1	First visual change in enamel (seen only after prolonged air drying or restricted to within the confines of a pit or fissure)
2	Distinct visual change in enamel
3	Localized enamel breakdown in opaque or discolored enamel (without visual signs of dentinal involvement)
4	Underlying dark shadow from dentine
5	Distinct cavity visible in dentine
6	Extensive distinct cavity visible in dentine involving more than half of the surface

2.14 What Are the Histopathological Features of Irreversible Pulpitis?

Acute irreversible pulpitis is characterized by gross inflammatory changes in the pulp. Vascular dilatation and oedema would also be visible histopathologically. In addition, a mild neutrophil predominant mixed inflammatory cell infiltration would be evident. Sometimes, pulpal abscesses and destruction of the odontoblasts adjacent to the focus of infection may present. This would progress into liquefactive necrosis of the entire pulp if left unattended.

2.15 How Would You Manage This Patient?

Irreversible pulpitis indicates that the pulp would eventually progress into a non-vital state irrespective of the modality of intervention aimed at preserving the pulp. This is mainly due to the unique anatomic location of the pulpal tissue, poor perfusion of the pulp to facilitate healing especially in mature teeth due to the miniscule end arteries perfusing the pulp and the relative lack of defense mechanisms to ward off inflammation. Thus, in managing this patient, the primary aim is to relieve pain and preservation of the tooth ensuring a long-term feasible restoration which would require pulp therapy or root canal treatment. If the tooth 25 is deemed to have a poor restorative outcome, extraction of it with a suitable prosthesis should be planned. The patient should be assessed in terms of the factors that contribute to caries such as excessive and frequent consumption of sweets, use of dentifrices and medicaments which help in the prevention of caries such as those containing fluorides. Preventative advice should be given with the aim of preventing caries affecting this and the other teeth. Regular reviews should be carried out based on the caries risk assessment to determine the success or failure of previous treatment and occurrence of new carious lesions (◘ Fig. 2.4).

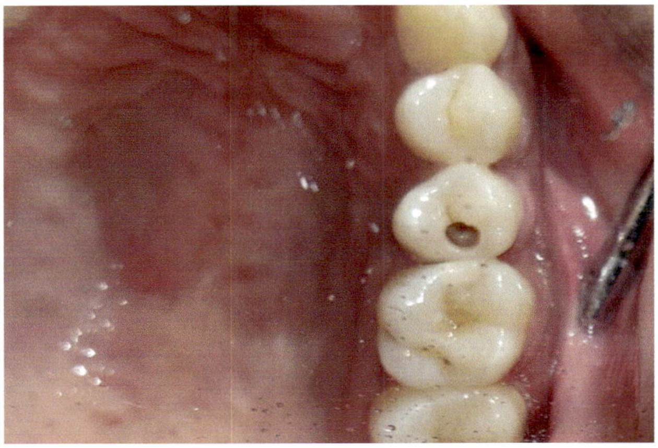

◘ **Fig. 2.4** Accessing the cavity reveals underlying caries

Pain relief is best achieved through removal of caries and extirpating the inflamed pulp. This is best carried out using local anaesthesia. Caries of 25 was removed under rubber dam isolation and the pulp chamber opened. There was profuse bleeding from the pulp (◘ Fig. 2.5), and around 2 mm of the inflamed pulp was removed with a stainless steel round bur following which the pulp was irrigated with 0.5% sodium hypochlorite. The bleeding was arrested (◘ Fig. 2.6), and the pulp chamber was closed with a mineralo-trioxide aggregate (MTA) plug (◘ Fig. 2.7). The tooth was restored with a light-cured composite restoration. The removal of the coronal pulp could be carried out in 2 mm increments to assess the reduction or removal of the inflamed pulp prior to the placement of an MTA plug. After the entire coronal pulp is removed and there is still bleeding from the radicular pulp, root canal treatment is indicated if the tooth is to be saved.

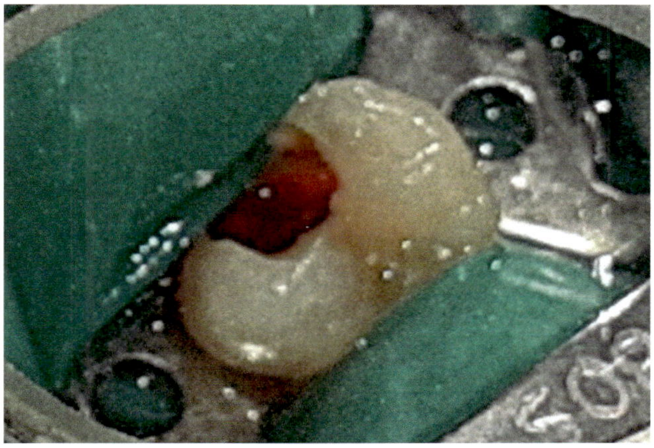

◘ **Fig. 2.5** Profuse bleeding or oozing of blood from the pulp indicates an irreversible pulpitis

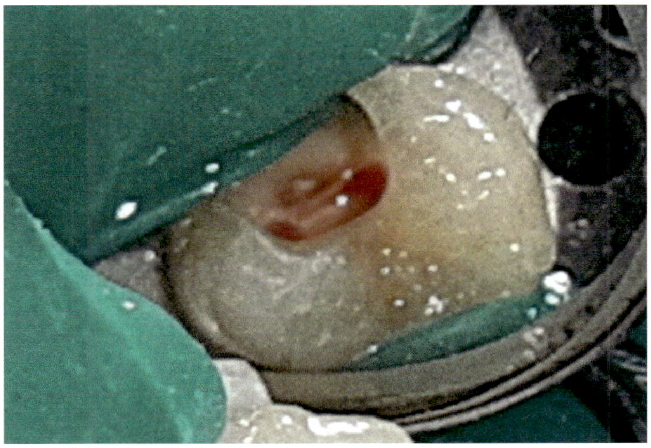

◘ **Fig. 2.6** Two mm of pulpal tissue is removed and examined. Note the lack of bleeding

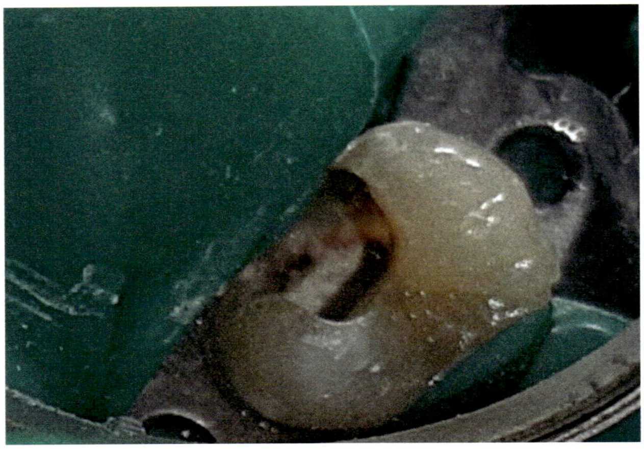

Fig. 2.7 An MTA plug is placed over the opened pulp

2.15.1 Review and Follow-Up

This is important in any chronic disease process, and caries is not an exception. The follow-up should be planned, depending on the caries risk, and a high-risk individual would require shorter follow-up intervals of about 6 months (Table 2.2). An annual reassessment of the patient in terms of the state of the restored teeth and observation of any new lesions developing is important to facilitate long-term reduction of caries. Advice on preventive measures and oral hygiene practices could be reinforced at these follow-up visits which would help motivate the patient towards achieving positive long-term results. This patient was followed up initially at 1 month and then every 6 months. The tooth showed no

Table 2.2 Recall intervals based on the caries risk (Adopted from the AAPD Guidelines for patients older than 6 years)

Risk Category	Diagnostics	Interventions			Restorative
		Fluoride	Diet	Sealants λ	
Low risk	- Recall every 6–12 months - Radiographs every 12–24 months	- Twice daily brushing with fluoridated toothpaste	No	Yes	- Surveillance
Moderate risk patient/parent engaged	- Recall every 6 months - Radiographs every 6–12 months	- Twice daily brushing with fluoridated toothpaste - Fluoride supplements [δ] - Professional topical treatment every 6 months	- Counseling	Yes	- Active surveillance[ε] of incipient lesions - Restoration of cavitated or enlarging lesions
Moderate risk patient/parent not engaged	- Recall every 6 months - Radiographs every 6–12 months	- Twice daily brushing with toothpaste - Professional topical treatment every 6 months	- Counseling, with limited expectations	Yes	- Active surveillance of incipient lesions - Restoration of cavitated or enlarging lesions
High risk patient/parent engaged	- Recall every 3 months - Radiographs every 6 months	- Brushing with 0.5% fluoride - Fluoride supplements [δ] - Professional topical treatment every 3 months	- Counseling - Xylitol	Yes	- Active surveillance of incipient lesions - Restoration of cavitated or enlarging lesions
	- Recall every 3 months - Radiographs every 6 months	- Brushing with 0.5% fluoride - Professional topical treatment every 3 months	- Counseling, with limited expectations - Xylitol	Yes	- Restore incipient, cavitated, or enlarging lesions

symptoms during the review, and no new carious lesions were detected clinically and radiographically.

2.16 Pulpitis

Pulpitis or inflammation of the pulp is a common sequalae of caries, traumatic injury to teeth, tooth wear, advanced periodontal disease and even due to excessive preparation of teeth for indirect restorations. Due to the unique anatomical locations of the pulp as a consequence of being surrounded by hard tissue, any inflammatory process of the pulp leading to an exudative response would result in severe pain. This is further complicated by the fact that the vessels that perfuse the pulp are terminal vessels with no collaterals. As a result, the inflammatory process leads to severe pain.

Clinically, pulpitis is subclassified into reversible, irreversible and a non-vital or necrotic pulp. In reversible pulpitis, pain occurs due to hot, cold or sweet stimulation and is sharp and short-lasting. The pain is relieved by removing the stimulation.

2.16.1 Reversible Pulpitis

A diagnosis of reversible pulpitis is made when the patient exhibits pain only on hot, cold or sweet stimulation, and the nature of pain is a sharp, shock-like pain. It lasts for a very short duration and does not occur spontaneously.

The sequalae of reversible pulpitis is quite favorable in terms of preservation of pulp vitality as the degree of inflammation is initial and has not affected a major portion of the pulpal tissue. Prior to management, a careful pain history must be elicited, and a detailed radiographic assessment should be carried out to determine the extent of caries towards the pulp, the presence of an area of sound dentine between the carious lesion and the pulp and the periapical and periodontal state especially in individual roots of multi-rooted teeth.

In the management, the primary aim is to alleviate pain and preserve the tooth. Pulp preservation strategies are adopted in this situation.

There are four (04) management strategies for reversible pulpitis:

1. One-stage selective caries removal and restoration:

   This is carried out when the carious lesion is deep and affecting up to the inner quarter of dentine. An attempt is made to remove all the soft and firm caries so that the cavity is rendered caries-free. Ideally, this should be carried out using rubber dam isolation with proper magnification and illumination. A layer of MTA or Glass Ionomer cement should be applied to the deep dentine in close proximity to the pulp and the tooth restored with light-cured composites. The patient should be followed up for any recurrence of symptoms and signs or degradation of the restoration. An 80% 5-year success rate is reported with this treatment modality.
2. Two-stage step-wise caries removal and restoration:

   This is carried out in deep or extremely deep caries (caries affecting the entire thickness of dentine). Caries removal is restricted to the soft dentine in the area closest to the pulp. However, complete removal of caries should be achieved around the margins of the cavity to ensure a hermetic seal from the restoration. MTA or setting calcium hydroxide should be placed on the remaining caries affected firm dentine and the tooth hermetically restored. Re-entry is suggested after 3 months to remove the remainder of the affected dentine as a pulpal barrier would be formed within this time preventing pulp exposure. However, most of the time re-entry is not necessary. A 60% 5-year success rate is reported for this treatment modality
3. Pulp capping and restoration:

   This is advocated for teeth with deep or extremely deep caries where there is a pinpoint pulp exposure. Total caries removal should be carried out and done under rubber dam isolation. The exposure should be disinfected with a cotton pellet soaked in 0.5% sodium hypochlorite and examined to ensure that there is no bleeding suggestive of more serious inflammation. An MTA layer is applied on the exposed pulp, and the tooth should be restored.
4. Partial pulpotomy or pulpotomy:

   This is advocated for many extremely deep carious lesions where there are carious pulp exposures. The success rate is deemed higher in this modality compared to pulp capping as the inflamed pulp is removed using high-speed round burs. A 2 mm portion of pulp tissue is removed as described for irreversible pulpitis and disinfected and bleeding arrested with sodium hypochlorite or chlorohexidine. MTA is placed within the pulp chamber, and the tooth is restored. The coronal pulp could be progressively removed in 2 mm increments if bleeding is persistent until uninflamed tissue is reached. This could be done until the entire coronal pulp is removed. If bleeding persists in the radicular pulp, pulpectomy and root canal treatment are indicated.

The decision of which strategy to adopt depends mostly on the clinical and radiologic assessment of the tooth but may have to be ultimately decided during the procedure. Thus, preparation for all the possible modalities of treatment may be a good practice.

Follow-up is necessary to determine the success of treatment. The patient should be free of symptoms and the tooth void of any clinical and radiographic signs of non-vitality or periapical pathology.

2.16.2 Irreversible Pulpitis

Irreversible pulpitis is triggered by the invasion of caries-related microorganisms into dentinal tubules and pulp. The degree of inflammation is proportional to the intensity and/or the severity of tissue damage. Inflammation of the pulp does not take place only when the bacteria in the carious lesion has reached the pulp; rather, bacterial products may reach the pulp at a much earlier stage and trigger an inflammatory response. The inflammatory response is acute at first and followed by chronic inflammation. Innate immunity of the pulp is non-specific but uses receptors to recognize molecular patterns common to microbes and initiate phagocytosis. Persistent infection leads to activation of adaptive immunity. A transition to an adaptive immune response will take place in the dental pulp as caries and bacteria approach the pulp. Antigens are recognized individually, and lines of lymphocytes are developed to produce specific antibodies which attach to the recognized cells and initiate their destruction. Phagocytes remove the remains. Both B cells and T cells are involved in the process.

A variety of cytokines have been observed in the pulp. Patients with symptomatic and asymptomatic irreversible pulpitis show an almost 23-fold increase in the cytokine IL-8 in the pulp. Cytokines in the pulp interact with each other. The ultimate effect on pulpal inflammation and healing is dependent upon the integrated actions of these inflammatory mediators.

According to the Brännström's hydrodynamic theory, nociceptors are activated as a result of fluid movement causing increased pressure within the pulp which is enclosed by hard tissue, and other irritants through the patent dentine tubules result in intense pulpal pain. The unmyelinated, slow-conducting C-fibres aid in the feeling of a slow, burning pain. On the other hand, the highly myelinated Aδ-fibres, which allow for fast conduction, are responsible for the sharp, shooting paining.

Pain mechanisms associated with irreversible pulpitis are similar to those of the rest of the body. Inflammatory mediators act on specific receptors relating to nociceptive neurons, leading to the production of second messengers and activation of phospholipases and protein kinases. The second messengers regulate receptors ion channels that deal with sensitization. The ion channels open based on pain stimuli propagating action potentials in sensory neurons.

Irreversible pulpitis could be managed through a partial pulpotomy as described in this case in the management of tooth 25. However, if the inflammation has progressed to the radicular pulp as evident by profuse bleeding from the radicular pulp through the root canal orifices after a complete pulpotomy, root canal treatment would have to be initiated.

In root canal treatment, the radicular pulp is extirpated through chemo-mechanical preparation of the root canal. The coronal two-thirds of the root canal/s are debrided using gates-glidden burs or shaping files, following which the working length has to be established using electronic apex locators. This could be confirmed through a working length radiograph. Once the length is established, canal preparation and disinfection could be carried out using endodontic files and 2% sodium hypochlorite irrigation.

Provided there is no suppuration or bleeding through the root canals following chemo-mechanical debridement, the obturation could be carried out on the same visit using gutta percha and root canal sealant. If there is suppuration or bleeding, an intra-canal medicament could be used. Non-setting calcium hydroxide or, in severely infected situations, a steroid/antibiotic paste such as ledermix or odontopaste could be used. The dressing can be kept for 7–14 days following which root canal obturation should be carried out. Once root canal treatment is completed, a hermetic coronal seal should be placed (◘ Fig. 2.8).

Endodontically treated posterior teeth are prone to fracture due to the extensive destruction of the coronal

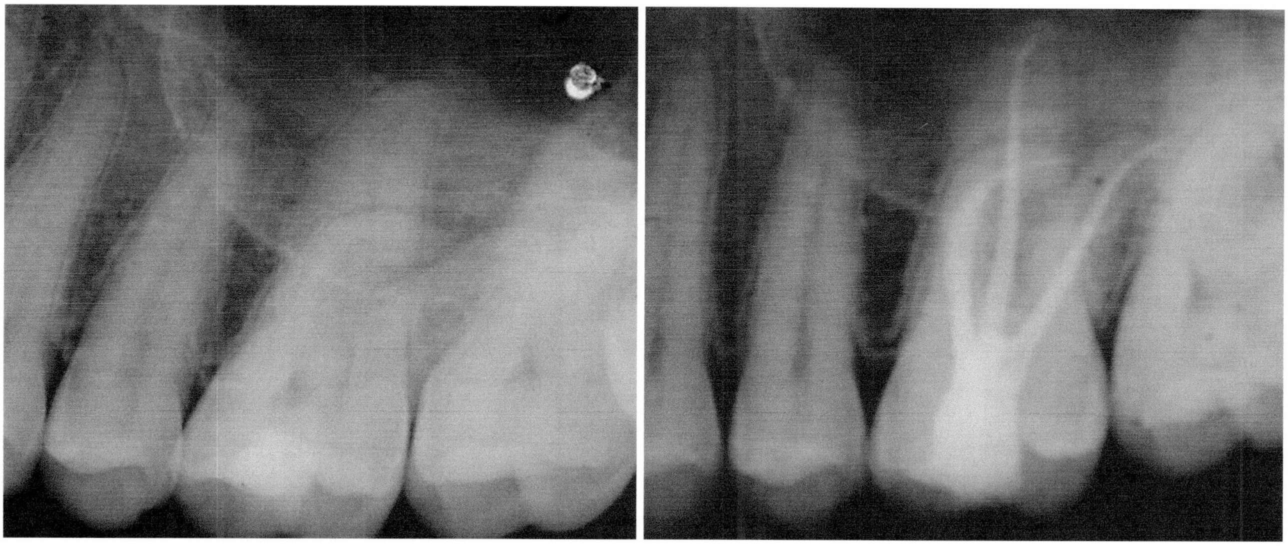

Fig. 2.8 Upper left first molar (26) with irreversible pulpitis treated with root canal treatment

tooth structure as a result of the disease process removal of tooth tissue for root canal access and the effects of medicaments. Thus, a cuspal coverage restoration such as an onlay or crown is recommended to ensure long-term survival.

2.16.3 Non-vital Pulp

In a state of a non-vital or necrotic pulp, there are no symptoms with or without stimulation. Histologically, reversible pulpitis can be characterized by the absence of bacteria and localized coagulation and liquefaction necrosis in the immediate surroundings of the irritant. In irreversible pulpitis, it is characterized by the presence of bacteria or by-products within the dental pulp and abundant acute inflammatory cells predominantly neutrophils in the tissue beneath the lesion suggesting chemotactic activity. Lysosomal enzymes discharged by neutrophils result in widespread tissue damage and suppuration. Treatment in this situation would only be root canal treatment of the affected tooth or extraction of it if the long term restorative prognosis is poor.

2.16.4 Histological Classification of Pulpitis

Pulpitis could also be classified depending on the histological appearance into acute pulpitis, chronic pulpitis and chronic hyperplastic pulpitis. Acute pulpitis is signified with severe pain and is the common cause for patients to seek treatment for dental pain. Histologically, a diffuse inflammatory infiltrate is seen within the pulpal tissue where neutrophils predominate. In chronic pulpitis, there is mild or minimal pain and may represent a quiescent period of acute pulpitis. Histologically, there could be a mono-nuclear cell infiltrate with evidence of fibroblastic activity with micro-abscesses and granulation tissue formation. Chronic hyperplastic pulpitis is commonly seen in deciduous teeth where low-grade irritation and bacterial infiltration of the pulp are seen. In addition, seeding of desquamated epithelial cells on the exposed pulpal tissue leads to development of a polyp. However, it is generally agreed that histologic and clinical classification of pulpal diagnosis still needs to be improved and refined to accurately represent the clinical presentation and determine the form of treatment.

Diagnostic and Management Algorithm

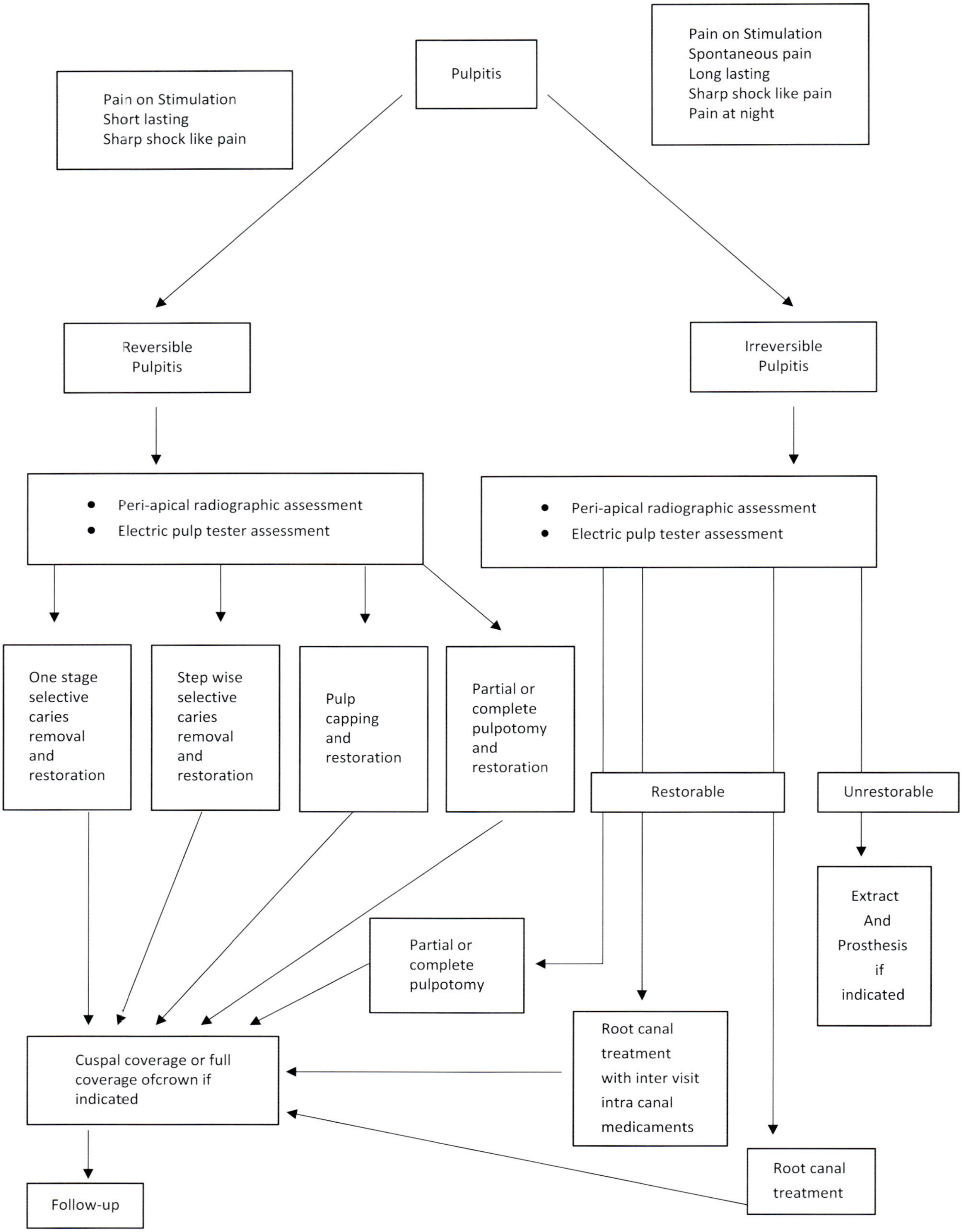

Self-Assessment Questions

1. List the clinical features of reversible and irreversible pulpitis.
2. State the important conditions that need to be included in the differential diagnosis.
3. List the important investigations and findings which would determine the management of pulpitis.
4. Explain the different strategies of management of reversible pulpitis.
5. Outline the importance of following up a patient with pulpitis due to caries.

Summary

Pulpitis is the most common cause for dental pain. Different clinical entities of pulpitis have subtle variations in their clinical presentation, and thus through careful patient assessment, an accurate diagnosis of the pulp state could be made. An accurate diagnosis is important as the management options vary depending on the status of the pulp. The selection of the treatment option should be based on clinical and radiological findings in addition to considering the prognostic factors such as the long-term survival of the tooth. A reasonable follow-up of the patient is also mandatory in minimizing complications and progression of caries.

Further Reading

Bjørndal L. In deep cavities stepwise excavation of caries can preserve the pulp. Evid Based Dent. 2011;12:68. https://doi.org/10.1038/sj.ebd.6400803.

Duncan HF, Galler KM, Tomson PL et al. European Society of Endodontology position statement: Management of deep caries and the exposed pulp. European Society of Endodontology (ESE).

Guideline on caries risk assessment and management of infants, children and adolescents American Academy of Paediatric Dentistry Guidelines. 2006.

Hargreaves KM, Berman LH, Rotstein I. Cohen's pathways of the pulp. 11th ed. Elsevier; 2016. p. 345–52.

Slayton RL, Urquhart O, Araujo MWB et al. Evidence-based clinical practice guideline on nonrestorative treatments for carious lesions. A report from the American Dental Association. https://doi.org/10.1016/j.adaj.2018.07.002.

Pus Discharging from the Gum: Periodontal Disease

Dhanushka Leuke Bandara and Aruni Tilakaratne

Contents

W. M Tilakaratne, T. G. Kallarakkal (eds.), *Clinicopathological Correlation of Oral Diseases*,
https://doi.org/10.1007/978-3-031-24408-7_3

Learning Goals

1. Devise the correct way of compiling the history of the disease presentation with appropriate questions
2. Develop differential diagnoses after history taking
3. Clinically recognize and differentiate periodontal disease presentations
4. Understand the pathogenesis of periodontitis and the role of risk factors
5. Learn the role of periodontal assessments and the investigations in the diagnosis and management of periodontal diseases
6. Outline a management plan for a patient presented with periodontal disease
7. Comprehend the importance of clinicopathological correlation in arriving at the correct diagnosis
8. Recognize the importance of a diagnostic algorithm in arriving at a diagnosis

3.1 Main Complaint

A 40-year-old lady complains of pus discharge from the gum margin in relation to several upper teeth (◘ Fig. 3.1a–c).

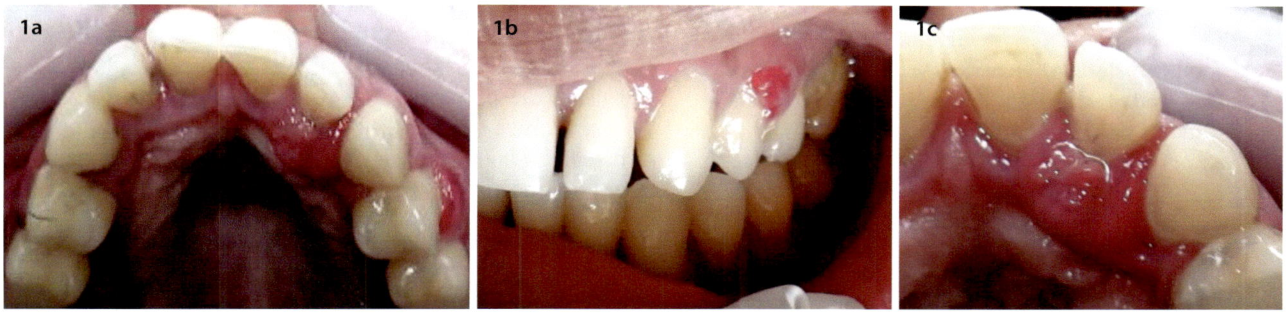

◘ **Fig. 3.1** Palatal view of the upper arch (**a**), labial and buccal view of upper left region (**b**), palatal close-up view of 22 (**c**). Photographs courtesy of Dr. K. M. C. P. Kahawaththa

3.2 History of Complaint

Question: How long have you noted the problem and have you experienced any other associated problems?

I have been experiencing swollen, painful gums followed by pus discharge from the gum margin of the affected teeth for the last three months. I have also noted bleeding while brushing and my teeth started shaking a couple of months ago.

Question: Have you undergone any treatment for the presenting problem?

I have been using some Ayurvedic medicine and tried a mouthwash also. However, the problem remained unresolved. I have not sought any other treatment, nor have I visited a dentist.

3.3 Additional Complaints

Question: Have you experienced any toothache prior to swelling of the gum?

I haven't had any history of toothache or other difficulties before.

3.4 Past Dental and Medical History

Question—Have you undergone any dental treatment before, and are you under treatment for any medical condition?

I haven't been to a dentist for years, and I have no other medical problem. However, I have not been on regular medical check-up.

3.5 Social History and Family History

Question: Are you employed, and if so, what is your occupation?

I am a housewife.

Question: Is there anyone in your family affected with similar problems in the mouth?

My elder brother has had a few shaky teeth which fell-off eventually.

[The importance of obtaining family history is that highly destructive types of periodontitis may support the notion of familial tendency due to genetic predisposition of individuals].

3.6 Oral Hygiene Practices

Question: What is the type of toothbrush that you are using, and how frequently do you brush?

I brush twice a day by using a toothbrush with medium-textured bristles.

[The importance of obtaining details of tooth brushing practices is that mechanical plaque control plays a key role in the prevention of periodontal diseases and also to minimize recurrence or relapse following treatment of disease. Therefore, it is important to assess the mechanical plaque control measures of the patient].

Question: Do you use any tools to clean in between teeth?

I don't use any such tools.

[The importance of interdental plaque control tools is that interdental sites are known to retain more plaque and carry a higher risk for developing periodontitis and proximal caries. Furthermore, brushing has demonstrated optimal cleaning on facial and oral surfaces of teeth compared to interdental sites. Therefore, appropriate interdental tools such as dental floss and interdental brushes could be recommended for better plaque control depending on the need of the patient].

3.7 With the Findings from History, What Is Your Differential Diagnosis?

1. Periodontitis
2. Oral abscess

3.8 How Do You Justify Your Differential Diagnosis After History Taking?

1. She has had bleeding from gums and had felt mobility of teeth during the past months. Bleeding from gums is a primary feature of inflammation of the periodontium. Mobility of teeth may indicate loss of periodontal support as well as unstable periodontium. Furthermore, she reveals the absence of

toothache prior to gingival swelling which would mostly exclude tooth-related causes for the presentation.

2. Pus discharge from the gum margin could be seen in an oral abscess draining through the gingiva. Oral abscess is a type of odontogenic infection resulting in a localized collection of pus associated with the structures surrounding the teeth. Depending on the aetiological factor, oral abscesses could vary on presentation. Main types of abscesses that could be considered in this presentation are periodontal abscesses and peri-apical abscesses. However, these presentations mostly reflect localized problems.

Considering the presented information, periodontitis is the most likely diagnosis. However, any underlying pathology and differential diagnoses should be excluded during the course of examination and investigations.

3.9 Clinical Examination

3.9.1 How Do You Assess the Periodontal Health of This Patient?

Basic periodontal examination (BPE) is a simple and rapid screening tool which recognizes the periodontal care needs of a patient and necessity for further detailed examination. Therefore, BPE must be carried out by using a WHO/CPI (Community Periodontal Index) probe, and the BPE codes for each sextant are as shown below.

4	4	4
3	4	3

3.9.2 How Do You Interpret the BPE Codes Recorded?

According to 2019 British Society of Periodontology guidelines for BPE, the codes are interpreted as shown below (Table 3.1).

3.9.3 Does This Patient Need Further Periodontal Assessment, and If So, Why?

A full-mouth detailed periodontal assessment is indicated for this patient (Fig. 3.2).

In general, for patients with BPE codes of 0, 1 and 2, no detailed periodontal assessment is indicated. However, BPE should be repeated at every routine dental visit/examination. Code 3 for any given sextant may require 6PPC only in that sextant. However, after

Table 3.1 Interpretation of BPE codes

Code	Probing depth (PD)	Examination findings (with a CPI probe)	Interpretation of further care needs
Code 0	PD <3.5 mm	No calculus/overhangs, no bleeding on probing (black band of the probe is entirely visible)	No need for periodontal treatment
Code 1	PD <3.5 mm	No calculus/overhangs, bleeding on probing (black band is entirely visible)	Oral hygiene instructions (OHI)
Code 2	PD <3.5 mm	Supra or subgingival calculus/overhangs (black band is entirely visible)	As for Code 1 and additionally, removal of plaque retentive factors including all supra and subgingival calculus
Code 3	Probing depth 3.5–5.5 mm	Black band is partially visible, indicating pockets of 4–5 mm	As for Code 2 and Root Surface Debridement (RSD) if required, after carrying out a detailed periodontal assessment [six-point-pocket-chart (6PPC)] in the relevant sextant
Code 4	Probing depth > 5.5 mm	Black band is completely invisible indicating a pocket of 6 mm or more	OHI, Scaling and RSD following 6PPC Assess the need for more complex treatment, and referral to a specialist may be considered
*		Furcation involvement	Treat according to BPE code 0–4. Assess the need for more complex treatment; referral to a specialist may be indicated

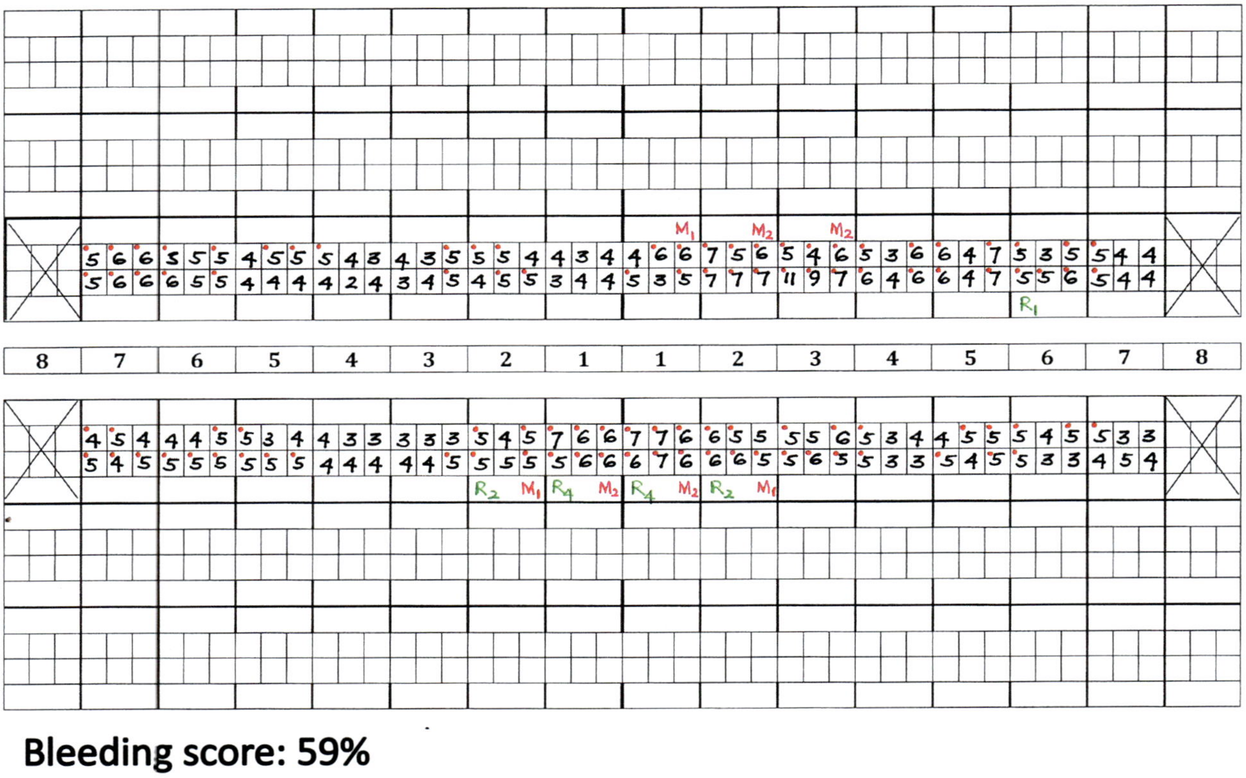

Fig. 3.2 Six-point pocket chart of the patient (6PPC)

carrying out initial therapy which includes oral hygiene instructions, scaling and control of risk/plaque retentive factors, 4–5 mm pockets may disappear. In such situations, the initial detection of 4–5 mm pockets can be attributed to false pocketing due to inflammatory swelling of gingiva. If the shallow pockets of 4–5 mm persist even in the absence of inflammatory gingival swelling, RSD is indicated in these sites. Nevertheless, for a BPE code of 4 in any sextant, a full-mouth 6PPC is indicated.

3.9.4 What Are the Other Relevant Findings?

It is very important to record the plaque score on a plaque chart preferably following disclosing plaque with a disclosing dye (Fig. 3.3). The patient in this case is free of caries. In occlusion, canine guidance is evident on the right side and group function on the left side.

The importance of obtaining a plaque score is that it aids in mapping the sites missed by the patient during brushing, as well as in providing guidance to pay more attention on such areas. Plaque disclosing, plaque demonstration and recording of plaque charts should also be used in motivation and education of the patient and in monitoring improvements.

3.9.5 What Is Your Clinical Differential Diagnosis?

- Generalized periodontitis
- Multiple periodontal abscesses
- Endodontic-periodontal lesions
- Periodontitis as a manifestation of systemic disease
- Systemic diseases or conditions affecting the periodontal supporting tissues

3.9.6 How Do You Exclude Other Conditions and Justify the Inclusion of the Diseases That You Have Mentioned in the Differential Diagnosis to Arrive at a Working Diagnosis?

1. **Periodontitis**

Periodontitis is a chronic inflammatory disease characterized by progressive destruction of tooth-supporting apparatus due to the immuno-inflammatory reactions initiated by pathogenic microorganisms in plaque biofilms. The level of

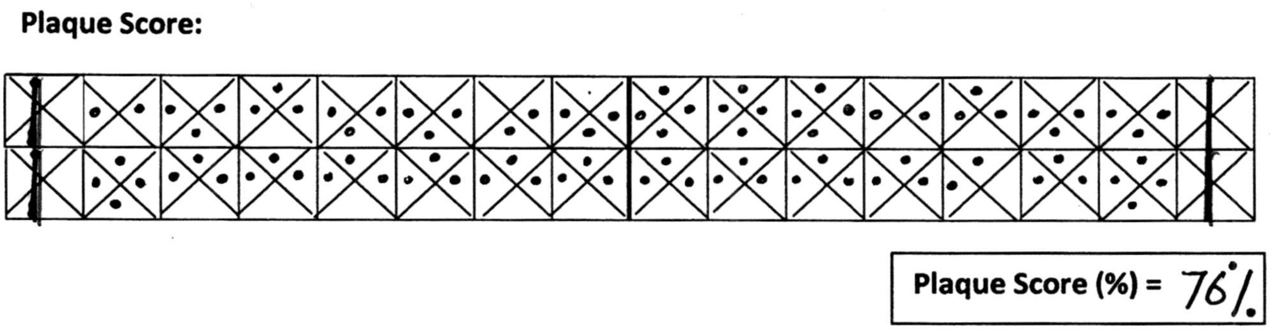

Fig. 3.3 Plaque chart of the patient

immuno-inflammatory reactions may be altered by risk factors, influencing the susceptibility of the individual for the disease. In this patient, the 6PPC indicates periodontal pockets with more than 6 mm in four sextants and mobility of several teeth which are severely affected. Furthermore, the plaque and bleeding scores are high in this patient.

2. **Abscesses**

   With the microbial insult, abscesses may develop in relation to deep periodontal pockets. Diagnosis of a periodontal abscess is based on the medical and dental history as well as oral/dental examination. An ovoid elevation of the gingiva spreading along the lateral part of the root in relation to the affected tooth and bleeding on probing are considered as primary signs of a periodontal abscess although suppuration, deep periodontal pocket and increased tooth mobility may coexist. However, according to reports, abscesses may occur in relation to previously healthy sites due to impacted foreign objects or in a pre-existing periodontal pocket, due to inadequate debridement/irrigation during debridement. Moreover, in patients with systemic-level risk factors such as uncontrolled diabetes mellitus, occurrence of multiple periodontal abscesses, recurrent abscesses and poor response to treatment are commonly reported.

3. **Endodontic-Periodontal Lesions**

   Due to the embryonic origins of the endodontium and the periodontium, both entities share a close connection. Therefore, there is high chance for spread of infection from one compartment to the other, and it is important to consider under differential diagnoses. The pathological communications between pulpal and periodontal tissues may occur either in acute or chronic forms and are defined as endodontic-periodontal lesions. Deep periodontal pockets extending to the root apex and/or negative/altered response to pulp sensibility tests are considered as the main signs in these lesions. Other signs and symptoms may include purulent exudate, sinus tract/fistula, radiographic evidence of apical bone loss/changes in the furcation areas, history of pulpal pain, pain on percussion, tooth mobility and discoloration of tooth.

4. **Influence of Systemic Diseases**

   The link between general health and the oral health is well documented. There are several systemic diseases/conditions that affect the periodontal health, and these have been recognized as systemic risk factors of periodontal disease. In the presence of systemic risk factors, the compromised periodontal health may be manifested out of proportion to the prime aetiological factor, dental biofilm. Furthermore, some systemic diseases such as Papillon–Lefèvre syndrome generally result in periodontitis, and these conditions/diseases are categorized under periodontitis as a manifestation of systemic disease. Nevertheless, conditions such as uncontrolled diabetes mellitus could increase the susceptibility of an individual altering the course of periodontitis.

Considering the clinical presentation of this patient, the above listed conditions are considered under differential diagnoses.

3.9.7 What Is the Most Likely Clinical Diagnosis?

Generalized periodontitis with periodontal abscesses.

3.10 Investigations

3.10.1 According to the BPE Codes Which Investigations Are Indicated?

Codes 3 and 4 denote that radiographic assessment should be proceeded. Bitewing radiographs, intra-oral peri-apical (IOPA) radiographs and/or dental panoramic tomograph (DPT) would be requested depending on the extent of the disease according to the clinical picture. Therefore, a DPT and an IOPA radiograph of 21–23 were obtained for this patient (◘ Fig. 3.4a and b).

3.10.2 How Do You Interpret the Radiographs?

On the IOPA radiograph of 21–23 region, about 70%-interdental bone loss on the distal aspect of 22 was evident. The DPT showed 30–60% generalized proximal bone loss and horizontally impacted 38 and 48. CAL was evident in >30% of sites. Bilateral horizontally impacted mandibular third molar teeth were incidentally noted.

3.10.3 What Are the Other Investigations That Could Be Carried Out to Aid Diagnosis?

To exclude the possibility of endodontic-periodontal lesions, pulp sensibility testing is indicated on the affected teeth. All teeth responded positively to the electric pulp tester. Furthermore, to exclude the presence of underlying systemic disease such as uncontrolled diabetes mellitus, necessary haematological investigations were requested. At the time of the first appointment, random blood glucose level was reported as 18.4 mmol/L, and fasting blood glucose level was later revealed to be 15.3 mmol/L.

3.10.4 What Is the Significance of High Glycaemic Levels Found in This Patient?

Diabetes is diagnosed at fasting blood sugar of greater than or equal to 7.0 mmol/L (126 mg/dL). Therefore, with high glycaemic level, this patient is considered as carrying an increased risk for periodontitis with high severity. Changes in the periodontal microbiome and impaired treatment response with uncontrolled diabetes may further compromise the periodontal health (◘ Fig. 3.5).

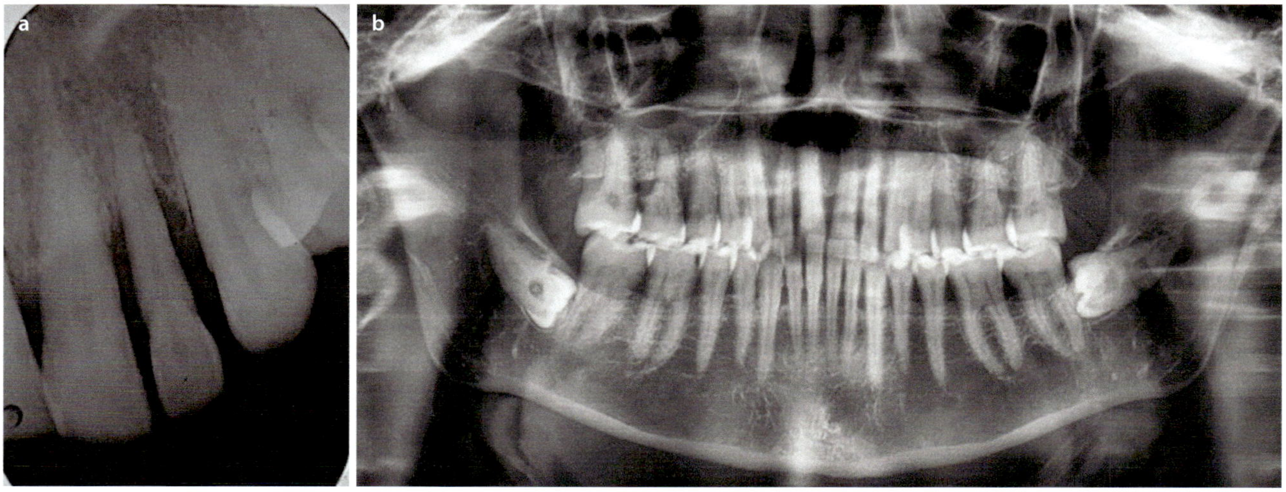

◘ **Fig. 3.4** IOPA radiograph of 21–23 region (**a**), DPT (**b**)

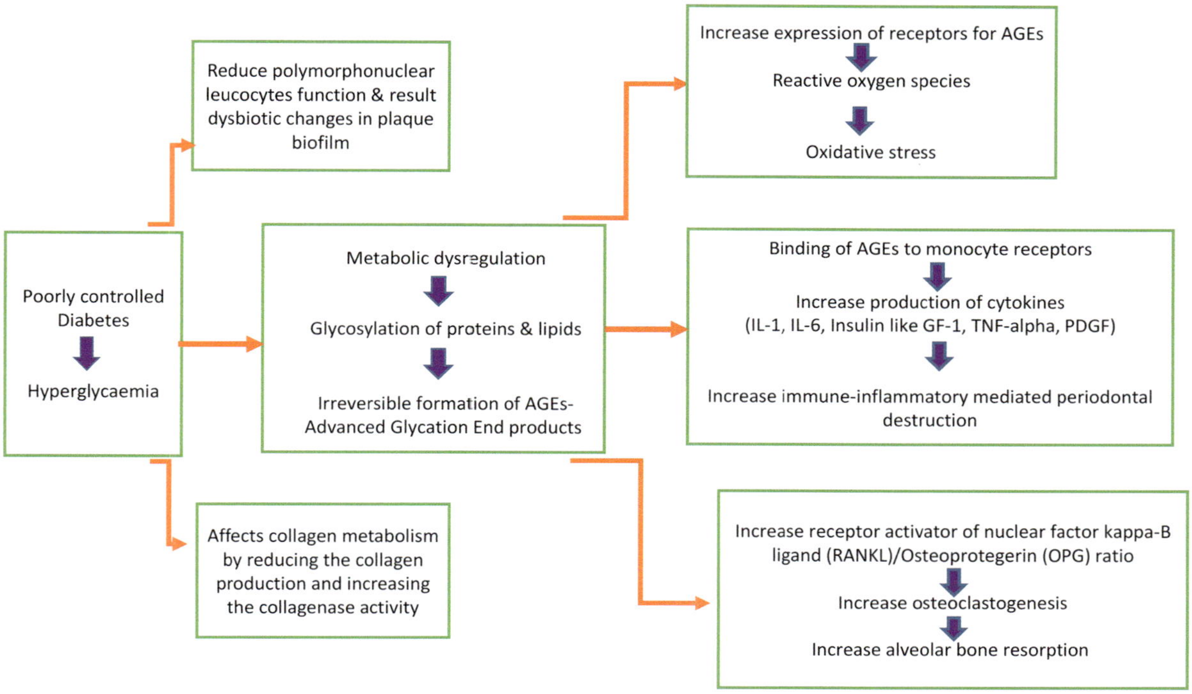

Fig. 3.5 The impact of poorly controlled diabetes on periodontal structures

Fig. 3.6 Multi-level periodontal risk assessment

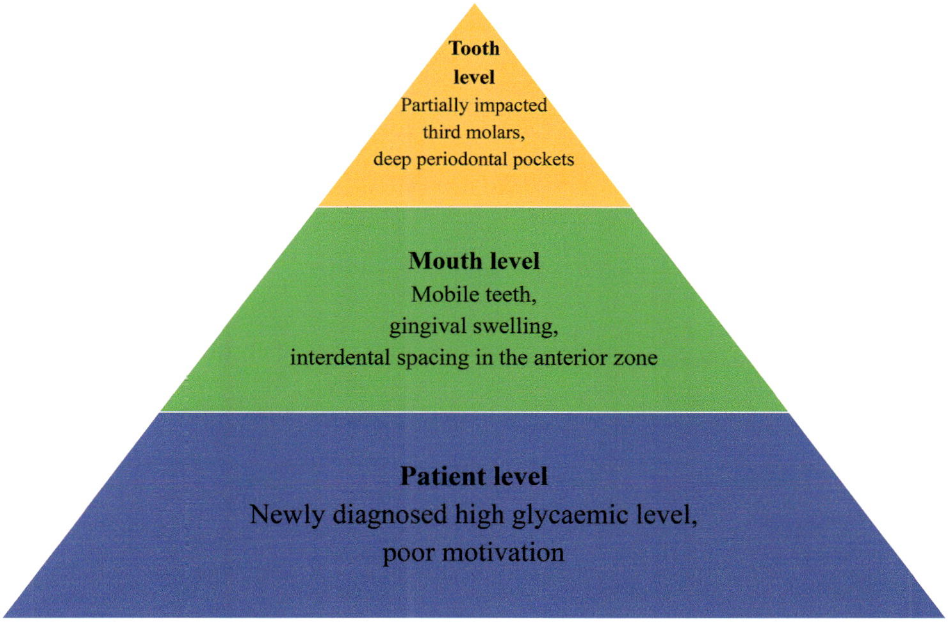

3.10.5 How Would You Carry Out a Systematic Multi-level Periodontal Risk Assessment on This Patient? (Fig. 3.6)

3.10.6 What Is the Definitive Diagnosis?

Generalized periodontitis stage III, grade C, currently unstable, associated with uncontrolled diabetes mellitus and periodontal abscesses in relation to 22, 24 and 25.

3.10.7 How Did You Arrive at the Diagnosis of Periodontitis?

According to the classification introduced by the American Academy of Periodontology & European Federation of Periodontology (AAP & EFP) for periodontal diseases and conditions-2017 (Table 3.2), diagnostic criteria to decide on the severity of periodontitis is either the presence of inter-proximal clinical

3

Table 3.2 2017 AAP & EFP classification for periodontal and peri-implant diseases and conditions

1. Periodontal Health, Gingival Diseases and Conditions	I. Periodontal Health and Gingival Health II. Gingivitis: Dental biofilm-induced III. Gingival Diseases: Non-dental biofilm-induced
2. Periodontitis	I. Necrotizing periodontal diseases II. Periodontitis III. Periodontitis as a manifestation of systemic disease IV. Periodontal abscesses and endodontic-periodontal lesions
3. Periodontal manifestations of systemic diseases and developmental and acquired conditions	I. Systemic diseases or conditions affecting periodontal supporting tissues II. Mucogingival deformities and conditions III. Traumatic occlusal forces IV. Tooth- and prosthesis-related factors
4. Peri-Implant diseases and conditions	I. Peri-implant health II. Peri-implant mucositis III. Peri-implantitis IV. Peri-implant soft and hard tissue deficiencies

attachment loss (CAL) of ≥2 mm or ≥3 mm at ≥2 non-adjacent teeth and by assessing the percentage of radiographic bone loss in comparison to the length of the root at the worst-affected tooth. In this patient, interproximal CAL of ≥2 mm was observed in all sites with a bleeding score of 59%. Staging of periodontitis was based on the maximum CAL observed in relation to 22. According to Fig. 3.4a and b, the radiographic bone loss of the worst-affected tooth (22) was found with involvement of middle one-third of the root. Therefore, the severity stage was decided as 'stage III' (Fig. 3.7).

The rate of disease progression depicted by grading is determined by dividing the maximum percentage of radiographic bone loss by the age of the patient. Since the maximum amount of bone loss at the worst-affected tooth was approximately 70%, and the age of the patient is 40 years, the ratio was derived as 1.75 (70/40 = 1.75). Accordingly, the corresponding grade of periodontitis was decided as grade C which designated rapid rate of progression (Fig. 3.7). The patient's risk profile was identified as uncontrolled diabetes due to poorly controlled glycaemic status.

3.10.8 What Specific Findings Help You in Arriving at the Diagnosis? (Table 3.3)

3.10.9 How Would You Assess the Prognosis of Teeth?

When assigning the prognostic category as favourable, questionable, unfavourable or hopeless (Table 3.4), the prognostic factors should be considered (Fig. 3.8). However, depending on the clinical presentation, the prognosis could be assessed in several aspects:

- intended treatment outcome
- short term vs long term
- individual teeth vs overall dentition

In this patient, uncontrolled diabetes is considered as a major prognostic factor which could affect the overall dentition. To assess the individual prognosis, individual tooth should be assessed with both general and local prognostic factors.

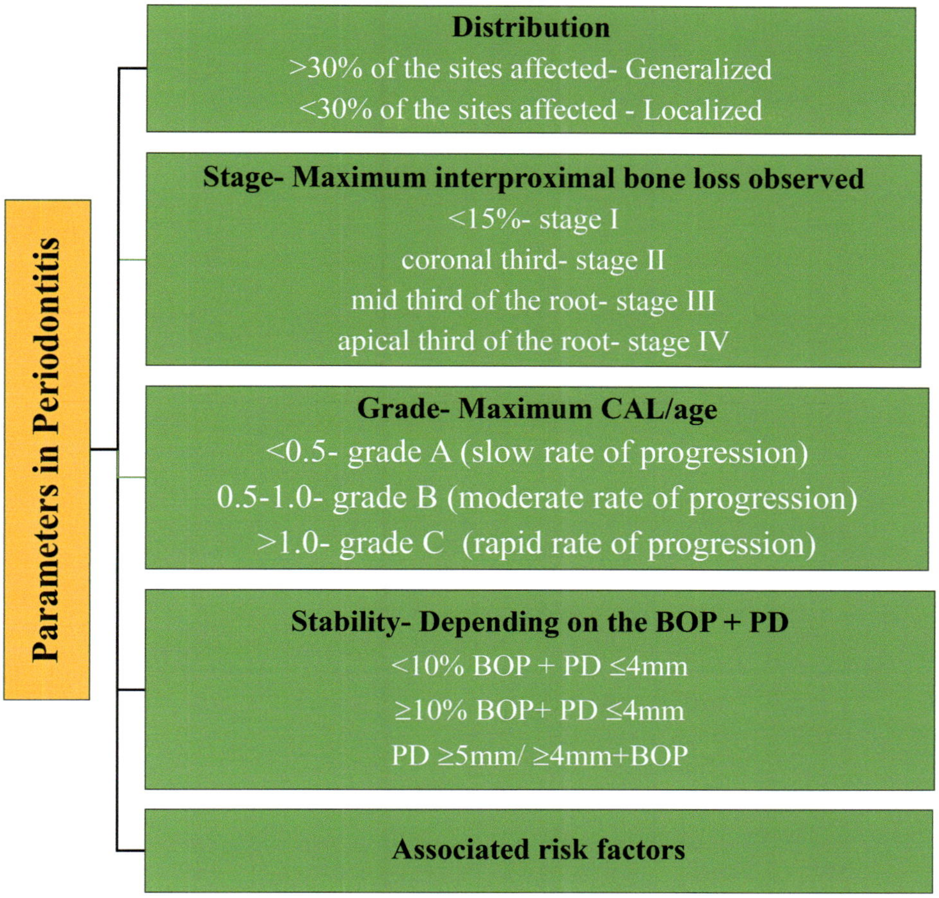

Fig. 3.7 Parameters of periodontitis (*PD* probing depths; *BOP* bleeding on probing; *CAL* clinical attachment loss)

Table 3.3 Findings leading to diagnosis

History	Findings from clinical examination	Findings from investigations
Pus discharge from gingiva	Periodontal pocket depth ranging from 4–11 mm, with BOP	Generalized bone loss
Bleeding during brushing	Mobile teeth due to loss of periodontal support	No apical pathologies/ endodontic infections
Recurrent gingival swelling	Periodontal abscesses	Vital pulp sensibility recording
Mobility of teeth	Poor plaque control	High glycaemic levels
Poor motivation, poor attendance for dental check-up visits		

Table 3.4 Prognostic categories

Parameter	Favourable	Questionable	Unfavourable	Hopeless
Control of local and systemic risk factors	Possible	May/may not be possible	Cannot be controlled	
Chance of achieving periodontal stability (minimal BOP, optimal improvements in PD and CAL and no progressive disease)	Likely to achieve	May be achieved	Unlikely to achieve	No chance to achieve. Therefore, most likely to decide for extraction
Chance of future periodontal destruction	Comparatively minimum	Depends on achieving periodontal stability. If achieved, future disease progression is less likely	Most likely to continue	Yes

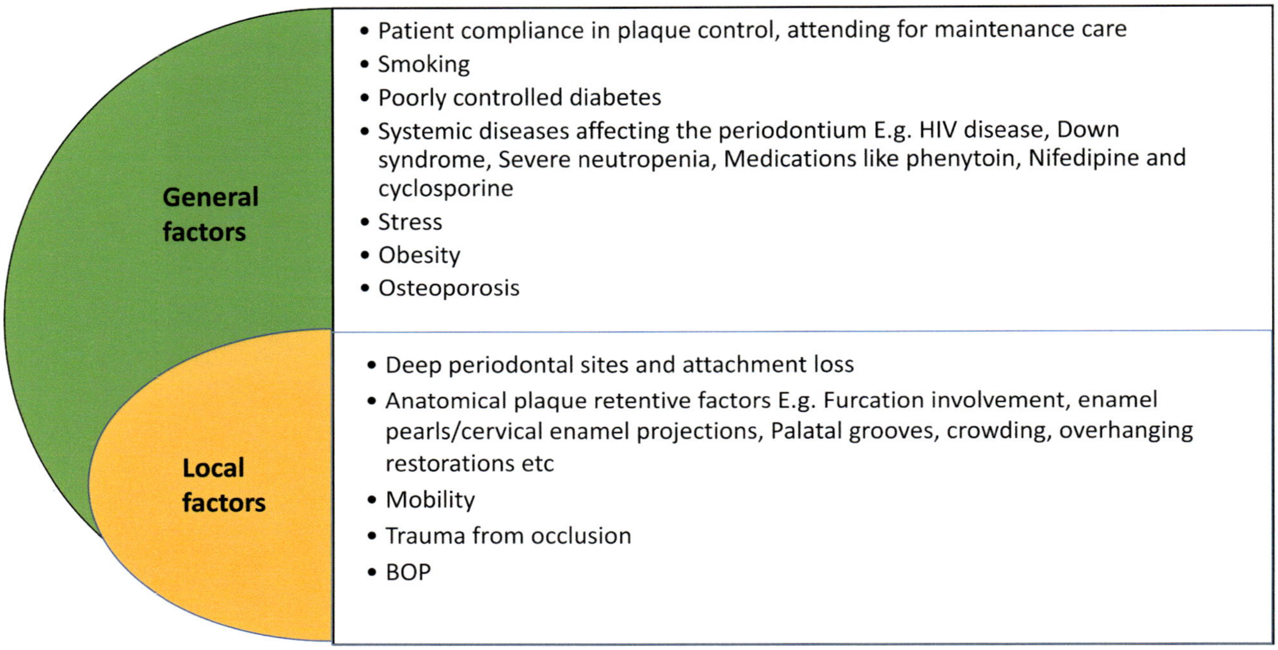

Fig. 3.8 General and local prognostic factors

For example:

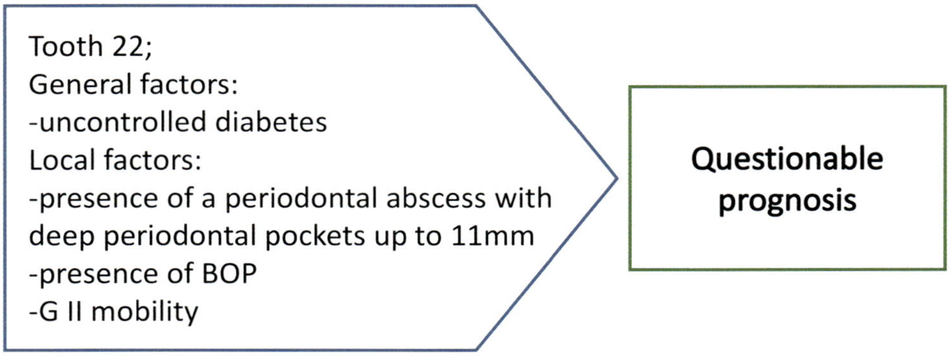

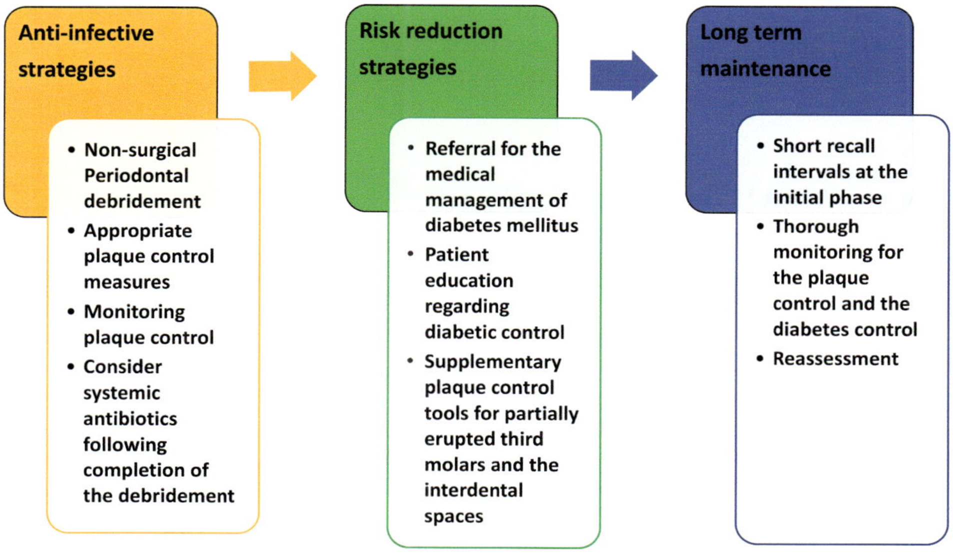

Fig. 3.9 Key strategies in patient management

3.10.10 How Would You Manage This Patient?

The following key areas need to be considered when managing this patient (Fig. 3.9):

1. Anti-infective strategies—reduce the microbial challenge
2. Risk reduction strategies—reduce the susceptibility of the patient for disease progression
3. Long-term maintenance care plan

These key areas could be incorporated into a treatment plan as follows:

1. Emergency phase:
   - Debridement of teeth affected with periodontal abscesses
   - Recommend analgesics
   - Direct the patient for medical management of diabetes mellitus

2. Preventive phase:
   - Tailored oral hygiene regime
     – Plaque disclosing and guided brushing instructions
     – Introducing supplementary plaque control tools; inter-dental brush and dental floss
   - Education of the patient regarding the link between oral health and general health
   - Specific oral health instructions to control both aetiological factors and identified risk factors

3. Stabilization phase:
   - Quadrant-wise non-surgical debridement (scaling and RSD)
   - Monitoring plaque control
   - Surgical removal of horizontally impacted, partially erupted mandibular third molars
4. Periodontal reassessment:
   - Evaluate the outcome of non-surgical phase of care and the glycaemic control
5. Definitive phase:
   - Assess the patient for residual problems as well as for any need for periodontal surgical procedures
6. Maintenance phase

3.10.11 What Is Meant by Non-surgical Debridement?

The main goal of non-surgical periodontal therapy is to control microbial periodontal infection by eliminating bacterial biofilm, calculus and toxins from the periodontally involved sites and to establish an oral environment conducive for maintenance of periodontal health. This could be mainly achieved by mechanical nonsurgical periodontal treatment which has shown to reduce inflammation and probing pocket depths.

Quadrant/sextant-wise instrumentation, full-mouth debridement (full-mouth scaling and root instrumentation within 24 h) and full-mouth disinfection (instrumentation of all pockets within a 24 h period and use of local antiseptics) are a few accepted protocols that could be followed to deliver mechanical non-surgical treatment. As adjunctive strategies, use of systemic antimicrobials, instrumentation in combination with laser or photodynamic therapy could be considered.

According to the 2015 XI European Workshop in Periodontology, the optimal endpoints of active periodontal therapy are:

- Reduction of BOP scores $\leq$15%
- Elimination of deep pockets which are $\geq$5 mm
- Having no signs of active infection—absence of suppuration
- Absence or minimal patient-level risk factors

Therefore, at the end of a non-surgical treatment phase, reassessing the outcomes along these parameters would help the clinician in determining future treatment needs of the patient.

3.10.12 What Is the Importance of Achieving a Convincing Glycaemic Control?

It has been reported that poor glycaemic control in type 2 diabetes is associated with poorer periodontal status and outcomes from periodontal therapy. Demonstrating a bidirectional relationship, periodontitis has shown to be associated with dysglycaemia, increased insulin resistance, increased risk for diabetes and its complications. Furthermore, periodontal therapy has shown to improve the metabolic control of diabetes, highlighting the importance of concurrent management of periodontitis and diabetes mellitus. Early detection of diabetes or pre-diabetes would warrant better chances for a successful outcome from periodontal therapy.

However, irrespective of the level of diabetes control, non-surgical periodontal therapy is essentially indicated for all patients as the first line of management.

3.10.13 How Would You Plan the Maintenance Phase for This Patient?

Maintenance phase is important to minimize recurrence of disease with timely detection of re-emerging problems. It has been evident that delivering the right level of maintenance care could either halt the disease process or at least slow down the progression and thereby could reduce the incidence of tooth loss. Maintenance phase usually commences following completion of active periodontal treatment and when the clinician decides that the patient should be recalled within suitable time intervals. Patients with high risk levels should be recalled at short recall intervals compared to those with a low-risk profile. During the maintenance visit, following an update of the medical and dental histories, extraoral and intraoral examination, periodontal evaluation, radiographic review, assessing the patient's ability in removing plaque, superficial debridement and selective root surface instrumentation on indicated sites and polishing of teeth are carried out.

Presence of recently detected diabetes mellitus with high glycaemic levels and grade C periodontitis may make this patient susceptible for future attachment loss. Thus, short recall intervals with monitoring of diabetes status and other local risk factors should be instituted.

3.11 Periodontal Diseases and Common Conditions Affecting the Periodontium

Periodontal diseases are primarily a result of pathogenic microorganisms in plaque biofilm although numerous risk factors could influence the susceptibility of the individual for the disease. Pathogenesis of periodontal disease is considered as multi-directional, and the immuno-inflammatory reactions could instigate destruction of periodontal structures (Fig. 3.10).

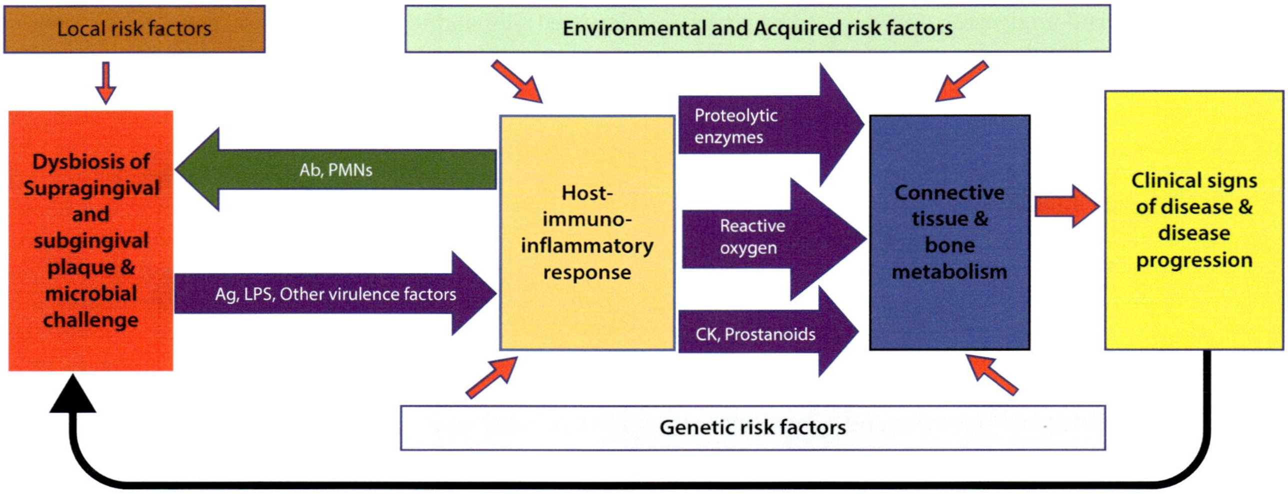

Fig. 3.10 Pathogenic process of Periodontitis. (*Ab* antibodies against the microbial challenge; *PMNs* polymorphonuclear leukocytes; *Ag* antigen produced against the microbial challenge; *LPS* lipopolysaccharides produced by Gram-negative bacteria, Proteolytic enzymes; e.g. Matrix metalloproteinases, CK-Cytokines; *IL-1*, *IL-6*, *TNF-α*, *PDGF*, Insulin-like growth factor-1, Prostanoids; e.g. Prostaglandin E2)

Periodontitis, a multi-factorial chronic inflammatory disease in the periodontium, mostly presents with an episodic nature. The disease is characterized by progressive destruction of the tooth-supporting apparatus resulting in clinical attachment loss and manifested as periodontal pocketing, gingival bleeding and radiographic bone loss. The severe-most form is estimated to affect 11.2% of the global adult population and is a major cause of tooth loss. Tooth loss could adversely affect the nutritional status, speech, self-esteem and overall quality of life of an individual.

Histopathologically, initiation and progression of periodontal disease have been categorized into initial, early, established and advanced lesions. The categorization is based on animal and human studies where experimental gingivitis was evident. While 'initial lesion' (1–2 days) is well localized to gingival crevice and bordering tissue, the 'early lesion' (4–7 days) is characterized by proliferation of both junctional epithelium and crevicular epithelium. However, the 'established lesion' (usually within 2–3 weeks) is known to extend further as proliferation of junctional and crevicular epithelium along with some amount of loss of collagen, although no loss of periodontal attachment would be evident. Next, the 'advanced lesion' which is usually beyond a period of 3 weeks is characterized by deep pocketing and loss of periodontal attachment where collagen and bone loss would be apparent.

It is important to note that an established lesion can persist for many years, and its shift to an advanced lesion marks the transition from a chronic reaction to a destructive immunopathological mechanism denoting periodontitis. Although the factors responsible for this progression are unclear, it is envisaged that either the host immune response or specific microorganisms in plaque biofilm with changing virulence are responsible for the development of the advanced lesion. The factors which are responsible for the transition from reversible gingivitis to destructive periodontitis are largely unknown. There is no factual evidence to suggest that destructive periodontitis is necessarily a result of pre-existing gingivitis. Some preceding gingival inflammation may lead to periodontitis, though it may not be a constant. The 'advanced' lesion is clinically identified as periodontitis, with classical features such as pocket formation, ulceration of the pocket epithelium, destruction of periodontal ligament and bone resorption. At this stage, there is irreversible loss of attachment of periodontal ligament and bone. These changes may lead to mobility of the tooth and eventual tooth loss. The extension of the inflammatory infiltrate both apically and laterally reduces the collagen content, and a dense accumulation of lymphocytes, plasma cells and macrophages would be evident. Peripherally, there could be reparative fibrosis.

3.11.1 Periodontal Abscess

A periodontal abscess is a localized collection of pus within the gingival wall of the periodontal pocket/sulcus, causing rapid destruction of underlying tissue. Thus, periodontal abscess is an acute destructive process in the periodontium. *Porphyromonas gingivalis, Prevotella intermedia, Tannerella forsythia* and *Fusobacterium nucleatum* have been identified as the most prevalent microorganisms in periodontal abscesses. Periodontal abscesses can develop in the milieu of persisting periodontitis, and conversely, abscesses can also occur in the absence of periodontitis. Periodontal abscess originating from chronic periodontitis could primarily be due to marginal closure of a periodontal pocket, or the pocket lumen may be too rigid to drain the increased suppurative fluid. The prevalence of periodontal abscess is relatively high which also affects the prognosis of the tooth. Early intervention is necessary in the management of periodontal abscesses to minimize rapid destruction of periodontal tissues as well as patient's discomfort and pain. It is of wide belief that for patients with periodontitis and acute periodontal abscesses, a complete phase of therapy would help in the management of the conditions in two stages. The first stage is aimed at the acute lesion, while the second stage is for appropriate comprehensive treatment for chronic or any residual lesions. The management of an acute periodontal abscess includes establishing drainage via pocket lumen, by carrying out thorough scaling and superficial debridement, following which compression of the pocket wall may be required to facilitate expression and drainage of pus from the pocket. If there is any foreign body impaction, it should be removed. In situations where drainage cannot be obtained through the pocket lumen, an incision to establish drainage followed by irrigation could be recommended. In extreme situations, a flap may be raised to help remove the suppuratives. Extraction of the tooth is the inevitable last resort, if the prognosis of the tooth is deemed hopeless. In case of systemic symptoms, antibiotics may be recommended following thorough debridement.

3.11.2 Endodontic-Periodontal Lesions

There are numerous pathways through which an inflammatory lesion in the endodontium could communicate with the periodontium, and vice versa. As an example, these lesions may occur due to traumatic and/or iatrogenic factors such as root perforation, fracture/cracking or external root resorption. Depending on the presence of root damage, they could be further classified into 'with root damage' and 'without root damage'. Periodontitis and endodontic pathologies due to caries/non-vital pulp are considered as the main aetiological factors for endodontic-periodontal lesions without root damage. Therefore, detection of endodontic-periodontal lesions and associated factors is essential as they will directly impact on the prognosis as well as the treatment.

Salient features of periodontal disease

	Healthy periodontium	**Gingivitis**	**Periodontitis**	**Periodontal stability achieved with adequate care**
Bleeding on probing	No/minimal	Yes	Yes	No/minimal
Gingival sulcus depth	Normal 1–3 mm	May increase	Increase and deep pockets found	May increase
Alveolar height	Radiographically an intact lamina dura seen with an average distance of 2 mm between alveolar bone crest to the cemento-enamel junction	Normal height. No evidence of bone loss	Reduced bone height. Radiographically bone loss detected	Reduced bone height
Presence of CAL	No	No	Yes	Yes
Local and systemic risk factors	No	May be present	Present	Mostly controlled

Early diagnosis minimizes further periodontal destruction. Meticulous plaque control and maintaining low-risk profile with regular long-term maintenance care are the key modes for management

- **Diagnostic and Management Algorithm for Periodontal Disease**

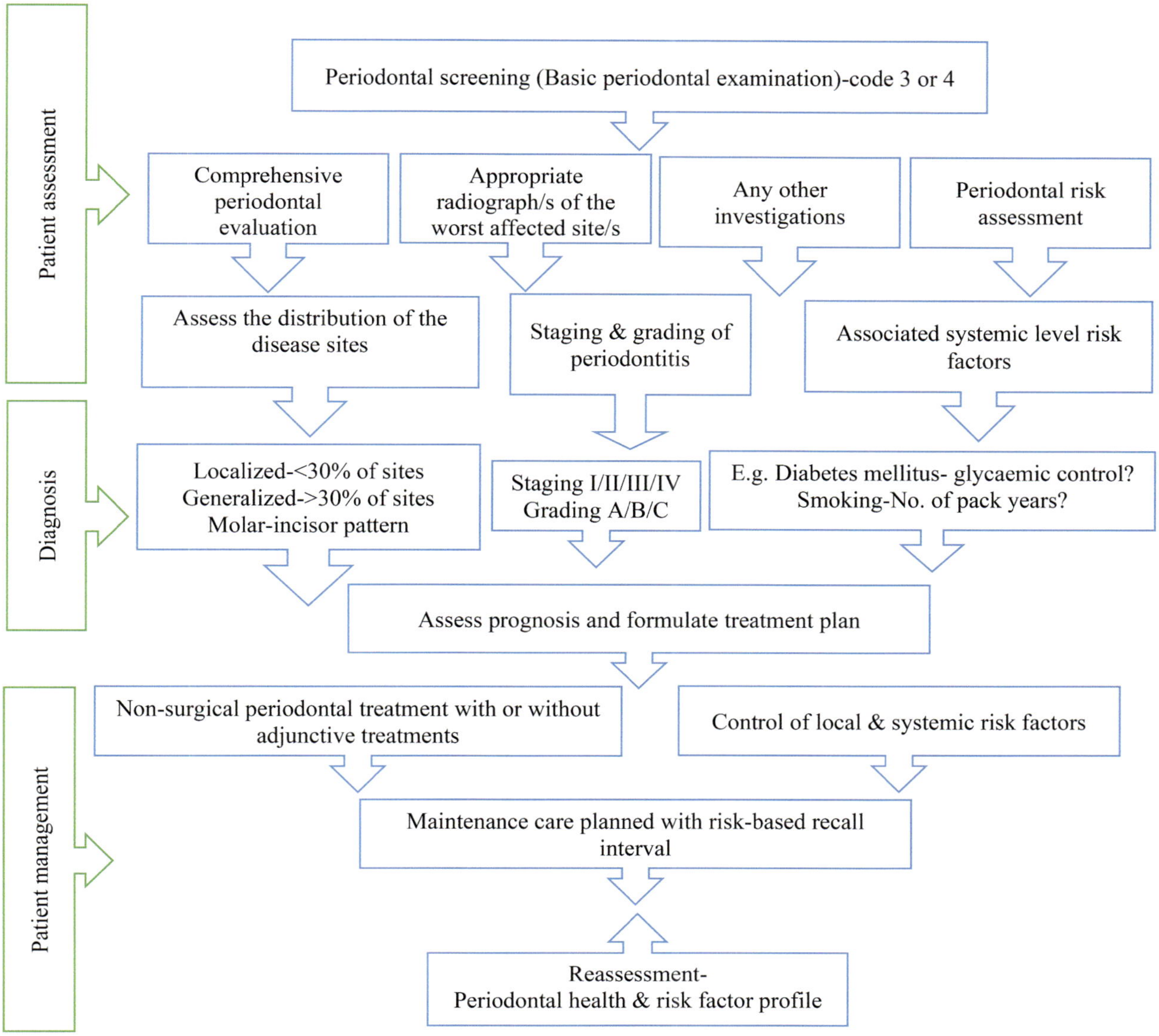

3

? Self-Assessment Questions

1. List the clinical periodontal parameters which can be associated with pus discharging periodontal pockets
2. List the aetiological factors and risk factors which may contribute for the development of a periodontal abscess
3. List the features to differentiate a periodontal abscess from a peri-apical abscess
4. Outline the importance of controlling periodontal infection in diabetic patients
5. Briefly explain the rationale for the Root Surface Debridement (RSD)
6. List the limitations of systemic antibiotic therapy in controlling periodontitis

Further Reading

Albandar JM, Susin C, Hughes FJ. Manifestations of systemic diseases and conditions that affect the periodontal attachment apparatus: case definitions and diagnostic considerations. J Clin Periodontol. 2018;45(Suppl 20):S171–89.

Caton J, Armitage G, Berglundh T, et al. A new classification scheme for periodontal and peri-implant diseases and conditions—introduction and key changes from the 1999 classification. J Clin Periodontol. 2018;45(Suppl 20):S1–8.

Cohen RE, Research, Science and Therapy Committee, American Academy of Periodontology. Position paper: periodontal maintenance. J Periodontol. 2003 Sep;74(9):1395–401.

Graziani F, Gennai S, Solini A, et al. A systematic review and meta-analysis of epidemiologic observational evidence on the effect of periodontitis on diabetes an update of the EFP-AAP review. J Clin Periodontol. 2018;45(2):167–87.

Lang NP, Bartold PM. Periodontal health. J ClinPeriodontol. 2018;45(Suppl 20):S9–S16.

Martinez-Canut P, Llobell A. A comprehensive approach to assigning periodontal prognosis. J Clin Periodontol. 2018;45(4):431–9.

Page RC, Kornman KS. The pathogenesis of human periodontitis: an introduction. Periodontol. 2000;1997(14):9–11.

Papapanou PN, Sanz M, et al. Periodontitis: Consensus report of Workgroup 2 of the 2017 World Workshop on the classification of periodontal and peri-implant diseases and conditions. J Clin Periodontol. 2018;45(Suppl 20):S162–70.

Tonetti MS, Eickholz P, Loos BG, Papapanou P, van der Velden U, Armitage G, Bouchard P, Deinzer R, Dietrich T, Hughes F, Kocher T, Lang NP, Lopez R, Needleman I, Newton T, Nibali L, Pretzl B, Ramseier C, Sanz-Sanchez I, Schlagenhauf U, Suvan JE. Principles in prevention of periodontal diseases: Consensus report of group 1 of the 11th European Workshop on Periodontology on effective prevention of periodontal and peri-implant diseases. J Clin Periodontol. 2015 Apr;42(Suppl 16):S5–11.

Tonetti MS, Greenwell H, Kornman KS. Staging and grading of periodontitis: Framework and proposal of a new classification and case definition. J Clin Periodontol. 2018;45(Suppl 20):S149–61.

Odontogenic and Non-Odontogenic Cysts

Contents

Hard Swelling in the Back of the Lower Jaw: Odontogenic Keratocyst

Yet Ching Goh, Siti Mazlipah Ismail, and Harsha Lal De Silva

Contents

W. M Tilakaratne, T. G. Kallarakkal (eds.), *Clinicopathological Correlation of Oral Diseases*,
https://doi.org/10.1007/978-3-031-24408-7_4

Learning Goals

1. Devise the correct way of compiling the history with appropriate questions.
2. Develop a differential diagnosis after history taking.
3. Deduce appropriate procedures in clinical examination.
4. Formulate a differential diagnosis combining findings in the history and clinical examination.
5. Justify the relevant investigations required to arrive at the diagnosis.
6. Comprehend the importance of clinicopathological correlation in arriving at the correct diagnosis.
7. Outline the management plan.
8. Recognize the importance of a diagnostic algorithm in arriving at a diagnosis.

4.1 Main Complaint

A 27-year-old male presented to the outpatient clinic complaining of a bony hard swelling in the left side of his lower jaw, having been referred by his dentist.

4.2 History of Complaint

He had recently visited a dentist for a routine dental check-up and a "cleaning". The dentist took an intraoral bitewing radiograph for caries detection and noticed a radiolucency distal to the left mandibular second molar tooth (◘ Fig. 4.1—Bitewing radiograph). On re-examination, the dentist found a painless swelling in the left posterior mandible. He decided to refer the patient for specialist consultation for further assessment.

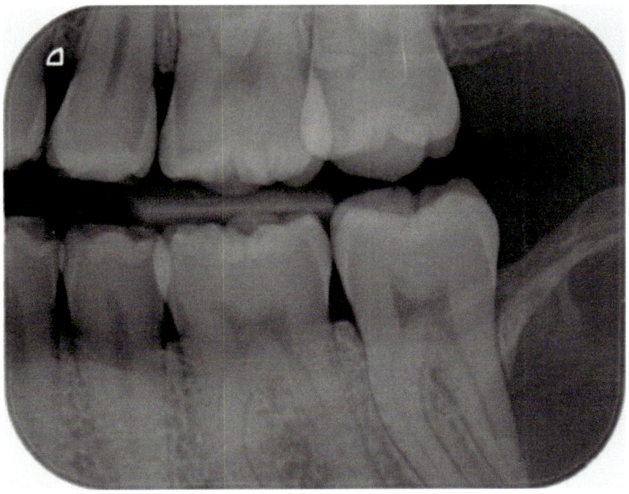

◘ **Fig. 4.1** A bitewing radiograph taken for a routine dental check-up shows a radiolucency distal to the left mandibular second molar tooth

? Question: Did you feel any pain, discomfort or anything unusual in your lower jaw or your neck any time, apart from the "bump"?

✓ No, I never felt anything unusual in my jawbone. I was surprised when my dentist told me what he saw in my mouth and the X-ray (radiograph).

4.3 Past Dental, Medical and Social History

? Question: Do you go for regular dental check-ups?

✓ I went for an annual dental check until I turned 18. Since entering the university and starting to work after graduation, I couldn't keep yearly visits.

? Question: What dental treatment have you had in the past?

✓ Once every few years, I get scaling of my teeth. My teeth and gums have been generally healthy, according to my dentists. In 2013, my dentist thought I had impacted wisdom teeth and referred me to an oral surgeon. He took a radiograph and told me I had a cyst in one of them. I had my four wisdom teeth removed under general anaesthesia. My surgeon told me they found a cyst with my right lower jaw wisdom tooth. He recommended visiting him annually to check whether the cyst will come back again. I went for three annual visits.

? Question: Why didn't you continue to go for follow-ups?

✓ I couldn't continue as a change in my employment made me come to this part of the country. My surgeon was happy with the final radiograph he took in 2016, saying that the cyst has completely resolved. Since I didn't notice anything unusual in my jaw, I didn't think it was necessary to notify my current dentist.

? Question: Do you have any general health problems?

✓ I consider myself fit and healthy. I have never been in the hospital except for the wisdom teeth surgery. I don't take regular medications or supplements and don't recall being allergic to any medicine, foods or other substances.

Question: Do you smoke or drink alcohol?

I am a non-smoker. I enjoy a glass of wine or a beer occasionally in social gatherings.

4.4 Clinical Examination

He appears an otherwise fit and healthy individual. There is no visible facial asymmetry, and he has a full range of jaw movements with no tenderness, clicking or crepitus in the temporomandibular joints. No neuro-sensory deficits are noted on clinical examination, and the cervical lymph nodes are not enlarged. On palpation, a non-tender, small bony-hard, expansile enlargement is felt beneath the lower border of his left mandible, immediately anterior to the left masseter muscle.

The dentition is complete except for third molars and is free of obvious untreated caries. None of his teeth is tender to gentle percussion. Oral hygiene appears satisfactory with no obvious gingival bleeding or periodontal pocketing. Intra-oral examination of the left mandible reveals a palpable, non-tender, bony-hard, smooth-surfaced, slight buccal cortical expansion located beneath the vestibule, extending posteriorly from the left mandibular second premolar region. There is a minimal palpable expansion of the lingual cortex felt in the medial aspect of the ramus, posteroinferior to the second molar tooth. No inflammation/ulceration of the overlying mucosa is noted, nor are other clinically obvious anomalies detected in the intra-oral examination.

A national health record database search reveals that the patient underwent surgical removal of four impacted wisdom teeth and exploration and enucleation and curettage of two lesions associated with mandibular wisdom teeth. The Dental Pantomograph (DPT) taken before surgery shows a unilocular radiolucent lesion associated with an unerupted right mandibular third molar (#48) and a smaller radiolucency associated with an unerupted left mandibular third molar (#38). Subsequent DPT taken in 2015 shows good bone healing resulting in complete resolution of the lesions mentioned above (Fig. 4.2a and b). The histopathology of the lesions removed in 2013 was reported to be consistent with:

1. An odontogenic keratocyst (reported as keratocystic odontogenic tumour according to WHO classification used in the year 2013) associated with (#48)
2. A hyperplastic dental follicle with no cystic degeneration associated with (#38)

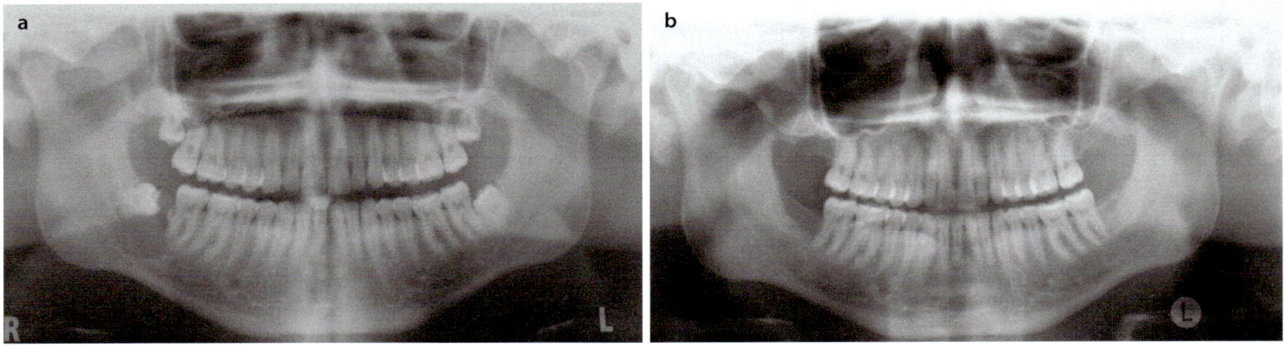

Fig. 4.2 DPTs showing the radiolucencies associated with mandibular third molars (**a**). Before surgery (**b**) 2 years post-surgery

4.5 What Is Your Differential Diagnosis with the Findings from the History and Clinical Examination? Give a Justification for Including Different Entities

1. Odontogenic Keratocyst (OKC)
2. Ameloblastoma
3. Other odontogenic tumour/cyst
4. Giant cell lesion/tumour

The lack of pain/tenderness related to this expansile lesion of the mandibular bone indicates the possibility of a cyst or a tumour growing within the bone instead of a lesion of inflammatory origin. Given that this is an incidental finding at a routine dental check-up, the lesion may have grown over time. The age group and the anatomical location favour OKC or ameloblastoma, but the possibility of any other tumour/cyst of the odontogenic origin or giant cell lesions of bone cannot be ruled out exclusively from history and clinical examination alone.

4.6 What Is the Most Likely Clinical Diagnosis?

OKC is the most likely clinical diagnosis. Despite being in the age group for both OKC and ameloblastoma, the former is more common and is more likely, given the clinical finding of minimal cortical expansion. The lack of tooth mobility and the absence of neurosensory disturbances in the ipsilateral lower lip further support a clinical diagnosis of an OKC. Root resorption leading to tooth mobility and the encroachment of inferior alveolar neurovascular bundle resulting in sensory disturbances in the ipsilateral lower lip are uncommon with OKC and other odontogenic cysts but are more likely to be associated with tumours showing a locally invasive growth pattern. Ameloblastomas tend to expand buccolingually to produce cortical thinning and extension into soft tissues, while OKCs have a preference to extend mesiodistally with little or no cortical expansion. The history of a previous OKC associated with the #48 too indicates a possibility of an OKC in the left side, given that multiple OKCs could be a feature of an underlying potential Basal Cell Naevoid Syndrome (BCCNS) in this patient.

Although dentigerous cysts and radicular cysts are more common than OKCs, there is no clinical evidence of a missing tooth or a non-vital tooth in the left mandibular quadrant to suggest the existence of these pathologies. Other tumours (odontogenic/non-odontogenic) and giant-cell lesions are relatively uncommon.

4.7 What Are the Necessary Investigations That Should Be Carried Out in a Logical Sequence?

4.7.1 Dental Panoramic Tomography (DPT)

A dental panoramic tomography (DPT) reveals the presence of a well-demarcated, multilocular radiolucency involving the left mandible (◘ Fig. 4.3). The radiolucency extends posteriorly from the periapical region of the left mandibular second premolar to the ipsilateral ramus. It involves the body of the mandible reaching inferiorly the lower border and superiorly through the bone proximal to the second molar to reach beyond the mandibular foramen. There are no unerupted teeth, displacement of erupted teeth or radiographically evident root resorption of teeth associated with the radiolucency. The inferior alveolar canal appears displaced towards the lower border, where cortical expansion and thinning are evident. No other lesions of significance is apparent in the DPT.

4.7.2 Pulp Sensibility Tests

Pulp sensibility was performed in the left lower quadrant. All teeth tested positive for "cold-testing". This helps exclude the possibility of an unlikely event of a radicular cyst arising from the left mandibular second molar tooth, which could have been made non-vital from iatrogenic damage at the time of surgical removal of #38. Further, it is a benchmark to monitor the vitality of teeth, which may be retained but with potentially compromised blood supply following future surgical interventions.

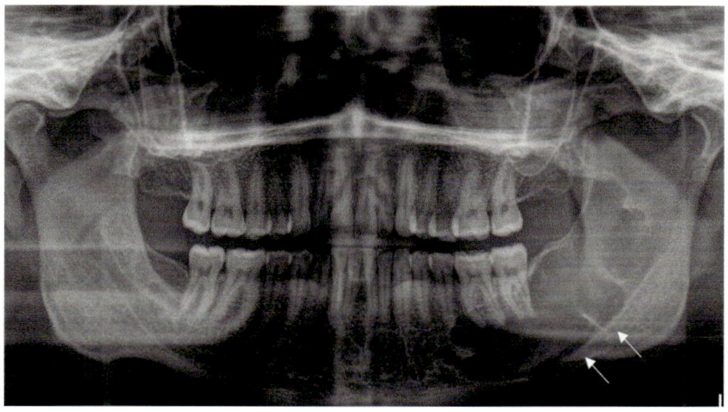

◘ **Fig. 4.3** The DPT obtained after the bitewing radiograph (shown in ◘ Fig. 4.1) shows a large multilocular radiolucency in the left mandible extending from the mandibular second premolar posteriorly into the ascending ramus. Arrows indicate the inferior displacement of the inferior alveolar canal

4.7.3 Aspiration Biopsy

An aspiration under a local anaesthetic performed using a syringe coupled to a wide-bore needle may help confirm the cystic/solid nature of the lesion and also to exclude the possibility of being a vascular anomaly. However, an aspiration wasn't undertaken for this patient since it would have needed drilling through the mandibular buccal cortex. Also, in contemporary practice, non-invasive three-dimensional (3-D) imaging modalities are often reliable in providing the aforementioned information.

Aspiration of non-purulent, creamy, yellowish material suggests the possibility of an OKC. An aspirate from an OKC, if examined under a microscope, may show an abundance of keratinaceous materials accompanied by squamoid appearing epithelial cells. Aspirate from any other odontogenic cyst or a tumour with cystic degeneration is likely to be a straw-coloured fluid with no keratin present.

4.7.4 Incisional Biopsy

Under local anaesthesia, a mucoperiosteal flap was raised to expose the buccal bone distal in the mandibular molar and retromolar region. A bony window was created to expose the lesion. Incising the soft tissue lining beneath the bone revealed a cyst cavity containing thick yellow material. The cyst lining was friable, and a sample was harvested fixed in formalin for dispatching for histopathological examination. Cystic areas were irrigated with saline. A decompression tube was inserted into the cyst cavity and was externalized into the oral cavity through a window in the mucoperiosteal flap. The mucoperiosteal flap was replaced using 3/0 Vicryl sutures, and the decompression tube was anchored at the mucosal opening with 2/0 proline sutures (Fig. 4.4).

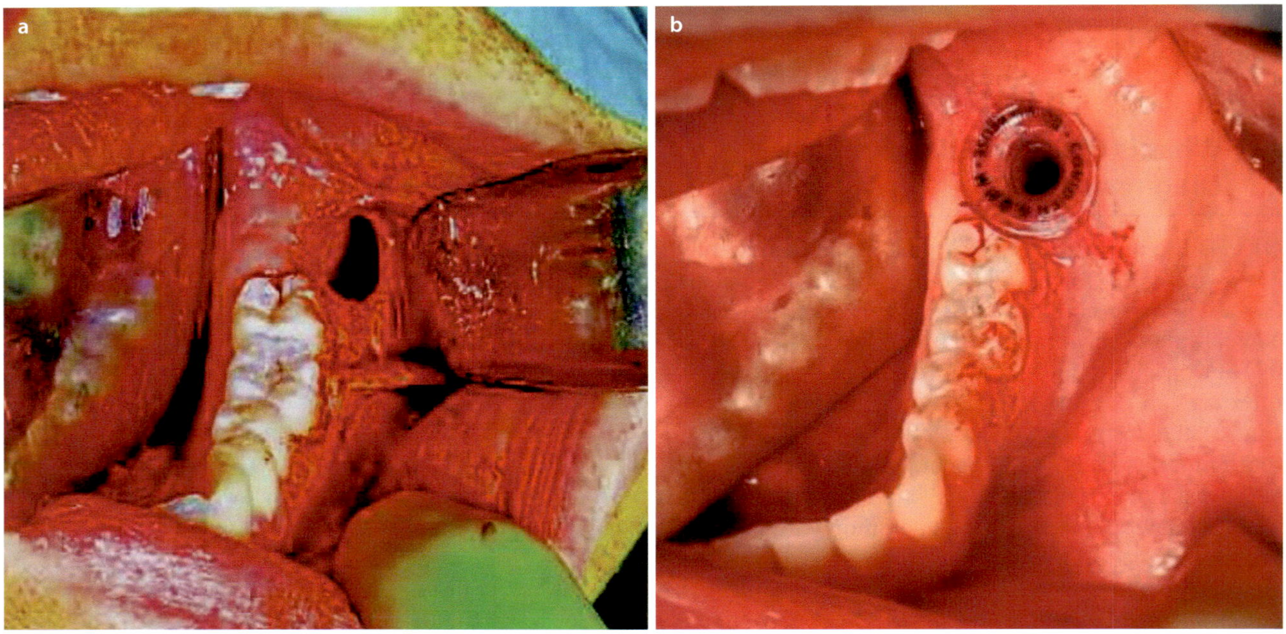

Fig. 4.4 Intra-operative photographs show (**a**) an opening made into the cyst cavity to obtain a sample of cyst lining for histopathology examination and (**b**) securing a silicone tube for decompression and for helping the patient to regularly irrigate the cyst cavity for hygiene maintenance

4.8 What Are the Histopathological Findings?

4.8.1 Histopathological Examination

The haematoxylin/eosin (H&E) stained sections show a small amount of mature fibrous connective tissue lined by parakeratinized stratified squamous epithelium with a prominent palisaded basal cell layer and reversed polarity of nuclei in some areas. The fibrous connective tissue is minimally inflamed (◘ Fig. 4.5). The epithelium and connective tissue interface is flat and is free of rete ridges. Detachment of the epithelial lining is seen in many regions. The histopathology is consistent with an odontogenic keratocyst (OKC).

4.8.2 3-D Imaging

A CT scan (computerized tomography) was performed to accurately assess the extent of the lesion to help plan definitive treatment. Imaging showed mild expansion of both buccal and lingual cortices of the body of the left mandible with thinning of the expanded cortex towards the lower border. There was significant cortical thinning in some areas but no evidence of cortical breaching and extension into overlying soft tissues.

Since this is the second primary OKC to be diagnosed in this patient, he was comprehensively assessed for other known manifestations of NBCCS. Both the clinical examination and the CT scan did not reveal any other features described with NBCCS (◘ Fig. 4.6).

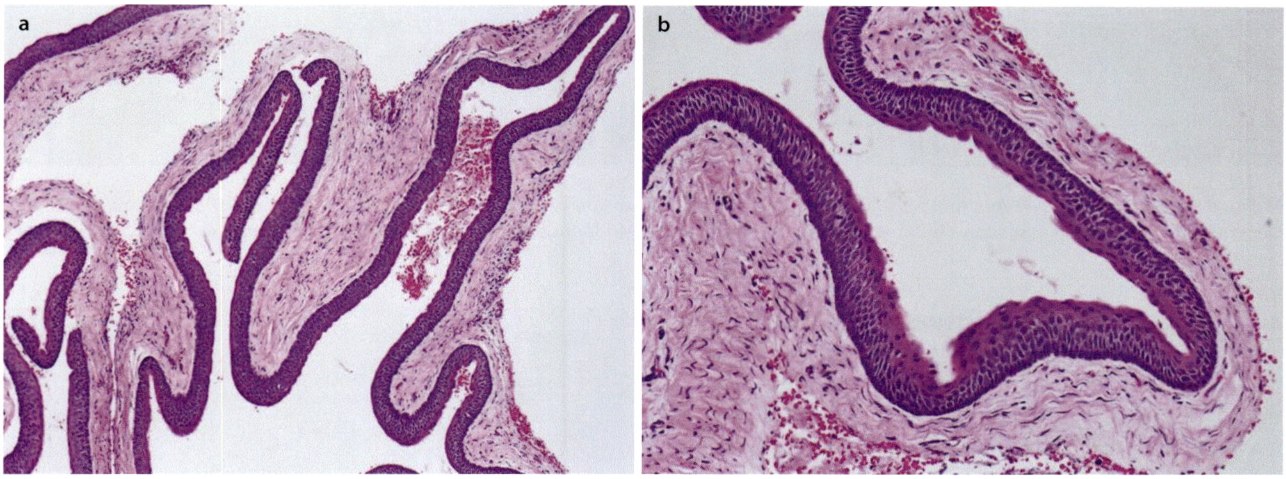

◘ **Fig. 4.5** (**a**) Cystic lesion lined by regular and thin parakeratinized stratified squamous epithelium exhibiting flat epithelium-connective tissue interface. (**b**) The basal-cell layer demonstrates palisaded hyperchromatic nuclei

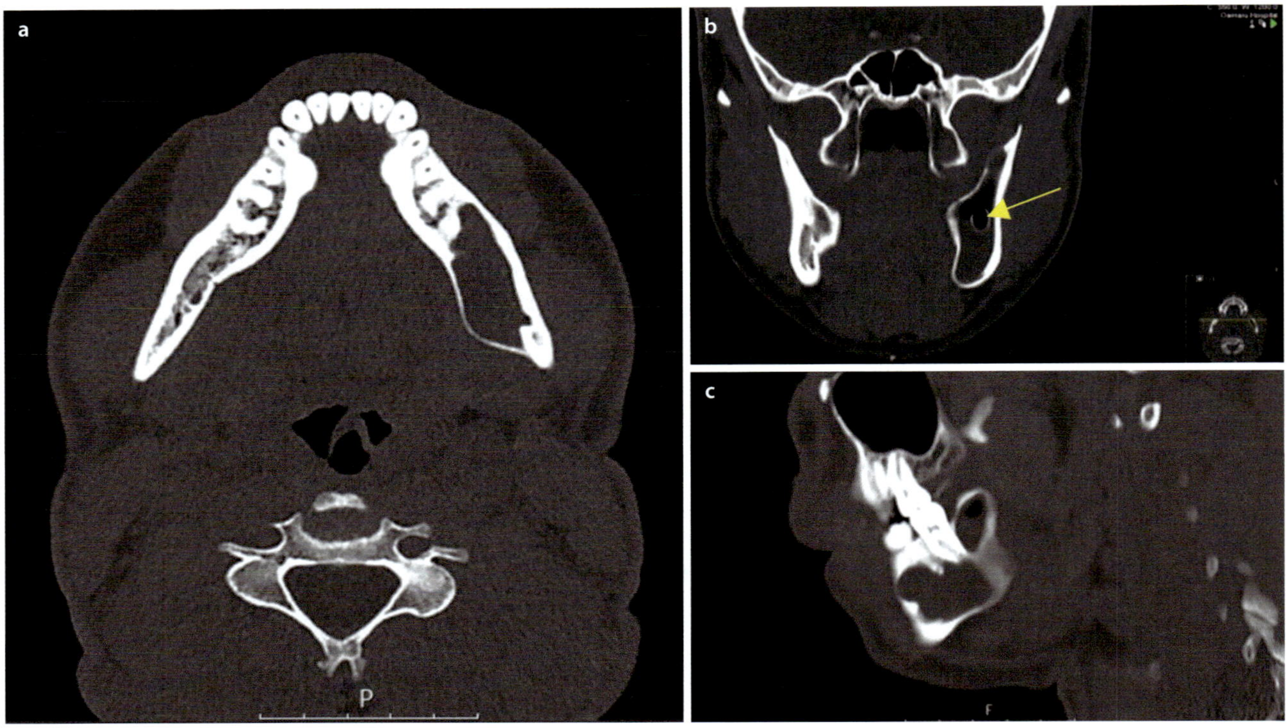

Fig. 4.6 Computerized tomography shows (**a** and **b**) minimal expansion of buccal and lingual cortices and (**c**) mutilocularity and no evidence of root resorption in mandibular second molar. The arrow in (**b**) indicates the position of the decompression tube

4.9 What Is the Definitive Diagnosis?

In the absence of other features described in NBCCS, the multilocular radiolucent lesion involving the left mandibular body and ascending ramus is consistent with a diagnosis of an odontogenic keratocyst (OKC) with no radiologically evident extra-osseous extension (Table 4.1).

Table 4.1 Features of naevoid basal-cell carcinoma syndrome

Major criteria	Minor criteria
• Multiple basal cell carcinoma or BCC arising before 20 years of age • A first degree relative with NBCCS • Abnormal calcification is seen radiographically in the head and neck region (e.g. calcification of falx cerebri) • Odontogenic keratocyst/s • Bifid/fused or splayed ribs • Multiple (>3) palmer and/or planter pits • PTCH1 mutation	• Macrocephaly/ Frontal bossing • Cleft lip/palateor polydactyly • Skeletal anomalies • Cardiac or ovarian fibroma • Medulloblastoma

An individual needs to have at least two major criteria or one major criterion with two minor criteria to be diagnosed with NBCCS

4.10 What Specific Findings Help You to Arrive at the Diagnosis?

The insidious nature of the swelling with minimal symptoms suggested a slow, potentially benign disease process also endorsed by the absence of tooth loosening and/or displacement. The involvement of the tooth-bearing region is strongly indicative of a lesion of an odontogenic origin. Multilocular radiolucency involving the posterior mandible in a male in his 30 s, with no clinical and radiological association with an unerupted tooth or a non-vital tooth, increases the likelihood of a diagnosis between ameloblastoma or OKC. The minimal cortical expansion amidst an extensive mesiodistal extension, absence of any neurosensory deficits in the distribution of the inferior alveolar nerve and the lack of tooth displacement and tooth mobility favour a clinical and radiological diagnosis of OKC over ameloblastoma. Like in many oral lesions, histopathology is the confirmatory diagnostic test for OKC. Despite known limitations of representation, an incision biopsy is a prudent option when dealing with a large lesion. Early histopathological confirmation of the diagnosis helps formulate an appropriate treatment plan to offer this patient.

4.11 How Will You Treat This Patient?

Following a detailed discussion with this patient, a decision was made to adopt a two-stage approach: to continue maintaining cyst decompression over 6–12 months followed by a definitive surgical treatment consisting of enucleation with curettage/peripheral ostectomy with the application of cryotherapy to the cyst cavity walls. The patient was advised on how to irrigate the cyst cavity through the decompression tube, the necessity to maintain good oral hygiene and attend regular periodic follow-ups for clinical and radiological monitoring of the lesion.

4.12 What Is the Rationale for Treatment?

OKC is a benign lesion but with a potential for locally aggressive behaviour coupled with a high tendency to recur following inadequate treatment. Historically treatment strategies were in favour of radical excisions/curettage to mitigate the high recurrence rates. This approach often resulted in significant intra and postoperative morbidity, including loss of vitality of the teeth in proximity to the lesion, loss of sensory innervation in the lower lip and teeth from damage to the inferior alveolar nerve and in some cases, to iatrogenic fracture of the mandible. However, a deeper understanding of the biological behaviour of the lesion and the recent reversal into a cyst category from its previous position among odontogenic tumours has promoted more conservative approaches to treatment. In contemporary practice, many clinicians have opted to initially decompress the cyst, which in most instances may lead to complete if not substantial regression of the size of the cyst over time. This permits subsequent definitive treatment to be planned and performed with minimal damages to vital structures (i.e. inferior alveolar bundle, tooth roots, etc.) and also significantly reduces the risk of iatrogenic, jaw fractures. However, such treatment decisions should be made through careful consideration of the patient's ability to comply with maintenance of good oral hygiene and attending periodic follow-up visits.

4.13 Follow-Up and Prognosis

This patient was reviewed in the outpatient clinic 3 months post-biopsy and decompression surgery to ensure he managed self-irrigation of the cyst cavity to maintain good hygiene. A DPT taken at the following review (6 months post-surgery) showed bone in-fill resulting in a significant shrinkage of the cyst cavity (◘ Fig. 4.7).

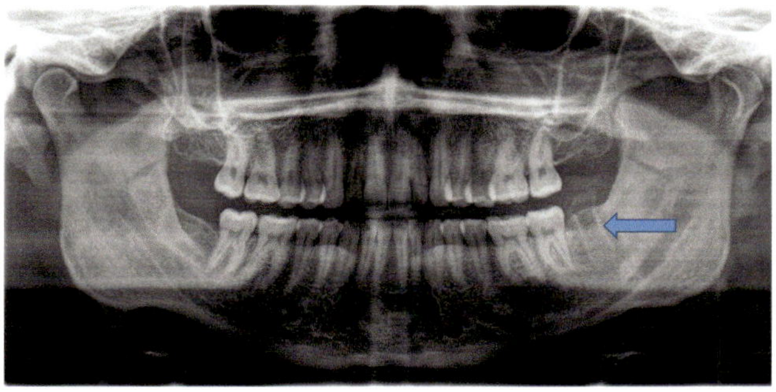

◘ **Fig. 4.7** The DPT at 6 months follow-up shows a good response to decompression. Note how the cyst has reduced in size (compare with ◘ Fig. 4.3) and the decompression tube in situ (arrow)

He will be reviewed again at 9 months post-surgery for definitive treatment of the OKC. The anticipated treatment would include removing the decompression tube, enucleation of the residual cyst lining, peripheral ostectomy/curettage and achieving primary closure to facilitate healing. On completion of the definitive surgery, a further 5–10-year follow-up with periodic clinical and radiological monitoring will be implemented for surveillance against potential recurrence and the emergence of any features indicative of BCCNS.

4.14 Odontogenic Keratocyst

Odontogenic keratocyst (OKC) is the third most common cyst of the jaws and accounts for approximately 10–20% of all odontogenic cysts. It is a benign, but locally aggressive developmental cyst due to its propensity to recur following treatment. The odontogenic keratocyst is defined by the fourth edition of WHO Head and Neck Tumours as "an odontogenic cyst characterized by a thin, regular lining of parakeratinized stratified squamous epithelium with palisading hyperchromatic basal cells". It was first described by Philipsen in 1956 as an odontogenic cyst exhibiting distinctive histopathological features and further investigated for its characteristics by Pindborg and Hanson in 1963. Gorlin and Goltz then described multiple OKCs as one of the manifestations of naevoid basal cell carcinoma syndrome.

Clinical behaviour and the high recurrence rate of OKCs have placed OKCs in a unique position within the spectrum of odontogenic lesions. The first and second editions of WHO classifications of Head and Neck tumours regarded OKC as a developmental odontogenic cyst. This lesion was then regarded as neoplasm because of its some unusual histological features, aggressive clinical behaviour and association with mutation or inactivation of PTCH gene which is a tumour suppressor gene. In the third edition of WHO classification of Head and Neck Tumours, this entity was classified as a neoplasm and renamed as keratocystic odontogenic tumour (KCOT). However, this lesion was reclassified as an odontogenic cyst in 2017 as published in the fourth edition of WHO classification of Head and Neck tumours as there was insufficient evidence to support the neoplastic origin of the lesion.

OKCs occur in patients over a wide age range with a peak in the second and third decades of life with a male predominance. The mandible is the most common site of occurrence for OKC, and more than half of the lesions involve the posterior body and ramus of the mandible. On the contrary, the anterior sextants, mainly the canine region, are the most common site of origin in the maxilla. OKC occurs in the posterior maxilla and has been associated with naevoid basal cell carcinoma syndrome.

Aetiologically, OKC is a developmental cyst that can be traced from remnants of dental lamina that involve in the development of gingiva and periodontal ligament. Researchers have also suggested that the basal layer of the oral mucosal epithelium may involve in the aetiology of OKC in consideration of the common presence of OKC at the posterior mandible region. The characteristic growth pattern of OKC along anteroposterior direction has been proposed to be in association with intraluminal hyperosmolarity, the collagenolytic activity of the cyst wall, epithelial proliferation and interleukin synthesis. Patched (PTCH) gene mutation has been implicated for the neoplastic capability and high recurrence rate of OKC. PTCH gene mutation activates the SHH signalling pathway leading to aberrant cell proliferation in the epithelium of OKC.

Clinically, OKC can manifest as single or multiple lesions. Small lesions are often asymptomatic and are found as incidental findings during radiographic investigations. Symptomatic lesions are frequently larger and cause displacement of adjacent structures. Most OKCs however, cause less bone expansion compared to ameloblastoma. It has a propensity to grow in an anteroposterior direction. Maxillary OKCs may displace the orbit and are more often associated with secondary infection. In the presence of multiple OKCs, the patient should be evaluated for the naevoid basal cell carcinoma syndrome. The syndromic OKC tends to occur in younger patients.

Radiographic investigations play an important role in the diagnosis and management of OKC. The radiological imaging techniques that are commonly used are conventional radiography (mainly dental panoramic tomograph), computed tomography (CT) and magnetic resonance imaging (MRI). Radiographically, OKC presents as a well-defined unilocular or multilocular radiolucency with well-corticated margins. OKC is often seen in association with a crown of a mandibular third molar, giving rise to a similar radiographic appearance to a dentigerous cyst. Radiographic features for small unilocular OKCs are not pathognomonic as they can show resemblance to other odontogenic and non-odontogenic cysts. The peculiar pattern of growth for large mandibular OKCs may determine an extensive radiolucent lesion with considerable mesiodistal dimensions without significant cortical expansion. Maxillary OKCs of large size may extend to involve adjacent structures such as the maxillary antrum and the nasal cavity. Displacement of any adjacent teeth and root resorption can occur with OKCs but are less frequently seen when compared to ameloblastomas and other locally aggressive tumours. Similarly, neurosensory defects are uncommon except when an OKC is secondarily infected or is extensively large. A discovery of multiple radiolucencies within the jawbone may be a syndromic manifestation and merits further investigation.

Histopathological features of OKCs are well characterized and pathognomonic. OKC exhibits thin and regular parakeratinized epithelium with a corrugated surface. It is about 5–8 cell layers in thickness without rete ridges. The basal cell layer is well defined and shows prominent nuclear palisading, with hyperchromatic nuclei and focal reversal polarity. The epithelial-connective tissue junction is often flat. The accompanying fibrous wall is often uninflamed unless secondarily infected. Inflamed OKCs may display loss of typical parakeratinized lining and may exhibit hyperplastic stratified squamous epithelium. Small islands or satellite cysts may be found within the cyst wall. The salient features of OKC are summarized in ◘ Table 4.2.

Table 4.2 Salient features of odontogenic keratocyst

Clinical	Small lesions, often asymptomatic and discovered during radiographic examination. Larger lesions may cause cortical expansion and displacement of adjacent structures. Multiple OKCs may be associated with NBCCS
Radiology	A well-defined unilocular or multilocular radiolucency with corticated margins
Histopathology	Uninflamed fibrous cyst wall lined by thin and regular parakeratinized stratified squamous epithelium with flat epithelium-connective tissue interface. The basal cell layer is often palisaded and exhibits hyperchromatic nuclei with reversal nuclei polarity. Daughter cysts may be found within the cyst wall
Treatment	Treatment is mostly by enucleation, decompression/marsupialization followed by enucleation or resection based on clinical and radiological assessment and the anticipated potential morbidity associated with different options

OKC is a developmental cyst and, if inadequately treated, is associated with a high recurrence rate. A long-term, regular periodic follow-up is essential to monitor potential recurrences

Treatment of OKC depends on the patient's age, size of the lesion, location of the cyst and involvement of surrounding structures. The treatment options can be classified as conservative and radical approaches. Traditionally, a conservative approach would have included a simple enucleation or a marsupialization, whereas a radical approach consists of peripheral osteotomy with or without chemical curettage with Carnoy's solution, cryotherapy, electrocautery and in some cases, an en-bloc resection. Simple enucleation is reportedly associated with a 30–60% high recurrence rate. Radical approaches show reduced recurrence rates but are frequently associated with significant postoperative morbidity, which could be unacceptable to some patients. A recent trend towards a more conservative yet comprehensive approach, including an initial decompression followed by enucleation and curettage/application of cryotherapy, is gaining popularity. This hybrid approach adopted in carefully selected patients helps achieve better clinical outcomes with less operative morbidity. In contemporary practice, radical resections are generally reserved for managing recurrent lesions.

The aggressive behaviour and high recurrence rate of OKC, despite its benign nature, have gained special attention over the years. The recurrence rate ranges from 25 to 60%, and most of the cases reportedly recur within 5 years post-treatment. The factors that are associated with recurrence of OKCs include incomplete removal of cystic lining, thin and fragile epithelial lining, budding in the basal layer of the epithelium, bony perforation, involvement of adjacent structures, split of the epithelial lining during manipulation and growth of new OKC from satellite cysts or remnants. The use of adjunctive methods such as liquid nitrogen cryotherapy and the application of Carnoy's solution to destroy residual cyst lining was a popular option to reduce potential recurrences. Despite its efficacy, the recent concerns on potential carcinogenicity have resulted in the discontinuation of Carnoy's solution in many countries. Recent reports on using a chloroform-free "Modified Carnoy's solution" haven't shown the same efficacy for reducing recurrences when used in the management of OKCs.

Diagnostic Algorithm

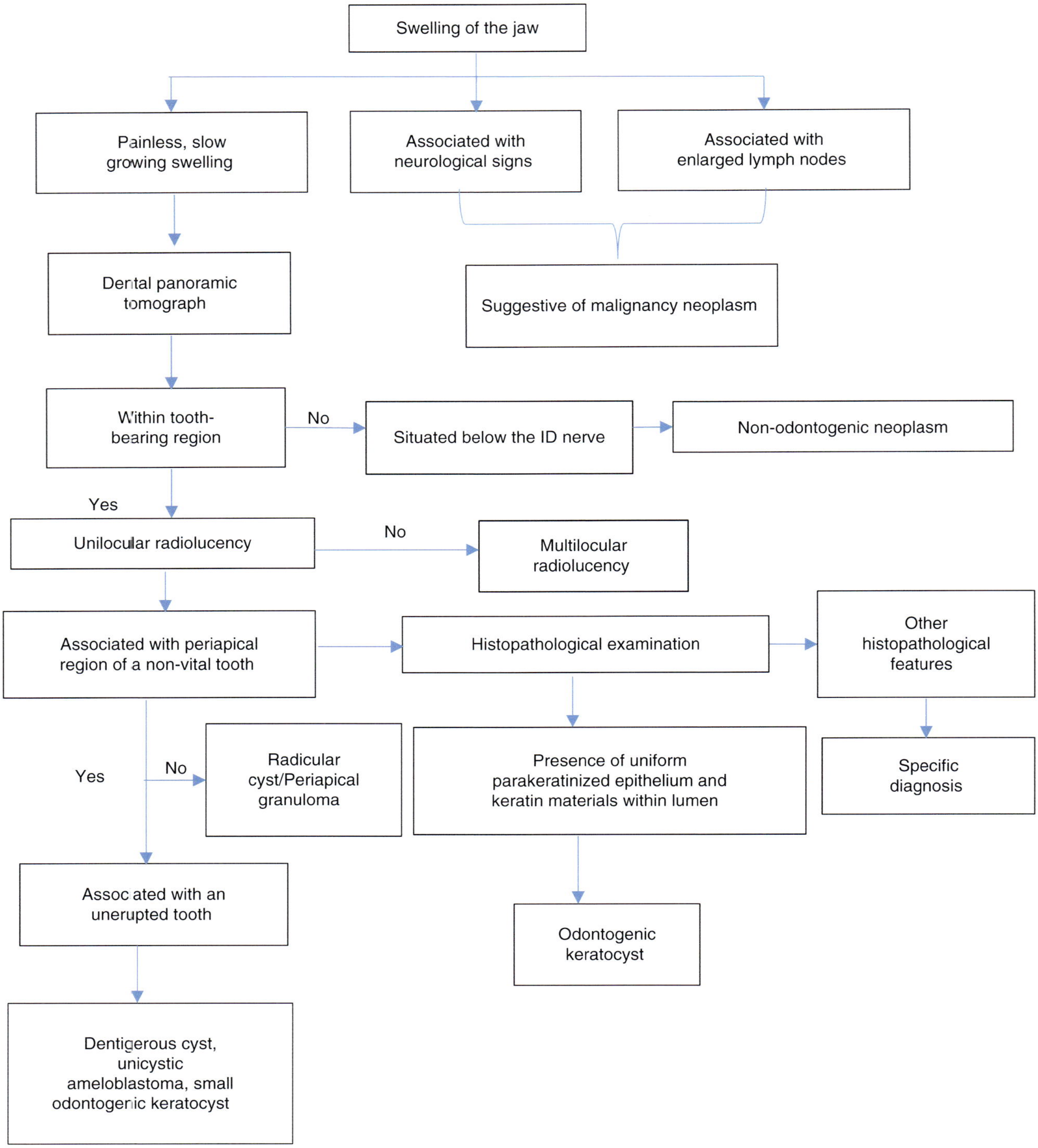

Self-Assessment Questions

1. State the clinical characteristics of odontogenic keratocyst.
2. Discuss the clinical significance of multiple odontogenic keratocysts occurring in an individual.
3. Describe the histopathological features of odontogenic keratocyst.
4. Discuss the treatment of odontogenic keratocyst.
5. Discuss the factors associated with the high recurrence rate of odontogenic keratocyst.

Summary

OKC is a developmental cyst and, if inadequately treated, is associated with a high recurrence rate. A long-term, regular periodic follow-up is essential to monitor potential recurrences.

Further Reading

Blanas N, Freund B, Schwartz M, Furst IM. Systematic review of the treatment and prognosis of the odontogenic keratocyst. Oral Surg Oral Med Oral Pathol Oral Radiol Endod. 2000;90(5):553–8.

Borghesi A, Nardi C, Giannitto C, Tironi A, Maroldi R, Di Bartolomeo F, Preda L. Odontogenic keratocyst: imaging features of a benign lesion with an aggressive behaviour. Insights Imaging. 2018;9(5):883–97.

Jung HD, Lim JH, Kim HJ, et al. Appropriate follow-up period for odontogenic keratocyst: a retrospective study. Maxillofac Plast Reconstr Surg. 2021;43:16.

Li TJ. The odontogenic keratocyst: a cyst, or a cystic neoplasm? J Dent Res. 2011;90(2):133–42.

Lo Muzio L. Nevoid basal cell carcinoma syndrome (Gorlin syndrome). Orphanet J Rare Dis. 2008;3:32. https://doi.org/10.1186/1750-1172-3-32.

Menon S. Keratocystic odontogenic tumours: etiology, pathogenesis and treatment revisited. J Maxillofac Oral Surg. 2015;14(3):541–7.

Nayak MT, Singh A, Singhvi A, Sharma R. Odontogenic keratocyst: what is in the name? J Nat Sci Biol Med. 2013;4(2):282–5.

Ribeiro-Júnior O, Borba AM, Alves CAF, Gouveia MM, Deboni MCZ, Naclério-Homem MDG. Reclassification and treatment of odontogenic keratocysts: a cohort study. Braz Oral Res. 2017;31:e98.

Dull Pain and Discoloration of Upper Front Tooth: Radicular Cyst

Anand Ramanathan and Yet Ching Goh

Contents

W. M Tilakaratne, T. G. Kallarakkal (eds.), *Clinicopathological Correlation of Oral Diseases*,
https://doi.org/10.1007/978-3-031-24408-7_5

5

Learning Goals

1. Devise the correct way of compiling the history with appropriate questions.
2. Develop a differential diagnosis after history taking.
3. Deduce appropriate procedures in clinical examination.
4. Formulate a differential diagnosis combining findings in the history and clinical examination.
5. Justify the relevant investigations required to arrive at the diagnosis.
6. Comprehend the importance of clinicopathological correlation in arriving at the correct diagnosis.
7. Outline the management plan.
8. Recognize the importance of a diagnostic algorithm in arriving at a diagnosis.

5.1 Main Complaint

A 30-year-old gentleman came to the dental clinic complaining of dull pain and tooth discoloration involving an upper front tooth.

5.2 History of Complaint

Question: When did you notice the discoloration?

The discoloration has been there for more than 1 year.

Question: Did you experience injury/accident related to the tooth?

I had a fall and knocked my front teeth a few years ago. Both upper front teeth had fractured at the edge.

Question: Did you seek dental treatment following the injury?

I visited a dental practitioner, and a few procedures were performed. I was informed that one of the tooth was dead and needed root canal treatment. However, I was not keen on having a root canal treatment.

Question: What happened after that?

After a few years, I realized that one of my fractured teeth was getting discoloured. Then I decided to visit a Dentist. He explained to me that the tooth is dead and needed root canal treatment. The tooth was treated accordingly.

Question: Did you have any problems in relation to that tooth after root canal treatment?

Not until recently when it started giving dull pain.

Question: Did the tooth change in colour despite the dental treatment performed?

I noticed the tooth with root canal treatment turning more yellowish after the treatment was completed.

Question: Did you have other symptoms besides the discoloration?

There was mild pain as I said earlier whenever I bite on hard food. Otherwise, there was no discomfort.

Question: Did you notice any swelling pertaining to the area?

I did not notice any swelling in that area but I felt some difference.

Question: Can you tell us more about the pain?

The pain was mild. The pain did not disturb my daily activities.

Question: Did you seek for treatment for the pain?

I did not visit dental clinic after the root canal treatment was completed.

5.3 Past Medical History

Question: Are you suffering from any other medical problems? If yes, what kind of medication have you been taking until now?

I am not suffering from any medical problems.

5.4 Findings of Intra-oral Examination

Question: What are the intra-oral findings that you see in this patient?

Tooth 21 is discoloured with unsatisfactory fractured restoration at the incisal aspect (Fig. 5.1a). The mesio-incisal edge of 11 is also fractured and restored with a tooth-coloured restoration. There is a large restoration noted at the palatal surface of 21 (Fig. 5.1b).

Question: What are your clinical differential diagnoses for this presentation? Provide justification for your differential diagnoses.

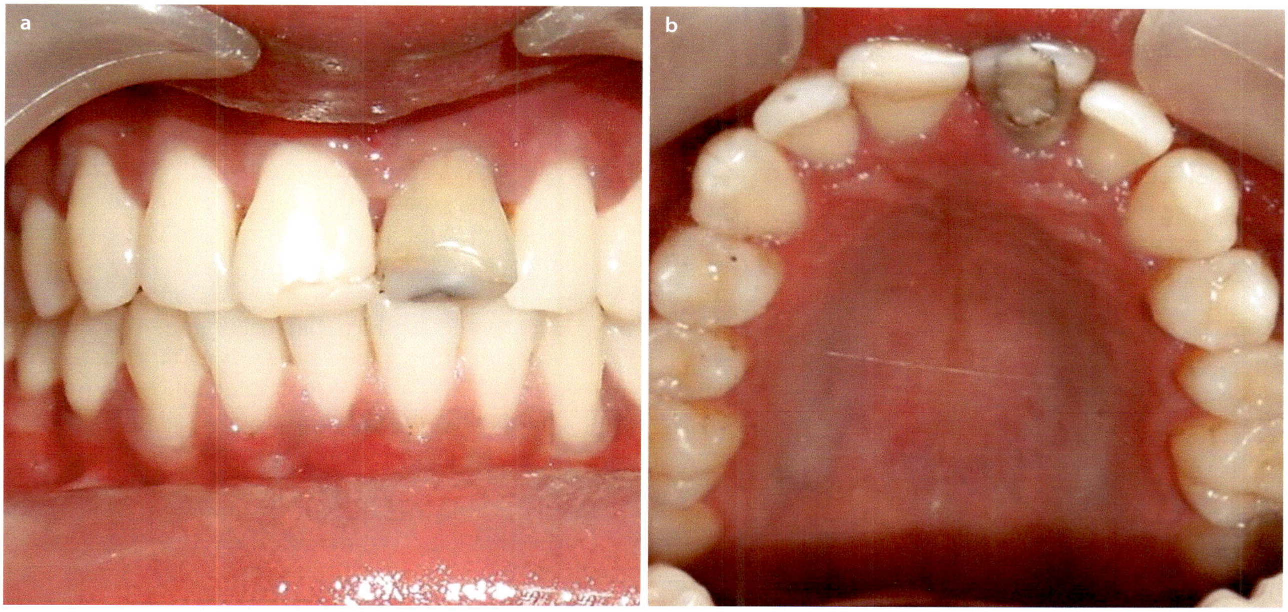

Fig. 5.1 Tooth 21 shows discoloration with fractured restoration at the incisal aspect (**a**). There is a large tooth-coloured restoration at the palatal surface of 21 (**b**). (Courtesy: Dr. Ruvinath Rajapaksa)

Chronic pain arising from periapical pathosis such as:
1. Chronic periapical abscess
2. periapical granuloma
3. Radicular cyst

An endodontically treated tooth is expected to be symptom-free following a successful root canal treatment. Inappropriate mechanical debridement, persistence of bacteria in the canals and apex, poor obturation quality, over and under extension of the root canal filling and coronal leakage are some of the commonly attributable causes of failure. It is also possible that a cystic lesion was present at the time of root canal treatment, and it has got inflamed or infected with time. In the present case, the tooth requires further assessment to work out any underlying causes for the chronic pain.

5.5 What Is the Most Likely Clinical Diagnosis for This Lesion?

Periapical pathosis (Chronic periapical abscess, periapical granuloma or radicular cyst).

5.6 What Investigations You Would Need to Carry Out for This Patient?

1. The associated tooth is endodontically treated. Hence, it is unjustifiable for a tooth sensibility test as the response may not be representative for the true status of the tooth. There may be exaggerated response from the periodontal ligament which may give rise to a false-positive reading; hence, pulp sensibility test is not needed.

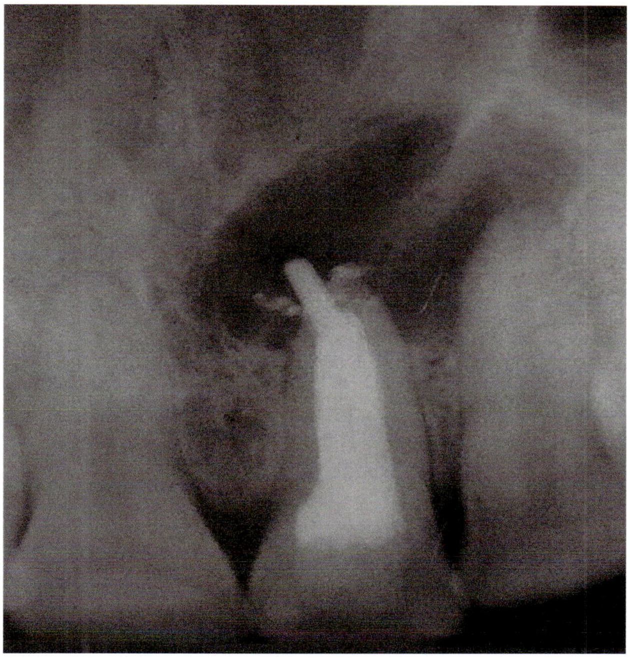

Fig. 5.2 IOPA revealed a radiolucency at the periapical region of tooth 21 with extruded root canal filling material. (Courtesy: Dr. Ruvinath Rajapaksa)

2. An intra-oral periapical radiograph (IOPA) of tooth 21 and 11 is required to investigate the presence of periapical pathology.

The IOPA radiograph showed a well-demarcated radiolucency with cortication at the periapical region of tooth 21 (Fig. 5.2). A radio-opacity within the root canal of tooth 21 consistent with root canal filling material was indicative of prior root canal treatment. The root canal filling material appeared extruded from the apical foramen.

5.7 What Is the Most Likely Working Diagnosis?

Radicular cyst.

Both the periapical granuloma and radicular cyst appear as radiolucency radiographically. However, radicular cyst usually has corticated border and attains larger size than periapical granuloma (more than 1.5 cm). In the present case, the features are more justifiable for a working diagnosis of a radicular cyst.

5.8 How Would You Manage This Patient?

If the tooth can be restored without the need for extraction, then the treatment of choice would be to carry out:

(a) Non-surgical root canal treatment followed by enucleation of the cystic lesion. Root canal retreatment for the central incisor involving the removal of existing root canal filling material and re-obturation. Enucleation of the cystic lesion can be performed after the retreatment of the associated tooth is completed.

(b) Periradicular surgery followed by enucleation of the cystic lesion. Apicectomy to remove the apical portion of the root with ill-filled root canal material and enucleation of the cystic lesion can be carried out concurrently.

For the present case, the periapical region of 21 was surgically explored. A cystic cavity was revealed during procedure (◘ Fig. 5.3a). Apicectomy followed by apical plug placement with mineral trioxide aggregate (MTA) was performed. A bone graft was placed after periapical curettage (◘ Fig. 5.3b). The enucleated tissue was submitted for histopathological examination. The post-operative periapical radiograph showed well-sealed root canal of 21 and bony defect that was packed with bone graft (◘ Fig. 5.3c).

The soft tissue which was curettage was sent for histopathological examination.

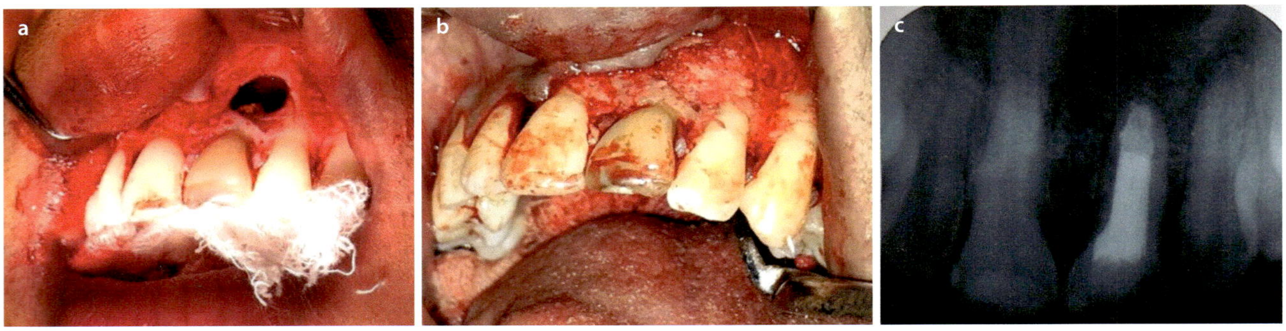

◘ **Fig. 5.3** Intraoral photographs show (**a**) an empty cavity consistent with cystic cavity was observed upon surgical exploration (**b**) bone graft was placed after periapical curettage and MTA apical barrier placement (**c**) post-operative periapical radiograph taken after a few months shows signs of healing of the cystic cavity. (Courtesy: Dr. Ruvinath Rajapaksa)

5.9 What Specific Histopathological Features Are Helpful to Arrive at a Definitive Diagnosis?

There is a cystic lesion lined by stratified squamous epithelium exhibiting exocytosis and spongiosis with an underlying fibrous connective tissue heavily infiltrated by chronic inflammatory cells (◘ Fig. 5.4a). In areas, the epithelium proliferates in an arcading pattern (◘ Fig. 5.4b). Aggregates of cholesterol clefts are observed in the cyst wall (◘ Fig. 5.4c).

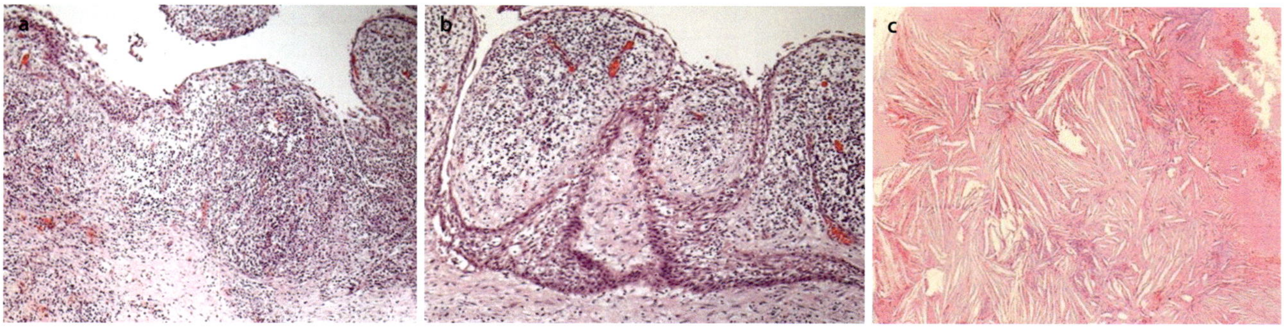

◘ **Fig. 5.4** Photomicrographs show (**a**) non-keratinized stratified squamous epithelium lining with an underlying inflamed connective tissue (**b**) hyperplastic lining epithelium proliferates in arcading pattern (**c**) foci of cholesterol clefts are present in the connective tissue wall

5.10 What Is the Definitive Diagnosis for This Lesion?

Radicular cyst (The synonyms for radicular cyst include dental cyst, periapical cyst and periodontal cyst).

5.11 What Specific Findings Would Help You to Arrive at the Diagnosis of Radicular Cyst?

1. Clinical findings: Clinically, a discoloured tooth indicated the pulp undergoing necrosis leading to a non-vital tooth.
2. Radiographic findings: IOPA radiograph showing the presence of a periapical radiolucency in relation to the central incisor. The radioloucency is well demarcated and corticated and more than 1.5 cm in diameter.
3. Histopathological findings: Histopathology examination reveals a cystic lesion lined by non-keratinized stratified squamous epithelial lining. The epithelium shows typical arcading pattern. Dense chronic inflammatory cell infiltrate is present in the connective tissue wall.

5.12 What Is the Prognosis for Radicular Cyst?

Usually, radicular cysts have a good prognosis without recurrence. Some radicular cysts persist as residual cysts even after the extraction of the associated tooth.

5.13 Radicular Cyst

A radicular cyst is defined as an odontogenic cyst of inflammatory origin associated with a non-vital tooth. A residual cyst is a radicular cyst that persists in the jaw after the extraction of the affected tooth. Radicular cyst is also called as an inflammatory dental cyst, dental cyst, periapical cyst or periodontal cyst. It is the most common cyst of jaws with 55% of all odontogenic cysts being radicular cysts. Its peak incidence is in the fourth and fifth decades of life, but it can occur over a wide range of ages. It shows a slight male predilection. About half of the cases occur in the anterior region of the maxilla. Radicular cyst is mostly located at the apex of the tooth. However, some radicular cysts do occur along the lateral side of the tooth when it is associated with a lateral root canal and is defined as inflammatory lateral periodontal cyst.

The pathogenesis of radicular cyst formation can be divided into three phases: (1) initiation, (2) cyst formation and (3) enlargement.

5.13.1 Initiation of Cyst

Radicular cyst is said to arise due to the proliferation of the cell rests of Malassez (remnants of Hertwig epithelial root sheath). These cell rests are present in the periodontal ligament that is present within the periapical granuloma which is associated with the necrotic and infected pulp. The key factors that initiate the proliferation of the epithelial rests of Malassez are the bacterial endotoxins and antigens released from the necrotic pulp. The necrosis of the pulp can occur either due to extension of dental caries into pulp or due to trauma. Areas of intense inflammation in the cyst contain numerous lymphocytes, polymorphonuclear leukocytes, plasma cells and Langerhan cells. T-lymphocytes predominate with both helper T-cells (CD4) and suppressor/cytotoxic T cells (CD8) in both the periapical granuloma and cyst. The helper T-cells are seen in the connective tissue around the epithelium, whereas suppressor/cytotoxic T-cells are present within the epithelium. Langerhan cells are antigen-presenting cells that present bacterial antigens which enter the periapical region of the tooth to helper T-cells, thus initiating an inflammatory response. The helper T-cells release cytokines such as interleukin-2 (IL-2) and γ-interferons (INF-γ). INF-γ further activates the macrophages which release cytokines such as IL-1, IL-6 and tumour-necrosing factor-α (TNF-α). IL-1 and IL-6 help in proliferation of the cell rests of Malassez. IL-2 helps in further proliferation of helper T cells and activation of B lymphocytes into plasma cells that produce antibodies such as IgG, IgA, IgE and IgM. These antibodies result in the formation of antigen–antibody complexes leading to coactivation of complement pathway and resulting in increased vascular permeability and leucotactic response which enhances inflammation and proliferation of the epithelium. The bacterial endotoxins may also activate the complement pathway. Endotoxins initiate an inflammatory response resulting in the production of cytokines with pro-inflammatory and bone-resorbing activities. Interleukin-1α (IL-1α), IL-1β, IL-6, IL-8, tumour-necrosing factor-α (TNF-α), γ-interferons (INF-γ) and transforming growth factor-β1 (TGF-β1) are the bone resorbing factors produced in radicular cysts. IL-6 and IL-8 also have a direct effect on epithelial proliferation. As the periapical granuloma increases in size, local changes such as decreased oxygen tension and increased carbon dioxide tension result in low pH and activate proliferation of the cell rests of Malassez.

5.13.2 Formation of Cyst

In this phase, the cavity of the cyst starts to line by proliferating epithelium. This can happen in two ways that are independent of each other. First, an abscess is formed in the centre around which the epithelium proliferates and covers the connective tissue of the abscess cavity or the cavity that is formed by the breakdown of the connective tissue as a result of proteolytic enzyme activity. Secondly, the epithelium proliferates and undergoes degeneration at its centre to produce a cystic cavity filled with fluid. This degeneration at the centre of the proliferating epithelium can occur in two ways. The central cells of the epithelium get degenerated due to immunological reaction or autolysis leading to the formation of the cystic cavity filled with fluid and lined by an epithelium. Due to lack of blood supply, the cells at the centre are further away from their nutrient source and undergo liquefactive necrosis, thus forming the cystic cavity filled by fluid and lined by an epithelium. As the epithelium proliferates, numerous microcysts form at different parts of the connective tissue and coalesce together to form a large cystic cavity.

5.13.3 Growth and Enlargement of the Cyst

There are several reasons postulated for the growth and enlargement of the cyst. Expansion of the radicular cyst may be due to the increased osmotic pressure within the cystic lumen. High protein content, inflammatory exudate, cell breakdown products and hyaluronic acid in the cystic fluid contribute to the increased osmotic pressure which results in further fluid accumulation within the cystic cavity, thus causing further expansion. In addition, increased hydrostatic pressure which is higher than the capillary pressure leads to bone resorption, thus resulting in expansion of the cyst. Further, resorption of bone takes place due to the presence of inflammatory cytokines such as IL-1, IL-6 and prostaglandins (PGE_2 and PGI_2) that are released from plasma cells, histiocytes, endothelial cells and fibroblasts. The cyst expansion is also facilitated due to the breakdown of connective tissue components by collagenases. In addition, continuing epithelial proliferation occurs as a result of inflammation also lead to further cyst growth and enlargement.

Usually, the radicular cysts are symptomless and are found as incidental findings on radiographic examination. They are always associated with a non-vital tooth, which is a pathognomonic feature for their diagnosis. Radicular cysts show a round or oval, unilocular, well-demarcated radiolucency at the apex of the tooth. The radiolucency is usually about 1–2 cm in diameter, but rarely it can be larger. A residual cyst shows a persistent well-demarcated radiolucency at the site of a previously extracted tooth. However, it is difficult to distinguish radicular cyst from periapical granuloma by radiographic examination alone. Large periapical lesions are more likely to be radicular cysts than granuloma. Radicular cyst can be differentiated from periapical granuloma by periapical fluid analysis by polyacrylamide gel electrophoresis, tomography and ultrasound real-time imaging. However, the definitive diagnosis can only be obtained by histopathological examination of the periapical tissue.

Radicular cysts show a cystic lining of non-keratinized stratified squamous epithelium which is proliferative with elongated rete-ridges forming an arcading pattern. The connective tissue wall consists of a mixed inflammatory cell infiltrate. The inflammatory cells that are predominantly present in the connective tissue wall are lymphocytes, plasma cells, neutrophils and foamy macrophages (tissue histiocytes). Foreign-body giant cells may also be present. Deposits of cholesterol crystals (clefts) may be present in heavily inflamed radicular cysts. Hyaline or Rushton bodies may be present in some cases, but they are not pathognomonic to radicular cysts (◘ Fig. 5.5). Mature radicular cysts or residual cysts may have a regular thin non-keratinized stratified squamous epithelium and less inflammation within the connective tissue wall.

Radicular cyst can be classified into true cysts and bay/pocket cysts based on the relationship of the cyst

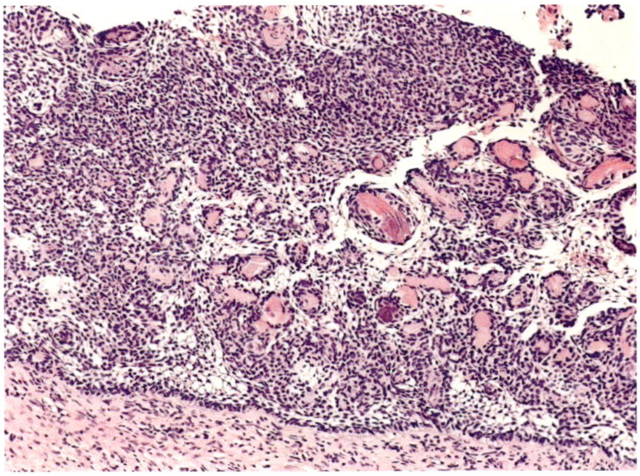

◘ **Fig. 5.5** Photomicrograph shows numerous hyaline or Rushton bodies present within the non-keratinized stratified squamous epithelium. (Courtesy Dr. Fairuz Abdul Rahman)

5

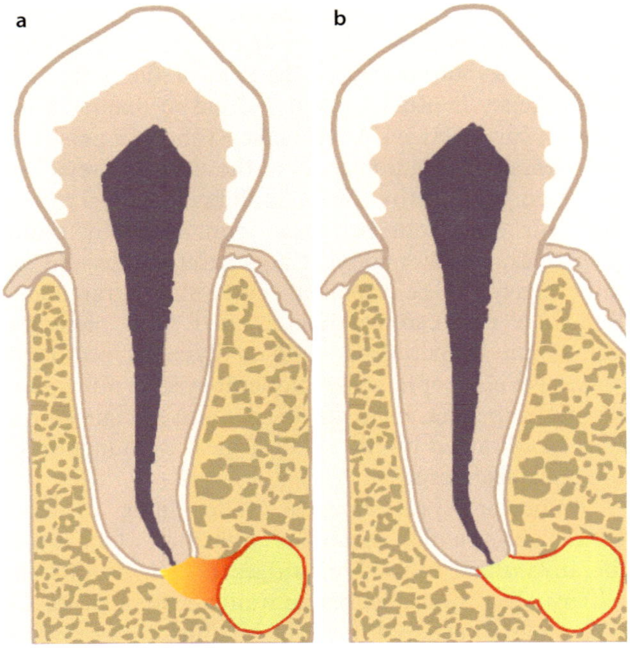

Fig. 5.6 Illustration shows (**a**) true cyst and (**b**) bay cyst

cavity to the root canal through the apical foramen. The true cysts are those radicular cysts with an independent cavity which has no communication with the root canal, whereas bay/pocket cysts are those radicular cysts showing a communication with the root canal through the apical foramen, and the root apex is protruded into the cavity (Fig. 5.6). The prevalence of true cysts ranges from 48 to 61.5%, whereas that of bay cysts ranges from 38.5 to 56% of all radicular cysts.

Radicular cysts may be treated by either non-surgical root canal treatment or periradicular surgery followed by apicectomy with enucleation of the cystic cavity or extraction of the associated tooth and enucleation of the cystic cavity. The true cysts are self-sustaining lesions that cannot heal by non-surgical root canal treatment, whereas the bay cysts especially the small ones heal after non-surgical root canal treatment. The reason being that the true cysts are independent from the root canal infection and therefore non-responsive to root canal treatment, whereas the bay cysts are in continuity with the root canals and therefore amenable to root canal infection control. However, this theory has been challenged as bay cysts can be more prone to infection from the bacteria that advances directly from the root canals into the cystic cavity and thus impairs healing even after proper intra-canal microbial treatment. Recent study has reported that there is no significant difference between true and bay cysts in clinical, radiographic, intra- or extra-radicular infections and severity of histological inflammation except for the morphological relationship of the cyst cavity with root canals, thus questioning the need to differentiate between the true and bay cysts. The failure of endodontic treatment of both types of cysts is attributed to either persistent or secondary intra-radicular bacterial infections and sometimes along with extra-radicular bacterial infections.

The prognosis of radicular cysts is good, but rarely the radicular cyst may persist even after the extraction of the associated tooth giving rise to a residual cyst.

Salient Features of Radicular Cyst	
Clinical	Dull pain, history of trauma, discoloured tooth, non-vital tooth (either carious or heavily restored). Swelling is observed when the lesion reaches considerable large size.
Radiological	Periapical radiolucency at the apex of the affected tooth which is well corticated.
Histopathology	Non-keratinized stratified squamous epithelium lining the cystic lumen and presence of chronic inflammatory cells in the connective tissue wall.
Treatment	Non-surgical root canal treatment or periradicular surgery with apicectomy and enucleation of the cystic cavity or extraction of the affected tooth followed by enucleation of the cyst.

■ Diagnostic Algorithm

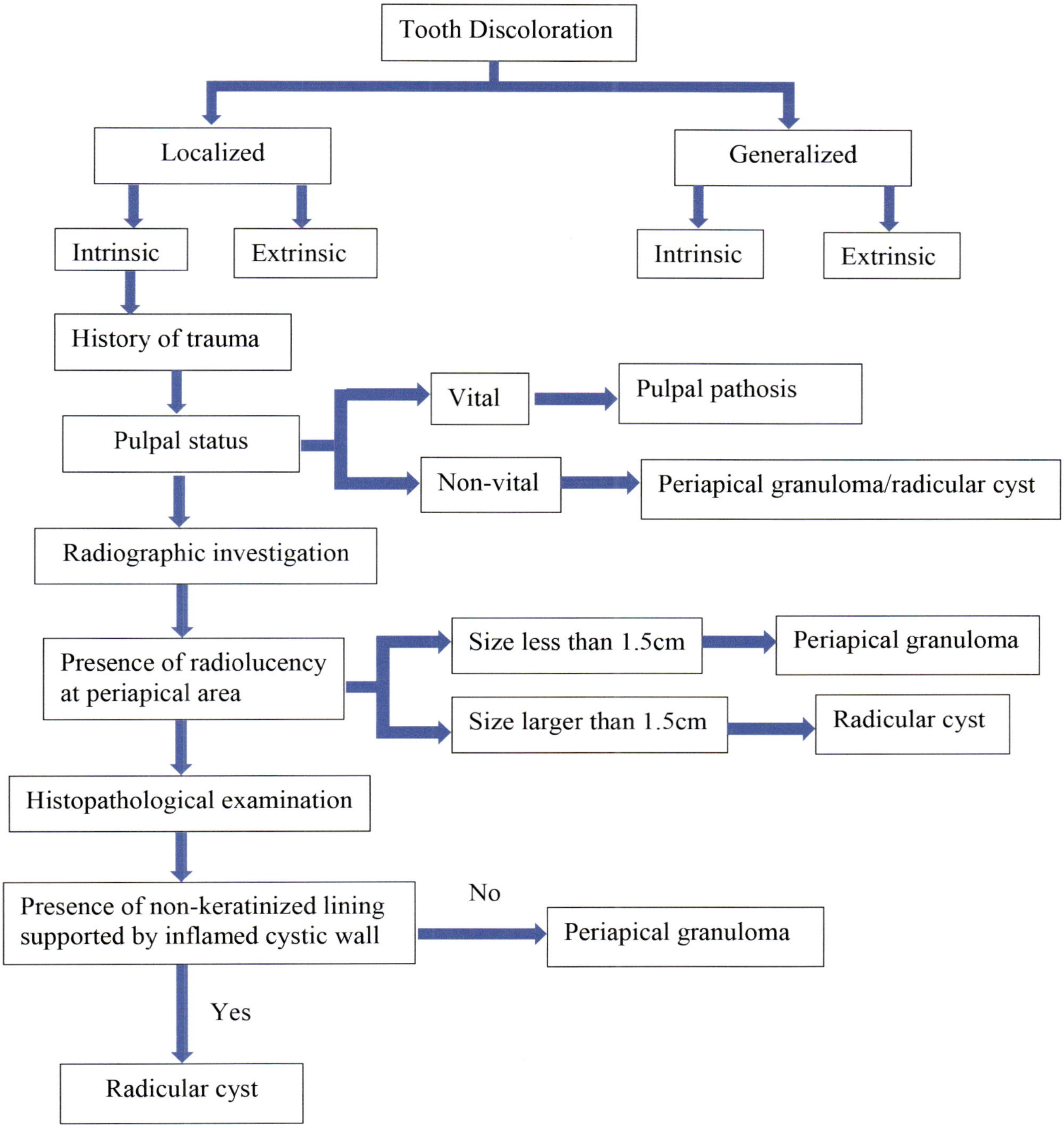

5

Self-Assessment Questions

1. List the pathognomonic clinical features of radicular cyst.
2. State THREE (3) differential diagnoses of radicular cyst.
3. Describe the THREE (3) phases in the pathogenesis of radicular cyst.
4. State the histopathological features of radicular cyst.
5. State the difference between "true" and "bay" cysts.
6. List the treatment of radicular cyst.

Summary

Radicular cyst is an inflammatory odontogenic cyst associated with non-vital tooth. This cyst may clinically and radiographically be indistinguishable with other periapical pathosis. Clinically, they may present with dull pain, history of trauma. But the pathognomonic clinical features for radicular cyst are discoloured and non-vital tooth (either carious or heavily restored). Swelling can be observed only when the lesion reaches considerable large size. Radiographically, there is the presence of a periapical radiolucency at the apex of the affected tooth which is well corticated. Histopathological radicular cyst is composed of non-keratinized stratified squamous epithelium lining the cystic lumen and presence of chronic inflammatory cells in the connective tissue wall. Non-surgical root canal treatment or periradicular surgery with apicectomy and enucleation of the cystic cavity or extraction of the affected tooth followed by enucleation of the cyst is the treatment option. Prognosis of radicular cysts is good, but rarely the radicular cyst may persist even after the extraction of the associated tooth to give rise to residual cyst.

Further Reading

El-Naggar AK, Chan JKC, Grandis JR, Takata T, Slootweg PJ. World Health Organization classification of head and neck tumours. 4th ed. Lyon: IARC; 2017.

Nair PNR. Non-microbial etiology: periapical cysts sustain post-treatment apical periodontitis. Endod Topics. 2003;6:96–113.

Ramachandran Nair PN, Pajarola G, Schroeder HE. Types and incidence of human periapical lesions obtained with extracted teeth. Oral Surg Oral Med Oral Pathol Oral Radiol Endod. 1996;81(1):93–102. https://doi.org/10.1016/s1079--2104(96)80156-9.

Ricucci D, Pascon EA, Ford TR, Langeland K. Epithelium and bacteria in periapical lesions. Oral Surg Oral Med Oral Pathol Oral Radiol Endod. 2006;101(2):239–49. https://doi.org/10.1016/j.tripleo.2005.03.038. Epub 2005 Sep 26

Ricucci D, Rôças IN, Hernández S, Siqueira JF Jr. "True" Versus "Bay" apical cysts: clinical, radiographic, histopathologic, and histobacteriologic features. J Endod. 2020;46(9):1217–27. https://doi.org/10.1016/j.joen.2020.05.025. Epub 2020 Jun 14

Siqueira JF Jr. Aetiology of root canal treatment failure: why well-treated teeth can fail. Int Endod J. 2001;34(1):1–10. https://doi.org/10.1046/j.1365-2591.2001.00396.x.

Simon JH. Incidence of periapical cysts in relation to the root canal. J Endod. 1980;6(11):845–8. https://doi.org/10.1016/S0099--2399(80)80039-2.

Mild Pain in the Left Lower Jaw: Dentigerous Cyst

Yet Ching Goh and Anand Ramanathan

Contents

W. M Tilakaratne, T. G. Kallarakkal (eds.), *Clinicopathological Correlation of Oral Diseases*,
https://doi.org/10.1007/978-3-031-24408-7_6

Learning Goals

1. Devise the correct way of compiling the history with appropriate questions.
2. Develop a differential diagnosis after history taking.
3. Deduce appropriate procedures in clinical examination.
4. Formulate a differential diagnosis combining findings in the history and clinical examination.
5. Justify the relevant investigations required to arrive at the diagnosis.
6. Comprehend the importance of clinicopathological correlation in arriving at the correct diagnosis.
7. Outline the management plan.
8. Recognize the importance of a diagnostic algorithm in arriving at a diagnosis.

6.1 Main Complaint

A 22-year-old female patient presented to the dental clinic with a complaint of mild pain in the left lower jaw.

6.2 History of Complaint

Question: How long have you noticed pain?

I started to feel the pain since 3 months ago.

Question: Can you describe the type of pain that you experienced?

The pain is mild in intensity.

Question: Can you tell me whether you get the pain at any specific times?

It is a kind of a dull pain throughout. I don't recognize any specific time as such.

Question: Are there any aggravating factors of your pain?

I don't recognize anything except a little increased pain when food particles touch the area.

Question: Does the pain radiate to other part of the face?

No, the pain is always felt behind the last tooth of my left lower jaw.

Question: Is there any redness, pus discharge or bleeding from the affected area?

I have not observed any pus discharge or bleeding from the affected area.

Question: Is there a history of injury to the affected area?

I don't recollect any injury in relation to the area.

Question: Is there history of extraction at that area?

No, I never had any erupted tooth in that area. I have a feeling that my wisdom tooth never erupted.

Question: Do you have difficulty in opening your mouth?

I can open my mouth normally with a little discomfort in the area that I have pain.

Question: Do you experience any alteration of sensation in the lower lip?

There is no alteration of sensation involving my lower lip.

6.3 Past Medical History

Question: Do you have any underlying medical problems?

I do not have any medical problems.

6.4 Past Dental History

Question: Have you undergone any dental treatment?

This is my first visit to a dental clinic.

6.5 Social History

Question: Do you smoke or drink alcohol?

I do not smoke or drink alcohol.

6.6 With the Findings from the History, What Is Your Differential Diagnosis and How Do You Justify Your Differential Diagnosis?

1. Odontogenic cyst: Either a dentigerous cyst or odontogenic keratocyst

   Dentigerous cyst is the favoured differential diagnosis as 75% of the dentigerous cysts are associated with unerupted mandibular third molar. Odontogenic keratocyst is one of the differential diagnoses considering the site of involvement, and it is not uncommon to develop it in association with an unerupted tooth. The age is also compatible with both lesions.
2. Benign odontogenic tumours

   The findings of the history are not suggestive of an odontogenic tumour. Ameloblastoma is the most likely differential diagnosis as angle of the mandible is the commonest site for Ameloblastoma. Especially, unicystic ameloblastoma associated with an unerupted tooth in a young patient is a possibility. Early stage of ameloblastoma is often asymptomatic and does not cause obvious swelling. The possibility of other odontogenic tumours cannot be excluded.

6.7 Findings of Extra-oral Examination

Question: What are the clinical extra-oral findings that you see in this patient?

Extra-oral examination reveals absence of facial swelling. There is no abnormality detected at the mandibular region. Submandibular lymph nodes are not palpable.

6.8 Findings of Intra-oral Examination

Question: What are the intra-oral clinical findings that you see in this patient?

Intra-oral examination of left posterior mandible shows presence of 35, 36 and 37. Tooth 38 is clinically absent. There is no obvious swelling observed. The overlying mucosa is normal in colour and does not show any discharge or bleeding (Fig. 6.1). There is slight tenderness of the surface mucosa behind the tooth 37. The adjacent 37 does not have any visible carious lesions.

Question: What are your clinical differential diagnoses with justification for this patient?

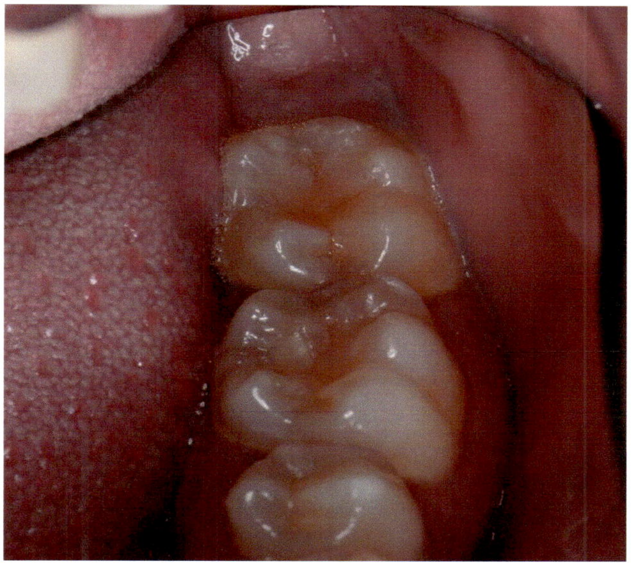

Fig. 6.1 Intraoral photograph of clinically missing 38 with normal overlying mucosa

1. Dentigerous cyst

   Dentigerous cyst is the most common developmental odontogenic cyst that commonly involves mandibular third molar. Small dentigerous cysts are completely asymptomatic and are discovered during radiographical investigation. Large dentigerous cyst can cause swelling and facial asymmetry. Presence of mild pain may be due to inflammatory changes of the cyst. Therefore, dentigerous cyst is the most likely diagnosis.
2. Odontogenic keratocyst

   Odontogenic keratocyst is an odontogenic cyst usually seen in young patients and affects the mandible in majority of the cases. Odontogenic keratocyst grows in an antero-posterior direction and is unlikely to cause obvious swelling when it is small in size. Therefore, this is a possible differential diagnosis.
3. Ameloblastoma

   Specially, unicystic ameloblastoma is often diagnosed in young adults and shows predilection for mandibular third molar area. It may be seen in association with an unerupted tooth. An early lesion is asymptomatic and shows no bony expansion.

Question: What investigations need to be carried out for this patient in arriving at the working diagnosis?

Dental panoramic tomogram (DPT) was taken for this patient, and it shows a unilocular, well-demarcated and well-corticated radiolucency surrounding the crown of the unerupted 38. There is no significant buccolingual or antero-posterior expansion. Resorption or displacement of adjacent teeth is not evident. Tooth 38 is slightly displaced posteriorly. The tooth 48 is also impacted (◘ Fig. 6.2).

? Question: What is the working diagnosis for this lesion?

✓ Dentigerous cyst is the most likely working diagnosis based on the history, clinical and radiographical findings.

? Question: What is the treatment performed following the DPT?

✓ The lesion was enucleated together with removal of the unerupted tooth 38. An empty cavity consistent with cystic cavity was evident (◘ Fig. 6.3). The enucleated specimen was sent to Oral Pathology Laboratory for histopathological examination. The enucleated specimen shows soft tissue attachment at the cemento-enamel junction of the molar tooth (◘ Fig. 6.4).

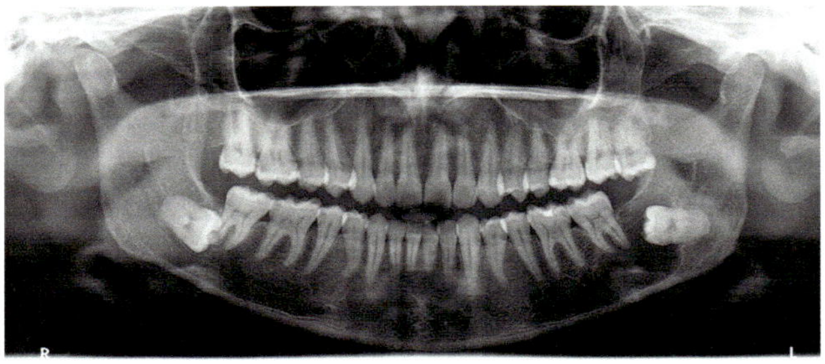

◘ **Fig. 6.2** Dental panoramic tomogram shows a unilocular, well-defined radiolucency surrounding the crown of unerupted 38

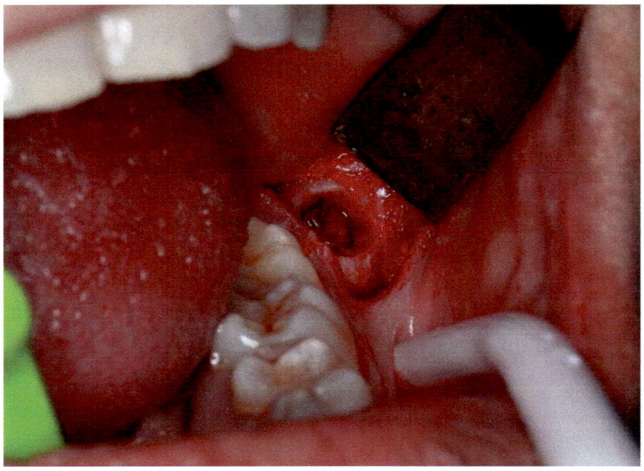

◘ **Fig. 6.3** An empty cavity consistent with cystic cavity is observed during the surgical procedure

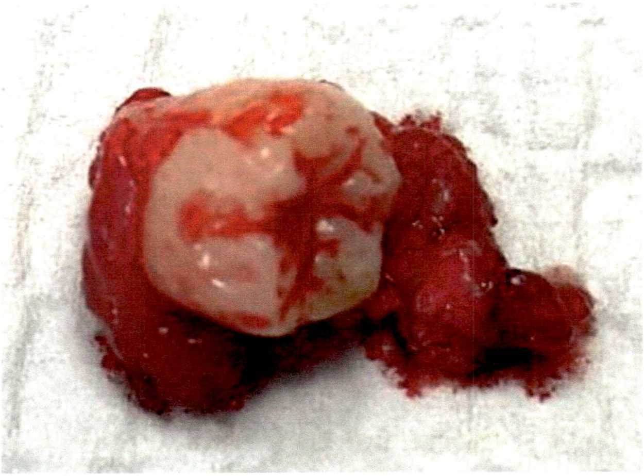

◘ **Fig. 6.4** Enucleated lesion with soft tissue attached to the CEJ region of the unerupted 38

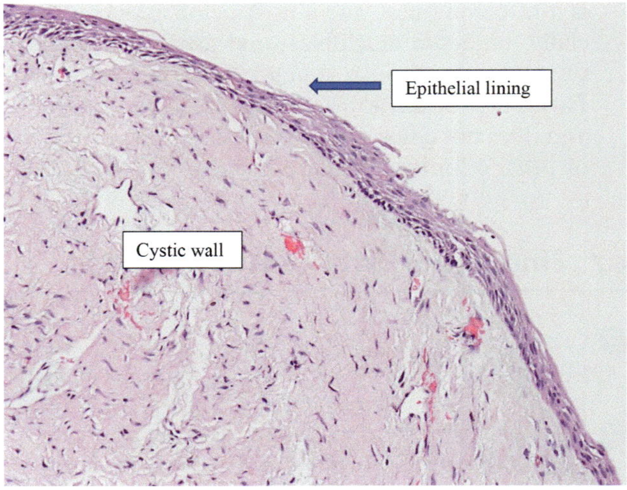

◘ **Fig. 6.5** The epithelial lining consists of thin non-keratinized stratified squamous epithelium with supporting fibrous connective tissue cyst wall, and this part of the cyst wall is minimally inflamed

? Question: What are the histopathological features of the submitted specimen?

✓ Haematoxylin and eosin sections show fibrous cystic capsule, lined by non-keratinized stratified squamous epitheliumranging from 2 to 4 cell layers in thickness in most areas (◘ Fig. 6.5). Some parts of the cyst wall are inflamed. In the presence of dense chronic inflammatory cell infiltration, the overlying epithelium shows varying amounts of hyperplasia and marked spongiosis (◘ Fig. 6.6).

? Question: What is the definitive diagnosis for this lesion?

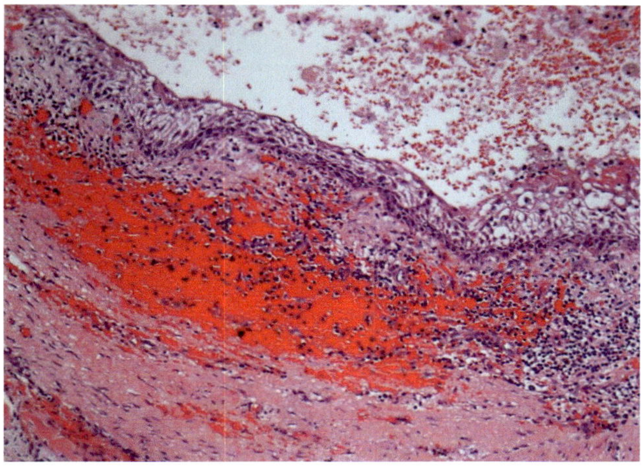

Fig. 6.6 The epithelium is hyperplastic and spongiotic due to inflammation

Dentigerous cyst

Question: What are the features that support the definitive diagnosis of a dentigerous cyst?

1. Clinical features that help in the diagnosis are the absence of the lower left third molar tooth (38).
2. DPT shows a unilocular, well-demarcated radiolucency surrounding the crown of the unerupted 38. On macroscopic/gross examination of the enucleated lesion, the cystic sac is seen attached to the neck of the impacted tooth.
3. Histopathological examination shows the presence of a cyst wall lined by thin epithelial lining comprising non-keratinized stratified squamous epithelium consistent with dentigerous cyst. Some areas showing inflammation explains the mild pain that the patient was complaining.

6.9 Follow-Up and Prognosis

Question: What is the prognosis of dentigerous cysts?

The prognosis of dentigerous cysts is good, and they do not recur. Very rarely, ameloblastoma may arise from a dentigerous cyst. Malignant transformation is exceptionally rare.

6.10 Dentigerous Cyst

Dentigerous cyst is defined as a developmental odontogenic cyst that is attached to the cervical region of an unerupted tooth and envelops the crown. It is also called as a follicular cyst. Dentigerous cysts are the second most common cysts of the jaw after radicular cysts. Dentigerous cysts account for about 20% of all odontogenic cysts. The peak incidence of dentigerous cyst is second to fourth decade of life, but they can occur over a wide age range. They show a male predilection with the male:female ratio of about 3:2. Multiple or bilateral cysts can be present in cleidocranial dysplasia and Maroteaux–Lamy syndrome.

The pathogenesis of dentigerous cyst is uncertain. It arises due to accumulation of cystic fluid between reduced enamel epithelium of the dental follicle and the crown of the unerupted tooth. Most of the dentigerous cysts are associated with unerupted mandibular third molars, followed by maxillary canine, maxillary third molars and mandibular second premolars. Dentigerous cysts are usually symptomless and discovered during radiological investigation for missing tooth. However, if the dentigerous cyst becomes large, it may manifest as a swelling which may affect the symmetry of the face or the mandible. If they get secondarily infected, pain and swelling are a usual presentation.

Radiographically, the dentigerous cyst shows a unilocular, well-demarcated radiolucency with corticated margins surrounding the crown of an unerupted tooth. The unerupted tooth may be displaced. The adjacent tooth may be displaced and may show root resorption. Three main radiographic variations of dentigerous cyst have been described, namely central type, lateral type and circumferential type (Fig. 6.7). The crown of an impacted tooth is enveloped symmetrically in central type, exerting pressure to the crown of the tooth and may push it away from its initial location. The lateral type often results from dilatation of the follicle on one aspect of the crown, whereas circumferential type appears as entire tooth being enveloped by the cyst.

Macroscopically, the dentigerous cyst shows a cystic sac covering the crown of the unerupted tooth. The cystic sac is attached to the cervical region of the unerupted tooth at the CEJ.

Histopathological features of dentigerous cyst consist of an uninflamed loose (myxoid) connective tissue wall lined by a non-keratinized stratified squamous epithelium of regular 2–4 cell layer thickness. There may be small quiescent rests of odontogenic epithelium within the connective tissue wall. Mucous cells and cilia may be present within the epithelial lining especially in those cysts that occur in the maxilla. When inflamed, the cystic lining epithelium is altered and becomes hyperplastic showing long rete-ridges along with cholesterol clefts. Hyaline bodies of Rushton may also be seen. When this happens, differentiation of a dentigerous cyst from a radicular cyst is impossible microscopically. Clinicopathological correlation is essential to arrive at the correct diagnosis in such cases as radicular cyst is always associated with a non-vital tooth, while a dentigerous cyst is associated with an unerupted tooth.

6

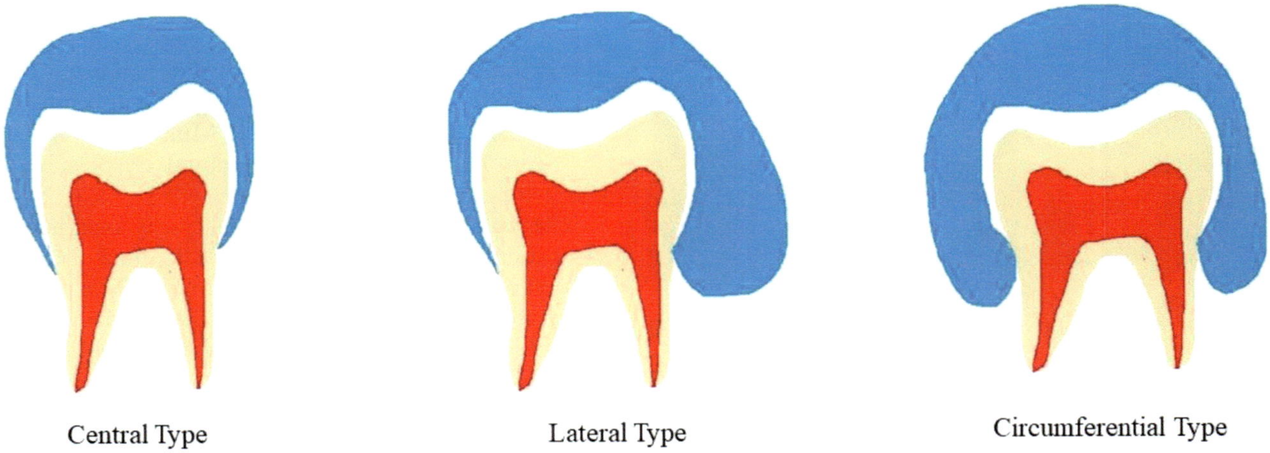

Fig. 6.7 Radiographic variations of dentigerous cyst

The treatment options are enucleation of the cyst or marsupialization. The latter is considered when the tooth has a possibility of eruption in a young patient. Sometimes, orthodontic treatment following conservative surgical treatment will be carried out to retain the involved impacted tooth and ensure the eruption into normal occlusion. The treatment approaches are based on patient's age, site of the cyst, size, involvement of vital structures and potential for normal eruption of the impacted tooth. The eruption potential is closely related to the root formation of the impacted tooth. Dentigerous cyst usually does not recur following complete removal. Malignant transformation has rarely been reported. Very rarely, ameloblastoma can arise from a dentigerous cyst.

Salient Features of Dentigerous Cyst	
Clinical features	Absence of a tooth (impacted) associated with the lesion.
Radiological features	Unilocular, well-demarcated radiolucency surrounding the crown of an unerupted (impacted) tooth.
Macroscopic features	A cystic sac attached to the neck of the impacted tooth and surrounding the crown of the impacted tooth.
Histopathological features	Non-keratinized stratified squamous epithelium about 2–4 cell layers in thickness attached to the CEJ of the tooth and lining the cystic lumen. The cyst wall is not inflamed.
Treatment	Enucleation of the cyst with removal of the impacted tooth.

6.11 Eruption Cyst

Eruption cyst is the soft tissue variant of a dentigerous cyst. It is found within the soft tissue overlying the erupting tooth. Eruption cyst occurs in children and accounts for <2% of cases. Eruption cysts occur over the deciduous mandibular incisors or permanent maxillary first molars. Clinically, the eruption cyst shows a soft, smooth swelling of the alveolar mucosa over the erupting tooth. The swelling may be translucent or if traumatized gives the appearance of a hematoma (reddish-blue in colour). Eruption cysts are usually treated by marsupialization of the cyst to allow the eruption of the unerupted tooth.

Diagnostic Algorithm

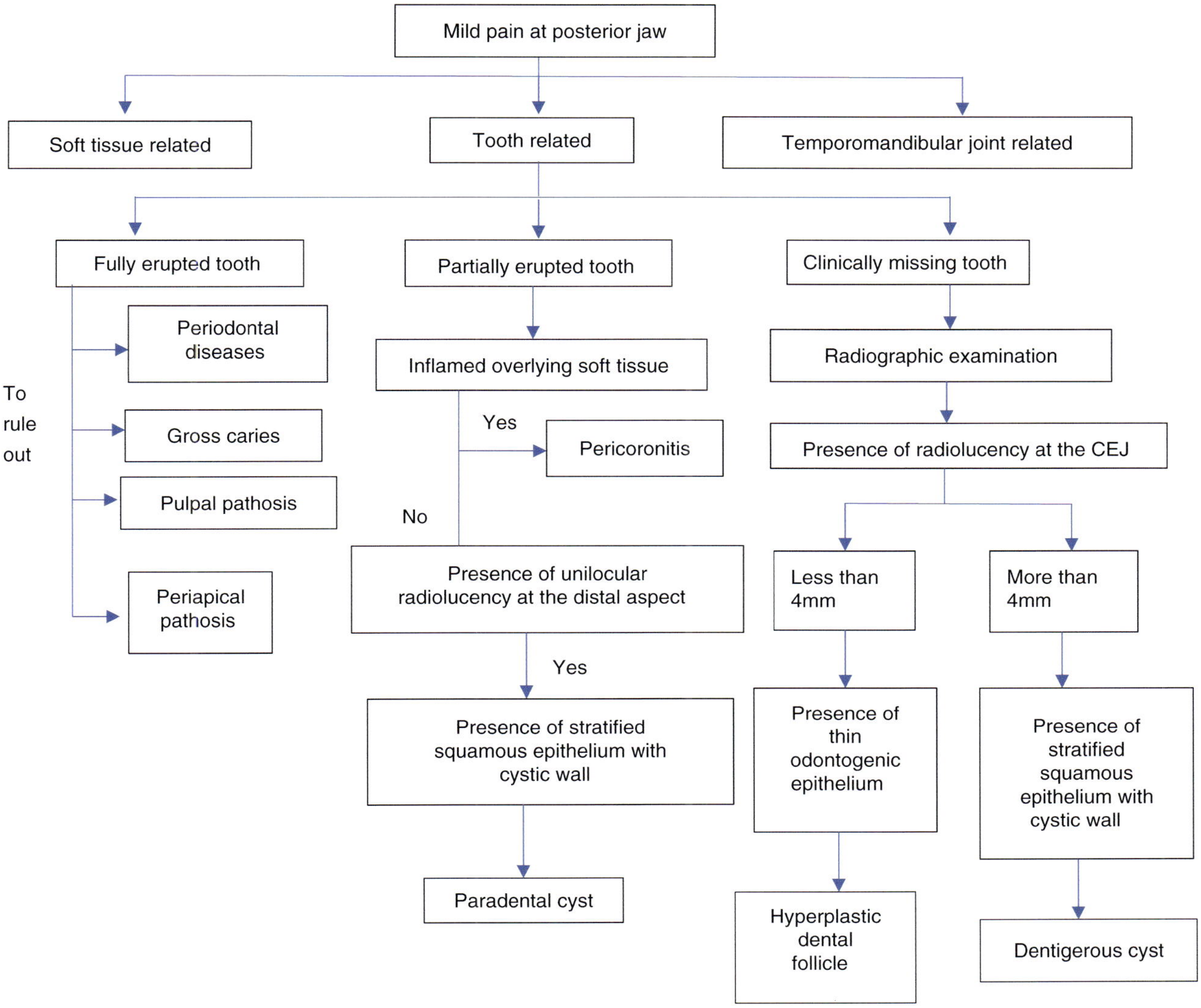

Self-Assessment Questions

1. State THREE (3) clinical differential diagnoses for a dentigerous cyst.
2. Describe the macroscopic features of a dentigerous cyst.
3. Describe the histopathological features of a dentigerous cyst.
4. Describe the aetiopathogenesis of a dentigerous cyst.
5. Outline the treatment of a dentigerous cyst.

Further Reading

El-Naggar AK, Chan JKC, Grandis JR, Takata T, Slootweg PJ. World Health Organization classification of head and neck tumours. 4th ed. Lyon: IARC; 2017.

Scholl RJ, Kellett HM, Neumann DP, Lurie AG. Cysts and cystic lesions of the mandible: clinical and radiologic-histopathologic review. Radiographics. 1999;19(5):1107–24. https://doi.org/10.1148/radiographics.19.5.g99se021107.

Shear M, Speight PM, Shear M. Cysts of the oral and maxillofacial regions. Oxford: Blackwell Pub; 2007.

Slater LJ. Dentigerous cyst versus paradental cyst versus eruption pocket cyst. J Oral Maxillofac Surg. 2003;61(1):149. https://doi.org/10.1053/joms.2003.50051.

Terauchi M, Akiya S, Kumagai J, Ohyama Y, Yamaguchi S. An analysis of dentigerous cysts developed around a mandibular third molar by panoramic radiographs. Dentistry J. 2019;7(1):13. https://doi.org/10.3390/dj7010013.

Wehr C, Cruz G, Young S, Fakhouri WD. An insight into acute pericoronitis and the need for an evidence-based standard of care. Dentistry J. 2019;7(3):88. https://doi.org/10.3390/dj7030088.

Lump in the Floor of the Mouth: Epidermoid/Dermoid Cyst

Anand Ramanathan and Yet Ching Goh

Contents

W. M Tilakaratne, T. G. Kallarakkal (eds.), *Clinicopathological Correlation of Oral Diseases*,
https://doi.org/10.1007/978-3-031-24408-7_7

Learning Goals

1. Devise the correct way of compiling the history with appropriate questions.
2. Develop a differential diagnosis after history taking.
3. Deduce appropriate procedures in clinical examination.
4. Formulate a differential diagnosis combining findings in the history and clinical examination.
5. Justify the relevant investigations required to arrive at the diagnosis.
6. Comprehend the importance of clinicopathological correlation in arriving at the correct diagnosis.
7. Outline the management plan.
8. Recognize the importance of a diagnostic algorithm in arriving at a diagnosis.

7.1 Main Complaint

A 34-year-old man came to the clinic complaining of a lump beneath his tongue.

7.2 History of Complaint

Question: When did you notice the lump?

I noticed the lump about 2 years ago. It started as a small swelling and gradually increased in size.

Question: Are there any symptoms such as pain in relation to this lump?

I don't feel any discomfort or pain.

Question: Do you have any difficulty in speech or swallowing?

I have slight difficulty in swallowing. I also have a slurred speech due to inability to move my tongue freely because of the increase in size of the swelling.

Question: Have you been experiencing any altered taste in the mouth?

I have not experienced any altered taste till now.

Question: Have you experienced dry mouth ever since you have noticed the lump?

I do not have any mouth dryness.

Question: Do you have any history of trauma involving the affected site?

I can't relate any traumatic incident involving the affected site.

Question: Is the swelling getting enlarged during meal time?

It remains the same size during meal time.

Question: Have you noticed any change in the colour of the swelling?

I have not noticed any change in the colour of the swelling.

Question: Have you felt any foul discharge from the affected site?

I have not felt any foul discharge from the affected site.

Question: Is the swelling hard when you touch?

It feels like a soft swelling when I press.

Question: Have you undergone any dental treatment?

I have undergone dental scaling and got a few fillings done. The last dental visit was 1 year ago for a routine dental checkup.

Question: Do you have any underlying medical problems?

I do not have any diagnosed medical problems.

Question: Are you a smoker?

I am a non-smoker.

Question: Do you take alcohol?

I take alcohol occasionally.

Question: With the findings from the history, what is your differential diagnosis?

1. Ranula
2. Dermoid/epidermoid cyst
3. Lymphangioma
4. Salivary calculus
5. Benign/malignant salivary gland neoplasm

7.3 How Would You Justify Your Differential Diagnosis After History Taking?

1. A ranula is a mucocele that occurs in the floor of the mouth due to ductal obstruction leading to accumulation of saliva. Clinically, a ranula manifests as a transparent swelling located in the floor of the mouth causing elevation of the tongue.
2. Intra-orally, an epidermoid or dermoid cyst affects the floor of the mouth frequently. An epidermoid/dermoid cyst is often asymptomatic when it is small in size. It causes swelling of the affected site when it reaches to a considerable size and presents in the midline. It appears yellowish and assumes a round shape clinically.
3. Lymphangioma/cystic hygroma arises from malformed lymphatics which fails to drain into other lymphatics or veins and hence accumulation of lymph forming enlarged and dilated lymphatics. It shows high predilection for head and neck region. Lymphangioma appears pebbly or multilobulated and with a translucent hue owing to its superficial location. It may appear erythematous or bluish if the vascular component within it ruptures due to trauma. It is common in childhood and rare in adults. It occurs in the submental and/or submandibular region extending into the midline of the neck. However, this is not high-priority differential diagnosis as the patient says that no colour change is observed.
4. A salivary calculus can form within the salivary gland due to mineralization of the inspissated mucin. Salivary calculus leads to swelling of the associated gland and discomfort during eating. Patient may also experience alteration in taste.
5. Benign/malignant salivary gland neoplasm can occur in the floor of the mouth involving either the sublingual or submandibular gland.

7.4 Findings of Extra-oral Examination

Extra-oral examination reveals a swelling in the submental region (Fig. 7.1). The overlying skin appeared unremarkable with the absence of erythema. On palpation, the swelling is soft, mobile, and it is not attached to surrounding tissue. The temperature of the affected site is normal. There is no sinus tract detected. It does not cause tenderness or discomfort during examination.

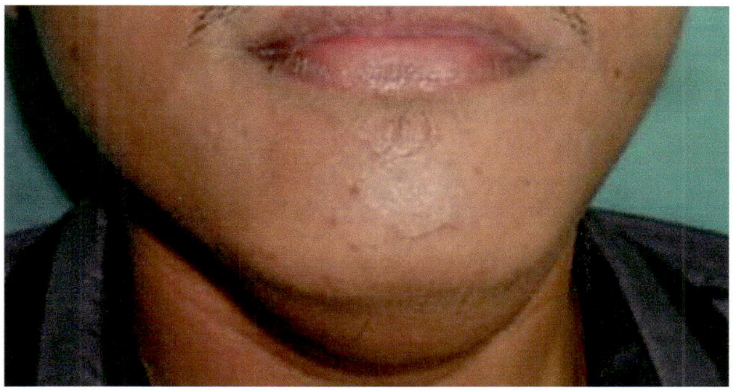

Fig. 7.1 Extra-oral photograph showing a swelling at the submental region. (Courtesy of Dr. Nadeena Jayasuriya)

7.5 Findings of Intra-oral Examination

Intra-oral examination reveals raised tongue with a swelling in the midline of the floor of mouth. The floor of the mouth space is obliterated. The overlying mucosa is normal in colour and shows surface telangiectasia (Fig. 7.2). The swelling is soft, mobile and not fixed to surrounding structures. There is no discharge or bleeding on the surface. Reduction of salivary flow is not observed in the submandibular salivary duct.

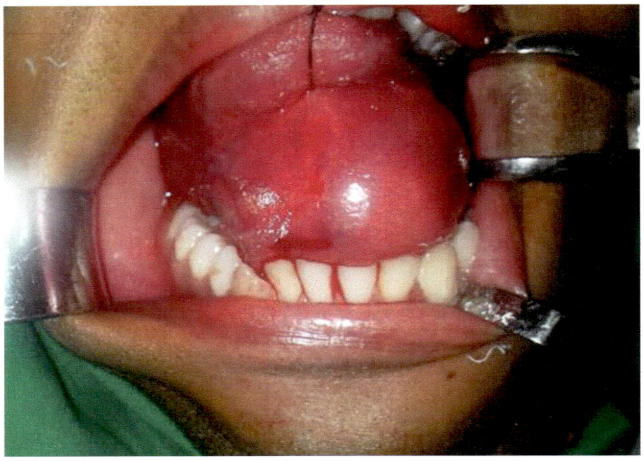

Fig. 7.2 Intra-oral photograph shows a swelling in the midline of the floor of the mouth with the tongue appearing raised. (Courtesy of Dr. Nadeena Jayasuriya)

7

7.6 What Are the Most Likely Clinical Diagnoses?

1. Ranula
2. Epidermoid/dermoid cyst

7.7 How Would You Investigate This Patient?

1. Fine needle aspiration cytology (FNAC): This can give rise to a reasonable diagnosis in most lesions. However, when the FNAC results are not pathognomonic, an incisional biopsy can be performed.
2. Radiographic investigations

   An ultrasound scan can be carried out in which the cyst may show a well-circumscribed predominantly hypoechoic mass. Larger lesions can be a little heterogeneous due to the presence of mucin, fat, calcification or pus. A computer tomography (CT) scan or a magnetic resonance imaging (MRI) can help in determination of the size and the anatomical relationship of the swelling.

7.8 What Are the Findings of FNAC in This Patient?

The FNAC of the swelling had thick pultaceous foul smelling material. The smear showed debris with mature squamous cells and numerous keratinaceous debris. There were occasional inflammatory cells.

7.9 What Is Your Working Diagnosis?

Epidermoid cyst/dermoid cyst.

7.10 What Is the Treatment for This Lesion?

Treatment is complete excision of the lesion as larger lesions of the floor of the mouth may cause airway obstruction and respiratory distress to the patient by pushing the tongue further upwards and backwards. The surgical approach in excising the lesion can be either an intra-oral or an extra-oral or a combined approach. After complete excision of the lesion, the excised tissue needs to be sent for histopathological examination (◘ Fig. 7.3).

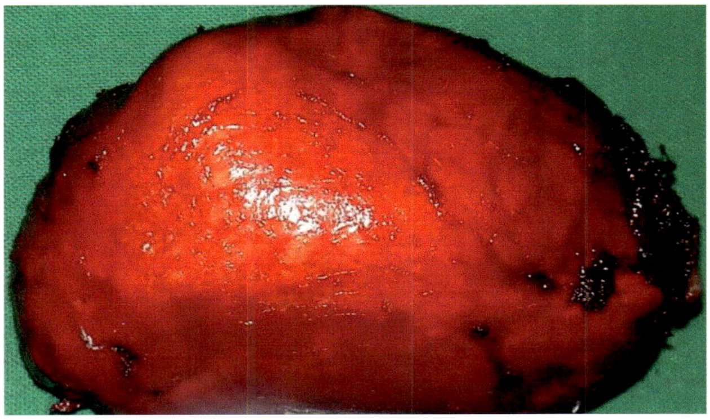

◘ **Fig. 7.3** Photograph shows an ovoid lesion that has been excised. (Courtesy of Dr. Nadeena Jayasuriya)

7.11 What Are the Macroscopic Features Seen in the Excised Lesion?

The lesion is a rounded and doughy mass that is enclosed within a cystic sac. The cut surface of the swelling shows cheesy yellowish material due to its keratinaceous content.

7.12 Biopsy Report Confirms That the Lesion Is an Epidermoid Cyst. What Are the Histopathological Features That Help in Arriving at the Diagnosis?

Histopathological examination shows fibrous cyst wall lined by thin and regular hyperorthokeratinized stratified squamous epithelium. The epithelial lining exhibits a prominent stratum granulosum layer. Keratinaceous material can be seen within the lumen. There are no skin appendages in the cyst wall (◘ Figs. 7.4 and 7.5).

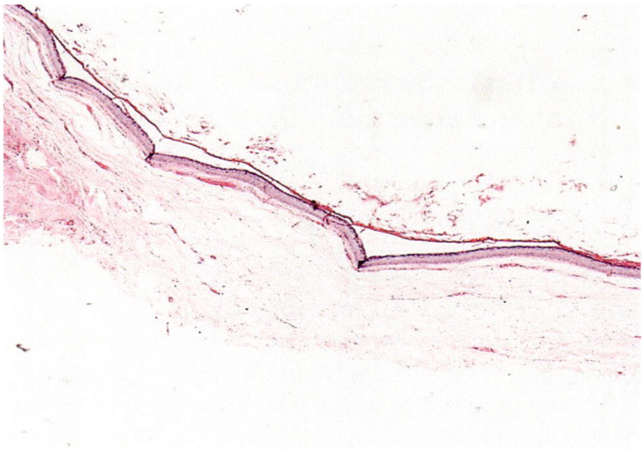

◘ **Fig. 7.4** Photomicrograph shows orthokeratinized stratified squamous epithelium lining the cystic lumen with keratinaceous material. The cyst wall is composed of loosely arranged collagen fibres

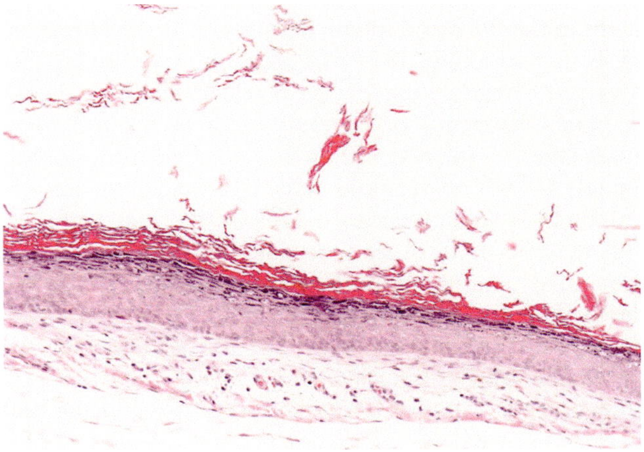

◘ **Fig. 7.5** Photomicrograph shows orthokeratinized stratified squamous epithelium lining the cystic lumen with a prominent stratum granulosum layer and keratinaceous material within the lumen

7.13 What Is the Definitive Diagnosis for This Lesion?

Epidermoid cyst.

7.14 What Specific Findings Help You to Arrive at the Diagnosis of Epidermoid Cyst?

Clinical features that help in the diagnosis are the presence of a swelling in the midline of the floor of the mouth causing elevation of the tongue. The occurrence of ranula may be lateral to the midline. Macroscopically, there is cheesy yellowish material within the lesion. Histopathologically, it shows orthokeratinized stratified squamous epithelium with a prominent granular cell layer. The cystic lumen contains abundant keratinous material. The cyst wall does not contain any skin appendages.

7.15 What Is the Prognosis of an Epidermoid Cyst?

The prognosis of an epidermoid cyst is good, and they do not recur once excised.

7.16 Epidermoid/Dermoid Cyst

Epidermoid cyst is mainly found on the face, trunk, neck, extremities and scalp. The prevalence of epidermoid cysts in the oral cavity and submental region is approximately 1.6% and 11.5%, respectively. They most frequently occur in the midline of the floor of the mouth. Buccal mucosa and tongue are rarely involved. Epidermoid cysts are reportedly more common in males. Although they may occur at any age, they are more prevalent in the third and fourth decades of life. Epidermoid cysts that are associated with syndromes such as Gardner syndrome have a younger age of occurrence.

The occurrence of dermoid cysts in the head and neck region is fairly common and accounts for approximately 34% of all dermoid cysts. Dermoid cysts are predominantly subcutaneous lesions in the head and neck but may occur in other mucosal sites. With respect to oral cavity, the floor of the mouth (◘ Fig. 7.6) is the most common location for dermoid cysts. Most dermoid cysts in the floor of the mouth occur during the second to fourth decades of life. There is no gender predilection reported for dermoid cysts involving the oral cavity. These cysts may be congenital or acquired. Dermoid cyst occurs more commonly in females.

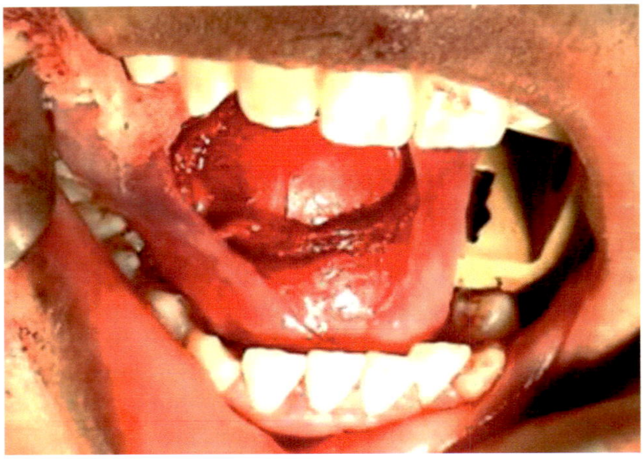

◘ **Fig. 7.6** Intraoral photograph shows the presence of a dermoid cyst in the midline of the floor of the mouth. (Courtesy Dr. Ahmad Fadhli)

There are three theories that have been proposed on the origin of these cysts. The most popular theory proposes that during the third or fourth week of the intrauterine life, the embryonic cells of the first and second branchial arch get entrapped within the mesenchyme of that region. However, the second theory proposes that these cysts arise due to the implantation of epithelial cells subsequent to accidental or surgical injury. This theory may explain the occurrence of the acquired variety of these cysts. The third theory suggests that these cysts are a variant of the thyroglossal duct cyst.

Clinically, both epidermoid and dermoid cysts present as a swelling in the midline of the floor of the mouth in most cases. In some cases, they might present as a unilateral swelling in the floor of the mouth. Rarely, they present as a swelling in other regions of the oral cavity such as the buccal mucosa or tongue. They tend to enlarge slowly. The patient may complain of difficulty in swallowing (dysphagia) and slurred speech (dysarthria). However, when the swelling increases in size, it may raise the tongue and make it fall back and cause difficulty in breathing (dysponea). The overlying mucosa appears normal. However, there might be telangiectatic blood vessels on the surface. Pain may occur if these cysts get secondarily infected. On palpation, the cyst may be semi-hard to fluctuant depending on their size. These may be classified as median genioglossal, median geniohyoid and lateral cyst based on the anatomical location of the cyst in relation to the muscles of the floor of the mouth. Based on their location in the floor of the mouth, they can be either central (midline) or lateral cysts.

If the cyst is present above the geniohyoid muscle, then the swelling is obvious intra-orally in the floor of the mouth. However, if the cyst is present below the geniohyoid muscle, then the swelling extends to the submental region and is seen as a double chin appearance extra-orally.

Scintigraphy scan with Tc^{99m} may help to differentiate these cysts from ectopic thyroid gland. Injection of endographine or lipiodol may help in delineating the boundaries of these cysts and defining their size. Ultrasound-guided FNAC might be useful to obtain a working diagnosis is some cases. In ultrasound imaging, multiple rounded lobulated echogenic structures within the cystic area can be seen. CT and MRI are helpful in precisely defining the anatomical location, size and the extent of the lesion.

Macroscopy of the excised cyst shows a well-defined swelling of red to brown colour, and the cut shows cheesy yellowish material (Fig. 7.7). Histopathologically, both dermoid and epidermoid cysts consist of orthokeratinized stratified squamous epithelium lining the cystic lumen containing keratinous material and fibrous connective tissue wall. The histopathological difference between dermoid and epidermoid cysts is the presence of cutaneous appendages such as hair follicles, hair, sweat glands and sebaceous glands (Fig. 7.8) in the dermoid cysts, whereas they are absent in the epidermoid cysts.

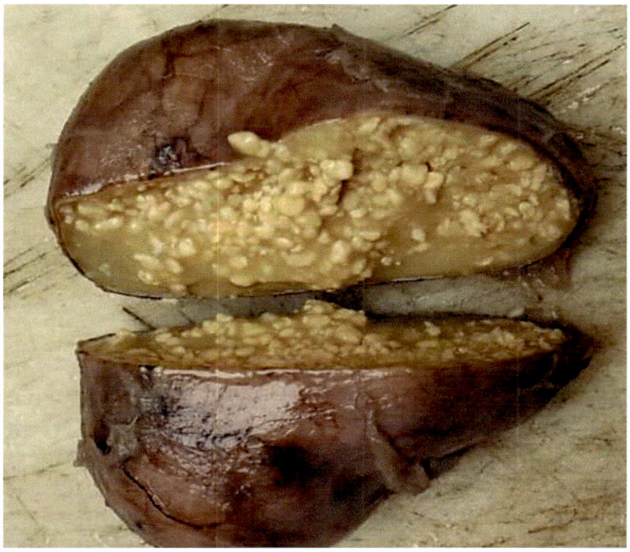

Fig. 7.7 Photograph shows the cut surface of a dermoid cyst with yellowish cheesy material. (Courtesy Dr. Fairuz Abdul Rahman)

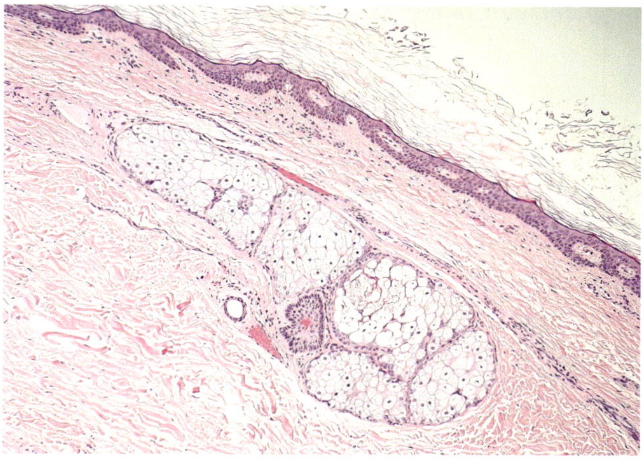

Fig. 7.8 Photomicrograph of a dermoid cyst shows orthokeratinized stratified squamous epithelial lining, cystic lumen filled with keratinous material and sebaceous glands within the connective tissue wall. (Courtesy Dr. Fairuz Abdul Rahman)

Salient Features of Epidermoid/Dermoid Cysts	
Clinical features	Rare in the oral cavity. Male predilection for epidermoid cyst. Age second to fourth decade of life. Occurs mostly in the midline of the floor of the mouth. Slow growing. Not painful. Dysphagia and dysarthria may be present. Dyspnea may present as the cyst increases in size intraorally. If it presents above the geniohyoid muscle results in an intraoral swelling in the floor of the mouth. If present below the geniohyoid muscle it causes a double chin appearance. Fluctuant to semi-hard in consistency.
Imaging features	Ultrasound imaging: Multiple rounded lobulated echogenic structures are found within the cystic area. CT scans and MRI help in showing the anatomical location, size and extent.
Treatment	Complete surgical excision of the cyst. Prognosis is good with no recurrence.
Macroscopy	Well-defined swelling of red to brown colour. The cut surface shows cheesy yellowish material.
Histopathological features	Epidermoid cysts consist of orthokeratinized stratified squamous epithelium lining the cystic lumen containing keratinous material and fibrous connective tissue wall without skin appendages. Dermoid cysts consist of orthokeratinized stratified squamous epithelium lining the cystic lumen containing keratinous material and fibrous connective tissue wall with skin appendages such as hair follicles, hairs, sweat glands and sebaceous glands.

7

■ Diagnostic Algorithm

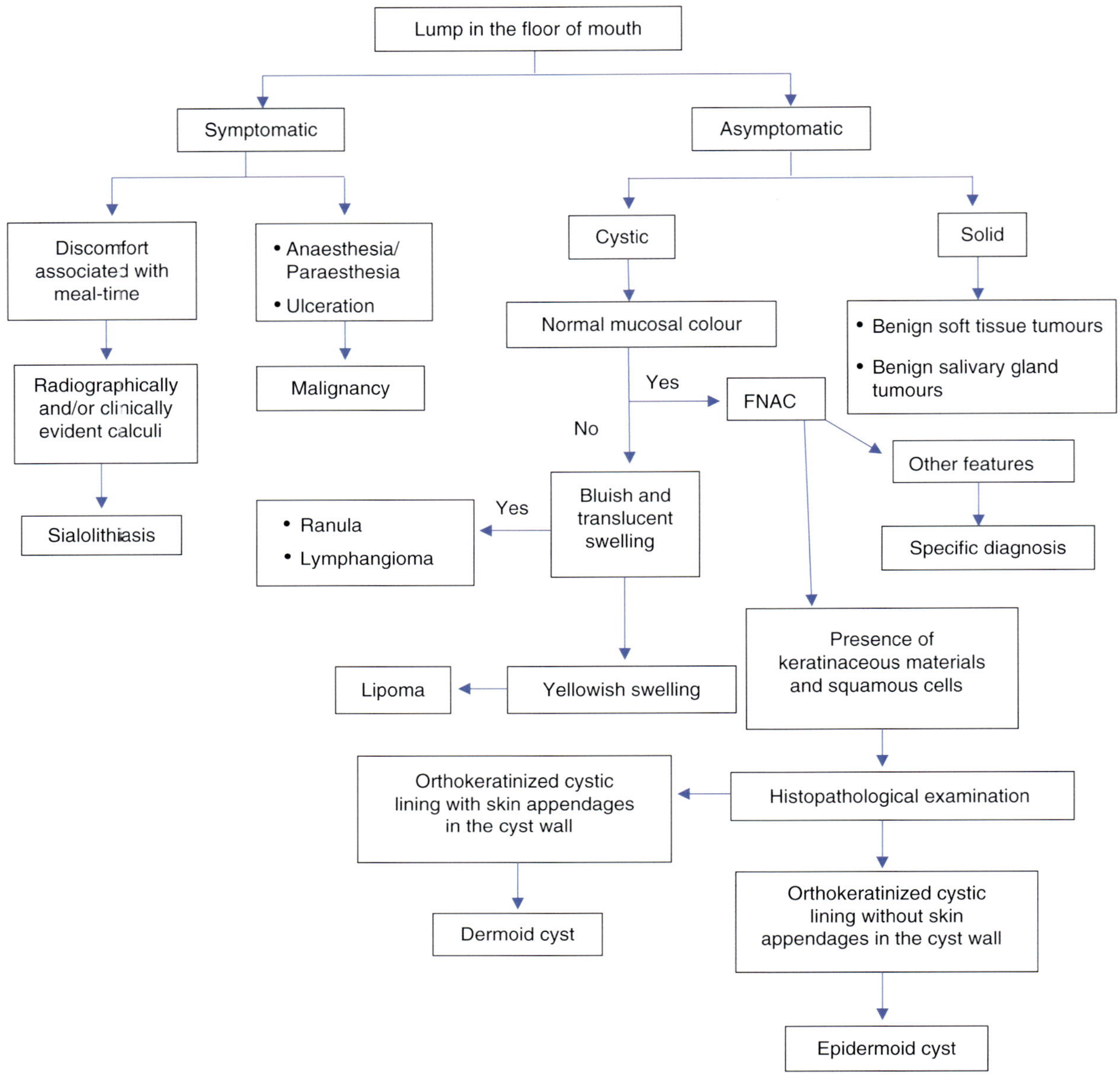

Self-Assessment Questions

1. Discuss the differential diagnoses for epidermoid/dermoid cysts.
2. Discuss the theories of origin of epidermoid/dermoid cysts.
3. Describe the clinical features of epidermoid/dermoid cysts.
4. Outline the treatment of epidermoid/dermoid cysts.
5. Describe the histopathological features of epidermoid and dermoid cysts.

Summary

Epidermoid cyst and dermoid cyst are cysts that tend to occur in the floor of the mouth. The cysts could reach relatively large size clinically and cause complications such as dysphagia and dysarthria or dyspnea. Ultrasound imaging shows that multiple rounded lobulated echogenic structures are found within the cystic area. Whereas, CT scans and MRI help in showing the anatomical location, size and extent of this cyst. Complete surgical excision of the cyst is the treatment. These cysts have a good prognosis and recurrences are uncommon. Histopathologically, epidermoid cysts consist of orthokeratinized stratified squamous epithelium lining the cystic lumen containing keratinous material and fibrous connective tissue wall without skin appendages, whereas dermoid cysts contain skin appendages within the connective tissue wall.

Further Reading

Dutta M, Saha J, Biswas G, Chattopadhyay S, Sen I, Sinha R. Epidermoid cysts in head and neck: our experiences, with review of literature. Indian J Otolaryngol Head Neck Surg. 2013;65(Suppl 1):14–21. https://doi.org/10.1007/s12070-011-0363-y.

Makos C, Noussios G, Peios M, Gougousis S, Chouridis P. Dermoid cysts of the floor of the mouth: two case reports. Case Rep Med. 2011;2011:362170. https://doi.org/10.1155/2011/362170.

Mervyn Shear and Paul Speight. Cysts of the oral and maxillofacial regions. 4th ed. Munksgaard: Blackwell; 2007.

Pupić-Bakrač J, Pupić-Bakrač A, Bačić I, Kolega MŠ, Skitarelić N. Epidermoid and dermoid cysts of the head and neck. J Craniofac Surg. 2021;32(1):e25–7. https://doi.org/10.1097/SCS.0000000000006834.

Santos HB, Rolim LS, Barros CC, Cavalcante IL, Freitas RD, Souza LB. Dermoid and epidermoid cysts of the oral cavity: a 48-year retrospective study with focus on clinical and morphological features and review of main topics. Med Oral Patol Oral Cir Bucal. 2020;25(3):e364–9. https://doi.org/10.4317/medoral.23388.

Trauma to the Lower Lip: Mucocele

Muhammad Kamil Hassan and Thomas George Kallarakkal

Contents

W. M Tilakaratne, T. G. Kallarakkal (eds.), *Clinicopathological Correlation of Oral Diseases*,
https://doi.org/10.1007/978-3-031-24408-7_8

Learning Goals

1. Devise the correct way of compiling the history with appropriate questions.
2. Develop a differential diagnosis after history taking.
3. Deduce appropriate procedures in clinical examination.
4. Formulate a differential diagnosis combining findings in the history and clinical examination.
5. Justify the relevant investigations required to arrive at the diagnosis.
6. Comprehend the importance of clinicopathological correlation in arriving at the correct diagnosis.
7. Outline the management plan.
8. Recognize the importance of a diagnostic algorithm in arriving at a diagnosis.

8.1 Main Complaint

A 16-year-old female patient presented to the dental clinic complaining of a lump on the lower left lip.

8.2 History of Complaint

Question: How long has this lump been there, and what problems are you facing with it?

It has been there for about 2 months now. I noticed it after a recent injury during a martial arts training, where I accidentally bit my lips. The lump has grown gradually but has reached a stage where it is not growing anymore.

8.3 Additional Complaints

Question: Does the lump cause any pain, bleeding, ulceration or difficulties with other functions such as eating, speaking or breathing?

The lump does not cause any pain, bleeding, ulceration or difficulties in eating and speech. There are no other abnormal sensations related to the lump. However, it has become more noticeable, and my close friends are aware of the lump when they look at me. I am also becoming more uncomfortable with the lump's presence.

Question: Do you have any other problems with regard to the face, head and neck?

I don't have other significant issues or complaints related to the face and head and neck.

Question: Do you have any blister-like lesions elsewhere on the body?

There are no other lesions elsewhere on my body.

Question: Do you have any other diseases, allergies and take medications?

I don't have any allergy and not on any medications.

Question: Have you had any surgery in the past?

I have not undergone any surgeries in the past.

Question: Have you had any dental treatment?

I have been getting 6 monthly dental check-ups with routine scaling and polishing.

Question: What is your social background?

I am in secondary school and will be sitting for final exams next year. I am active in sports and outdoor activities.

Question: Do you have any habits?

I don't smoke cigarettes or drink alcohol. I was a thumb sucker as a toddler but stopped the habit before entering school. I used to bite pens and have a tendency to bite the lower lip.

8.4 What Is Your Differential Diagnosis with the Findings from the History?

1. Mucocele
2. Fibroepithelial polyp

8.5 How Do You Justify Your Differential Diagnosis After History Taking?

1. The patient developed the lump on the lower lip following an episode of trauma. This suggests a correlation between the trauma and development of the lesion. Mucocele is known to result from extravasation or spillage of mucus into the tissues caused by trauma to minor salivary glands.
2. The slow growth and absence of features such as bleeding and ulceration suggest that the lesion is likely to be benign.
3. The habit of lip biting also acts as contributing factor for the development of mucocele and fibroepithelial polyp.

8.6 Findings of Clinical Examination

There is a raised, soft and fluctuant lump on the labial mucosa of the lower left lip. It is about 1.5 cm in diameter (◘ Fig. 8.1). It appears to be slightly bluish in colour compared to the surrounding mucosa. It does not blanch on palpation. The lump has no signs of inflammation or infection.

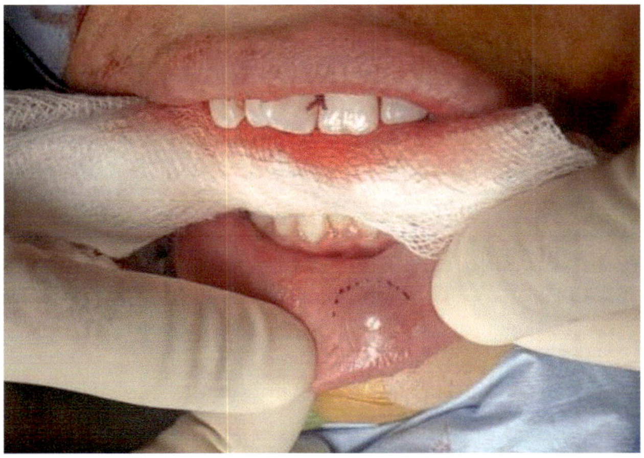

◘ **Fig. 8.1** Dome-shaped swelling on the lower lip

8.7 What Other Relevant Features Would You Look For?

Transillumination of the lesion by directing a focused light source onto the lesion. It helps to determine whether the lesion is solid or a cystic lesion containing fluid.

8.8 What Is Your Clinical Diagnosis?

Mucocele.

8.9 What Is Your Justification for the Clinical Diagnosis?

A slightly bluish colour and fluctuant nature of the lesion together with the history of trauma to the lip are suggestive of the diagnosis of a mucocele. Fibroepithelial polyp presents as a firm nodule with the same colour as the surrounding mucosa, while a haemangioma blanches on application of pressure.

8.10 How Would You Investigate This Patient?

Excisional biopsy for confirmation of the diagnosis.

8.11 How Would You Perform an Excisional Biopsy for This Patient? What Are the Important Considerations?

Mucoceles can be removed by surgical excision of the whole lesion. This is normally done under local anaesthesia (LA) for cooperative children or adults or can be combined with sedation when necessary. Depending on the site of mucocele, the incision mark is made prior to injection of local anaesthesia (◘ Fig. 8.1). This is done to ensure the marking is not distorted by the local anaesthetic solution. LA is given as infiltration or nerve block, depending on the location of the lesion.

LA was given as infiltration around the lesion. Alternatively, it could also be administered as a mental nerve block.

Following anaesthesia, an incision was made on the site of marking. The incision was made through the superficial mucosa and away from the lesion to avoid rupture of the mucocele which can make the complete removal of the lesion difficult (◘ Fig. 8.2).

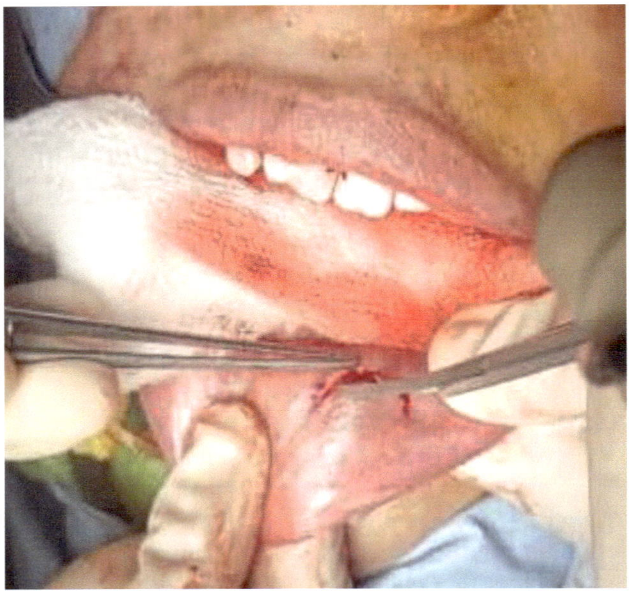

Fig. 8.2 The incision is made around the lesion

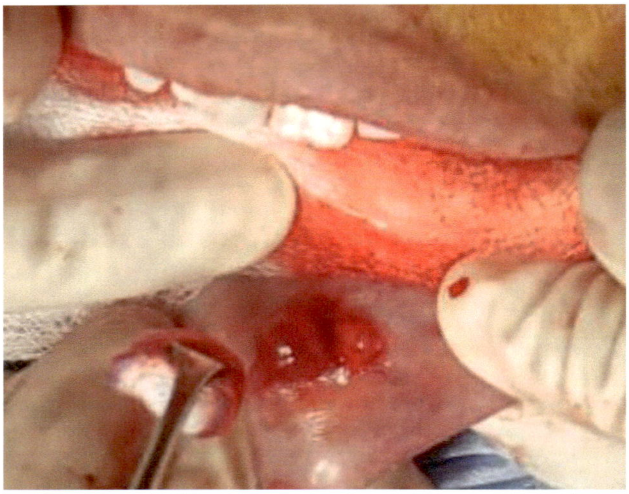

Fig. 8.3 Mucocele herniating through the incision

Following incision, the mucocele was bluntly dissected out using a small curved artery forceps or tenotomy scissors. When most of the lesion was dissected from the underlying tissues, it was possible to see the mucocele 'herniating' through the surgical site, as the lesion was not ruptured (Fig. 8.3).

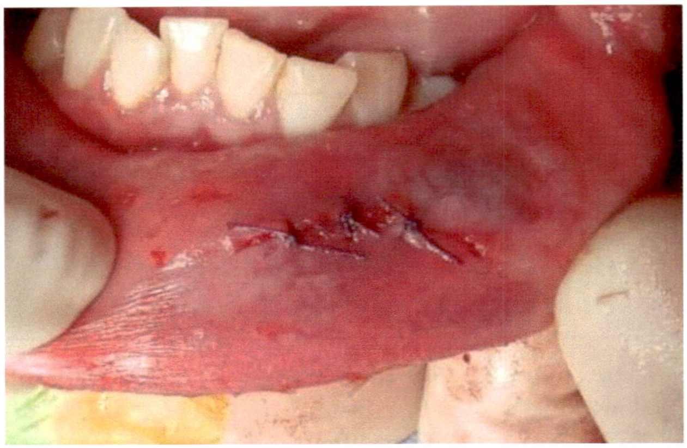

Fig. 8.4 Closure of the surgical wound with Vicryl (Polyglactin) suture

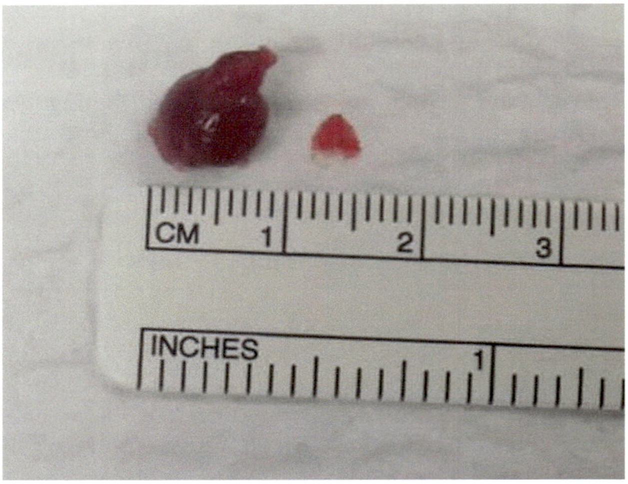

Fig. 8.5 Excised lesion

The lesion was then dissected out fully from the lower lip. It is common to see other minor salivary glands surrounding the mucocele. They can be removed or left in situ. Some surgeons remove the exposed salivary glands to avoid recurrence or to prevent injury to the glands and ducts when suturing.

The surgical site was then closed primarily with resorbable sutures, 4-0 Vicryl (Polyglactin) suture material (Fig. 8.4). Haemostasis was achieved, and the dissected specimen (Fig. 8.5) was sent for histopathological examination.

8.12 Mucocele

Mucocele ('muco' meaning mucus and 'coele' meaning cavity), by definition, is a cavity filled with mucin. This occurs as a result of either accumulation of mucin within an obstructed duct (mucous retention cyst) or extravasation of mucin into surrounding tissue (mucous extravasation cyst). The latter usually occurs as a result of trauma and is the common type out of the two.

Mucoceles arise from minor salivary glands, in the palate, buccal mucosa, labial mucosa and floor of the mouth. When a mucocele occurs in the floor of mouth, it enlarges to a significant size prominently showing the small blood vessels on the surface mimicking the appearance of a frog's belly, hence the term ranula. This may grow into a larger size occupying a significant area of the floor of the mouth. Further, it can herniate through the mylohyoid muscle into the neck. Then the term plunging ranula is used. The lower lip is the most common site of occurrence as it is a common site of trauma. The close proximityto the teeth is also seen as a risk factor due to lip biting or recurrent trauma from sharp edges of the teeth.

The lesion presents as a soft and painless swelling. The colour ranges from pink to deep blue. The variation of colour results from tissue cyanosis or vessel congestion associated with the swelling of the lesion. The size of a mucocele except a ranula varies from 0.7 to 1.5 cm in diameter. However, those arising from deeper areas such as the sublingual gland can grow much larger.

Mucoceles develop by two different mechanisms. Accordingly, they are named as mucous extravasation or retention cysts. Extravasation implies that there is spillage of mucus from the salivary glands into the surrounding tissues. This results in an inflammatory response from the surrounding tissues, resulting in granulation tissue lining surrounded by condensed fibrous connective tissue.

The retention mechanism results from an obstruction or narrowing of the salivary gland duct opening. This causes an inadequate path for exit of the saliva, thus leading to dilatation of the duct and swelling.

On histopathological examination, the haematoxylin and eosin stained sections show extravasated mucin surrounded by compressed granulation tissue (◘ Fig. 8.6). The extravasated mucin is infiltrated by

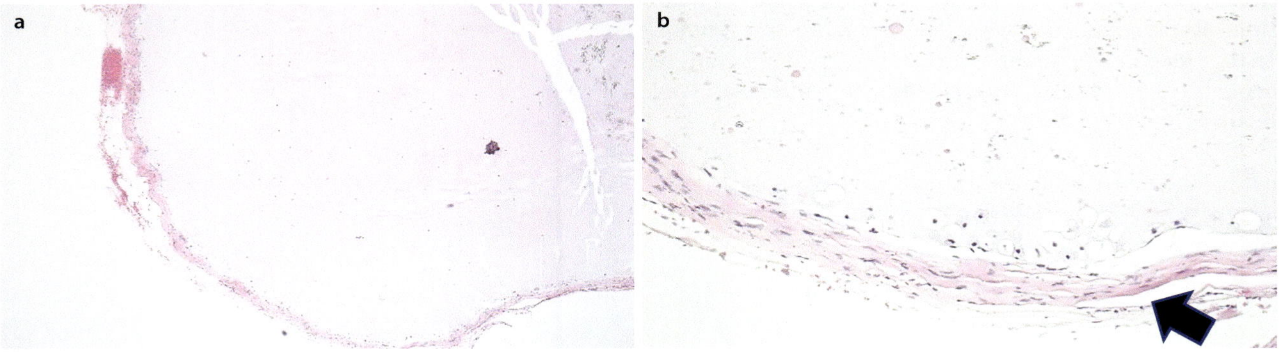

◘ **Fig. 8.6** Extravasated mucin surrounded by compressed granulation tissue (**a**). High-power view shows compressed granulation tissue at the periphery (black arrow) (**b**)

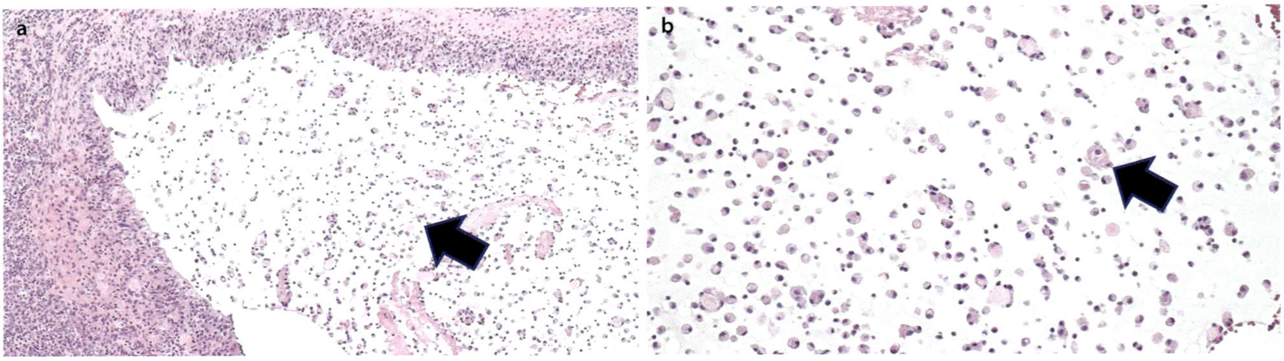

Fig. 8.7 Extravasated mucin infiltrated by chronic inflammatory cells (black arrow) (**a**). High-power view shows mucinophages (black arrow) (**b**)

chronic inflammatory cells. Numerous mucinophages (macrophages which have ingested mucin) are seen (Fig. 8.7).

Mucoceles are conventionally treated with surgical excision of the whole lesion. Smaller lesions are commonly removed as a whole, while with larger ones, marsupialization of the lesion may avoid damage to other vital anatomical structures. Other treatment modalities include cryosurgery, CO_2 laser ablation and intralesional steroids. Cryosurgery is relatively successful with about 6% recurrence rate. CO_2 laser is shown to be precise and causes minimal haemorrhage and inflammatory reaction. Recurrence rate with this modality is minimal. Irrespective of the treatment modality, it is important to avoid further trauma to the region in order to avoid recurrence.

The management of mucoceles depends on the size and location

Size	Clinical presentation	Investigations	Management
Small <1.5 cm	Commonly presents on the lip, buccal mucosa, palate, floor of mouth. Soft, fluctuant. Variable surface colour, depending on depth of lesion and proximity to other structures e.g. veins	Clinical correlation with history	1. No treatment, if contra-indicated by medical history/status. Monitor lesion 2. Surgical excision or other treatment modalities e.g. CO2 laser or cryotherapy
Large >1.5 cm	Similar clinical presentation as smaller lesions	Clinical correlation with history When suggestive of involvement of major salivary glands, other radiographical investigation maybe helpful e.g. MRI When doubtful of diagnosis, aspiration and soft tissue biopsy is required prior to further intervention	1. No treatment, if contra-indicated by medical history/status. Monitor lesion. 2. Surgery: (a) Marsupialization (b) Marsupialization with excision (c) Surgical excision (with or without involved salivary gland)

Salient Features of Oral Mucocele

Clinical	Commonly asymptomatic, soft, fluctuant swelling on the oral mucosa (lips, buccal mucosa, palate, floor of mouth), with pink or bluish colour, smooth surface and well-defined borders (when superficial)
Histopathology	Extravasated mucin surrounded by compressed granulation tissue with chronic inflammation in mucous extravasation cyst and collection of mucin surrounded by ductal epithelium in retention cyst
Treatment	Surgical excision, CO2 laser ablation, cryotherapy, or marsupialization for larger lesions

Mucoceles are benign lesions that are commonly asymptomatic and do not cause any functional issues. However, it may cause aesthetic concerns if located on the lips. It is commonly removed surgically but can also be monitored when indicated or contraindicated for surgery

Diagnostic Algorithm for Small Swellings/Lesions in the Oral Cavity

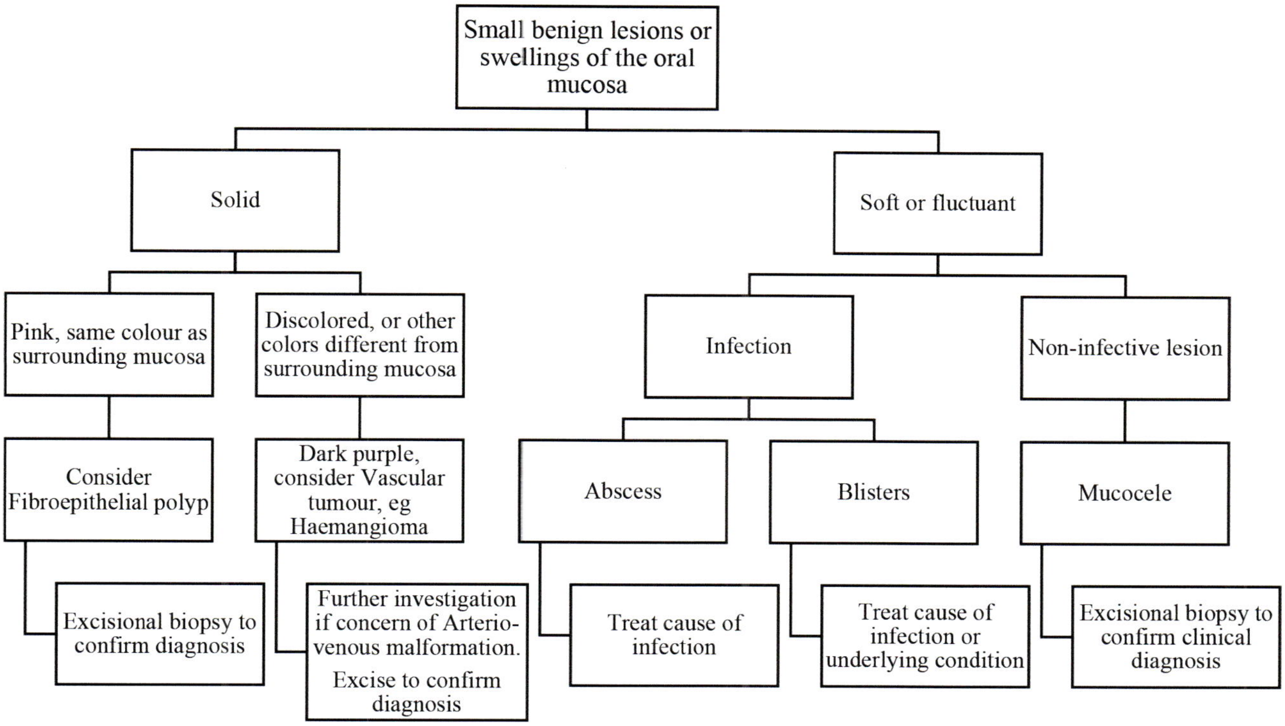

Self-Assessment Questions

1. Discuss the clinical features of an oral mucocele.
2. Describe the pathogenesis of a mucocele.
3. State the important conditions that need to be included in the differential diagnosis for a mucocele.
4. Describe the histopathological features of mucocele.
5. Outline the management plan in treating patients with oral mucocele.

Further Reading

Baurmash HD. Mucoceles and ranulas. J Oral Maxillofac Surg. 2003;61(3):369–78. https://doi.org/10.1053/joms.2003.50074.

de Camargo Moraes P, Bönecker M, Furuse C, Thomaz LA, Teixeira RG, de Araújo VC. Mucocele of the gland of Blandin-Nuhn: histological and clinical findings. Clin Oral Investig. 2009;13(3):351–3. https://doi.org/10.1007/s00784-009-0252-x.

Huang IY, Chen CM, Kao YH, Worthington P. Treatment of mucocele of the lower lip with carbon dioxide laser. J Oral Maxillofac Surg. 2007;65(5):855–8. https://doi.org/10.1016/j.joms.2006.11.013.

More CB, Bhavsar K, Varma S, Tailor M. Oral mucocele: A clinical and histopathological study. J Oral Maxillofac Pathol. 2014;18(Suppl 1):S72–7. https://doi.org/10.4103/0973-029x.141370.

Re Cecconi D, Achilli A, Tarozzi M, Lodi G, Demarosi F, Sardella A, Carrassi A. Mucoceles of the oral cavity: a large case series (1994-2008) and a literature review. Med Oral Patol Oral Cir Bucal. 2010;15(4):e551–6. https://doi.org/10.4317/medoral.15.e551.

Yeh CJ. Simple cryosurgical treatment for oral lesions. Int J Oral Maxillofac Surg. 2000;29(3):212–6.

Oral Mucosal Pigmented Lesions

Contents

Greyish Black Patch on the Cheek: Amalgam Tattoo

Anand Ramanathan

Contents

W. M Tilakaratne, T. G. Kallarakkal (eds.), *Clinicopathological Correlation of Oral Diseases*,
https://doi.org/10.1007/978-3-031-24408-7_9

Learning Goals

1. Devise the correct way of compiling the history with appropriate questions.
2. Develop a differential diagnosis after history taking.
3. Deduce appropriate procedures in clinical examination.
4. Formulate a differential diagnosis combining findings in the history and clinical examination.
5. Justify the relevant investigations required to arrive at the diagnosis.
6. Comprehend the importance of clinicopathological correlation in arriving at the correct diagnosis.
7. Outline the management plan.
8. Recognize the importance of a diagnostic algorithm in arriving at a diagnosis.

9.1 Main Complaint

A 36-year-old female patient presented to the dental clinic with a complaint of grey to black patch on the left buccal mucosa.

9.2 History of Complaint

Question: How long have you noticed the grey/black patch on your left cheek mucosa?

The patch has been there for a few years.

Question: Has the patch increased in size?

It has not increased in size.

Question: Have you noticed any colour changes in the patch?

There have been no colour changes.

Question: Does the patch disappear when you press?

It does not disappear when pressed.

Question: Do you bite on things such as pencils?

I do not have such habits.

Question: Do you have pain or other associated symptoms?

I do not have pain or any other associated symptoms.

9.3 Past Medical History

Question: Do you have any underlying medical problems?

I do not have any medical problems.

9.4 Past Dental History

Question: Have you undergone any dental treatment?

I have got a few amalgam fillings done, few crowns and cleaning of my teeth in the past.

Question: When was the amalgam filling in the tooth near the black patch done?

It was done about 10 years ago.

9.5 Social History

Question: Do you smoke or drink alcohol?

I do not smoke or drink alcohol.

9.6 With the Findings From the History, What Is Your Differential Diagnosis?

1. Amalgam tattoo
2. Graphite tattoo
3. Melanotic macule
4. Melanocytic naevus
5. Hemangioma
6. Varix

9.7 Amalgam Tattoo

The pigmented lesion on the left buccal mucosa could be an amalgam tattoo since it is a solitary pigmented lesion which is grey/black in colour, and there is a history of multiple amalgam fillings. Pieces of amalgam from the filling might have got impregnated into the buccal soft tissue. Amalgam tattoo can be a well-demarcated or diffuse lesion. They occur commonly on the buccal mucosa or gingiva.

9.8 Graphite Tattoo

Graphite tattoo is a solitary pigmented lesion that can be irregular and grey in colour. Habit of biting pencil which might accidently injure the mucosa and the graphite might get implanted into the mucosa. They commonly occur in the palate and are more common in younger age group. However, this patient denied the habit.

9.9 Melanotic Macule

A solitary well-demarcated flat and black lesion on the oral mucosa which is not more than 1.0 × 1.0 cm is usually the presentation of a melanotic macule. They occur commonly on the lips.

9

9.10 Melanocytic Naevus

A naevus is also a well-demarcated and black/brown/blue in colour. It is usually very slightly raised form the surrounding mucosa. It can occur on the palate, lips and buccal mucosa.

9.11 Hemangioma

Hemangioma can be well-circumscribed or diffuse red or bluish-red swellings in the oral cavity. It is a hamartoma showing local proliferation of blood vessels. It can occur on the lips, tongue, buccal mucosa and the palate. There are different types of haemangiomas. Congenital hemangiomas are present at birth, whereas infantile hemangiomas develop during the first 2 months of age and proliferate between 6 months and 12 months of age. Most of the hemangiomas regress, whereas 10–20% persist into adult life. Clinically, hemangiomas show blanching with diascopy test (pressure test). The diascopy test is carried out by applying pressure on the hemangioma with either a glass slide or a blunt instrument.

9.12 Varix

Oral varix is an elevated blue or bluish-red swelling in the oral cavity. It occurs in increasing frequency with age. It can be a dilated vein or a few venules. It also shows blanching with diascopy test as hemangiomas. It is common on the ventral surfaces of the tongue, floor of the mouth, lips and buccal mucosa.

9.13 Findings of Intra-oral Examination

There is a small, well-demarcated grey/black pigmented oval-shaped lesion present on the left buccal mucosa. The colour of the lesion is uniform. The lesion is very slightly elevated. The size of the pigmentation is about 1.0 × 0.5 cm. The adjacent lower molar tooth has a large amalgam filling on the buccal surface (▣ Fig. 9.1). The diascopy test is carried out by applying pressure on the lesion, but there is no blanching.

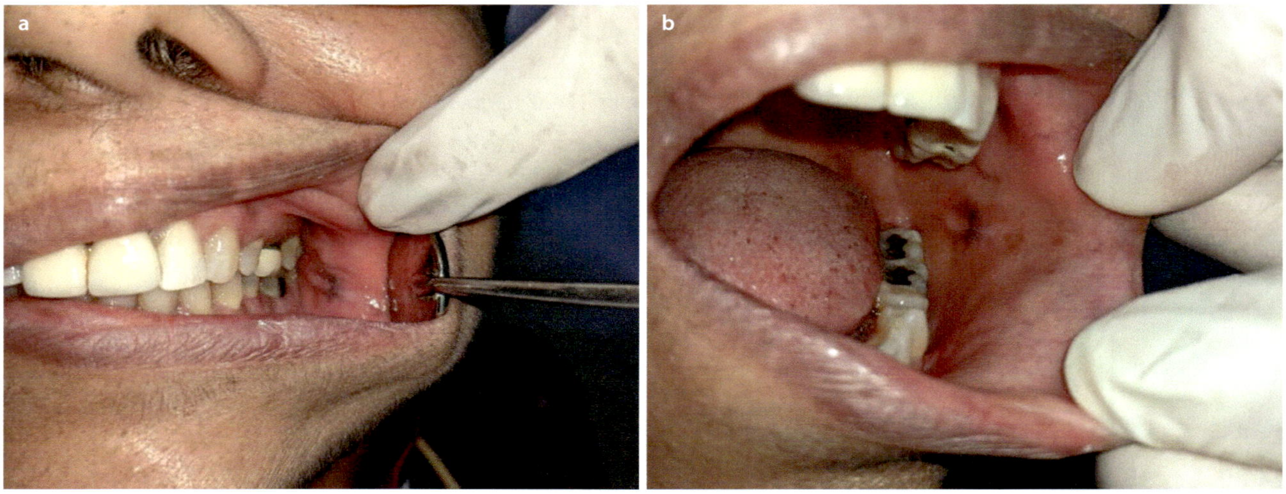

▣ **Fig. 9.1** Intra-oral photograph shows grey/black well-demarcated pigmented lesion on the left buccal mucosa (**a**) with an amalgam filling (**b**) in the adjacent lower molar tooth. (Courtesy of Mr. Muhamad Adi Hassan Rofiqi bin Saifullrizal)

9.14 What Other Relevant Features Would You Look for with the Findings You Have So Far?

It is necessary to look for any similar pigmentations elsewhere in the body to rule out other focal or diffuse pigmented lesions.

9.15 What Is the Most Likely Clinical Diagnosis?

Amalgam tattoo.

9.16 How Would You Justify Your Clinical Diagnosis?

It is an amalgam tattoo since it is a well-demarcated grey/black pigmented oval-shaped lesion present on the left buccal mucosa adjacent to a large amalgam restoration. The amalgam restoration was done about 10 years ago. The negative result for diascopy suggests that it may not be a haemangioma. Moreover, the patient is not young and does not have the habit of biting pencils. Although melanocytic naevus is a possibility, buccal mucosa is a rare site to be involved, and the lesion should preferably be slightly raised. Melanocytic malignancy can be ruled out as this is a well-demarcated lesion which has been there for many years.

9.17 What Investigations Need to Be Carried Out for This Patient?

An excisional biopsy of the pigmented lesion may be required if aesthetics is affected or if the definitive diagnosis needs to be determined when it is a concern for the patient, especially if the patient is cancerphobic.

9.18 What Are the Histopathological Features of the Excised Lesion?

On histopathological examination, the section shows deposits of black material in the connective (▫ Fig. 9.2) and around blood vessels (▫ Fig. 9.3). There are a few inflammatory cells. The overlying epithelium is normal (▫ Fig. 9.2).

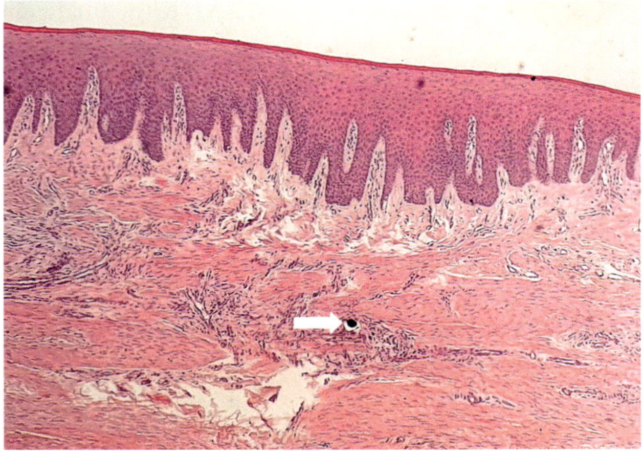

▫ **Fig. 9.2** Photomicrograph shows a black deposit (white arrow) within the connective tissue. (Courtesy Dr. Fairuz Abdul Rahman)

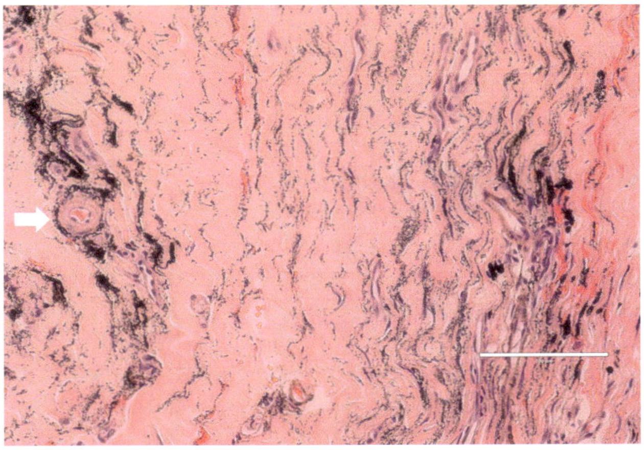

▫ **Fig. 9.3** Photomicrograph shows scattered black deposits within the lamina propria along collagen fibres and around blood vessels (white arrow)

9.19 What Is the Definitive Diagnosis for This Lesion?

Amalgam tattoo.

9.20 What Specific Findings Help You to Arrive at the Diagnosis of Amalgam Tattoo?

Clinical features that help in diagnosis are the presence of a well-demarcated grey/black pigmented lesion present on the left buccal mucosa adjacent to the lower molar tooth that is heavily restored with amalgam. Histopathologically, there are numerous deposits of black material scattered within the connective tissue along the collagen fibres and around the blood vessels.

9.21 What Is the Treatment for This Lesion?

Treatment is not required unless the patient is cancerphobic or needs to get it removed for aesthetic reasons. The patient needs to be assured that amalgam tattoo does not cause any problems.

9.22 What Is the Prognosis for Amalgam Tattoo?

Prognosis of amalgam tattoo is excellent as they do not recur once excised. However, most of the time amalgam tattoos are not excised if they do not cause any functional or aesthetic problems.

9

9.23 Amalgam Tattoo

Amalgam tattoo is defined as the presence of exogenous amalgam fragments within the oral mucosa which causes a brown to black pigmentation. It was formerly called localized argyria.

They may be caused by accidental deposition of amalgam material into the open wound during dental extraction of the tooth restored by amalgam. They may be impregnated into the oral mucosa while inserting or removing amalgam fillings. It can occur while using amalgam-contaminated dental floss, remnants of amalgam trapped in the surgical site following retrograde endodontic procedures (Fig. 9.4). They may also occur when two dissimilar metals are used for restoration on opposing teeth which results in galvanic currents that dissolve and precipitate these metals as inorganic salts within the oral mucosa. Once deposited within the oral mucosa, these metals are transported by lymphatic vessels and along the collagen fibres resulting in the increase in size of the lesion mimicking a melanoma.

Amalgam tattoos are localized blue, grey or black pigmentations on the oral mucosa which may manifest as a well-defined flat macule or slightly raised lesion measuring a few millimetres. Sometimes they can be diffuse lesions measuring a few centimetres in size. Multiple lesions may be present in some cases. These lesions show negative diascopy as they do not blanch with pressure. They are common on alveolar mucosa followed by gingiva, palate and buccal mucosa. They are usually asymptomatic and do not cause any pain and are discovered on routine oral examination. Sometimes amalgam tattoos may be present on the gingiva or buccal mucosa of an edentulous area where previously a tooth with large amalgam restoration was present.

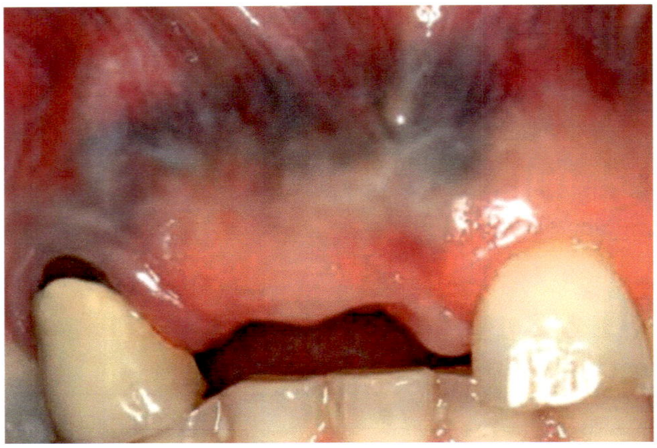

Fig. 9.4 Intra-oral photograph shows a diffuse grey/black pigmented lesion on the upper anterior labial gingiva with a history of retrograde amalgam root filling. (Courtesy Dr. Karthik Rajaram)

The differential diagnosis for amalgam tattoos that are solitary and well-defined are other solitary pigmented lesions such as graphite tattoo, melanotic macule, melanocytic nevus, hemangioma and varix. Clinically, it is difficulty to differentiate between amalgam and graphite tattoos. The most helpful feature that can differentiate the two is the presence of amalgam restoration or history of amalgam restoration in relation to the pigmented lesion whereas, for graphite tattoo, it is the history of pencil biting with accidental injury in younger age group. Moreover, graphite tattoos are more common on the palate, whereas amalgam tattoos are more common on the buccal mucosa.

Clinically, amalgam tattoo may mimic melanotic macule when it is flat. When they are slightly raised, they mimic a naevus. The diffuse amalgam tattoo may mimic melanoma as they may seem to be increasing in size. Therefore, histopathology can give the definitive diagnosis in cases where there is a doubt. Hemangiomas and varix can be differentiated from amalgam tattoo as they are more bluish or reddish in colour and blanch with diascopy test. Whereas amalgam tattoo, melanotic macule, naevus and melanoma do not blanch with diascopy test.

Since most of the amalgam tattoos are incidental findings, a thorough dental history and clinical oral examination are required to differentiate these lesions form other similar pigmented lesions as stated above. If in doubt, an excisional or incisional biopsy is required to obtain the definitive diagnosis. Sometimes, periapical or DPT radiographs may help in identifying the radio-opaque amalgam material that is lodged within the oral mucosa.

The treatment for amalgam tattoo is complete excision of the lesion if aesthetics is an issue. At times, the amalgam fragments might get embedded within the alveolar mucosa of the edentulous ridge and may cause tenderness or pain when the denture is worn over them. This might also warrant for excision of the lesion. Otherwise, these lesions do not cause any trouble for the patients and do not require any treatment. The prognosis of amalgam tattoo is very good, and they do not recur once excised.

Salient Features of Amalgam Tattoo	
Clinical features	Solitary or multiple small blue-grey/black pigmented lesion that occurs on the alveolar mucosa, gingiva, palate or buccal mucosa. Most lesions are flat but some may be raised. They can have well-defined or have diffuse margins. An amalgam restoration is usually present on the adjacent tooth.
Radiological features	Usually there is no radiopacity found in the periapical radiograph or DPT. However, some cases may show a radiopaque mass embedded within the oral soft tissues.
Histopathological features	Presence of scattered deposits of black materials within the connective tissue along the collagen fibres and around the blood vessels.
Treatment	Treatment is not required unless aesthetic or functional concerns are present.

Diagnostic Algorithm

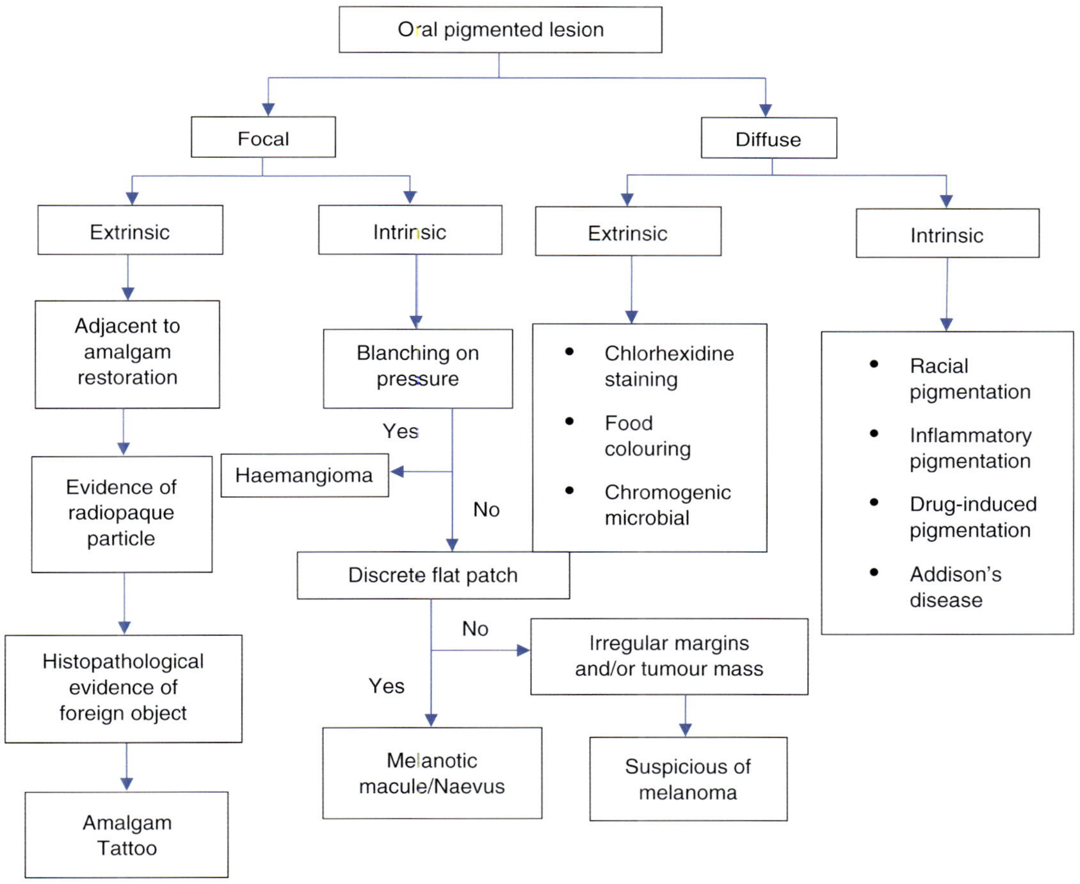

Self-Assessment Questions

1. Discuss the differential diagnoses for amalgam tattoo.
2. State the ways in which amalgam can get embedded in the tissues.
3. State the clinical features of amalgam tattoo.
4. State the histopathological features of amalgam tattoo.
5. Outline the treatment of amalgam tattoo.

Summary

Amalgam tattoo is a pigmented lesion which clinically is either a solitary or multiple small blue-grey/black pigmented lesions that occur on the alveolar mucosa, gingiva, palate or buccal mucosa. Most lesions are flat, but some may be raised. They can have well-defined or have diffuse margins. An amalgam restoration is usually present on the adjacent tooth. Some cases may show a radiopaque mass embedded within the oral soft tissues. Histopathologically, there is the presence of scattered deposits of black materials within the connective tissue along the collagen fibres and around the blood vessels. Treatment is not required unless aesthetic or functional concerns are present.

Further Reading

Lau JC, Jackson-Boeters L, Daley TD, Wysocki GP, Cherian MG. Metallothionein in human gingival amalgam tattoos. Arch Oral Biol. 2001;46(11):1015–20.

Buchner A, Hansen LS. Amalgam pigmentation (amalgam tattoo) of the oral mucosa: A clinicopathologic study of 268 cases. Oral Surg Oral Med Oral Pathol. 1980;49(2):139–47.

Amano H, Tamura A, Yasuda M, Yamanaka M, Takeuchi Y, Sasaoka K, et al. Amalgam tattoo of theoral mucosa mimics malignant melanoma. J Dermatol. 2011;38(1):101–3. https://doi.org/10.1111/j.1346-8138.2010.01007.x.

Tan QS, Pandarathodiyil AK, John J, Karthick Sekar, Palaniappan PL RS, Ramanathan A. Ignored amalgam pigmentation leading to discomfort upon denture wearing: a case report. Int J Dentistry Oral Sci. 2021;8(6):2723–6. https://doi.org/10.19070/2377-8075-21000534.

Kauzman A, Pavone M, Blanas N, Bradley G. Pigmented lesions of the oral cavity: review, differential diagnosis, and case presentations. J Can Dent Assoc. 2004;70(10):682–3.

A Fast-Growing Black Patch on the Upper Front Gum: Malignant Melanoma

Pilana Vithanage Kalani Shihanika Hettiarachchi and Wanninayake M Tilakaratne

Contents

W. M Tilakaratne, T. G. Kallarakkal (eds.), *Clinicopathological Correlation of Oral Diseases*,
https://doi.org/10.1007/978-3-031-24408-7_10

Learning Goals

1. Devise the correct way of compiling the history with appropriate questions.
2. Develop a differential diagnosis after history taking.
3. Deduce appropriate procedures in clinical examination.
4. Formulate a differential diagnosis combining findings in the history and clinical examination.
5. Justify the relevant investigations required to arrive at the diagnosis.
6. Comprehend the importance of clinicopathological correlation in arriving at the correct diagnosis.
7. Outline the management plan.
8. Recognize the importance of a diagnostic algorithm in arriving at a diagnosis.

10.1 Main Complaint

A 55-year-old male patient presented to the clinic complaining of a blackish pigmented lesion in relation to the area of upper anterior teeth.

10.2 History of Complaint

Question: When did you first notice this?

It has been there for 9 months. Initially, I noticed a change in the colour of the gums and the palate. Three months later, a swelling appeared in the same region. I did not seek any medical advice until the swelling was fast increasing in size.

10.3 Additional Complaints

Question: Do you have any pigmented lesions elsewhere on the body?

I don't have any other, pigmented lesions on the body.

Question: Have you experienced loss of appetite and loss of weight recently?

I have not experienced any loss of appetite or weight; however, I feel tired after daily work. I can manage my routine work without much of a problem.

Question: Do you feel dizzy when you change your positions? For example, standing up from a sitting position.

I do not have any dizziness.

Question: Are you suffering from any other medical problems such as heart disease, high blood pressure, diabetes, bleeding disorder, respiratory diseases? If yes, what kind of medications have you been taking until now?

I have a history of recurrent respiratory infections. There are no other significant medical problems.

Question: Have you experienced coughing and shortness of breath or abdominal pain with altered bowel habits?

I have been experiencing mild cough and intermittent shortness of breath from time to time, but without any associated gastrointestinal symptoms.

Question: Have you noticed any swellings in any part of your body (especially in the arms, legs, face or scrotum)?

I haven't noticed any such abnormal swellings.

Question: Have you undergone any dental treatment?

I have undergone several fillings and extractions for decayed teeth.

Question: What is your occupation?

I am a farmer.

Question: Do you have any specific chewing habits?

I do not have the habit of betel quid chewing.

Question: Are you a smoker?

Yes, I am a smoker and smoke about 10–15 cigarettes per day for the past 20 years.

Question: Do you take alcohol?

I am not into the habit of drinking alcohol.

10.4 With the Findings from the History, What Is Your Differential Diagnosis?

1. Oral malignant melanoma.
2. Kaposi sarcoma.
3. Vascular malformation.
4. Melanosis associated with smoking.
5. Amalgam tattoo.
6. Melanotic-macule.

10.5 How Do You Justify Your Differential Diagnosis After History Taking?

1. Pigmented lesions in the oral cavity may occur due to many reasons and include melanotic macule, smoking-associated melanosis, amalgam tattoo, drug-induced pigmentation, malignant melanoma and vasculartumours such as Kaposi sarcoma. Since he does not have a suggestive drug history, the possibility of drug-induced pigmentation can be excluded.
2. Benign pigmented lesions such as melanotic macule or smoker's melanosis can be seen in different regions of the oral mucosa, such as gums, palate and lips. Since melanotic macule is a common benign lesion, this can be considered in the differential diagnosis. Smoker's melanosis is also a possibility as this patient is a chronic heavy smoker. Further, as this patient has multiple restorations, amalgam tattoo could also be a possible differential diagnosis. However, as the lesion has started growing fast recently, above lesions are unlikely differential diagnoses.
3. The rapid nature of the growth raises the suspicion of a tumour, and therefore, the possibility of malignant melanoma and Kaposi sarcoma should be considered. Since the patient has a cough with shortness of breath and recurrent respiratory tract infection, compromised immunity could be suspected. Therefore, the possibility of Kaposi sarcoma as a result of HIV infection is included in the differential diagnosis.

10.6 Findings of Clinical Examination

There is a pigmented growth on the buccal gingivae in relation to the edentulous upper left canine region measuring about 2.5 cm in width which extends to the palatal mucosa. The lesion smoothens out into a pigmented irregular patch on the palate (◘ Fig. 10.1a and b).

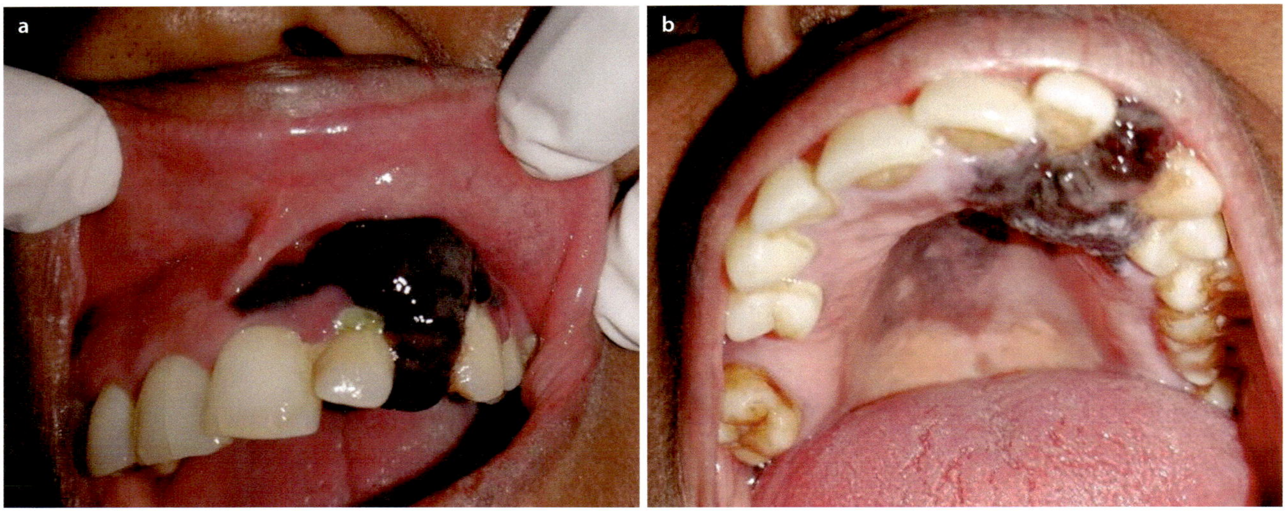

◘ **Fig. 10.1** (**a**) Pigmented growth on the buccal gingivae extending to the palatal aspect through the upper left edentulous area in the canine region. (**b**) The pigmented lesion extended on to the palate with irregular margins

10.7 What Other Relevant Features Would You Look for with the Findings You Have So Far?

There are no other areas of pigmentation present in the oral cavity. The lesion is not ulcerated, and there is no bleeding (◘ Fig. 10.1a). It did not blanch under pressure. There are no palpable cervical lymph nodes.

10.8 What Is Your Clinical Differential Diagnosis?

1. Oral Malignant Melanoma.
2. Kaposi Sarcoma.

10.9 How Would You Exclude Other Conditions and Justify the Inclusion of the Diseases That You Have Mentioned in the Differential Diagnosis to Arrive at a Working Diagnosis?

10.9.1 Melanosis Associated with Smoking (Smoker's Melanosis)

Oral pigmentation is increased significantly in heavy smokers. Exposure to polycyclic amines (such as nicotine and the benzpyrenes) has been shown to stimulate melanin production by stimulating melanocytes. Although this patient has a heavy smoking history, the type of the lesion present in the mouth is not consistent with melanosis associated with smoking. Even though, any mucosal surface may be affected (◘ Fig. 10.2), resulting in a growth as presented in this case. Therefore, melanosis associated with smoking or smoker's melanosis is unlikely to be the diagnosis for his complaint.

10.9.2 Amalgam Tattoo

Amalgam tattoo is a common benign pigmented lesion caused by deposition of amalgam particles in the oral mucosal tissue. This presents as a painless, bluish-grey or black and flat lesion commonly located on the gingivae close to an amalgam restoration or at a site not related to any fillings such as the inside of the cheeks, lips, tongue and the palate. Even though this patient had undergone several restorations, none of them were amalgam restorations. Moreover, amalgam tattoos usually manifest as macular lesions. Therefore, the possibility of an amalgam tattoo can be excluded.

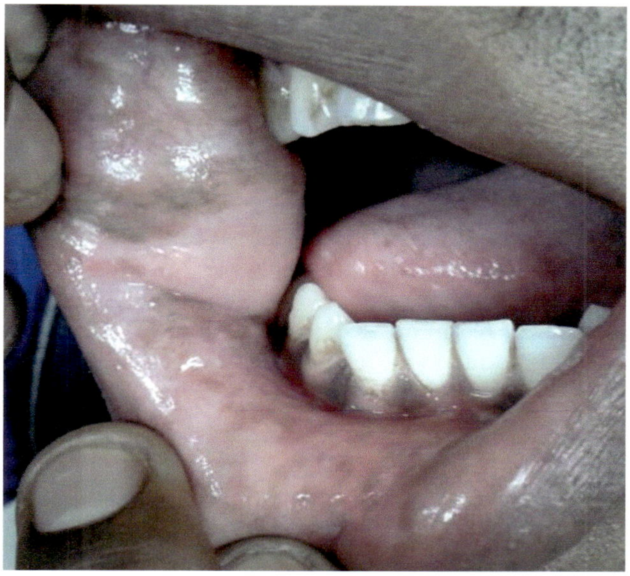

◘ Fig. 10.2 Oral pigmentation seen in smokers, note the mild staining on the teeth due to smoking

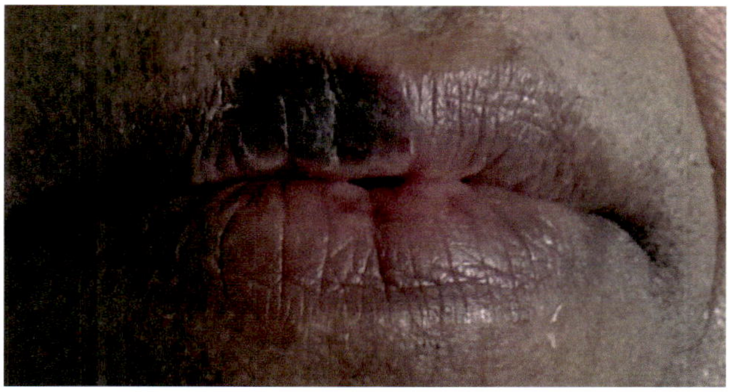

◘ Fig. 10.3 Focal pigmented lesion on the upper lip consistent with an oral melanotic macule

10.9.3 Oral Melanotic Macule

Oral melanotic macule is a benign hyperpigmentation of mucous membranes occurring in approximately 3% of the general population. There is an increase in focal melanin deposition without an increase in the number of melanocytes. These lesions are commonly found on the lips (◘ Fig. 10.3); however, gingiva and the palate may also get affected. As the name denotes, these are typical "macular lesions" and are very unlikely to be present as an extensive nodular lesion of this nature. Therefore, oral melanotic macule is an unlikely differential diagnosis in this case.

10.9.4 Vascular Malformations

These are structural anomalies of blood vessels with normal endothelial cell turnover. By definition, in contrast to hemangiomas, vascular malformations (Fig. 10.4) are present at birth and persist throughout life. They can be categorized according to the type of vessel involved (capillary, venous or arteriovenous) and according to hemodynamic features (low flow or high flow). This lesion was not pulsatile, didn't blanch under pressure and was of recent onset. Hence, the possibility of a vascular malformation is remote.

10.9.5 Kaposi Sarcoma

Kaposi sarcoma (KS) is a vascular tumour of lymphatic endothelial origin. It is the most common neoplasm that occurs in patients with HIV infection and is considered as an AIDS defining disease. Typically, the early lesions manifest as red, purplish, flat or macular lesions on the skin or intra-orally or more frequently may present as multiple lesions. The most common sites in the oral cavity affected by KS are palate and the gingivae. KS is believed to be caused by Human herpes virus-8 (HHV-8). This patient manifested a cough with shortness of breath which may be due to respiratory involvement associated with KS. However, the patient did not have any other features suggestive of HIV infection or involvement of other systems especially cervical lymphadenopathy which occurs due to dissemination of the disease. The present findings of a solitary, non-ulcerated lesion with no other associated oral or systemic manifestations of HIV could exclude KS to be the primary diagnosis for his complaint.

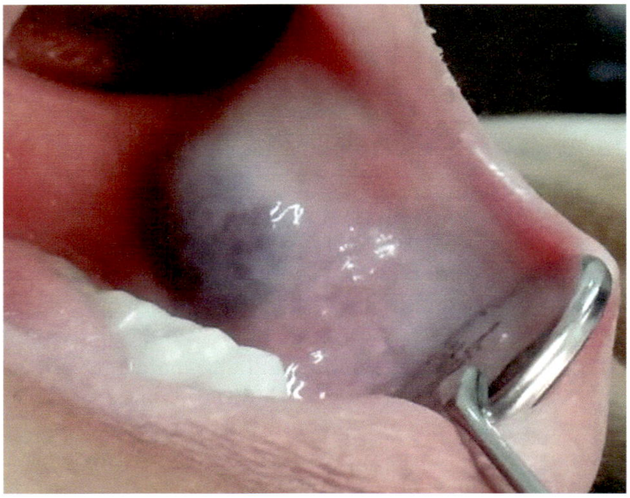

Fig. 10.4 Vascular malformation on the left buccal mucosa

10.10 What Is the Most Likely Diagnosis?

Oral malignant melanoma.

10.11 How Would You Investigate This Patent?

- Incisional biopsy for the confirmation of diagnosis and to plan long-term management.
- Imaging for the assessment of the extension of the lesion and neck node status.

10.12 How Would You do an Incisional Biopsy for This Patient? What Are the Important Considerations?

Biopsy is mandatory for confirmation of the diagnosis. The present guidelines for the surgical management of primary cutaneous melanoma recommend a diagnostic excisional biopsy of the lesion followed by a wide local excision once the diagnosis is proven. However, in the oral cavity, the size of the lesion or anatomical limitations, particularly the presence of teeth, may preclude performing an excisional biopsy. Therefore, it is proposed to perform an excisional biopsy with a 1–2-mm margin for small lesions in amenable locations, but an incisional biopsy, through the thickest or the most suspicious part of the tumour, in case of a large lesion or a lesion located in sites where an excisional procedure would involve extensive and mutilating surgery. The rationale for suggesting an excisional biopsy is that cutting into the lesion during an incisional biopsy could result in accidental dissemination of malignant cells within the adjacent tissues ("seeding") or even into the blood or lymphatic stream, with the subsequent risk of local recurrence or regional or distant metastasis.

10.13 Biopsy Report Confirms the Previous Clinical Diagnosis of Oral Malignant Melanoma. What Are the Histopathological Features That Help in the Diagnosis?

The tumour comprises atypical epithelioid and spindle cells arranged into solid sheets (Fig. 10.5). The cells show cellular atypia including hyperchromatism, nuclear and cellular pleomorphism and frequent mitoses (Fig. 10.5). Occasional abnormal mitotic figures and foci of necrosis are also observed. Proliferating melanocytes extend into the epithelium as single cells and nests.

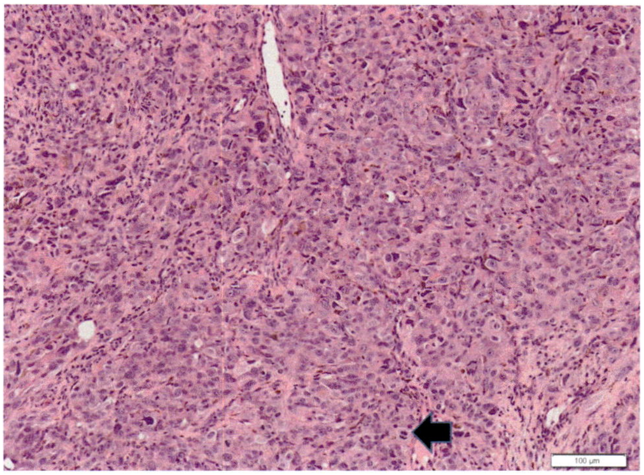

Fig. 10.5 Atypical epithelioid and spindle cells arranged into solid sheets. The cells show cellular atypia including hyperchromatism, nuclear and cellular pleomorphism and frequent mitoses (black arrow)

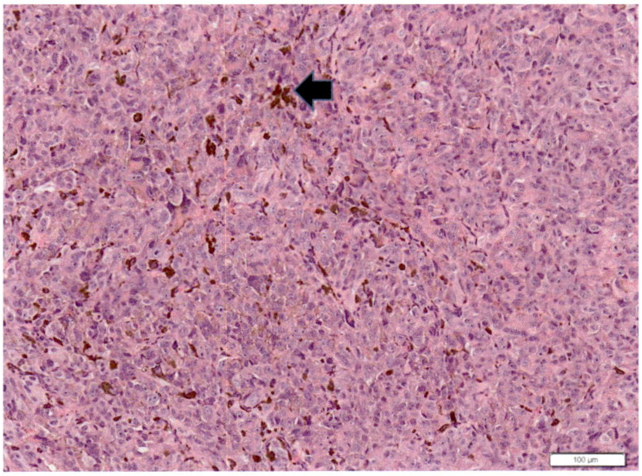

Fig. 10.6 The tumour cells contain melanin pigment (black arrow)

The tumour cells contain fine granules of melanin pigment (Fig. 10.6).

10.14 How Would You Manage This Patient?

Radical surgery is indicated and often is combined with adjunctive radiation therapy. Radical resection of the primary lesion preferably using an intra-oral approach and involving at least 1.5 cm of healthy tissue followed by reconstruction is recommended. Postoperative radiotherapy is recommended if poor prognostic pathologic features such as multiple positive nodes or extranodal spread of metastastic melanoma or positive excision margins are evident histopathologically. The patient has to be followed up once a month in the clinic postoperatively.

Targeted therapy and immunotherapy are also being used for the treatment of malignant melanomas. Immunotherapy, also called biologic therapy, is designed to boost the body's natural defenses to fight the cancer. It uses materials made either by the body or in a laboratory to improve, target or restore immune system function. In recent years, there have been major advances in treating stage III and stage IV melanomas with immunotherapy. Targeted therapy is a treatment that targets the cancer's specific genes, proteins or the tissue environment that contributes to cancer growth and survival. The discovery that about 50% of melanomas have a mutated or activated *BRAF* gene has provided an important new direction in targeted therapy for melanoma.

10.15 Oral Malignant Melanoma (OMM)

Melanomas are malignant neoplasms arising from melanocytes, which originate from the neural crest. Oral lesions are relatively uncommon than their skin counterparts and are considered to be one of the deadliest human neoplasms.

In contrast to cutaneous melanomas, the exact aetiology of OMM is unknown. These melanomas have no apparent relationship to chemical, thermal or physical events (e.g. smoking; alcohol intake; poor oral hygiene; irritation from teeth, dentures or other oral appliances) to which the oral mucosa is constantly exposed. Benign, intraoral melanocytic proliferations (nevi) exceptionally rarely transform into oral melanomas. However, the sequence of events is poorly understood in the oral cavity. Presently, most oral melanomas are thought to arise de novo, from apparently normal mucosa.

Oral malignant melanoma was first described by Weber in 1859. This tumour affects more often the hard palate and the gingiva. In the head and neck region, nasal and paranasal melanomas are three times more common than OMM. Primary OMM is rare, representing 0.2–8% of all melanomas and accounting for 0.5% of all oral malignancies. Further, these neoplasms are more common in some countries such as Japan and Africa but uncommon in Western countries.

The clinical presentations of this neoplasm vary widely. OMM is usually insidious in onset, with few symptoms until it has progressed. Typically, these may present as pigmented macules or nodular lesions, with uniformly brown or black colour. Alternatively, they may show variation of colour, with black, brown, grey, purple and red shades. They may also present as non-pigmented neoplasms that may be solitary or multiple. Often satellite foci may surround the primary tumour and the tumour surface may be smooth, with an intact overlying mucosa, or may be ulcerated. Other presenting signs and symptoms include bleeding, pain, increased mobility of teeth and delayed healing of extraction sockets. Regional lymphadenopathy may be present and connotes a poor prognosis. Based on the clinical presentation, five types of OMM are identified.

- Pigmented nodular type
- Non-pigmented nodular type
- Pigmented macular type
- Pigmented mixed type
- Non-pigmented mixed type.

OMM is reported to have a male predilection and mostly occurs in the age range of 20–80 years, with a mean age of 56 years. However, occurrence of OMM is rare before the age of 20 years. Apart from the hard palate and maxillary gingiva, other oral sites including the mandibular gingiva, buccal mucosa and floor of the mouth may be involved. Intra-oral malignant melanomas are easy to diagnose clinically as they are mostly pigmented and have an irregular shape and outline. The ABCD checklist ("Asymmetry", "Border" irregularities, "Colour" variegation and "Diameter" > 6 mm) that is commonly used in the identification process of cutaneous melanoma could also be of some help in the diagnosis of oral melanoma. These lesions usually remain asymptomatic and may be detected only when there is ulceration of the overlying epithelium and/or haemorrhage. When an oral pigmentation cannot be confidently diagnosed as benign on clinical grounds, a biopsy is mandatory in order to exclude OMM. Radiological examination including computed tomography (CT), magnetic resonance imaging (MRI) or positron emission tomography (PET) could be useful for evaluation of primary tumour and regional or distant metastases. Delayed detection may be the reason for poor prognosis of oral malignant melanomas with the 5-year survival rate being 15–38%. Invasion of the bone may occur, increasing the likelihood of metastasis. In addition, the rich vascular supply present in the oral cavity may further contribute to the dissemination of melanomas.

10

Histopathologically, malignant melanoma is characterized by atypical epithelioid and spindle cells arranged into solid sheets showing marked cellular atypia including, hyperchromatism, nuclear and cellular pleomorphism, and frequent mitoses. Proliferating melanocytes extend into the epithelium as single cells and nests. The tumour cells contain fine granules of melanin pigment. Melanomas have two growth phases, namely radial and vertical. Radial growth phase is usually followed by vertical growth. There is no frank invasion of tumour cells into connective tissue during radial growth phase as it is mostly restricted to the epithelium. This is classically seen in the skin in relation to superficially spreading, acral lentiginous and lentigo malignant melanoma subtypes.

The management of OMM poses the clinician with great challenge. This task becomes more challenging as the treatment is still controversial, and there is lack of consensus with regard to the best therapeutic approach. The preferred treatment option is considered to be ablative surgery, if the tumour is considered resectable. Excision of the primary lesion, preferably using an intraoral approach and involving at least 1.5 cm of healthy tissue, is recommended. Surgery could be combined with radiotherapy, chemotherapy or immunotherapy even though the effectiveness of such therapies either as primary or in association with the surgical treatment is mostly unknown. In patients with primary OMM, the risk for lymph node metastasis is approximately 25%. Neck dissection should be reserved for cases with preoperatively confirmed lymph node metastases, and the choice of the modality of neck dissection should be guided by the extent and the level of the involved nodes. Postoperative radiotherapy is generally recommended if poor prognostic pathologic features are present, such as multiple positive nodes, or extranodal spread of metastastic melanoma, even though OMMs are regarded as poorly radiosensitive.

OMM is a highly aggressive tumour with a high mortality rate. The reported prognosis of oral melanoma is poor, the 5-year survival rate for OMM ranges from 9.4 to 15.6% even after radical treatment. The survival rate decreases parallel to the time that elapses from diagnosis to treatment. The median survival for all oral mucosal melanomas is slightly more than 2 years from the time of diagnosis. One reason for the poor prognosis of OMM is early invasion of the underlying tissue, increasing the likelihood of metastasis.

The present case presentation emphasizes the importance of early diagnosis and treatment, because of its aggressive behaviour and extremely poor prognosis. The clinician must therefore carefully examine the head, neck and oral cavity and maintain a high index of suspicion for any pigmented lesion within the oral cavity especially those occurring in high-risk sites such as palate and maxillary gingivae.

Salient Features of Oral Malignant Melanoma	
Clinical	Asymptomatic, asymmetric pigmented lesions with variation in colour from red to black to brown with an irregular outline
Histopathology	Epithelioid and spindle cells showing high degree of cellular atypia with melanin production. Varying degrees of radial and vertical growth with prominent junctional activity
Treatment	Surgery remains the preferred treatment option

Diagnorithm

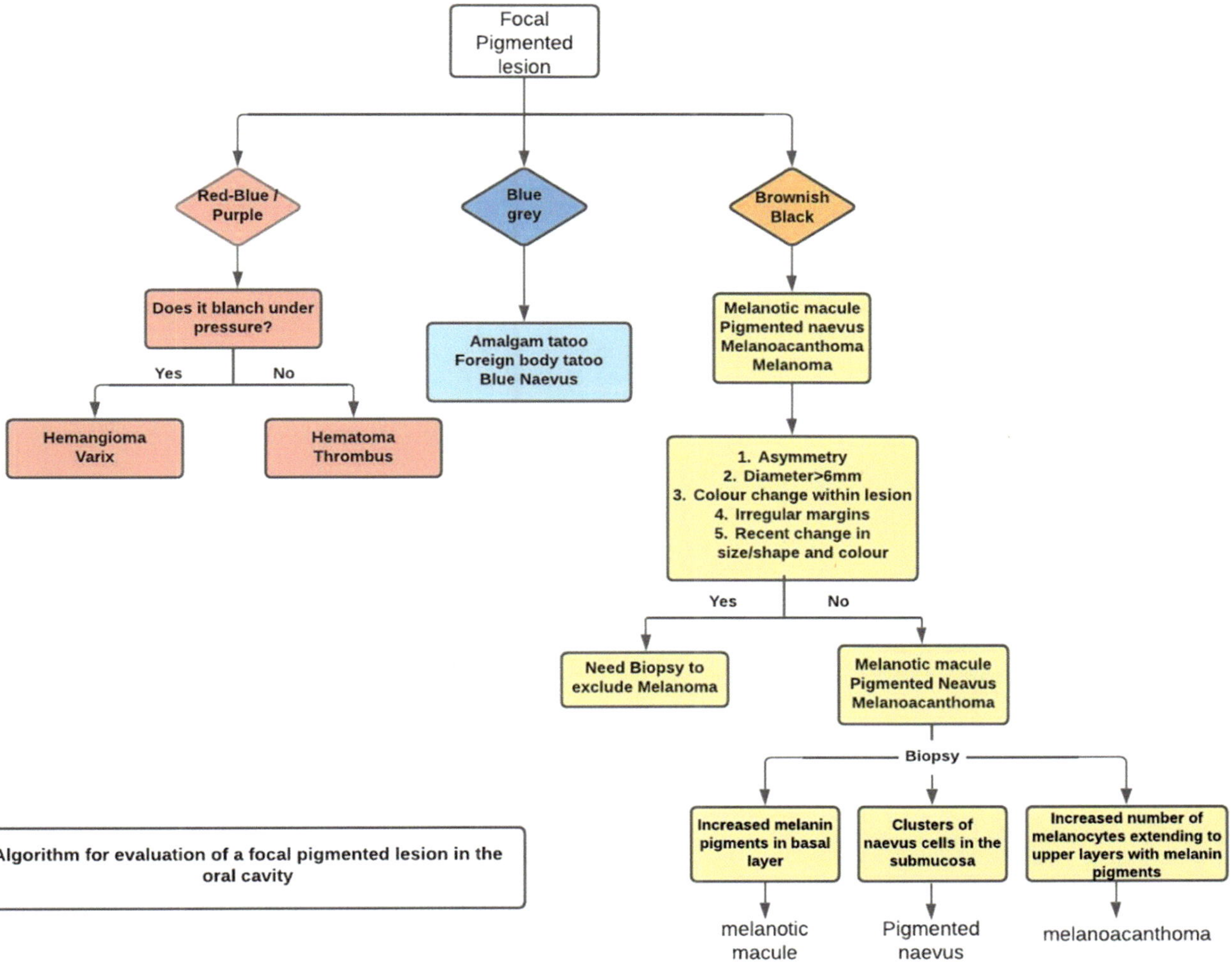

Algorithm for evaluation of a focal pigmented lesion in the oral cavity

Self-Assessment Questions

1. State the important conditions that need to be included in the differential diagnosis of a pigmented lesion in the oral cavity.
2. Explain the clinical features of oral malignant melanoma.
3. Describe the histopathological features of OMM.
4. List the different melanocytic markers helpful for diagnosis.
5. Outline the management of OMM.

Further Reading

Ascierto PA, Accorona R, Botti G, Farina D, Fossati P, Gatta G, et al. Mucosal melanoma of the head and neck. Crit Rev. Oncol Hematol. 2017;112:136–52. https://doi.org/10.1016/j.critrevonc.2017.01.019.

Boulaadas M, Benazzou S, Mourtada F, Sefiani S, NazihN EL, Kzadri M. Primary oral malignant melanoma. J Craniofac Surg. 2007;18:1059–61.

Neville BW, Damm DD, Allen CM, Chi AC. Oral and maxillofacial pathology. 2016.

Natarajan E. Black and brown oro-facial mucocutaneous neoplasms. Head Neck Pathol. 2019;13(1):56–70.

Femiano F, Lanza A, Buonaiuto C, Gombos F, Di Spirito F, Cirillo N. Oral malignant melanoma: a review of the literature. J Oral Pathol Med. 2008;37(7):383–8.

A Black Spot on the Upper Gum for Many Years: Melanotic Macule

Pilana Vithanage Kalani Shihanika Hettiarachchi and Wanninayake M Tilakaratne

Contents

W. M Tilakaratne, T. G. Kallarakkal (eds.), *Clinicopathological Correlation of Oral Diseases*,
https://doi.org/10.1007/978-3-031-24408-7_11

Learning Goals

1. Devise the correct way of compiling history with appropriate questions.
2. Develop a differential diagnosis after history taking.
3. Deduce appropriate procedures in clinical examination.
4. Formulate a differential diagnosis combining findings in the history and clinical examination.
5. Justify the relevant investigations required to arrive at the diagnosis.
6. Comprehend the importance of clinicopathological correlation in arriving at the correct diagnosis.
7. Outline the management plan.
8. Recognize the importance of a diagnostic algorithm in arriving at a diagnosis.

11.1 Main Complaint

A 25-year-old female patient, complaining of a black spot on the upper gum presented to the clinic.

11.2 History of Complaint

Question: When did you first notice this?

It has been there for many years and I have not sought any medical advice to date but now I am worried as it has been there for a long duration. However, the black patch remains asymptomatic.

11.3 Additional Complaints

Question: Was this lesion present since birth?

According to my mother, this lesion has been present since I was around 10 years old. She cannot recall its presence since birth.

Question: Do you have any other pigmented lesions elsewhere on the body, especially on the hands and feet?

I don't have any other, pigmented lesions on other areas of the body.

Question: Does any of your family members have similar lesions?

None of my other family members have similar lesions.

Question: Did you notice any recent enlargement of the lesion or any change in color?

There hasn't been any recent change in color or size of the lesion and it has remained the same size since I initially noticed this.

Question: Are you experiencing any symptoms associated with the gastrointestinal system like abdominal pain, vomiting, diarrhea, or rectal bleeding?

I am suffering from mild gastritis. Apart from that I do not have any other symptoms.

Question: Are you on any medications for any medical problems?

I am not on any medications.

Question: Have you undergone any dental treatment?

I have had several fillings and extractions done for decayed teeth.

Question: What is your occupation?

I am a banker in the private sector.

11.4 With the Findings from the History, What Is Your Differential Diagnosis?

1. Melanotic macule
2. Amalgam tattoo
3. Melanoacanthoma
4. Melanocytic naevus

11.5 How Do You Justify Your Differential Diagnosis After a History Taking?

1. This is a long-standing pigmented lesion. As this patient does not have a suggestive drug history nor a smoking history, the possibility of drug-induced pigmentation and melanosis associated with smoking was excluded.
2. Melanotic macule is a common benign lesion. Hence this was considered in the differential diagnosis. Further, as this patient has multiple restorations amalgam tattoo also becomes another possible diagnosis.

3. Despite the fact, that this lesion has been there for a long period of time, it being asymptomatic is in favor of a diagnosis of a benign disease process such as an oral melanoacanthoma.

11.6 Findings of Clinical Examination

There is a well-demarcated, localized macule on the labial gingivae measuring about 4 mm in maximum diameter in between the upper two central incisors (Fig. 11.1).

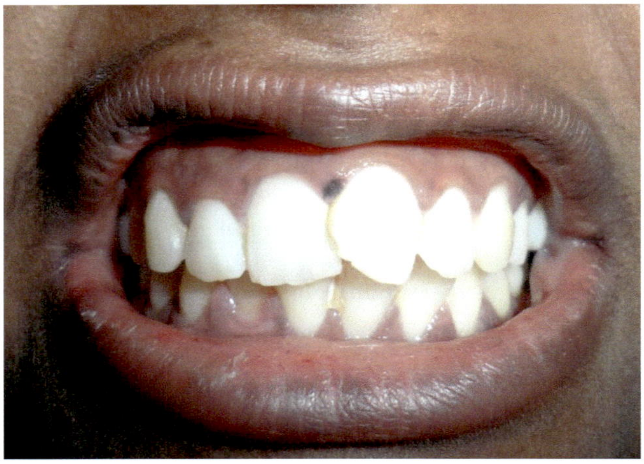

Fig. 11.1 Well-localized pigmented flat lesion on the labial gingiva between the two upper central incisors measuring about 4 mm in maximum diameter

11.7 What Other Relevant Features Would You Look for with the Findings You Have So Far?

The patient had undergone multiple restorations. However, none of them are amalgam restorations. The lesion present is a primary solitary lesion and she does not have any other areas of pigmentation in the oral cavity. The lesion is not ulcerated and there is no bleeding. Further, this lesion does neither blanch under pressure nor is any pulsation noted.

11.8 What Is Your Clinical Diagnosis?

Melanotic macule.

11.9 How Would You Exclude Other Conditions and Justify the Inclusion of the Diseases That You Have Mentioned in the Differential Diagnosis to Arrive at a Working Diagnosis?

11.9.1 Amalgam Tattoo

Amalgam tattoo is a common benign pigmented condition caused by the deposition of amalgam (silver filling) particles in the oral mucosal tissue (Fig. 11.2a). This presents as a painless, bluish-gray or black, flat lesion commonly on the gingivae close to an amalgam restoration or at a site not related to any fillings such as the inside of the cheeks, lips, tongue, and the palate. This patient had undergone several restorations. However, none of them were amalgam restorations. Therefore, the possibility of an amalgam tattoo was excluded as it is unlikely to be the primary diagnosis for her complaint.

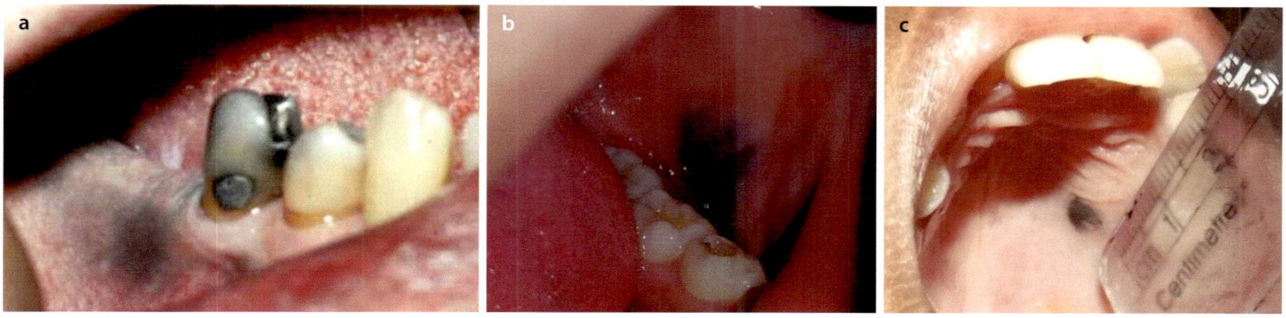

Fig. 11.2 Clinical differential diagnosis for a long-standing pigmented lesion. An amalgam tattoo (**a**) melanoacanthoma (**b**) oral melanocytic naevus (**c**)

11.9.2 Oral Melanoacanthoma

Oral melanoacanthoma is a rare, benign, reactive process that occurs at a mean age of 29 years. These are usually asymptomatic, pigmented lesions characterized clinically by the sudden appearance and rapid growth of a macular brown-black lesion. Even though, clinically, the lesion is a flat or slightly raised black or brown macule (Fig. 11.2b), the absence of an initial rapid growth phase, in this case, excludes the possibility of an oral melanoacanthoma.

11.9.3 Oral Melanocytic Naevus

Oral melanocytic nevi are benign proliferations of nevus cells in the epithelial layer, the submucosal layer, or both. They are classified as junctional, intramucosal, and compound nevi. Nevi may also be classified as congenital or acquired. Unlike their cutaneous counterparts, oral melanocytic nevi are rare. These are mainly seen on the palate (Fig. 11.2c) and gingiva and are usually slightly raised papules, compared to melanotic macules which are invariably flat. As naevus is relatively rare in the oral cavity and the presented lesion is flat, the possibility of an oral melanocytic naevus is less likely.

11.10 What Is the Most Likely Diagnosis?

Oral melanotic macule.

11.11 How Would You Investigate This Patent?

Usually investigations are not warranted for oral melanotic macule, as these lesions are considered to be benign in nature with no malignant potential. However, an incisional or excisional biopsy may be performed in order to confirm the diagnosis.

11.12 How Would You Do an Incisional Biopsy for This Patient? What Are the Important Considerations?

Lesions with a typical history and appearance need not be biopsied. Even though biopsy is not mandatory for the diagnosis, early-stage melanomas can have a similar clinical appearance. Depending on the size of the lesion an incisional or excisional biopsy is advised to rule out the possibility of malignancy.

11.13 Biopsy Report Confirms the Previous Clinical Diagnosis of Oral Melanotic Macule. What Are the Histopathological Features That Will Help in the Diagnosis?

The stratified squamous epithelium on the surface is normal in appearance. Increased melanin production is seen in the basal and parabasal layers of the epithelium. Melanocyte numbers may also be increased in some cases. Melanin pigmentary incontinence is also evident in the upper corium (Fig. 11.3).

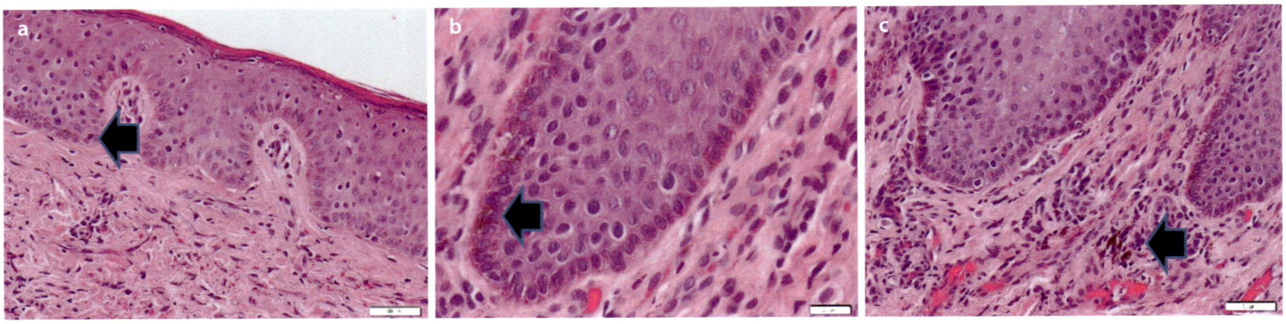

Fig. 11.3 The basal and parabasal layers of the epithelium show increased melanin production (**a**) and (**b**) (black arrows). Melanin incontinence is seen in the superficial connective tissue (black arrow) (**c**)

11.14 How Would You Manage This Patent?

Generally, these are considered as benign lesions with no malignant potential. Therefore, these lesions can be kept under observation. However, removal may be desirable especially for a labial melanotic macule where aesthetics is a concern. Excisional biopsy is the preferred treatment method. Further, electrocautery, laser ablation, or cryosurgery can also be considered.

11.15 Oral Melanotic Macule (Focal Melanosis)

An oral melanotic macule is a benign hyperpigmentationwhich appears as a flat, brown discoloration of the mucous membrane. This occurs in approximately 3% of the general population. There is an increase in focal melanin deposition. Melanotic macules are most commonly found on the vermillion border of the lip, more often on the lower lip than the upper lip. Lesions can also be found on the gingiva or palate or in the vulva, and they may be multiple. Some experts refer to lesions on the lip as "labial melanotic macules" and to lesions in the vulva as "vulvar melanosis," although histopathology is identical at any mucosal site.

Oral melanotic macule is common in patients with darker skin phototypes and may appear at any age, with the average age of presentation to the physician being 43 years. There is also a female preponderance with a female: male ratio of 2:1. However, in patients with darker skin phototypes, onset typically occurs in adolescence. Usually these lesions appear as single, well-demarcated, uniformly pigmented oval or round macules with the greatest diameter of 7 mm or less. Usually, the color may vary from tan to dark brown. However, rarely it may be either blue or black in color.

Although typically reported as a benign lesion with no malignant transformation, all oral pigmented macules of recent onset, large size, irregular pigmentation, unknown duration, or recent enlargement should be submitted for microscopic examination to exclude a diagnosis of melanoma. Clinical differential diagnosis includes amalgam tattoo, melanacanthoma, melanocytic naevus, and malignant melanoma.

Although these lesions may be followed up in areas where aesthetics is not a concern, treatment is often requested with the involvement of the labial mucosa. In such cases, excision would be the best option. However, other treatment modalities like electrocautery, laser ablation, or cryosurgery are effective but, the limitation is that no proper tissue is available for histopathologic examination after these procedures.

Further, rarely these flat pigmented lesions may be associated with systemic, genetic disorders such as Peutz-Jegher syndrome, McCune-Albright syndrome, Addison disease, Neurofibromatosis type I or with certain medications including chloroquine and other quinine derivatives, phenolphthalein, estrogen and AIDS-related medications.

Salient features of oral melanotic macule	
Clinical	Asymptomatic round or oval macule, solitary pigmented lesion, well-demarcated, uniformly tan to dark-brown in color. Usually, will not exceed 7 mm in diameter. Once maximum diameter is achieved, it may remain constant
Histopathology	Normal surface epithelium and increased melanin pigmentation in basal and parabasal layers. There may be an increase in the number of melanocytes
Treatment	Excision remains the preferred treatment option. Electrocautery, laser ablation, or cryosurgery is also effective
Oral melanotic macule is a benign lesion, however, it is crucial to differentiate this entity from other possible malignant lesions that occur in the oral cavity especially, malignant melanoma	

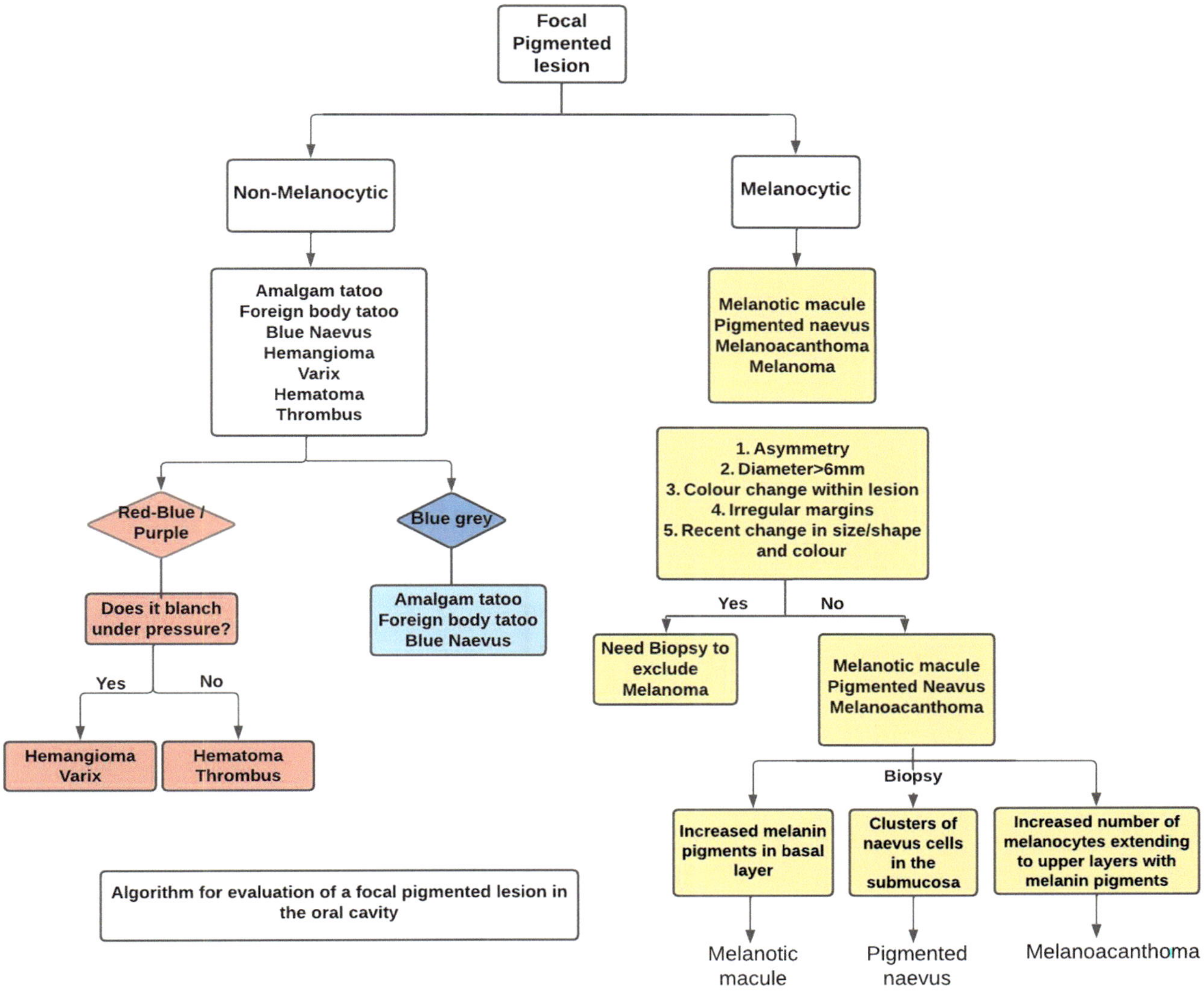

Algorithm for evaluation of a focal pigmented lesion in the oral cavity

Self-Assessment Questions

1. List different benign pigmented lesions in the oral cavity.
2. Describe the important findings in the history that is essential to differentiate melanotic macule from other causes of pigmentation.
3. Discuss the characteristic clinical features of oral melanotic macule.
4. Describe the histopathological features of oral melanotic macule.
5. Outline the management plan for oral melanotic macule.

Further Reading

Buchner A, Merrell PW, Carpenter WM. Relative frequency of solitary melanocytic lesions of the oral mucosa. J Oral Pathol Med. 2004;33:550–7.

Duan N, Zhang YH, Wang WM, Wang X. Mystery behind labial and oral melanotic macules: Clinical, dermoscopic and pathological aspects of Laugier-Hunziker syndrome. World J Clin Cases. 2018;6(10):322–34.

Neville BW, Damm DD, Allen CM, Chi AC. Oral and maxillofacial pathology. 2016.

Shen ZY, Liu W, Bao ZX, et al. Oral melanotic macule and primary oral malignant melanoma: epidemiology, location involved, and clinical implications. Oral Surg Oral Med Oral Pathol Oral Radiol Endod. 2011;112:e21–5.

Blue-Purple Lump on the Lip: Haemangioma/Vascular Anomaly

Harsha Lal De Silva and Benedict Seo

Contents

W. M Tilakaratne, T. G. Kallarakkal (eds.), *Clinicopathological Correlation of Oral Diseases*,
https://doi.org/10.1007/978-3-031-24408-7_12

Learning Goals

1. Understand the presentation and pathogenesis of vascular lesions in the head and neck region.
2. Clinically recognise and differentiate vascular lesions.
3. Classify vascular lesions to help plan their management.
4. Recognise and appreciate the clinical challenges in their management.
5. Learn the use of modern imaging technology in the diagnosis and assessment of vascular lesions.

12.1 Main Complaint

A 65-year-old female patient presents to your clinic with a complaint of a dark blue/purplish lump on her left lower lip (Fig. 12.1).

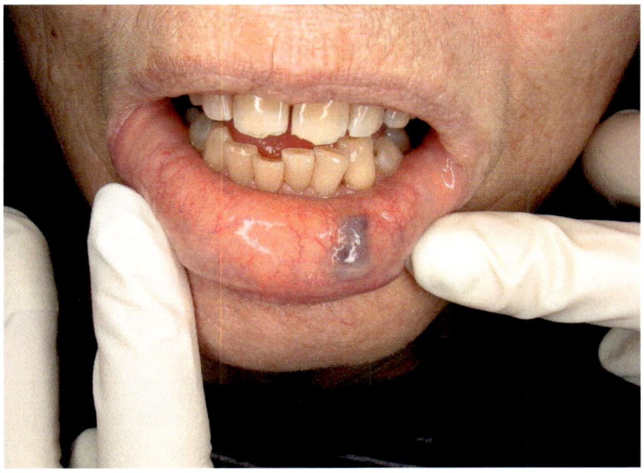

Fig. 12.1 A bluish-purple lump in the lower lip mucosa

12.2 History of Complaint

Question: How long have you had this lump?

It is difficult for me to be precise but I believe it had been there for at least 10 years if not more.

Question: Have you experienced any issues with this lump?

It seldom gave me any concerns. I can't remember it being painful or giving me much discomfort. Perhaps, that may be why I cannot recall how and when it first appeared.

Question: Have you ever noticed it change in colour or size?

No, I don't think it has increased in size from the time I first noticed. It may be getting darker over time.

Question: Have you had any injury or some form of trauma to your lip?

I do not recall any specific incidents. However, sometimes it does get in the way of my daily routines such as eating and tooth brushing. Occasionally it gets accidentally bitten or scratched with some foods like crusty bread.

Question: What happens when it is traumatised?

It bleeds quite badly and also becomes a little sore and may develop an ulcer on its surface. It heals on its own and I can't remember having to take any medications to relieve the discomfort or to promote healing.

Question: What do you do for a living? Do you work mainly indoors or outdoors?

I recently retired from being a gardener. Yes, I have worked outdoors all my life and I still spend a lot of time in my garden.

Question: Do you smoke or drink alcohol?

In the past, I have smoked cigarettes a few times, and that too when I am enjoying an occasional social drink with my friends. Since retirement, I usually enjoy a glass of wine on a Friday evening but certainly no smoking.

Question: Do you have any other medical issues of note?

No, I have been fit and healthy throughout. My only hospitalisation was for a small fracture in my right ankle from a cycling accident, several years ago.

12.3 From the findings of the history, what is your Differential Diagnosis?

1. Vascular anomaly (malformation/haemangioma)
2. Pyogenic granuloma
3. Mucocoele/other salivary gland lesions
4. Melanocytic naevus

12.4 How do you justify your Differential Diagnosis reached from the findings of the history?

1. The lesion is papular in appearance and is darkly coloured (blue-purple). Darkly pigmented purplish lesions with dome-shaped elevated surface is a common presentation of vascular lesions and anomalies. In addition, vascular lesions may develop secondary to chronic sun exposure or trauma in adults. These lesions tend to bleed profusely if traumatised.
2. Pyogenic granuloma is a red-purple benign reactive hyperplastic vascular lesion that can occur in the lip. They commonly occur following low-grade irritation or trauma or as a result of hormonal imbalances or alterations.
3. Mucocoele is the most common lump in the lip region, especially in the lower lip. They are commonly seen in young and middle-aged individuals, usually presenting as pale blue, dome-shaped swellings. They may be fluctuant but do not empty on compression and do not bleed excessively if traumatised. In this case, the patient is of advanced age but mucocoele cannot be conclusively ruled out on clinical examination alone. The lower lip is an uncommon location for salivary neoplasms.
4. Naevomelanocytic lesions may also be considered as they are typically pigmented and may be raised. The head and neck is not uncommon site for naevi.

12.5 Clinical Examination Findings

She had a full range of jaw movements with no pain, clicking or tenderness in her temporomandibular joints. There was no associated palpable cervicofacial lymphadenopathy. Extra-oral and intra-oral examinations revealed no remarkable findings over and beyond the current lesion. Minor malocclusion and sharp tooth edges were noted but appeared non-contributory concerning the localisation of the current lesion.

The lesion in her lower lip measured approximately 10 × 15 mm in size, was dark bluish/purple with no surface ulceration. It felt soft and compressible to palpation with no evident induration at its base or the periphery. The lesion didn't feel pulsatile and showed partial blanching when compressed. No other oral or facial lesions of similar nature was detected on clinical examination.

12.6 What other features would you look for in formulating a Clinical Diagnosis?

- Surface characteristics such as presence or absence of ulceration and uniformity in colour.
- Texture and tactile characteristics such as degree of fluctuance, blanching upon compression, pulsatility, induration and fixation.
- Current symptoms and reported variations in shape and size with function.

12.7 What is your Clinical Diagnosis?

Vascular anomaly (malformation).

12.8 How would you exclude other conditions and justify the linclusion of the disease entity that you have mentioned as the Clinical Diagnosis?

Mucocoeles represent a mucous extravasation phenomenon whereby an incidence of trauma leads to severance of associated duct/s with mucin seeping out into the surrounding soft tissues. Confirmed history of trauma is often helpful but not essential. Some mucocoeles may fluctuate in size corresponding to the degree of salivation during mastication. Mucocoeles are biopsied to include the damaged ducts and associated gland/s within the excision. This form of a biopsy would be both diagnostic and most often curative. The absence of any history of trauma and long duration is not supportive of diagnosing this as a mucocoele.

Pyogenic granuloma (vascular anomaly/tumour) is a reactive vascular hyperplastic lesion that is reactionary to local or systemic stimuli. They occur as sessile or pedunculated masses often with surface ulceration. In this patient, there is no surface ulceration and the lesion appears more deeply blue/purple in, as opposed to the typical reddened appearance expected of pyogenic granuloma.

Melanocytic naevus tends to be more flat and non-fluctuant/compressible. Naevi however may self-involute over time and older people tend to have less. Dimensionally naevi are usually smaller than 6 mm in diameter. Naevoid lesions typically show a spectrum of brownish pigmentation although some may show a more profoundly dark brown to a blue hue, due to the Tyndall effect. For example, blue naevus presents as a dark blue pigmented lesion due to more deeply seated pigmentary melanin particles. History of profuse bleeding after trauma, compressibility and raised popular nature are not the features of a naevus.

12.9 What is the most likely working diagnosis?

Vascular anomaly (malformation).

12.10 How would you investigate this patient?

Vascular anomalies are an extensively heterogeneous group of lesions that may be difficult to distinguish solely based on the clinical appearance. Consideration should be given for excisional biopsy upon discussion with the patient. Complete excision is expected to be both diagnostic and curative.

12.11 If a biopsy was to be performed, what are the important considerations?

Potential peri-operative haemorrhage is the most important consideration. The small lesions are best excised with a small cuff of normal tissue to avoid profuse haemorrhage. This patient's lip lesion is small, appears superficially located and therefore is best managed with a total excision which should be both diagnostic and curative. However, given the vascular nature of the lesion, referral to a specialist or planning the biopsy in a controlled environment is advisable.

If the lesion was larger, an incision biopsy could still be considered provided adequate surgical skills and facilities are available to manage a potential profuse perioperative haemorrhage. Electrocautery is a useful adjunct to control bleeding. However, lesions with clinical suspicion to be more deeply seated or extensive than what appears on the surface, need specialised imaging to delineate the nature and extent of the pathology before attempting any invasive surgical interventions, to reduce the potential risk of profuse perioperative haemorrhage.

12.12 The biopsy report confirms the previous Clinical Diagnosis of Vascular Malformation. What are the Histopathological Features that help in confirming the diagnosis?

Histologically vascular malformations may look relatively diverse depending on the type of the anomaly and the vessels involved. Typically oral mucosal vascular malformations tend to involve low flow capillary/venous vessels rather than high flow vascular malformations. The involved blood vessels may appear to be markedly dilated (cavernous, ◘ Fig. 12.2a) or maybe small or normal-sized capillaries that are more numerous (capillary, ◘ Fig. 12.2b) for the given anatomical location. Often, both cavernous and capillary features may be observed in a single lesion. The vessels involved do not show active proliferation or stacking appearance observed in true haemangiomas and other neoplastic vascular growths.

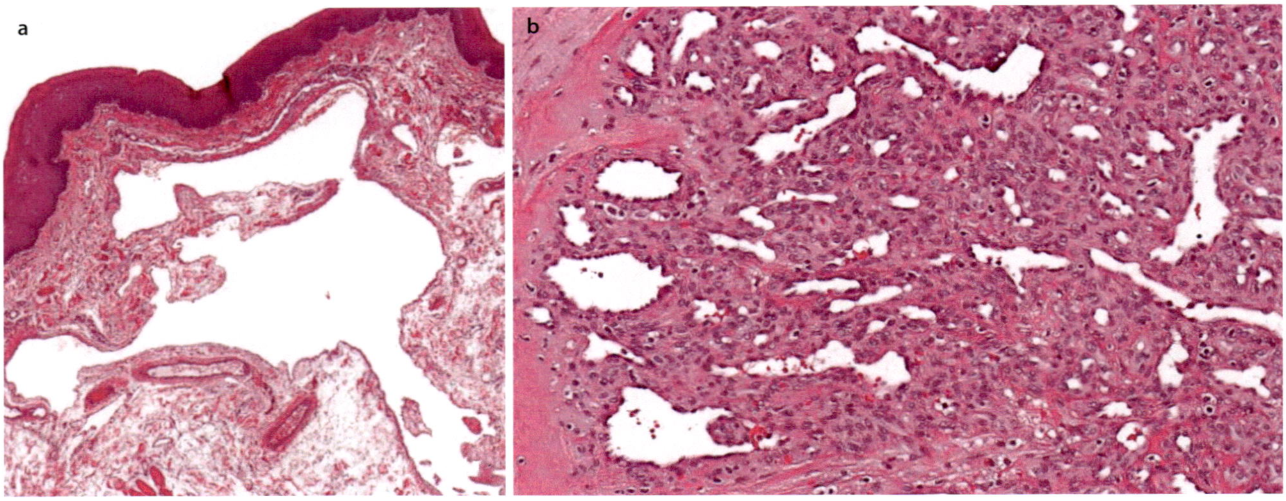

Fig. 12.2 Vascular malformations show (**a**) regions of widely dilated endothelial-lined blood vessels, often described as a cavernous haemangioma, and (**b**) areas showing numerous small thin-walled blood vessels, some with indistinct lumina, which has been described as a capillary haemangioma

12.13 How could you manage this patient?

This patient appears to have a relatively small vascular lesion located superficially on her lower lip. While it has not caused any significant trouble she reports the lesion being inadvertently traumatised a few times during daily routines resulting in profuse bleeding and some ulceration. Hence, it is prudent to discuss with the patient the merits and demerits of actively treating this lesion. Given the smaller size of the lesion, it can be easily and safely treated to minimise potential complications that may cause inconvenience to her in the future.

This lesion, being small and superficial, could be treated with photocoagulation using a diode laser. Photodynamic ablation with a diode laser is likely to give an excellent outcome with minimal post-surgery discomfort and scarring. It may be necessary to repeat the treatment once or twice to achieve a complete cure. Alternatively, sclerotherapy using an intralesional injection of a sclerosing agent is equally effective in inducing fibrosis and involution. However, the latter technique may cause more local inflammation and pain during the healing period. Both these techniques, however, will not provide a tissue specimen for histopathological confirmation of the diagnosis.

Alternatively, given the small size of the lesion and its superficial location, it can be safely excised using a conventional surgical scalpel. The bleeding can be managed effectively by excising the lesion with a peripheral cuff of normal tissue and by using local haemostatic adjuncts. This approach has the value of providing a tissue sample for histopathological confirmation of the clinical diagnosis.

12.14 Vascular Anomalies/Haemangioma

Vascular anomalies can be regarded as a group of lesions arising from congenital errors in angiogenesis. The current understanding of pathogenesis and molecular makeup remains incomplete. However, much progress has been made in the past two decades resulting in a better understanding of their biological behaviours, imaging protocols, novel therapies and improvement of the conceptual framework on pathogenesis to underpin treatment decisions.

The classification and nomenclature for vascular anomalies are complex and encompass a diverse range of lesions of different origins, locations and pathogenesis. The International Society for the study of Vascular Anomalies (ISSVA) Classification divides the lesions into Tumour and Malformation categories with numerous subcategories under each section (Table 12.1). Vascular 'tumours' include benign, locally aggressive/borderline and malignant lesions which include neoplastic, non-neoplastic and those with controversial pathogenesis. Infantile haemangioma (IF) in this category is a relatively common benign vascular endothelial proliferation on the skin of infants which tend to self-involute over time with a prevalence estimated to be 4–5%. Recent molecular studies show that the IF endothelial cells express glucose transporter type 1 (GLUT-1) protein (also known as solute carrier family 2, facilitated glucose transporter member 1, encoded by gene *SLC2A1*), and this protein can act as an immunohistochemical biomarker of IF. Congenital haemangiomas on the other hand are present and fully developed at birth in neonates. Congenital haemangiomas (CH) can

Table 12.1 The International Society for the study of Vascular Anomalies (ISSVA) Classification of vascular lesions

Vascular Tumours	Vascular malformations			
Benign • Infantile haemangioma • Congenital haemangioma pyogenic granuloma • Others	**Simple** • Capillary • Lymphatic • Venous • Arteriovenous malformation • Arteriovenous fistula	**Combined** • Combination of the simple types	**Of major named vessel**[a] • Lymphatics, veins and arteries and include various anomalies (origin, course, number, length, diameter, valves, communication and persistence)	**Associated with other anomalies** • Sturge Weber syndrome • Others
Locally aggressive/ borderline • Kaposi sarcoma • Others				
Malignant • Angiosarcoma • Others				

[a] Refers to malformations involving large axial conducting vessels, for example, aorta

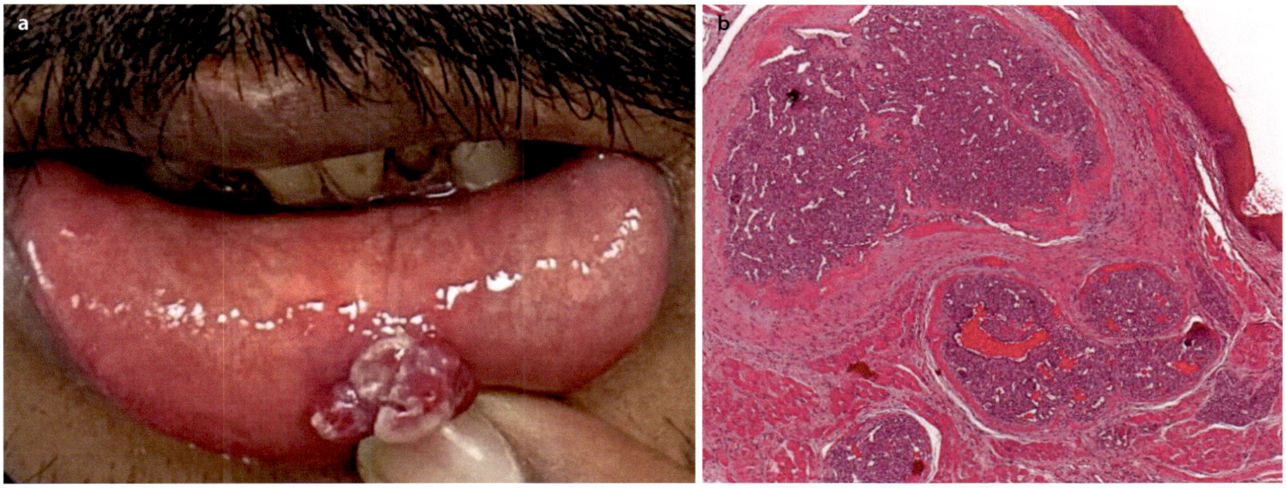

Fig. 12.3 A patient everts his lower lip to show the pyogenic granuloma presenting as an exophytic dark red/purple lesion with surface ulceration in his lower labial mucosa (**a**). Histological evidence of lobulation of the hyperplastic vascular connective tissue (**b**)

be further subclassified into 'rapidly involuting' (RICH), 'non-involuting' (NICH) and 'partially involuting' (PICH) types.

It is of note that the term haemangioma has been used historically and conventionally to describe a range of vascular lesions, in an almost indiscriminate fashion. As such most non-specific vascular lesions in the oral regions have been described as haemangiomas with subclassification based on their histopathologic appearances—into 'capillary' and 'cavernous'. This terminology should not be used vaguely to describe benign vascular lesions as they may refer to specific types of 'haemangiomas' such as IF and CH. Additionally, the term haemangioma implies, somewhat confusingly, a possible neoplastic process. Whilst some lesions termed haemangiomas may be truly neoplastic, many others such as infantile and congenital haemangiomas regress spontaneously. True neoplasms, by definition, will not spontaneously regress. Pyogenic granuloma (Fig. 12.3a) is another common vascular lesion that represents a reactive hyperplastic vascular growth forming as a result of physiological or external stimuli. Some pyogenic granulomas show distinct lobulation of the vascularlesional tissues and the term 'lobular capillary haemangioma' has been used (◘ Fig. 12.3b). This phenomenon is more commonly observed on the skin rather than the oral cavity, and the term is considered to be a synonym for pyogenic granuloma. Although it is implied that the precipitating causation is more readily identifiable in cases of pyogenic granuloma than true developmental vascular malformations and anomalies.

The vascular 'malformation' category on the other hand include lesions supposedly of developmental nature and can be sub-classified based on the types of vessels involved, their anatomical location and association with any other anomalies. Of the lesions classified under the vascular malformations category, the simple type, involving a singular vasculature, is the most common form, particularly those involving capillary vessels. These lesions usually present as pink to violaceus papules on the skin often persisting for life. Terms such as 'port-wine stains' have been used to describe these lesions based on their clinical appearance. Whilst such malformations may be isolated and limited in extent, they may also be a presenting indication of a broader spectrum of syndromes that include other forms of anomalies. For example, Sturge-Weber syndrome (SWS) encompasses such port-wine staining of the skin of the head and neck, typically along the first and second divisions of the trigeminal nerve. SWS is a congenital neurovascular syndrome involving a somatic mutation of *GNAQ* gene which leads to malformations of the vasculature, as well as disturbances in the development of the eye, skin and brain.

Age- and sun-induced vascular anomalies also share some of the histological features of 'haemangiomas/vascular malformations. Lesions such as venous lakes present as a darkly pigmented maculopapular lesion on the sun-exposed sites, commonly on the lip of elderly patients (◘ Fig. 12.4a). Histologically the lesion shows markedly dilated thin-walled blood vessels in the background of sun-damaged skin (◘ Fig. 12.4b). Features of sun-induced changes include epithelial dysplasia on the surface and solar elastosis in the underlying fibrous connective tissue. Some of the dilated and often congested lesional vessels may also show thrombosis and eventual granulation tissue formation within the lumen.

The oral cavity and the head and neck region are sites of predilection for lymphatic malformations. The term lymphangioma has been used to describe such lesions but currently, it is thought that most of these lesions are better described as lymphatic malformations or benign hamartomatous malformations. Intraorally, lymphangiomas most commonly occur in the anterior tongue and present with somewhat pebbled surface architecture and may grow to a large size. Histologically, lymphangiomas have been described as capillary, cavernous, or cystic (macrocystic, microcystic or mixed), depending on the size of the vessel/s involved but often different subcategories may be present at the same time. With secondary haemorrhage, lymphatic vessels may be difficult to distinguish from blood vessels and proteins such as D2-40 (podoplanin, encoded by *PDPN*) and lymphatic vessel endothelial hyaluronic acid receptor 1 (LYVE-1, encoded by *LYVE1*) have been proposed as helpful distinguishing molecular markers.

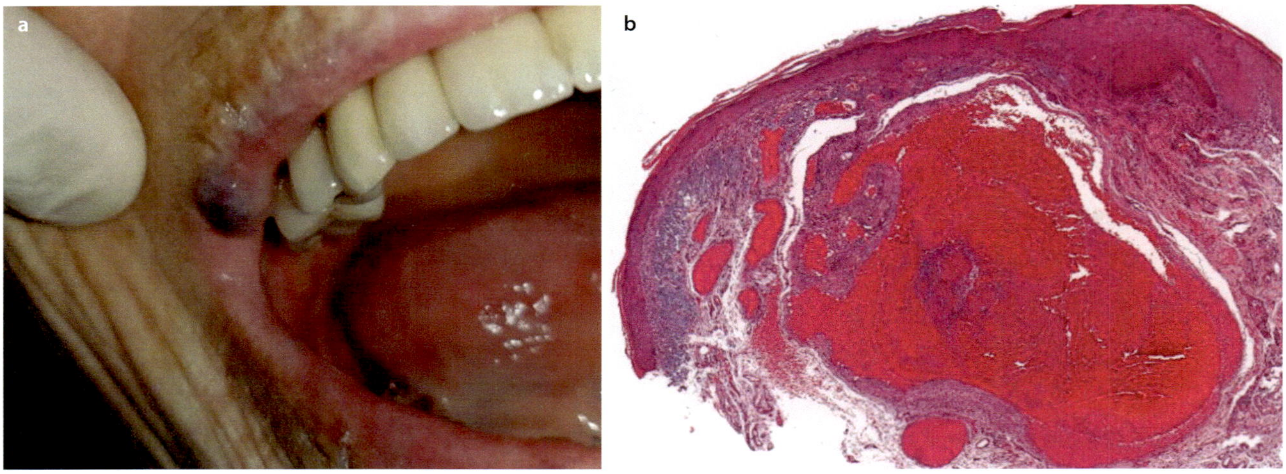

◘ **Fig. 12.4** An example of a vascular anomaly commonly referred to as 'venous lake' on the upper lip of an elderly patient (**a**). Histologically there is a widely dilated thin-walled blood vessel with evidence of thrombosis. The fibrous connective tissue shows evidence of solar elastosis (**b**)

12.15 Management of Vascular Lesions

12.15.1 Haemangiomas

The most important determinant is the history confirmation of whether the lesion was present at birth (Congenital Haemangioma) or developed in early infant life (Infantile haemangioma). The infantile haemangiomas tend to appear very early in life and almost all cases will follow a cycle of proliferative phase (increasing in size), a stable phase and thereon to an involuting phase which will result in involution and may lead to complete resolution of the lesion. Hence, most can be managed by careful observation only to allow natural regression. In the instances of an infantile haemangioma interfering with the structural integrity of a vital organ (i.e., an infantile haemangioma in the orbit interfering with the globe) or compromise function (tendency to bleed during feeding) an early therapeutic intervention becomes necessary to mitigate the adverse implications. The majority of congenital haemangiomas too undergo a similar path and rarely warrant treatment. A small proportion of non-involuting lesions may merit active intervention.

Where treatment is indicated medical management with beta-blockers or steroids (intralesional or oral administration) is the preferred option. Sclerotherapy can be used for accessible lesions. For larger and deep-seated lesions, magnetic resonance imaging (MRI) is the preferred diagnostic investigation to demarcate the extent of the lesion and its spatial relationships to vital structures. MRI may also facilitate therapeutic embolisation procedures, used rarely to trigger the involution of a large lesion. Recently, laser photocoagulation has been used to treat small, accessible lesions. Surgery is reserved for smaller lesions or any smaller residual lesions which may remain following the use of non-surgical interventions.

12.15.2 Vascular Malformations

Vascular malformations are the commonest group presenting in adults. The vascular malformations in adults are best divided into low-flow and high-flow varieties to help manage decisions. The low-flow vascular malformations include capillary, venous, lymphatic or mixed types featuring a combination of more than one vessel type.

Capillary malformations are commonly seen in the head and neck region. They may occur both superficially and in deep locations. Superficial lesions may cause discolouration of the skin or the mucosa giving a colour ranging from pink to blue or purple hue. Some capillary malformations may be a part of syndromes and may occur alongside other clinical manifestations. One such example is the Sturge–Weber syndrome which may have cutaneous capillary haemangiomas producing a characteristic Port–Wine stain and may also have lesions in the leptomeninges resulting in focal neurological disturbances.

Not all capillary malformations need treatment. Treatment is usually offered for those causing cosmetic disfigurement or clinical symptoms due to a mass effect. Superficial capillary malformations are best treated with pulsed-dye lasers. Laser therapy induces selective photothermolysis of superficial vascular lesions where haemoglobin absorbs the laser light and converts it to heat causing coagulation of the vessels while preserving the integrity of other skin/mucosal components. Complications are rare and may include transient hyperpigmentation and mild skin atrophy/scarring.

Venous malformations account for almost 50–60% of all vascular malformations. Nearly 40% of them occur in the head and neck region. The vast majority of them occur as sporadic lesions and are the commonest low-flow vascular malformations seen in the oral cavity. Some may be seen at birth but many become obvious in adult life. They vary in colour from being hardly detectable to bluish-purple, largely dependent on how deep the lesion is located. They can be compressed and may become engorged through the Valsalva manoeuvre; both features help to distinguish them from lymphatic malformations. The low-flow malformations rarely cause symptoms except when they are large or are easily traumatised. They may occasionally cause pain due to intra-lesional haemorrhage, thrombosis and subsequent inflammation.

Lymphatic malformations are seen more in younger children and adults. Lesions are commonly found in the head and neck region and within the oral cavity may frequently involve lips, tongue or the buccal mucosa. Histologically they may show two distinct patterns namely microcystic or macrocytic.

Larger lesions may need three-dimensional imaging to assess the true extent of the pathology. MRI is the primary imaging modality to assess both venous and lymphatic malformations. Used in conjunction with MRI, Doppler ultrasonography further enhances the characterisation of the vascular anomaly and venous flow.

Asymptomatic low-flow venous and lymphatic anomalies may not need any active interventions and can be managed conservatively through periodic clinical observation and monitoring. Where treatment is indicated due to symptoms or for cosmetic disfigurement, superficial venous malformations can be treated effectively with pulse-dye laser photocoagulation or with cryotherapy. Sclerotherapy using intralesional injections of sclerosing agents is the gold standard for managing moderate and larger lesions. A plethora of different agents have been used that include ethanol, sodium tetradecyl sulphate, polidocanol, bleomycin and doxycycline. Sclerotherapy causes inflammation of the vascular endothelium leading to luminal obliteration through fibrosis and healing. Large lesions may need more than one application.

High-flow malformations include arteriovenous fistulas (AVFs) and arteriovenous malformations (AVMs). AVFs may occur following trauma but the pathogenesis of AVMs remains obscure. AVMs may be present at birth but may manifest only in later life with bleeding, pain and tissue destruction secondary to mass effect. The clinical examination may reveal a vascular blush in the overlying skin or mucosa. The lesion commonly exhibits pulsatility and may also have an audible bruit. High-flow vascular lesions need further evaluation through specialised imaging studies. MRI and angiography along with Doppler ultrasonography help the characterisation of the lesion and facilitate treatment decisions. Selective therapeutic embolisation of the feeding vessels performed by a skilled interventional radiologist is the gold standard of care. Surgery can be potentially hazardous and is usually undertaken only for lesions that are very small or have been embolised in advance to produce shrinkage in size and flow rates (▣ Fig. 12.5).

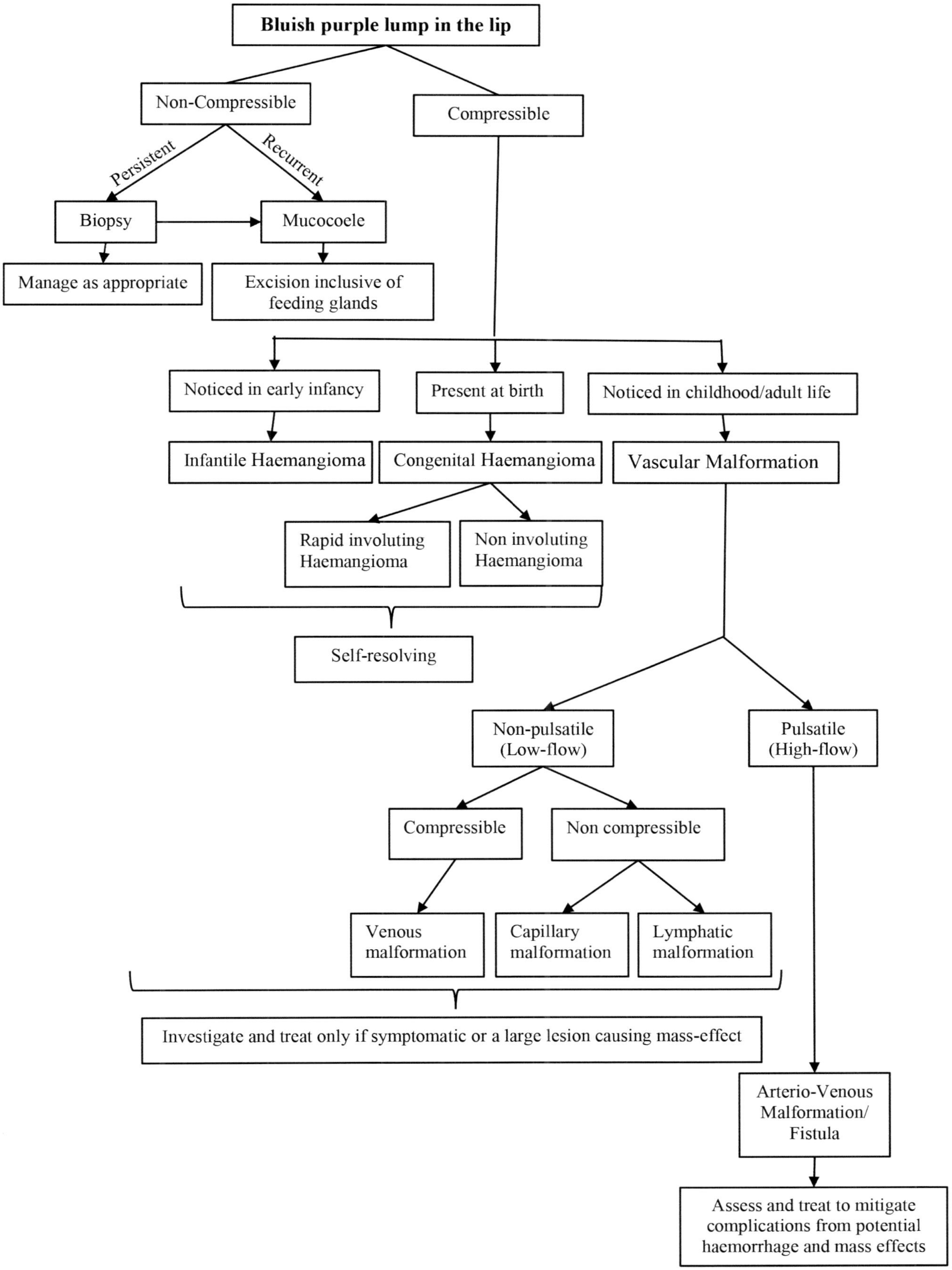

Fig. 12.5 A suggested algorithm for managing a bluish-purple lump in the lower lip

Self-Assessment Questions

1. How do common vascular lesions in children differ from those occurring in adults?
2. Why do you have to be cautious when performing a biopsy of a bluish lesion in the lower lip?
3. How can you clinically differentiate between a mucocoele and a venous malformation?
4. How can you clinically differentiate between an arteriovenous malformation and a venous malformation?
5. What are the potential dental implications of Sturge–Weber syndrome?

Summary

Vascular anomalies tend to occur in the head and neck region and may present as congenital or infantile lesions or develop later in life. Some may self-resolve but others may warrant treatment for the potential risk of being accidentally traumatised leading to troublesome, potentially life-threatening haemorrhage. It is important to recognise, assess and evaluate them carefully before undertaking invasive procedures for diagnosis or treatment. Modern imaging technologies and novel therapies based on their biological behaviours have improved safety and better therapeutic outcomes.

Further Reading

Buckmiller L, Richter G, Suen J. Diagnosis and management of hemangiomas and vascular malformations of the head and neck. Oral Dis. 2010;16:405–18. https://doi.org/10.1111/j.1601-0825.2010.01661.x.

Izadpanah A, Izadpanah A, Kanevsky J, et al. Propranolol versus corticosteroids in the treatment of infantile hemangioma: a systematic review and meta-analysis. Plast Reconstr Surg. 2013;131:601–13.

Mulligan PR, Prajapati HJ, Martin LG, Patel TH. Vascular anomalies: classification, imaging characteristics and implications for interventional radiology treatment approaches. Br J Radiol. 2014;87(1035):20130392. https://doi.org/10.1259/bjr.20130392.

Mulliken JB, Glowacki J. Hemangiomas and vascular malformations in infants and children: a classification based on endothelial characteristics. Plast Reconstr Surg. 1982;69:412–22.

Munden A, Butschek R, Tom WL, et al. Prospective study of infantile haemangiomas: incidence, clinical characteristics and association with placental anomalies. Br J Dermatol. 2014;170(04):907–13.

North PE, Waner M, Mizeracki A, et al. GLUT1: a newly discovered immunohistochemical marker for juvenile hemangiomas. Hum Pathol. 2000;31:11–22.

Shirley MD, Tang H, Gallione CJ, Baugher JD, Frelin LP, Cohen B, North PE, Marchuk DA, Comi AM, Pevsner J. Sturge-Weber syndrome and port-wine stains caused by somatic mutation in GNAQ. N Engl J Med. 2013;368(21):1971–9.

Reddish Growths on the Hard Palate: Kaposi Sarcoma

Yet Ching Goh

Contents

W. M Tilakaratne, T. G. Kallarakkal (eds.), *Clinicopathological Correlation of Oral Diseases*,
https://doi.org/10.1007/978-3-031-24408-7_13

Learning Goals

1. Devise the correct way of compiling the history with appropriate questions.
2. Develop a differential diagnosis after history taking.
3. Deduce appropriate procedures in clinical examination.
4. Formulate a differential diagnosis combining findings in the history and clinical examination.
5. Justify the relevant investigations required to arrive at the diagnosis.
6. Comprehend the importance of clinicopathological correlation in arriving at the correct diagnosis.
7. Outline the management plan.
8. Recognize the importance of a diagnostic algorithm in arriving at a diagnosis.

13.1 Main Complaint

A 34-year-old gentleman was referred to the oral and maxillofacial surgery clinic for management of erythematous growths on the hard palate.

13.2 History of Complaint

Question: How long since you have noticed the growths in the mouth?

I noticed a growth about 1 month ago. It started as a small red patch on the palate and gradually increased in size and number.

13

13.3 Additional Complaints

Question: Did you notice a blister on the palate before the red patch?

I did not notice any blister on the hard palate.

Question: Did you have similar lesions before?

I cannot remember having similar lesions in the past.

Question: Are they painful?

They are not painful.

Question: Have you noticed or felt any other changes or difficulties in the mouth?

I felt roughness on the palatal region and bleeding during brushing teeth. I was not able to eat hard food as it would cause discomfort to my palate.

Question: Do you have any lesions elsewhere on the body?

I noticed a violaceous papule on the left chest about 2 weeks ago. There was no associated discomfort or itchiness.

Question: Are you suffering from other medical problems like heart disease, high blood pressure, diabetes, bleeding disorder, or respiratory diseases? If yes, what kind of medications, have you been taking until now?

Review of the medical history revealed that he is a medically compromised patient. He was HIV positive since 2010 and had pulmonary tuberculosis in 2011. Apart from carrying thalassemia trait, the patient was also diagnosed with oropharyngeal candidosis (Fig. 13.1) and latent syphilis. He was seen in psychiatric clinic as he was feeling stressed and hopeless. He was started with highly active antiretroviral therapy (HAART) 7 years ago but discontinued due to financial issues. He had completed tuberculosis treatment and was undergoing treatment for syphilis and oropharyngeal candidosis. Blood investigation showed CD4+ T lymphocyte count of 35 cells/mm^3 (3%).

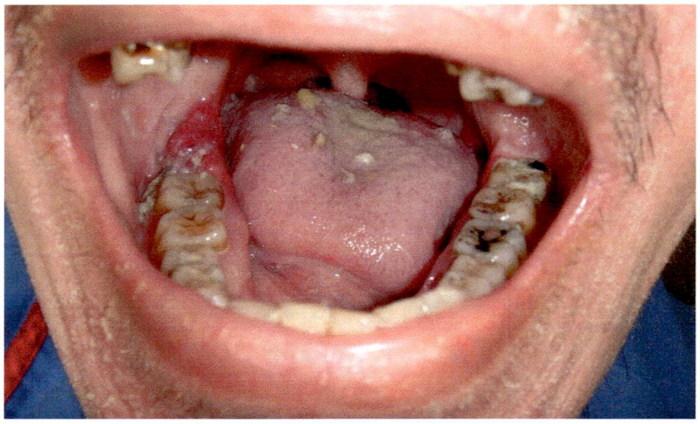

Fig. 13.1 Whitish papules suggestive of candidosis was evident on the dorsal surface of the tongue. Also present was an erythematous lesion on lower right retromolar region. (Courtesy of Dr. Tan Chuey Chuan)

Question: Do you have any idea as to how you acquired HIV infection?

I was a homosexual and had sexual relationships with multiple partners. I was a drug abuser and was on crystal methamphetamine (ice). I stopped the habit 6 months ago.

Question: Are you a smoker?

I don't practice any smoking habits.

Question: Do you take alcohol?

I am not an alcohol user.

13.4 With the Findings of the History, What Is Your Differential Diagnosis?

1. Kaposi sarcoma
2. Haematological malignancies including leukaemia and lymphoma
3. Erythematous candidosis

13.5 How Would You Justify Your Differential Diagnosis After History Taking?

1. He had noticed a violaceous papule on the left chest. Multiple erythematous papules or nodules on skin or oral mucosa are typical manifestations of Kaposi Sarcoma. A positive history of retroviral disease is a contributory finding as Kaposi sarcoma is highly associated with HIV infection. It can manifest intraorally involving the hard palate, gingiva and tongue.
2. The preponderance of HIV-infected patients to develop haematological disorders, particularly non-Hodgkin lymphoma is significantly higher.
3. Oral candidosis is the most common intraoral manifestation of HIV infection. Erythematous candidosis is associated with broad spectrum antibiotic therapy and immunosuppression. He is a medically compromised patient and was diagnosed with oropharyngeal candidosis at the same time. Early lesions of Kaposi sarcoma before developing into tumour stage can present as red areas mimicking erythematous candidosis.

13.6 Findings of Clinical Examination

The general oral hygiene is poor with a lot of plaque accumulation. Whitish papules are observed on the posterior third of tongue. There is an erythematous lesion on the right lower retromolar region (Fig. 13.1). An erythematous to violaceous plaque-like lesion with ill-defined margins measuring 1 cm × 1 cm is seen on the left palate (Fig. 13.2). The lesion is soft in consistency and not tender. Multiple erythematous macules are also observed (Fig. 13.2). A similar red to the violaceous lesion with a slightly raised surface is observed on the left chest (Fig. 13.3).

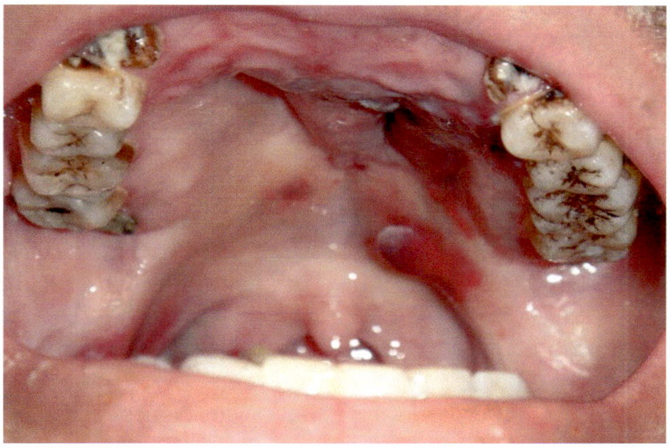

Fig. 13.2 Several erythematous to purplish poorly demarcated lesions on the left hard palate. (Courtesy of Dr. Tan Chuey Chuan)

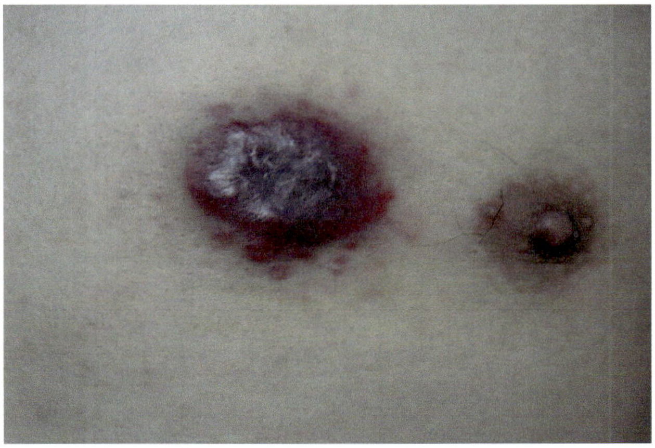

Fig. 13.3 Red and irregular lesion on the patient's left chest has increased in size and thickness recently. (Courtesy of Dr. Tan Chuey Chuan)

13.7 What Other Relevant Features Would You Look for with the Findings You Have So Far?

The neck nodes are not palpable. There is no petechiae noticed elsewhere. The oral cavity is moist and no extreme dryness is seen.

13.8 What Is Your Clinical Diagnosis?

Kaposi sarcoma.

13.9 How Would You Exclude Other Conditions and Justify Your Clinical Diagnosis?

1. Erythematous candidosis
   Erythematous candidosis is frequently seen in patients with immunological defects. The clinical presentation is often of irregular erythematous macules or patches distributed on the tongue, hard palate or buccal mucosa. The lesions seen in this patient are multiple and violaceous, a few of them being nodular and do not match the glossitis or "thumbprint lesions" described for erythematous candidosis.
2. Haematological malignancies (lymphoma/leukaemia)
   Although lymphoma is not an uncommon association of HIV positive patients, the presentation in this patient is not characteristic of a lymphoma. Lymphoma is usually a single lesion in the oral cavity and cervical lymph nodes may also be involved usually. The presence of multiple reddish growths and skin involvement is unusual for lymphoma. Hence, the diagnosis of a lymphoma is unlikely. Leukaemia usually presents in the oral cavity as reddish and fleshy gingival growths. In addition, leukaemia is associated with other systemic manifestations such as fever, hepatosplenomegaly and general weakness. The diagnosis of leukaemia is unlikely as this patient did not have these features.

13.10 What Is the Most Likely Diagnosis?

Kaposi sarcoma.

13.11 How Would You Investigate This Patient?

1. Swab from palatal lesion to exclude candidal infection
2. Incisional biopsy for the confirmation of diagnosis.

13.12 How Would You Do an Incisional Biopsy for This Patient? What Are the Important Considerations?

The lesion is highly vascular and carries a risk of bleeding. Special precautions should be observed in order to achieve proper haemostasis. A biopsy from a representative area is crucial for a definitive diagnosis. Operative procedure in HIV/AIDS patients pose risk of HIV transmission to health care workers. Bodily fluid-contaminated substances should be regarded as hazardous.

13.13 Biopsy Report Confirms the Previous Clinical Diagnosis of Kaposi Sarcoma. What Are the Histopathological Features That Would Help in the Diagnosis?

Histopathological examination shows proliferation of spindle-shaped cells arranged in long and short interlacing fascicles exhibiting mild cytological atypia (Fig. 13.4a). A moderate vascularity is observed with numerous endothelium-lined vascular channels (Fig. 13.4b). Occasional capillaries demonstrating staghorn pattern are observed. In areas, slit-like spaces containing erythrocytes are noted between proliferating spindle cells. Extravasated red blood cells and hyaline globules are present (Fig. 13.4c). Immunohistochemical staining reveals CD34 positivity (Fig. 13.4d).

One week after the biopsy, the patient presents with enlarged palatal lesion and several lobulated purplish swellings on upper and lower gingival region (Fig. 13.5). The lesion on the patient's left chest has also increased in size and thickness.

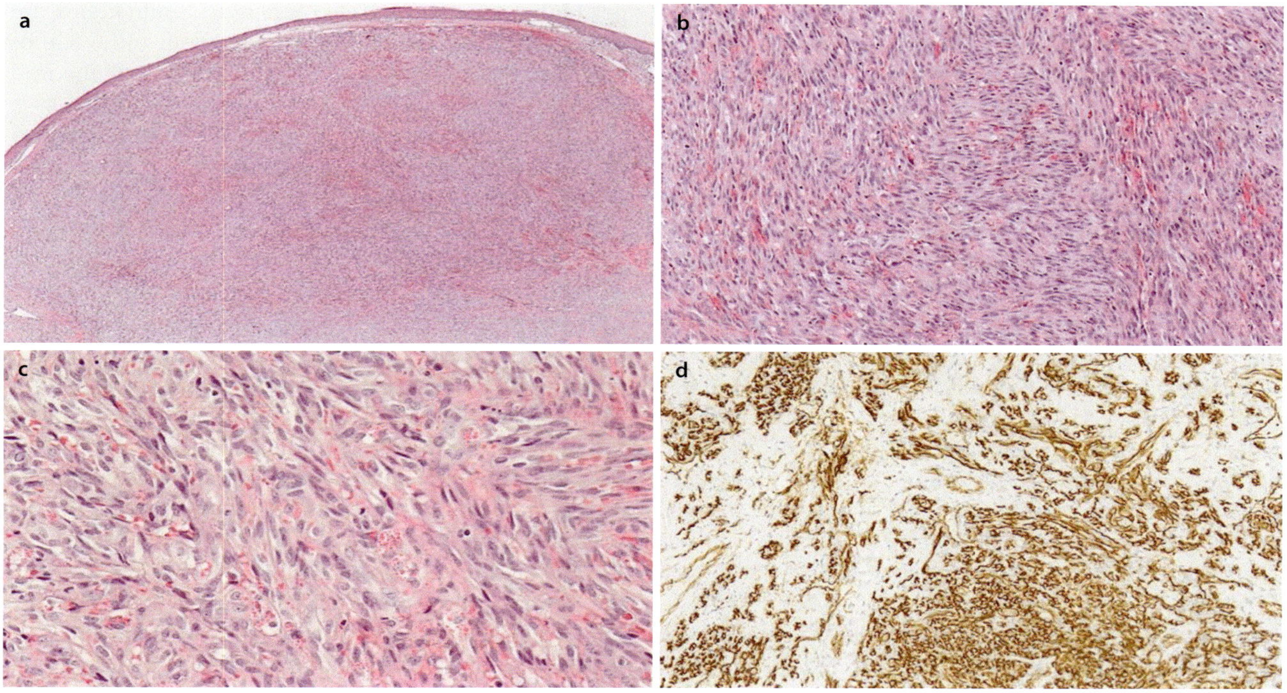

Fig. 13.4 Proliferation of spindle-shaped cells beneath the surface covering of parakeratinised stratified squamous epithelium (**a**). Moderate vascularity with numerous endothelium-lined vascular channels (**b**). Extravasated erythrocytes and hyaline globules (**c**). Immunohistochemical staining with CD34 yields intense positivity (**d**)

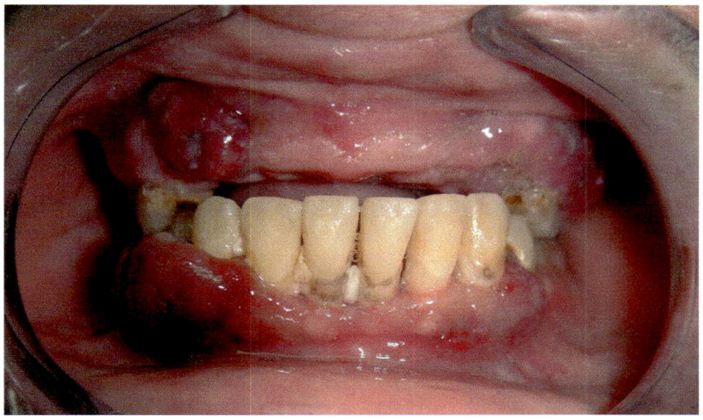

Fig. 13.5 Several lobulated purplish nodular swellings on upper and lower gingival region. (Courtesy of Dr. Tan Chuey Chuan)

13.14 How Would You Manage This Patient?

Patient was referred to medical department for further management. He was started on HAART therapy and prescribed tenofovir (nucleoside/-tide reverse transcriptase inhibitor, NRTI), emtricitabine (NRTI), lopinavir (protease inhibitor) and ritonavir (protease inhibitor) for 24 months. He was also referred to the oncology department for the management of oral and skin lesions of Kaposi sarcoma. Ten cycles of radiotherapy 20 Gy were administered and the patient was coping well with the radiotherapy. Subsequent follow-up revealed complete resolution of palatal, gingival and left chest lesions.

13.15 Kaposi Sarcoma

According to the World Health Organization (WHO) Classification of Head and Neck Tumours, Kaposi sarcoma, also known as Kaposi disease, is defined as a locally aggressive vascular neoplasm of intermediate grade, frequently associated with HHV-8 infection. Kaposi sarcoma (Classic type) was first described by a Hungarian dermatologist, Moritz Kaposi in the nineteenth century as a vascular tumour affecting the lower extremities of elderly men from the Mediterranean region.

Four distinct epidemiological categories have been described, namely classic type, endemic (African) type, iatrogenic/transplant-associated type and AIDS-related type. Another form of Kaposi sarcoma in HIV-negative men having sex with men (MSM) has been described recently. Classic Kaposi sarcoma occurs predominantly in elderly men. The lesions are usually cutaneous and restricted to lower extremities. The lesions primarily present as multiple purplish-red pigmented plaques on the skin of arms, legs and trunk and tend to progressively enlarge spreading to the more proximal sites. Classic Kaposi sarcoma carries a benign indolent course and often spares viscera.

Endemic (African) Kaposi sarcoma is a variant of the disease affecting human immunodeficiency virus-seronegative children and middle-aged men. The clinical course of endemic Kaposi sarcoma is variable and includes indolent skin disease (cutaneous plaques and nodules), locally infiltrative lesions of extremities (deep lesion with dense fibrosis), and aggressive visceral involvement with potentially fatal sequelae. Oral mucosa is infrequently affected in endemic Kaposi sarcoma. This type of Kaposi sarcoma carries a poor prognosis. Iatrogenic Kaposi sarcoma is associated with the use of steroids, immunosuppressive agents and drugs with anti-tumour necrosis factor (TNF) activity in patients with autoimmune disorders, inflammatory conditions, or solid tissue transplantation. Iatrogenic Kaposi sarcoma predominates in males and may involve mucocutaneous tissues, lymph nodes or viscera. It is reportedly more common in liver transplant patients than recipients of kidney or heart allografts. This form of Kaposi sarcoma may present as solitary or multifocal cutaneous lesions with or without visceral involvement.

Epidemic or acquired immunodeficiency syndrome (AIDS)-related Kaposi sarcoma is the most common variant and carries a more aggressive clinical course. The incidence of epidemic Kaposi sarcoma is reportedly in correlation with the mode of HIV acquisition in which HIV-seropositive male homosexuals are five to ten times at risk for Kaposi sarcoma compared to other groups with high-risk behaviours. Although epidemic Kaposi sarcoma may develop throughout the entire spectrum of HIV disease, it is more likely to occur in the context of immunosuppression and could represent the first manifestation of HIV infection in some patients. Lesions of epidemic Kaposi sarcoma tend to enlarge, multiply in number, become more nodular and coalesce in association with immune deterioration and drop in CD4 cell count.

In the oral cavity, hard palate and gingiva are the most characteristic sites for the presentation of Kaposi sarcoma. Presence of Kaposi sarcoma in the oral cavity is of great prognostic importance as it can be the initial manifestation of generalized Kaposi sarcoma and the first indication of HIV infection. It is reported that the presence of oral Kaposi sarcoma in AIDS patients signifies higher mortality rates compared to individuals presenting with cutaneous Kaposi sarcoma only. Kaposi sarcoma can serve as a prognostic marker for the individual's response to HAART treatment.

Kaposi sarcoma is proposed to be of lymphatic origin with the spindle tumour cells shown to belong to the lymphatic endothelial cell lineage. Presence of inflammatory cells and vascular spaces can also be seen histologically. The interaction of these histological components is hypothesized as the key factor in initiation and progression of Kaposi sarcoma. Kaposi sarcoma's progression requires activation of various pathogenic mechanisms. The primary role of this process is played by human herpes virus-8 (HHV-8). HHV-8 is believed to be the infectious agent necessary for development of all clinical subtypes of Kaposi sarcoma irrespective of the differences in presentation, clinical history, or prognosis. It has also been suggested that HHV-8 is an opportunistic pathogen that benefits from the severe immunosuppression during HIV infection and promotes the invasiveness and aggressiveness of Kaposi sarcoma. It has also been postulated that HIV-mediated immune suppression promotes the synthesis of T-helper type-1 cytokines, such as TNF-alpha, interleukin-1β (IL-1β) and IL-6 which in turn promote the invasiveness and aggressiveness of Kaposi sarcoma. HIV-infected cells produce HIV-Tat protein that further contributes to release of pro-inflammatory cytokines, vascular endothelial growth factors (VEGFs), and matrix metalloproteinases (MMPs), facilitating the proliferation of endothelial cells and development of Kaposi sarcoma.

Microscopic features of Kaposi sarcoma are diagnostic and shared by all variants of the disease. The features include abundance of proliferating mononuclear inflammatory and spindle cells, ill-defined vascular channels, haemorrhage and oedema. Kaposi sarcoma histopathologically closely mirrors the clinical evolution of the lesions. Histologically, the features of Kaposi sarcoma become more prominent with clinical progression from early patch to plaque and more advanced nodular form of the disease. As the lesions increase in size, an increase in vascularity and cellularity is noted. The proliferation of new blood vessels lacking pericytes accounts for the extravasational haemorrhage. The haemorrhage is usually seen accompanying deposition of haemosiderin and scattered amorphous hyaline globules within and between lesional cells. The microscopic diversity of oral Kaposi sarcoma and the high prevalence of coexistent pathology pose diagnostic challenges often perpetuated by inadequate clinical details. The diagnosis of oral Kaposi sarcoma should be diligently followed by serologic investigations when a patient's retroviral status is unknown.

Selection of treatment interventions for Kaposi sarcoma depends on the location and variant of Kaposi sarcoma, the rate of progression and distribution of the lesions, presence of symptoms, efficacy and potential side effects of therapy, presence of HIV infection and comorbidities, and degree of host immune competence. Therapy for Kaposi sarcoma aims to palliate symptoms, reduce tumour-associated oedema, and improve aesthetics and functions. Therapeutic approaches for Kaposi sarcoma include no treatment to surgical excision, local interventions and radiotherapy. It has been reported that epidemic Kaposi sarcoma often regresses with HAART and potent antiretroviral medications have led to reduced incidence of Kaposi sarcoma among patients infected with HIV. Radiotherapy has been documented as a highly effective modality for local Kaposi sarcoma causing pain, bleeding, or oedema and the remission rate is in excess of more than 90% for AIDS-associated Kaposi sarcoma.

Salient Features of Kaposi Sarcoma	
Clinical	• Typically manifests as multiple lesions on skin or oral mucosa. • Intraorally, hard palate, gingiva and tongue are frequently affected sites. • It usually begins as macular lesions that do not blanch with pressure. • As the lesions progress, the lesions appear raised and may present as solid lesions.
Histopathology	• Three stages: Patch, plaque and nodular • Proliferation of vascular channels in a background of spindle cells. • Numerous extravasated erythrocytes are present.
Treatment	• HAART therapy • Intralesional injection of chemotherapeutic agent/sclerosing agent • Laser ablation or electrosurgery • Radiotherapy

Oral lesions clinically suggestive of Kaposi sarcoma should be biopsied and patients with biopsy-proven Kaposi sarcoma should be tested for HIV infection

Diagnostic Algorithm for Kaposi Sarcoma

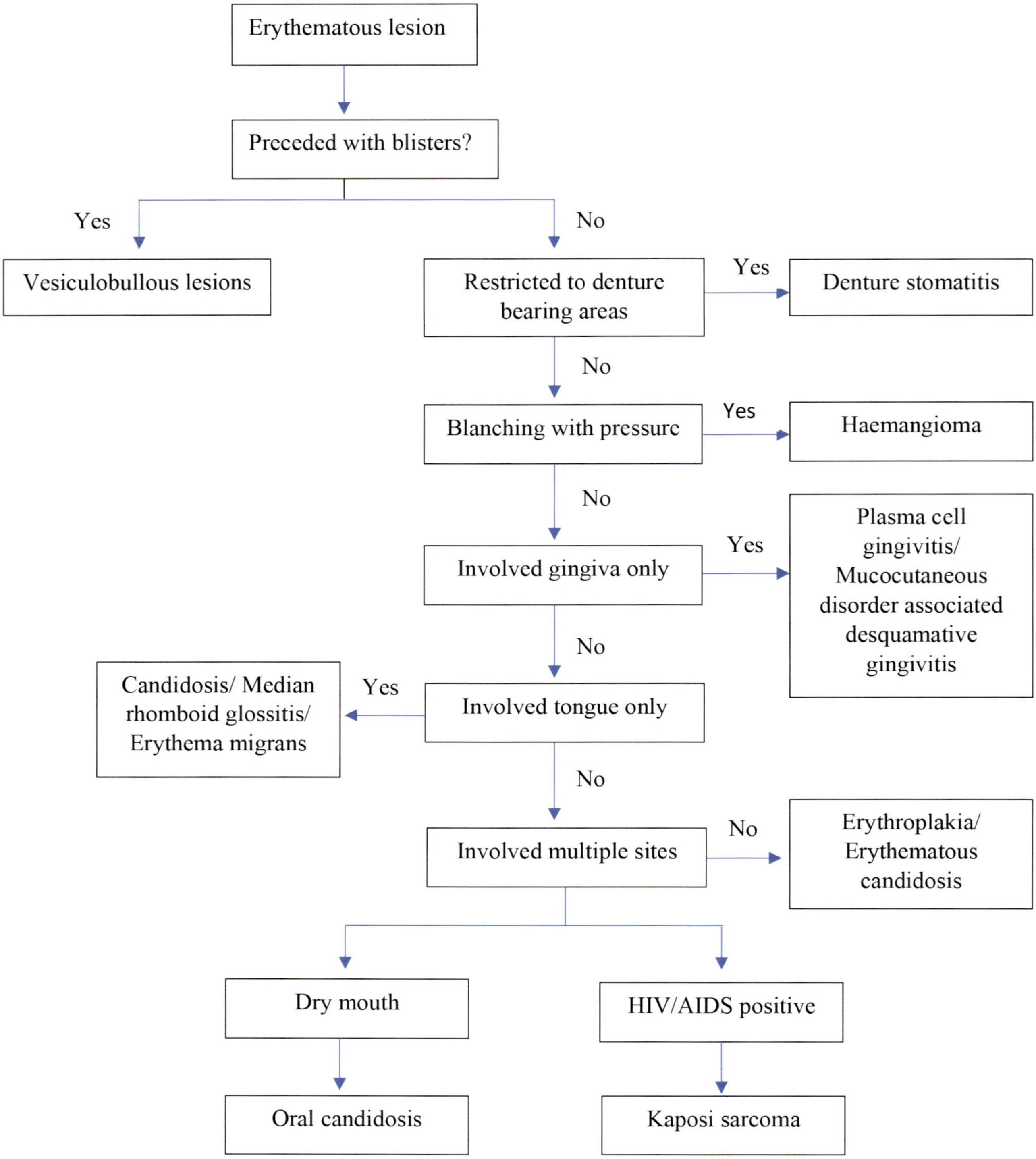

13

Self-Assessment Questions

1. List the pathognomonic clinical features of Kaposi Sarcoma.
2. State the important conditions that need to be included in the differential diagnosis.
3. State the histopathological features of Kaposi sarcoma.
4. List the aetiologic factor of Kaposi sarcoma.
5. Explain the principles of management of Kaposi sarcoma.

Summary

Kaposi sarcoma is a locally aggressive vascular neoplasm of intermediate grade associated with HHV-8 infection. Presence of Kaposi sarcoma in the oral cavity is of great prognostic importance as it can be the initial manifestation of generalized Kaposi sarcoma and the first indication of HIV infection. The treatment interventions for Kaposi sarcoma depend on the location and variant of Kaposi sarcoma, the rate of progression and distribution of the lesions, presence of symptoms, efficacy and potential side effects of therapy, presence of HIV infection and comorbidities, and degree of host immune competence.

Further Reading

Bunn BK, Carvalho MDV, Louw M, Vargas PA, Van Heerden WF. Microscopic diversity in oral Kaposi sarcoma. Oral Surg Oral Med Oral Pathol Oral Radiol. 2013;115(2):241–8.

Fatahzadeh M. Kaposi sarcoma: Review and medical management update. Oral Surg Oral Med Oral Pathol Oral Radiol. 2012;113(1):2–16.

Lager I, Altini M, Coleman H, Ali H. Oral Kaposi's sarcoma: A clinicopathologic study from South Africa. Oral Surg Oral Med Oral Pathol Oral Radiol Endod. 2003;96(6):701–10.

Ramírez-Amador V, Anaya-Saavedra G, Martínez-Mata G. Kaposi's sarcoma of the head and neck: A review. Oral Oncol. 2010;46(3):135–45.

Scully C. Human immunodeficiency virus infection. In: Oral & maxillofacial medicine: the basis of diagnosis and treatment. 3rd ed. Elsevier Churchill Livingstone; 2013. p. 346–256.

Shetty K. Management of oral Kaposi's sarcoma lesions on HIV-positive patient using highly active antiretroviral therapy: case report and a review of the literature. Oral Oncol Extra. 2005;41(9):226–9.

Shetty K. Disseminated oral Kaposi sarcoma lesion with extensive visceral involvement. Oral Oncol Extra. 2006;42(1):18–21.

Simon V, Ho D, Karim Q. HIV/AIDS epidemiology, pathogenesis, prevention and treatment. Lancet. 2010;368(9534):489–504.

Thompson LDR, Ro JY, Wenig BM. Soft tissue and neural tumours. In: El-Naggar AK, Chan JKC, Grandis JR, Takata T, Slootweg PJ, editors. WHO classification of head and neck tumours. 4th ed. Lyon: IARC Press; 2017. p. 124–5.

Fibro-Cemento Osseous Lesions

Contents

Slow Growing Hard Lump over the Cheek: Fibrous Dysplasia

Thomas George Kallarakkal and Wei Cheong Ngeow

Contents

W. M Tilakaratne, T. G. Kallarakkal (eds.), *Clinicopathological Correlation of Oral Diseases*,
https://doi.org/10.1007/978-3-031-24408-7_14

Learning Goals

1. Devise the correct way of compiling the history with appropriate questions.
2. Develop a differential diagnosis after history taking.
3. Deduce appropriate procedures in clinical examination.
4. Formulate a differential diagnosis combining findings in the history and clinical examination.
5. Justify the relevant investigations required to arrive at the diagnosis.
6. Comprehend the importance of clinicopathological correlation in arriving at the correct diagnosis.
7. Outline the management plan.
8. Recognize the importance of a diagnostic algorithm in arriving at a diagnosis.

14.1 Main Complaint

A 22-year-old female patient presented to the clinic complaining of a slow-growing swelling over the right side of her face.

14.2 History of Complaint

Question: How long have you been having this swelling?

The swelling was first noticed by my mother when I was 17 years old. The swelling has been gradually increasing in size since then. I have been finding it difficult to wear my spectacles for the last 2 months.

Question: Did you have any treatment for the problem?

I never sought any medical treatment for my complaint until now.

14.3 Additional Complaints

Question: Have you noticed or felt any other changes or difficulties in the mouth?

My upper and lower teeth seem to have changed their position. I feel that my teeth do not meet in the same position as previously.

Question: Do you experience any pain in your jaws or teeth when eating?

I do not have any pain in the mouth during eating.

Question: Do you have any swellings elsewhere in the body?

I have been noticing a slight swelling over the left side of my face since 3 months. Apart from that I do not have any swellings elsewhere in my body.

Question: Do you have any brown discolourations on your skin?

I do not have any brownish discolourations on my skin.

Question: When did you start wearing spectacles?

I have difficulty in seeing objects clearly that are far away. I was diagnosed with myopia when I was 16 years old and have been wearing spectacles since then.

Question: Have you noticed any other disturbances in your vision recently?

I have not noticed any changes in my vision recently.

Question: Do you have any difficulty in hearing?

I do not have any hearing problems.

Question: Do you have nasal congestion or any other symptoms of sinusitis such as headache, nasal discharge or pain in your upper teeth?

I do not have any symptoms of sinusitis.

Question: Have you been experiencing any symptoms such as weight loss, irregular heartbeats, increased sweating, increased bowel movements, fatigue, anxiety or tremor?

I do not have any such symptoms.

Question: Are your menstrual periods normal?

I do not have any menstrual problems.

Question: Do you have any other medical problems like heart disease, high blood pressure, diabetes, bleeding disorders or respiratory diseases?

I do not have any other medical problems.

Question: Do you have any history of trauma to your face?

I have not suffered from any trauma involving my face or jaws.

Question: Have you undergone any surgery?

I have not undergone any surgery in the past.

Question: Have you undergone any dental treatment?

I have had multiple restorations. I also had three of my lower teeth extracted due to caries.

Question: Does anybody in your family have a similar problem?

All my immediate family members are fit and healthy.

Question: Do you have any risk habits such as smoking or drinking alcohol?

I do not have any risk habits.

Question: Are you employed?

I am a final year graduate student.

14.4 With the Findings from the History, What Is Your Differential Diagnosis?

1. Craniofacial fibrous dysplasia (CFFD)
2. Florid cemento-osseous dysplasia (FCOD)
3. Multiple central giant cell granulomas (CGCGs)
4. Familial gigantiformcemetoma (FGC)
5. Multiple cemento-ossifying fibromas
6. Multiple odontogenic cysts or tumours
7. Cherubism

14.5 How Do You Justify Your Differential Diagnosis After History Taking?

She has a slow-growing painless swelling over the right side of her face that has been present for almost 5 years. Besides she also complains of a similar slow-growing swelling over the left side of her face since 3 months. She has difficulty in getting her teeth to meet properly that is suggestive of a malocclusion due to alveolar bone involvement. Involvement of multiple craniofacial bones characterized by facial asymmetry is highly suggestive of congenital benign fibro-osseous lesions such as craniofacial fibrous dysplasia (CFFD), florid cemento-osseous dysplasia (FCOD) and cherubism.

1. The symptoms of CFFD may manifest only during childhood or adolescence as seen in this patient. Moreover, the absence of symptoms such as endocrinopathy and skin pigmentation ruled out the possibility of McCune Albright syndrome.
2. FCOD is a benign fibro-osseous lesion that shows a marked tendency for bilateral and symmetrical swelling of all four quadrants of the jaw bones.
3. Central giant cell granulomas (CGCGs) are benign tumours that tend to involve the jaw bones, the mandible is more commonly involved than the maxilla. They are usually asymptomatic and tend to occur more commonly in females. Similar lesions occur in patients with hyperparathyroidism.
4. Familial gigantiform cementoma (FGC), typically presents as slow-growing, multifocal expansile lesions involving both jaws. In advanced cases, the lesions can cause remarkable painless swelling and facial deformity.
5. Cemento-ossifying fibroma commonly occurs in females between the second and fourth decades of life. It usually presents as a progressive, painless, slow-growing swelling of the tooth-bearing area of the posterior jaws. Multifocal involvement may occur in hyperparathyroidism-jaw tumour syndrome and gnathodiaphyseal dysplasia. Hyperparathyroidism-jaw tumour syndrome is a rare hereditary disorder inherited as an autosomal dominant trait characterized by parathyroid adenoma or carcinoma and bilateral kidney cysts, hamartomas, or Wilms tumours while gnathodiaphyseal dysplasia is an orthopaedic condition in which sclerosis, bowing of tubular bones, and overall bone fragility occurs.

6. Odontogenic cysts and tumours usually occur as solitary lesions. However bilateral and multiple odontogenic cysts and tumours such as dentigerous cysts, odontogenic keratocysts (OKCs) and adenomatoid odontogenic tumours (AOTs) have been reported in both syndromic and non-syndromic patients. Multiple OKCs and AOTs occur in Gorlin-Goltz syndrome and Schimmelpenning syndrome (SS) respectively.
7. She complains of a bilateral painless swelling of the face with malocclusion. Bilateral facial swelling limited to the lower two-thirds of the face is characteristic of cherubism, a benign fibro-osseous lesion with a typical age of onset of 2–10 years. Therefore this is not a very likely differential diagnosis.

14.6 Findings of Clinical Examination

She has a diffuse, bilateral, non-tender maxillary swelling and a right mandibular swelling which is bony hard in consistency. The maxillary swelling is more pronounced on the right side of the face (■ Fig. 14.1). The margins of the swellings are not well-defined. The overlying skin is normal. There is no limitation in mouth opening. Intra-orally there is bilateral buccolingual expansion of the body of the mandible and buccal and palatal expansion of the maxilla. There is generalized displacement of the teeth with anterior open bite. There are no abnormalities involving the rest of the skeleton.

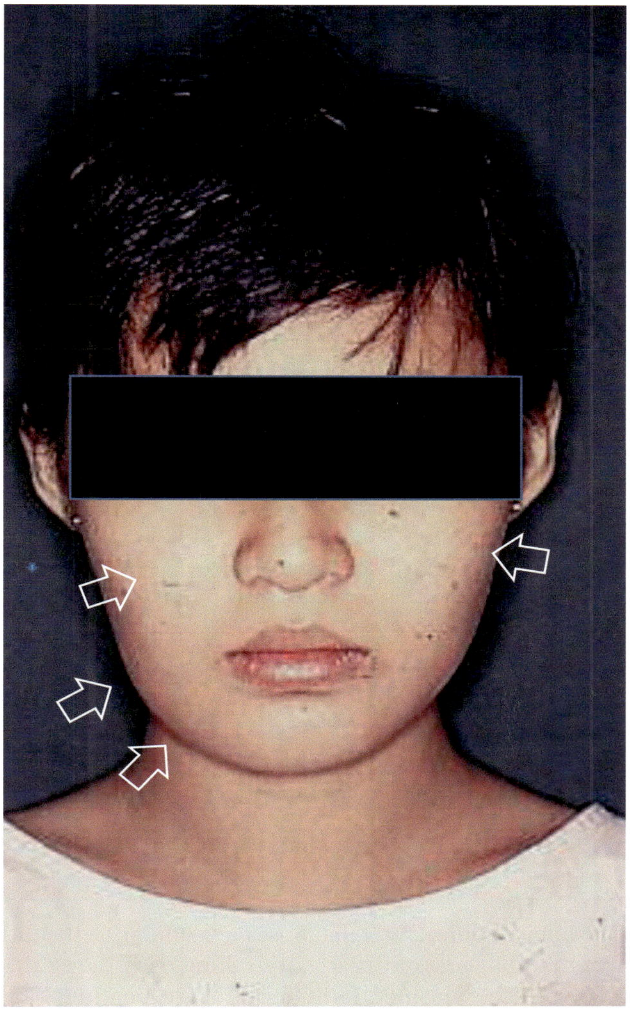

■ **Fig. 14.1** Diffuse bilateral maxillary swelling which is more pronounced on the right side and right mandibular swelling

14.7 What Other Relevant Features Would You Look for with the Findings You Have so Far?

She does not have any numbness or paresthesia over the face. There are no significantly enlarged lymph nodes in the neck. She does not have multiple nevi or pigmentations on the skin.

14.8 What Is Your Clinical Differential Diagnosis?

1. Craniofacial fibrous dysplasia (CFFD)
2. Multiple central giant cell granulomas (CGCGs)
3. Florid cemento-osseous dysplasia (FCOD)
4. Familial gigantiform cementoma (FGC)
5. Multiple cemento-ossifying fibromas
6. Multiple odontogenic cysts or tumours

14.9 How Would You Exclude Other Conditions and Justify the Inclusion of the Diseases That You Have Mentioned in the Differential Diagnosis to Arrive at a Working Diagnosis?

The clinical differential diagnoses are similar to the differential diagnoses after history taking with the exception of cherubism. Radiological investigations are necessary to exclude other differential diagnoses due to their overlapping clinical features.

14.10 What Radiologic Investigations Would You Need to Exclude Other Conditions and Justify the Inclusion of the Diseases That You Have Mentioned in the Differential Diagnosis to Arrive at a Working Diagnosis?

Posteroanterior (PA) view (Skull).

Dental panoramic tomography (DPT).

A skull PA view and a DPT are mandatory basic imaging investigations for this patient to arrive at a working diagnosis. The PA view provides an overview of the entire skull without highlighting any specific region while a DPT is valuable for a general full mouth survey including review of the antra and the temporomandibular joint.

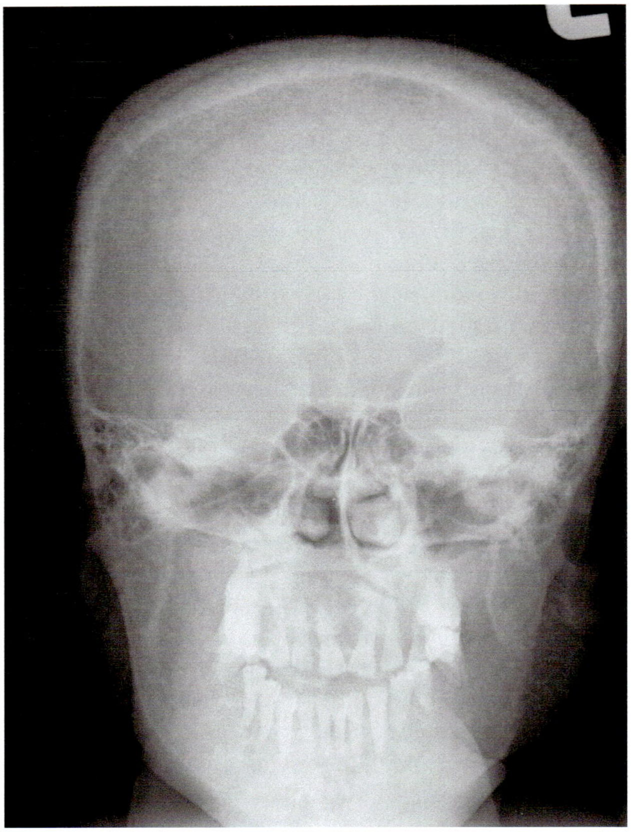

Fig. 14.2 PA view of the skull shows a diffuse radiopacity with ill-defined margins involving the craniofacial skeleton

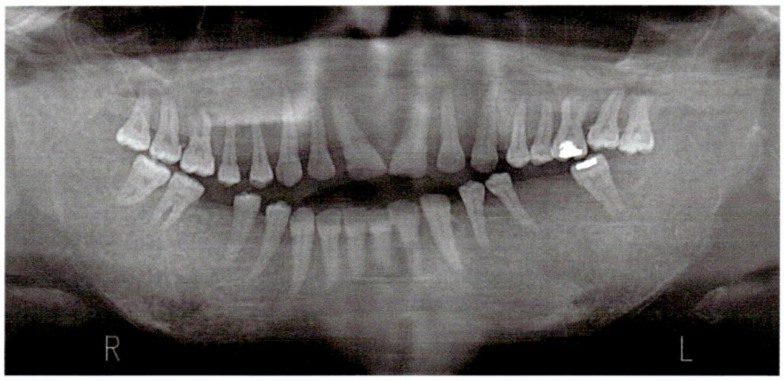

Fig. 14.3 The DPT shows a diffuse "ground glass" and "peau-de-orange appearance with generalized loss of lamina dura and periodontal ligament space around the teeth

The PA view (Fig. 14.2) of the patient's skull shows a diffuse radiopacity of the skull bones. The DPT (Fig. 14.3) displays a diffuse "ground glass" and "peau-de-orange" appearance with ill-defined margins that merge imperceptibly with the surrounding normal bone. There is a generalized absence of the periodontal ligament space around the teeth and loss of lamina dura with an alteration of the normal bone pattern (Fig. 14.3).

CFFD presents as a gradual, painless enlargement of the craniofacial region, leading to facial asymmetry. Lesions involving the craniofacial bones are not sharply demarcated and very commonly affect the zygomatico-maxillary complex and sphenoid bones. The form of fibrous dysplasia affecting the craniofacial region is not restricted to a single bone but is in fact confined to a single anatomical site. The observed radiological findings are consistent with the clinical diagnosis of CFFD.

Cherubism usually manifests as a bilateral painless swelling of the lower two-thirds of the face resulting in full round cheeks, with the upward cast of the eyes, giving the patients a cherubic appearance. The affected patients may demonstrate various dental abnormalities such as tooth agenesis, tooth displacement, and failure of tooth eruption often leading to malocclusion. The condition generally regresses around the time of pubescence resulting in a decrease in facial deformity. The present case did not have a cherubic appearance and dental abnormalities characteristic of cherubism. Moreover, the symptoms in this patient manifested only after pubescence which is unlike in cherubism where the symptoms usually regress after puberty. Radiologically the characteristic features include jaw lesions that are usually radiolucent, multilocular, with well-defined margins and usually associated with tooth displacement, root resorption, or agenesis. These features were not evident in the present case.

CGCG of the jaws is usually a non-neoplastic bone lesion accounting for fewer than 7% of all jaw lesions affecting mainly children or young adults. It is generally confined to the tooth-bearing areas of the jaws. The radiologic features of the CGCG comprise a unilocular or a multilocular radiolucency and varying degrees of expansion of the cortical plates. Multiple CGCGs of the jaws are rare and have been reported to occur in association with syndromes such as Noonan syndrome, Neurofibromatosis type 1 and the LEOPARD syndrome or with cherubism. Brown tumours of the jaw bones are focal bony lesions that arise as a result of primary or secondary hyperparathyroidism and are more common in women aged 50 years and above. The mandible is affected more commonly than the maxilla. They have a similar clinical and histological picture as CGCG. The biologic behaviour of CGCG ranges from a slowly growing asymptomatic swelling to an aggressive process associated with pain, cortical bone destruction, root resorption and displacement of teeth. CGCG is an unlikely differential diagnosis based on the clinical and radiological findings seen in this case.

Cemento-osseous dysplasia (COD) represents a group of benign fibro-osseous lesions characterized by the replacement of normal bone by fibrous connective tissue. They are subdivided into three variants; periapical, focal, and florid COD affecting mainly the jaws in the tooth-bearing or edentulous alveolar ridges. Periapical COD occurs in the anterior mandible, focal COD in isolated areas within the jaws except in the anterior mandible, and florid COD (FCOD) occurs multifocally, often in both the mandible and the maxilla. CODs including FCOD produce minimal clinical or radiographic evidence of bone expansion. Radiographically, FCOD shows multifocal confluent radiolucencies and mixed or radiopaque images surrounding the teeth root apices. The lesions are well-defined and have a radiolucent rim. They have a tendency to increase in size and to become predominantly radiopaque. In the early stage, the radiographic appearance can mimic an inflammatory periapical lesion. In the present case, the patient had a bilateral maxillary swelling and a mandibular swelling on the right side. The radiographs displayed a diffuse "ground glass" appearance with ill-defined margins that lacked a peripheral radiolucent rim and merged imperceptibly with the surrounding normal bone. Hence FCOD can be excluded from the list of differential diagnoses.

FGC is an uncommon fibro-osseous lesion, which occurs predominantly in young patients and has the potential to cause considerable jaw expansion. All cases are not familial and sporadic cases have been reported. The early radiological features of FGC include a radiolucent and mixed radiolucent–radio-opaque appearance. During maturation, significant expansion, tooth displacement and progressive opacification occur. Mature FGCs cease to enlarge and manifest as a lobular radio-opacity with a radiolucent rim. This appearance has been likened macroscopically to the appearance of ginger roots. The radiographic findings in the present case did not show the characteristic multilobular radio-opaque appearance with a radiolucent rim. There was also no evident familial history. Hence a differential diagnosis of FGC and sporadic gigantiformcementoma may be deemed unacceptable.

Cemento-ossifying fibroma is a benign tumour that commonly occurs in females between the second and fourth decades of life. It usually presents as a progressive, painless, slow-growing swelling of the tooth-bearing area of the posterior jaws affecting the mandible more commonly than the maxilla. Expansion of the buccal and lingual cortices is usually observed. Large lesions can cause bowing of the inferior border of the mandible. Radiographically, they appear as well-defined round or oval lesions that appear radiolucent in the early stages which eventually becomes radiopaque as the lesion attains complete maturity. Displacement and resorption of teeth are a common findings. They are usually solitary lesions but bilateral as well as multiple familial cemento-ossifying fibromas occurring in the jaws have been reported. In the present case, the radiographic findings did not manifest as multiple well-demarcated radiolucent/radiopaque lesions. Hence a differential diagnosis of multiple cemento-ossifying fibromas is excluded. There were also no features to support a diagnosis of hyperparathyroidism-jaw tumour syndrome and gnathodiaphyseal dysplasia in this patient.

Odontogenic keratocyst (OKC) is a developmental cyst that occurs over a wide age range with a bimodal peak incidence in the second to third decades of life and the sixth to seventh decades of life. OKCs are most frequently found in the posterior body and ramus of the mandible. Radiology shows a well-demarcated radiolucent lesion with a corticated margin that may be unilocular or multilocular. Multiple odontogenic keratocysts may occur as part of nevoid basal cell carcinoma syndrome (Gorlin–Goltz syndrome). In addition to multiple OKCs, these patients also manifest multiple basal cell carcinomas and other developmental anomalies. Dentigerous cysts are usually solitary lesions that may manifest as a slowly enlarging expansion of the jaw associated with unerupted mandibular third molars. However multifocal presentation has been reported. Radiographs show a unilocular, well-demarcated radiolucency often with a corticated margin that surrounds the crown of an unerupted tooth. The radiological features of the patient were not consistent with the diagnosis of multiple OKCs and multiple dentigerous cysts. The patient also did not have any clinical manifestations suggestive of nevoid basal cell carcinoma syndrome.

Adenomatoid odontogenic tumours (AOTs) tend to occur twice as common in females with a strong predilection for individuals in their first three decades of life. They tend to involve the anterior maxilla more commonly. On the radiograph they are usually seen associated with an unerupted tooth in a pericoronal relationship appearing as a well-defined unilocular radiolucency having a corticated margin. Multiple AOTs are a rarity and are a manifestation of SS. SS is a congenital neurocutaneous disorder characterized by the presence of linear nevus sebaceous, ophthalmic, neurologic, skeletal, urologic, and cardiovascular alterations. Multiple AOTs are excluded from the differential diagnosis due to the lack of supporting associated radiographic findings in this case. Besides multiple OKCs, dentigerous cysts and AOTs, odontoma a benign odontogenic tumour can also rarely present as multifocal lesions manifesting as slow-growing expansion of the jaws. However, they have specific radiographic findings characterized by amorphous radiopaque or well-formed tooth-like structures surrounded by a radiolucent halo that distinguishes them from the lesion seen in the present case.

14.11 What Is the Most Likely Diagnosis?

Craniofacial fibrous dysplasia (CFFD).

14.12 How Would You Further Investigate This Patent?

1. Thorough evaluation of the extent of skeletal disease to determine if the disease is polyostotic or monostotic and the presence of extraskeletal manifestations. Monostotic fibrous dysplasia is defined as the presence of fibrous dysplasia in one skeletal site only. Polyostotic fibrous dysplasia is defined as the presence of fibrous dysplasia in more than one skeletal site without extra-skeletal manifestations. In the craniofacial skeleton the maxilla and frontal bones are most commonly involved. When the maxilla is affected, other adjacent bones separated by sutures (zygoma, sphenoid, frontal, nasal) are often also involved and hence cannot be considered as monostotic in the true sense. Similarly, when the frontal bone is affected, involvement of the adjacent sphenoid, temporal, and zygomatic bones is common.
2. Thorough evaluation to rule out McCune-Albright syndrome (MAS) is necessary. MAS is defined as the combination of fibrous dysplasia and one or more extraskeletal features, OR the presence of two or more extra skeletal features. Extra-skeletal features include;
   - Café-au-lait skin macules with characteristic features of jagged, irregular borders.
   - Gonadotropin-independent sex steroid production resulting in precocious puberty or recurrent ovarian cysts.
   - Thyroid lesions.
   - Growth hormone excess.
3. Intraoral (periapical) radiographs to assess maxillary and mandibular arches, as well as adjacent anatomic structures including maxillary sinuses, nasal cavity, mental foramina and mandibular canals.
4. CBCT to determine the proximity of the lesions to the eyes, optic nerves and other vital structures in the vicinity.
5. Incisional biopsy

   Additional investigations if indicated;
6. Evaluation of thyroid-stimulating hormone (TSH), free thyroxine (T4), and total triiodothyronine (T3) levels to determine the presence and severity of the

thyroid lesions, as well as radioactive iodine uptake and scan of the thyroid gland to determine its cause.
7. Hormone tests to assess growth hormone excess and imaging such as MRI to diagnose pituitary abnormalities.
8. Genetic testing for *GNAS* mutation in patients with an uncertain clinical diagnosis.

14.13 How Would You Perform an Incisional Biopsy for This Patient? What Are the Important Considerations?

Biopsy with histological evaluation of fibrous dysplasia is usually only necessary in unusual or questionable cases, and/or if malignancy is suspected. The risks and benefits of a biopsy should be clearly explained to patients including that a biopsy does not typically lead to the regrowth of fibrous dysplasia. An ideal biopsy should include the margins of the lesion. This will enable the pathologist in interpreting the histology with confidence as the lesional tissue blends with the adjacent cancellous bone and the overlying cortex in FD unlike other fibro-osseous lesions. The lesional tissue in the other fibro-osseous lesions tend to be separated from the normal cancellous bone and overlying cortical bone by a rim of fibrous tissue. Most of the time the pathologist is presented with curetted fragments making distinction from other fibro-osseous lesions impossible. Correlation of clinical and radiographic information with histological features lead to a final diagnosis in such instances.

14.14 Biopsy Report Confirms the Previous Clinical Diagnosis of Craniofacial Fibrous Dysplasia. What Are the Histopathological Features That Will Help in the Diagnosis?

The H & E sections show cellular fibrous tissue composed of spindled fibroblasts in a moderate.

amount of collagen. The fibrous tissue contains fine branching, curvilinear trabeculae of woven bone and mature lamellar bone with very little evidence of osteoblast rimming (◘ Fig. 14.4a). The lesional bone merges with adjacent cancellous bone and overlying cortex (◘ Fig. 14.4b).

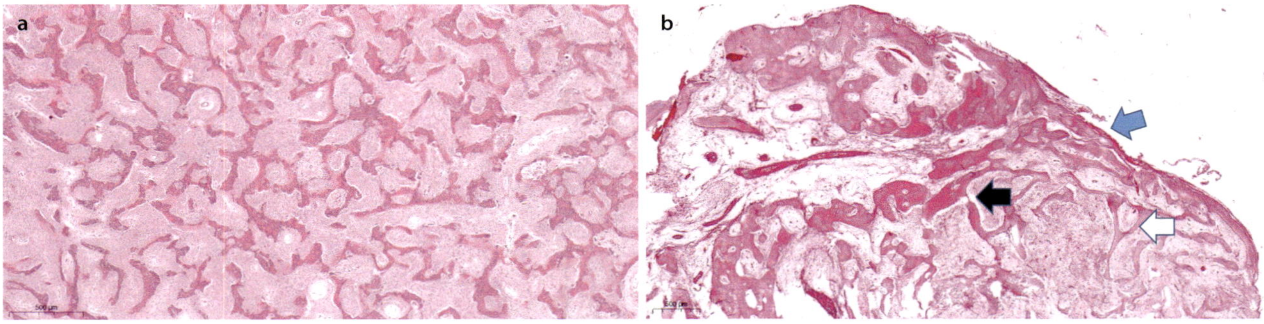

◘ **Fig. 14.4** (**a**) Curvilinear trabeculae of woven bone in a fibrous tissue stroma. (**b**) Lesional bone (white arrow) merging with normal trabecular (black arrow) and cortical bone (blue arrow)

14.15 How Would You Manage This Patent?

CFFD is a rare disease which may be associated with debilitating manifestations. There is no specific cure and approved treatment for this condition. The patient and her family should be provided with sufficient information about the disease with the aim to empower and support them. They should be informed of the non-inherited genetic nature of disease and the relatively rare risk of malignant transformation in these cases. Generally, a "wait and watch" approach is preferred as the long-term outcome is generally unpredictable. A multidisciplinary team (MDT) including surgeons and physicians should be involved in caring for patients with CFFD. Surgical treatment should be carefully coordinated with all specialists involved in the care of the patient. The primary goal of treatment of patients with CFFD should include:

(a) Prevention of functional loss—especially hearing and vision
(b) Arrest or reduction of physical disfigurement;
(c) Prevention of secondary deformity and
(d) Minimization of long-term morbidity from CFFD and its treatment.

It is recommended to avoid surgery in the absence of functional deficits or aesthetic concerns. All CFFD patients should be reviewed at least annually or more frequently depending on the extent of their disease and risk of complications. Baseline and periodic CT scans of the head should be performed based on symptoms and at least once in every 5 years in asymptomatic patients.

14.16 Fibrous Dysplasia (FD)

Fibro-osseous lesions are a group of lesions characterized by the replacement of bone with cellular fibrous tissue containing foci of mineralization that vary in amount and appearance. Fibrous dysplasia (FD) is a fibro-osseous lesion caused by sporadic mutation of the α-subunit of the Gs stimulatory protein (*GNAS*). The disease may be classified as monostotic FD when the disease process is localized to a single bone and polyostotic FD when multiple bones are involved. McCune-Albright syndrome (MAS) and Jaffe Lichtenstein syndrome refers to FD that is associated with extra-skeletal abnormalities. The presence of endocrine involvement differentiates MAS from Jaffe Lichtenstein syndrome. Mazabraud syndrome denotes FD with associated intramuscular myxomas. *GNAS mutations* lead to activation and inappropriate cyclic adenosine monophosphate (cAMP) overproduction. This results in bone marrow stromal cells with an impaired capacity to differentiate towards mature osteoblasts, adipocytes, and haematopoietic cells eventually resulting in a stroma devoid of haematopoietic marrow. The monostotic form never progresses to polyostotic FD or McCune–Albright syndrome (MAS), and spontaneous resolution of FD does not occur.

Majority of the cases of FD are diagnosed before 30 years of age. A female predilection has been reported in the polyostotic form of the disease. Craniofacial bones are very commonly involved in FD. In the gnathic bones, the maxilla is affected more commonly than the mandible. Clinically CFFD presents as a gradual, painless enlargement of the craniofacial region, leading to facial asymmetry (◘ Fig. 14.5). Lesions involving the craniofacial bones are not sharply demarcated and very commonly affect the zygomaticomaxillary complex and sphenoid bones. Hence the form of fibrous dysplasia affecting the craniofacial region is not restricted to a single bone but is in fact confined to a single anatomical site. This type of fibrous dysplasia does not meet the precise criteria for the monostotic or polyostotic forms and has been termed craniofacial fibrous dysplasia. These slowly growing mass lesions appear in childhood, cause facial deformity and distortion of adjacent structures such as the optic and vestibulocochlear nerves, eye/globe, nasal airway, middle ear ossicles and teeth.

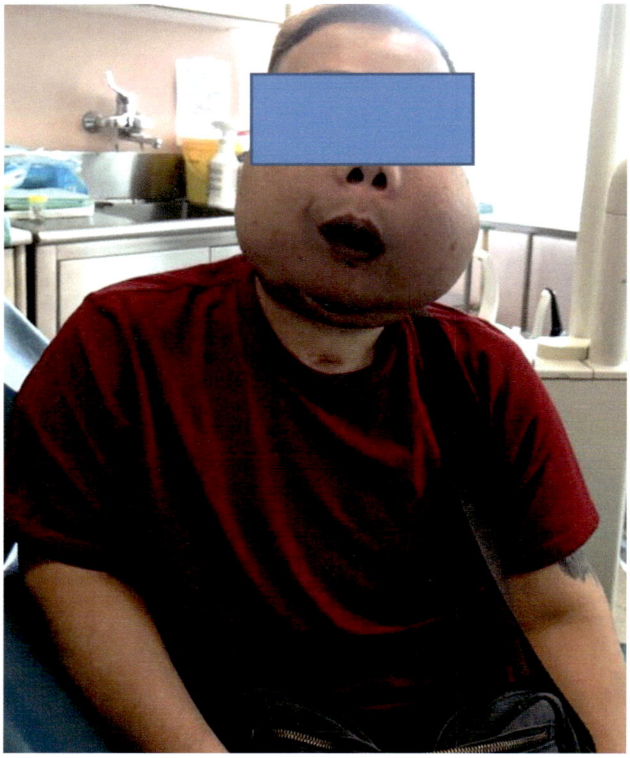

◘ **Fig. 14.5** Massive bilateral progressive painless enlargement of the face leading to facial asymmetry. (Picture courtesy: Dr. Thomas Abraham, Sentosa Specialist Hospital, Selangor, Malaysia)

However, asymptomatic lesions are often detected incidentally on dental radiographs, computed tomography (CT), or magnetic resonance imaging.

Approximately 2–3% of patients with FD have MAS. Bone changes in MAS are often more severe than in polyostotic FD without extra-skeletal manifestations. These patients regularly experience multiple fractures and require adequate surgical treatment. Patients diagnosed with MAS manifest precocious puberty usually in females along with other endocrinopathies including hyperparathyroidism, hyperthyroidism and Cushing syndrome. Cafe au lait skin pigmentation is also a common finding. These macular lesions often occur along the midline of the body commonly occurring on the chest, neck and superior portion of the intergluteal cleft. The borders of these lesions tend to be jagged, resembling the "coast of Maine" (in contrast to the smooth-bordered "coast of California" lesions seen in neurofibromatosis). The variation in the severity of the disease between FD and MAS may be explained by the fact that the mutation is postzygotic in FD and is dependent on the stage of embryogenesis. Mutations occurring in the early stage of embryogenesis results in more generalized disease as seen in MAS. In Jaffe Lichtenstein syndrome, polyostotic FD manifests with cafe au lait skin pigmentation in the absence of endocrinoathies.

Radiologically FD appears as a poorly defined radiolucency when compared to the surrounding bone. As the lesion matures, it becomes more radiopaque, the classical radiological description being an orange peel or ground glass appearance. Narrowing of the periodontal ligament space and alteration of the lamina dura to an abnormal bone pattern are characteristic features (◘ Fig. 14.6). These changes are a reflection of a programmed field effect of abnormal bone development in a congenitally predisposed bone matrix. FD occurring in other parts of the skeleton are well demarcated with a sclerotic rim while the gnathic lesions tend to be more radiopaque and poorly defined, blending into the surrounding bone. The primary reason for this can be attributed to the fact that the craniofacial bones develop as a result of intramembranous ossification.

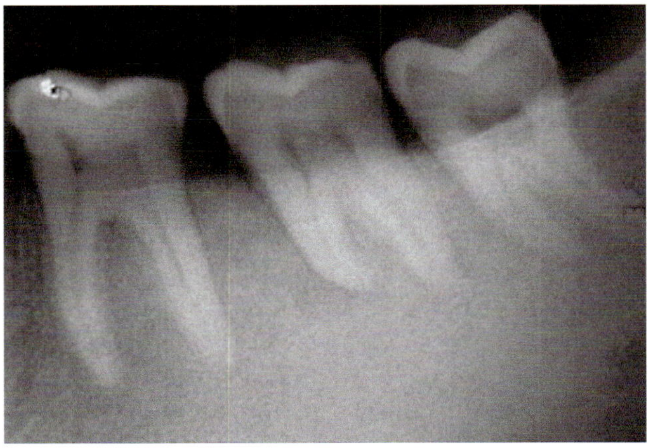

◘ **Fig. 14.6** Narrowing of the periodontal ligament space and alteration of the lamina dura. (Picture courtesy: Dr. Mahima V. Guledgud, JSS Dental College & Hospital, Mysuru, India)

Microscopically FD shows a monotonous pattern of irregularly shaped trabeculae of woven bone with little evidence of osteoblastic rimming in a cellular, loosely arranged fibrous stroma. These trabeculae are not connected to one another. Occasional tiny calcified spherules may also be seen interspersed with the bony trabeculae. In longstanding lesions involving the craniofacial skeleton, trabeculae composed of mature lamellar bone arranged in parallel arrays may be evident.

Diagnosis of FD is always based on a combination of clinical, radiographic, pathologic and molecular information. The radiographic presentation of a characteristic ground glass appearance is essentially confirmatory for the diagnosis of FD and may not necessitate a biopsy. The gold standard for diagnosis of FD is GNAS mutation testing. However, this is complicated by the level of mosaicism (some cells in the tissue may not carry the mutation) in the affected tissue that demands the use of highly sensitive techniques such as next-generation sequencing. MAS is diagnosed based on either the presence of polyostotic bone disease or the presence of two or more clinical features of the syndrome. A diagnosis of FD or MAS should be followed up by a comprehensive screening evaluation to identify any additional manifestations. This should include bone scintigraphy to identify polyostotic disease, biochemical analysis, and thyroid and gonadal ultrasonography to identify endocrine involvement.

A potential complication in long-standing fibrous dysplasia of craniofacial skeleton is sarcomatous transformation which has been reported in at least 4% of MAS patients and a very low proportion of FD patients. Most of the cases with reported malignant transformation have had exposure to radiotherapy. The affected patients develop malignancies which include osteosarcoma, fibrosarcoma, chondrosarcoma and undifferentiated pleomorphic sarcoma. Radiographic features that raise the suspicion of a sarcomatous transformation in FD include permeative and ill-defined borders of the lesion, irregular cortical outline, spiculated periosteal new-bone formation and widening of the entire periodontal ligament space.

Management of FD is based on the symptoms. The growth rate of FD of long bones usually ceases following puberty. As for the polyostotic and craniofacial FD, these lesions can continue growing even after osseous maturity is reached. CFFD lesions can be categorized into quiescent, non-aggressive, or aggressive types. As their names suggest, quiescent lesions show no growth, non-aggressive lesions grow slowly, while the aggressive lesions grow rapidly and may be associated with pain, paraesthesia, and rarely malignant transformation. Medications such as bisphosphonates or denosumab have been shown to reduce pain. As the skeleton matures, stabilization of FD happens, hence often clinicians will opt to wait and observe until the patients have reached puberty before deciding more definitive treatment. Bone contouring or debulking may be undertaken to improve aesthetics, but patients must be warned of the risk of recurrence. Occasionally, complete removal is indicated for the recalcitrant lesions. The prognosis of FD is generally good.

Salient features of craniofacial fibrous dysplasia	
Clinical features	Onset at a young age between the second and fourth decades of life Slow growing, painless enlargement of the craniofacial bones most commonly the mandible resulting in facial asymmetry Displacement of teeth leading to malocclusion
Radiological features	Poorly defined radiolucency in the early stages Mature lesions appear more radiopaque with a characteristic orange peel or ground glass appearance Lesions blend into the surrounding bone
Histopathological features	Monotonous pattern of irregularly shaped trabeculae of woven bone that are not connected to one another Minimal evidence of osteoblastic rimming Cellular, loosely arranged fibrous stroma
Genetic features	*GNAS* mutation
Treatment	There is no definitive treatment Current management is based on the symptoms Bisphosphonates or denosumab (RANKL inhibitor) to reduce pain in symptomatic cases Bone contouring or debulking may help to improve aesthetics Recommended to delay surgical intervention until puberty when the lesion stabilizes

Diagnostic Algorithm

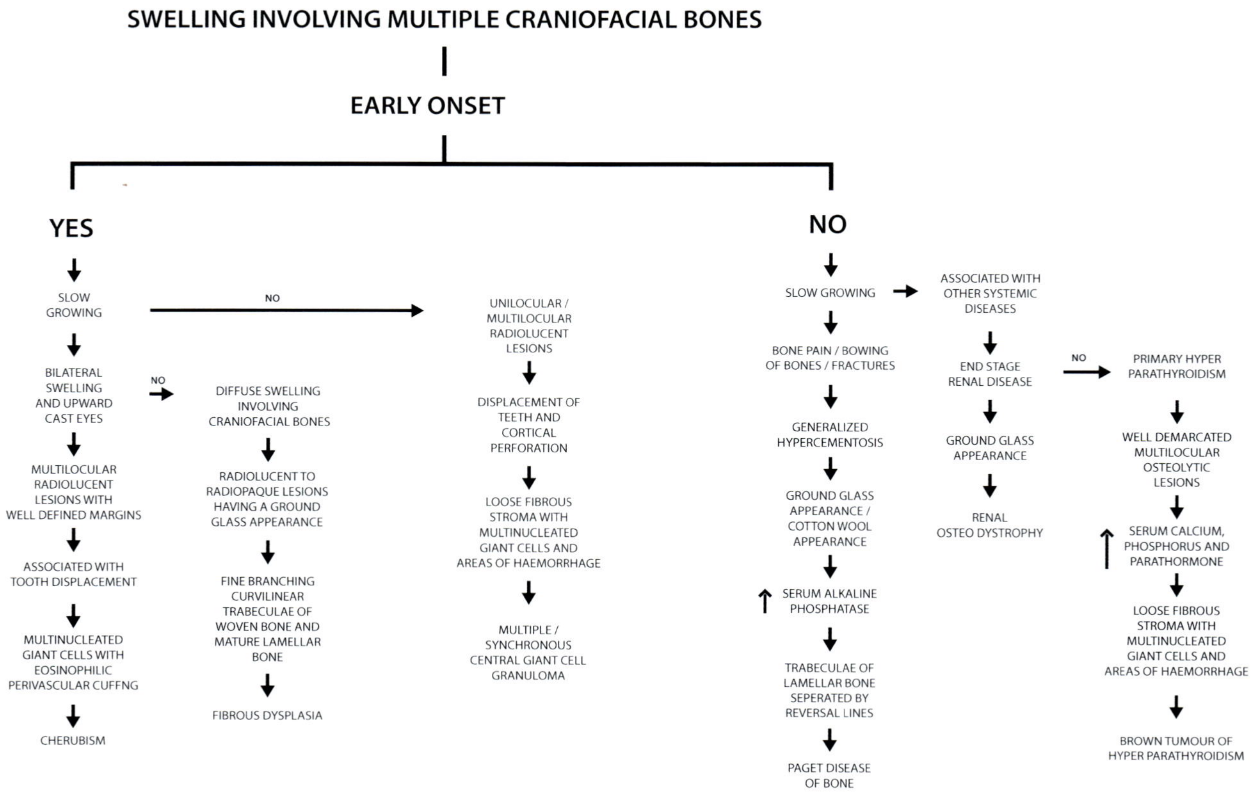

Self-Assessment Questions

1. List the pathognomonic clinical features of CFFD.
2. Describe the radiological features of CFFD.
3. Discuss the differential diagnoses for CFFD.
4. Explain the histopathological features of CFFD.
5. Explain the pathogenesis of FD.

Summary

Fibrous dysplasia (FD) is a fibro-osseous lesion. Lesions involving the craniofacial bones are not sharply demarcated and very commonly affect the zygomaticomaxillary complex and sphenoid bones. This type of fibrous dysplasia is termed craniofacial fibrous dysplasia (CFFD). CFFD presents as a gradual, painless enlargement of the craniofacial region, leading to facial asymmetry. As the skeleton matures, stabilization of CFFD happens, hence often clinicians will opt to wait and observe until the patients have reached puberty before deciding more definitive treatment. Bone contouring or debulking may be undertaken to improve aesthetics, but patients must be warned of the risk of recurrence. Occasionally, complete removal is indicated for the recalcitrant lesions. The prognosis of FD is generally good.

Further Reading

Boyce AM, Collins MT. Fibrous dysplasia/McCune-Albright syndrome: a rare, mosaic disease of Gα s activation. Endocr Rev. 2020;41(2):345–70.

Burke A, Collins MT, Boyce AM. Fibrous dysplasia of bone: craniofacial and dental implications. Oral Dis. 2017;23(6):697–708.

Cawson RA, Odell EW. Cawson's essentials of oral pathology and oral medicine e-book. Elsevier Health Sciences; 2017.

Chrcanovic BR, Guimarães L, Gomes C, Gomez RS. Cherubism: a systematic literature review of clinical and molecular aspects. Int J Oral Maxillofac Surg. 2021;50(1):43–53.

Holley TJ, Giannini PJ, Narayana N, Desa VPJ. Early detection of cherubism with eventual bilateral progression: a literature review and case report. Oral Surg Oral Med Oral Pathol Oral Radiol. 2019;127(3):e77–83.

Javaid MK, Boyce A, Appelman-Dijkstra N, Ong J, Defabianis P, Offiah A, Arundel P, Shaw N, Dal Pos V, Underhil AJO. Best practice management guidelines for fibrous dysplasia/McCune-Albright syndrome: a consensus statement from the FD/MAS international consortium. Orphanet J Rare Dis. 2019;14(1):1–17.

Kushchayeva YS, Kushchayev SV, Glushko TY, Tella SH, Teytelboym OM, Collins MT, Boyce AM. Fibrous dysplasia for radiologists: beyond ground glass bone matrix. Insights Imaging. 2018;9(6):1035–56.

Neville BW, Damm DD, Allen C, Chi AC. Oral and maxillofacial pathology. Elsevier Health Sciences; 2015.

Sivapathasundharam B. Shafer's textbook of oral pathology-e book. Elsevier Health Sciences; 2016.

Warnakulasuriya S, Tilakaratna WM, editors. Oral medicine & pathology: a guide to diagnosis and management. JP Medical Ltd.; 2013.

Fast Growing Bony Hard Lump: Cemento-ossifying Fibroma

Thomas George Kallarakkal and Wei Cheong Ngeow

Contents

W. M Tilakaratne, T. G. Kallarakkal (eds.), *Clinicopathological Correlation of Oral Diseases*,
https://doi.org/10.1007/978-3-031-24408-7_15

15.1 Main Complaint

A 24-year-old female patient presented to the clinic complaining of a swelling over the lower right side of her face.

15.2 History of Complaint

Question: How long have you been having this swelling?

I first noticed the swelling about 3 months ago. The swelling has been increasing in size since then. I feel that the swelling has further increased in size since the last 2 weeks. I have been seeking traditional medical treatment for the swelling since 1 month. However, I have not observed any improvement in my condition.

15.3 Additional Complaints

Question: Have you noticed or felt any other changes or difficulties such as numbness or paresthesia over the right side?

I do not have any other difficulties such as numbness or paresthesia over the right side of my face and mouth.

Question: Do you experience any pain in your jaws or teeth when eating?

I initially had pain when I first noticed the swelling 3 months ago. Subsequently, the pain decreased in intensity. Currently, I do not have any pain over the right side of my face in relation to the swelling when eating.

Question: Do you have any swellings in the neck on the right side?

I do not have any swellings in the neck.

Question: Have you noticed that your teeth on the right side have moved out of position recently?

I have not noticed any changes in the way I bite on my teeth.

Question: Have you been experiencing any symptoms such as loss of appetite and loss of weight?

I do not have any such symptoms.

Question: Do you have any other medical problems like heart disease, high blood pressure, diabetes, bleeding disorder or respiratory diseases?

I do not have any other medical problems.

Question: Do you have any history of trauma to your face?

I do not have any history of trauma involving my face or jaws.

Question: Have you undergone any surgery?

I have not undergone any surgery in the past.

Question: Have you undergone any dental treatment?

I have had multiple restorations. I have also had one of my lower left tooth extracted due to caries.

Question: Does anybody in your family have a similar problem?

All my immediate family members are fit and healthy.

Question: Do you have any risk habits such as smoking or alcohol intake?

I am a smoker and smoke about five to six cigarettes a day.

Question: Are you employed?

I am currently pursuing my Master degree at a local university.

15.4 With the Findings from the History, What Is Your Differential Diagnosis?

1. Odontogenic cysts such as dentigerous cyst and odontogenic keratocyst (OKC)
2. Benign odontogenic tumours including cemento-ossifying fibroma (COF)
3. Monostotic fibrous dysplasia (MFD)
4. Central giant cell granuloma (CGCG)
5. Osteoblastoma
6. Malignant maxillofacial bone tumours such as chondrosarcoma and osteosarcoma.
7. Malignant odontogenic tumours such as ameloblastic carcinoma and primary intraosseous carcinoma (PIOC).

15.5 How Do You Justify Your Differential Diagnosis After History Taking?

She has a rapidly growing swelling over the lower right side of her face that has been present for about 3 months. The clinical presentation of a rapidly growing swelling is highly suggestive of an aggressive lesion or a malignancy. The patient is healthy otherwise and does not have any associated generalized manifestations such as loss of appetite, loss of weight and cachexia that are characteristic of a malignancy. Moreover signs of nerve involvement such as paresthesia and numbness suggestive of malignant tumours are absent in this patient. She also doesn't have any teeth mobility that may be a consequence of a destructive malignant jaw bone tumour. Nevertheless a malignant tumour should be included in the differential diagnosis in view of the rapid and progressive nature of the tumour growth. Similarly other jaw bone lesions that can cause cortical expansion resulting in a facial swelling should be included in the differential diagnoses.

1. Odontogenic keratocysts (OKCs) predominate in the third decade of life with the posterior mandible being most commonly involved. Dentigerous cysts primarily occur in the second to third decades of life within the posterior mandible and are usually associated with impacted mandibular third molars. Large dentigerous cysts and OKCs can become symptomatic causing bony expansion with resulting facial asymmetry. However, a swelling of 3 months duration resulting in facial asymmetry as seen in this patient is not in favour of a cystic lesion.
2. Complex odontomes are frequently found in the right posterior mandible whereas compound odontomes occur more commonly in the anterior jaws. Generally, they are small lesions measuring 3 cm in maximum dimension but larger lesions measuring more than 6 cm referred to as giant odontomes have been reported in the literature. Odontomes however generally tend to grow very lowly. Ameloblastomas commonly affect the right posterior mandible with a peak incidence in the third and fourth decades of life. The usual presentation is that of a slow, painless growth but may exhibit accelerated growth in the later stages. Odontogenic myxomas and cementoblastomas occur between the second and fourth decades of life with no specific gender predilection and the posterior mandible is commonly involved. Clinically they manifest slow growth, cortical expansion, root resorption and tooth movement. Calcifying epithelial odontogenic tumours (CEOTs) like the other benign odontogenic tumours included in the differential diagnosis also involve the posterior mandible. They usually occur in the third to fourth decades of life and demonstrate no specific gender predilection. Cemento-ossifying fibroma (COF) is a benign odontogenic fibro-osseous neoplasm that commonly occurs in females between the second and fourth decades of life. It usually presents as a progressive, painless, slow-growing swelling of the tooth-bearing area of the posterior jaws affecting the mandible more commonly than the maxilla.
3. Monostotic fibrous dysplasia (MFD) is usually diagnosed before 30 years of age. Patients usually complain of pain, swelling and numbness on the affected side.
4. Central giant cell granulomas (CGCGs) are benign tumours that tend to involve the jaw bones, the mandible is more commonly involved than the maxilla. They are usually asymptomatic and tend to occur more commonly in females.
5. Osteoblastoma mostly occurs in the second or third decades of life and has a predilection for the posterior mandible in men.
6. Osteosarcomas and chondrosarcomas of the jaw bones are relatively rare tumours which tend to occur more commonly in the third decade of life. They usually develop spontaneously and manifest non-specific symptoms such as swelling and loosening of teeth. Pain is infrequently associated with a chondrosarcoma in contrast to an osteosarcoma.
7. Ameloblastic carcinoma is the most common among malignant odontogenic tumours. The affected patients complain of a rapidly growing painful swelling in the posterior mandible. Primary intraosseous carcinoma (PIOC) presents with non-specific symptoms suggestive of malignancy such as pain, ulceration, loosening of teeth, pathologic fractures and signs of nerve involvement.

15.6 Findings of Clinical Examination

Extra-orally she has a diffuse swelling at the right body of the mandible. The overlying skin is normal (◘ Fig. 15.1). There is no limitation in mouth opening. Intra-orally expansion of the buccal and lingual cortical plate is observed from tooth 43 to 48. The swelling is bony hard on palpation. The teeth are not displaced in the region of the swelling. There is no perforation of the cortical plates and involvement of the adjacent soft tissue.

15

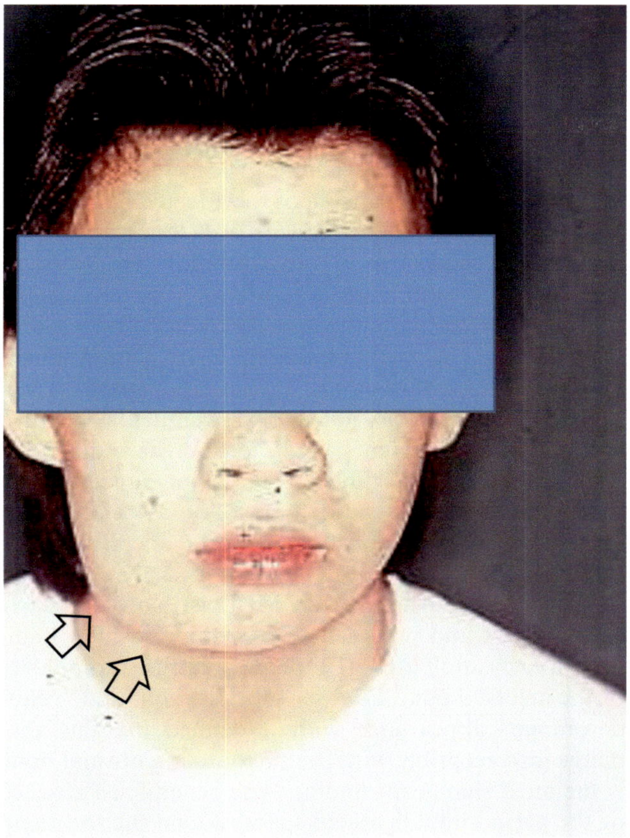

Fig. 15.1 A diffuse swelling involving the right lower third of the face causing bowing of the inferior border of the mandible

15.7 What Other Relevant Features Would You Look for with the Findings You Have So Far?

There are no enlarged submandibular or cervical lymph nodes. The sensory function of the trigeminal nerve on the affected side is intact.

15.8 What Is Your Clinical Differential Diagnosis?

1. Benign odontogenic tumours including COF
2. Odontogenic cysts such as dentigerous cyst and OKC
3. CGCG
4. MFD
5. Osteoblastoma

15.9 How Would You Exclude Other Conditions and Justify the Inclusion of the Diseases That You Have Mentioned in the Differential Diagnosis to Arrive at a Working Diagnosis?

The patient did not present any characteristic features of a malignancy such as ulceration, loosening of teeth and involvement of the adjacent soft tissues. The trigeminal nerve function on the affected side was intact with no evidence of numbness or paraesthesia. There were no palpable submandibular and cervical lymph nodes. Moreover, ameloblastic carcinomas, PIOCs and other odontogenic malignancies are usually seen in individuals in or above the fifth decade of life. It is also relatively common for patients diagnosed with ameloblastic carcinoma to have a history of long-standing benign ameloblastoma or have undergone treatment for the same. This was not seen in the present case. Hence malignant bone tumours and malignant odontogenic tumours can be excluded from the clinical differential diagnosis. The rest of the clinical differential diagnoses are similar to the differential diagnoses after history taking. A working diagnosis cannot be established based only on the history and findings from the clinical examination. Radiographic investigations are essential to establish a working diagnosis.

15.10 What Radiologic Investigations Would You Need to Exclude Other Conditions and Justify the Inclusion of the Diseases That You Have Mentioned in the Differential Diagnosis to Arrive at a Working Diagnosis?

1. Dental panoramic tomograph (DPT) to assess the mandibular arch as well as adjacent anatomic structures such as mental foramina and mandibular canal.

A DPT shows a partly circumscribed mixed radiolucent to radiopaque lesion involving the right body of the mandible extending from tooth 41 to the angle of the mandible (Fig. 15.2). Teeth 41–47 show root resorption. The inferior border of the mandible is intact but demonstrates a bowing of the inferior cortex.

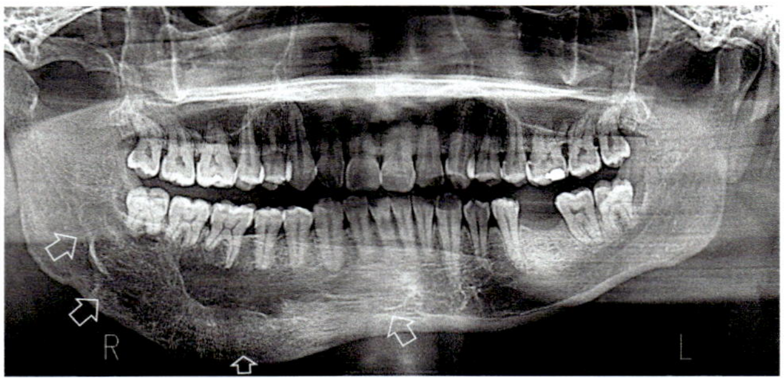

Fig. 15.2 The DPT shows a partly circumscribed, mixed radiolucent to radiopaque lesion with focal peripheral osteocondensation involving the right body of the mandible. Teeth 41–47 exhibit root resorption

Mature complex odontomes appear as a well-defined radiopacity surrounded by a radiolucent halo. They are frequently associated with unerupted teeth. Ameloblastomas manifest as a multilocular radiolucency with scalloped margins. Displacement and root resorption of the adjacent teeth is a common finding. Odontogenic myxomas also appear as a unilocular or multilocular radiolucency with scalloped margins. Displacement of teeth rather than root resorption is the most frequently observed finding in an odontogenic myxoma. Radiographically, a cementoblastoma typically demonstrates a well-circumscribed, radiopaque mass attached to the root of the involved tooth with a surrounding thin radiolucent zone. Attachment to the root of the involved tooth with root resorption and loss of root outline is pathognomonic. CEOTs present as unilocular or multilocular radiolucencies with varying degrees of radiopacity causing tooth displacement and root resorption. The radiographic features of the present case did not conform to the characteristic features of benign odontogenic tumours and can be excluded from the differential diagnoses. Moreover most of the benign odontogenic tumours do not demonstrate a rapid growth phase as seen in the present case.

15

OKCs have a characteristic radiographic appearance of a well-demarcated radiolucent lesion with a corticated margin that may be either unilocular or multilocular. Dentigerous cysts show a unilocular, well-demarcated radiolucency often with a corticated margin that surrounds the crown of an unerupted tooth. OKCs and dentigerous cysts are excluded from the differential diagnosis based on the radiographic presentation and the clinical history of rapid growth of the present case. CGCGs vary in behaviour from a slowly growing asymptomatic swelling to an aggressive process associated with pain, cortical bone destruction, root resorption and displacement of teeth. CGCG is also excluded from the differential diagnosis as they present as a unilocular or multilocular radiolucency associated with teeth displacement and root resorption which is not seen in this case.

COFs present as a slow-growing progressive enlargement of the affected bone. However, it can occasionally behave in an aggressive manner characterized by progressive and rapid expansion of the affected bone. COFs appear as well-defined round or oval lesions that predominantly appear as a mixed radiolucent to radiopaque lesion with a sclerotic border. They eventually become completely radiopaque surrounded by a radiolucent rim as the lesion attains maturity. Displacement and resorption of teeth is a common finding. Even though the lesion did not appear well-defined with a sclerotic margin evident only in focal areas, a diagnosis of COF cannot be excluded as the lesion appeared as a mixed radiolucent to radiopaque lesion associated with displacement and resorption of teeth and history of rapid growth.

The natural history of an MFD is that of an early age of onset and progressive slow growth which stabilizes in early adult life. MFD shows a diffuse radiopacity of the involved bone. Diffuse "ground glass" and "peau-de-orange" appearance with ill-defined margins that merge imperceptibly with the surrounding normal bone is the most significant finding. The generalized absence of the periodontal ligament space around the teeth and loss of lamina dura with an alteration to the abnormal bone pattern is also pathognomonic. MFD is excluded from the differential diagnosis due to the absence of pathognomonic clinical and radiographic findings consistent with MFD in this case.

Osteoblastomas most often arise in the vertebral column. Mandible is the second most common site of involvement followed by the other craniofacial bones. The affected patients may be either asymptomatic or may exhibit significant pain and swelling. A subset of osteoblastomas characterized by aggressive behaviour is designated as aggressive osteoblastoma. Radiographic features of an osteoblastoma are variable but usually show a relatively defined mixed radiolucent to radiopaque lesion with a radiolucent rim. A diagnosis of osteoblastoma cannot be excluded from the differential diagnosis based on the clinical and radiographic findings. A confirmatory diagnosis can be established only by histopathological examination.

15.11 What Is the Most Likely Working Diagnosis?

Cemento-ossifying fibroma.

Osteoblastoma (less likely).

15.12 How Would You Further Investigate This Patent?

1. Intraoral (periapical) radiographs to assess the relationship of the lesion with the teeth and adjacent anatomic structures including mental foramen and mandibular canal.
2. CBCT to determine the proximity of the lesion to the inferior alveolar nerve and other vital structures in the vicinity.

15.13 How Would You Arrive at a Definitive Diagnosis?

1. Fine needle aspiration cytology (FNAC)
2. Incisional biopsy for histopathological examination

Aspiration of the lesion did not yield any fluid. Thus FNAC was not relevant in this case.

15.14 How Would You Perform an Incisional Biopsy for This Patient? What Are the Important Considerations?

Biopsy with histological evaluation is necessary. An ideal biopsy should include the margins of the lesion. The lesional tissue in COF tend to be separated from the normal cancellous bone and overlying cortical bone by a fibrous tissue capsule. The finding of a fibrous capsule is very important as the rest of the histopathological features seen in COF is similar to those seen in all other fibro-osseous lesions. Correlation with clinical and radiographic information is essential to arrive at a final diagnosis.

15.15 Biopsy Report Confirms the Previous Clinical and Radiological Diagnosis of Cemento-ossifying Fibroma. What Are the Histopathological Features That Help in the Diagnosis?

The H & E sections show a highly cellular moderately collagenous connective tissue surrounded by a capsule. The stromal cells are composed of plump to spindle-shaped fibroblasts. There is no cytological atypia either in the stromal cells or in osteoblasts. Mitoses are absent. Trabeculae of woven bone and globular calcifications are interspersed within the stroma. The trabeculae of woven bone exhibit a brush border at the periphery (◘ Fig. 15.3). Sparsely cellular basophilic rounded cementum-like calcifications may also be present (◘ Fig. 15.4). There is moderate vascularity and minimal inflammatory infiltrate within the stroma.

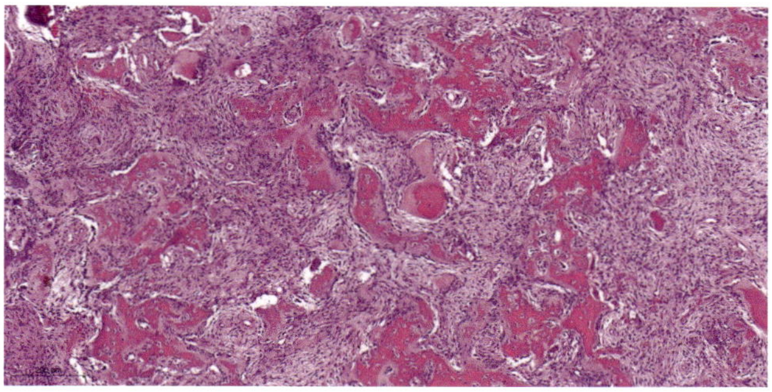

◘ **Fig. 15.3** Trabeculae of woven bone with osteoblastic rimming in a fibrocellular stroma

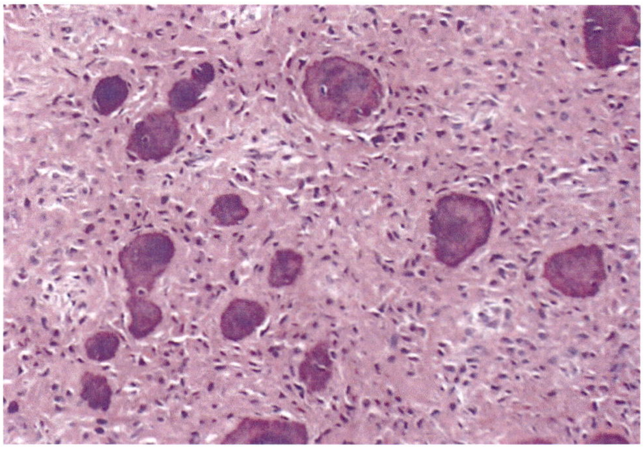

◘ **Fig. 15.4** Basophilic rounded cementum-like calcifications in a fibrocellular stroma

15.16 What Is the Final Diagnosis?

Cemento-ossifying fibroma.

15.17 How Would You Manage This Patent?

The treatment of COF is by surgery. Surgical treatment by conservative local excision or enucleation with curettage is the treatment of choice for well-delineated non-invasive tumours. In case of more extensive disease with invasion into adjacent structures, radical resection is the treatment of choice. Clinical and radiological follow-up after the excision of the lesion is recommended to identify possible early relapses.

15.18 Cemento-ossifying Fibroma (COF)

Fibro-osseous lesions are a group of diverse lesions in which the normal bone architecture is replaced by fibroblasts, collagen fibres and variable amounts of mineralized material. Benign fibro-osseous lesions in the oral and maxillofacial region broadly includes (1) fibrous dysplasia, (2) cemento-osseous dysplasias, (3) segmental odontomaxillary dysplasia, (4) fibro-osseous neoplasms; juvenile trabecular ossifying fibroma and psammomatoid ossifying fibroma and (5) familial gigantiformcementoma. Cemento-ossifying fibroma (COF) is a benign odontogenic fibro-osseous neoplasm arising from the pluripotential cells of the periodontal ligament that can form bone, cementum and fibrous tissue. Juvenile trabecular ossifying fibroma (JTOF) is a benign fibro-osseous neoplasm with a predilection for children and adolescents and tendency for rapid growth. Histologically JTOF is characterized by trabeculae of cellular osteoid and woven bone. Psammomatoid OF (PsOF) is characterized histologically by spherical ossicles and affects patients over a wide age range with a mean age range of 16–33 years while the mean age range for JTOF is 8–12 years.

The term COF was introduced in the fourth edition of World Health Organization (WHO) classification of Head and Neck Tumours under odontogenic tumours. Cemento-ossifying fibromas have been synonymously referred to as ossifying fibroma and cementifying fibroma. The pathogenesis of COF is unclear but it can be considered to arise from congenital defects during the maturation of dental tissues which are able to form cementum and bone. Trauma to the affected area by way of teeth extraction and the presence of chronic infections such as periodontitis has been reported to be triggering factors.

Clinically, COFs tend to occur in patients aged between 20 and 40 years of age. Occurrence in children and adolescents has also been reported. Women are significantly affected more commonly than men in a ratio of 5:1 with the mandibular posterior region being the most commonly involved site. The clinical behaviour varies from an indolent course manifesting as painless and progressive expansion of the affected bone to an aggressive behaviour characterized by pain and rapid cortical expansion of the involved bone and an increased tendency for recurrence. As the lesion progressively increases in size, cosmetic deformities ensue. Displacement of teeth is an early clinical feature. The affected teeth remain vital and the overlying mucosa remains intact with no evidence of ulceration. COFs demonstrate a centrifugal growth pattern that causes bowing of the inferior border of the mandible eventually leading to pathological fractures. Cortical perforation and paraesthesia have generally not been reported with COF. COF usually presents as a solitary lesion. However, multiple lesions can arise as part of the hyperparathyroidism-jaw tumour syndrome which is a rare autosomal dominant disorder characterized by bilateral cysts, hamartomas or Wilms tumours in kidneys and parathyroid neoplasms. In addition, gnathodiaphyseal dysplasia, a very rare skeletal disorder also shows fibro-osseous lesions in jaw bones including psammomatoid type COF.

Radiologically, COF appears initially as a radiolucent lesion followed by gradual transformation into a mixed radiolucent to radiopaque lesion. Eventually, a mature lesion may demonstrate complete radiopacity surrounded by a radiolucent rim (Fig. 15.5). CT images show a well-differentiated mass with the same density as a bone while the centre of the lesion shows low density.

COFs are neoplasms that are well-delineated and separated from adjacent cancellous bone or soft tissue by an expanded and attenuated layer of cortical bone. During surgery, they can be removed with relative ease from the surrounding normal bone and may demonstrate a capsule grossly (Fig. 15.6a and b) and microscopically.

Histologically COF is characterized by the presence of calcified material in a fibrocellular stroma. The calcified material is composed of bony trabeculae that may be either separated from one another or demonstrate a retiform arrangement. The bony trabeculae show osteoblastic rimming. Occasional osteoclasts may also be seen. Lobulated cementum-like calcifications that may show the characteristic "brush border" pattern may be seen scattered throughout the whole lesion. The fibrocellular stroma consists of spindle-to-stellate fibroblasts that may occasionally exhibit a storiform pattern. A major diagnostic challenge lies in differentiating COF from focal cemento-osseous dysplasia (FocCOD). FocCOD represents one of the far more common fibro-osseous lesions of the jaws compared to the other lesions in the group and occurs most commonly in the tooth-bearing area of the posterior jaws. The calcified material in FocCODs takes the form of anastomosing, thick curvilinear, relatively acellular bony trabeculae that are either seen focally or within the centre of the lesion. These trabeculae have been likened to the appearance of ginger roots. The bony trabeculae in COF are thin, single and separate and are localized to the periphery of the lesion. Another difference between the two lesions is

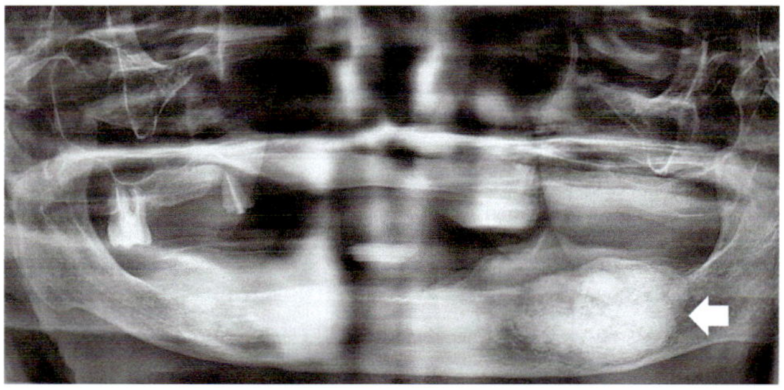

Fig. 15.5 A mature COF manifesting as a radiopaque lesion surrounded by a radiolucent rim (white arrow)

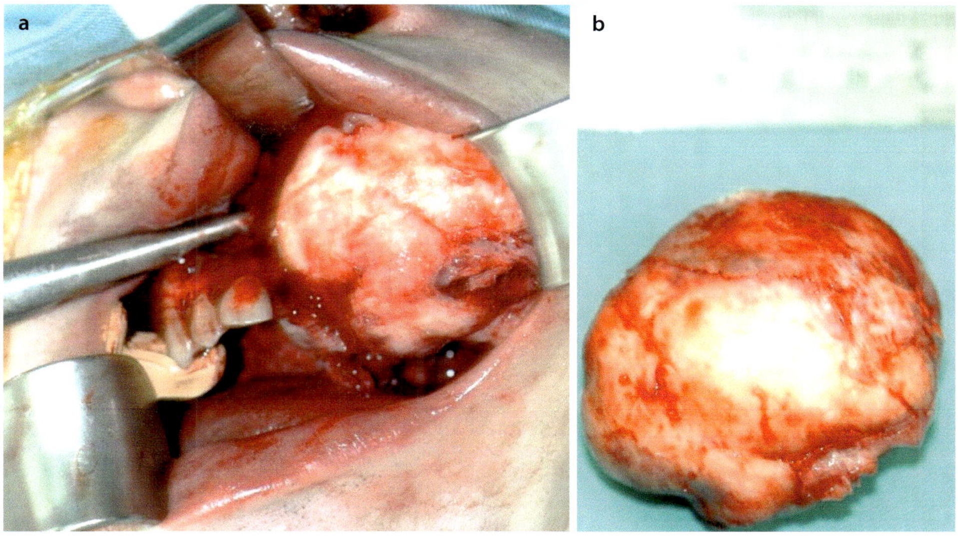

Fig. 15.6 A COF involving the right maxilla being enucleated out easily from the surrounding bone (**a**). Macroscopically COF appears as an encapsulated lesion (**b**). (Picture courtesy: Dr. Thomas Abraham, Sentosa Specialist Hospital, Selangor, Malaysia)

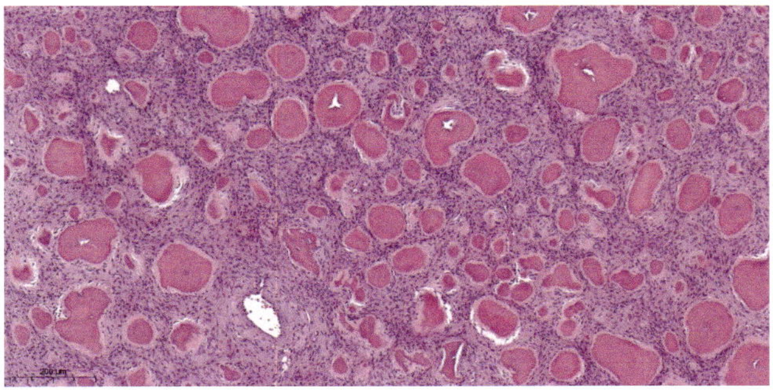

Fig. 15.7 Small uniform spherical ossicles in Psammomatod ossifying fibroma

the nature of haemorrhage within the lesions. Free haemorrhage tends to be more frequent and distributed throughout the lesion in FocCOD whereas it is confined to the periphery in COF. PsJOF is characterized by small uniform spherical ossicles resembling psammoma bodies (Fig. 15.7). These spherical masses are uniform in size and are dispersed in a fibroblastic stroma. JTOF is recognised by the presence of trabeculae of fibrillary osteoid and woven bone.

The recommended clinical management for COF is conservative surgical excision or enucleation until healthy bone margins are achieved. Larger lesions that demonstrate an infiltrative behaviour into the adjacent bones will require radical resection. COFs generally shell out easily at the time of surgery as they are well circumscribed and tend to be separated from the surrounding bone by a fibrous capsule. Generally, maxillary COFs are more difficult to be removed completely when compared to mandibular COFs primarily due to the difference in the nature of the bone structure between the maxilla and mandible. A recurrence rate varying between 6 and 28% has been reported for patients with COF involving the mandible. Radiotherapy is ineffective and is contraindicated owing to an increased incidence of malignant transformation. Long-term follow-up is recommended regardless of the treatment advocated. A recurrence if noted should be treated by a second conservative excision.

Salient features of cemento-ossifying fibroma	
Clinical features	Onset in young patients between 20 and 40 years of age Slowly progressive painless expansion of the involved jaw bones Female to male ratio is 5:1 Posterior mandible is the most commonly involved site Demonstrates a centrifugal growth pattern that causes bowing of the inferior border of the mandible
Radiological features	Well-circumscribed mixed radiolucent to radiopaque lesion surrounded by a peripheral radiolucent rim Displacement and resorption of teeth on the affected side
Histopathological features	Bony trabeculae showing osteoblastic rimming and lobulated cementum-like calcifications demonstrating characteristic brush borders in a fibrocellular stroma Fibrocellular stroma is composed of spindle to stellate shaped fibroblasts
Treatment	Conservative surgical excision Enucleation

Diagnostic Algorithm

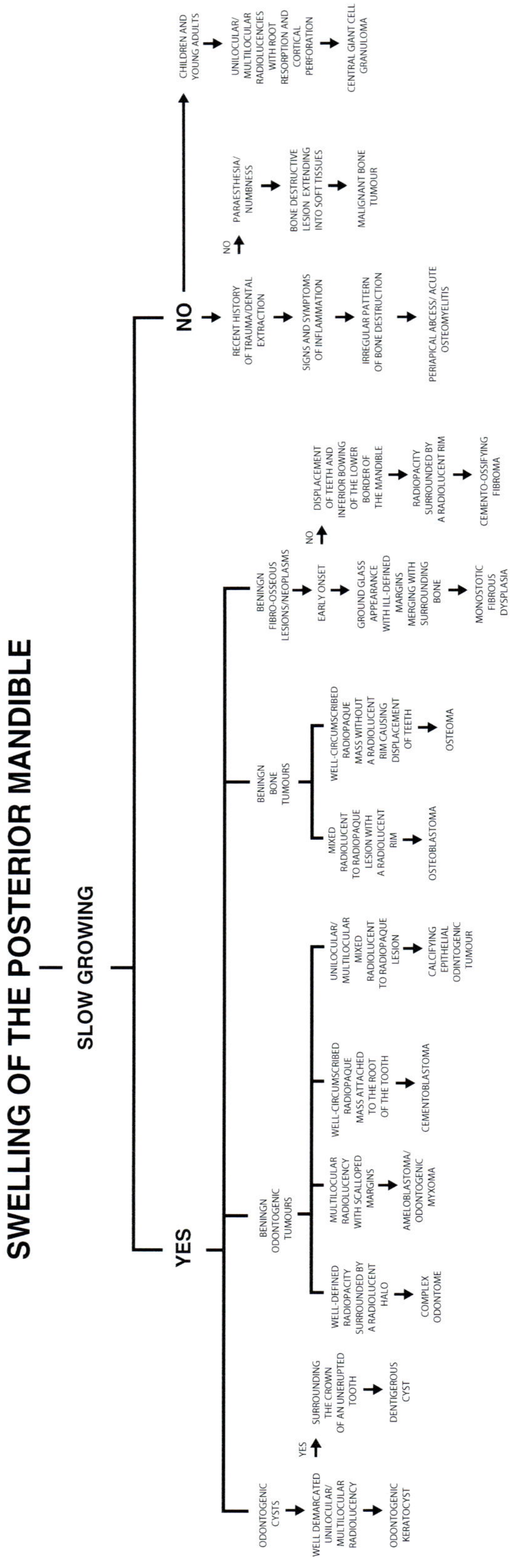

15

Self-Assessment Questions

1. List the pathognomonic clinical features of cemento-ossifying fibroma.
2. Describe the radiological features of cemento-ossifying fibroma.
3. Discuss the differential diagnoses for cemento-ossifying fibroma.
4. Explain the histopathological features of cemento-ossifying fibroma.
5. Describe the histological features of juvenile cemento-ossifying fibroma.

Summary

Cemento-ossifying fibroma (COF), a benign odontogenic fibro-osseous neoplasm arises from the pluripotential cells of the periodontal ligament that can form bone, cementum and fibrous tissue. COFs present as a slow-growing progressive enlargement of the affected bone. However, it can occasionally behave in an aggressive manner characterized by progressive and rapid expansion of the affected bone. COFs appear as well-defined round or oval lesions that predominantly appear as mixed radiolucent to radiopaque lesions with a sclerotic border. They eventually become completely radiopaque surrounded by a radiolucent rim as the lesion attains maturity. The recommended clinical management for COF is conservative surgical excision or enucleation until healthy bone margins are achieved. Larger lesions that demonstrate an infiltrative behaviour into the adjacent bones will require a radical resection. COFs generally shell out easily at the time of surgery as they are well circumscribed and tend to be separated from the surrounding bone by a fibrous capsule. A recurrence rate varying between 6 and 28% has been reported for patients with COF involving the mandible. Radiotherapy is ineffective and is contraindicated owing to an increased incidence of malignant transformation. Long-term follow-up is recommended regardless of the treatment advocated. A recurrence if noted should be treated by a second conservative excision.

Further Reading

Cawson RA, Odell EW. Cawson's essentials of oral pathology and oral medicine e-book. Elsevier Health Sciences; 2017.

Chang C-C, Hung H-Y, Chang JY-F, Yu C-H, Wang Y-P, Liu B-Y, Chiang C-P. Central ossifying fibroma: a clinicopathologic study of 28 cases. J Formos Med Assoc. 2008;107(4):288–94.

Gondivkar SM, Gadbail AR, Chole R, Parikh RV, Balsaraf S. Ossifying fibroma of the jaws: report of two cases and literature review. Oral Oncol. 2011;47(9):804–9.

Neville BW, Damm DD, Allen C, Chi AC. Oral and maxillofacial pathology. Elsevier Health Sciences; 2015.

Sivapathasundharam B. Shafer's textbook of oral pathology-e book. Elsevier Health Sciences; 2016.

Su L, Weathers DR, Waldron CA. Distinguishing features of focal cemento-osseous dysplasias and cemento-ossifying fibromas: I. A pathologic spectrum of 316 cases. Oral Surg Oral Med Oral Pathol Oral Radiol Endod. 1997;84(3):301–9.

Tortorici S, Buzzanca ML, Burruano F, Difalco P. Juvenile central ossifying fibroma of the mandible: a case report. J Pediatr Surg. 2010;45(10):e1–4.

Trijolet J-P, Parmentier J, Sury F, Goga D, Mejean N, Laure B. Cemento-ossifying fibroma of the mandible. Saudi Med J. 2011;128(1):30–3.

Warnakulasuriya S, Tilakaratna WM, editors. Oral medicine & pathology: a guide to diagnosis and management. JP Medical Ltd.; 2013.

Zupi A, Ruggiero A, Insabato L, Senghore N, Califano L. Aggressive cemento-ossifying fibroma of the jaws. Oral Oncol. 2000;36(1):129–33.

Accidental Finding on the Radiograph: Periapical Cemento-osseous Dysplasia

Thomas George Kallarakkal and Wei Cheong Ngeow

Contents

W. M Tilakaratne, T. G. Kallarakkal (eds.), *Clinicopathological Correlation of Oral Diseases*,
https://doi.org/10.1007/978-3-031-24408-7_16

16.1 Main Complaint

A 34-year-old female patient, presented to the clinic complaining that her teeth appeared discolored.

16.2 History of Complaint

Question: How long have you been having this complaint?

I have been having this complaint for the past 6–7 months.

16.3 Additional Complaints

Question: Is the discoloration localized to only a single tooth or generalized involving many teeth?

I feel that the discoloration is generalized but is more pronounced on the lower anterior teeth.

Question: Have you noticed any pain in your teeth or jaw?

I have not noticed any pain in my teeth or jaws. However, I occasionally feel a slight discomfort in my lower anterior teeth.

Question: Do you experience any pain in your teeth or jaws when taking cold drinks or sweet food?

I don't experience any pain in my teeth or jaws when taking cold drinks or sweet food.

Question: What is the nature of the discomfort felt in your lower anterior teeth?

I feel a dull ache occasionally in the region of my lower anterior teeth.

Question: Do you have any history of trauma to your teeth or the jaws?

I don't recall any trauma to my teeth or jaws.

Question: Have you ever been diagnosed with metabolic diseases such as alkaptonuria, congenital porphyria, and congenital hyperbilirubinemia?

I have never been diagnosed with any such diseases.

Question: Do you have any other medical problems like heart disease, high blood pressure, diabetes, bleeding disorder, respiratory diseases? If yes, what kind of medications, have you been taking until now?

I was diagnosed with diabetes mellitus 2 years ago. I am currently on Tab Metformin 500 mg bid for 2 years. I am also currently on oral contraceptives; Tab Desogestrel 1 Tablet (75 mcg) OD.

Question: Have your parents ever told you that you were diagnosed with any childhood diseases that necessitated the administration of certain drugs such as tetracycline that can cause discoloration of teeth?

I was not diagnosed with any childhood diseases.

Question: Have you undergone any surgery?

I have not undergone any surgery in the past.

Question: Do you have any decayed teeth?

I think I have a couple of decayed lower teeth.

Question: Have you undergone any dental treatment?

I visited my dentist a year ago for a fixed bridge to replace my upper anterior teeth and for multiple tooth-coloured fillings on my lower posterior teeth.

Question: How often do you brush your teeth daily?

I brush my teeth only once daily in the morning.

Question: Do you floss your teeth daily or after every meal?

I rarely floss my teeth.

Question: Do you use any mouthwashes?

I have been using chlorhexidine mouthwash every morning for 1 year.

Question: Does anybody in your family have a similar problem?

My family members do not have any such problems. Both my parents are diabetics and are on medication. My mother had mobile teeth. She had all her teeth extracted and is currently wearing dentures. My husband and my two children also do not have any similar problems.

❓ Question: Did your mother have any diseases during her pregnancy that could have affected your teeth?

✅ My mother has never told me about any such diseases during her pregnancy.

❓ Question: Did you live your childhood years in an area associated with increased levels of fluoride in the local drinking water supply or groundwater supply?

❓ Question: I lived my childhood years in a neighbourhood that had access to a good drinking water supply without any increased levels of fluoride in the water supply according to the available information.

❓ Question: Did you as a take a lot of fluoride supplements during your childhood?

✅ I don't remember taking any fluoride supplements as a child.

❓ Question: Do you have any risk habits such as smoking or drinking alcohol?

✅ I smoke about five to six cigarettes a day. I am a social drinker and usually consume alcoholic drinks on the weekends.

❓ Question: Do you have any betel quid chewing habits?

✅ I don't chew betel quid.

❓ Question: Do you consume a lot of fruits that can cause staining of teeth such as blueberries?

✅ I eat moderate amounts of fruits daily, particularly bananas and apples.

❓ Question: Do you drink a lot of tea or coffee?

✅ I usually drink five to six cups of coffee every day.

❓ Question: Are you employed?

✅ I work as a sales executive in an automobile dealership.

16.4 With the Findings from the History, What Is Your Differential Diagnosis?

1. Extrinsic discoloration of the teeth
2. Dental fluorosis
3. Dental caries and periapical pathology involving the lower anterior teeth

16.5 How Do You Justify Your Differential Diagnosis After History Taking?

She complains of generalized discoloration of her teeth since 6 months which is more prominent in the lower anterior region. Teeth discoloration may follow a change to the structural composition of the enamel which may be observed in a number of metabolic diseases and systemic factors that affect the developing dentition or it may be due to extrinsic stains derived from dietary components that may be adsorbed on to the tooth surfaces. She does not have a history of any pre-natal or childhood diseases as well as any maternal diseases in her mother during pregnancy that may have caused any structural alterations in her developing dentition. Her family members do not have any similar problems which rule out any inherited diseases such as amelogenesis imperfecta or dentinogenesis imperfecta. She does not have any history of trauma to her lower anterior teeth that could have caused pulpal necrosis resulting in pain/discomfort and discoloration of her lower anterior teeth. She has been using chlorhexidine mouthwash regularly for the past 1 year. The use of chlorhexidine mouth rinse has been linked to generalized staining of teeth surfaces. She is a smoker and drinks five to six cups of coffee every day which could contribute to a generalized staining of teeth surfaces. The patient complains of a more pronounced discoloration and slight discomfort related to lower anterior teeth. Dental caries leading to pulpal necrosis and periapical pathology could give rise to these symptoms. Dental fluorosis manifests as characteristic opacities in mild cases. The clinical appearance may vary from few faint white flecks to more generalized involvement of tooth surfaces referred to as snowcapping or snowflaking. Severe cases are characterized by dark brown staining and large enamel defects. The patient did not give any history of living in an area endemic to fluorosis during early childhood. However, fluorosis is included in the differential diagnosis in keeping with the patient's chief complaint of discoloured teeth.

16.6 Findings of Clinical Examination

Extra-orally her face is symmetrical. There are no abnormalities on her facial skin and vermillion border. There is no limitation in mouth opening. There are no enlarged submandibular or cervical lymph nodes. Intraorally there is generalized brown staining on all teeth surfaces which is slightly more pronounced on her lower anterior teeth (◘ Fig. 16.1). There is a mild to moderate degree of dental fluorosis characterized by faint white

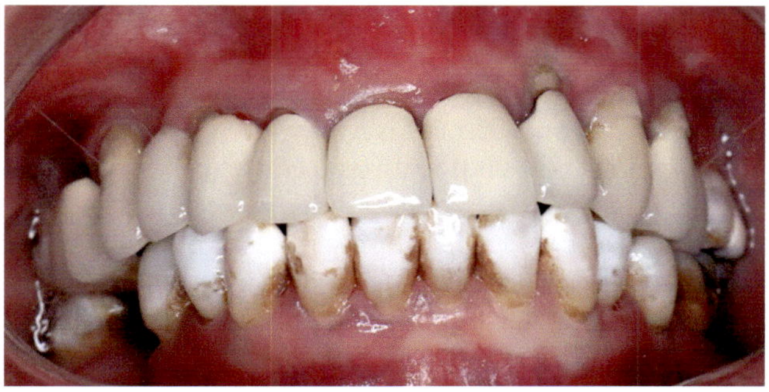

Fig. 16.1 Generalized brown staining on the lower anterior teeth

flecks on teeth 34 and 35 to more prominent opacities involving greater surfaces of teeth 44 and 45. Oral hygiene is fair. She has a fixed partial denture extending from teeth 16 to 25. There are multiple tooth-coloured restorations. There is no mucosal abnormality, bony swelling or teeth displacement involving her lower anterior region. There is no caries and periodontal disease involving the lower anterior teeth. The lower anterior teeth are not tender to percussion.

16.7 What Other Relevant Features Would You Look for with the Findings You Have So Far?

There is no draining sinus or paresthesia involving her lower anterior region. The lower anterior teeth are vital and responded positively to hot and cold tests and pulp sensibility tests.

16.8 What Is Your Clinical Differential Diagnosis?

1. Extrinsic discoloration of the teeth
2. Dental fluorosis

16.9 How Would You Exclude Other Conditions and Justify the Inclusion of the Diseases That You Have Mentioned in the Differential Diagnosis to Arrive at a Working Diagnosis?

The patient did not have any clinical findings suggestive of active dental caries or periodontal disease related to the lower anterior teeth. They were no restorations on the lower anterior teeth. The teeth responded positively to hot and cold tests and pulp sensibility tests thus ruling out any pulpal and periapical pathology.

16.10 How Would You Investigate This Patient?

1. Intraoral (periapical) radiograph of the lower anterior region to rule out any periapical pathosis as the patient complained of a slight discomfort in her lower anterior teeth.

An intraoral periapical radiograph (IOPA) shows multiple apical radiopaque lesions involving the anterior teeth with vital pulp (Fig. 16.2). The periodontal ligaments of the involved teeth appeared intact and the lesions were not fused to the roots.

The differential diagnosis for well-defined radiopaque lesions in the anterior mandibular region should include:

- Periapical cemento-osseous dysplasia (PCOD)
- Idiopathic osteosclerosis (IO)
- Condensing osteitis (CO)
- Odontoma
- Cementoblastoma
- Cemento-ossifying fibroma (COF)
- Osteoma
- Osteoblastoma
- Osteoid osteoma (OO)

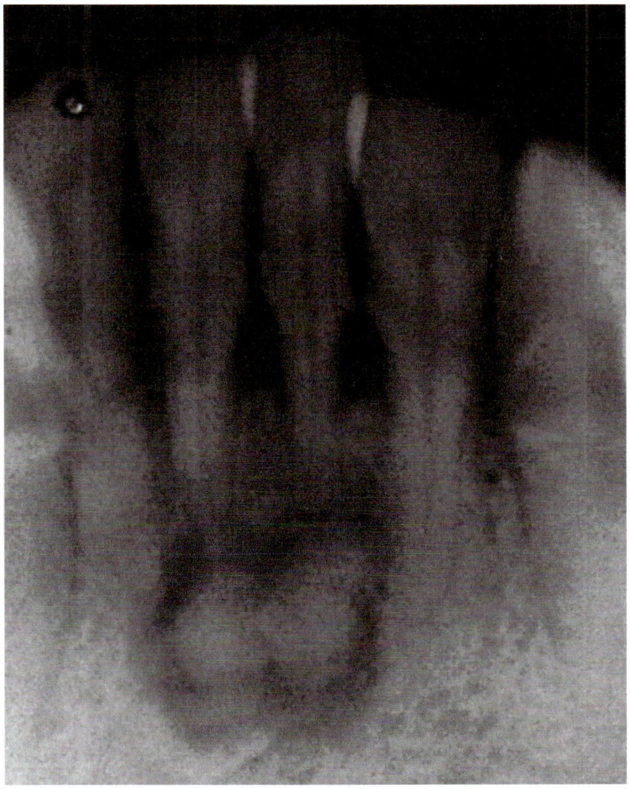

Fig. 16.2 Multiple well-defined radiopacities within a radiolucent lesion associated with teeth 31 and 41. The surrounding bone appeared normal

PCOD is an uncommon type of fibro-osseous lesion (FOL) that affects the anterior mandible in middle aged women. The affected patients are usually asymptomatic but can present with vague pain or discomfort involving the affected area. Radiographic investigations are essential to establish a definitive diagnosis. PCOD arises from the periodontal ligament and affects the tooth bearing, cancellous areas of the jaw bones. PCOD is associated with vital teeth and rarely manifests any significant clinical symptoms. Majority of these cases are accidentally diagnosed during radiographic examination which are ordered for other reasons. PCOD manifests radiographically as a radiolucent, radiopaque or a mixed lesion. In the early stages, a PCOD may mimic a periapical granuloma or a cyst. The characteristic radiographic appearance is the presence of calcifications within a radiolucent lesion that involves multiple vital teeth. These lesions progressively mature to form increasing number of radiopaque areas with a lobular, ginger root-like appearance surrounded by a radiolucent rim.

Idiopathic osteosclerosis (IO) of the jaws is a localized radiopacity of unknown origin. They are usually asymptomatic and are discovered incidentally on radiographs taken for other reasons. IO is also synonymously referred to as dense bone island, enostosis, and focal periapical osteopetrosis. On the radiographs, they appear as a well-defined radiopacity located adjacent to sound teeth, teeth with small restorations or away from the teeth. They are usually round or elliptical in shape with the absence of a radiolucent rim and are more than 3 mm in size. The most common location of IO is the first molar and premolar region of the mandible (◘ Fig. 16.3). In the present case, the intraoral periapical radiograph demonstrated, well-defined radiopacities within a radiolucent lesion involving the mandibular central incisors which was consistent with the radiographic appearance of PCOD.

Condensing osteitis (CO) of the jaws represents a focal periapical osseous reaction resulting in new bone formation. CO mostly arises as a sequelae of pulpal inflammation and or necrosis. However, it may also be seen in relation to vital teeth as a consequence of occlusal trauma. On the radiographs or on CBCT, CO appears as a focal well-circumscribed or ill-defined area of sclerosis with the absence of a radiolucent halo surrounding the apices of teeth with necrotic or inflamed dental pulp (◘ Fig. 16.4). They may be either single or multiple lesions affecting the mandibular premolar or molar teeth and are more commonly seen in children and young adults. A diagnosis of CO was not considered in the present case as the involved teeth were vital and responded positively to pulp sensibility testing.

Odontomes are the most common benign odontogenic tumours. Majority of all odontomes are associated with an impacted tooth. Odontomes are classified into compound and complex types. Compound odontomes generally occur in the anterior maxilla. They are usually 1–2 cm in diameter and appear as multiple radiopaque tooth-like structures surrounded by a thin radiolucent rim separating it clearly from the adjacent bone. Complex odontomes tend to involve the posterior mandible more commonly and are characterized by amorphous calcifications composed of dysplastic dentin covered by enamel. They have a distinct radiographic pattern having an amorphous radiopaque structure with a fine radiopaque periphery surrounded by a radiolucent rim. The radiographic appearance in the present case did not reveal any tooth-like structures suggestive of a compound odontome. A complex odontome was not a likely diagnosis in this case as the lesion appeared as a well-defined round to ovoid radiopaque lesion in the anterior mandible rather than having an amorphous radiopaque structure.

Cementoblastoma is a benign odontogenic tumour accounting for less than 1% of all odontogenic tumours.

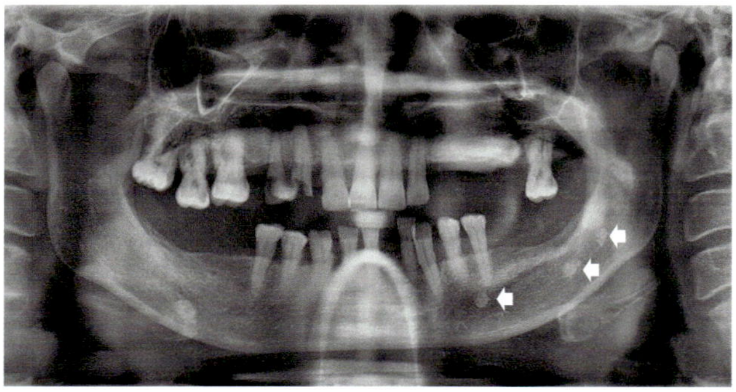

◘ **Fig. 16.3** Well-defined round radiopaque lesions without a radiolucent rim (white arrows). (Picture courtesy: Prof. Dr. Ruwan D. Jayasinghe Faculty of Dental Sciences, University of Peradeniya, Sri Lanka)

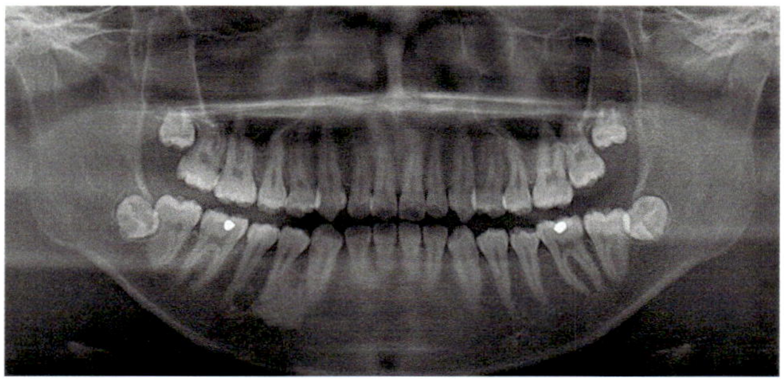

◘ **Fig. 16.4** Ill-defined sclerosis associated with tooth 44 due to pulpal inflammation as a result of occlusal trauma. (Picture courtesy: Prof. Dr. Norliza Binti Ibrahim, Faculty of Dentistry, Universiti Malaya, Kuala Lumpur, Malaysia)

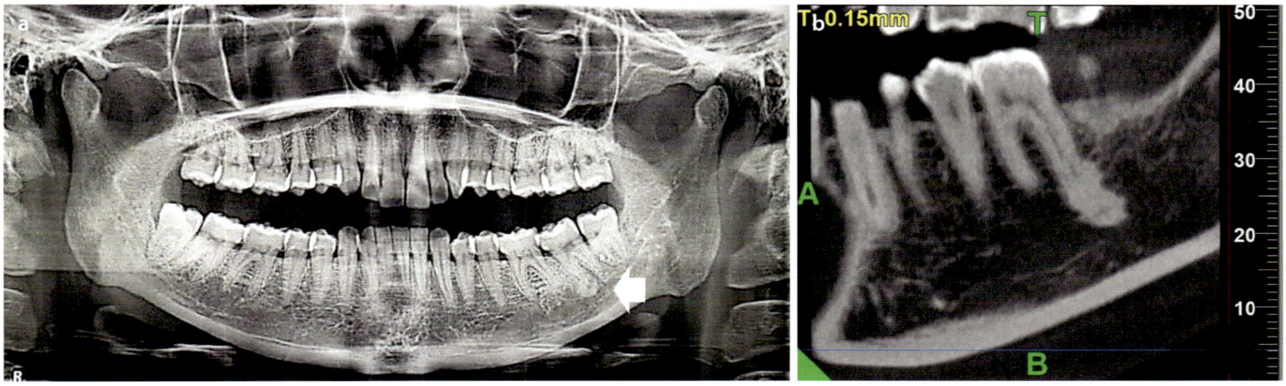

Fig. 16.5 (**a**) A periapical radiopaque lesion with a radiolucent rim fused to the mesial root of tooth 36 (white arrow). (Picture courtesy: Prof. Dr. Norliza Binti Ibrahim, Faculty of Dentistry, Universiti Malaya, Kuala Lumpur, Malaysia). (**b**) A cone beam computed tomography (CBCT) image showing the intimate relationship of cementoblastoma to the root of tooth 36 and obscuring its morphology. (Picture courtesy: Prof. Dr. Ruwan D. Jayasinghe Faculty of Dental Sciences, University of Peradeniya, Sri Lanka)

They predominantly occur within the mandible in the molar or premolar region in children and young adults. On imaging, they appear as a periapical, radiopaque sharply defined lesion surrounded by a radiolucent margin which is fused to the roots of the tooth (Fig. 16.5a). Root resorption and the intimate relationship of the lesion with the roots of the involved tooth presents the most pathognomonic feature of cementoblastoma (Fig. 16.5b). In addition more aggressive features including bony expansion, perforation of cortical plates, displacement of adjacent teeth, invasion into pulp chamber and root canals and extension to incorporate adjacent teeth are also observed. A cementoblastoma was excluded from the differential diagnosis as the lesion did not appear to be fused to the roots of the involved teeth unlike in a cementoblastoma.

Ossifying fibroma (OF) is a benign FOL of neoplastic behaviour. OF is classified into i) cemento-ossifying fibroma (COF), ii) juvenile trabecular ossifying fibroma (JTOF), and iii) juvenile psammomatoid ossifying fibroma (JPOF). COF is of odontogenic origin and occurs exclusively in the tooth-bearing areas of the jaws. The incidence of COF peaks in the third and fourth decades of life where it tends to occur more commonly in females. The mandibular premolar and molar regions are most commonly involved. It appears as a round or ovoid expansive painless mass that may displace or cause resorption of the roots of the adjacent teeth. Early lesions are primarily radiolucent. As they mature, they assume a mixed radiolucent and radiopaque appearance. Mature lesions are described as having an eggshell appearance with asymmetric opacities forming concentric bony trabeculae, surrounded by peripheral osteocondensation. Majority of the COFs in younger patients also have a radiolucent periphery suggestive of a capsule. The absence of any clinically evident expansion in the anterior mandible and the radiographic appearance of multiple well-defined radiopacities within radiolucencies associated with mandibular anterior teeth ruled out the possibility of a COF.

Osteomas of the jaws are benign osteogenic neoplasms. They are classified into peripheral osteomas which arise from the periosteal surfaces and are attached to the cortical plates. Central osteomas arise from the endosteal bone surfaces. Multiple osteomas are a hallmark of Gardner syndrome, an autosomal dominant disease caused by mutation in APC tumour suppressor gene. Apart from multiple central and peripheral osteomas, patients with Gardner syndrome also manifest colorectal adenomas that may undergo malignant transformation if left untreated. Peripheral osteomas more commonly involve the mandibular condyle than the maxilla and appear as a radiopaque often mushroom-shaped mass protruding from the surface of the jawbone. Central osteomas are not related to the teeth and manifest as a well-circumscribed radiopaque mass causing expansion of the bone and displacement of the teeth. A perilesional radiolucent halo is absent. The lesion in the present case showed a radiolucent halo and appeared to be closely related to the teeth making it distinct from osteoma.

Osteoblastoma is a benign bone tumour that rarely occurs in the facial bones but most often arises in the vertebral column, long bones of the appendicular skeleton and small bones of the hands and feet. The mandible is affected more commonly than the maxilla where the lesions more often tend to involve the body of the mandible. The affected patients may be either asymptomatic or complain of a localized, dull, aching pain that is insidious in onset and does not respond to aspirin. Radiographic features of an osteoblastoma are variable but usually show a relatively defined mixed radiolucent to radiopaque lesion with a radiolucent rim.

Osteoid osteomas (OO) occur in the long bones and rarely involve the jaw bones. Females in their second and third decades are more commonly affected. Majority of these cases involve the posterior mandible, particularly the molar region. A characteristic feature of OO is a dull or boring pain which may be either continuous or intermittent. The pain tends to be more severe at night and is relieved by aspirin. On the radiograph OO appears as a radiopaque mass characterized by a radiolucent or radiopaque nidus with surrounding reactive radiopacity and a radiolucent rim. The patient neither had any clinical features such as swelling or pain nor any radiographic features to suggest an OO in the present case.

16.11 What Is the Most Likely Diagnosis?

Periapical cemento-osseous dysplasia.

16.12 What Further Investigations Would You Recommend for This Patient?

1. CBCT to determine the exact extent of the lesion and its internal architecture.

16.13 Biopsy Report Confirms the Previous Clinical Diagnosis of Periapical Cemento-osseous Dysplasia. What Are the Histopathological Features That Help in the Diagnosis?

The haematoxylin and eosin (H & E) sections show a non-encapsulated, variably cellular moderately collagenous connective tissue. The cellularity is primarily composed of plump to spindle-shaped fibroblasts. Cellular pleomorphism and mitoses are absent. The stroma contains mineralized tissues consisting of osteoid, bone and cementum-like material. There is pronounced vascularity with areas of haemorrhage within the lesion. There is minimal inflammatory infiltrate within the stroma (Fig. 16.6).

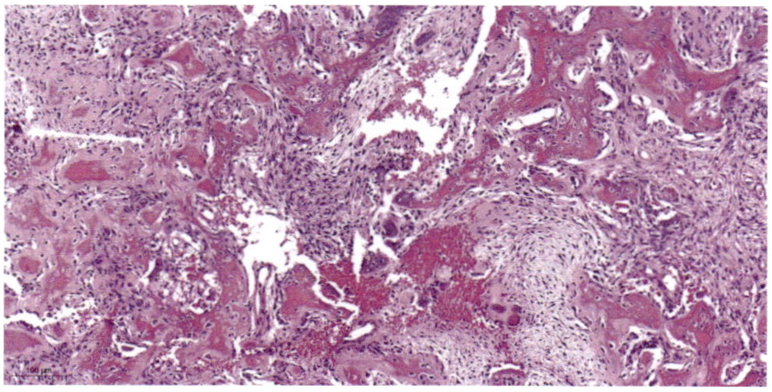

Fig. 16.6 A cellular and vascular connective tissue stroma containing osteoid and bony trabeculae

16

16.14 What Is the Final Diagnosis?

Periapical cemento-osseous dysplasia.

16.15 How Would You Manage This Patient?

The patient should be advised to brush and floss the teeth two times a day to remove the extrinsic stains. The patient does not require any specific treatment for fluorosis as it is only mild. PCOD does not require any active treatment. However, it is recommended to keep the patients on long-term follow-up. The development of symptoms like bone expansion and displacement of teeth may be an indication that the initial lesion could have been an early stage of florid cemento-osseous dysplasia, fibrous dysplasia or cemento-ossifying fibroma. The early stages of PCOD may mimic a periapical pathology such as a periapical granuloma or a periapical cyst on the radiograph. A thorough clinical evaluation should be carried out to determine the vitality of the involved teeth to avoid unnecessary endodontic treatments. In the present case, the patient complained of a dull ache in the anterior mandibular region that necessitated a biopsy. Upon a definitive diagnosis of PCOD based on radiographic and clinicopathological correlation, the patient was reassured and placed on follow-up without any further intervention.

16.16 Periapical Cemento-osseous Dysplasia (PCOD)

FOLs of the jaws represent a unique process that is characterized by the replacement of normal bone with fibrous tissue. The newly formed fibrous tissue contains varying amounts of mineralized tissue composed of bone or cementum-like tissue. There has been a considerable variability in the literature regarding the classification and nomenclature of fibro-osseous lesions. The classification proposed by Waldron in 1993 categorized FOLs into three groups i) fibrous dysplasia, ii) reactive dysplastic lesions and iii) fibro-osseous neoplasms. Cemento-osseous dysplasias (CODs) are categorized as reactive or dysplastic FOLs that occur in the tooth-bearing area of the jaws and are presumably of periodontal ligament origin or of unknown aetiology. According to the fifth edition of the World Health Organisation (WHO) Classification of Tumours, benign fibro-osseous lesions in the oral and maxillofacial region broadly includes (1) fibrous dysplasia, (2) cemento-osseous dysplasias, (3) segmental odontomaxillary dysplasia, (4) fibro-osseous neoplasms; juvenile trabecular ossifying fibroma and psammomatoid ossifying fibroma and (5) familial gigantiform cementoma.

CODs are classified into three variants primarily on the basis of their anatomical location. PCOD is associated with the apical areas of the mandibular anterior teeth while focal cemento-osseous dysplasia (FocCOD) is associated with a single tooth. Florid cemento-osseous dysplasia (FCOD) manifests multifocal involvement usually involving multiple quadrants. CODs are more commonly seen in middle-aged African American females and women of Asian descent. CODs occur sporadically in the tooth-bearing area of the jaws. Familial occurrence has been reported. Familial cases unlike non-hereditary cases do not occur in middle-aged African females and Asian women. Familial inheritance is generally seen in FCOD. PCODs typically present as well-defined, radiolucent, and mixed radiolucent to radiopaque or a radiopaque lesion associated with single or multiple mandibular anterior teeth that are vital.

Diagnosis of PCOD is usually incidental when radiographs are taken for other reasons as they are usually asymptomatic. PCOD has been traditionally described as progressing through three distinct radiological and histological stages. The osteolytic stage represents the early stage of PCOD which is characterized by well-defined radiolucencies surrounding the root apex of one or more mandibular anterior teeth. This stage of PCOD poses a diagnostic challenge to clinicians as they are frequently misdiagnosed as periapical inflammatory lesions of pulpal origin leading to unnecessary endodontic treatment. Histologically the osteolytic stage is primarily composed of cellular connective tissue containing mineralized structures that replace the normal trabecular bone. The mineralized structures are of insufficient size to be demonstrated radiographically accounting for the well-defined radiolucent appearance at this stage. The osteolytic phase is followed by the cementoblastic stage and is signified by the presence of radiolucent areas containing nodular radiopaque deposits. A mixture of spherical calcifications and irregularly shaped deposits of osteoid and bone in a cellular connective tissue constitutes the salient histopathological features seen in this stage. In the mature or late stage, the typical radiographic appearance includes well-defined, dense radiopacities usually surrounded by a radiolucent rim. In this stage, the lesional tissue is primarily composed of spherical calcifications and mineralized bone with a paucity of connective tissue.

FocCOD develops in relation to a single tooth with vital pulp, in the region of extractions or an edentulous area in the molar region. They are usually diagnosed only on radiographs and presents as a radiolucent or mixed radiolucent to radiopaque lesion. They occur more commonly in women in the fourth and fifth decades of life. FocCOD rarely causes expansion of the bone and is an important feature that distinguishes it from COF.

FCOD involves both the maxilla and the mandible affecting multiple quadrants synchronously where it causes expansion of the bone. The affected patients are symptomatic and complain of pain and paresthesia. FCOD can compromise the blood supply of the affected bone as it replaces the normal bone structure with fibrous tissue containing mineralized structures. This predisposes the patient to increased risk of infections such as chronic osteomyelitis following surgical interventions like tooth extraction, biopsy and implant placement in the affected area. FCOD can arise as a familial disease and is inherited as an autosomal dominant trait.

The histological characteristics of all the distinct types of COD are identical. They are non-encapsulated and consist of cellular and vascular fibrotic tissue with calcified structures composed of spherical calcifications and irregularly shaped deposits of osteoid and mineralized bone. As the lesion matures, it is composed primarily of coalesced spherical calcifications and sclerotic mineralized bone with scant connective tissue. CODs have been found to be associated with simple bone cysts (SBCs) in a minority of cases. SBC is a pseudocyst as it lacks an epithelial lining and is surrounded by a hard bony wall. The cystic cavity may either be empty or may contain fluid. They tend to be solitary and are found within the marrow spaces not confined to the tooth-bearing areas. More than half of all SBCs are found to be associated with a traumatic event. Development of cystic lesions in CODs is currently labelled as haemorrhagic cystic degeneration rather than true SBCs or aneurysmal bone cysts. CODs can become secondarily infected as they are located close to the apices of the teeth. This may follow a periapical or periodontal infection involving the teeth affected with COD. The infected calcified masses within the COD are prone to necrosis. Cases with necrosis cannot be successfully treated with the administration of antibiotics alone because of the ensuing foreign body reaction to the dead tissues and will require surgical intervention.

PCOD is a self-limiting disease. Diagnosis is primarily based on characteristic radiographic findings of well-defined radiopacities surrounded by a radiolucent halo confined to the periapical regions of the anterior mandibular teeth. Surgical intervention is recommended only for symptomatic cases. Unnecessary surgical intervention may precipitate secondary infection and necrosis within the calcified deposits in the lesion leading to osteomyelitis. Asymptomatic cases which are diagnosed on routine radiographic investigations for other reasons should be kept on long-term follow-up as PCOD and FocCOD could in fact be an early or unifocal manifestation of FCOD. However, a PCOD or FocCOD does not transform into an FCOD.

Salient Features of Periapical Cemento-osseous Dysplasia	
Clinical features	Predilection for middle-aged black females Painless, non-expansile lesions located in the anterior mandible
Radiological features	One or more circumscribed lesions usually 0.5 cm or less in the periapical areas of vital teeth Radiolucent, radiopaque, or mixed radiolucent to radiopaque appearance with a radiolucent rim
Histopathological features	Cellular fibrous stroma containing mineralized tissues consisting of osteoid, bone and cementum-like material. Pronounced vascularity with areas of haemorrhage within the lesion
Treatment	No active treatment Long term follow-up

Diagnostic Algorithm

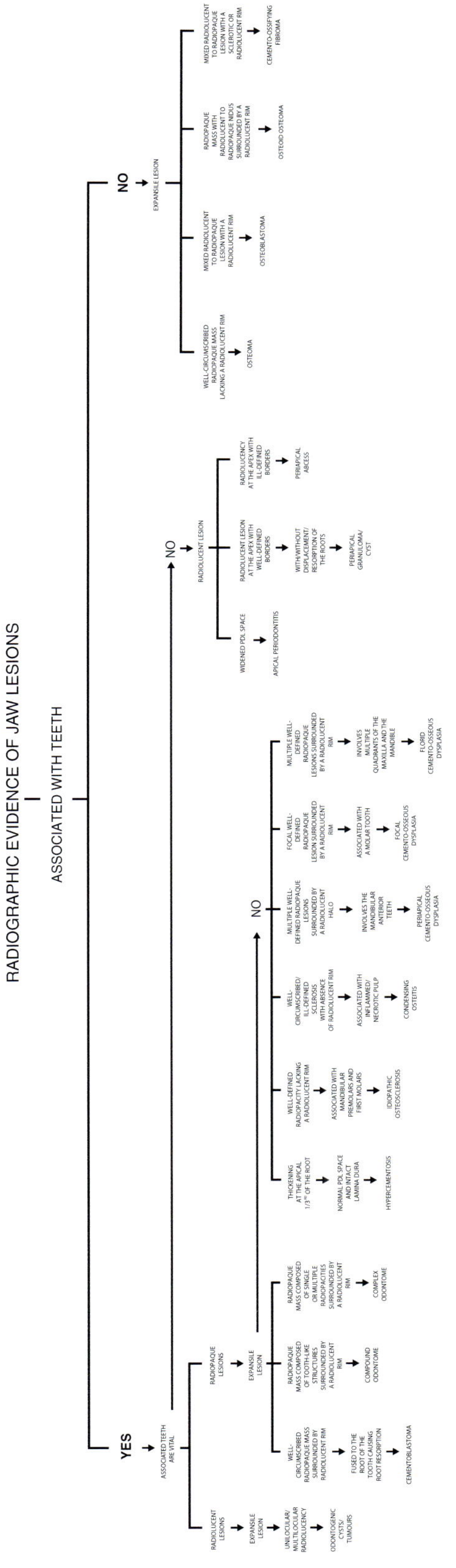

Self-Assessment Questions

1. Describe the pathognomonic clinical and radiological features of PCOD.
2. Classify CODs.
3. Discuss the differential diagnoses for PCOD.
4. Describe the histopathological features of PCOD.
5. Discuss the management of PCOD.

Summary

Periapical cemento-osseous dysplasia (PCOD) is an uncommon type of fibro-osseous lesion (FOL) that affects the anterior mandible in middle-aged women. The affected patients are usually asymptomatic but can present with vague pain or discomfort involving the affected area. Radiographic investigations are essential to establish a definitive diagnosis. PCOD arises from the periodontal ligament and affects the tooth-bearing, cancellous areas of the jaw bones. PCOD is associated with vital teeth and rarely manifests any significant clinical symptoms. Majority of these cases are accidentally diagnosed during radiographic examination which is ordered for other reasons. PCOD manifests radiographically as a radiolucent, radiopaque or a mixed lesion. In the early stages, a PCOD may mimic a periapical granuloma or a cyst. The characteristic radiographic appearance is the presence of calcifications within a radiolucent lesion that involves multiple vital teeth. PCOD is a self-limiting disease. Diagnosis is primarily based on characteristic radiographic findings of well-defined radiopacities surrounded by a radiolucent halo confined to the periapical regions of the anterior mandibular teeth. Surgical intervention is recommended only for symptomatic cases. Unnecessary surgical intervention may precipitate secondary infection and necrosis within the calcified deposits in the lesion leading to osteomyelitis.

Further Reading

Brody A, Zalatnai A, Csomo K, Belik A, Dobo-Nagy C. Difficulties in the diagnosis of periapical translucencies and in the classification of cemento-osseous dysplasia. BMC Oral Health. 2019;19(1):1–8.

Cawson RA, Odell EW. Cawson's essentials of oral pathology and oral medicine e-book. Elsevier Health Sciences; 2017.

Kawai T, Hiranuma H, Kishino M, Jikko A, Sakuda M. Cemento-osseous dysplasia of the jaws in 54 Japanese patients: a radiographic study. Oral Surg Oral Med Oral Pathol Oral Radiol Endodontol. 1999;87(1):107–14.

Neville BW, Damm DD, Allen C, Chi AC. Oral and maxillofacial pathology. Elsevier Health Sciences; 2015.

Ogunsalu CO, Lewis A, Doonquah L. Benign fibro-osseous lesions of the jaw bones in Jamaica: analysis of 32 cases. Oral Dis. 2001;7(3):155–62.

Sivapathasundharam B. Shafer's textbook of oral pathology-e book. Elsevier Health Sciences; 2016.

Warnakulasuriya S, Tilakaratna WM, editors. Oral medicine & pathology: a guide to diagnosis and management. JP Medical Ltd.; 2013.

16

Multiple Radiopaque Masses in the Lower Jaw: Florid Cemento-Osseous Dysplasia

Thomas George Kallarakkal and Wei Cheong Ngeow

Contents

W. M Tilakaratne, T. G. Kallarakkal (eds.), *Clinicopathological Correlation of Oral Diseases*,
https://doi.org/10.1007/978-3-031-24408-7_17

17.1 Main Complaint

A 55-year-old female patient was referred to the oral surgery specialist clinic by her general dentist for an incidental finding of multiple radiopacities involving her lower jaw bilaterally.

17.2 History of Complaint

Question: When did your dentist notice the abnormal radiographic findings?

I was informed about the abnormal radiographic findings when I went for my dental treatment 3 months ago.

Question: What kind of dental treatment did you undergo previously?

I had a few of my upper and lower teeth extracted due to dental caries many years ago. I underwent root canal treatment for two of my upper and lower right posterior teeth. I also had a fixed denture done to replace my missing anterior teeth.

17.3 Additional Complaints

Question: Do you have any pain or tenderness in your lower jaw?

I don't have any pain in my lower jaw at present. I also have not felt any tenderness upon touching my lower jaw. Previously I experienced pain in my lower jaw on the right and left side when taking hot, cold, and sweet food. My dentist extracted my lower right and left posterior teeth as they had extensive caries and could not be salvaged.

Question: Do you have any pain in other areas of the body such as your thighs, waist, and back?

I have never experienced any severe pain involving other areas of my body. I am currently taking calcium and vitamin D supplements as directed by my physician.

Question: Have you had any bone fractures?

I fractured my arm when I was in secondary school due to a fall during a basketball match. I have not suffered any fractures since then.

Question: Do you have any history of trauma to your face?

I have not suffered from any trauma involving my facial region.

Question: Have you noticed any swelling on your face or in the mouth in relation to your upper or lower jaws?

I have not observed any swelling on my face or in my mouth in relation to my upper and lower jaws.

Question: Do you have any swellings in other parts of the body?

I have not noticed any swellings in other parts of my body.

Question: Do you feel that your face is asymmetrical?

I have never noticed any facial asymmetry.

Question: Do you experience any foul discharge or an unpleasant taste in your mouth?

I have not felt any foul discharge or unpleasant taste in my mouth.

Question: Do you have any difficulty in opening your mouth?

I don't have any difficulty in opening my mouth wide.

Question: Do you have any abnormal sensations over the face or in the mouth in relation to your upper or lower jaws?

I do not have any abnormal sensations such as numbness or tingling sensation on my gums or my face.

Question: Have you noticed any symptoms such as progressive loss of vision, tinnitus, deafness, or epiphora?

I do not have any such symptoms.

Question: Have you been diagnosed with any skin lesions such as epidermoid cysts?

I have not been diagnosed with any skin lesions before.

Question: Have you noticed that your teeth have moved out of position recently?

I have not noticed any such changes. I can chew without any problem.

Question: Have you been experiencing any symptoms such as loss of appetite and loss of weight?

I do not have any such symptoms.

Question: Do you have any other medical problems like heart disease, high blood pressure, diabetes, bleeding disorder, renal diseases, gastrointestinal disorders, and respiratory diseases?

I don't have any medical problems. During my last annual health checkup, my low density cholesterol level (LDL) was border line high (142 mg/dL) while my high density cholesterol level (HDL) was border line low (54 mg/dL). My general physician advised me to exercise regularly and eat a healthy diet. However, I was not prescribed any medications.

Question: Are you taking any other medications?

I am not taking any medications other than the calcium and vitamin D supplements mentioned earlier.

Question: Have you undergone any surgery?

I have not had any surgery in the past.

Question: Does anybody in your family have a similar problem?

All my family members are fit and healthy.

Question: Do you have any risk habits such as smoking or drinking alcohol?

I am not a smoker or an alcohol drinker.

Question: Are you employed?

I am a house wife.

17.4 With the Findings From the History, What Is Your Differential Diagnosis?

1. Condensing osteitis (CO).
2. Idiopathic osteosclerosis (IO).
3. Florid cemento-osseous dysplasia (FCOD).
4. Chronic diffuse sclerosing osteomyelitis (CDSO).
5. Multiple osteomas associated with Gardner syndrome (GS).
6. Paget disease of bone.

17.5 How Do You Justify Your Differential Diagnosis After History Taking?

The patient is asymptomatic. She was referred by her general dentist for an incidental radiographic finding of bilateral multiple radiopacities involving her lower jaw.

Condensing osteitis (CO) also known as focal sclerosing osteomyelitis is characterized by the formation of periapical sclerotic bone consequent to an inflammatory stimulus or a local low-intensity trauma. They are usually asymptomatic or present with mild pain without any evidence of cortical bone expansion. On the radiograph they appear as focal well-circumscribed or ill-defined radiopaque lesions without a radiolucent halo associated with apices of teeth with inflamed or necrotic dental pulp, teeth with periodontal disease, previously restored teeth, or teeth undergoing occlusal trauma. They may be either single or multiple lesions most commonly affecting the mandibular premolar or molar teeth and are more commonly seen in children and young adults. The patient has a history of severe dental caries and extraction of multiple mandibular teeth. There are bilateral radiopaque lesions in the mandible without any noticeable facial swelling which supports the diagnosis of CO involving the mandible.

Idiopathic osteosclerosis (IO) of the jaws are asymptomatic lesions discovered incidentally on radiographs taken for other reasons. The lesions appear as well-defined radiopacities in the jaw bones that are round or elliptical in shape and not more than 3 mm in size. They are located above the mandibular canal associated with sound teeth, teeth with small restorations, or separated from teeth most commonly in the region of the mandibular first molars. IO is considered in the differential diagnosis in the present case as the patient was asymptomatic and the radiographic finding was discovered accidentally during the course of her dental treatment.

Florid cemento-osseous dysplasia (FCOD) is a benign fibro-osseous lesion that characteristically affects middle-aged black women aged above 45 years but may also occur in Caucasian and Asian women. FCOD is usually asymptomatic and is discovered on routine radiographs taken for other reasons. Occasionally the affected patients report a dull or intermittent aching sensation in the affected region. In severe cases, focal cortical expansion can occur secondary to infection. FCOD typically results in pagetoid (bottom to top) round or lobulated radiopaque masses often with a circumferential radiolucency restricted to the alveolar region. These radiopaque masses tend to be symmetrically distributed in multiple quadrants of the jaw with the mandible being affected more severely than the maxilla. A differential diagnosis of FCOD is considered in the present case as the patient is an elderly asymptomatic woman with an incidental finding of multiple radiopacities involving the mandible bilaterally.

Chronic diffuse sclerosing osteomyelitis (CDSO) is an inflammatory process that presents with clinical features of swelling and episodes of intermittent pain and tenderness. The pain and tenderness are associated with periods of exacerbation. It is always unilateral and confined to the mandible. CDSO has a protracted course that may last for a duration of up to 10 years. Radiographically CDSO appears as a poorly demarcated mixed radiopaque to radiolucent segment that involves the body of the mandible extending from the alveolus to the inferior border which may also involve the ramus. Subperiosteal bone formation may also be evident. The clinical features in the present case do not support a diagnosis of CDSO as the patient did not have any history of swelling, or pain and tenderness. However, an inflammatory disease process such as CDSO cannot be totally ruled out in view of the patient's history of multiple dental extractions of grossly decayed teeth.

Gardner syndrome (GS) is a hereditary disorder inherited as an autosomal dominant trait and complete penetrance with a locus on chromosome 5 (5q21–22). It represents one end of the spectrum of the disorder known as familial adenomatous polyposis (FAP). The clinical manifestations of GS include intestinal polyps which are predominantly adenomas that may occur in any part of the gastrointestinal tract and have 100% potential for malignant change. Other manifestations include osteomas, compound odontomes, supernumerary teeth, hypodontia, abnormal tooth morphology, impacted or unerupted teeth, multiple epidermoid cysts, and desmoid tumours. Multiple osteomas in GS commonly involve the mandible and may be classified as peripheral or central osteomas. Peripheral osteomas appear as a radiopaque often mushroom-shaped mass protruding from the surface of the jawbone. Central osteomas are not related to the teeth and manifest as a well-circumscribed radiopaque mass causing expansion of the bone and displacement of the teeth. A perilesional radiolucent halo is absent. The patient did not complain of any features suggestive of GS such as gastrointestinal symptoms, cutaneous lesions, or soft tissue swellings during history taking. However, multiple osteomas associated with GS are included in the differential diagnosis owing to the radiographic evidence of multiple radiopacities in her mandible.

Paget disease of bone (PDB) is a metabolic bone disease which rarely occurs in individuals before 40 years of age. Involvement of jaw bones is characterized by progressive enlargement of maxilla and mandible, widening of alveolar ridges, spacing between teeth, and flattening of the palate. The radiographic features include loss of lamina dura, hypercementosis, and calcified pulp chambers. Depending on the stage of bone remodeling, the radiographic appearance varies from a ground glass appearance during the early osteolytic stage to a "cotton wool" appearance during the osteoblastic stage. In the present case, the patient did not have any clinical features suggestive of PDB. However, for an elderly woman with multiple radiopacities involving the jaws, PDB should be included as a differential diagnosis.

17.6 Findings of Examination

Extra oral examination shows no abnormal findings. The skin of the face appears normal. The lips are competent and the face is symmetrical with no evidence of any facial swelling. There is no limitation in mouth opening and there are no enlarged lymph nodes in the neck. On intra oral examination, there are multiple missing teeth in all the four quadrants of the jaw and extensive restorations on multiple upper and lower teeth on the right side. There is a fixed partial denture extending from the right canine to the left canine on the maxillary arch. The oral hygiene is fair. A mild expansion of the cortical plates is seen in the left posterior body of the mandible.

17.7 What Other Relevant Features Would You Look for with the Findings You Have So Far?

There is no evidence of inflammation or infection involving the oral cavity. There are no draining sinuses or paresthesia involving her lower jaws.

17.8 What Is Your Clinical Differential Diagnosis?

1. Florid cemento-osseous dysplasia (FCOD).
2. Chronic diffuse sclerosing osteomyelitis (CDSO).
3. Multiple osteomas associated with Gardner syndrome (GS).
4. Paget disease of bone.

17.9 How Would You Justify the Inclusion of the Diseases That You Have Mentioned in the Differential Diagnosis to Arrive at a Working Diagnosis?

The patient has a mild bony swelling in relation to the left posterior body of the mandible. CO and IO are excluded from the differential diagnoses, as they do not produce any cortical expansion. The remaining clinical differential diagnosis is essentially the same as the diagnosis after history taking. Radiographic investigations are essential to narrow down the differential diagnosis.

17.10 What Is the Most Likely Diagnosis?

Florid cemento-osseous dysplasia (FCOD).
Paget disease of bone (PDB).

17.11 How Would You Investigate This Patient?

1. Dental panoramic tomograph (DPT) for a general full mouth survey.
2. Intraoral (periapical) radiographs to assess the relationship of the lesion with the teeth.
3. Cone beam computed tomography (CBCT) to determine the exact extent of the lesion and its internal architecture.
4. Serological investigations for PDB.

Biochemical markers of bone turnover
(Markers of bone formation)
- Total alkaline phosphatase (ALP).
- Bone-specific alkaline phosphatase (BSAP).
- Osteocalcin (OC).

17

(Markers of bone resorption)
- Hydroxyproline (Hyp).
- Pyridinoline (PYD).

An analogous increase in both of these markers confirms the association of bone formation and resorption seen in Paget disease.

A DPT revealed multiple sclerotic masses in the upper and lower jaws (Fig. 17.1). The sclerotic mass in the left posterior mandible appeared better defined with a peripheral radiolucent rim while the radiopacities in the right posterior mandible and the left upper maxilla appeared poorly defined with evidence of a radiolucent rim noticed only focally.

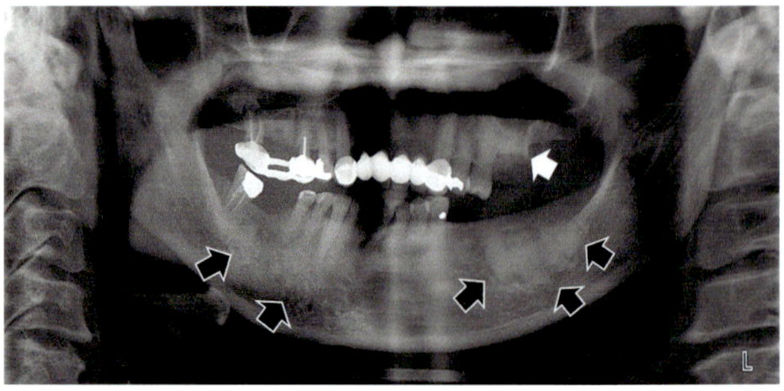

Fig. 17.1 Multiple dense sclerotic masses observed in the upper (white arrows) and lower jaws (black arrows). (Picture courtesy: Prof Dr Sumanth Kumbargere Nagraj, Faculty of Dentistry, Manipal University College Malaysia)

A characteristic feature of FCOD is its symmetrical distribution in multiple posterior quadrants of the mandible and less commonly the maxilla. The dense radiopaque masses in FCOD are usually limited to the alveolar processes and limited by a peripheral radiolucent rim. The radiographic features in the present case are consistent with a diagnosis of FCOD. CDSO was included in the differential diagnosis due to the patient's history of extensive dental caries and the possibility of an inflammatory process involving the jaws. A poorly demarcated mixed radiolucent and radiopaque lesion lacking a radiolucent rim with a periosteal reaction or external bone resorption is the typical radiographic manifestation of CDSO. In the present case, the lesions are confined to the alveolar process and involve multiple quadrants which is characteristic of FCOD. There is also no evidence of periosteal bone reaction. Multiple central osteomas, a feature of GS, are not restricted to the alveolar process and manifest as well-circumscribed radiopaque masses causing expansion of the bone and displacement of the teeth. A perilesional radiolucent halo is absent. PDB is characterized by a ground glass or a "cotton wool" appearance depending on the stage of bone remodeling. In addition, features such as loss of lamina dura and hypercementosis involving the teeth in the affected area of the jaws are noticed. The radiographic features do not support a diagnosis of PDB in the present case. Nevertheless, it is optimal to investigate further to rule out PDB owing to the evolving nature of the disease.

The results of the serological investigations were within the normal limits thus excluding the diagnosis of PDB.

17.12 Would You Do an Incisional Biopsy for This Patient? What Are the Important Considerations?

A diagnosis of FCOD relies primarily on correlation of clinical and radiographic features alone. Histological features alone are not conclusive. A biopsy is not recommended in asymptomatic patients with typical radiographic features such as symmetrical radiopaque masses in multiple quadrants as seen in the present case. Elective procedures including biopsies for histopathological analyses are not indicated due to the risk of secondary infection.

17.13 What Are the Histopathological Features That Help in the Diagnosis?

The histologic features of FCOD are indistinguishable from a cemento-ossifying fibroma and to some extent from other fibro-osseous lesions. Histologically, FCOD is characterized by calcified deposits within a cellular stroma. This stroma can vary from slightly myxoid to densely collagenous. The calcifications are of irregular shape which are variably sized and consist of bony trabeculae with osteocytes or acellular cementum-like tissue. The bony trabeculae are rimmed by plump osteoblasts in focal areas. Areas of resorption with multinucleated osteoclasts are also seen. Mature lesions are relatively avascular and are composed of dense masses of cementum and bone (◘ Fig. 17.2).

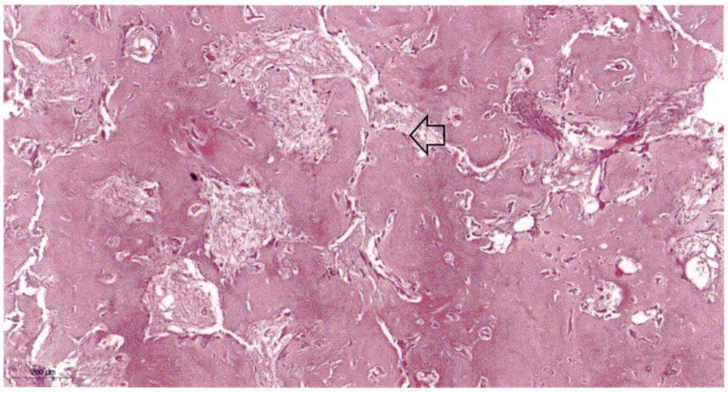

◘ **Fig. 17.2** Bony trabeculae rimmed by osteoblasts (arrows) in a fibrocellular stroma

17.14 What Is the Final Diagnosis?

Florid cemento-osseous dysplasia.

17.15 How Would You Manage This Patient?

The treatment of FCOD is continuous observation using imaging modalities. Surgical treatment is not advisable unless symptomatic. Owing to the avascular nature of this lesion, antibiotics alone may not be sufficient and surgical debridement and sequestrectomy may be required when treating symptomatic cases.

17.16 Florid Cemento-osseous Dysplasia (FCOD)

Florid cemento-osseous dysplasia (FCOD) is a fibro-osseous lesion (FOL) in which the normal bone is replaced by fibrous connective tissue containing varying amounts of mineralized material. The mineralized component is composed of variable amounts of osteoid, bone, or cementum-like tissue. FOLs include (i) fibrous dysplasia; (ii) cemento-osseous dysplasias; (iii) segmental odontomaxillary dysplasia; (iv) fibro-osseous neoplasms; juvenile trabecular ossifying fibroma, and psammomatoid ossifying fibroma; and (v) familial gigantiform cementoma (◘ Table 17.1). Cemento-

◘ **Table 17.1** Classification of benign fibro-osseous lesions

Fibrous dysplasia
Fibrous dysplasia (monostotic, polyostotic, or syndromic)
Craniofacial fibrous dysplasia
Reactive dysplastic lesions (cemento-osseous dysplasias)
Acquired origin (non-hereditary)
Periapical cemento-osseous dysplasia
Focal cemento-osseous dysplasia
Florid cemento-osseous dysplasia
Hereditary origin
Familial gigantiform cementoma
Fibro-osseous neoplasms
Juvenile trabecular ossifying fibroma
Psammomatoid ossifying fibroma

osseous dysplasias (CODs) which include periapical cemento-osseous dysplasia (PCOD), focal cemento-osseous dysplasia (FocCOD), and florid cemento-osseous dysplasia (FCOD) are classified as reactive dysplastic lesions. CODs occur in the tooth-bearing area of the jaws and presumably arise from the periodontal ligament. The abnormal and disorganized tissue that replaces the normal bone in FCOD results in pagetoid globular osteosclerosis involving two or more quadrants of the jaws. In contrast, PCOD is associated with the apical areas of the mandibular anterior teeth while FocCOD is associated with a single tooth predominantly in the molar region. FCOD is strictly restricted to the alveolar process, in dentulous and edentulous jaws. It is not associated with any other bones in the skeleton.

FCOD often affects middle-aged African or Asian women. It is usually asymptomatic and is normally discovered as an incidental finding during radiologic examination. FCOD is usually symmetrically distributed in a bilateral fashion. The mandible is always affected, while the maxilla is affected in two-thirds of cases. Radiographically, FCOD classically presents as multiple, well-defined, sclerotic radiopaque masses with ill-defined borders. A peripheral radiolucent rim with a sclerotic border surrounds the radiopaque masses. These lesions may start as a small radiolucency or multiple small mixed radiolucent/radiopaque lesions, which coalesce to form large, irregularly shaped sclerotic masses. Expansion of the cortical plates can rarely occur in FCOD due to secondary infection. This may lead to pain and facial swelling. It is important to establish a differential diagnosis in instances when there is bone expansion as other jaw lesions can have a similar radiographic appearance as FCOD. These include familial gigantiform cementoma (FGC), Paget disease of bone (PDB), and fibrous dysplasia (FD).

FGC is a rare benign FOL of the jaws that has an autosomal dominant mode of inheritance and variable phenotype. It is more common in Asian patients. FGC has an early onset with multifocal or multiple quadrant involvement of the jaws. The lesions are progressive and expansive reaching massive proportions causing significant facial deformity. Extensive, well-circumscribed, mixed radiolucent-radiopaque masses surrounded by a peripheral radiolucent rim involving the maxilla and mandible signify the radiographic appearance of FGC.

PDB is predominantly found in Caucasians with the highest prevalence reported among the populations from Great Britain, Australia, and New Zealand. The prevalence of PDB doubles for every decade subsequent to the age of 50 years. The pathogenesis of PDB of jaws includes focal areas of increased bone remodeling leading to rapid bone resorption and excessive and disorganized bone formation. The disease can be confined to a single bone or involve multiple bones. The bones most commonly affected are lumbar vertebra, pelvis, skull, and femur. Jaw involvement is relatively rare and maxilla is affected more commonly than the mandible. The patients usually complain of a constant dull, aching type of pain. Other symptoms include paresthesia, abnormal gait, non-specific headache, impaired hearing, and tinnitus depending upon the bones involved. The involved bones become enlarged, thickened, and weak with increased susceptibility to bowing deformity and fractures. When the jaws are involved, there is progressive enlargement of the maxilla and mandible. The radiographic appearance varies from a ground glass appearance to a "cotton wool" appearance involving multiple quadrants of the jaws depending on the stage of the disease (Fig. 17.3).

The histopathological features of FCOD are not unique and do not differ from other FOLs including periapical cemento-osseous dysplasia (PCOD), focal cemeto-osseous dysplasia (FocCOD), cemento-ossifying fibroma (COF), and fibrous dysplasia (FD). All these FOLs are characterized by replacement of normal bone architecture with a benign fibrous tissue matrix that contains varying degrees of mineralization in the form of woven bone or cementum-like round acellular, basophilic structures. A diagnosis of FCOD cannot be made based on the histological features alone, and in the absence of adequate clinical and radiological information, a pathologist can only suggest that the features in the given biopsy are consistent with a benign FOL. Clinico-pathological correlation is a must in order to arrive at the definitive diagnosis of fibro-osseous lesions (Fig. 17.4).

FCOD may persist indefinitely without any symptoms. Oral prophylaxis is of utmost importance, with

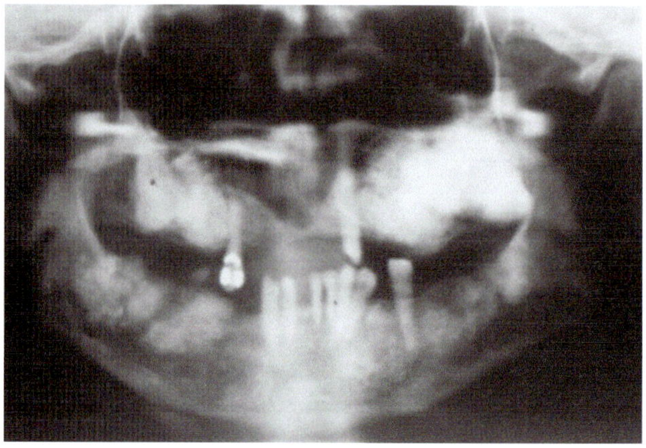

Fig. 17.3 A cotton wool appearance involving all the quadrants of the jaws

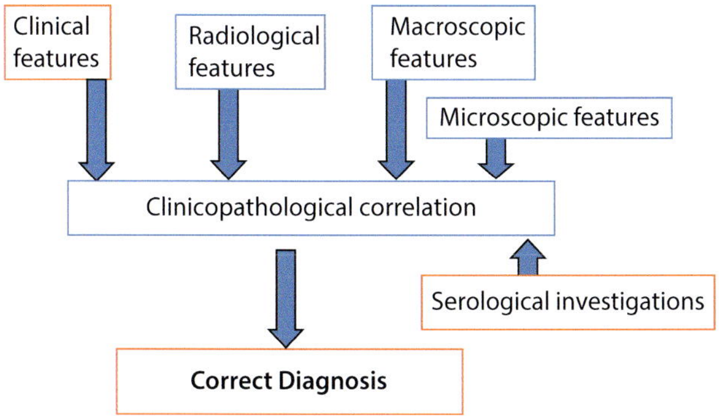

Fig. 17.4 A scheme of work-up for diagnosis of fibro-osseous lesions

stress on the control of periodontal disease and the prevention of tooth loss. The management of FCOD can become complicated and unsatisfactory in symptomatic patients, the most common symptom being dull pain. Surgical intervention is indicated in patients with severe symptoms but they are at risk for secondary infection and osteomyelitis. Exposure of the sclerotic masses into the oral environment can also occur secondary to alveolar ridge atrophy, advanced periodontal disease, odontogenic infections, or following dental extractions. The exposed poorly vascularized bone is highly susceptible to osteomyelitis. Treatment with antibiotics is always not satisfactory as the tissue perfusion by the drug is poor due to its relatively avascular nature. In the absence of any clinical symptoms, it is recommended to keep the patient on regular follow-up with periodic radiographic evaluation to detect any changes.

Salient features of florid osseous dysplasia	
Clinical features	Primarily seen in middle-aged African but also in middle- to older-aged Caucasian and Asian women Female to male ratio is 2.6:1 Involvement of jaw bones, with bilateral symmetrical occurrence Extensive involvement of all the four quadrants The adjacent teeth remain vital
Radiological features	Multiple, well-defined, sclerotic radiopaque masses with ill-defined borders A peripheral radiolucent rim with a sclerotic border surrounds the radiopaque masses Cortical expansion or displacement of the inferior alveolar nerve can occur with an expansive lesion
Histopathological features	Calcified deposits within a cellular stroma The stroma can vary from slightly myxoid to densely collagenous The calcifications are of irregular shape and variably sized and consist of bony trabeculae with osteocytes or acellular cementum-like tissue. Vascularity is lost in mature lesions
Treatment	Continuous radiographic observation (2–3 years) with no surgical intervention Biopsy is indicated only when the radiographic findings are suggestive of rapid bone changes in order to avoid complication from its poor healing capacity

▪ Diagnostic Algorithm

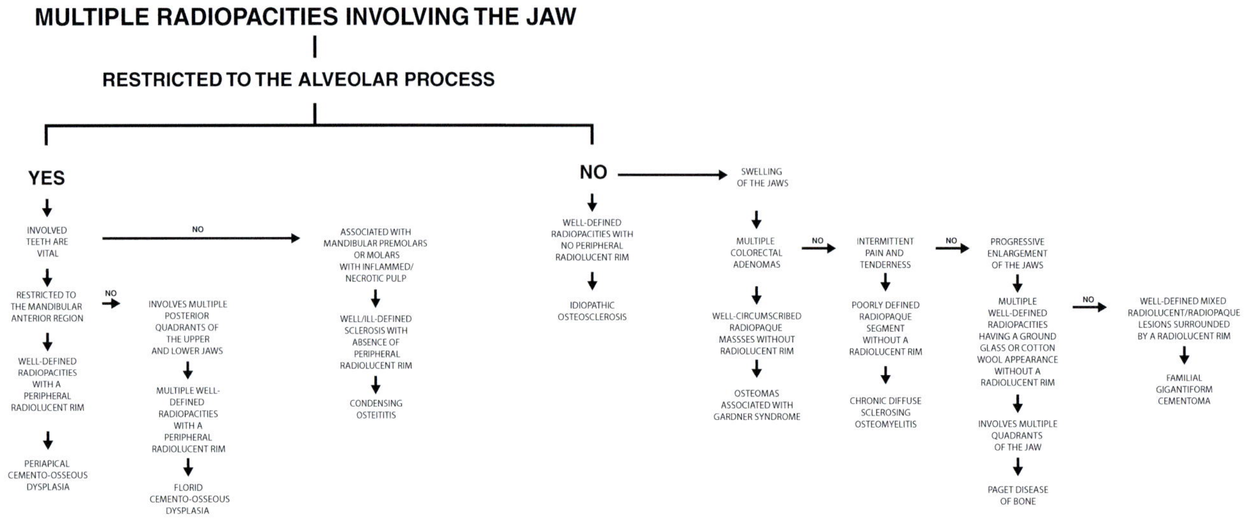

Self-Assessment Questions

1. List the clinical features of FCOD.
2. Describe the pathognomonic radiological features of FCOD.
3. Discuss the differential diagnoses for FCOD.
4. Explain the histopathological features of FCOD.
5. Describe the treatment plan for patients with FCOD.

Summary

Florid cemento-osseous dysplasia (FCOD) is a benign fibro-osseous lesion that characteristically affects middle-aged black women aged above 45 years but may also occur in Caucasian and Asian women. FCOD is usually asymptomatic and is discovered on routine radiographs taken for other reasons. Occasionally the affected patients report a dull or intermittent aching sensation in the affected region. In severe cases, focal cortical expansion can occur secondary to infection. FCOD typically results in pagetoid (bottom to top) round or lobulated radiopaque masses often with a circumferential radiolucency restricted to the alveolar region. These radiopaque masses tend to be symmetrically distributed in multiple quadrants of the jaw with the mandible being affected more severely than the maxilla. The management of FCOD can become complicated and unsatisfactory in symptomatic patients, the most common symptom being dull pain. Surgical intervention is indicated in patients with severe symptoms but they are at risk for secondary infection and osteomyelitis. Exposure of the sclerotic masses into the oral environment can also occur secondary to alveolar ridge atrophy, advanced periodontal disease, odontogenic infections, or following dental extractions. The exposed poorly vascularized bone is highly susceptible to osteomyelitis. Treatment with antibiotics is always not satisfactory as the tissue perfusion by the drug is poor due to its relatively avascular nature. In the absence of any clinical symptoms, it is recommended to keep the patient on regular follow-up with periodic radiographic evaluation to detect any changes.

Further Reading

Cawson RA, Odell EW. Cawson's essentials of oral pathology and oral medicine e-book. Elsevier Health Sciences; 2017.

de Santana Sarmento DJ, de Brito Monteiro BV, de Medeiros AMC, da Silveira EJD. Severe florid cemento-osseous dysplasia: a case report treated conservatively and literature review. Oral and Maxillofacial Surgery. 2013;17(1):43–6.

Delai D, Bernardi A, Felippe GS, da Silveira Teixeira C, Felippe WT, Felippe MCS. Florid cemento-osseous dysplasia: a case of misdiagnosis. Journal of Endodontics. 2015;41(11):1923–6.

Jerjes W, Banu B, Swinson B, Hopper C. Florid cemento-osseous dysplasia in a young Indian woman. A case report. British Dental Journal. 2005;198(8):477–8.

Musella AE, Slater LJ. Familial florid osseous dysplasia: a case report. Journal of Oral and Maxillofacial Surgery. 1989;47(6):636–40.

Neville BW, Damm DD, Allen C, Chi AC. Oral and maxillofacial pathology. Elsevier Health Sciences; 2015.

Sivapathasundharam B. Shafer's textbook of oral pathology-E book. Elsevier Health Sciences; 2016.

Warnakulasuriya S, Tilakaratna WM, editors. Oral medicine & pathology: a guide to diagnosis and management. JP Medical Ltd; 2013.

Reactive Lesions and Benign Tumours of the Oral Mucosa

Contents

Painless Nodule on the Cheek: Fibroepithelial Polyp

Zakiah Mat Ripen and Nurul Izyan Zainuddin

Contents

W. M Tilakaratne, T. G. Kallarakkal (eds.), *Clinicopathological Correlation of Oral Diseases*,
https://doi.org/10.1007/978-3-031-24408-7_18

Learning Goals

1. Devise the correct way of compiling the history with appropriate questions.
2. Develop a differential diagnosis after history taking.
3. Deduce appropriate procedures in clinical examination.
4. Formulate a differential diagnosis combining findings in the history and clinical examination.
5. Justify the relevant investigations required to arrive at the diagnosis.
6. Comprehend the importance of clinicopathological correlation in arriving at the correct diagnosis.
7. Outline the management plan.
8. Recognize the importance of a diagnostic algorithm in arriving at a diagnosis.

18.1 Main Complaint

A 50-year-old female patient presented to the clinic with a complaint of growth on her left cheek.

18.2 History of Complaint

Question: How long since have you noticed this growth?

I have noticed this growth for more than 5 years.

Question: Did you notice any increase in its size?

It started as a small nodule and lately I realized that it is very slowly increasing in size.

18.3 Additional Complaints

Question: Was there any history of trauma to the region?

I do not recall any such event.

Question: Is the growth causing any pain?

The growth does not cause any pain. However, when I accidentally bite on the lesion, it ulcerates leading to mild pain.

Question: Were there any episodes of bleeding or any other fluid discharge from the growth?

I cannot recall any fluid discharge or bleeding from the growth.

Question: Is the growth disturbing your normal function?

I do not have any pain or bleeding associated with the growth. It disturbs me while I chew as I accidentally bite on the growth.

Question: Were there any similar growths in the oral cavity earlier?

I do not have any previous history of similar lesions.

Question: Have you undergone any dental treatment before?

I am not a regular dental attendee. I have had extractions and restorations done previously without complications.

Question: Do you have any medical problems?

I do not have any medical illnesses. I am not allergic to any medications.

Question: Have you undergone any surgery?

I do not have any previous history of surgery or hospital admission.

Question: What is your occupation?

I am a housewife.

Question: Do you have habits of smoking, betel quid chewing, or taking alcohol?

I do not have any habit of betel quid chewing, smoking cigarettes, or drinking alcohol.

18.4 What Is Your Differential Diagnosis After History Taking?

- Fibroepithelial polyp (FEP)
- Benign tumours including salivary gland tumour
- Squamous cell papilloma
- Mucocele

18.5 How Do You Justify Your Differential Diagnosis After History Taking?

18.5.1 Fibroepithelial Polyp (FEP)

The nature of the nodule is of a chronic lesion that becomes symptomatic when it is traumatized. There was no fluid discharge from the lesion. The lesion remained the same without any increase in size for a long time suggesting that it could be a benign lesion. FEP is a common oral lesion that occurs on the buccal mucosa, tongue, or gingiva.

18.5.2 Squamous Cell Papilloma

Squamous cell papilloma presents as a small, slowly growing lesion, with no pain unless secondary to trauma.

18.5.3 Mucocele

A mucocele arises as a result of trauma to the minor salivary glands located in the buccal mucosa. However, if it is due to minor trauma, the patient may not be able to recall the incident. The patient will usually recall a history of rupture of the lesion with a clear salty discharge followed by recurrence of the lesion.

18.5.4 Benign Tumours Including Salivary Gland Tumour

Minor salivary glands are present within the submucosa in almost every part of the oral cavity. The history of an unremarkable slow-growing lesion on the buccal mucosa could possibly be due to a benign tumour arising from the minor salivary glands or soft tissues.

18

18.6 Findings of Clinical Examination

The lesion is located on the left buccal mucosa (Fig. 18.1). The size of the lesion is less than 1 cm. The overlying mucosa appears normal with a smooth surface and a focal area of increased keratinization. Upon palpation, the lesion is nontender and not fluctuant. There is no discharge from the lesion. The lesion is mobile and not attached to underlying structures. The location of the lesion coincides with the occlusal plane of the upper and lower teeth.

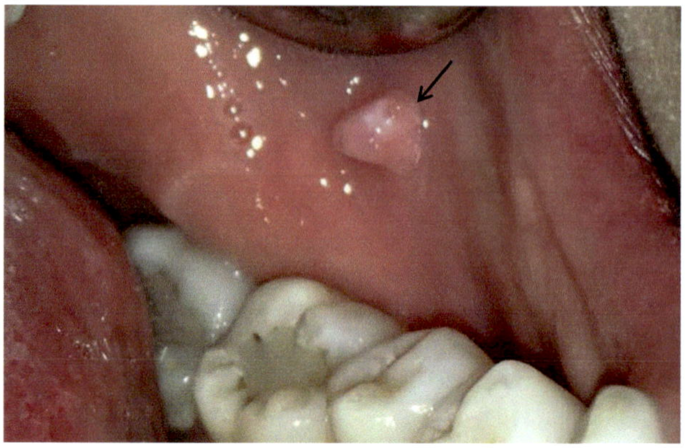

Fig. 18.1 Left buccal mucosa showing a lesion with overlying normal mucosa with a smooth surface and a focal keratotic surface (arrow)

18.7 What Is Your Clinical Differential Diagnoses?

1. Fibroepithelial polyp
2. Enlarged papilla of the parotid duct
3. Squamous cell papilloma
4. Mucocele
5. Benign tumours including salivary gland tumours

18.8 How Do You Justify the Inclusion of the Diseases That You Have Mentioned in the Differential Diagnosis to Arrive at a Working Diagnosis?

18.8.1 Fibroepithelial Polyp

It is a common oral lesion that occurs on the buccal mucosa, tongue, or gingiva. It is a reactive lesion that usually arises in response to chronic irritation such as sharp edges of the tooth, restorations, or prosthesis. Clinically it is painless unless preceded by trauma. The overlying mucosa is normal in colour. The clinical presentation of an exophytic lesion that is of normal mucosal colour and along the occlusal plane of the upper and lower teeth is highly suggestive of a reactive lesion such as FEP.

18.8.2 Squamous Cell Papilloma

A squamous cell papilloma presents as a small, slow-growing lesion, with no pain unless secondary to trauma. The lesion is pedunculated with numerous finger-like projections. Depending on the keratin build-up around the lesion, the projections may appear long and pointed or short and rounded. Heavily keratinized lesions appear white, while less keratinized lesions appear pink or red with a raspberry-like appearance. The absence of pointed or short and rounded projections on the surface of the lesion in this patient precludes the diagnosis of a squamous cell papilloma.

18.8.3 Enlarged Papilla of the Parotid Duct

The lesion is small in size with a normal mucosal appearance that might mimic the papilla of the parotid duct. The papilla of the parotid duct is a small elevation where the parotid duct opens into the oral cavity next to the maxillary second molar tooth. However, the lesion was not anatomically closely related to the opening of the Stenson's duct. In addition, the enlarged parotid papilla is usually associated with inflammatory signs.

18.8.4 Mucocele

A mucocele arises as a result of trauma to the minor salivary glands located in the buccal mucosa. The patients will recall a history of rupture of the lesion with a clear salty discharge followed by recurrence of the lesion. The clinical appearance of the lesion is dome-shaped and appears translucent or bluish. Upon palpation, it is fluctuant and nontender. The absence of the above features in this lesion eliminates the diagnosis of a mucocele.

18.8.5 Benign Tumours Including Salivary Gland Tumours

Although reactive lesions like an FEP tend to occur more commonly, the possibility of a benign tumour arising from the soft tissue or minor salivary glands cannot be excluded from the clinical findings. This is because benign tumours arising from the soft tissues or minor salivary glands can also present clinically as a slow-growing and mostly submucosal nodule and therefore requires excisional biopsy and histopathological findings for a definitive diagnosis. However, the clinical presentation of a small exophytic lesion as seen in this patient is unlikely to be a benign tumour but more consistent to be a reactive lesion.

18.9 What Is the Most Likely Diagnosis?

Fibroepithelial polyp

18.10 How Would You Investigate This Patient?

A thorough clinical examination should be carried out to eliminate any possible causes of trauma such as:
- Sharp tooth edges
- Faulty restorations
- Ill-fitting dentures
- Malocclusion
- Evidence of chronic cheek biting

18.11 How do You Confirm the Diagnosis for This Lesion?

The lesion is small and there are no features to suggest malignancy. Hence an excisional biopsy should be performed to arrive at the definitive diagnosis.

18.12 What Specific Findings Help You to Arrive at the Diagnosis (History, Clinical Findings and Investigations)?

The lesion is reported to be slow growing and asymptomatic. Clinically, the lesion is sessile and located along the occlusal plane of the upper and lower teeth indicating a possibility of trauma. There is no discharge or bleeding from the lesion.

The histopathological features of the lesion show a mucosal nodule containing dense coarse collagen fibres covered by parakeratinized stratified squamous epithelium (◘ Fig. 18.2). The corium contains little to no inflammatory cells (◘ Fig. 18.3).

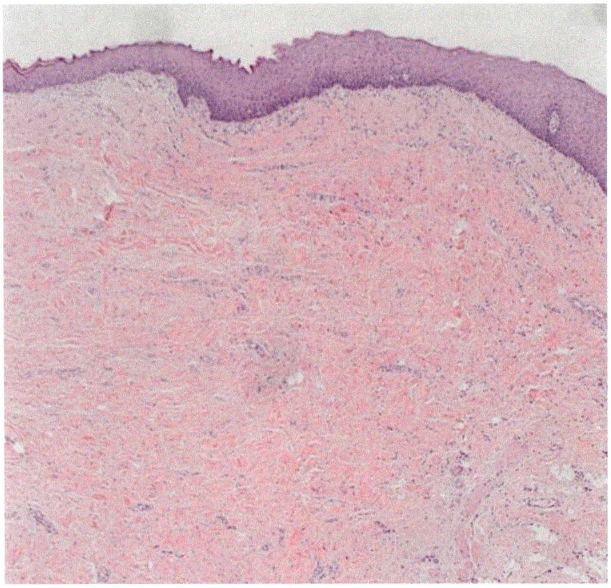

Fig. 18.2 Mucosa containing densely packed collagen fibres covered by parakeratinized stratified squamous epithelium of variable thickness

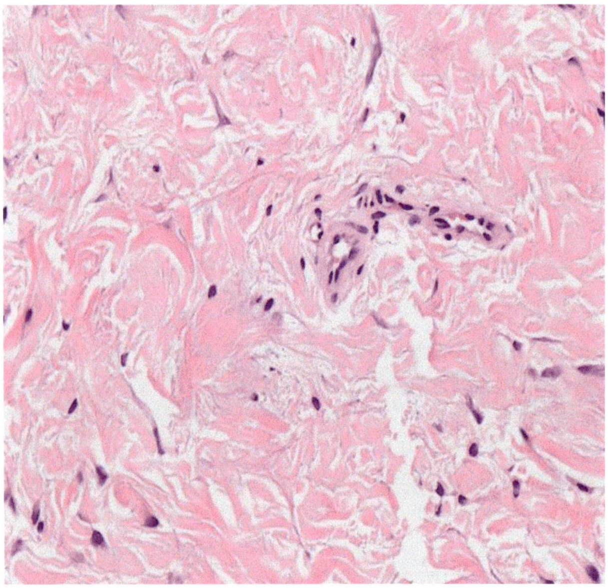

Fig. 18.3 Higher magnification shows the corium containing coarse collagen fibres with sparse inflammatory cell infiltrate

18.13 What Is Your Definitive Diagnosis?

Fibroepithelial polyp

18.14 What Is the Treatment?

Surgical excision of the lesion and removal of the source of trauma/friction is the treatment of choice. Surgical excision is necessary to prevent further functional disturbance. It can also prevent continuous trauma/irritation to the lesion as the patient tends to accidentally bite on the lesion. Removal of the source of trauma/friction can prevent recurrence of the lesion. Any small lesion that appears reactive or benign needs to be surgically excised for diagnostic and curative purposes.

18.15 Fibroepithelial Polyp

FEP is a reactive epithelial lesion of the oral cavity. It commonly occurs on the buccal mucosa, tongue and labial mucosa. Most of the time, it presents as a single, whitish to pink (similar colour as surrounding mucosa), painless growth that may be sessile or pedunculated. The size of the lesion may vary but most of them are within 0.5–1 cm. The lesion is firm in consistency.

FEP is a reactive lesion that arises in response to chronic irritation. It results from repeated cheek/lip biting, irregular denture borders, faulty restorations, sharp tooth edges or another oral prosthesis. Depending on the size and site of the lesion, it may disturb the patient's normal functions such as speech and mastication. The closest clinical differential diagnosis is a squamous cell papilloma. However, it has a characteristic papillomatous/verrucous surface. Another common differential diagnosis that should be included is an organizing mucocele due to the loss of its characteristic colour and texture thereby mimicking an FEP.

Histopathologically, it is a mucosal nodule covered by parakeratinized stratified squamous epithelium containing dense bundles of collagen. The cellularity may vary with some lesions.

Multiple FEPs can be a feature of Cowden syndrome, a rare inherited condition caused by a mutation in the PTEN tumour suppressor gene located on chromosome 10q23.31. It is characterized by several hamartomas in a variety of tissues arising from all three germ layers. The intraoral manifestations of Cowden syndrome usually show polyps on the gingiva and buccal mucosa. On occasions, they may coalesce showing a characteristic cobblestone appearance. As Cowden syndrome is associated with an increased risk of developing malignancies such as breast, thyroid and endometrial cancer, clinicians should be able to recognize this syndrome by performing genetic testing.

The treatment of choice is the surgical removal of the lesion. The chances for recurrence are less if the source of irritation is removed. Therefore, it is mandatory to look for any cause of trauma in the region and should be corrected accordingly.

Salient features of fibroepithelial polyp	
Clinical	Firm swelling on the mucosa. The colour of the lesion is very close to normal mucosa. It is usually not ulcerated unless traumatized. Does not bleed easily, and there is no fluid discharge. It is usually related to chronic local irritation
Histopathology	Corium containing dense collagen fibres covered by para-/ortho-keratinized stratified squamous epithelium
Treatment	Surgical removal of the lesion and removal of the source of irritation
This is a benign lesion. However, long-term irritation of the lesion may cause the growth to increase in size. A large FEP can disturb normal function of the patient.	

▪ Diagnostic and Management Algorithm for FEP

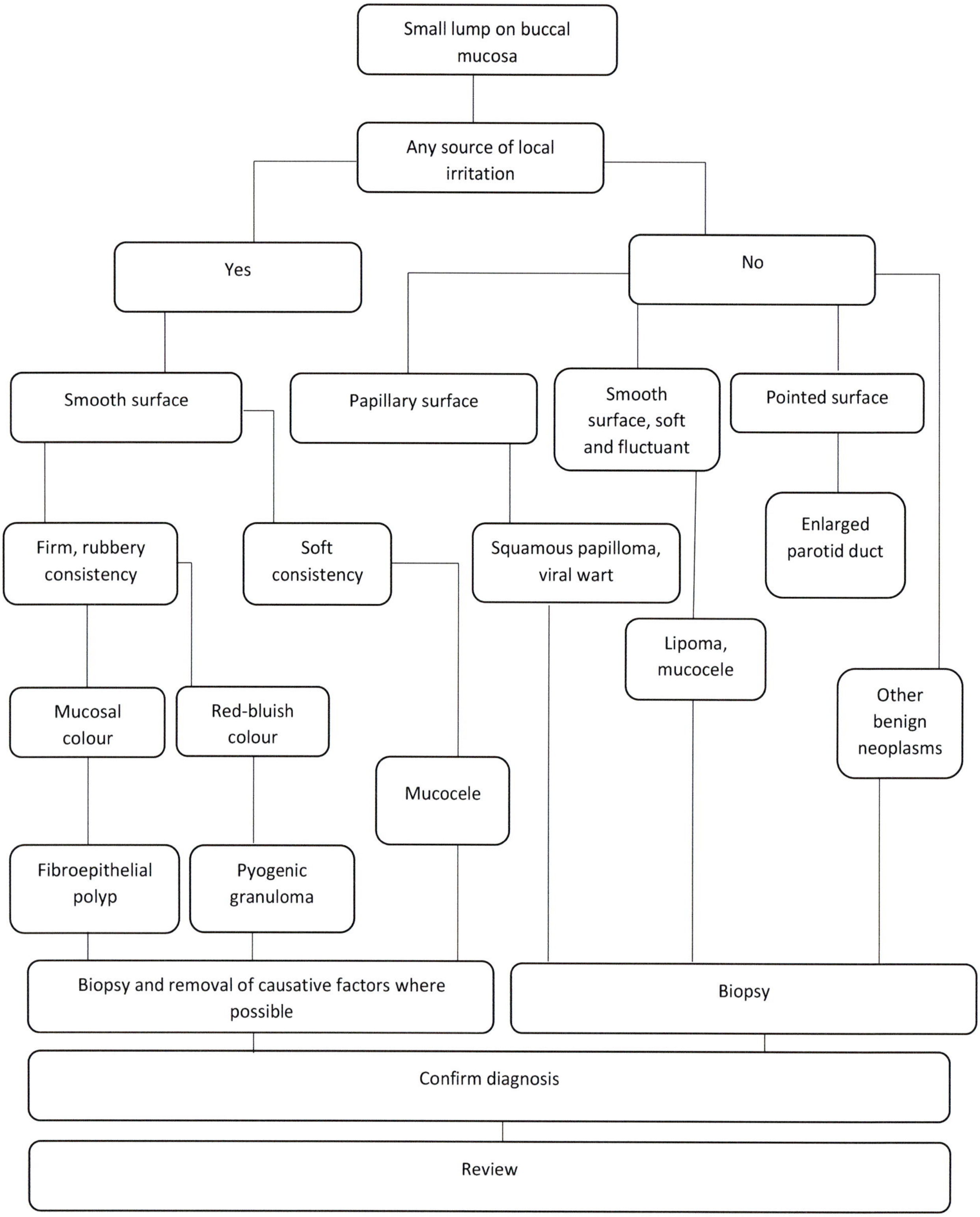

Self-Assessment Questions

1. Describe the important clinical features that will aid you in making the diagnosis of FEP.
2. Describe the histopathological features of FEP.
3. Describe the management plan for FEP.
4. Discuss the differential diagnosis for FEP.
5. Describe the features of the syndrome associated with multiple FEP.

Further Reading

Farooq A, Walker LJ, Bowling J, Audisio RA. Cowden syndrome. Cancer Treat Rev. 2010;36(8):577–83.

Mishra A, Pandey RK. Fibro-epithelial polyps in children: a report of two cases with a literature review. Intractable Rare Dis Res. 2016;5(2):129–32.

Neville BW, Damm DD, Allen CM, Chi AC. Oral and maxillofacial pathology. 4th ed. Amsterdam: Elsevier Health Sciences; 2015.

Odell EW. Clinical problem solving in dentistry. Elsevier: Churchill Livingstone; 2014.

Odell EW. Cawson's essentials of oral pathology and oral medicine. 9th ed. London: Elsevier Health Sciences; 2017.

Sharma P, Kochar D, Sachdeva S, Goyal J, et al. Recurring sessile fibroepithelial polyp of palatal gingiva—A case report. Int J Periodontol Implantol. 2021;2(3):98–100.

Red Lump on the Gum: Pyogenic Granuloma

Nurul Izyan Zainuddin

Contents

W. M Tilakaratne, T. G. Kallarakkal (eds.), *Clinicopathological Correlation of Oral Diseases*,
https://doi.org/10.1007/978-3-031-24408-7_19

Learning Goals

1. Devise the correct way of compiling the history with appropriate questions.
2. Develop a differential diagnosis after history taking.
3. Deduce appropriate procedures in clinical examination.
4. Formulate a differential diagnosis combining findings in the history and clinical examination.
5. Justify the relevant investigations required to arrive at the diagnosis.
6. Comprehend the importance of clinicopathological correlation in arriving at the correct diagnosis.
7. Outline the management plan.
8. Recognize the importance of a diagnostic algorithm in arriving at a diagnosis.

19.1 Main Complaint

A 35-year-old female patient presents to the dental clinic with the complaint of a painless red lump on her lower left gingiva.

19.2 History of Complaint

Question: How long has this lesion been present?

I noticed the lesion about a month ago.

Question: Explain the nature of the lump.

It gradually increased in size and bleeds easily when I brush my teeth. However, I did not experience any pain. I hoped it will go off by itself but the lesion persists.

Question: Is this the first time you experienced this condition or is this a recurrence?

Yes, this is the first time I experienced it.

Question: Do you have any medical illnesses or conditions, or currently taking any medications?

I do not have any medical illnesses but currently I am 3 months pregnant. I do not take any medications except a few supplements as prescribed by my doctor.

Question: Is this your first pregnancy?

Yes, this is my first pregnancy.

Question: Do any of your family members have any diagnosed medical conditions?

Both my parents and siblings are fit and free of any medical illness.

Question: When was the last time you visited the dentist? What treatment was carried out and was there any complication following the treatment?

I visited the dentist 5 months ago for a tooth extraction. I was told that the tooth was mobile and couldn't be saved. I was also told to come again for scaling, but I was preoccupied with work and haven't been to the dentist since then. There weren't any complications after the extraction.

Question: What is your occupation?

I work as a teacher hence this lesion has affected my self-confidence as it is visible when I speak.

Question: Do you smoke or take alcohol? Do you have any parafunctional habits?

I do not smoke or take alcohol and is not aware of having any parafunctional habits.

From the history, what is your differential diagnosis?

1. Pyogenic granuloma
2. Peripheral giant cell granuloma
3. Fibrous epulis
4. Hemangioma
5. Neoplasm

19.3 How Do You Justify Your Differential Diagnoses After History Taking?

1. The lump is on her gingiva and bleeds easily as she brushes her teeth or upon gentle manipulation. These are the characteristic clinical features of a pyogenic granuloma.
2. The patient is pregnant and pyogenic granuloma is commonly seen in pregnant patients due to the hor-

monal imbalance. High levels of estrogen and progesterone are present in this group of patients.
3. Lumps that are present on the gingiva can either be due to reactive lesions (pyogenic granuloma, peripheral giant cell granuloma or fibrous epulis) or neoplastic lesions (hemangiona or any other epithelial or mesenchymal neoplasms).
4. The lump has been there for 1 month indicating the chronicity of the lesion. Hence, acute reactive lesions such as periodontal abscesses are not included in the differential diagnoses.

19.4 Findings of Clinical Examination

On extraoral examination, there is no facial asymmetry and no palpable cervical lymph nodes. Intra-orally there is a pink to red nodular mass on the labial gingiva of the left mandibular canine and incisor area, which is slightly tender on palpation and soft in consistency. The size is approximately 10 mm × 9 mm. A small area of ulceration is also seen on the surface of the lump. The lump bleeds on manipulation. The patient's overall oral hygiene is fair (Fig. 19.1).

19.5 What Is Your Most Likely Clinical Diagnosis?

1. Pyogenic granuloma
2. Peripheral giant cell granuloma
3. Ulcerated fibrous epulis

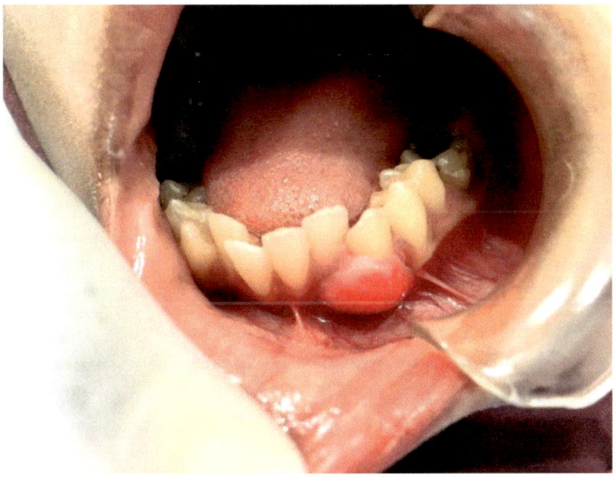

Fig. 19.1 Irregular pink, reddish lump on lower left gingiva covering one-third of the full height of the crown of lower left lateral incisor and canine. (Courtesy Dr Nurul Ruziantee)

19.6 How Would You Investigate This Patient?

1. Intra-oral periapical radiograph
2. Excisional biopsy for histopathological examination

19.7 What Are the Specific Findings to Help You Arrive at the Diagnosis (History, Clinical, and Investigations)?

The history given by the patient regarding the nature of the lump and the clinical features are indicators that it is reactive. The fact that the patient is pregnant and only experienced this during her pregnancy period is also an indicator of a reactive lesion, specifically pyogenic granuloma or pregnancy epulis.

On clinical examination, the lesion appears pink to red in colour, was soft in consistency and occasionally bled. The overall oral hygiene of the patient was fair. These are the common findings in patients with pyogenic granuloma.

The intra-oral periapical radiograph showed widening of the periodontal ligament space with no significant crestal bone loss. The radiographic presentation excluded bony lesions. Malignancy is also unlikely.

The histopathological findings reveal a polypoid mass of mucosa containing large areas of granulation tissue and dense mixed inflammatory cells. There is an area of ulceration, and it is covered by fibrinopurulent membrane (Fig. 19.2). The fibrous connective tissue is hypercellular. Numerous endothelial cell proliferations and small blood vessels are also present (Fig. 19.3).

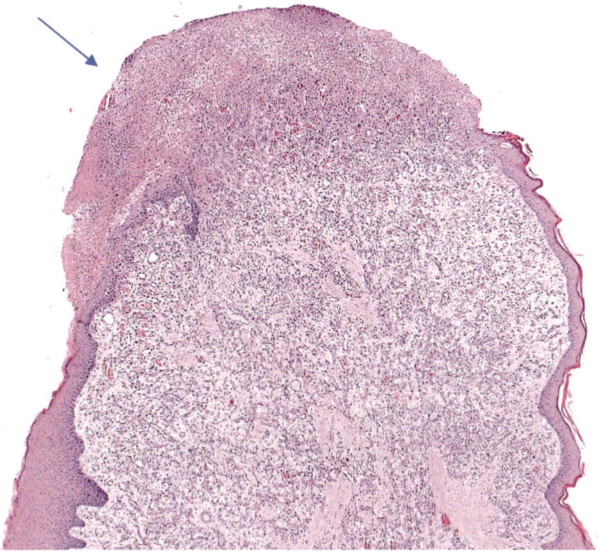

Fig. 19.2 An area of surface ulceration in a pyogenic granuloma (blue arrow). The fibrous connective tissue is hypercellular and contains granulation tissue

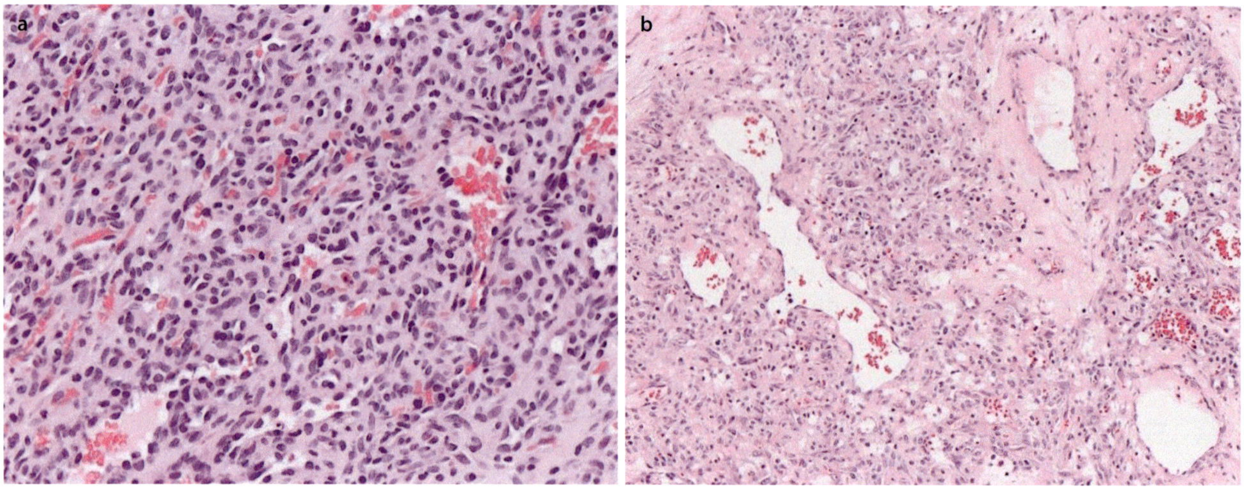

Fig. 19.3 Higher magnification shows numerous endothelial cells (**a**) and proliferation of newly formed blood vessels (**b**)

19.8 What Is the Definitive Diagnosis?

Pyogenic granuloma (pregnancy epulis)

19.9 Why Are the Differential Diagnoses Stated Earlier Excluded?

19.9.1 Peripheral Giant Cell Granuloma

Clinically, peripheral giant cell granuloma would appear more purplish than pyogenic granuloma, which is more vascular and hence appears more red. The diagnosis of peripheral giant cell granuloma is confirmed through histopathological examination. The histology of this lesion would show numerous multinucleated giant cells in a background of haemorrhage and proliferating plump polygonal and spindle cells.

19.9.2 Fibrous Epulis

Epulis refers to a growth on the gingiva. Clinically, fibrous epulis appears more pink/fibrotic than pyogenic granuloma. Histological examination of fibrous epulis would reveal fibrous connective tissue containing densely packed collagen fibres usually covered by an acanthotic surface epithelium. The fibrous connective tissue contains little to no inflammation.

19.9.3 Hemangioma

Hemangioma manifests during birth, shows rapid growth until 6–8 months and would involute at 8–9 years of age. Thus the behaviour of hemangioma, a true vascular tumour, is not fitting to the patient's history which suggests that it is of recent onset.

19.9.4 Neoplasm

This lesion is slow growing. The patient also did not report any systemic signs and symptoms or loss of appetite or weight, which is a common finding in patients with malignancy. Furthermore, histological findings are not consistent with any benign or malignant neoplasm.

19.10 What Is the Treatment for This Patient?

During the initial visit, the treatment for this patient is to remove the potential causative factors which are dental plaque and calculus. They have to be eradicated through oral prophylaxis followed by oral hygiene instructions and motivation. The patient has to be reviewed and the lump has to be monitored. Since the patient is pregnant, she should be given options either to remove the lump after her delivery or to do it as soon as possible. In instances where the size of the lump significantly reduces following oral prophylaxis, excisional biopsy of the lesion might not be necessary. However, as the size of the lump in this case is relatively large and has compromised her aesthetics, it is worthwhile to excise the lesion. The excision has to extend to the periosteum to prevent recurrences in the future. The patient is also entering her third month of pregnancy, making this the right time to have the lesion excised and have her treatment and review appointments completed during her second trimester. In this case, an excisional biopsy is performed as a diagnostic and therapeutic measure. Following the excisional biopsy, the patient should be constantly motivated to keep good oral hygiene.

19.11 Pyogenic Granuloma

Pyogenic granuloma is a common reactive lesion in the oral cavity. Despite the term 'pyogenic', this lesion is not caused by pyogenic organisms but is thought to represent an exuberant tissue response to local irritation. There are several aetiological factors related to this lesion. Besides reaction to low-degree stimuli as stated earlier, poor oral hygiene, hormonal factors and certain drugs have also been associated with pyogenic granuloma. High incidence of this lesion during pregnancy is known to be associated with elevated levels of estrogen and progesterone.

Pyogenic granuloma can occur at any age, but it is most common in young adults. There is a definite female predilection presumably because of the effects of the female hormones. Gingiva is the most common site for pyogenic granuloma and poor oral hygiene is the causative factor in many patients when it involves the gingiva (◘ Fig. 19.1). Some lesions extend to the interproximal areas and involve lingual and facial aspects of the gingiva. Other common sites include lips, tongue and buccal mucosa. Patient may also report history of trauma prior to the emergence of the lesion.

The pyogenic granuloma typically presents as smooth, lobulated mass which can either be sessile or pedunculated. The colour usually ranges from pink to red or purple. A young pyogenic granuloma frequently appears as more red due to its high vasculature while an older lesion tends to be more pink as a result of it becoming more collagenized. It is also not uncommon to find surface ulcerations in pyogenic granuloma.

The size of oral pyogenic granuloma can range from few millimetres to several centimetres in diameter. As it may demonstrate rapid growth in some occasions, this creates fear in both the clinician and the patient who would think that the lesion is malignant in nature. Pyogenic granuloma, when it occurs on the gingiva of a pregnant patient, is termed pregnancy epulis or granuloma gravidarum. The patient may notice this lesion to start developing during the first trimester. In some cases, these pyogenic granulomas resolve without treatment or undergo fibrous maturation after pregnancy.

The histopathological features of pyogenic granuloma include highly vascular granulation tissue with endothelial cell proliferation and newly forming vascular channels in an inflammatory background. Pyogenic granuloma can be classified as lobular capillary hemangioma (LCH) and nonlobular capillary hemangioma (non-LCH). The microscopic examination of LCH reveals numerous endothelial-lined channels of variable sizes engorged with red blood cells which are arranged in lobular arrangement (◘ Fig. 19.4), whereas for non-LCH, the vascular proliferation resembles granulation tissue without lobular arrangement (◘ Fig. 19.3b). A mixed acute and chronic inflammatory cell infiltrate is evident in the connective tissue of pyogenic granuloma, where neutrophils are more commonly found towards the ulcerated surface. In a more mature pyogenic granuloma, the granulation tissue is replaced by densely packed collagen fibres which gives it a more fibrotic appearance.

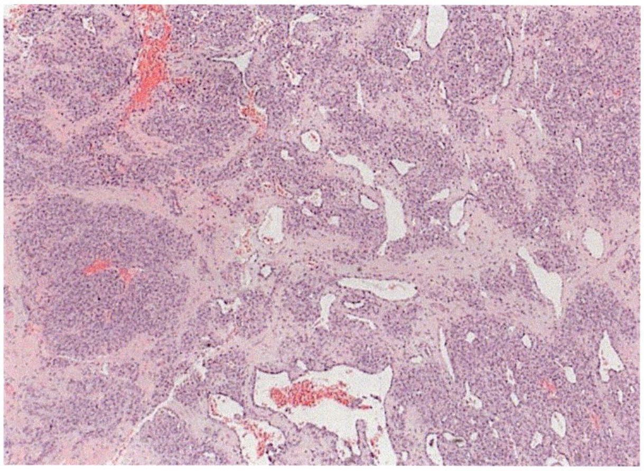

◘ **Fig. 19.4** Granulation tissue arranged in a lobular pattern as seen in lobular capillary hemangioma

The standard treatment for pyogenic granuloma is conservative surgical excision of the lesion. Incisional biopsy is mandatory in very large lesions. If the lesion is small in size, painless and does not bleed, clinical examination and follow-up are recommended. Among other treatments that can be suggested include cryotherapy technique and laser surgery which have been known to reduce the risk of bleeding.

Salient features of pyogenic granuloma	
Clinical	Smooth, sometimes ulcerated lobulated mass, pink to dark red/purple in colour
Histopathology	Highly vascularized granulation tissue beneath an area of surface ulceration It can be divided into lobular capillary hemangioma (LCH) where the granulation tissue is organized in a lobulated pattern or nonlobulated capillary hemangioma (non-LCH) when granulation tissue is present without the lobular arrangement
Treatment	Excision/complete surgical removal

Self-Assessment Questions

1. Describe the clinical features of pyogenic granuloma.
2. Name few lesions that can mimic the clinical presentation of pyogenic granuloma.
3. Describe the histopathological features of pyogenic granuloma.
4. Outline the treatment for pyogenic granuloma.

■ Diagnostic and Management Algorithm for Pyogenic Granuloma

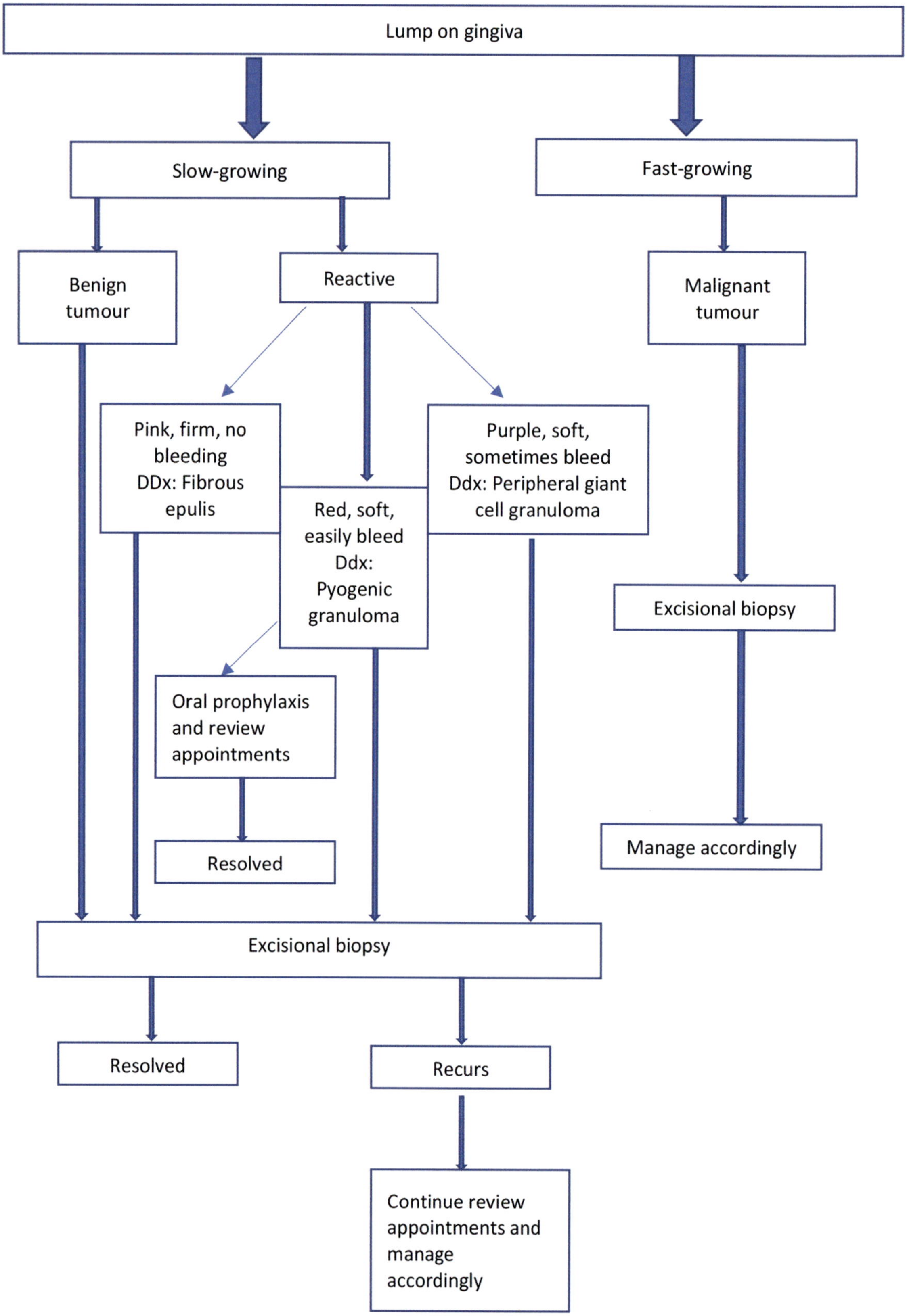

Further Reading

Amirchaghmaghi M, Falaki F, Mohtasham N, Mozafari PM. Extragingival pyogenic granuloma: a case report. Cases J. 2008;1(1):371.

Chandrashekar B. Minimally invasive approach to eliminate pyogenic granuloma: a case report: case reports. Dentistry. 2012;2012:909780. https://doi.org/10.1155/2012/909780.

Greenberg MS, Glick M. Burket's oral medicine: diagnosis and treatment. 10th ed. Hamilton: BC Decker; 2003. p. 141–2.

Jafarzadeh H, Sanatkhani M, Mohtasham N. Oral pyogenic granuloma: A review. J Oral Sci. 2006;48(4):167–75.

Neville BW, Damm DD, Allen CM, Chi AC. Oral and maxillofacial pathology. Elsevier Health Sciences; 2015.

Sills ES, Zegarelli DJ, Hoschander MM, Strider WE. Clinical diagnosis and management of hormonally responsive oral pregnancy tumor (pyogenic granuloma). J Reprod Med. 1996;41:467–70.

Lump on the Tongue: Schwannoma

Nurul Izyan Zainuddin

Contents

W. M Tilakaratne, T. G. Kallarakkal (eds.), *Clinicopathological Correlation of Oral Diseases*,
https://doi.org/10.1007/978-3-031-24408-7_20

Learning Goals

1. Devise the correct way of compiling the history with appropriate questions.
2. Develop a differential diagnosis after history taking.
3. Deduce appropriate procedures in clinical examination.
4. Formulate a differential diagnosis combining findings in the history and clinical examination.
5. Justify the relevant investigations required to arrive at the diagnosis.
6. Comprehend the importance of clinicopathological correlation in arriving at the correct diagnosis.
7. Outline the management plan.
8. Recognize the importance of a diagnostic algorithm in arriving at a diagnosis.

20.1 Main Complaint

A 20-year-old male patient came to the Oral and Maxillofacial Surgery Clinic complaining of a lump on his tongue. He appeared fit and healthy but requested further investigations and treatment for the lump.

20.2 History of Complaint

Question: How long have you been noticing this lesion?

I have been noticing it for nearly 6 months. I did not have any problem in the beginning nor did I experience any pain, but I have been noticing that it is gradually increasing in size. Occasionally I bite on the lesion thus causing pain.

Question: Describe the nature of the lesion?

I am experiencing this condition for the first time. It is a hard lump and the colour is the same as the rest of the tongue surface.

20.3 Additional Complaints

Question: Are there similar lumps present elsewhere, either in the oral cavity or in other parts of the body?

I don't have any lumps elsewhere on my body.

Question: Has the lump ruptured?

The lump has never ruptured.

Question: Do you remember any episode of trauma prior to the emergence of the lesion?

I cannot recall any history of trauma before the lesion appeared.

Question: Do you have any medical conditions or history of hospitalization?

I have no significant medical conditions. I have only been hospitalized once when I was a child due to high fever and was treated with antibiotics. I have never undergone any surgery. However, I did a blood test recently as I was having a fever that lasted for a few days. The laboratory test results were normal.

Question: Have you experienced any abrupt weight loss within the last 6 months?

I have not experienced any significant weight loss within the last 6 months.

Question: Have you undergone any dental treatment?

I had a full scaling done last week. That was when the dentist suggested me to go to an oral and maxillofacial clinic to get the lump removed after further investigations.

Question: What do you do for a living?

I am a student.

Question: Do you smoke or drink alcohol?

I do not smoke or drink alcohol.

Question: Do you have any parafunctional habits such as clenching, lip-biting or tongue-biting?

I don't have any parafunctional habits.

20.4 With the Findings From the History, What Are Your Differential Diagnoses?

The differential diagnoses for tongue swellings include:

Reactive lesions:

- Fibroepithelial polyp
- Pyogenic granuloma
- Traumatic neuroma
- Mucous extravasation cyst

Benign tumours:

- Papilloma

- Lipoma
- Schwannoma
- Granular cell tumour
- Neurofibroma
- Leiomyoma
- Rhabdomyoma
- Salivary gland tumour

20.5 How Would You Justify Your Differential Diagnoses After History Taking?

The lesion has been there for 6 months. This denotes the slow-growing nature and chronicity of the lesion suggesting that it is a chronic reactive lesion or a benign neoplasm. Malignant neoplasms are not included in the differential diagnoses as malignant neoplasms rapidly increase in size. The patient is fit and healthy, and he does not report any significant weight loss associated with malignancy or significant underlying medical conditions.

The lesion is localized, with no lumps present elsewhere in the oral cavity or other parts of the body. The patient has not experienced a similar condition previously. If there are multiple lumps present, this may also suggest syndromes like neurofibromatosis, Cowden syndrome or multiple endocrine neoplasia (MEN) syndrome.

Fibroepithelial polyp is considered to be one of the provisional diagnoses as it is the most common reactive lesion in the oral cavity. This lesion could be precipitated by trauma even though the patient could not exactly recall any traumatic incident to the area before the emergence of this lesion. However, he did admit that he occasionally bit on the area, hence this may have caused the lesion to slightly increase in size.

Another common lump that can present in the oral cavity is a pyogenic granuloma. Pyogenic granuloma is also reactive in nature and commonly occurs as a response to stimuli such as chronic local irritation and trauma. Although it most commonly occurs on the gingiva, it can also occur on the lips, buccal mucosa and tongue.

Traumatic neuroma is commonly found on the tongue. It is a reactive proliferation of neural tissue after transection or damage of an adjacent nerve bundle and would present as a well-defined, sessile, fibrous lump.

If the lesion is not preceded by a history of trauma or irritation, it may suggest the possibility of a neoplasm, either benign or malignant. A malignant neoplasm can be ruled out due to the chronic nature of the lesion and the lack of any significant malignancy symptoms. The common benign neoplasms occurring on the tongue include schwannoma, granular cell tumour and neurofibroma. Benign salivary gland tumours are exceptionally rare on the tongue.

A mucocele, haemangioma and lipoma are unlikely as the patient mentions that the lump is hard in nature and has the same colour as the rest of the tongue surface; whereas these lumps are more soft with variable surface mucosal colour.

20.6 Findings of Clinical Examination

There is a well-circumscribed lump of normal mucosal colour, firm in consistency with a smooth surface on the left lateral border of the tongue. The size is approximately 1.5 cm × 1.5 cm. The surrounding mucosa is normal. The oral hygiene is fair (Fig. 20.1).

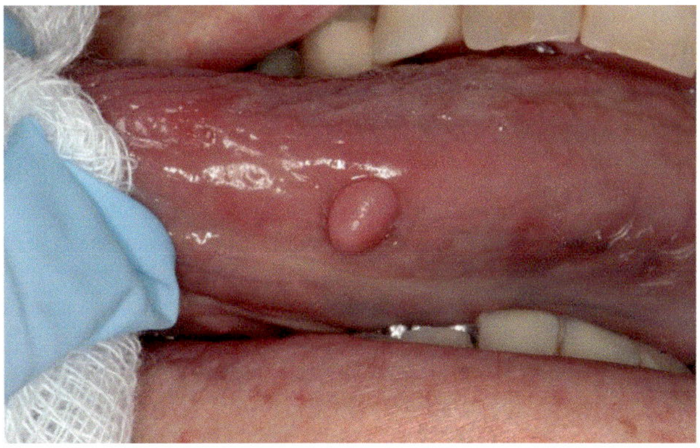

Fig. 20.1 Sessile, solitary, smooth-surfaced lump on the left lateral border of the tongue. (Courtesy Oral Medicine Clinic, Faculty of Dentistry, University of Otago)

20.7 What Other Relevant Features Would You Look for with the Findings You Have So Far?

It is a sessile, solitary lump and no other lumps are present elsewhere in the oral cavity. The colour of the lump is not reddish or purplish. There is no evidence of ulceration on the lump. The lump is not tender, is firm in consistency, with no blanching and associated anaesthesia or paraesthesia present.

20.8 What Is Your Clinical Differential Diagnosis?

1. Reactive lesion
   - Fibroepithelial polyp
   - Traumatic neuroma
2. Benign soft tissue tumour
   - Schwannoma
   - Neurofibroma
   - Granular cell tumour
   - Leiomyoma
   - Rhabdomyoma

20.9 How Would You Exclude Other Conditions and Justify the Inclusion of the Diseases That You Have Mentioned in the Differential Diagnoses to Arrive at a Working Diagnosis?

20.9.1 Pyogenic Granuloma

The clinical features of pyogenic granuloma are not fitting to the clinical appearance seen in the present case. Clinically, a pyogenic granuloma would present as a well-defined, red to purplish solitary lump, which is sometimes ulcerated. It is usually soft in consistency.

20.9.2 Lipoma

Lipoma is a benign tumour of adipocytes. Clinically, it presents as a solitary lump, with a yellowish hue, and is soft in consistency. These clinical features are not concurrent with the findings seen in this patient.

20.9.3 Haemangioma/Mucocele

The clinical appearance, especially the colour is not consistent with these lesions and haemangioma shows evidence of blanching.

20.10 What Is the Most Likely Diagnosis?

At this stage, the diagnosis can include any reactive lesions or a benign soft tissue tumour as stated previously. Absence of a history of trauma or surgery at the site may exclude the possibility of a fibroepithelial polyp or a traumatic neuroma. Therefore, the possibility of the lesion being a benign tumour is very likely.

20.11 How Would You Investigate This Patient in Order to Arrive at the Final Diagnosis?

Since this is a small solitary lump, an excisional biopsy of the lesion and subsequent histopathological examination is appropriate.

20.12 What Does the Histopathological Examination Reveal?

The H&E sections show encapsulated tumour with proliferation of spindle-shaped Schwann cells in fascicles within the background of a delicate collagenous stroma. There are hypercellular areas composed of palisaded nuclei and intervening accumulation of eosinophilic cell processes forming Verocay bodies (Antoni A) (◘ Fig. 20.2), whereas the hypocellular area reveals a non-specific pattern of arrangement of cells within a loose stroma (Antoni B). There is no cytological atypia involving the spindle cells.

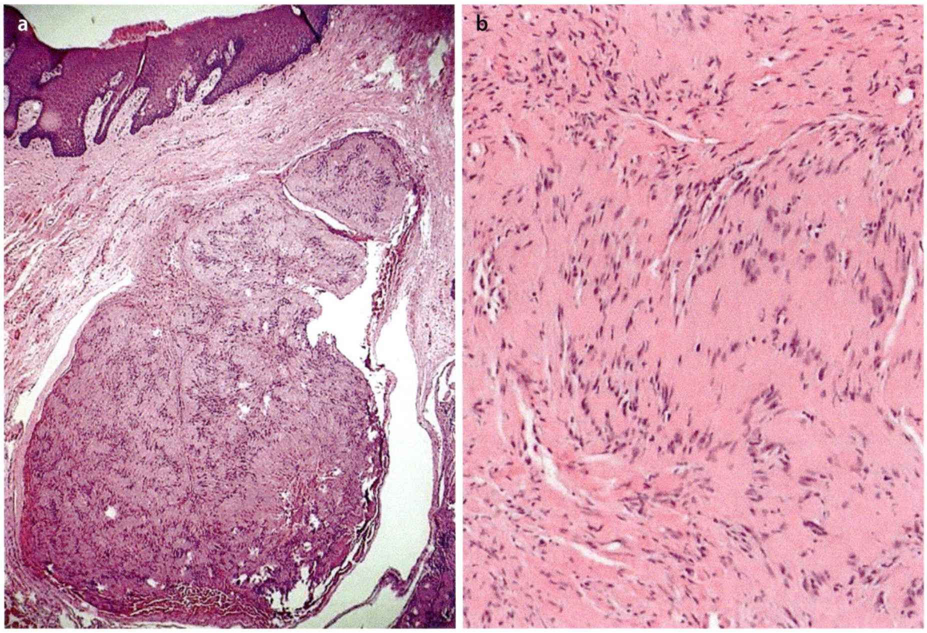

Fig. 20.2 H&E section shows an encapsulated tumour demonstrating a hypercellular zone with fusiform cells and nuclei arranged in a palisading manner forming parallel rows of Verocay bodies (**a**). There is no evidence of pleomorphic cells. Higher magnification of the lesional area (**b**). (Courtesy Dr Fairuz Rahman)

20.13 Schwannoma

Schwannoma or neurilemmoma is a benign tumour that arises from peripheral, cranial (excluding cranial nerves 1 and 2) or autonomic nerves that contain Schwann cells. The aetiology of schwannoma is not very much understood. However, several theories have been proposed regarding its onset. It has been postulated that it is an ectodermal tumour derived from Schwann cells while another theory proposed that it is a mesodermal tumour arising from perineurium. Although rare, trauma has also been considered as an aetiological factor for schwannoma.

About 25–45% of all schwannomas are found in the head and neck region and only between 1% and 12% of them have an intraoral origin. The tongue is known to be the most common site for intraoral schwannoma. There is no specific gender predilection for intraoral schwannoma. Schwannomas are more commonly seen in the second and third decades of life.

Intraoral schwannoma typically presents as a firm, lobulated mass of variable size. It is usually asymptomatic but some patients may also report paraesthesia in long-standing lesions. It can be solitary but multiple schwannomas have also been reported, which, if occur, may require the evaluation for neurofibromatosis type 2 (NF-2). Neurofibromatosis 1 (NF-1), formerly termed von Recklinghausen's disease, is an autosomal dominant disorder. The NF1 gene is located on chromosome 17q11.2 and the protein product termed neurofibromin acts as a tumour suppressor. NF-1 is associated with multiple neurofibromas and other associated features such as café au lait spots, axillary freckling, Lisch nodules in iris and bone deformities. In NF-2, multiple schwannomas are usually found in relation to the vestibulocochlear nerve. NF-2 is an autosomal dominant disease caused by inactivating mutations of the NF2 gene and is characterized by the development of nervous system tumours, ocular abnormalities and skin tumours.

Most of the schwannomas are painless and slow growing. However, it may rapidly increase in size if there is an internal haemorrhage. There have also been reports of tongue schwannoma becoming symptomatic when they approach 3 cm in greatest dimension.

Histologically, schwannoma is an encapsulated tumour consisting of cells arranged in two patterns namely Antoni A and Antoni B. Antoni A area is hypercellular and consists of closely packed spindle cells organized in rows with palisading, elongated nuclei. There is an acellular eosinophilic area between the rows of the nuclei termed as Verocay bodies (Fig. 20.3). Antoni B is less cellular and is composed of loosely arranged spindle cells in a myxoid or hyalinized stroma. Collagen fibres are delicate and scarce inflammatory cells are usually present. The tumour cells of schwannoma show S100, SOX10 and GFAP positivity when subjected to immunohistochemical staining.

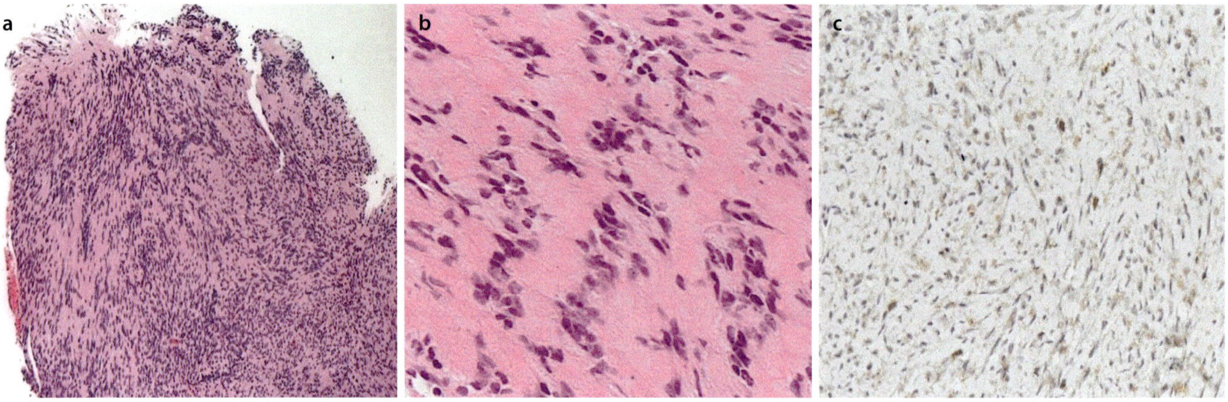

Fig. 20.3 Histopathology of Schwannoma: Low-power view showing a representative section of a schwannoma containing hypercellular areas (Antoni A) and hypocellular areas (Antoni B) (**a**). High-power view of Antoni A shows fusiform spindle cells with palisading nuclei and Verocay bodies (**b**). S100 is diffusely positive (**c**). (Adapted from Cohen & Wang)

There are four major histological types of schwannoma which are termed as conventional, plexiform, cellular and ancient variants. The conventional variant mostly has Antoni A areas and occasionally Antoni B. Additionally, conventional variant would also have areas of hyalinization, thin vessels and acute and/or chronic inflammatory cells. The cellular variant is characterized by a predominant Antoni A pattern, increased connective tissue cellularity, spindle cells organized in compact fascicles with some degree of nuclear hyperchromatism and pleomorphism, and lack of Verocay bodies. The mitotic activity is also increased in this variant. The cellular variant of schwannoma is often confused with sarcoma because of these features. The ancient variant has more degenerative changes such as mild pleomorphic and bizarre nuclei, microcyst formation, calcification and dilated vessels. The plexiform type contains both Antoni A and B regions with prominent Verocay bodies. However, the Schwann cells show a nodular arrangement with capsular delineation.

In some cases, a neurofibroma also shows some histological resemblance to a schwannoma. However, a neurofibroma lacks encapsulation and does not contain Antoni A and Antoni B areas. Immunohistochemistry studies for schwannoma and neurofibroma reveal strong positivity for S100, but calretinin has been increasingly utilized as an aid that can distinguish these two entities, as it shows diffuse positivity with schwannoma.

The treatment of choice for schwannoma is complete surgical removal of the lesion with the preservation of neighbouring structures. Excision done by the surgeon for diagnostic examination is always curative. Schwannoma rarely recurs once it is entirely removed. Despite being a benign neoplasm, malignant transformation of intraoral schwannoma, albeit very rare, has also been reported.

Salient features of schwannoma	
Clinical	Firm, asymptomatic, lobulated mass and of variable size
Histopathology	Encapsulated lesion and mainly consisting of two patterns, namely Antoni A and Antoni B. Antoni A is hypercellular and contains closely packed spindle cells organized in rows with palisading, elongated nuclei with Verocay bodies in between the rows. Antoni B is composed of loosely arranged spindle cells within a background of hyalinized stroma
Treatment	Complete surgical removal/excision

Self-Assessment Questions

1. Discuss the clinical differential diagnoses for swellings on the tongue.
2. Describe the characteristic histopathological features of schwannoma.
3. State other lesions which may resemble the histological presentation of schwannoma.
4. State the immunohistochemical markers used to diagnose schwannoma.
5. Explain four major histological types of schwannoma.

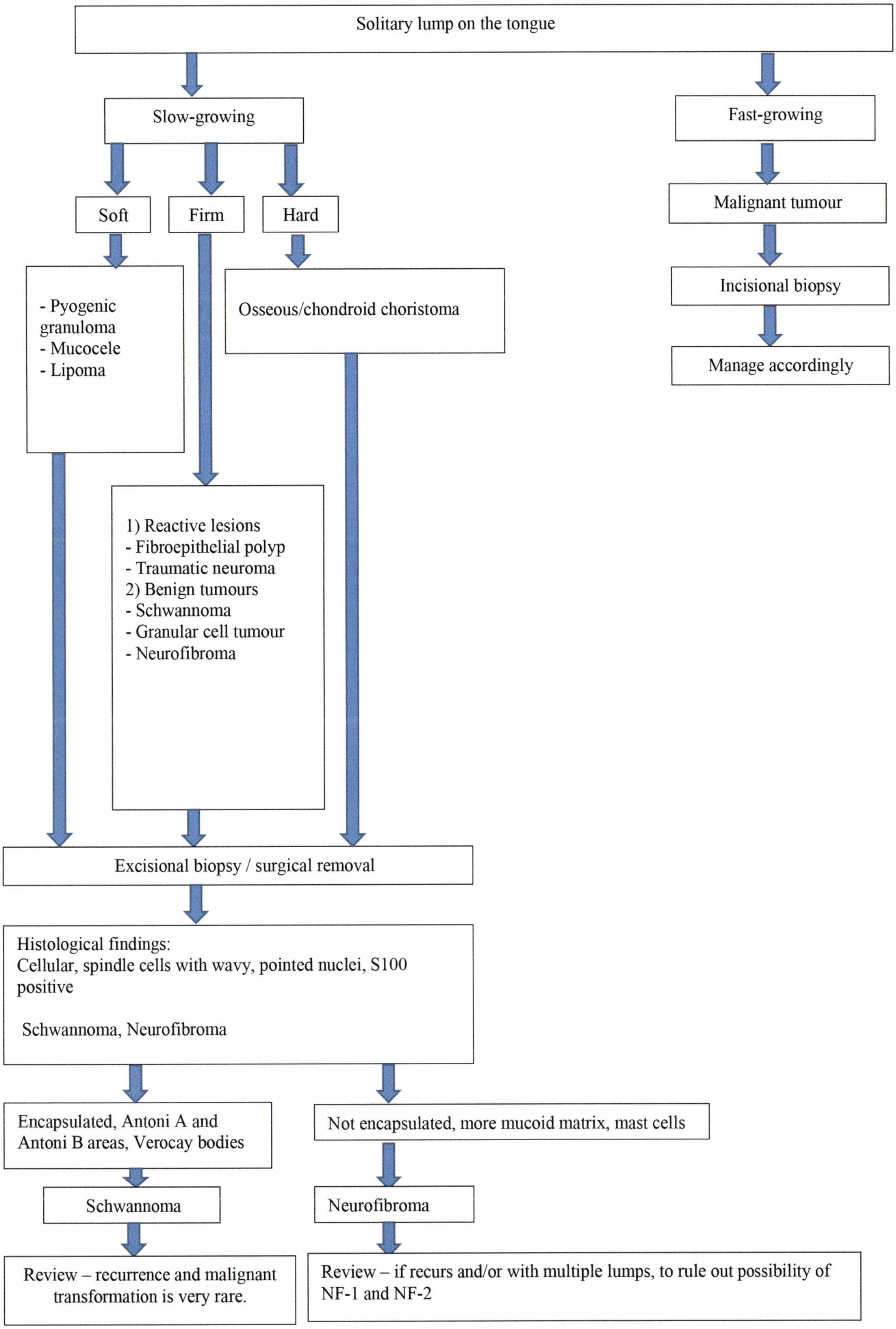
Solitary lump on the tongue
Slow-growing
Fast-growing
Soft
Firm
Hard
Malignant tumour
Incisional biopsy
Manage accordingly
- Pyogenic granuloma
- Mucocele
- Lipoma
Osseous/chondroid choristoma
1) Reactive lesions
- Fibroepithelial polyp
- Traumatic neuroma
2) Benign tumours
- Schwannoma
- Granular cell tumour
- Neurofibroma
Excisional biopsy / surgical removal
Histological findings:
Cellular, spindle cells with wavy, pointed nuclei, S100 positive
Schwannoma, Neurofibroma
Encapsulated, Antoni A and Antoni B areas, Verocay bodies
Not encapsulated, more mucoid matrix, mast cells
Schwannoma
Neurofibroma
Review – recurrence and malignant transformation is very rare.
Review – if recurs and/or with multiple lumps, to rule out possibility of NF-1 and NF-2

Further Reading

Colreavy MP, Lacy PD, Hughes J, et al. Head and neck schwannomas–a 10 year review. J Laryngol Otol. 2000;114(02):119–24.

Cohen M, Wang MB. Schwannoma of the tongue: two case reports and review of the literature. Eur Arch Otorhinolaryngol. 2009;266(11):1823–9. https://doi.org/10.1007/s00405-008-0907-2.

Dokania V, Rajguru A, Mayashankar V, Mukherjee I, Jaipuria B, Shere D. Palatal schwannoma: an analysis of 45 literature reports and of an illustrative case. Int Arch Otorhinolaryngol. 2019;23(3):e360–70.

Fine SW, McClain SA, Li M. Immunohistochemical staining for calretinin is useful for differentiating schwannomas from neurofibromas. Am J Clin Pathol. 2004;122(4):552–9. https://doi.org/10.1309/AGBG-TBRJ-4W0B-C7LN. PMID: 15487453

López-Carriches C, Baca-Pérez-Bryan R, Montalvo-Montero S. Schwannoma located in the palate: clinical case and literature review. Med Oral Patol Oral Cir Bucal. 2009;14(09):e465–8.

Lopez-Jornet P, Bermejo Fenoll-Ambrosio. Neurilemmoma of the tongue. Oral Oncol Extra 2005; 41:154-157.

Santos PPA, Freitas VS, Pinto LP, Freitas RA, de Souza LB. Clinicopathologic analysis of 7 cases of oral schwannoma and review of the literature. Ann Diagn Pathol. 2010;14(4):235–9.

Woo SB. Oral pathology E-book: a comprehensive atlas and text. Elsevier Health Sciences; 2016.

Oral Potentially Malignant Disorders and Oral Cancer

Contents

Burning Sensation to Spicy Food: Oral Submucous Fibrosis

Ruwan Jayasinghe and Wanninayake M Tilakaratne

Contents

W. M Tilakaratne, T. G. Kallarakkal (eds.), *Clinicopathological Correlation of Oral Diseases*,
https://doi.org/10.1007/978-3-031-24408-7_21

Learning Goals

1. Devise the correct way of compiling the history with appropriate questions.
2. Develop a differential diagnosis after history taking.
3. Deduce appropriate procedures in clinical examination.
4. Formulate a differential diagnosis combining findings in the history and clinical examination.
5. Justify the relevant investigations required to arrive at the diagnosis.
6. Comprehend the importance of clinicopathological correlation in arriving at the correct diagnosis.
7. Outline the management plan.
8. Recognize the importance of a diagnostic algorithm in arriving at a diagnosis.

21.1 Main Complaint

A 35-year-old male patient presents to the clinic complaining of a burning sensation in the mouth, especially for spicy food.

21.2 History of Complaint

Question: How long have you been having this feeling and what is the nature of it?

It has been there for 1-year duration. Initially it was tolerable but now I find it difficult to eat any food containing spices. I used to eat a lot of spices in the past, but now it has been reduced to a minimum. I do not enjoy the food at all and am worried about the quality of the food that I am eating.

21.3 Additional Complaints

Question: Have you noticed or felt any other changes or difficulties in the mouth?

I experience recurrent oral ulceration. I am finding it difficult to eat hard or rough food as it gives rise to ulceration. My mouth opening has reduced. I feel roughness in my inner cheeks and find it difficult to brush teeth as inserting and moving the toothbrush in the sulcus is difficult and painful. I also experience altered taste and difficulty in swallowing. In addition, I noticed a whitish area on the cheek.

Question: Do you have any lesions elsewhere in the body? Do you experience any pain or a burning sensation when urinating?

I have no additional problems other than the difficulties present in the mouth. Further, I do not have any other lesions elsewhere in the body. There is no pain or burning sensation while urinating.

Question: Do you get tired easily?

I feel tired during routine work but can manage without much of a problem.

Question: Tell me about your meals. What kind of food you eat for your regular meals?

My diet is mostly composed of food containing high amounts of starch with minimum protein.

Question: Are you suffering from any other medical problems like heart disease, high blood pressure, diabetes, bleeding disorder, or respiratory diseases? If yes, what kind of medications have you been taking until now?

I don't have any other medical problems. However, I had a course of antibiotics for 2 weeks due to a painful throat problem in the recent past.

Question: Have you undergone any surgery?

I have not undergone any surgery in the past.

Question: Have you undergone any dental treatment?

I had an extraction for a grossly broken tooth 2 months ago. It was a difficult extraction which took more than 1 hour. I had severe pain for 3 days after the extraction and it took more than 10 days to heal.

Question: How was your mouth opening before the extraction?

As I remember, it was there even before, and it became worse after the extraction.

Question: What is your occupation?

I am a daily wage manual labourer.

Question: Do you have any specific chewing habits?

I chew around ten betel quids a day for more than 15 years. I use betel quid containing betel leaf, tobacco, areca nut, and slaked lime. I keep the quid in the buccal sulcus for about 1 hour; after that I spit it out.

Question: Are you a smoker?

I am a past smoker. I used to smoke 10 cigarettes a day for 5 years and stopped the habit 2 years ago.

Question: Do you take alcohol?

I do not drink alcohol.

21.4 With the Findings in the History, What Is Your Differential Diagnosis?

1. Oral submucous fibrosis (OSF).
2. Scleroderma.
3. Anaemia.
4. Candidosis.
5. Oral lichen planus (OLP).

21.5 How Do You Justify Your Differential Diagnosis After History Taking?

1. He has restricted mouth opening with rough cheeks. These are characteristic features of OSF or scleroderma to some extent. His habit of betel chewing is the aetiology for OSF. White patches (leukoplakia) can be present in up to 25% of OSF patients. He had undergone a difficult dental extraction, which may have resulted in a temporomandibular disorder such as anterior disc displacement without reduction or myofibrotic contracture, leading to reduced mouth opening. However, restricted mouth opening has been there even before the extraction. Myofibrotic contracture usually results in trismus 2–3 days after the trauma and is associated with pain. Combination of the presenting symptoms and history of betel chewing suggests OSF as a likely differential diagnosis.
2. He has burning sensation for spicy food, which may be due to many diseases affecting the oral mucosa, including OSF, oral lichen planus (OLP), anaemia, and candidosis. Since he feels tired when working, and is not on a balanced diet, it suggests the possibility of him having anaemia. Further, oral ulceration is a frequent manifestation of anaemia. In addition, presence of whitish areas and burning sensation should lead to the suspicion of OLP.
3. He was on a course of antibiotics which may have predisposed him to develop candidosis leading to burning sensation. Further, the presence of a white patch may be due to a candidal infection.

21.6 Findings of Clinical Examination

Extra oral examination does not reveal any significant findings. The colour and texture of the skin appear normal. He has a pale mucosa with leathery feeling on palpation. There are multiple small ulcers on both buccal mucosae with erythematous surroundings.

21.7 What Other Relevant Features Would You Look for with the Findings You Have So Far?

There is depigmentation on lips and depapillation of the tongue. The palate is pale in colour with shrunken soft palate. Fibrous bands are palpable in the faucial region, retro molar area, and buccal mucosa. His maximum inter incisal mouth opening is 25 mm (Fig. 21.1). Tongue movements are restricted. Mouth appears to be dry. Brown-coloured stains are present on teeth. A white homogenous lesion measuring 3 × 2 cm is observed on the left side buccal mucosa extending from commissure to retro-molar area, which cannot be rubbed off (Fig. 21.1b).

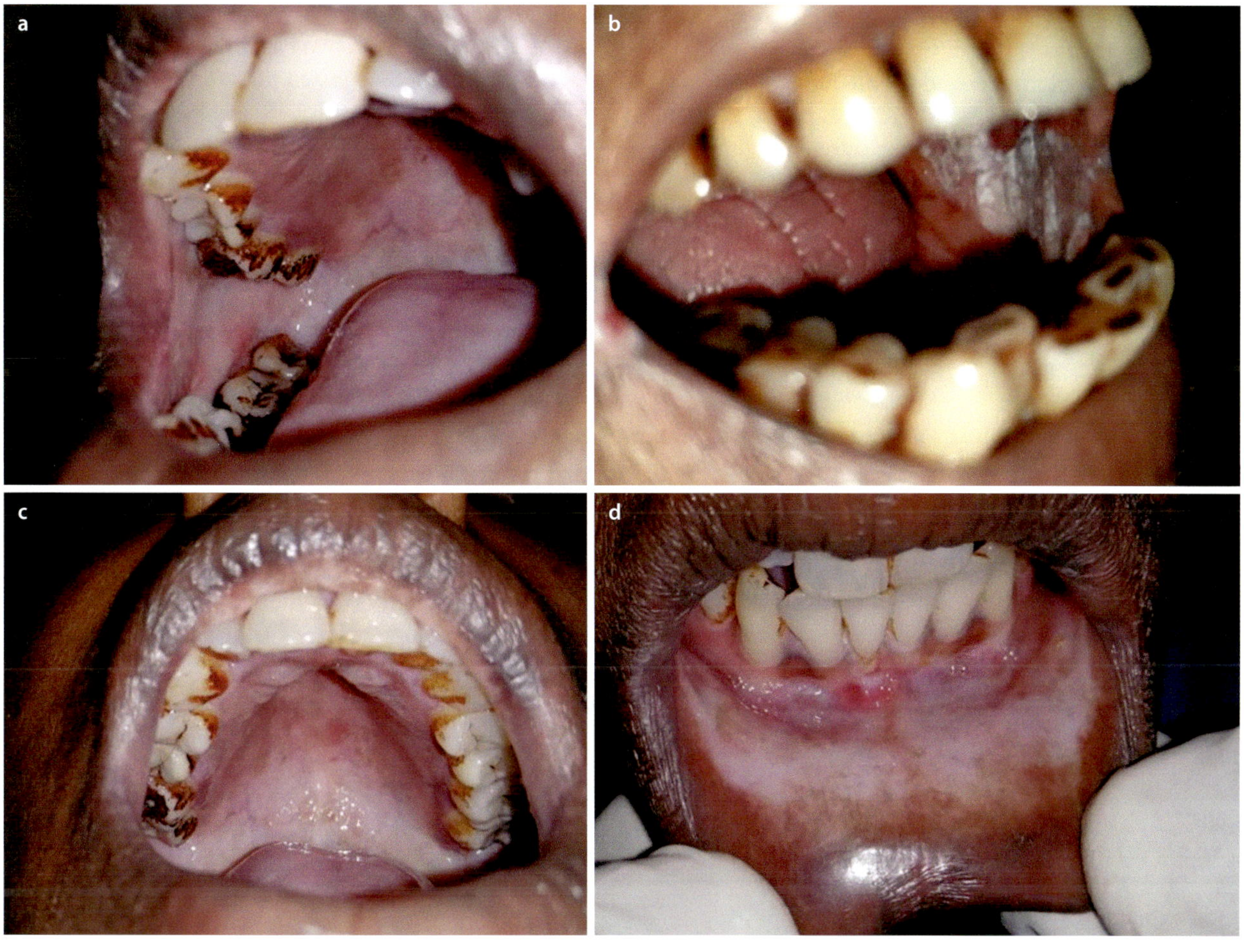

Fig. 21.1 Right buccal mucosa showing pale and blanched appearance due to fibrosis. Restricted mouth opening is visible (**a**, **b**), left buccal mucosa showing homogenous white patch (**b**), palatal mucosa is pale with shrunken soft palate (**c**), and lower labial mucosa with depigmentation (**d**)

21.8 What is Your Clinical Diagnosis?

Oral submucous fibrosis (OSF).

21.9 How Would You Exclude Other Conditions and Justify Your Clinical Diagnosis?

21.9.1 Candidosis

This is usually present in people who have predisposing factors for opportunistic infection. Although this patient has a history of antibiotic use, the type of white patch is not consistent with pseudomembranous candidosis, which is associated with antibiotics. It presents as a white plaque, which can be wiped off without causing pain or burning sensation. Chronic hyperplastic candidosis (CHC) usually appears as a thick white plaque commonly in the commissural region with no pain or burning sensation. This patient's white lesion on the buccal mucosa can be CHC, but considering the other findings of the oral mucosa, it is unlikely to be the primary diagnosis for his complaints.

21.9.2 Scleroderma

This is characterized by multi-organ involvement. The tongue becomes stiff and board-like due to fibrosis and may result in dysphagia. Gingival tissues are pale and unusually firm. Increased fibrosis in the perioral tissues leads to microstomia. Characteristic furrows radiating from mouth lead to "purse string" appearance. This patient doesn't seem to show most of these features and there was no evidence of skin involvement. Therefore, scleroderma is an unlikely differential diagnosis.

21.9.3 Oral Lichen Planus and Anaemia

OLP is usually characterized by bilateral white patches and most patients can have skin involvement. Although burning sensation is a common feature, presenting clinical features do not support OLP as a differential diagnosis. Both intra and extra oral findings together with clinical findings are not in favour of anaemia as a differential diagnosis.

21.9.4 OSF

The characteristic diagnostic feature of this disease is the presence of palpable fibrous bands. The presence of fibrous bands on lips, cheek, and hard palate is considered as the hallmark of the disease. He was found to have most of the other characteristic features of the disease, such as restricted mouth opening, depapillation and restricted movements of the tongue, and excessive brown staining, suggestive of very frequent practice of the habit of betel chewing. In addition, prevalence of leukoplakia is also a frequent finding in OSF. Therefore, the most likely working diagnosis can be considered as OSF.

21.10 What is the Most Likely Diagnosis?

Oral submucous fibrosis.

21.11 How Would You Investigate This Patient?

1. Full blood count (FBC) to exclude anaemia.
2. Swab from the white lesion on the buccal mucosa to exclude candidal infection.
3. Incisional biopsy for the confirmation of diagnosis and to plan long-term management.

21.12 How Would You Do an Incisional Biopsy for This Patient? What are the Important Considerations?

Advanced cases of OSF can be diagnosed with clinical features alone, but early and intermediate cases may pose difficulties in clinical diagnosis. However, biopsy can lead to fibrosis, which may complicate clinical problems. As this patient is having a white patch in the buccal mucosa which is a recognized potentially malignant disorder, a biopsy is mandatory. It has to be taken from the area of the white lesion with minimal trauma. Additional diagnostic aids like toluidine blue and velscope can be used to decide on the biopsy site. His FBC was normal. Biopsy report confirms the diagnosis of OSF.

21.13 What are the Histopathological Features That Help in Arriving at the Diagnosis?

H&E sections show mucosa covered by atrophic stratified squamous epithelium with sub-epithelial hyalinization and fibrosis of the corium. Fibrosis extends downwards depending on the severity of the disease, and in severe cases, it extends to the muscles, replacing the muscles with fibrosis. The density of the inflammatory cell infiltrate in the corium varies according to the stage of the disease. Vascularity of the corium reduces significantly with the progress of the disease. The epithelium shows varying degrees of dysplasia in some cases. The present patient has mild epithelial dysplasia in the background of OSF (◘ Fig. 21.2).

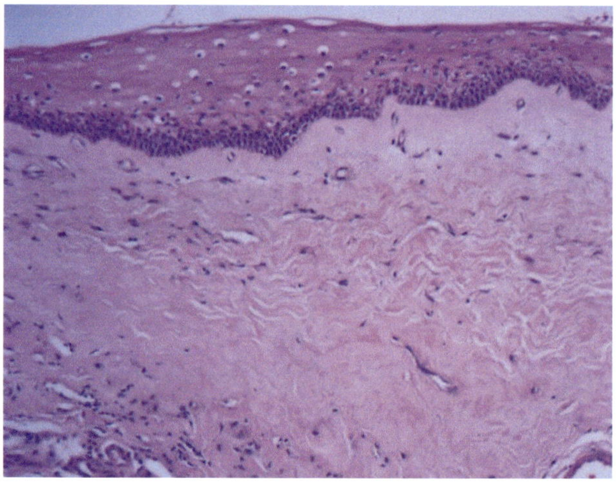

◘ **Fig. 21.2** Histopathological features of OSF: mucosa covered by atrophic epithelium showing mild epithelial dysplasia. The upper corium is hyalinized and fibrosed. Fibrosis extends into deeper tissues

21.14 What is the Significance of the Presence of Epithelial Dysplasia in OSF?

OSF is an oral potentially malignant disorder. The severity of dysplasia has a direct relationship with malignant transformation into oral squamous cell carcinoma (OSCC). The follow-up interval should be decided according to the degree of epithelial dysplasia.

21.15 How Would You Manage This Patient?

OSF is caused by the use of areca nut, and malignant transformation can be enhanced by tobacco and alcohol. Habit intervention is the most important step in the management. Since he is a betel quid chewer, advice on smokeless tobacco and areca nut cessation needs to be given. Antioxidants are very useful in reducing the symptoms and minimizing malignant transformation. Lycopene is a helpful drug in this respect. Intra-lesional steroid injections are recommended to improve the symptoms, especially mouth opening. Methyl prednisolone injection to the areas of fibrous bands can be given monthly. Physical interventions including various physical exercise regimens, splints, or other devices may also be helpful in maintaining the mouth opening.

Leukoplakia present in the buccal mucosa needs careful follow-up as it already shows mild epithelial dysplasia. Repeated toluidine blue or velscope tests are indicated to identify newly developed suspicious areas. If there is any change, a repeat biopsy is indicated. High-risk dysplasia is an indication for removal with laser or surgery followed by reconstruction and physical exercises. Improvement of oral hygiene is also necessary.

This patient has to be followed up once every 3 months in the clinic as he is at a risk of malignant transformation of developing an OSCC.

21.16 Oral Submucous Fibrosis (OSF)

Oral submucous fibrosis is a chronic, insidious disease that affects the lamina propria of the oral mucosa, and as the disease advances, it involves tissues deeper in the submucosa with loss of fibro-elasticity. OSF falls within a group of conditions that is classified under oral potentially malignant disorders. The disease manifests itself with blanching and stiffening of the oral mucosa, leading to limitation in the opening of the mouth. The presence of fibrous bands in the lips, cheeks, and soft palate is a hallmark of the disease. The disease is histopathologically characterized by fibrosis that affects the oral cavity, pharynx, and upper third of the oesophagus. The prevalence of the disease is on the rise as a result of increased use of commercially available areca nut preparations. The disease is mostly seen in South and Southeast Asia where the habit of betel chewing is practiced. OSF was first described in 1952 by Schwartz as atrophia idiopathica tropica mucosa oris. Several other descriptive terms such as idiopathic scleroderma of the mouth, idiopathic palatal fibrosis, and sclerosing stomatitis have also been used. The main aetiological factor for OSF is arecoline present in areca nut. In addition to arecoline, areca nut also contains other active components, including alkaloids (arecaidine, guvacine, guvacoline, and arecolinidine), polyphenols (catechin, flavonoids, and tannins), and trace elements (sodium, magnesium, chlorine, calcium, vanadium, manganese, copper, and bromine). Polyphenols in areca nut cause collagen fibres to abnormally cross-link, thereby making them less susceptible to degradation by collagenases. The resulting decrease in collagen breakdown, in turn, leads to increased fibrosis. In addition, fibrogenic cytokines such as TGF-β1 play a major role in activating fibroblasts to produce collagen. At the same time, collagen homeostasis is disturbed by increased amounts of tissue inhibitors of matrix metalloproteinases (TIMPs) and decreased levels of matrix metalloproteinases (MMPs), leading to accumulation of collagen. In addition to the local factors, various systemic factors have been suggested to play a role in causing the disease. These include anaemia, chronic iron and vitamin B complex deficiency, and genetic predisposition. Current evidence suggests that OSF occurs in genetically susceptible individuals who use areca nut. Onset of the disease is directly proportionate to the prevalence, concentration, and duration of areca nut chewing. However, younger patients develop clinical features early.

Clinical presentation depends on the stage of the disease. Initially, most patients present with burning sensation or intolerance to spicy food and may have vesicles, particularly on the palate. Ulceration and dryness of the mouth is followed by fibrosis of the oral mucosa, which leads to rigidity of oral structures and trismus. Involvement of the floor of the mouth and gingivae is rare.

Early forms of the disease present with burning sensation exacerbated by spicy food, vesiculation, blanching of the mucosa, and leathery mucosa, while late presentation includes woody changes of the mucosa and tongue, fibrous bands within mucosa, limitation of mouth opening, and narrowing of oropharyngeal orifice with distortion of uvula and sunken cheeks (▫ Fig. 21.3). Changes of OSF are similar to those of systemic sclerosis (scleroderma), but the features of OSF are limited to

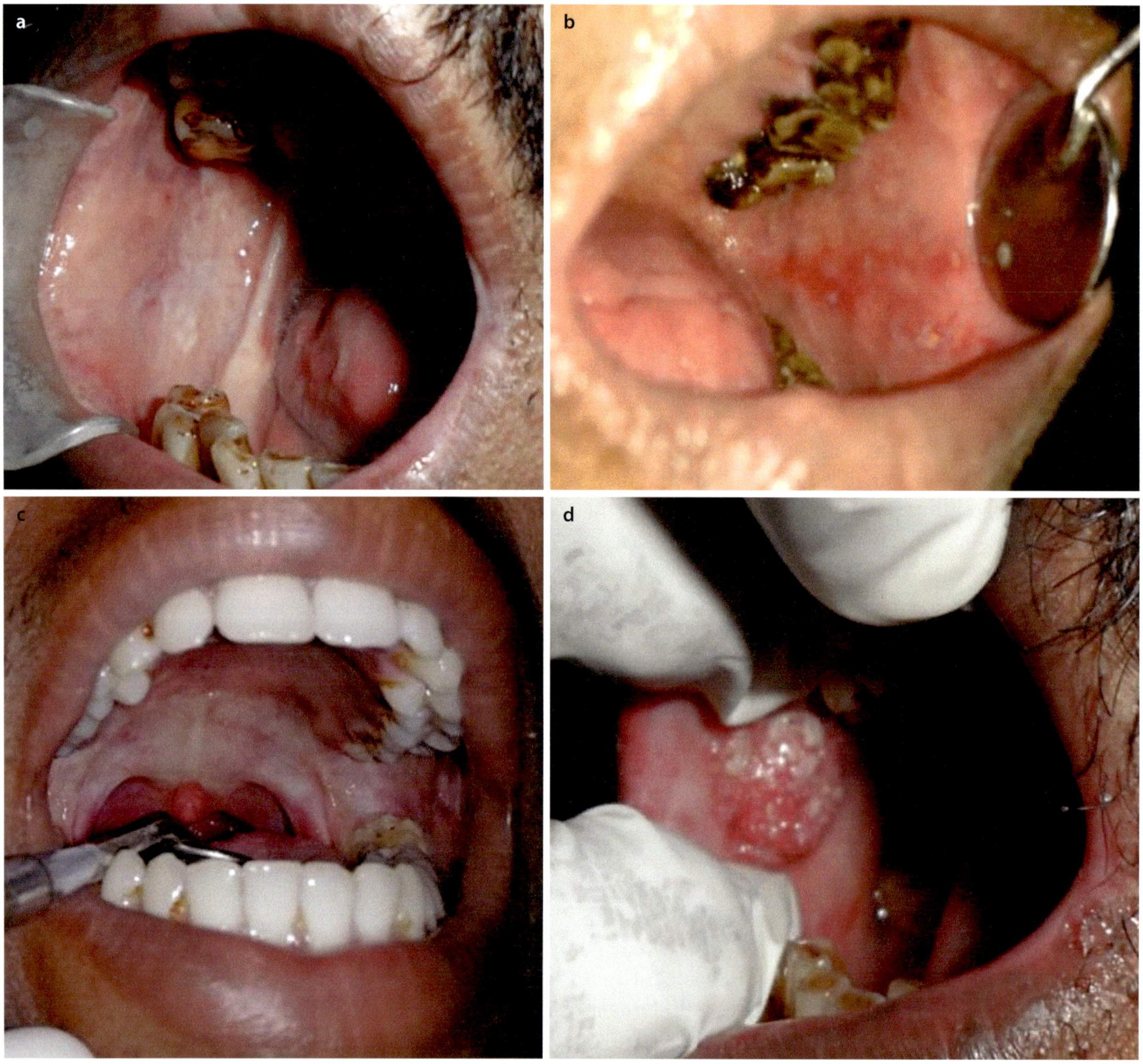

Fig. 21.3 Right-side buccal mucosa showing early changes, pale mucosa with normal mouth opening (**a**), left buccal mucosa showing multiple oral ulceration (**b**), fibrosed hard palate and shrunken uvula (**c**), and exophytic lesion indicating malignant transformation (**d**)

oral tissues. The more advanced stage of the disease is characterized by fibrous bands, both vertical and horizontal restricting the mouth opening and causing difficulty in oral functions such as mastication, speech, and swallowing. Restricted mouth opening, together with burning sensation, reduced elasticity, and ulcerations cause difficulties in maintaining oral hygiene. When fibrosis involves nasopharynx or oesophagus, patients may experience referred pain in the ear, nasal voice, and dysphagia to solid foods. Restricted mouth opening interferes with the examination of the oral mucosa and makes early diagnosis of cancer in the case of malignant transformation difficult.

OSF is diagnosed by its characteristic clinical features. However, an incisional biopsy may be needed in order to confirm the diagnosis and to assess the degree of epithelial dysplasia. The main histopathological features include atrophy of the surface epithelium, juxta epithelial hyalinization, and fibrosis and, depending on the stage of the disease, varying degrees of replacement of muscle by fibrous tissue. Vascularity of the corium is drastically reduced (Fig. 21.4). The surface epithelium develops epithelial dysplasia and the degree of epithelial dysplasia is a key indicator to draw the management plan. Clinical criteria for the diagnosis of OSF include mucosal blanching, hardening, and

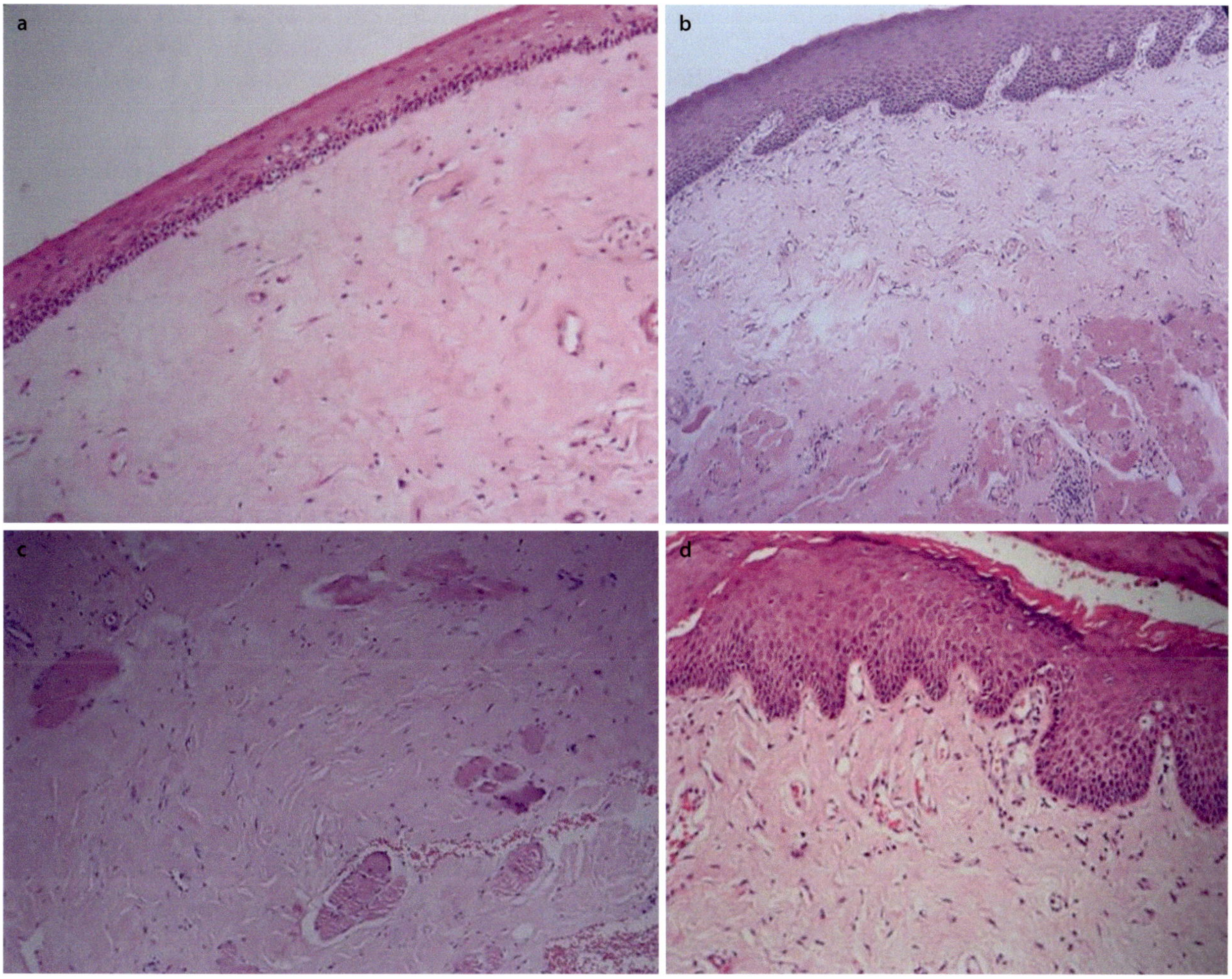

Fig. 21.4 Histopathological features with progression of OSF. Atrophic epithelium with fibrosis in the corium (**a**) followed by extension of fibrosis into superficial muscle (**b**) and replacement of muscle by fibrous tissue (**c**). Development of epithelial dysplasia in the surface epithelium (**d**)

the presence of characteristic vertical fibrous bands. However, these features may be absent or not prominent in early cases of OSF giving rise to a difficulty in accurate clinical diagnosis. Degree of mouth opening can be used as an objectively verifiable criterion to assess the severity of the disease (functional stage) whereas the site of the fibrous bands can be used to classify the disease clinically (clinical stage). The disease affects not only the oral cavity but also the upper-third of the oesophagus.

Differential diagnosis of OSF includes scleroderma, vitiligo, and anaemia. In scleroderma, multi-organ involvement may be present, and the tongue, soft palate, and larynx are the intraoral structures that are usually involved. Tongue becomes stiff and board-like due to fibrosis and may result in dysphagia. Gingival tissues are pale and unusually firm. Increased fibrosis in the perioral tissues leads to microstomia. Characteristic furrows radiating from mouth leads to "purse string" appearance. Another important feature of scleroderma is the widening of the periodontal ligament space. Vitiligo is an acquired hypopigmentary disorder with a possible autoimmune aetiology. Hypopigmentation present in OSF may mimic vitiligo, but involvement of the oral cavity by the latter is very rare.

There are many classifications for the disease staging and grading of OSF, but the grading system proposed by Kerr et al., 2011 is widely accepted.

- Grade 1 (mild) – Burning or depapillation or blanching/leathery mucosa and mouth opening >35 mm.
- Grade 2 (moderate) – Above features + mouth opening 20–35 mm.
- Grade 3 (severe) – Above features + mouth opening <20 mm.
- Grade 4A – OSF + other OPMD on clinical examination.
- Grade 4B – OSF + epithelial dysplasia on biopsy.
- Grade 5 – OSF + oral cancer.

The main complication in OSF is the possibility of malignant transformation to OSCC, which has been estimated to be around 5%. Frequency and duration of betel/areca nut chewing habit, combination of tobacco with areca nut, use of alcohol, presence of other potentially malignant disorders (especially leukoplakia and oral lichen planus), age, gender, changes in epithelial thickness, and presence of dysplasia at the initial biopsy are the main factors associated with malignant transformation in OSF. Poor nutritional status, immunologic abnormalities, altered cytokine levels, presence of mechanical trauma, and genetic susceptibility of the patient may further increase the risk of malignant transformation. Areca nut has been identified and labelled as a group I carcinogen and is primarily responsible for the malignant transformation in OSF. There are four identified carcinogens derive from arecoline, guacine, and guacoline, which are present in areca nut. A strong synergistic effect is reported with tobacco and alcohol increasing the risk of malignant transformation. Oral cancer that occurs in the background of OSF is OSCC. However, less frequently, verrucous carcinomas have also been reported. The prognosis of oral cancer occurring in the background of OSF is better as there is less metastasis compared to conventional OSCC.

Although OSF is considered to be a disease of the oral cavity, several studies have identified some extra oral manifestations such as liver cirrhosis, oesophageal fibrosis, and anaemia. Fibrosis in the oesophagus may cause difficulty in swallowing. Development of liver cirrhosis has been reported by several studies and is considered to be associated with high copper content in areca nut. Development of anaemia may be secondary to the disease due to difficulty in eating as a result of burning sensation, ulceration, and difficulty in swallowing.

There is no completely successful treatment for OSF at present. Aims of management are to reverse or alleviate signs and symptoms, to stop the progression of the disease, and to minimize the risk of malignant transformation. Current protocol for the management of OSF can be divided into three broad groups: medical, physical, and surgical treatments. Medical modalities include steroids (dexamethasone, methyl prednisolone, triamcinolone, and hydrocortisone), either topical or intra lesional enzymes (hyaluronidase, chymotrypsin, and collagenase), drugs (vitamin B complex, antioxidants, vitamins A, E, and C, interferon-gamma. and pentoxifylline), and nutritional interventions (turmeric oleoresin, turmeric oil, and turmeric extract, immune milk powder, lycopene, allicin and aloe vera). There are different types of surgical procedures that can be used in the management of OSF including split-thickness skin graft, nasolabial flaps, buccal fat pad, CO_2 laser, and coronoidectomy. Physical interventions including various physical exercise regimen, splints or other devices, and microwave diathermy have been used.

Treatment of patients with OSF depends on the extent of clinical involvement. If the disease is detected at a very early stage, cessation of the habit and follow-up is sufficient. Most patients with moderate to severe disease are difficult to treat successfully. Combined therapy with holistic approach can help the patient. The management of the disease depends on the stage of the disease and the degree of dysplasia (Table 21.1).

Table 21.1 Management of OSF

Disease stage	Clinical presentation	Investigations	Management
Early OSF	Burning sensation exacerbated by spicy food, vesiculation, blanching of mucosa, and leathery mucosa	FBC to exclude anaemia	Habit intervention, nutritional supplements if required, follow up with 3–6 month follow-up intervals Improvement of oral hygiene, topical steroids
Late OSF	Woody changes of mucosa and tongue, fibrous bands within mucosa, limitation of mouth opening, and narrowing of oropharyngeal orifice with distortion of uvula and sunken cheeks	FBC to exclude anaemia, biopsy if clinical diagnosis is not clear or dysplasia is suspected	Habit intervention and antioxidants, nutritional therapy, topical or intra lesional steroids, or physical therapy or surgery or combination therapy and follow up
OSF with other OPMD	Above features+ white or red patch	FBC to exclude anaemia, biopsy to identify the grade of dysplasia	Habit intervention and antioxidants, nutritional therapy, surgery (scalpel or laser) and follow up
OSF with oral cancer	Above features+ non-healing ulcer or proliferative lesion	FBC to exclude anaemia, biopsy to exclude cancer	Habit intervention and conventional treatment modalities for oral cancer and follow up

Table 21.1 (continued)

Salient features of oral submucous fibrosis	
Clinical	Burning sensation of oral mucosa, blanching, depigmentation, depapillation of the tongue, fibrous bands, and reduced mouth opening
Histopathology	Atrophic epithelium, sub-epithelial hyalinization and fibrosis, replacement of muscle by fibrous tissue, reduced vascularity, and varying degrees of epithelial dysplasia
Treatment	Habit intervention, physical, medical, and surgical
This is an oral potentially malignant disorder. It is important to plan vigorous follow-up for cases with epithelial dysplasia in order to identify early malignant transformation.	

Self-Assessment Questions

1. List the pathognomonic clinical features of OSF.
2. State the important conditions that need to be included in the deferential diagnosis.
3. Describe the histopathological features of OSF.
4. List different mechanisms of pathogenesis.
5. Explain the importance of identifying epithelial dysplasia in OSF.
6. Outline the management plan according to the stage of the disease.

Diagnostic and Management Algorithm for OSF

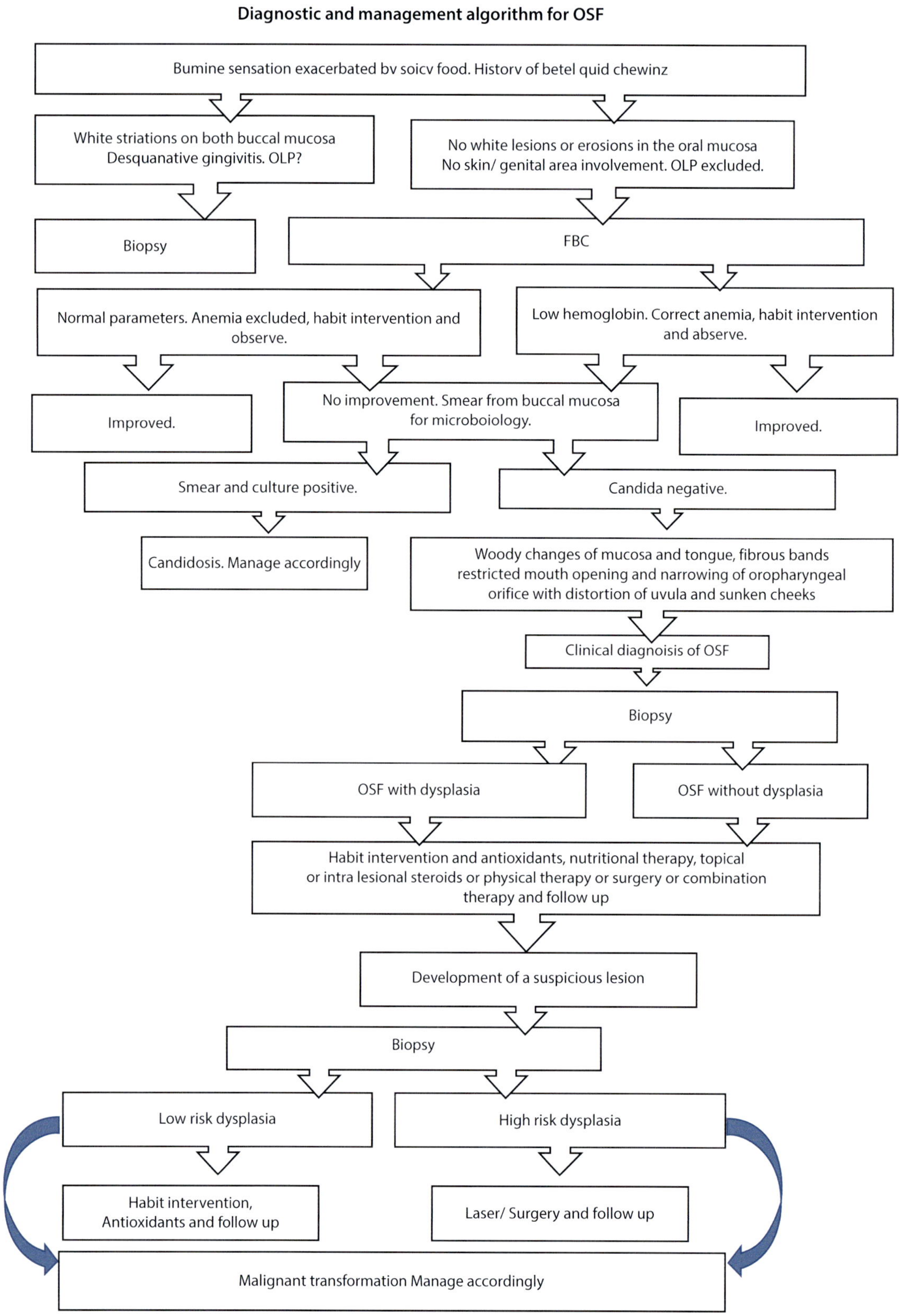

Summary

Oral submucous fibrosis (OSF) is a potentially malignant chronic, insidious disease. It is caused by the use of areca nut. The disease is characterized by blanching and stiffening of the oral mucosa due to fibrosis, which leads to restricted mouth opening. Clinical presentation depends on the stage of the disease. Some cases of OSF show different grades of epithelial dysplasia, showing its malignant transformation potential. Management is difficult at advanced stages and there is no completely successful treatment.

Further Reading

Ekanayaka RP, Tilakaratne WM. Oral submucous fibrosis: review on mechanisms of malignant transformation. Oral Surg Oral Med Oral Pathol Oral Radiol. 122(2):192–9.

Rao NR, Villa A, More CB, et al. Oral submucous fibrosis: a contemporary narrative review with a proposed inter-professional approach for an early diagnosis and clinical management. J Otolaryngol Head Neck Surg. 2020;49:3.

Tilakaratne WM, Ekanayaka RP, Saman W. Oral submucous fibrosis: a historical perspective and a review on etiology and pathogenesis. Oral Surg Oral Med Oral Pathol Oral Radiol. 122(2):178–19.

Tilakaratne WM, Klinikowski MF, Saku T, Peters TJ, SamanWarnakulasuriya. Oral submucous fibrosis: review on aetiology and pathogenesis. Oral Oncol. 2006;42:561–8.

Warnakulasuriya S, Ross K. Oral submucous fibrosis: a review of the current management and possible directions for novel therapies. Oral Surg Oral Med Oral Pathol Oral Radiol. 122(2):232–41.

White Patch on the Buccal Mucosa: Leukoplakia

Anand Ramanathan and Zuraiza Mohamad Zaini

Contents

W. M Tilakaratne, T. G. Kallarakkal (eds.), *Clinicopathological Correlation of Oral Diseases*,
https://doi.org/10.1007/978-3-031-24408-7_22

Learning Goals

1. Devise the correct way of compiling the history with appropriate questions.
2. Develop a differential diagnosis after history taking.
3. Deduce appropriate procedures in clinical examination.
4. Formulate a differential diagnosis combining findings in the history and clinical examination.
5. Justify the relevant investigations required to arrive at the diagnosis.
6. Comprehend the importance of clinicopathological correlation in arriving at the correct diagnosis.
7. Recognize the importance of a diagnostic algorithm in arriving at a diagnosis.
8. Outline the management plan.
9. Recognize the role of the dentist in the diagnosis, management and prevention of oral cancer.

22.1 Main Complaint

A 66-year-old female presented to the dental clinic complaining of a white patch on her left buccal mucosa.

22.2 History of Complaint

Question: How long have you had this white patch?

I think I had it for many years.

Question: Has the white patch changed in size?

It started small and grew slowly to its present size.

Question: Do you have any other issues associated with this white patch such as pain or a burning sensation?

No, I haven't had any trouble except I was becoming concerned why it is not going away and is also increasing in size.

Question: Are you able to wipe or scrape off the white patch?

No, it didn't get wiped off when I scraped it with a tooth brush.

Question: Do you tend to chew your cheeks?

No, I don't.

Question: Do you have any other white patches in your mouth?

No, I haven't noticed any.

Question: Do you have any white patches or skin rashes in any other parts of your body?

No, I don't have any skin lesions of similar nature.

22.3 Past Medical History

Question: Do you have any significant medical problems?

No, I don't. I consider myself generally healthy for my age.

Question: Are you taking any medications such as steroids?

I don't take any regular medications.

Question: Did you undergo any organ or bone marrow transplant?

No. As I said earlier, I haven't had any major medical issues.

22.4 Past Dental History

Question: Have you had any dental treatment?

I have had extractions of all my natural teeth and wear set of upper and lower full dentures for the past 4 years. I recently changed my dentures.

Question: Why did you change your dentures?

The teeth became worn in the previous set of dentures.

Question: Are the new dentures comfortable?

Yes, they are.

Question: Do you have any silver (amalgam) fillings in your mouth, closer to the white patch?

I have one silver colour filling, but it is on the opposite of the white patch.

Question: Did you recall keeping any crushed tablets, ointment or any oil inside your mouth?

I have never done that.

22.5 Social History

Question: Do you smoke or use other tobacco products?

I am a non-smoker and don't use any form of tobacco.

Question: Do you drink alcohol?

No, I am a teetotaller.

Question: Do you chew betel quid, areca nut or tobacco?

I do not chew betel, areca nut or tobacco.

22.6 Findings of Extra-Oral Examination

She had normal mouth opening, full range of jaw movements with no tenderness, clicking or crepitus in her TMJs. There were no palpable lymph nodes in the head and neck region. She had no skin lesions and her finger nails appeared clinically normal.

22.7 Findings of Intraoral Examination

There is a homogenous, non-scrapable white patch measuring approximately about 2.0 × 1.5 cm located on the left buccal mucosa that did not disappear on stretching the cheek (Fig. 22.1). There is no induration (firmness) or palpable fibrous bands beneath the buccal mucosa. The surrounding mucosa appeared clinically normal. The dentures were free of any sharp edges that could irritate the buccal mucosa.

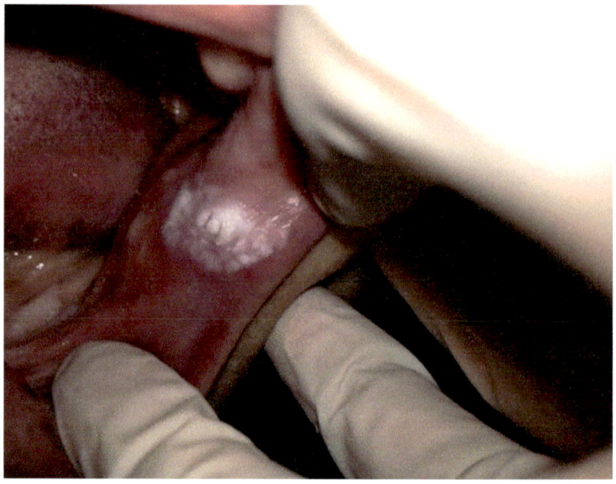

Fig. 22.1 Intraoral photograph showing a white patch on the left buccal mucosa. (Courtesy Dr. Fauziani Zainul Abidin)

22.8 What Are Your Differential Diagnoses for This White Patch on the Left Buccal Mucosa After History Taking and Clinical Examination?

Oral leukoplakia.

Frictional keratosis.

Oral lichen planus.

Oral lichenoid lesion.

Chronic hyperplastic candidosis.

Oral cancer.

Frictional keratosis presents as a whitish area on the mucosa that is non-scrapable and directly related to a traumatic agent (e.g. a sharp cusp of tooth or broken restoration or broken denture). Once the causative factor is eliminated, the lesion would usually resolve. The lesion seen in this patient does not show cause–effect relationship, with her dentures being free of any sharp edges. Hence, this white patch is unlikely to be a frictional keratosis.

Oral lichen planus (OLP) can be broadly classified into white and red forms. The white forms of oral lichen planus include (i) reticular type, (ii) papular type and (iii) plaque type. The reticular type has white distinct striae forming linear/reticular/annular patterns. The papular type has numerous tiny papules whereas the plaque type presents as a white patch. Oral lichen planus is usually bilateral or multifocal in distribution. Buccal mucosa is the commonest site but the tongue is no exception. OLP lesions cannot be scrapped off and may cause burning sensation especially when eating spicy food.

The persistent white lesion in this patient has some semblance to plaque form of oral lichen planus. However, the plaque type of oral lichen planus is usually accompanied by the other forms of lichen planus in other subsites in the mouth, which this patient does not have. Moreover, the lack of burning sensation too makes it less likely for the lesion being oral lichen planus.

Oral lichenoid lesions (OLL) include oral lichenoid contact lesions (OLCL), drug-induced lichenoid reactions (OLR) and chronic graft versus host disease (cGVHD). Oral lichenoid lesions due to dental materials are called OLCL. These lesions are usually solitary white patches or mixed red and white lesions with white striae which cannot be rubbed off and are located on the mucosa in contact with a large amalgam restoration. The white patch seen in this patient has a similar appearance to a lichenoid lesion but there is no associated amalgam restoration to call it an OLCL.

Oral lichenoid lesions due to betel quid occur in the area where the betel quid is placed in the mouth and are also considered OLCL They are usually white lesions with striae that do not crisscross, cannot be rubbed off and are usually seen in the buccal mucosa and lower buccal sulcus. However, this patient does not chew betel.

Oral lichenoid reactions (OLR) induced by drugs occur as white lesions with striae mimicking oral lichen planus. These white lesions cannot be scraped off and are seen in patients who are on or have taken medications known to be associated with lichenoid reactions in the recent past. The patient does not take such medications and the white lesion is free of striae. Hence OLR is an unlikely diagnosis for this patient.

Chronic graft versus host disease (cGVHD) usually presents as widespread oral lichenoid lesions. It occurs as either red and white mixed lesions or as white lesions with striae that mimicked oral lichen planus. These lesions cannot be scraped off and the patient may complain of burning sensation. To diagnose cGVHD, a patient should have a history of either organ or bone marrow transplantation. However, this patient lacks any history of organ or bone marrow transplantation.

Chronic hyperplastic candidosis is primarily a candidal infection which occurs as a white patch that cannot be scraped off. The white lesion in this patient fits into this description, justifying the inclusion of this condition in the differential diagnosis.

Oral cancer can clinically present as a persistent white patch. The common sites include lateral border of the tongue, buccal mucosa, ventral tongue and on the soft palate. This case could be oral cancer since the lesion is a white patch on the buccal mucosa that is non-scrapable. However, cancerous white lesions usually exhibit induration (firmness—attached to the underlying tissue) on palpation and also often have non-homogenous surface appearance; both features are missing in this patient.

This patient has a white patch that cannot be defined as any other lesion as mentioned above. Therefore, by exclusion, a clinical diagnosis of leukoplakia appears appropriate for the white patch in her left buccal mucosa. Oral leukoplakia is considered a potentially malignant disorder with a recognized risk for malignant transformation. Furthermore, this patient does not have any risk habits known to be associated with oral leukoplakia.

22.9 What Is the Most Likely Clinical Diagnosis for This White Patch on the Buccal Mucosa?

Idiopathic oral leukoplakia (homogenous type).

22.10 What Investigations Need to Be Carried Out for This Patient?

Idiopathic oral leukoplakia (homogenous type) is an oral potentially malignant disorder. The white patch was biopsied and the specimen was sent for histopathological examination to establish a definitive diagnosis.

22.11 What Are the Histopathological Features of the Submitted Specimen?

Hematoxylin and eosin-stained section shows mucosa covered by parakeratinized stratified squamous epithelium. The epithelium shows mild degree of architectural disturbances and cytological atypia. The architectural abnormalities present include loss of polarity of basal cells and bulbous and drop-shaped rete ridges. The cytological features present are abnormal variations in nuclear and cell size, abnormal variation in nuclear and cell shape, increased nuclear-cytoplasmic ratio and nuclear hyperchromatism. The atypical cytological features are confined to the lower one-third of the epithelium that has an intact basement membrane zone (◘ Fig. 22.2a and b).

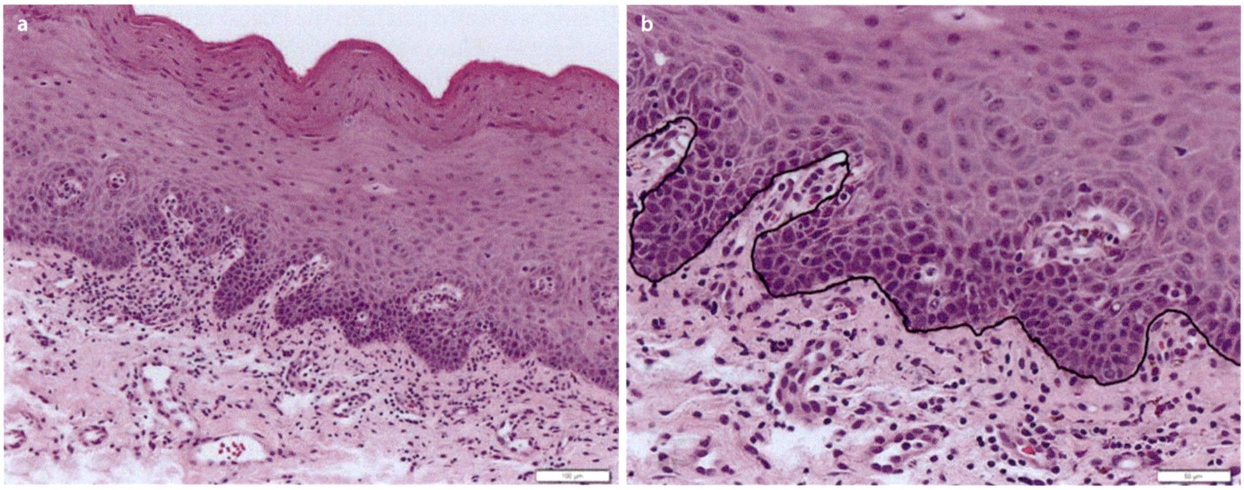

Fig. 22.2 Photomicrographs (a) and (b) show the cytological atypical features extending up to the lower one-third of the epithelium with intact basement membrane zone (black line), thus indicating mild epithelial dysplasia. (Courtesy: Dr. Nadia Najwa Shuhairi)

22.12 What Is the Definitive Diagnosis for This Lesion?

Oral leukoplakia (homogenous type) with mild epithelial dysplasia.

22.13 What Specific Findings Helped You to Arrive at the Diagnosis of Oral Leukoplakia with Mild Epithelial Dysplasia?

There is no history of trauma, immunocompromised status and drug history in this patient. There is no amalgam fillings directly related to the lesion. The presence of a homogenous white patch on the left buccal mucosa that cannot be scraped off and is not indurated suggests a diagnosis of leukoplakia. In addition, this lesion does not fit into any other definable lesions such as linea alba, leukoedema, frictional keratosis, pseudomembranous candidiasis, oral lichen planus, oral lichenoid lesion, white spongy naevus, chemical burn and oral cancer. The lesion is clinically diagnosed as idiopathic oral leukoplakia (homogenous type) after all other definable oral lesions have been excluded. On histopathological examination, there is no pathognomonic features suggestive of other known disease entities. Presence of dysplastic parakeratinized squamous epithelium showing intact basement membrane zone with architectural and cytological atypical features restricted to the lower one-third of the epithelium is consistent with a diagnosis of mild epithelial dysplasia.

22.14 How Do You Manage This Patient?

Clinically diagnosed idiopathic oral leukoplakia (homogenous type) should be biopsied to arrive at a definitive diagnosis as in this case. Therefore, it is best for the patient to be referred to an oral surgeon or an oral medicine specialist. In the light of current evidence, base an oral leukoplakia with mild epithelial dysplasia does not merit surgical intervention and could be managed conservatively and be kept under periodic surveillance. The patient should also be advised to avoid any risk habits such as use of tobacco in any form, betel quid chewing and alcohol use. Follow-up examinations at every 3–6 months is considered acceptable. If the lesion shows increase in size or change in surface appearance/texture, a re-biopsy is required to assess disease progression.

22.15 What Is the Prognosis for Homogenous Oral Leukoplakia with Mild Epithelial Dysplasia?

Leukoplakia has an overall malignant transformation rate of 9.5% with an annual malignant transformation rate of 1.56%. Homogenous leukoplakia tends to have lower malignant transformation rate compared to non-homogenous leukoplakia. The clinical features that are associated with malignant transformation risk in this patient are (i) female gender (female = medium risk), (ii) age (66 years old = medium risk), (iii) size of the lesion (>200 mm^2 = strong risk), (iv) habits (no habits/idiopathic = higher risk) and (v) presence of mild epithelial dysplasia (weak risk). Oral leukoplakia with mild epithelial dysplasia has a 15-year malignant transformation rate of 6%.

22.16 Oral Leukoplakia

Leukoplakia is defined as a white plaque of questionable risk of malignant transformation, having excluded other definable conditions. Hence it is a clinical diagnosis by exclusion and is considered an oral potentially malignant disorder. By definition, an oral potentially malignant disorder is an oral mucosal abnormality that is associated with a statistically increased risk of developing oral cancer. ◘ Table 22.1 shows the list of oral potentially malignant disorders.

The global prevalence of all OPMDs is approximately 4.47%, with males affected more than females. Asians tend to be more affected by OPMDs with a prevalence of 10.54%. Among the OPMDs, oral leukoplakia is the most common with a global prevalence rate ranging from 2.6 to 4.11%. In the western world, the prevalence rate of leukoplakia is 1–4% whereas its prevalence is higher in South and South-east Asian countries.

Oral leukoplakia is considered six times more common among smokers than in non-smokers. Leukoplakia is associated with the use of both smoked and smokeless tobacco. The number of cigarettes smoked per day is closely associated with the risk of developing oral leukoplakia. Oral leukoplakia may regress after discontinuation of the use of tobacco. Alcohol consumption is regarded as an independent risk factor for oral leukoplakia. Oral leukoplakia also occurs in persons with betel quid or areca nut chewing habit and can occur in the background of oral submucous fibrosis. It can also occur in individuals who do not have any risk habits such as tobacco, alcohol and betel quid use. Such lesions are called idiopathic leukoplakias. It is believed that human papillomavirus (HPV) may have a potential role in a minority of oral leukoplakia.

◘ Table 22.1 List of oral potentially malignant disorders

No.	Oral potentially malignant disorders
1.	Erythroplakia
2.	Leukoplakia
3.	Proliferative verrucous leukoplakia
4.	Oral submucous fibrosis
5.	Palatal lesions associated with reverse smoking
6.	Oral lichenoid lesions
7.	Oral lichen planus
8.	Actinic keratosis
9.	Smokeless tobacco keratosis
10.	Oral graft versus host disease
11.	Lupus erythematosus
12.	Familial cancer syndromes including Fanconi anaemia, dyskeratosis congenita, xeroderma pigmentosum, Li-Fraumeni syndrome, Blooms's syndrome, ataxia telangiectasia and Cowden's syndrome

22.16.1 Clinical Features

Oral leukoplakia is usually diagnosed after the fourth decade of life and is more common in males. It can be classified into two types: (i) homogenous leukoplakia and (ii) non-homogenous leukoplakia and the latter can be further subdivided into (i) speckled/erythroleukoplakia, (ii) nodular leukoplakia and (iii) verrucous leukoplakia. Proliferative verrucous leukoplakia is a distinct form of oral leukoplakia which is multifocal and has high malignant transformation rate.

In western population, oral leukoplakia is commonly seen on lateral margins of the tongue and on the floor of mouth whereas it is common on the buccal mucosa and lower buccal sulcus in Asian populations due to betel quid chewing habit. Gingival leukoplakia is uncommon. Most leukoplakias, especially the homogenous type, are usually asymptomatic. However, non-homogeneous leukoplakia such as the speckled variety may cause few symptoms that include discomfort when consuming spicy food, tingling and sensitivity to touch. Homogenous leukoplakia presents as a whitish plaque/patch on the oral mucosa. These patches are usually flat but sometimes slightly raised above the surrounding mucosa. The surface may show shallow cracks and wrinkles (◘ Fig. 22.3). Speckled leukoplakia is a type of non-homogenous leukoplakia, also known as erythroleukoplakia. The lesion is predominantly white with one or more red/erythematous areas (◘ Fig. 22.4). The red component indicates possible colonization by *Candida* species or an increased risk for the presence of epithelial dysplasia and/or malignancy. Nodular leukoplakia is predominantly a white lesion with multiple red/white nodular or granular areas, small polypoid outgrowths, rounded red or white excrescences on the oral mucosa (◘ Fig. 22.5). Verrucous leukoplakia is a type of non-homogenous leukoplakia which is predominantly a white lesion with warty or irregular blunt/pointed projections.

Proliferative verrucous leukoplakia (PVL) is a distinct entity of leukoplakia that is multifocal, has a pro-

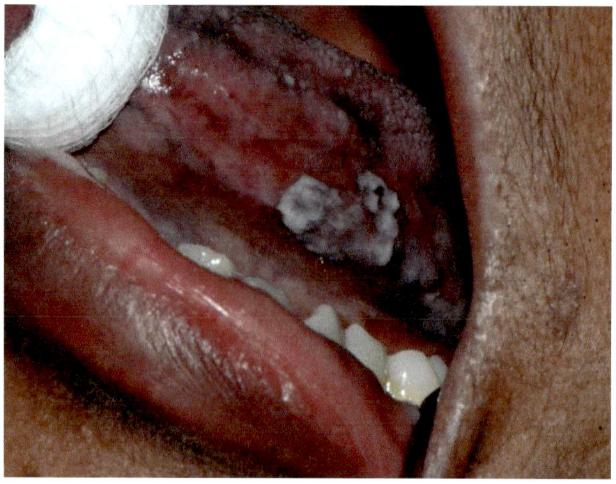

Fig. 22.3 Intraoral photograph shows homogenous leukoplakia on the left lateral surface of the tongue

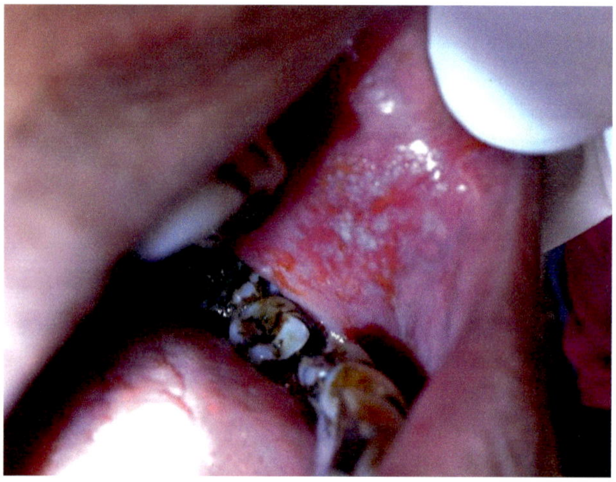

Fig. 22.4 Intraoral photograph shows a non-homogenous leukoplakia (speckled variety) on the left buccal mucosa in a betel quid chewer

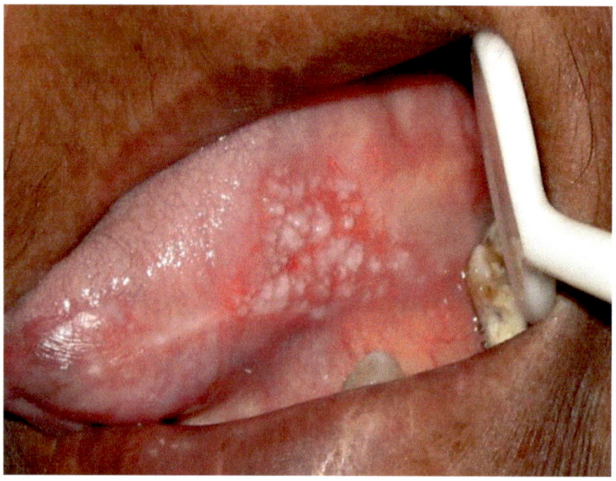

Fig. 22.5 Intraoral photograph shows a non-homogenous leukoplakia (nodular type) on the left lateral border of the tongue

gressive course and is associated with high recurrence and malignant transformation rates (50%). It is rare compared to conventional leukoplakia, common in elderly patients (>60 years), has strong female predilection (M/F: 1:4) and occurs most commonly in non-smokers. Proliferative verrucous leukoplakia has an unknown aetiology. It is not associated with any known risk habits such as tobacco smoking or alcohol consumption. Further there in no association with HPV or other viruses. It occurs commonly on gingiva, alveolar mucosa and palate, while the lateral and ventral surfaces of the tongue are rarely involved. It consists of four clinical stages: (i) focal flat white keratosis; (ii) diffuse, multifocal white patches (Fig. 22.6a); (iii) slowly progressive horizontal white lesions and exophytic growth resulting in warty (verrucous) surface with focal erythematous areas (Fig. 22.6b and c); and (iv) development of verrucous carcinoma or squamous cell carcinoma. However, these four stages do not occur in all cases of PVL.

The clinical differential diagnosis for homogenous leukoplakia includes linea alba, leukoedema, frictional keratosis, pseudomembranous candidosis, chemical burn, oral lichen planus, oral lichenoid lesion and oral cancer. Other differential diagnoses that may be considered are white spongy naevus, chronic hyperplastic candidosis, oral hairy leukoplakia, actinic keratosis and smokeless tobacco keratosis.

Linea alba is a white line on the buccal mucosa occurring in association with pressure, frictional irritation or sucking trauma from facial surfaces of the teeth. It is usually seen bilaterally, but can also be a unilateral presentation. It presents as a scalloped, persistent white line at the level of the occlusal plane.

Leukoedema is a diffuse white or greyish-white, smooth, oedematous appearance usually seen bilaterally on the buccal mucosa. It is prominent in smokers and dark-skinned persons. It has delicate vertical folding of the mucosal surface that disappears when stretched only to re-appear upon release. Leukoedema does not require treatment.

Chemical burns appear as a white lesion in the area where a caustic substance such as a drug (e.g. aspirin or other analgesics or pain killer balms) is applied in the mouth. The drug is usually crushed and applied on to the oral mucosa adjacent to a painful tooth for pain relief. The chemical damage from such applications makes the surface oral mucosa fragile and easy to peel off.

White spongy naevus is a hereditary disorder. It usually affects the buccal mucosa and is a large white lesion. It may occur in other mucous membranes such as the genital mucosa.

Chronic hyperplastic candidosis occurs as thick white lesions that cannot be scrapped off. These lesions

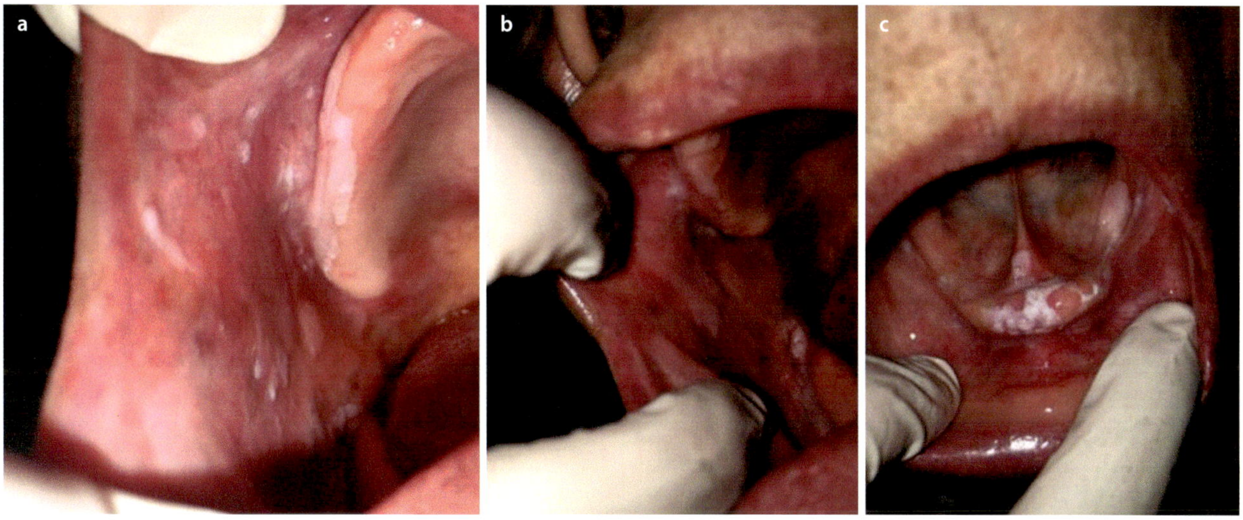

Fig. 22.6 Intraoral photographs of PVL showing (a) diffuse, multifocal white patches; slowly progressive horizontal white lesions (b); and exophytic growth resulting in warty (verrucous) surface with focal erythematous area (c). (Courtesy Dr. Fauziani Zainul Abidin)

occur due to the ability of certain *Candida* species to colonize and penetrate the superficial layers of the oral mucosa. Chronic hyperplastic candidosis should be differentiated from candidal leukoplakia. They are two different lesions. Candidal leukoplakia is primarily an oral leukoplakia, which is secondarily infected by *Candida* due to the presence of local or systemic immunosuppression, whereas in chronic hyperplastic candidiasis, it is primarily *candidal* infection that gives rise to the development of the lesion. However, the distinction between the two entities is difficult and some clinicians use them synonymously.

Oral hairy leukoplakia presents as whitish corrugated streaks at the lateral border of the tongue and is often bilateral. It cannot be scraped off and does not disappear with anti-fungal treatment. Oral hairy leukoplakia is caused by Epstein-Barr virus (EBV) and is common in immunocompromised persons having either human immunodeficiency viral (HIV) infections or when they tend to develop acquired immunodeficiency syndrome (AIDS).

Actinic keratosis is a rough, scaly white patch seen on the skin especially in areas that are exposed to sunlight. Hence the lesions are seen on the face, ears, forearm, scalp, neck and back of the hands. When it involves the vermilion of the lips, it is considered an oral potentially malignant disorder. Smokeless tobacco keratosis is a white to grey mucosal patch with wrinkled or fissured surface seen in the area where smokeless tobacco products such as chewing tobacco or moist/dry snuff are placed. These lesions appear as thin, translucent and granular mucosa or as wrinkled mucosa, usually on the buccal and labial mucosa. Later they become hyperkeratotic, thicker and opaque white lesions with surface fissures and folds. This lesion too is considered as an oral potentially malignant disorder. However, the lesions tend to disappear on stopping the smokeless tobacco habit.

The clinical differential diagnosis of non-homogenous leukoplakia of speckled variety includes mixed red and white lesions such as chemical burns, geographic tongue, stomatitis nicotina palatini, oral lichenoid lesions, oral lichen planus and oral cancer. Geographic tongue occurs on the dorsal surface of the tongue with atrophy of the lingual papillae. There are well-demarcated reddish areas of depapillation with peripheral whitish/yellowish, serpiginous lines that give the tongue a map-like appearance. These red areas heal spontaneously and disappear over time only to reappear in another area on the dorsal surface of the tongue, thus earning it the name erythema migrans. Speckled leukoplakia occurs more commonly on the buccal mucosa or lateral surface of the tongue. Stomatitis nicotina palatini or smoker's palate is also a mixed red and white lesion that occurs on the palatal mucosa of smokers. The palatal mucosa becomes blanched and white with tiny red spots representing the orifices of inflamed minor salivary gland ducts. This lesion tends to regress once the person quits smoking. Oral lichen planus, especially the erosive form, may present as mixed red and white lesions with striae in some areas. Oral cancers can present as indurated mixed red and white lesions.

22.16.2 Investigations

There are many diagnostic adjuncts that may be used to help early detection of oral cancer and oral potentially malignant disorders. They can be broadly classified into (i) visualization/optical adjuncts, (ii) vital staining, (iii) oral cytology and (iv) salivary adjuncts.

Visualization-based or optical adjuncts are either devices or machines that may use the changes in various optical properties such as absorption, reflection, refraction, autofluorescence and scattering associated with carcinogenesis in the oral mucosa. They generate real-time images or optical signals as a result of interaction of light with the tissue. Tissue reflectance and autofluorescence are visualization-based or optical adjuncts used in clinical practice.

Tissue reflectance is performed as a two-step process: (a) topical application of acetic acid on the oral mucosa and (b) direct illumination of the oral mucosa using low-wavelength (blue-white) light. In some of these processes, the light source is generated by a chemical reaction and is therefore called chemiluminescence, whereas others have LED lights. Vital staining adjunct diagnostic tools use dyes or markers that can stain the oral mucosa to provide macroscopic information.

Autofluorescence devices are hand-held devices which generate a blue-violet light (400–450 nm range). This range of light excites the tissue fluorophores such as nicotinamide adenine dinucleotide (NADH) and flavin adenine dinucleotide (FAD) that are present in the epithelium, collagen or elastin cross-linking in the submucosa to reveal a fluorescence emission. The normal mucosa emits an apple green fluorescence whereas the abnormal mucosa appears dark, defined as loss of fluorescence visualization (FVL) (◘ Fig. 22.7a and b).

Vital staining involves the application of a dye to an OPMD, which helps to characterize and better visualize the lesion. The mechanism by which it works is not fully understood. It probably works due to the increased permeability and affinity of toluidine blue to nuclear material in high-grade dysplasia and oral squamous cell carcinoma (OSCC). Toluidine blue 1% or 2% solution is commonly used (◘ Fig. 22.7c). Other dyes used for vital staining include Lugol's iodine, methylene blue and rose bengal.

Oral cytology refers to microscopic examination of surface epithelial cells harvested by non-invasive methods such as brush, spatula or curettes. Harvested cells are fixed on to a glass slide, stained and examined under the microscope for presence of cellular atypia. Oral cytology has high specificity and sensitivity in identifying oral cancer and oral epithelial dysplasia. However, it cannot replace the current gold standard of tissue biopsy and histopathological diagnosis since it is unable to distinguish between OSCC and oral epithelial dysplasia (OED) in some cases and also between the different grades of OED.

Although different salivary adjuncts are available, their reliability in routine diagnostics has not been proven. The sensitivity, specificity, positive predictive value, negative predictive value and accuracy of these adjunct tools vary considerably. Thus, tissue biopsy for histopathological examination still remains the gold standard in the diagnosis of OPMDs and early detection of oral cancer.

22.16.3 Tissue Biopsy

The types of tissue biopsy include (i) punch biopsy, (ii) incisional biopsy and (iii) excisional biopsy. The type of tissue biopsy performed depends on various factors such as size and location of the lesion and patient comfort. Punch biopsy uses a circular blade with rotary motion. Tissue punches are available in different diameters. Incisional and excisional biopsies use either scalpel or lasers to harvest the tissue specimen. Scalpel biopsy is preferred for diagnostic purposes since laser can distort tissue and make histopathological examination and interpretation difficult. Punch and incisional biopsies are usually performed for lesions larger than 1.0 cm in size to obtain a tissue sample deemed the best representative of the lesion. It is best if the biopsy includes a portion of adjacent normal tissue in the specimen. Multiple biopsies can be considered for larger lesions. Necrotic areas should be avoided. On the contrary, an excision biopsy is used for smaller lesions (usu-

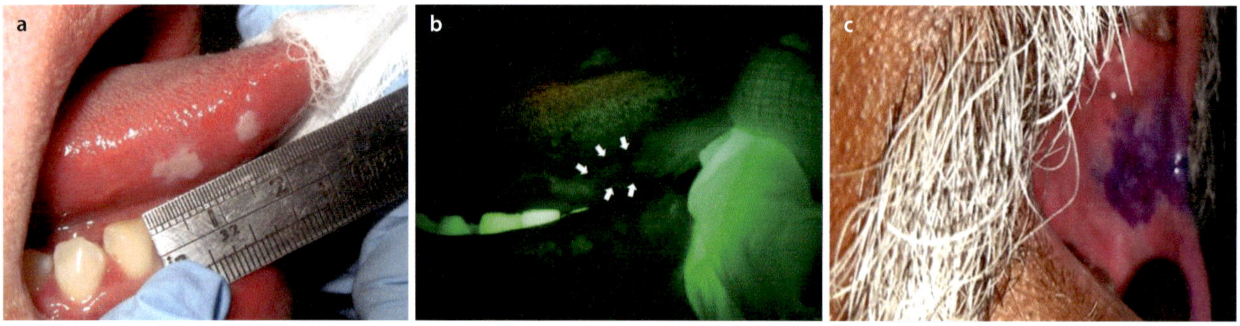

◘ **Fig. 22.7** Intraoral photographs show leukoplakia on the right lateral surface of the tongue (**a**); autofluorescence image of the right lateral surface of the tongue with areas of loss of fluorescence (white arrows), which turned out to be moderate epithelial dysplasia (**b**); and left buccal mucosa of another patient with increased uptake of the toluidine blue stain indicating dysplastic changes on the surface epithelium (**c**)

ally less than 1.0 cm in size) to remove the entire lesion for histopathological examination. Once the biopsy tissue has been taken, it is transferred into neutral buffered formalin, labelled and sent to the pathology laboratory for histopathological examination.

22.16.4 Histopathological Features

Histopathology of oral leukoplakia may range from hyperplastic or hyperkeratotic epithelium to dysplasia to invasive oral squamous cell carcinoma. Homogenous leukoplakia having thin smooth surface may show epithelial hyperplasia/hyperkeratosis and acanthosis of the surface epithelium with few chronic inflammatory cells within the fibrous connective stroma. The thick fissured leukoplakia may show hyperkeratosis, acanthosis and varying degrees of oral epithelia dysplasia. Verrucous leukoplakia shows irregular hyperkeratosis with bulbous rete ridges, varying degrees of epithelial dysplasia occasionally with superimposed candidal hyphae and moderate inflammatory infiltration in the connective tissue stroma. However, these histopathological features may vary to a greater extent in different cases of oral leukoplakia. Reportedly, 85% of oral leukoplakias show no dysplasia. Mild dysplasia is present in about 8%, moderate dysplasia in 5% and severe dysplasia in 2% of all oral leukoplakias.

Oral epithelial dysplasia is defined as a spectrum of architectural and cytological epithelial changes caused by accumulation of genetic changes and is reportedly associated with an increased risk of progression to squamous cell carcinoma. Oral epithelial dysplasia, particularly the severity of dysplasia, is widely believed to be the best predictor of malignant transformation.

Architectural features are the changes seen in the organization of maturation and normal layering of the epithelium whereas atypical cytological features are those seen at the individual cell level. The architectural and atypical cytological features seen in OED are listed in ◘ Table 22.2. However, the recent WHO classification on Head and Neck tumours has added more features to the list of dysplastic features.

In mild epithelial dysplasia, the cytologic and/or architectural alterations are confined to the lower third of the epithelium (basal and parabasal layers) (◘ Fig. 22.10a). In moderate epithelial dysplasia, the cytologic and/or architectural alterations extend from the basal layer to the mid-portion of the spinous layer (middle third) (◘ Fig. 22.10b), while in severe epithelial dysplasia, such changes extend from basal cells to a level beyond the midpoint of the epithelium (upper third) or the entire thickness of the epithelium (◘ Fig. 22.10c). Further, the degree of severity should be upgraded to severe dysplasia if marked cytological atypia is present in the lower and middle third of the epithelium.

◘ **Table 22.2** Architectural features and atypical cytological features present in oral epithelial dysplasia

Architectural features:	
(i)	Loss of polarity of basal cells (◘ Fig. 22.8a)
(ii)	Irregular epithelial stratification (◘ Fig. 22.8b)
(iii)	Drop-shaped rete ridges (◘ Fig. 22.8c)
(iv)	Increased number of mitotic figures (◘ Fig. 22.8d)
(v)	Abnormally superficial mitotic figures (◘ Fig. 22.8d)
(vi)	Premature keratinization in single cells (dyskeratosis) (◘ Fig. 22.9a)
(vii)	Keratin pearls within rete ridges (◘ Fig. 22.9b)
(viii)	Loss of epithelial cell cohesion (◘ Fig. 22.9c)
Atypical cytological features:	
(i)	Abnormal variation in nuclear size
(ii)	Abnormal variation in nuclear shape
(iii)	Abnormal variation in cell size
(iv)	Abnormal variation in cell shape
(v)	Increased nuclear-cytoplasmic ratio
(vi)	Atypical mitotic figures
(vii)	Increased number and size of nucleoli
(viii)	Nuclear hyperchromatism

The histopathology of PVL varies depending on the clinical stage of the lesion. The dysplastic features are usually not marked and mostly show architectural disturbances despite high malignant transformation rate. Flat to verrucous hyperkeratosis may show minimal to no dysplasia, which may lead to underestimation of the risk of malignant transformation. Dysplasia develops in late stages, before progressing to either verrucous carcinoma or squamous cell carcinoma. Definitive diagnosis of PVL requires clinicopathological correlation.

22.16.5 Treatment

Patients with risk habits such as smoking, alcohol drinking and betel quid chewing habits should be advised and counselled to quit such habits immediately. All oral leukoplakias should be referred to either an oral surgeon or to an oral medicine specialist for assessment, biopsy and further management. Non-homogenous leukoplakias, especially erythroleukoplakia, requires urgent referral for assessment and biopsy. Histopathological examination remains the gold standard for diagnosis, risk assessment and planning further management of oral leukoplakia. Oral leukoplakias with either hyperplasia,

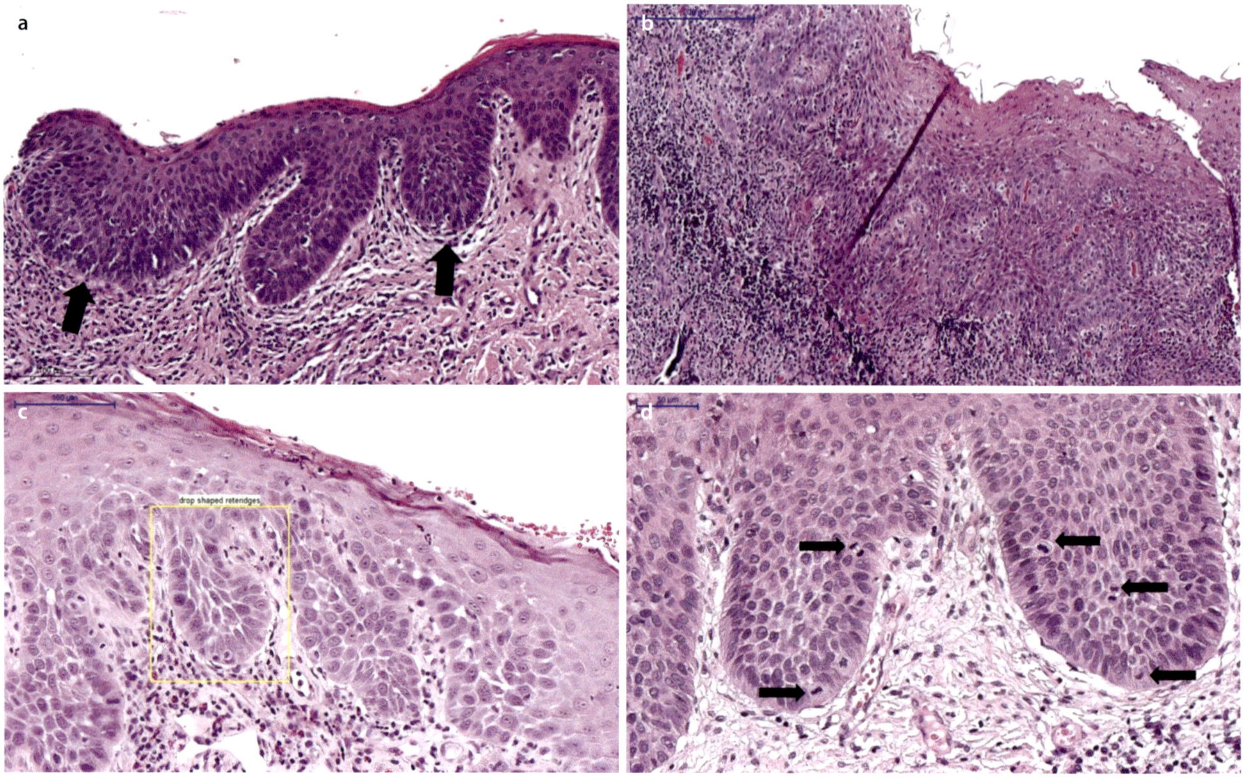

Fig. 22.8 Photomicrographs show (**a**) loss of polarity of basal cells (black arrows), (**b**) irregular epithelial stratification, (**c**) drop-shaped rete ridges and (**d**) increased number of mitotic figures and abnormally superficial mitotic figures (black arrows). (Courtesy: Assoc. Prof. Dr. Thomas George)

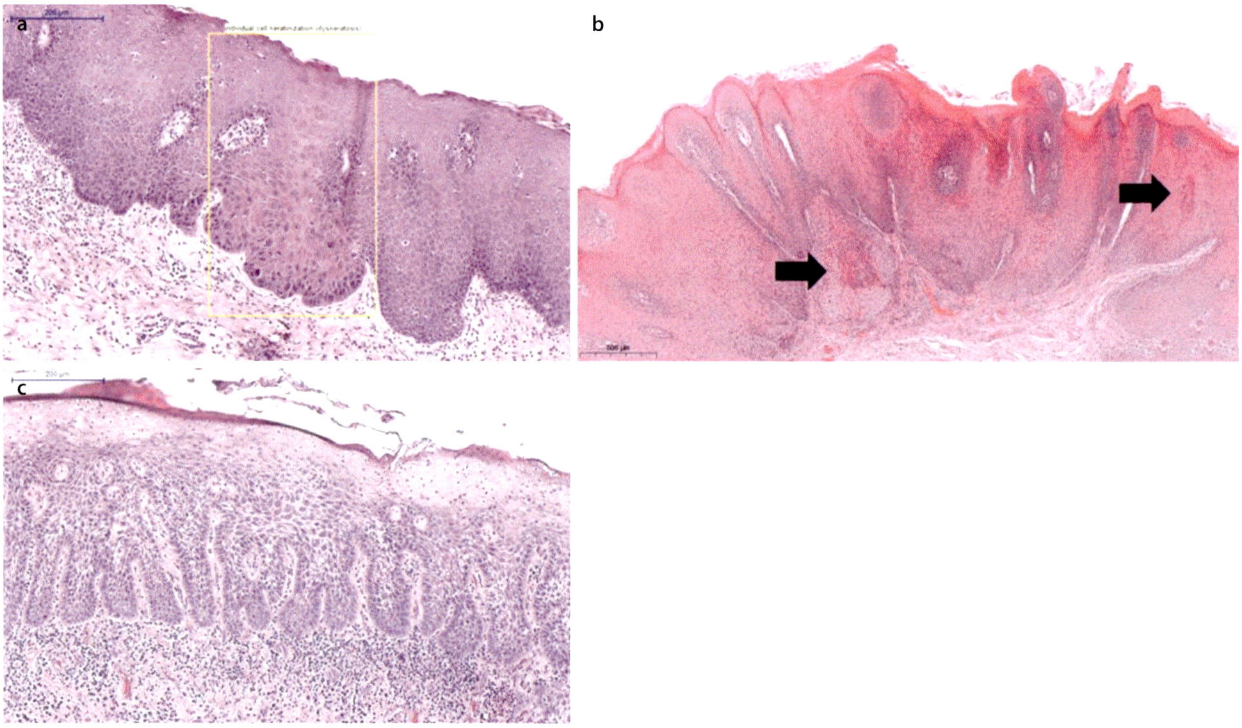

Fig. 22.9 Photomicrographs show (**a**) premature keratinization in single cells, (**b**) intraepithelial keratin pearls (black arrows) and (**c**) loss of epithelial cell cohesion. (Courtesy: Asst. prof. Dr. Thomas George)

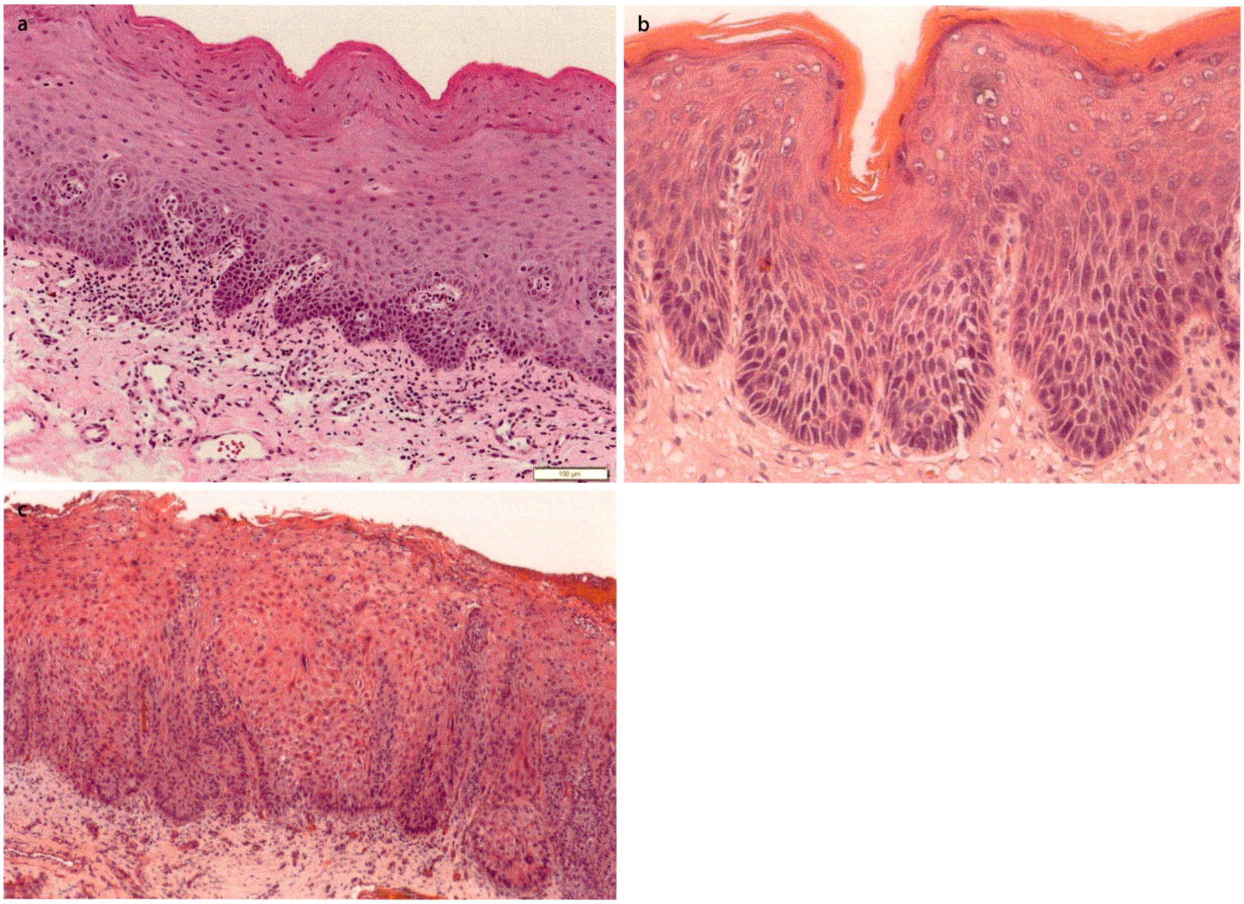

Fig. 22.10 Photomicrographs show (**a**) mild epithelial dysplasia, (**b**) moderate epithelial dysplasia and (**c**) severe epithelial dysplasia

hyperkeratosis or mild epithelial dysplasia are usually managed conservatively with regular periodic follow-up at every 3–6 months. If the lesion shows an increase in size and change in surface morphology, then a re-biopsy is recommended. Oral leukoplakia with a diagnosis of severe epithelial dysplasia is best managed by wide surgical excision. Following the excision, a monthly follow-up is recommended for the first year. If there is no recurrence, then the review intervals may be extended to 3–6 monthly intervals. However, the management of oral leukoplakia with moderate epithelial dysplasia shows a wide variation. Some oral surgeons recommend surgical excision of the lesion with wide margins whereas others tend to wait and watch with periodic follow-up. If the histopathological diagnosis is consistent with verrucous carcinoma, then the management is by wide surgical excision, while a diagnosis of conventional oral squamous cell carcinoma requires escalation of the management to involve surgery with or without neck dissection, radiotherapy, chemotherapy or combination of the aforementioned therapies.

Photodynamic therapy, beta-carotene, lycopene and vitamin A have been used as non-surgical treatment modalities for the management of oral leukoplakia. Their effectiveness needs to be validated by proper randomized clinical trials.

Patients with oral leukoplakia should maintain good oral hygiene. It is the responsibility of the general dentist to deliver oral hygiene education to these patients. Non-surgical oral prophylaxis (scaling and polishing) to maintain the dental and periodontal health is very important. Restoration of decayed teeth, extraction of non-restorable teeth and replacement of missing teeth should be provided as required to maintain good oral hygiene. If patients are wearing dentures, then oral hygiene instructions should cover denture cleanliness and maintenance.

22.16.6 Prognosis

Oral leukoplakia has a malignant transformation rate of 9.5% with an annual malignant transformation rate of 1.56%. The malignant transformation of oral leukoplakia depends on various factors. The factors predictive for an increased malignant transformation risk are classified based on history, clinical features and histopathological features.

History

1. Habits (idiopathic leukoplakia: strong association).
2. History of a previous head and neck carcinoma (present: strong association).

Clinical Features

3. Gender (female: medium association).
4. Age (>50 years: medium association).
5. Site (floor of mouth and tongue: strong association).
6. Colour (redness within the oral leukoplakia: strong association).
7. Texture (non-homogenous: strong association).
8. Size (>200 mm^2: strong association).

Histopathological features:

9. Grade of oral epithelial dysplasia (severe grade: strong association).

PVL rarely regresses even with therapeutic interventions. Moreover, PVL lesions are difficult to eradicate surgically as they tend to recur and/or develop in new sites. The malignant transformation rate of PVLs is around 49.5% with an annual malignant transformation rate of 9.3% and a mortality rate of 55%. Thus, PVL has high malignant transformation rate and is resistant to available treatment modalities.

Salient features of oral leukoplakia	
Clinical features	White or mixed red and white lesions. Broadly classified as homogenous and non-homogenous leukoplakia.
Histopathological features	May range from hyperplasia and/or hyperkeratosis to any grade of dysplasia to squamous cell carcinoma.
Treatment	Depends on the histopathological diagnosis. Epithelial hyperplasia/hyperkeratosis/mild epithelial dysplasia—conservative management with regular 3- to 6-month interval follow-ups. Moderate epithelial dysplasia—either conservative management or wide local excision and periodic close follow-up. Severe epithelial dysplasia—immediate intervention with wide surgical excision followed by periodic close follow-up. All patients should be advised regarding cessation of risk habits.

Self-Assessment Questions

1. List the different types of oral leukoplakia.
2. Discuss the differential diagnosis for homogenous leukoplakia.
3. Discuss the differential diagnosis for non-homogenous leukoplakia.
4. Discuss the clinical features that help in differentiating between plaque type of oral lichen planus and homogenous oral leukoplakia.
5. State the key histopathological features of oral epithelial dysplasia and oral squamous cell carcinoma.
6. State the factors that are associated with malignant transformation of oral leukoplakia.
7. Discuss the management of oral leukoplakia.

Diagnostic Algorithm for Diagnosis of White Lesions

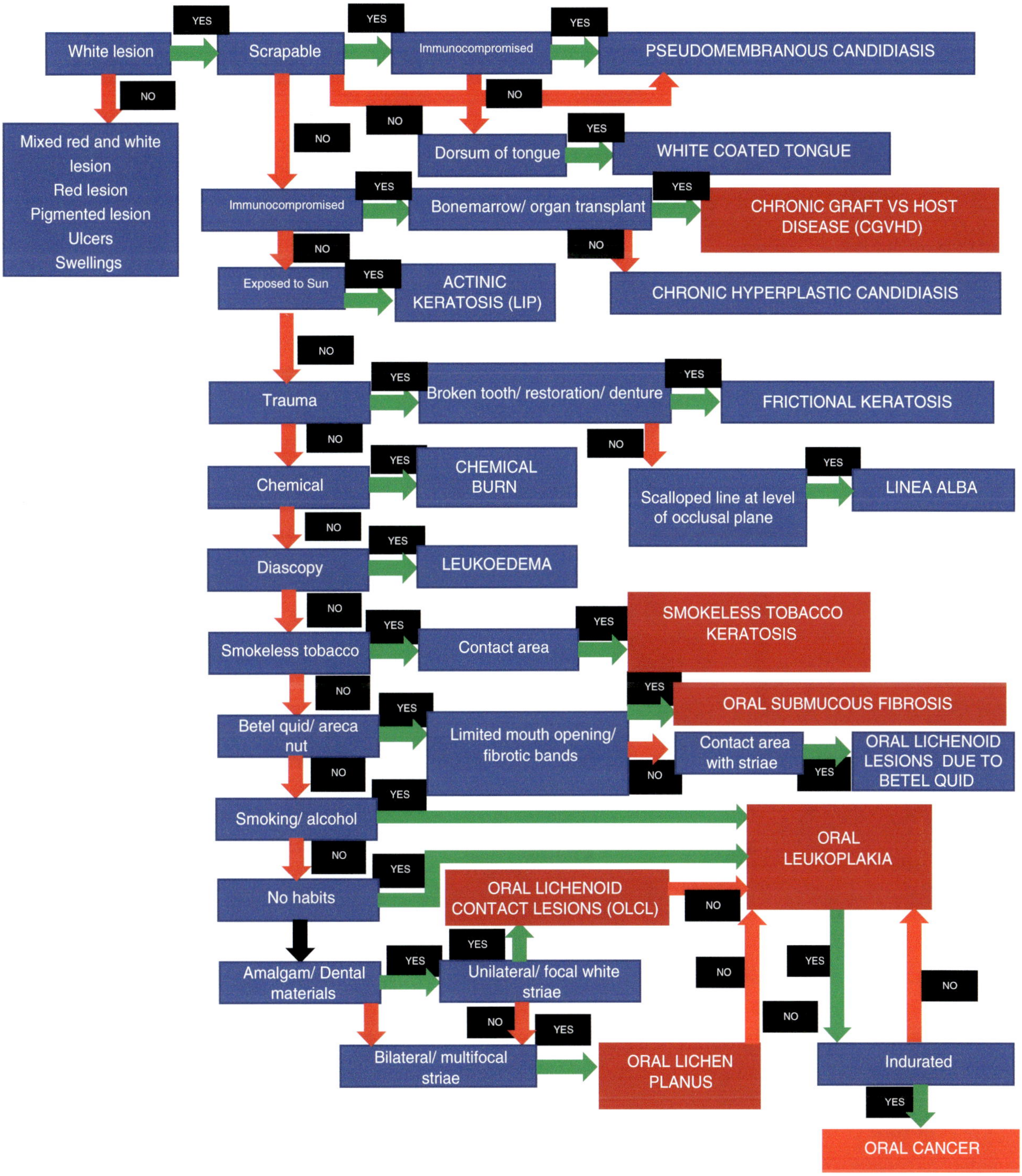

■ Diagnostic Algorithm for Diagnosis of Mixed Red and White Lesions

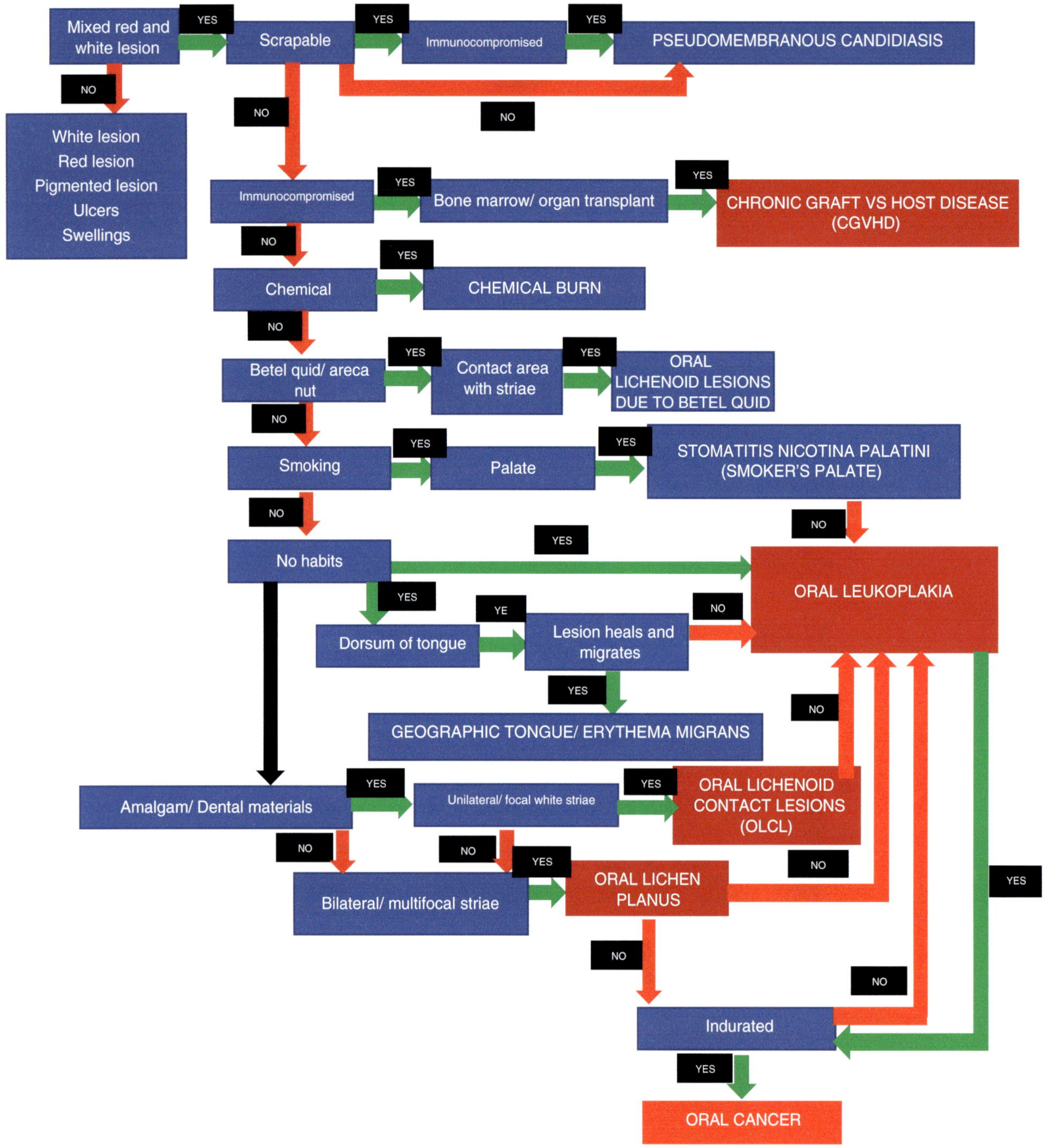

Summary

Leukoplakia is the most common oral potentially malignant disorder (OPMD) seen more commonly in smokers than in non-smokers. It is associated with both smoked and smokeless tobacco use. Histopathology of oral leukoplakia may range from hyperplastic/hyperkeratotic epithelium to dysplasia to invasive oral squamous cell carcinoma. Some oral leukoplakia may show the presence of oral epithelial dysplasia (OED). OED is the best predictor of malignant transformation of OPMDs. Dental practitioners play an important role in prevention, early detection of leukoplakia, giving proper advice and counselling to the patients to quit their habits and timely referral of these patients to the specialist for the management of leukoplakia. Moreover, the upkeep of the oral hygiene of these patients falls in the hands of the dental practitioners.

Further Reading

Iocca O, Sollecito TP, Alawi F, Weinstein GS, Newman JG, De Virgilio A, Di Maio P, Spriano G, Pardiñas López S, Shanti RM. Potentially malignant disorders of the oral cavity and oral dysplasia: a systematic review and meta-analysis of malignant transformation rate by subtype. Head Neck. 2020;42(3):539–55. https://doi.org/10.1002/hed.26006.

Neville B, Damm DD, Allen C, Chi A. Oral and maxillofacial pathology. 4th ed. Elsevier; 2015.

Reibel J, Gale N, Hille J, et al. Oral potentially malignant disorders and Oral epithelial dysplasia. In: El-Naggar AK, Chan JKC, Grandis JR, Takata T, Slootweg PJ, editors. WHO classification of head and neck tumours, vol. 9. 4th ed. Lyon: IARC; 2017. p. 112–5.

Warnakulasuriya and Greenspan. Textbook of oral cancer prevention, diagnosis and management. Springer; 2020.

Warnakulasuriya S, Tilakaratne WM. Oral medicine & pathology. A guide to diagnosis and management. 1st ed. New Delhi: Jaypee.

A Red Patch on the Cheek: Erythroplakia

Ruwan Jayasinghe and Wanninayake M Tilakaratne

Contents

W. M Tilakaratne, T. G. Kallarakkal (eds.), *Clinicopathological Correlation of Oral Diseases*,
https://doi.org/10.1007/978-3-031-24408-7_23

Learning Goals

1. Devise the correct way of compiling the history with appropriate questions.
2. Develop a differential diagnosis after history taking.
3. Deduce appropriate procedures in clinical examination.
4. Formulate a differential diagnosis combining findings in the history and clinical examination.
5. Justify the relevant investigations required to arrive at the diagnosis.
6. Comprehend the importance of clinicopathological correlation in arriving at the correct diagnosis.
7. Outline the management plan.
8. Recognize the importance of a diagnostic algorithm in arriving at a diagnosis.

23.1 Main Complaint

A 48-year-old male patient presents with a complaint of a reddish patch in the mouth on the right side of the cheek for 2 months' duration.

23.2 History of Complaint

Question: What other features did you notice in relation to the lesion? Do you remember any history of trauma to the region?

I saw it accidentally in the mirror when I tried to remove a food particle trapped between my teeth. It remained in the same size over the past 2 months. I do not have any pain and burning sensation in relation to the lesion when I eat spicy food. I do not remember any trauma to the affected area.

23.3 Additional Complaints

Question: Have you had similar red patches in the mouth in the past?

I have not experienced any lesions of this nature in the mouth in the past.

Question: Have you noticed or felt any other changes or difficulties in the mouth?

I do not have any other problems. I can open my mouth normally and I do not have any difficulty in talking or eating.

Question: Do you have any lesions elsewhere in the body?

I do not have any lesions elsewhere on my body. I have an ulcer on my leg. I am currently being treated with antibiotics by my physician.

Question: Are you suffering from any other medical problems like heart disease, high blood pressure, diabetes, bleeding disorder, or respiratory diseases? If yes, what kind of medications have you been taking until now?

I have high blood sugar levels and I am on oral medications for the same.

Question: Have you undergone any surgery?

I have not undergone any surgery in the past.

Question: Have you undergone any dental treatment?

I have not undergone any dental treatment in the past.

Question: What is your occupation?

I am a long-distance bus driver.

Question: Do you have any specific chewing habits?

I am a betel chewer. I have been chewing 10–15 quids a day with betel leaf, tobacco, areca nut and slaked lime for at least 15 years. I keep the quid in the mouth for a long time mostly on the right side of the cheek.

Question: Are you a smoker?

I am not a smoker.

Question: Do you take alcohol?

I do not consume alcohol.

Question: Tell me about your family details.

I am married and have four children.

23.4 With the Findings From the History, What Is Your Differential Diagnosis?

1. Erythroplakia.
2. Oral cancer.
3. Oral lichen planus/lichenoid reaction.

4. Discoid lupus erythematosus (DLE).
5. Erythematous candidosis.
6. Traumatic lesion.

23.5 How Do You Justify Your Differential Diagnosis After History Taking?

1. He complains of a non-painful red patch on the buccal mucosa since 2 months. He is a heavy betel chewer using 10–15 quids a day for more than 15 years and he keeps his quid for a long duration in the buccal sulcus on the right side. Buccal mucosa is a common site for epithelial changes in betel chewers. Erythroplakia needs to be excluded as it is a high-risk oral potentially malignant disorder.
2. He has a red patch on the buccal mucosa since 2 months. There is no pain or discharge from the lesion. He is a heavy betel chewer. As oral cancer is common especially in people with risk habits, it has to be considered in the differential diagnosis. Early cases of oral cancer can appear as a red patch which ulcerates eventually. Buccal mucosa is a common site for oral cancer in betel chewers and this patient has a history of keeping the quid for longer periods in the same site.
3. Oral lichen planus (OLP) is a common mucocutaneous disorder. It can present as an erythematous patch associated with white striations. OLP may present with or without burning sensation but most erythematous lesions are symptomatic. OLP is usually bilateral and commonly seen on the buccal mucosa followed by the tongue and the gingiva. Similar clinical presentation can present as a reaction to medications known as lichenoid reaction (LR). This patient is a known diabetic patient and is on oral anti-hypoglycemic drugs, which can also cause LR. Lichenoid reactions may also be precipitated as a reaction to the components of the betel quid.
4. Erythematous candidosis (antibiotic sore mouth) is seen in patients on broad spectrum antibiotics or long-term steroid therapy. This is a painful condition and the patient finds it difficult to eat or speak. The patient is on oral antibiotics for an ulcer on the leg, which could have resulted in erythematous candidosis.
5. Chronic irritation/trauma can result in a red patch/erosion/ulceration. It is important to exclude any form of trauma.
6. DLE may present as well-defined, erythematous areas with broad, slightly raised whitish margins from which arise numerous radiating delicate lines.

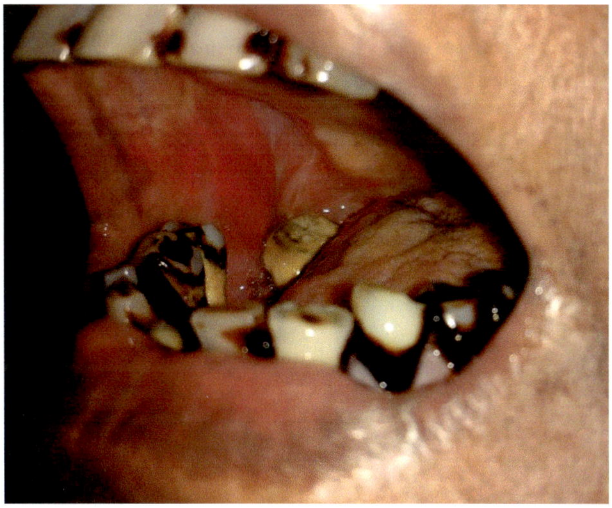

Fig. 23.1 Irregular reddish area on the right buccal mucosa with faint red colour on the anterior aspect

23.6 Findings of Clinical Examination

He has an irregular single reddish area measuring 3 × 3 cm in size on the right buccal mucosa (Fig. 23.1). A slight alteration of the colour is visible on the anterior part of the red lesion and it extends towards the commissural area. Betel stains are visible on the right lateral border of the tongue and on the remaining few teeth. There are no other lesions elsewhere in the mouth. The lower right first molar tooth shows severe attrition with sharp edges.

23.7 What Is Your Clinical Differential Diagnosis?

1. Oral cancer.
2. Erythroplakia.
3. Traumatic lesion.

23.8 How Would You Justify the Inclusion of the Diseases That You Have Mentioned in the Differential Diagnosis to Arrive at a Working Diagnosis?

23.8.1 Oral Cancer

Oral cancer is associated with risk habits such as betel chewing, smoking and alcohol consumption. Oral cancer usually presents as a non-healing, painless ulcer but early lesions can present as a reddish patch or as nodular/speckled areas. Pre-existing erythroplakia can undergo malignant transformation and become cancer. Oral cancer is a likely differential diagnosis as the patient keeps the quid for long hours on the same side where the lesion is present. Therefore, oral cancer has to be considered in the differential diagnosis and needs to be excluded by doing a biopsy.

23.8.2 Erythroplakia

He has an irregular red patch on the buccal mucosa and is a heavy betel chewer. Erythroplakia needs to be excluded, as it is a high-risk oral potentially malignant disorder seen in individuals with high-risk habits. The diagnosis of erythroplakia is made by excluding other red patches which can be classified as definable diseases. However, the attributes of the present lesion does not support definable disorders. Most erythroplakias exhibit a moderate to severe degree of dysplasia upon histopathological examination.

23.8.3 Traumatic Lesion

Chronic irritation/trauma can result in epithelial damage causing a red patch/erosion/ulceration. The lower right first molar tooth of this patient has sharp edges that could have caused trauma to the associated soft tissue. Chronic irritation can result in epithelial hyperplasia as a protective mechanism resulting in a whitish area, but later when the trauma is more severe and persistent, the epithelium undergoes erosion or ulceration. Traumatic lesions are always compatible with the source of trauma. However, in this patient, the red patch is much larger than the traumatic source. However, it is important to exclude any form of trauma in this kind of cases.

23.9 What Is the Most Likely Clinical Diagnosis?

Erythroplakia.

23.10 How Would You Investigate This Patent?

An incisional biopsy should be performed.

His biopsy report supported the clinical diagnosis of erythroplakia. The lesion has severe epithelial dysplasia.

23.11 What Are the Histopathological Features That Help in the Diagnosis?

Erythroplakia is a clinical diagnosis, which is arrived at by excluding other red lesions including traumatic lesions, vascular lesions, discoid lupus erythematosus (DLE), erosive lichen planus and erythematous candidosis. It should be diagnosed without any delay as most of the cases identified as erythroplakia clinically would have already transformed into squamous cell carcinoma. More than 50% of the cases are diagnosed as invasive squamous cell carcinoma whereas about 40% are diagnosed as severe epithelial dysplasia. The haematoxylin and eosin-stained sections show full-thickness epithelial dysplasia with both architectural and cytological atypia. The reason for the red colour clinically is due to supra-papillary atrophy of the epithelium bringing the underlying vasculature very close to the surface (◘ Fig. 23.2).

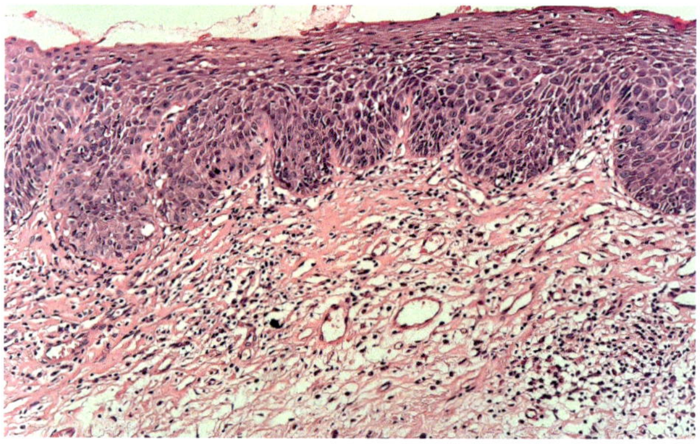

◘ **Fig. 23.2** Histopathological appearance showing stratified squamous epithelium exhibiting severe epithelial dysplasia

23.12 How Would You Manage This Patent?

Erythroplakia has a very high risk of malignant transformation and more than 90% of the cases have been identified as invasive squamous cell carcinoma or severe epithelial dysplasia at the time of biopsy. Early and effective treatment for erythroplakia is mandatory. The recommended treatment is surgical excision of the lesion. It can also be done using laser therapy and cryotherapy. Habit intervention, improvement of oral hygiene and careful follow-up are essential. There is no effective treatment in preventing malignant transformation of erythroplakia.

23.13 Erythroplakia

Erythroplakia is an oral potentially malignant disorder defined as a fiery red patch that cannot be characterized clinically or histopathologically as any other definable disease. It presents as a sharply demarcated, flat or depressed, erythematous area of mucosa with a matt appearance. Inflammatory conditions that may result in a red clinical appearance should be excluded prior to arriving at the diagnosis. The solitary presentation of erythroplakia helps to distinguish it from other more widespread conditions such as erosive lichen planus, lupus erythematosus, erythematous candidosis autoimmune disorders, infections and vascular hamartomas. Patients with erythroplakia usually present without any symptoms but rarely can cause burning sensation. It is a rare condition. It occurs commonly in middle-aged and elderly people. There is no gender predilection. Soft palate, floor of the mouth and buccal mucosa are the commonest sites for erythroplakia. Clinically it appears as a flat/depressed reddish lesion. Usually erythroplakia has a smooth and velvety surface but occasionally it can present as an irregular, red granular surface. Erythroplakia is commonly seen as a single lesion and only very rarely it presents as multiple lesions. It is usually small in size with an average diameter of 1 cm and rarely involves extensive areas of the mouth. The solitary nature of erythroplakia is important to differentiate it from other red lesions of the mouth such as erosive lichen planus, lupus erythematosus and atrophic candidosis. Erythroplakia is soft to palpation and does not become indurated or hard until malignant transformation occurs.

Non-homogeneous leukoplakias can manifest as mixed red and white lesions and should not be misdiagnosed as erythroplakia (◘ Fig. 23.3). There may be numerous, small irregular foci of leukoplakia dispersed in an erythematous background and such lesions are also defined as erythroleukoplakia or speckled leukoplakia (◘ Fig. 23.4).

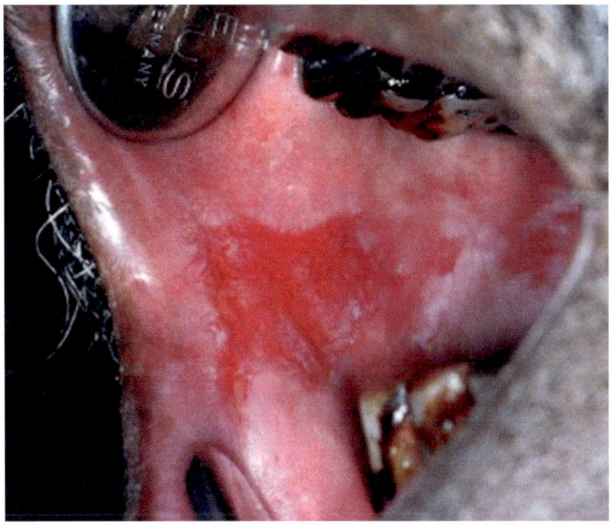

◘ **Fig. 23.3** Non-homogeneous leukoplakia on the right buccal mucosa

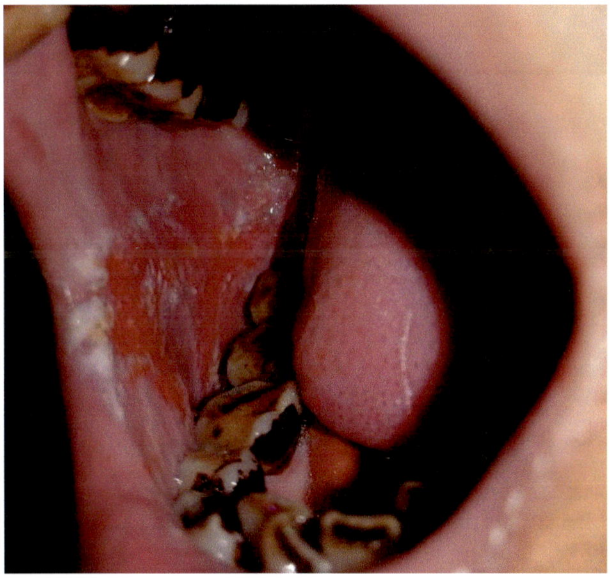

◘ **Fig. 23.4** Non-homogeneous leukoplakia (erythroleukoplakia/speckled leukoplakia) on the right buccal mucosa

The differential diagnosis for erythroplakia includes erythematous candidosis, early oral cancer, chronic local irritation, mucositis, oral lichen planus/lichenoid reaction, discoid lupus erythematosus, drug reaction and median rhomboid glossitis when on the tongue.

Acute erythematous candidosis (◘ Figs. 23.5 and 23.6) is also referred to as antibiotic sore mouth. It tends to develop following a reduction in the levels of the bacterial component of the normal oral microflora after the use of broad-spectrum antibiotics or steroid therapy, especially the inhaler form, as it can create a localized area of immune suppression that permits overgrowth of *Candida*. A decrease in bacterial counts results in

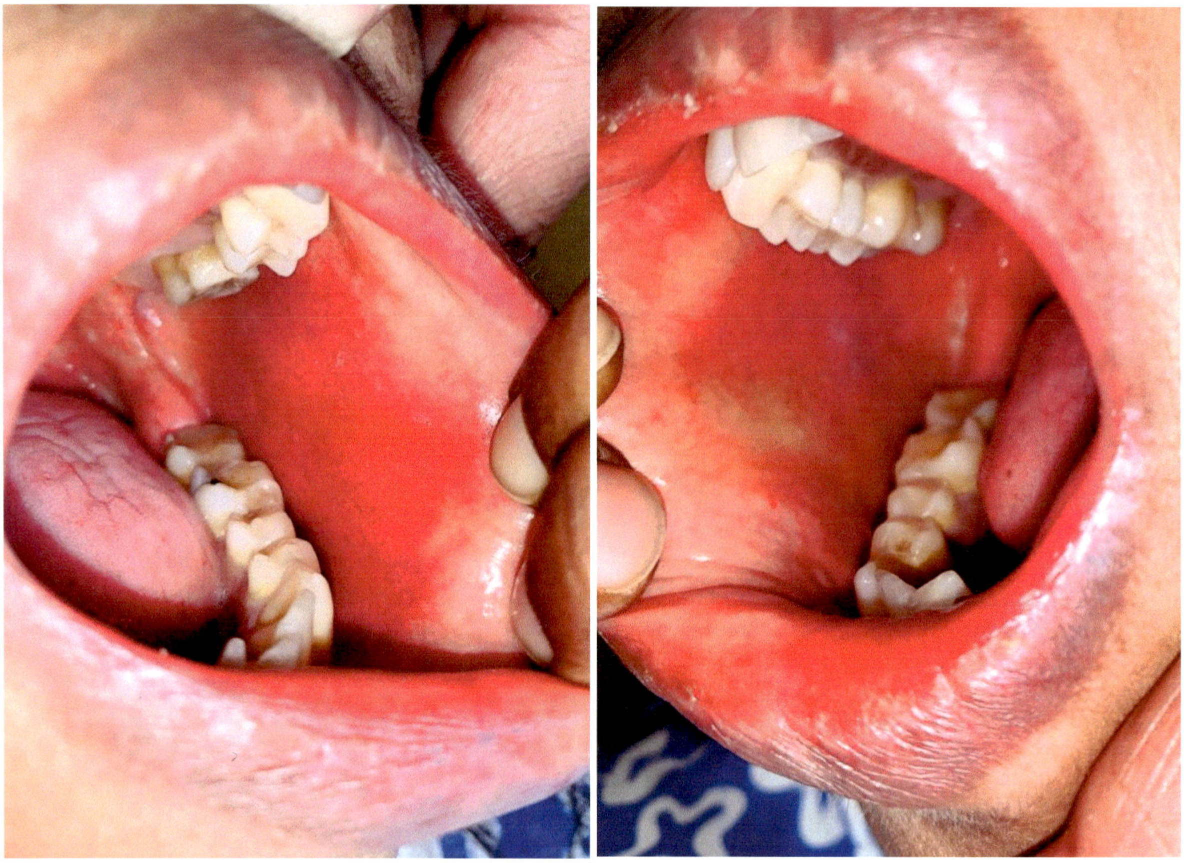

Figs. 23.5 and 23.6 Acute erythematous candidosis involving buccal mucosa showing erythematous areas with diffuse margins

reduced microbial competition for *Candida* in terms of nutrition and adherence sites resulting in a direct consequence of an ecological shift in normal homeostatic balance of the microbial community. It presents as a painful red lesion with diffuse margins. Although palate or buccal mucosa may be involved, the most common site of infection is the dorsum of the tongue. Cessation of antibiotic therapy results in the return of normal levels of bacteria, which subsequently resolves the candidosis without intervention. This can be easily differentiated from erythroplakia with the history and remission of the lesions with antifungal treatment.

Traumatic lesions can be differentiated easily as they are associated with trauma/chronic irritation. Careful history and examination are essential in this regard. OLP presents with bilateral but not always symmetrical lesions. Erosive lesions in OLP present with areas of reticular pattern in other areas of the oral mucosa, which is helpful in differentiating OLP from erythroplakia (Fig. 23.7).

Lupus erythematosus is a chronic autoimmune disease, which can be subdivided into three forms: (1) systemic, (2) drug induced and (3) discoid. Oral lesions may manifest in approximately 20% patients with systemic lupus. The disease is driven by an immune complex depo-

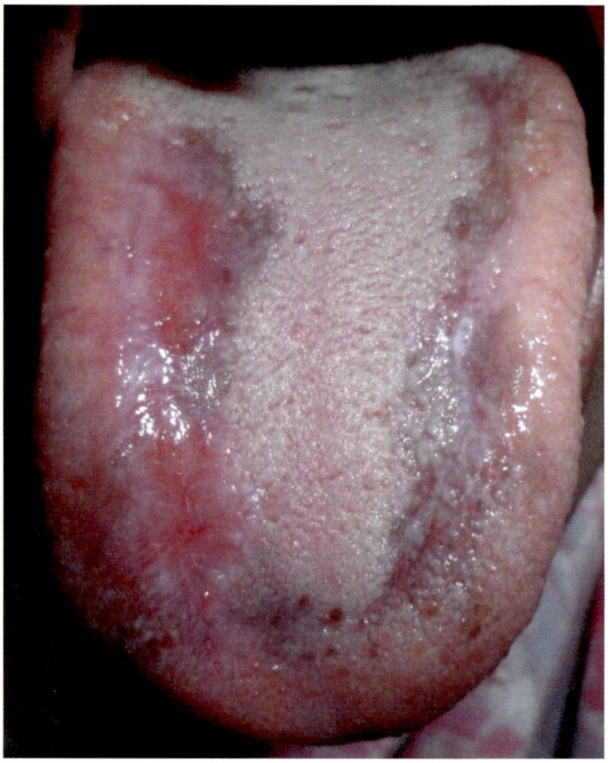

Fig. 23.7 Erosive lesions of OLP on the dorsal surface of the tongue

sition in the affected sites, leading to vasculitis. The discoid variety typically affects the sun-exposed areas of the face and neck and may present with the typical butterfly rash across the nasal bridge. The oral lesions consist of central zones of ulceration or erythema (representing vasculitis) surrounded by white striations, bearing a close resemblance to OLP. Immunofluorescence studies demonstrate subepithelial immunoglobulin and complement deposition (the lupus band), which assists in distinguishing DLE from oral lichen planus. Oral lesions typically affect the buccal mucosa, palate and lips.

Median rhomboid glossitis (MRG) is considered to be due to candidal infection. It has a characteristic rhomboid appearance seen on the dorsum of the tongue just anterior to the circumvallate papillae but at times it can have an oval, round or irregular shape. The affected area is devoid of papillae; however, it may sometimes present as an exophytic growth (◘ Figs. 23.8 and 23.9). Sometimes reciprocal lesions are present on the hard palate, which are known as "kissing lesions". Typical appearance, location, presence of kissing lesions and response to antifungal agents help in differentiating MRG from erythroplakia.

Angina bullosa haemorrhagica (ABH) is an idiopathic condition also known as blood blister (◘ Figs. 23.10 and 23.11). It is characterized by sudden appearance of a blood-filled blister on the oral mucosa, commonly on the soft palate, which ruptures spontaneously due to trauma, leaving a shallow ulcer that heals in a few days without any scarring. History of blood-filled blister and spontaneous healing seen in ABH helps to differentiate it easily from erythroplakia.

The malignant transformation potential in erythroplakia is very high. Hence, an immediate biopsy is indicated in all cases of erythroplakia. Potential causes like candidal infection and trauma need to be eliminated. Habit cessation instructions need to be given and re-evaluation of the patient is essential. Majority of the cases of erythroplakia undergo malignant transformation (◘ Fig. 23.12), hence urgent treatment is indicated. Surgery is the recommended treatment modality. Long-term follow-up is mandatory.

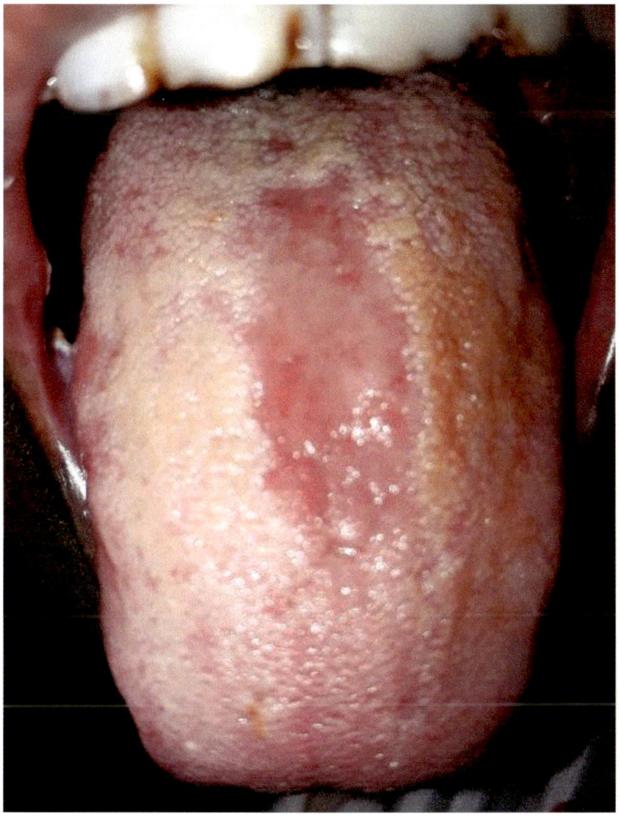

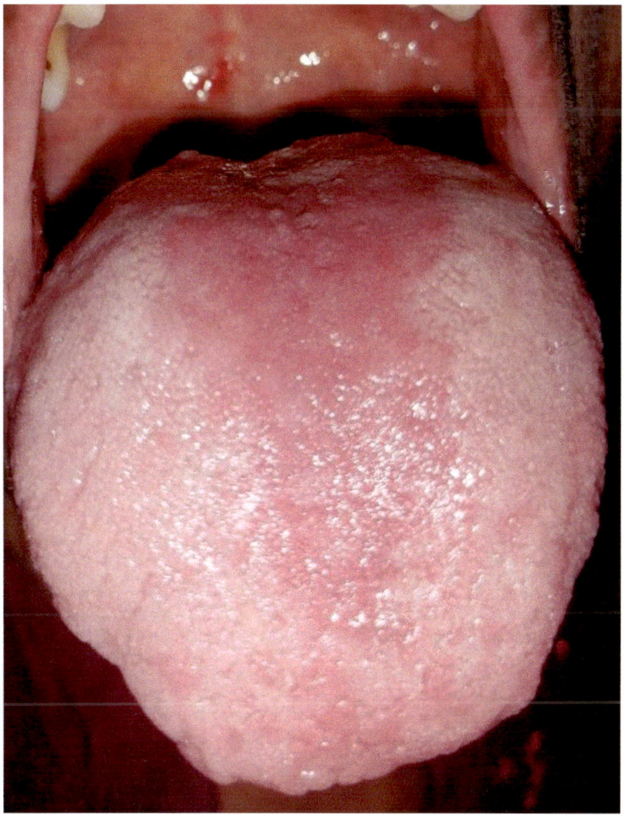

◘ **Figs. 23.8 and 23.9** Atrophic lesion of MRG on the dorsal surface of the tongue

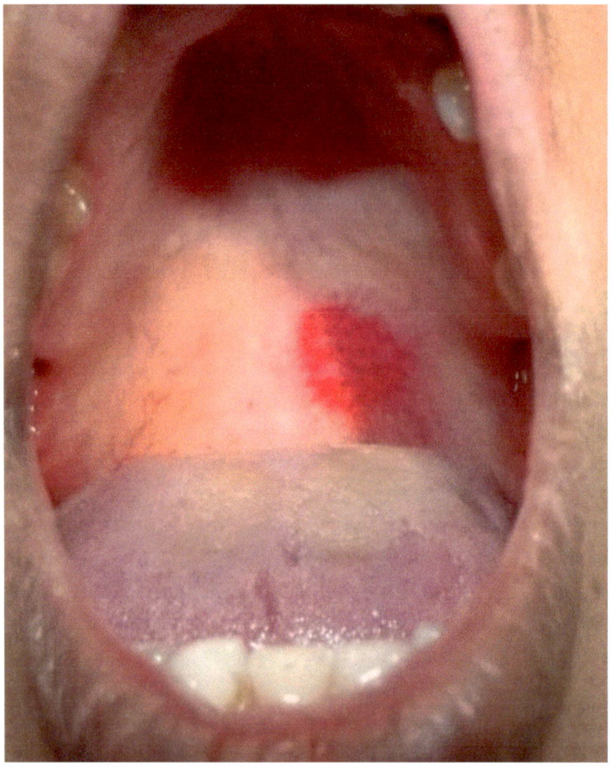

Fig. 23.10 ABH presenting as an erosive lesion

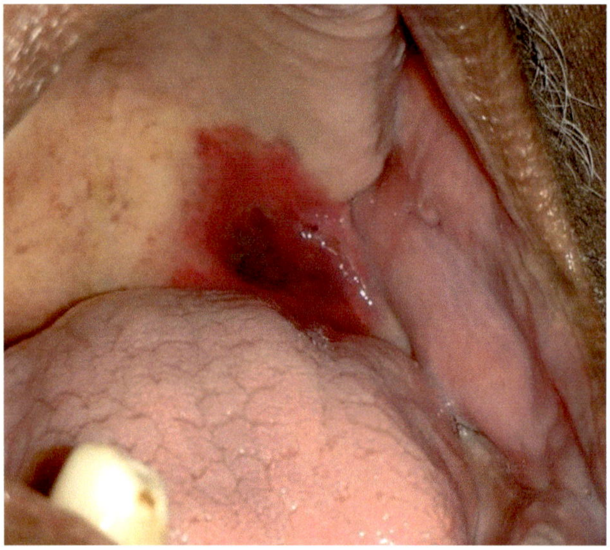

Fig. 23.11 ABH showing blood-filled blister

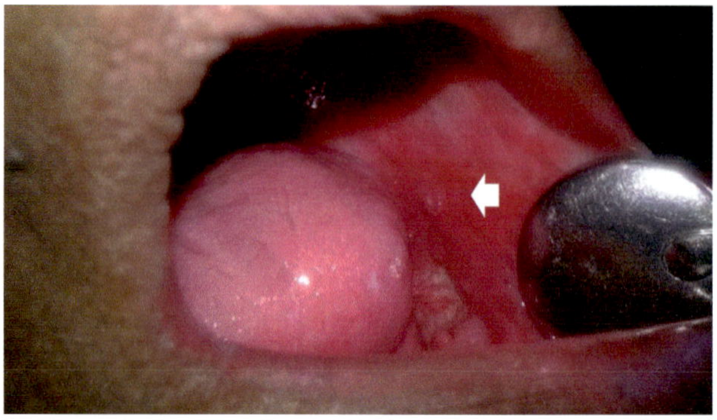

Fig. 23.12 Malignant transformation in erythroplakia characterized by an indurated lesion in the centre (white arrow)

Salient features of oral erythroplakia (OE)	
Clinical	Majority are symptomless, but it can rarely cause burning sensation. It occurs commonly in middle-aged and elderly people without any gender predilection. Soft plate, floor of the mouth and buccal mucosa are the common sites. Clinically it appears as a flat/depressed reddish lesion with a smooth and velvety surface. OE is commonly seen as a single lesion. It is usually small in size and rarely involves extensive areas of the mouth. It is soft to palpation. Differential diagnosis includes erythematous candidosis, oral cancer, local irritation, mucositis, oral lichen planus/lichenoid reaction, discoid lupus erythematosus, drug reaction and median rhomboid glossitis
Investigations	Diagnosis of OE is by exclusion. It should be diagnosed without any delay. Biopsy and histopathological confirmation are mandatory.
Treatment	Surgery is the recommended treatment modality. Long-term follow-up is mandatory.

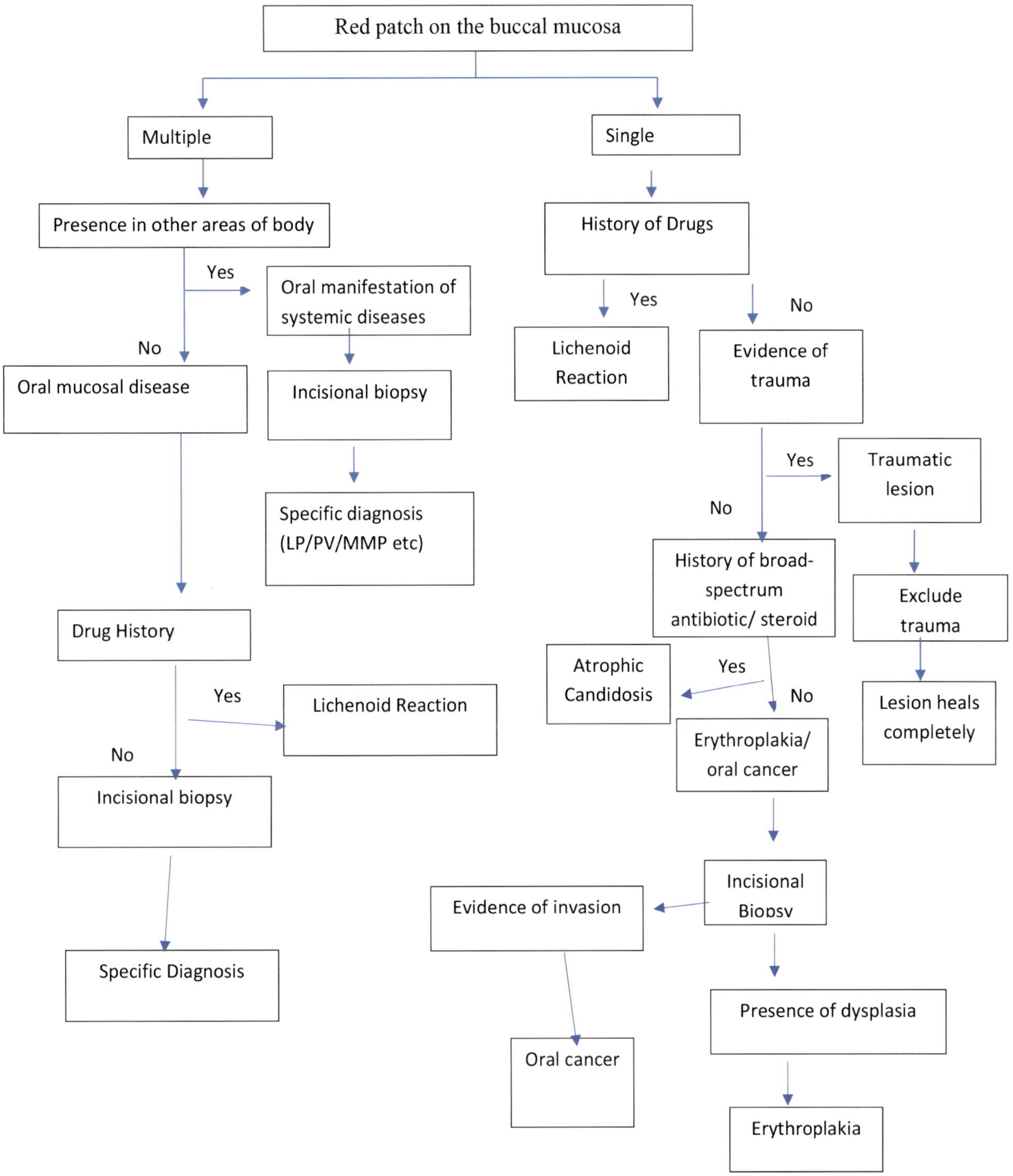
Red patch on the buccal mucosa
Multiple
Single
Presence in other areas of body
Yes
No
Oral manifestation of systemic diseases
Oral mucosal disease
Incisional biopsy
Specific diagnosis (LP/PV/MMP etc)
Drug History
Yes
No
Lichenoid Reaction
Incisional biopsy
Specific Diagnosis
History of Drugs
Yes
No
Lichenoid Reaction
Evidence of trauma
Yes
No
Traumatic lesion
Exclude trauma
Lesion heals completely
History of broad-spectrum antibiotic/ steroid
Yes
No
Atrophic Candidosis
Erythroplakia/ oral cancer
Incisional Biopsy
Evidence of invasion
Oral cancer
Presence of dysplasia
Erythroplakia

Self-Assessment Questions

1. Discuss the clinical differential diagnosis for erythroplakia.
2. Describe the rationale of diagnosing erythroplakia.
3. Describe the rationale for performing an immediate biopsy in suspected erythroplakia.
4. Describe the histopathological features of erythroplakia.
5. Outline the management of erythroplakia.

Summary

Erythroplakia is a rare oral potentially malignant disorder with a very high malignant transformation potential. Clinically it appears as a single, flat and depressed reddish lesion with a smooth and velvety surface. An immediate biopsy is indicated to diagnose it early. Surgery is the recommended treatment modality. Habit intervention and long-term follow-up are mandatory.

Further Reading

Reichart PA, Philipsen HP. Oral erythroplakia—a review. Oral Oncol. 2005;41:551–61.

Villa A, Villa C, Abati S. Oral cancer and oral erythroplakia: an update and implication for clinicians. Aust Dent J. 2011;56:253–6.

Tilakaratne WM, Jayasinghe RD. Oral potentially malignant disorders (OPMDs). Atlas of dermatoses in pigmented skin. Singapore: Springer; 2021. p. 879–902.

McNamara KK, Kalmar JR. Erythematous and vascular oral mucosal lesions: a clinicopathologic review of red entities. Head Neck Pathol. 2019;13(1):4–15. https://doi.org/10.1007/s12105-019-01002-8.

Warnakulasuriya S, Tilakaratna WM, editors. Oral medicine & pathology: a guide to diagnosis and management. New Delhi: JP Medical Ltd.; 2013.

Painful Mouth: Oral Lichen Planus

Zuraiza Mohamad Zaini

Contents

W. M Tilakaratne, T. G. Kallarakkal (eds.), *Clinicopathological Correlation of Oral Diseases*,
https://doi.org/10.1007/978-3-031-24408-7_24

Learning Goals

1. Devise the correct way of compiling the history with appropriate questions.
2. Develop a differential diagnosis after history taking.
3. Deduce appropriate procedures in clinical examination.
4. Formulate a differential diagnosis combining findings in the history and clinical examination.
5. Justify the relevant investigations required to arrive at the diagnosis.
6. Comprehend the importance of clinicopathological correlation in arriving at the correct diagnosis of OLP.
7. Outline the management plan.
8. Recognize the importance of a diagnostic algorithm in arriving at a diagnosis.

24.1 Main Complaint

A 52-year-old lady complains of painful and sore mouth particularly when eating.

24.2 History of Complaint

Question: When did it start and what is the nature of the sore mouth?

The symptoms started about 7 months ago. Initially I felt soreness when taking spicy and acidic food or drink that resolved spontaneously. Recently, the pain has become worse. It occurs with any type of food and only gradually fades away but sometimes persists. Often, I drink cold water to help ease the pain. Lately, I have started experiencing soreness even without taking food.

Question: Have you noticed any changes in the mouth?

I notice that both sides of my cheeks appear red and sometimes with ulcerations. The pain is unbearable when there are ulcers. Occasionally I get pain even without ulcers and there are periods where I am pain-free. I recently noticed white patches on my tongue which worries me as my friends informed that mouth cancer could arise from white lesions.

Question: Did you have any treatment for the pain and the lesions?

I put some oral cream over the redness and ulcers that I bought from a pharmacy but it didn't help ease the pain nor healed the ulcers.

Question: Are you experiencing any change in taste sensation?

I am not aware of any significant difference in taste sensation.

Question: Do you have any lesions elsewhere in the body? Have you had any lesions on the skin, scalp, or nails?

I have skin rashes on my right wrists, and they are very itchy. A few of my fingernails appear slightly darkened with prominent grooves.

Question: Do you have any medical problems like heart disease, high blood pressure, diabetes, joint problems, or respiratory diseases? Are you on any medications for the problems that you have? Is there any new drug that being prescribed recently?

I have been on amlodipine for hypertension over the past 5 years. I was diagnosed with diabetes 3 years ago and is currently being treated with metformin. I have not been prescribed with any new drugs.

Question: Do you have any food or drug allergies?

I have no allergies that I'm aware of.

Question: When was your last dental visit and what was the treatment done?

I had scaling done a year ago without any complications.

Question: Are you a smoker?

I am not a smoker.

Question: Do you take alcohol?

I do not consume alcohol.

24.3 With the Findings From the History, What Is Your Differential Diagnosis?

1. Oral lichen planus.
2. Oral lichenoid reaction (OLR).
3. Discoid lupus erythematosus (DLE).
4. Candidosis.
5. Vesiculobullous disorder.

24.4 How Do You Justify Your Differential Diagnosis After History Taking?

1. Symptom of soreness when taking spicy and acidic food may be due to erosions and ulcerations, which clinically appear as red oral mucosa. There is a wide range of oral mucosal diseases and underlying systemic conditions that may lead to painful mouth. The common oral disorders include but are not limited to oral lichen planus, oral lichenoid reaction, oral vesiculobullous lesions, and oral infection, primarily candidosis.
2. Oral lichenoid reaction can result from medications including antihypertensives and drugs used to treat diabetes mellitus. This condition has clinical and histopathological features similar to oral lichen planus.
3. Presence of mixed white and reddish mucosa with intermittent ulcerations is highly suggestive of oral lichen planus, oral lichenoid reaction, discoid lupus erythematosus, and oral vesiculobullous diseases.
4. Oral candidosis may present clinically as scrapable white lesions or painful red lesions. The affected patients usually complain of altered taste sensation and a burning sensation in the mouth.

24.5 Findings of Clinical Examination

Extra orally there are some changes in her nails including grooving and ridging. In addition, a few itchy areas are present in her arms. There are no palpable and no enlarged head and neck lymph nodes. Intraorally she has diffused white lesions mixed with erythematous areas and multiple ulcers on the buccal mucosae bilaterally (◘ Fig. 24.1a and b). White lesions are also present on the lateral and ventral tongue bilaterally (◘ Fig. 24.1c and d). Both oral mucosa and eyes don't show any signs of dryness.

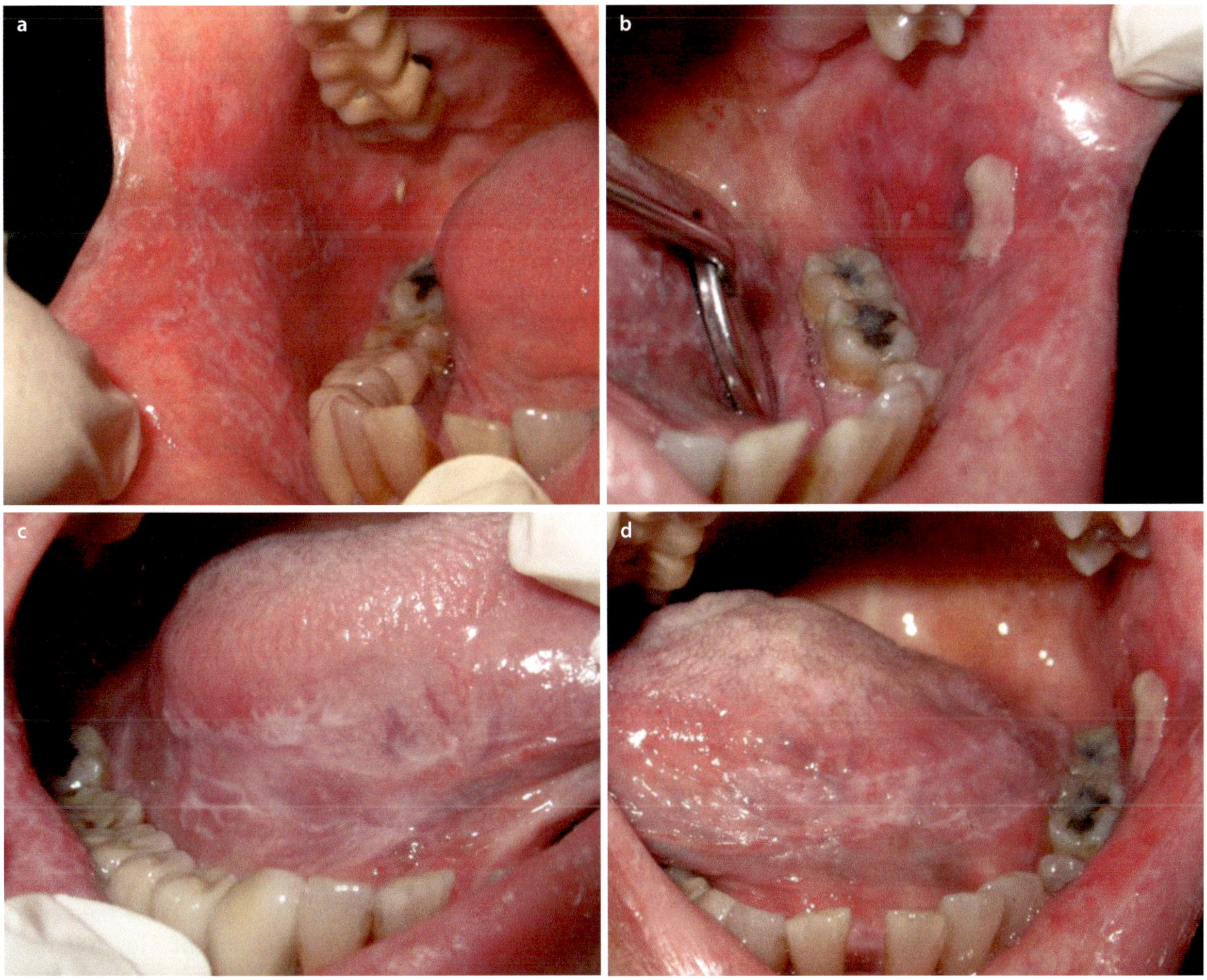

◘ **Fig. 24.1** Right and left buccal mucosae showing white reticular striae with erythematous areas (**a** and **b**). Striations on bilateral lateral ventral tongue (**c** and **d**)

The white lesions are ill-defined extending from the commissure to the posterior buccal mucosa and show fine reticular keratotic striations. These patterns are also seen on the ventral tongue bilaterally. Erythematous areas and multiple shallow ulcerations of variable sizes with yellowish ulcer beds are located posteriorly on the buccal mucosae bilaterally. She has multiple amalgam restorations and prosthetic crowns. Her oral hygiene is moderately poor, and the mouth is acceptably moist.

24.6 What Is Your Most Likely Clinical Diagnosis?

Oral lichen planus (OLP)

24.7 How Would You Exclude Other Conditions and Justify Your Clinical Diagnosis to Arrive at a Working Diagnosis?

24.7.1 Oral Lichenoid Reaction

Oral lichenoid reactions (OLRs) are indistinguishable from idiopathic OLP, clinically and histologically. Unlike OLP, OLRs are caused by drugs and dental materials and develop in patients with graft-versus-host disease (GVHD). OLR in relation to dental materials is localized to the mucosal site that is in contact with the dental restoration. Most cases of OLR resolve after discontinuation of the causative agent. However, the presence of itchy skin rashes and nail changes support the diagnosis of lichen planus over lichenoid reaction. The presence of bilateral, more or less symmetrical lesions in a lace-like network of slightly raised grey-white lines (reticular pattern) as seen in this patient strongly supports the diagnosis of OLP. Moreover, the erosive and atrophic lesions seen in this patient are accompanied by the presence of reticular lesions on the bilateral buccal mucosa, which is clinically consistent with OLP.

24.7.2 Lupus Erythematosus

Lupus erythematosus (LE) is an autoimmune disease characterized by autoantibodies and immune complexes that may affect several organ systems (systemic LE) or manifests as an isolated skin disease (cutaneous LE). Oral involvement is seen in 5–54% of systemic LE and 3–25% of cutaneous LE. While oral ulceration is commonly seen in each of these two types of LE, patients with discoid lupus erythematosus (DLE), a chronic form of cutaneous LE, frequently present with oral discoid lesions. Oral discoid lesion or oral DLE represents the typical clinical presentation of its skin analogue. It is characterized by well-defined, disc-like (discoid) or irregular erythematous patch that can be centrally depressed or ulcerated, with white radiating keratotic striae and telangiectasis. Oral DLE may mimic OLP/OLR. However, unlike OLP/OLR, the lesions are often asymmetric in distribution with buccal mucosa, gingiva, palate, and vermilion border being most commonly involved. OLP and OLR also rarely affect the palatal region and are more commonly found intraorally than LE. The clinical presentation of this patient does not support the diagnosis of LE.

24.7.3 Mucous Membrane Pemphigoid (MMP)

The patient did not report any blister formation. However, oral vesiculobullous lesions should be considered in the differential diagnoses of chronic multiple oral ulcerations or erosions. The patient may have been unaware of the presence of a blister as oral vesicles/bullae are short-lived and prone to burst rapidly, leaving only ulcers that can be seen clinically. Mucous membrane pemphigoid is the most common blistering disease involving predominantly the oral and ocular mucous membranes in which oral cavity is often the first affected site. The characteristic features include shallow ulcers with ragged margins. Epithelial tags are sometimes seen at the ulcer margins. Desquamative gingivitis is a common manifestation of MMP and was not evident in this patient. In addition, other intraoral and skin manifestations are not supportive of MMP.

24.7.4 Candidosis

Pseudomembranous candidosis, a subtype of oral candidosis, presents clinically as white patches, which can be scraped off using a gauze. Another subtype of candidiasis, chronic hyperplastic candidiasis (CHC) usually appears as a thick white plaque often involving the commissural region with no pain or burning sensation. Considering the principal clinical findings of bilateral white striations and white patches on the dorsum of the tongue that are nonscrapable, candidosis is unlikely to be the primary diagnosis for this patient. However, there is a possibility of super-infection with candida in this patient because she has diabetes.

24.8 How Would You Investigate This Patient?

1. Swab from the white lesions on the tongue to exclude superimposed candidal infection.
2. Incisional biopsy for the confirmation of diagnosis and to plan long-term management.

24.9 How Would You Do an Incisional Biopsy for This Patient? What Are the Important Considerations?

When selecting a biopsy site, the area that is the most representative of the suspected condition must be included. The centre of an ulcer will histologically show inflammation without surface epithelium and should be avoided. Incisional biopsy for this patient is best performed using scalpel to sample the lesion on her right buccal mucosa, which has white striae, and should include some adjacent normal appearing mucosa. OLP of plaque type clinically presents as white patches and should be biopsied to rule out epithelial dysplasia. Ideally the specimen should be elliptical in shape with approximately 1 cm in length, 3–6 mm in width, and 3–4 mm in depth into the submucosa.

24.10 The Specimen Was Sent for Histopathological Examination. What Are the Histological Findings?

Microscopic images of haematoxylin and eosin (H&E)-stained sections show a non-ulcerated surface epithelium that is parakeratinized (◘ Fig. 24.2a). A dense band-like infiltrate of lymphocytes is present in the superficial lamina propria, beneath the epithelium. The epithelium has variable thickness and exhibits basal cell degeneration, apoptotic bodies, and thickened basement membrane (◘ Fig. 24.2b). Several foci of adipose tissue, striated muscles, and neurovascular bundles are observed at the deeper connective tissue (◘ Fig. 24.2a). Periodic acid-Schiff (PAS)-stained smear does not show any evidence of fungal hyphae.

24.11 What Is Your Definitive Diagnosis Based on the Clinical and Histopathological Findings?

Oral lichen planus

24.12 How Would You Manage This Patient?

The treatment of OLP depends on whether the patient is symptomatic or not. Topical corticosteroid is the first line of therapy to treat symptomatic oral lichen planus. This patient must be initially followed up frequently for at least once monthly aiming to reduce the symptoms while helping the patient understands the characteristics of OLP, which comes with period of exacerbations and quiescence. Triggers of symptoms such as spicy and acidic food or drink should be avoided. The use of topical corticosteroids should be limited to only when OLP is symptomatic, and stopped when the condition has improved. A long-term use of corticosteroids may lead to opportunistic candidal infections. Although debatable, the patient should be followed at every 6 months to monitor the risk of malignant transformation.

24.13 Oral Lichen Planus

Oral lichen planus (OLP) is a chronic inflammatory disease associated with dysregulated T cell-mediated immune response. The disease has been estimated to

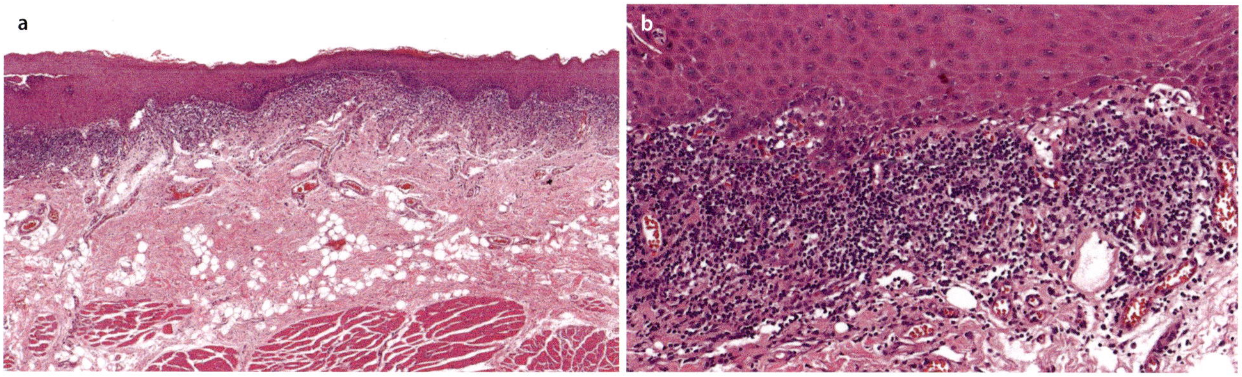

◘ **Fig. 24.2** Non-ulcerated parakeratinized surface epithelium and underlying connective tissue. A dense band-like infiltrate of lymphocytes is present in the superficial lamina propria (**a**) and lymphocytes extending to the epithelium with basal cell destruction and apoptosis (**b**)

affect 1–2% of the population worldwide. It affects more females in a ratio of 2.1:1 with age ranging from 40 to 70 years. Immune-mediated basis of OLP is defined by a cytotoxic T-cell infiltration of the basal lamina zone resulting in apoptosis of basal keratinocytes and degeneration of basal cells. Until today, the agents that initiate or perpetuate oral lichen planus remain unknown. Oral microbiota and mucosa-associated invariant T (MAIT) cells may act as a trigger for OLP. Though the precise aetiology is unknown, there are several predisposing factors that have been linked to the pathogenesis of OLP including stress, medication, hepatitis C virus infection, and diabetes.

OLP can be the sole manifestation of the disease, or it can present simultaneously with cutaneous lesions and/or lesions on other mucosal sites such as genital, eye, or gastrointestinal mucosa. Intraorally, the buccal mucosa, tongue, and gingiva are commonly involved although other sites may rarely be affected. The most common affected site is the buccal mucosa, which is seen in 80–90% of cases. Typically, OLP is characterized by the presence of white papules that can enlarge and coalesce to form reticular, annular, or plaque-like patterns. It can present as desquamative gingivitis when gingiva is involved. Other clinical variants include erosive-ulcerative, atrophic, plaque-like, and bullous forms, which are primarily based on clinical appearances. Patients with OLP may present with a single form or a combination of multiple subtypes. Reticular pattern is the most common subtype and present as white striae, known as "Wickham striae" that are usually bilateral, symmetrical, and often asymptomatic but may eventually progress to more severe, erosive subtypes.

Papular OLP usually shows small pinpoint papules and is considered as the initial, transient phase of OLP which causes it to be missed occasionally. Plaque-like OLP shows homogenous white patches, which clinically appear like oral leukoplakia. This variant is also commonly seen among smokers and in long-standing lesions. The atrophic subtype commonly involves the gingiva. Erosive OLP is considered as the most severe among the subtypes. It clinically appears as erosions or ulcerations of the mucosa with faint radiating white striae. Pseudomembranous slough can occasionally be seen covering the ulcers. Erythematous, erosive, or ulcerative lesions often cause pain and discomfort. Mechanical trauma on the mucosa such as friction from sharp cusps, trauma from dental procedures, and habits such as lip chewing can cause exacerbations of signs and symptoms of OLP.

The diagnosis of OLP is often based on clinical findings with a characteristic bilateral reticular pattern present but can be challenging as there are various conditions that can have this feature. The main clinical differential diagnoses include oral lichenoid drug reaction (OLDR), lupus erythematosus (LE), and graft-versus-host disease (GVHD). OLDR resembles OLP both clinically and histopathologically. The best method to establish the diagnosis is by withdrawal of the offending drugs resulting in resolution of the lesions. However, this method is potentially risky as resolution may take months. Oral lesions of LE present as ulcerated or erythematous areas surrounded by radiating white reticulation. Unlike OLP, LE is typically distributed in an asymmetrical pattern and often involves the hard palate. Lacy reticulations, thickened plaques, or erosions mimicking OLP are seen in around 80% of allogenic hematopoietic stem cell or bone marrow transplant recipients, known as GVHD. The lesions, however, are more widespread and often seen along with xerostomia. Extensive erosive and ulcerative presentation may raise the suspicion of diseases such as pemphigus vulgaris and mucous membrane pemphigoid. The history should be investigated by asking the patient whether the ulcer was preceded by a blister and a search for any intact fluid-filled lesions should be made during clinical examination.

In cases without a typical appearance or obvious bilateral presentation, diagnosis may be confirmed with biopsy. It would help to rule out epithelial dysplasia and malignancy. The histopathological criteria for diagnosis of OLP were originally published by WHO in 1978 (◘ Table 24.1). However, there was a lack of consensus on clinical and histopathological diagnosis of OLP. Hence, a modified WHO diagnostic criteria was established in 2003 that differentiates between OLP and oral lichenoid lesions (OLL) with high correlation of both clinical and histopathological criteria in diagnosing OLP (◘ Table 24.1). Diagnostic histological criteria of OLP include a dense band-like infiltration of lymphocytes and histiocytes along the superficial lamina propria and close to the epithelium, liquefactive degeneration of the basal cells, pyknotic nuclear fragments in shrunken epithelial cells (Civatte/colloid bodies) in the epithelium–connective tissue interface, and hyperkeratosis. The thickness of the epithelium varies, but atrophy is often seen, and erosive epithelium is evident in some cases. Liquefaction degeneration of the basal epithelial cells may often be replaced by an eosinophilic band. In the modified WHO criteria, the term OLL is used for cases that are clinically characteristic but histologically compatible, or clinically compatible but histologically characteristic, or clinically and histologically only compatible with OLP. The proposed criteria developed in 2016 provide more detailed clinical criteria to diagnose OLL and two histopathological criteria have been added that were not present in 2003 criteria (◘ Table 24.1).

Direct immunofluorescence (DIF) is a test used to support the diagnosis of OLP. It is especially useful in

Table 24.1 Clinical and histopathological diagnostic criteria of oral lichen planus

WHO 1978[a]	Modified WHO 2003[b]	AAOMP 2016[c]
Clinical criteria		
Presence of white papule, reticular, annular, plaque-type lesions, grey-white lines radiating from the papules	Presence of bilateral, more or less symmetrical lesions	Multifocal symmetric distribution
Presence of lace-like network of slightly raised grey-white lines (reticular pattern)	Presence of a lace-like network of slightly raised grey-white lines (reticular pattern)	White and red lesions exhibiting one or more of the following forms: – Reticular/papular – Atrophic (erythematous) – Erosive (ulcerative) – Plaque – Bullous
Presence of atrophic lesions, with or without erosion, and possibly also bullae	Erosive, atrophic, bullous, and plaque-like lesions are only accepted as a subtype in the presence of reticular lesions elsewhere in the oral mucosa	Lesions are not localized exclusively to the sites of smokeless tobacco placement
	In all other lesions that resemble OLP but not complete with the aforementioned criteria, the term "clinically compatible with" should be used	Lesions are not localized exclusively adjacent to and in contact with dental restorations
		Lesion onset does not correlate with the start of a medication
		Lesion onset does not correlate with the use of cinnamon-containing products
Histopathological criteria		
Presence of thickened ortho- or parakeratinized layer in sites that are normally keratinized, and if site is normally non-keratinized, this layer may be thin	Presence of well-defined band-like zone of cellular infiltration that is confined to the superficial part of the connective tissue, consisting mainly of lymphocytes	Band-like or patchy, predominately lymphocytic infiltrate in the lamina propria confined to the epithelium–lamina propria interface
Presence of Civatte bodies in basal layer, epithelium, and superficial part of connective tissue	Signs of "liquefaction degeneration" in the basal cell layer	Basal cell liquefactive (hydropic) degeneration
Presence of a well-defined band-like zone of cellular infiltration that is confined to the superficial part of the connective tissue, consisting mainly of lymphocytes	Absence of epithelial dysplasia	Lymphocytic exocytosis
Signs of liquefaction degeneration in the basal cell layer	When the histopathological features are less obvious, the term "histopathologically compatible with" should be used	Absence of epithelial dysplasia
	Final diagnosis of OLP or OLL To achieve a final diagnosis, clinical as well as histopathological criteria should be included 1. OLP: A diagnosis of OLP requires fulfilment of both clinical and histopathological criteria 2. OLL: The term OLL will be used under the following conditions: – Clinically typical of OLP but histopathologically only "compatible with" OLP – Histopathologically typical of OLP but clinically only "compatible with" OLP – Clinically "compatible with" OLP and histopathologically "compatible with" OLP	Absence of verrucous epithelial architectural change

[a] Kramer et al Oral Surg Oral Med Oral Pathol. 1978;46:518–539
[b] van der Meij & van der Waal
[c] Cheng et al are included in further reading

distinguishing OLP from autoimmune blistering diseases that manifest as desquamative gingivitis. The characteristic pattern of DIF seen in OLP is deposition of fibrinogen in a shaggy pattern along the basement membrane zone, with lack of immunoglobulin deposition (except for cytoid bodies) and complement deposition. However, this DIF findings may not be specific for OLP as there are reports of malignant and potentially malignant oral lesion with deposition of fibrinogen at the basement membrane. Algorithmic approach to reach a definitive diagnosis of OLP is shown in ◘ Fig. 24.3.

One of the most concerning issues regarding OLP is the risk of transformation to oral squamous cell carcinoma. OLP is recognized as an oral potentially malignant disorder. Despite this, there are many debates in the literature regarding not only the malignant potential of OLP, but also oral lichenoid reaction. A major factor in this controversy is the lack of universally accepted diagnostic criteria for OLP and OLR. The risk factors for malignant transformation include gender, clinical forms of erythematous atrophic or erosive OLP, site of lesion particularly the tongue, *Candida* or hepatitis C infections, and genetic factors. Malignant transformation is approximately 1.28%.

There is no curative treatment for OLP. Patients usually undergo symptomatic treatment to reduce or eliminate the symptoms as the disease is characterized by spontaneous remission and exacerbation. Foods, beverages, and oral hygiene products which trigger symptoms should be avoided. It is helpful to keep a good oral hygiene with regular dental scaling to minimize plaque accumulation and gingival inflammation that potentially aggravate OLP. Most patients with white or reticular lesions are usually asymptomatic but atrophic and ulcerative forms are painful. Corticosteroids are the most widely used treatment for OLP/OLL and the algo-

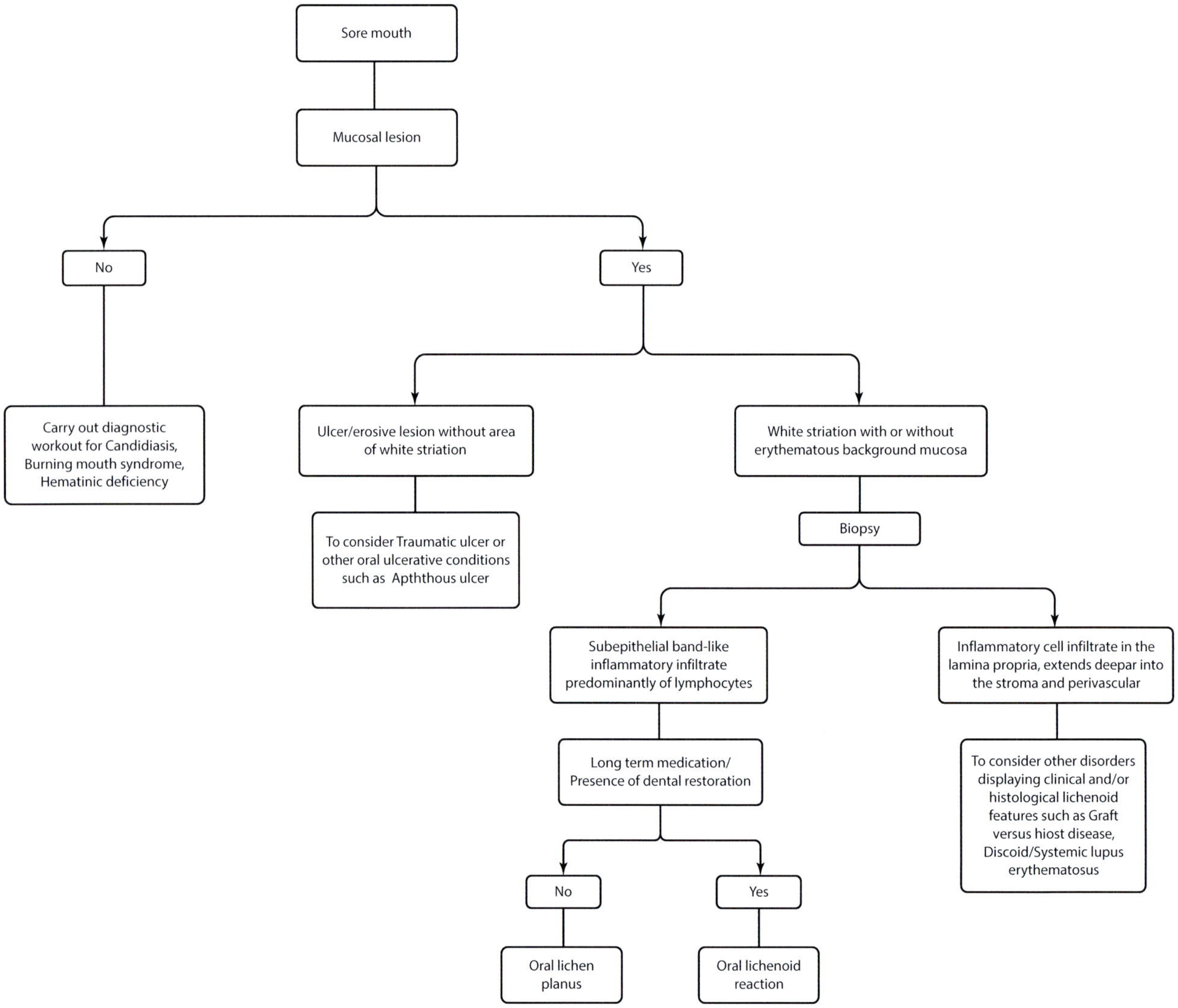

◘ **Fig. 24.3** Diagnostic algorithm of oral lichen planus

rithmic approach in using this therapy is illustrated in ◘ Fig. 24.4. Corticosteroids are available in the forms of topical, systemic, and intralesional injection and prescribed depending on the severity of the disease. The first line of treatment is topical agents, although there are no standard regimens on potency, formulation, concentration, or dosage. In principle, mid-potency steroids like triamcinolone acetonide and betamethasone valerate in topical forms are used to achieve a rapid response at the beginning of treatment for symptomatic lesions. Systemic corticosteroid is reserved for lesions that do not respond to topical therapy or in widespread cases involving other sites such as skin and other mucosa. Prednisolone with initial dosage of 40–80 mg daily is given for the shortest duration possible, for example, approximately 5–7 days and is then followed by tapering down the dosage. Second-line therapy for treating recalcitrant cases are calcineurin inhibitors including cyclosporine, tacrolimus, and pimecrolimus. Immunosuppressants and immunomodulators that have shown to be effective are retinoids, dapsone, and mycophenolates. Other alternative therapies suggested for OLP treatment include hyaluronic acid, curcuminoids, carbon dioxide laser vaporization, photodynamic therapy, and cryotherapy.

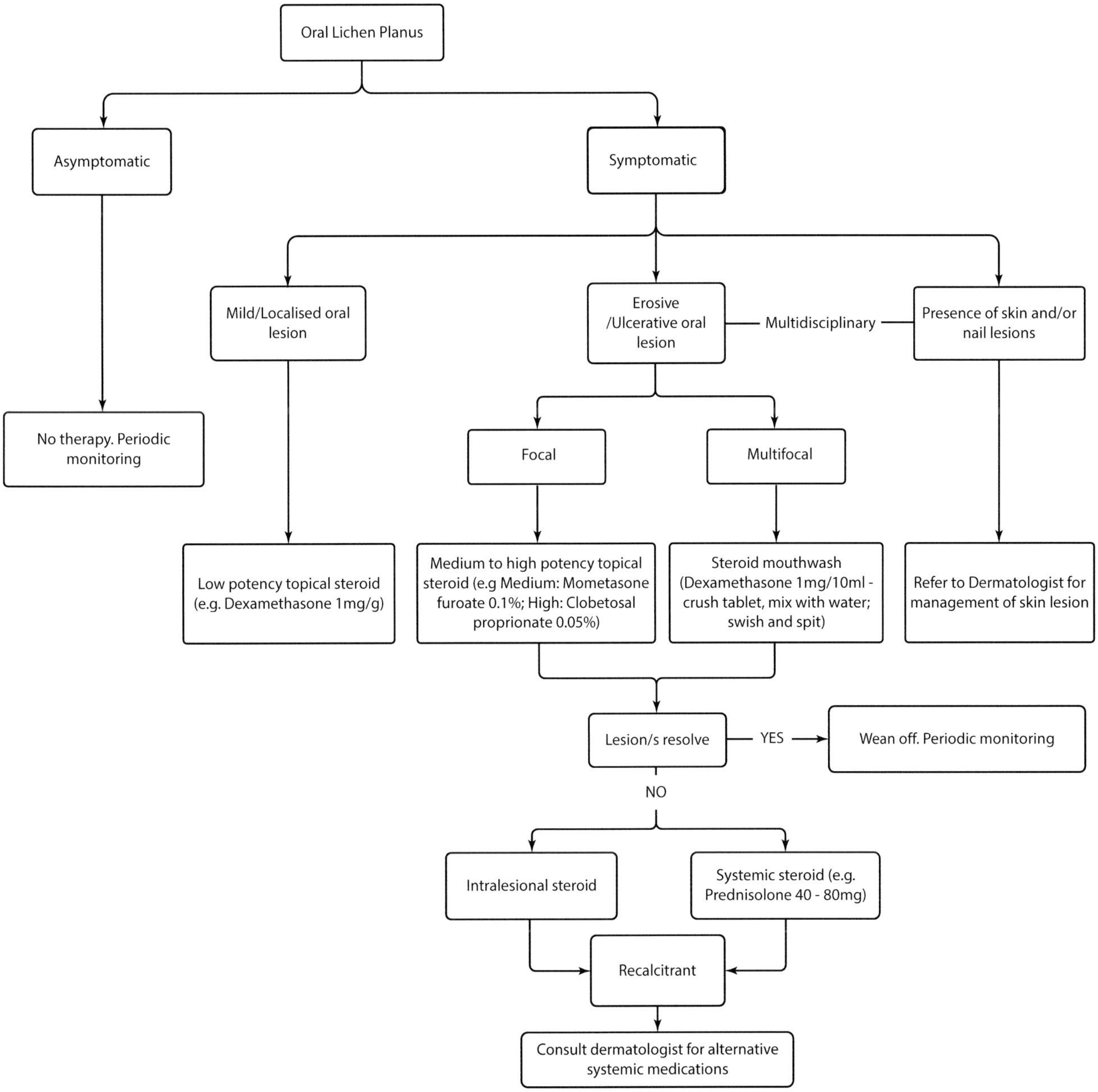

◘ **Fig. 24.4** Simplified management algorithm of oral lichen planus using corticosteroid as the first line of treatment

Self-Assessment Questions

1. Describe the aetiopathogenesis of OLP.
2. Describe the clinical features of OLP.
3. State the important conditions that need to be included in the differential diagnosis of OLP.
4. Describe the histopathological features of OLP.
5. Outline the management plan of OLP.

Further Reading

Alrashdan MS, Cirillo N, McCullough M. Oral lichen planus: a literature review and update. Arch Dermatol Res. 2016;308(8):539–51.

Cheng YS, Gould A, Kurago Z, Fantasia J, Muller S. Diagnosis of oral lichen planus: a position paper of the American Academy of Oral and Maxillofacial Pathology. Oral Surg Oral Med Oral Pathol Oral Radiol. 2016;122(3):332–54.

Neville BW, Damn DD, Alen CM, Chi AC. Oral and maxillofacial pathology. 4th ed; 2015. Elsevier Health Sciences

Van der Meij E, Van der Waal I. Lack of clinicopathologic correlation in the diagnosis of oral lichen planus based on the presently available diagnostic criteria and suggestions for modifications. J Oral Pathol Med. 2003;32(9):507–12.

Warnakulasuriya S, Tilakaratne WM, editors. Oral medicine and pathology; a guide to diagnosis and management. JP Medical Ltd.; 2013.

Non-healing Ulcer in the Right Lateral Surface of the Tongue: Oral Cancer

Anand Ramanathan, Siti Mazlipah Ismail, and Harsha Lal De Silva

Contents

W. M Tilakaratne, T. G. Kallarakkal (eds.), *Clinicopathological Correlation of Oral Diseases*,
https://doi.org/10.1007/978-3-031-24408-7_25

Learning Goals

1. Devise the correct way of compiling the history with appropriate questions.
2. Develop a differential diagnosis after history taking.
3. Deduce appropriate procedures in clinical examination.
4. Formulate a differential diagnosis combining findings in the history and clinical examination.
5. Justify the relevant investigations required to arrive at the diagnosis.
6. Comprehend the importance of clinicopathological correlation in arriving at the correct diagnosis.
7. Recognize the importance of a diagnostic algorithm in arriving at a diagnosis.
8. Outline the management plan.
9. Recognize the role of the dentist in the diagnosis, management and prevention of oral cancer.

25.1 Main Complaint

A 52-year-old male presented to the outpatient clinic, complaining of a persistent painful wound on the right side of his tongue.

25.2 History of Complaint

Question: When did you first notice this wound?

I think I have had this for more than 4 months. It was very small to begin with, but seems to be slowly growing in size.

Question: How did you notice it? Is it painful?

I never had much pain initially. It would sting when I ate something very spicy. But for the past 10 days or so, the pain seems to have become more intense and longer lasting.

Question: Is the pain limited to the tongue, or does it spread to other parts of your mouth or the face?

The pain is only confined to the right side of my tongue. It is not unbearable and eases with paracetamol.

Question: Did you notice any bleeding?

I can't recall seeing it bleed.

Question: Do you think you may have injured your tongue at any point of time?

Occasionally, the side of my tongue gets accidentally bitten but heals within a few days. But this wound hasn't healed as usual, and I am not sure whether it arose from a tongue bite.

Question: Do you recall having any ulcers in other parts of your mouth?

I don't get ulcers in my mouth except for an occasional biting of my tongue or the cheek during eating.

Question: Do you recall seeing any red or white patches on your tongue or other parts of your mouth?

I don't recall seeing any red or white patches in my tongue or other parts of my mouth.

Question: Do you have any significant health issues?

No, I am generally fit and healthy. I have never been admitted to a hospital in my life.

Question: Do you take any regular medications for an illness?

No regular medicines except for occasional painkillers if and when needed.

Question: Do you think you have lost appetite or weight recently?

I haven't noticed any change in my appetite except that I couldn't enjoy a spicy meal for the past 4 months. My wife thinks I have lost some weight but I haven't measured my weight for some time.

Question: Do you go for regular dental check-ups and treatments?

No, this is my first visit to a dental clinic.

Question: Do you smoke?

I do smoke.

❓ Question: How long and how heavy is your smoking?

✔ I have been smoking 15–20 cigarettes a day for the past 30 years or more.

❓ Question: Do you drink alcohol?

✔ I enjoy spirits. I would have a glass or two of spirits practically every night for the past 20 years or more. Sometimes I take beer and wine too.

❓ Question: Do you chew betel quid?

✔ I do not chew betel quid. I have never tried it in the past.

25.3 Findings of Extra-Oral Examination

The patient appears otherwise healthy. No pallor or jaundice is noted in his conjunctivae. There is no obvious facial swelling or skin rashes. He has clearly articulated speech and a full range of jaw movements and could protrude his tongue and move it to both left and right with no apparent restriction in mobility. A slightly tender, enlarged, solitary lymph node is noted on palpation in the right submandibular region, measuring approximately 1 cm and being freely movable and with no signs of tethering to skin or deep tissues.

25.4 Findings of Intraoral Examination

His oral hygiene is reasonably good. An irregular shaped ulcer with rolled margins, measuring 2 × 1 cm in its largest dimensions, is noted in the right lateral border of the anterior two-thirds of his tongue (◘ Fig. 25.1). The surface of the ulcer has a whitish slough, and both the base and the margins felt indurated on palpation. There is no pus or discharge, but the ulcer is slightly tender to palpate. The remainder of his oral mucosa appears clinically normal on examination.

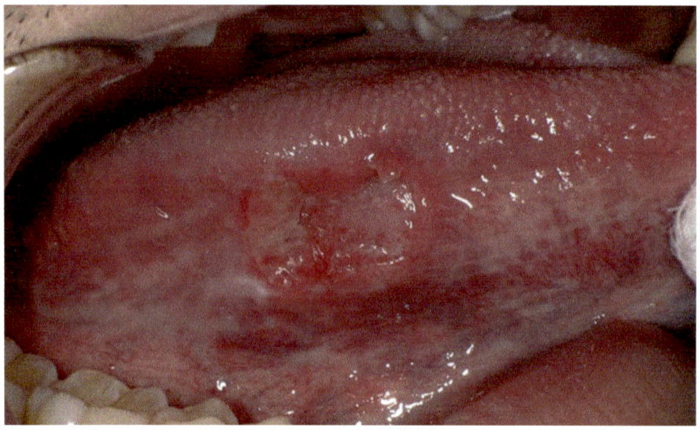

◘ **Fig. 25.1** Intraoral photograph of the non-healing ulcer in the right lateral surface of the tongue showing rolled margins with the base covered with white slough

25.5 What Is Your Clinical Differential Diagnoses?

The following entities were considered in the differential diagnosis based on the history and clinical examination findings.

- Neoplastic ulcer
- Traumatic ulcer
- Traumatic ulcerative granuloma with stromal eosinophilia (TUGSE)
- Major aphthous ulcer

25.6 What Is Your Justification for the Differential Diagnoses?

A persistent ulcer occurring in the lateral border of the tongue of a male in his fifties, having a significant history of smoking and alcohol consumption, increases the likelihood of oral malignancy. Oral cancer could initiate as non-painful ulceration, which persists and may become painful at later stages due to secondary infection or from an invasion of a sensory nerve. Moreover, the rolled margins, the indurated base and the failure to heal over 4 months further support a clinical diagnosis of a malignant ulcer.

A traumatic ulcer is usually associated with an injury from a sharp tooth, denture or a poorly contoured jagged edge of a dental restoration giving a cause-to-effect association. Traumatic ulcers are more common on the lateral surface of the tongue due to trauma from sharp lingual cusps of adjacent teeth. In this patient, sharp cusps are evident in the adjacent mandibular teeth, which matches the size of the ulcer. However, traumatic ulcers are usually painful from the start, seldom have an indurated base and readily heal if the causative stimulus is removed. Although this patient has some sharp cusped teeth in the ipsilateral mandibular dentition, cuspal grindings to eliminate trauma and waiting for 2–3 weeks for healing to exclude the possibility of a traumatic ulcer were not pursued in the light of strong clinical evidence supporting probable malignancy. Furthermore, a long-standing traumatic ulcer may occasionally mimic neoplasia and may require histopathology to exclude malignancy.

Traumatic ulcerative granuloma with stromal eosinophilia (TUGSE) is a rare self-limiting condition of the oral mucosa. It is an isolated ulcer that is commonly present on the lateral surface of the tongue. It may either be asymptomatic or causes mild to severe pain and may occasionally mimic neoplasia.

Major aphthous ulcers are larger than 1 cm in size and may occur in the lateral border of the tongue. Usually, there would be a history of recurrences, presence of multiple ulcers at a point of time, extremely painful and healing within 4–8 weeks. Despite having no history of recurrent ulceration, a major aphthous ulcer could be considered a valid differential as occasionally they may take longer than usual to heal following persistent trauma, inflammation and fibrosis.

25.7 What Is Your Working Diagnosis?

The clinical evidence strongly supported the probable diagnosis of the non-healing ulcer to be a malignancy. The patient's age, smoking and alcohol consumption argue for a provisional clinical working diagnosis of oral squamous cell carcinoma (OSCC) of the anterior two-thirds of the tongue. Oral squamous cell carcinoma is the commonest malignancy affecting the oral cavity. However, the clinical diagnosis of the malignancy needs endorsement from histopathological examination for grading, staging and planning appropriate treatment.

25.8 How Would You Investigate This Patient?

An incision biopsy was performed under local anaesthesia. An elliptical-shaped wedge of tissue down to the intrinsic muscle layer of the tongue and across the periphery of the ulcer to include clinically normal tissue in addition to the lesion was taken to obtain a representative sample for histopathological examination. The harvested tissue was dispatched to the laboratory immersed in formal saline along with documentation detailing the relevant clinical information. The wound was closed with 3/0 Vicryl resorbable sutures after obtaining haemostasis.

It is best to sample the edge of the ulcer avoiding the centre, as the latter is likely to contain necrotic tissue and inflammatory cells that may mask important histopathological features. Including clinically normal tissue at the periphery of the ulcer helps pathologists examine the transition from normal to malignancy. An adequate depth of the sample is of paramount importance to examine for depth of invasion and the nature of the advancing front of the tumour.

25.9 What Are the Histopathological Features of the Submitted Specimen?

Histopathological examination of H & E sections prepared from the biopsy specimen shows an ulcerated surface. The dysplastic parakeratinized squamous epithelium shows a break in the basement membrane zone and invasion of islands, nests and cords of squamous epithelial cells into the underlying corium and muscle. Numerous dyskeratotic epithelial tumour cells and a few keratin pearls are evident. The tumour cells exhibit moderate nuclear and cellular pleomorphism, increased nuclear:cytoplasmic ratio, hyperchromatic nucleus, increased mitotic figures (10 mitosis/10 high-power field) and increase in the number and size of the nucleoli (▫ Fig. 25.2a). The depth of invasion is 8 mm and is measured from a line through the surface of the adjacent normal mucosa (basement membrane) to the deepest point of the tumour (▫ Fig. 25.2b). The pattern of invasion (advancing front) is type IV (non-cohesive type). The lymphocytic host response is graded as intermediate.

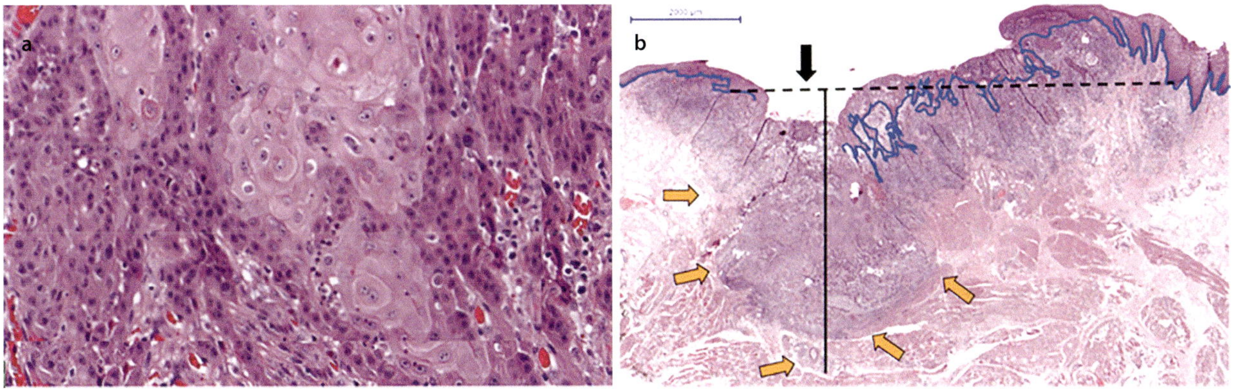

▫ **Fig. 25.2** Photomicrographs show (**a**) moderately differentiated epithelial tumour cells with dyskeratosis, moderate nuclear and cellular pleomorphism, increased nuclear:cytoplasmic ratio and hyperchromatic nucleus (**b**) invasion of the moderately differentiated epithelial tumour cells into the underlying connective tissue (orange arrows), the reconstructed surface (dotted line) and the depth of invasion (black line) (Courtesy: Prof. Dr Rosnah Binti Zain)

25.10 What Is Your Definitive Diagnosis

Moderately differentiated oral squamous cell carcinoma.

25.11 What Specific Findings Help You to Arrive at the Diagnosis of Oral Squamous Cell Carcinoma?

A non-healing ulcer persisting on the lateral border of the tongue over 4 months' duration triggers suspicions of malignancy. The regular, heavy, prolonged use of smoking and alcohol for more than two decades, the advanced age (50+ years) and the male gender are well-known risk factors for developing oral cancer. Furthermore, the rolled irregular edges and the indurated base are features usually associated with malignant ulcers. However, the confirmatory evidence comes from histopathology showing an ulcerated and dysplastic surface parakeratinized squamous epithelium with breach in the basement membrane zone and invasion of islands, nests and cords of moderately differentiated neoplastic epithelial cells into the underlying connective tissue stroma. Hence, the history, clinical findings and histopathological features align to confirm the diagnosis of moderately differentiated OSCC.

25.12 How Would You Manage This Patient?

On histopathological confirmation of the diagnosis, the malignancy has to be graded and staged to help determine prognosis and plan appropriate treatment. This may involve further targeted investigations.

25.12.1 Imaging

MRI is a preferred choice for assessing tongue lesions. The contemporary practice is to obtain a MRI scan of the head, neck, thorax and upper abdomen. The imaging provides information on the three-dimensional (3D) size and location of the primary tumour, the status of the cervical lymph nodes and the presence of distant metastases. The primary tumour measured 1.5 cm × 0.8 cm on MRI, and no significant cervical lymphadenopathy or distant metastases were detected.

The patient was then presented at the multidisciplinary head and neck meeting attended by the oral medicine and oral pathology specialists, oral and maxillofacial surgeons, ENT surgeons, plastic and reconstructive surgeons, radiologists and oncologists to discuss prognosis and decide on appropriate treatment options and their sequencing. The clinical, radiological and histopathological evidence were consistent with a diagnosis of stage 2 (T1N0M0) moderately differentiated squamous cell carcinoma of the right lateral border of the anterior two-thirds of the tongue. The patient was presented with the options of surgical excision or radiotherapy to treat the primary tumour. Following discussions with the patient and his immediate family, a decision was made to treat using radiotherapy with curative intent.

Surgery and radiotherapy remain the primary modalities for the treatment of OSCC, while chemotherapy is used as an adjuvant in selected cases. The use of different modalities, either as a standalone treatment or in combination with each other, is a treatment decision based on the stage of the disease and on other recognized prognostic markers.

An early lesion in the tongue (TNM stage 2) with no clinical or radiological evidence of regional or distance metastasis could be treated equally well with both radiotherapy and with surgery. Ablative surgery in the form of wide-local excisions and selective/radical neck dissections may carry significant postoperative morbidity and may also necessitate complex reconstructive surgery to replace excised tissue and restore function. Radiotherapy too results in chronic local complications that may affect the patient's oral health and function.

The radiation treatment field included both the primary lesion and the ipsilateral neck down to the level of clavicle to account for potential occult micro-metastatic regional spread of the disease. The decision to include the neck within the radiation treatment field was based on the histopathological findings of a discohesive advancing front (type IV), depth of invasion > 8 mm and the increased mitotic figures per microscopic field. All those features are believed to increase the likelihood of occult lymphatic spread.

25.13 What Is the Definitive Treatment Given for This Patient?

The patient underwent a comprehensive dental check-up to identify and treat all caries and optimize periodontal health in preparation for the radiation treatment. He was counselled on the importance of preventive dental care and was introduced to the use of fluoridated toothpaste and advised on efficient tooth brushing and flossing techniques. The radiotherapy administered consisted of a radiation dose of 70 Gy delivered, fractionated over 8 weeks. Fractionation allows time for tissue recovery and is important to reduce radiation side-effects. Patient developed oropharyngeal radiation mucositis by the third week of therapy and had to be nursed with a nasogastric feeding tube. The mucositis gradually resolved towards the end of the therapy, and the patient was directed to use alcohol-free chlorhexidine mouth rinses, miconazole oral gel and lignocaine viscous gel to ease oral discomfort.

25.14 How Would You Follow-Up This Patient and What Is the Prognosis?

The decision to treat with curative intent was based on the fact that the disease was diagnosed at an early stage (TNM stage 2), and the patient was in otherwise good health to be able to tolerate the aggressive therapy required for achieving a cure. The absence of clinically or radiologically detectable cervical lymph node involvement and the smaller size of the primary tumour (less than 2 cm in its largest dimension) signal a favourable prognosis. However, OSCC is well known to recur even following apparently effective treatment. Therefore, the patient needs close monitoring against potential primary and nodal recurrent disease. The patient will be followed up quarterly for 2 years and at six-monthly intervals for a further 3 years. Arrangements were also made for biannual dental check-ups to maintain his oral hygiene and also take advantage of the opportunity to perform an opportunistic clinical review for identifying potential recurrent disease.

25.15 Oral Squamous Cell Carcinoma

Oral cancer is defined as cancers that arise in the inner lip, tongue, gingiva, floor of the mouth, hard palate and rest of the mouth, excluding the base of the tongue and salivary glands. More than 90% of all oral malignancies are histopathologically diagnosed as OSCCs and are commonly referred to as oral cancer. Oral squamous cell carcinoma is defined as carcinoma with squamous differentiation arising from the mucosal epithelium. GLOBOCAN data for 2020 reported 377,713 new cases of OSCC worldwide, with an estimated 177,757 cancer-related deaths. The prevalence of oral cancer shows geographical variation. Asian countries record a comparatively higher incidence. Oral squamous cell carcinoma is common in the fifth and sixth decades of life. However, recently there has been an increasing trend for OSCC in younger people (<45 year old). There is a male predilection of 2:1, but an increasing incidence is reported amongst females in countries where females have taken to tobacco smoking and alcohol drinking. Oral cancer is usually common among the lower socio-economic sectors of the population.

Tobacco (smoking or smokeless), betel quid chewing and drinking alcohol are well-recognized risk factors. The risk conferred by bidi smoking (a cheap form of a cigarette) is the highest, followed by cigar smoking, cigarette smoking and pipe smoking. Betel quid contains a mixture of areca nut catechu and slaked lime wrapped in a betel leaf with or without tobacco. Betel quid with tobacco poses a higher risk for the development of oral cancer. The risk increases with the amount, frequency and duration. The effects of tobacco smoking, alcohol consumption and betel quid chewing are cumulative and raise the risk profile. Infection with papillomavirus (HPV) infection is a well-recognized risk factor for oropharyngeal cancers but its role in oral cancer remains unclear.

Oral squamous cell carcinoma may occur *de novo* or may be preceded by the presence of various oral potentially malignant disorders (OPMDs). The overall malignant transformation rate of all OPMDs is 7.9%. Leukoplakia is the most common OPMD encountered and has an overall malignant transformation rate of 9.5% and an annual malignant transformation rate of 1.56%. However, some OPMDs reportedly have a significantly higher malignant transformation rate (◘ Table 25.1).

Oral squamous cell carcinoma could affect any area of the oral cavity and quite often is related to the risk

◘ Table 25.1 Some oral potentially malignant disorders and their estimated malignant transformation risk

Oral Potentially Malignant Disorders	Estimated malignant transformation rate (%)	Estimated annual malignant transformation rate (%)
Homogenous leukoplakia	9.5	1.56
Erythroplakia	33.1	
Proliferative verrucous leukoplakia	49.5	9.3
Oral submucous fibrosis	5.2	0.98
Discoid lupus erythematosus	6.9	
Oral lichen planus	1.4	0.28
Oral lichenoid lesions	3.8	0.57
Palatal keratosis (associated with reverse smoking)	2.1-6.9	
Actinic cheilitis	3.07	

habits practised by an individual. Oral cancer most commonly occurs in the lateral surface of the tongue, the floor of the mouth and gingiva in smokers whereas, in betel quid chewers with or without tobacco, the common sites affected appear to be the buccal mucosa, buccal sulcus and the gingiva.

Early lesions may resemble an area of homogenous leukoplakia, nodular leukoplakia, oral lichen planus, erythroplakia or erythroleukoplakia. The only significant clinical feature that may help in differentiating between early lesions of OSCC and OPMDs is the partial loss of mucosal elasticity and hardened texture of these lesions, clinically referred to as induration. Early lesions are usually painless. They tend to become increasingly nodular, exophytic and may ulcerate. They may sometimes clinically mimic a traumatic ulcer or a pyogenic granuloma and may occasionally become painful due to secondary trauma and infection. The presence of rolled margins and induration are the important clinical features that suggest probable malignancy (◘ Fig. 25.3).

Advanced OSCC is defined as primary lesions measuring over 4 cm in size or infiltrating into the adjacent/deeper structures with or without evidence of regional/distant metastasis. Clinically the advanced-stage OSCC may present as extensive ulcers or exophytic growths with verrucous features or combined features of ulcer and exophytic growths (◘ Fig. 25.4 a–c). Advanced lesions may present with pain or paraesthesia that could be either from secondary infection or from a tumour involving adjacent sensory nerves. The lesions may be friable and bleed easily. Teeth within the lesion may be mobile because of tumour invasion into the periodontium and the supporting alveolar bone.

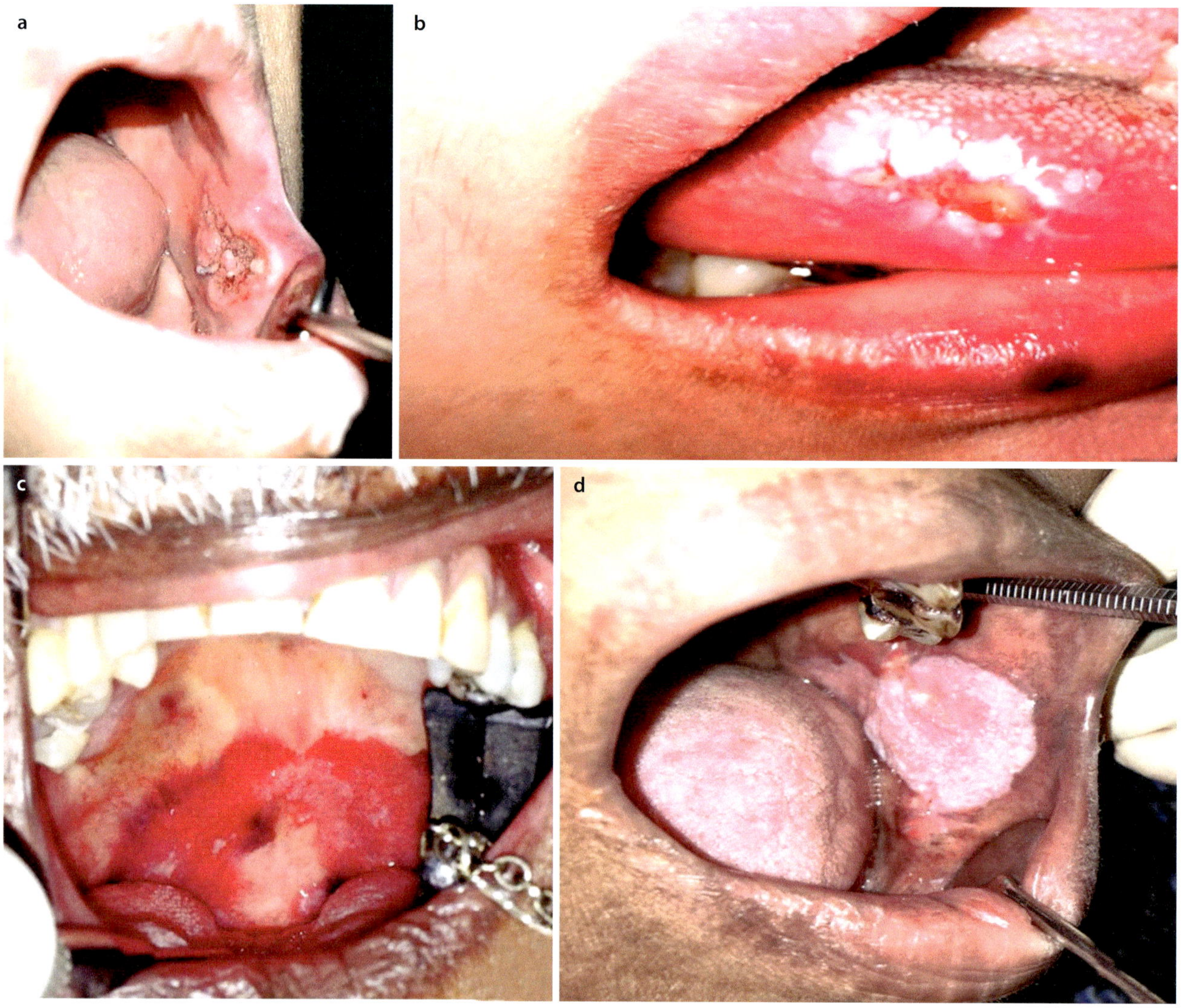

◘ **Fig. 25.3** Photographs showing early lesions of OSCC: (**a**) a non-healing ulcer on the left buccal mucosa, (**b**) a non-healing ulcer within a white leukoplakic patch on the right lateral border of the tongue, (**c**) a large erythematous flat red lesion (erythroplakia) involving the hard and soft palate and (**d**) a verrucopapillary lesion on the left buccal mucosa. (Courtesy: Dato' Prof. Dr Zainal Ariff)

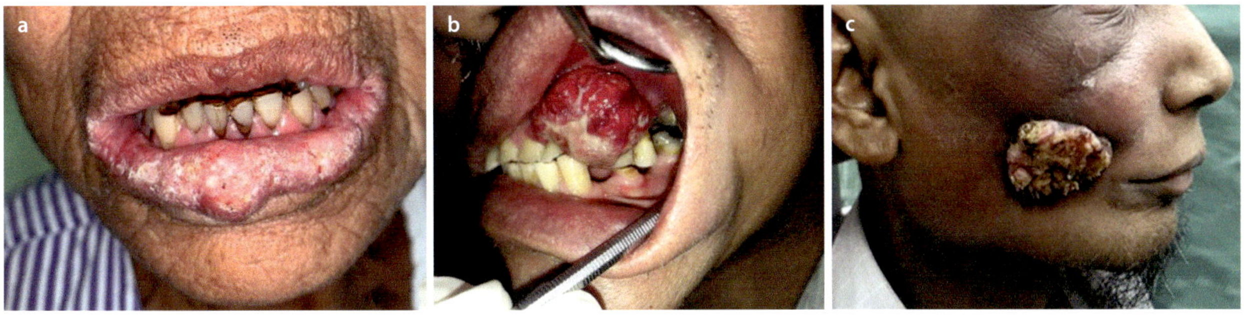

Fig. 25.4 Photographs showing advanced OSCC lesions: (**a**) an ulceroproliferative lesion extending from the right commissure to the left commissure region involving the full lower lip, (**b**) a large reddish growth on the upper labial gingiva and (**c**) a large ulceroproliferative lesion on the right cheek. (Courtesy: Dr Saravanan Gopalan)

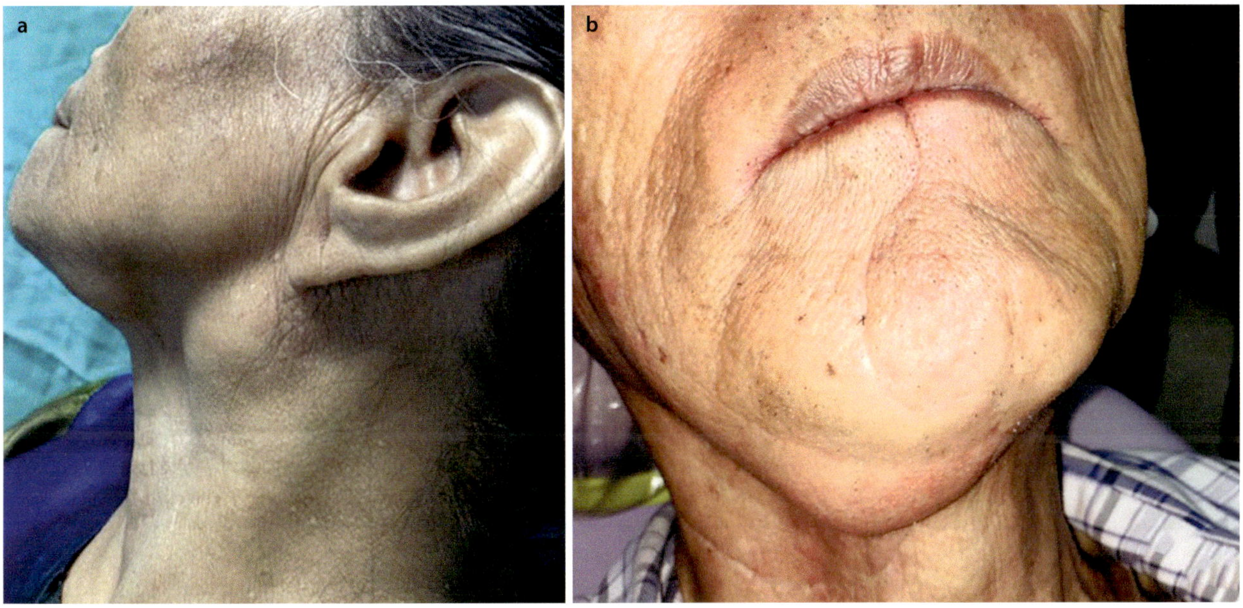

Fig. 25.5 Extra-oral photograph shows a lymph node swelling on (**a**) left side of the neck (Courtesy: Dr Saravanan Gopalan) and (**b**) right submandibular region

25.15.1 Metastasis to Neck Nodes

Oral squamous cell carcinoma tends to spread to cervical lymph nodes and may cause neck swellings at various levels (Fig. 25.5 a and b), producing malignant cervical lymphadenopathy. While advanced lesions have a higher likelihood of producing cervical lymphadenopathy, the early stage tumours are not totally exempt from causing regional spread. Notably, OSCCs arising in the floor of the mouth, tongue and mandibular gingiva have a greater tendency for early lymphatic spread. Primary lesions transgressing the midline may spread to involve lymph nodes on both sides of the neck.

25.16 Investigations

Clinical features alone are inconclusive of OSCC as they may mimic a variety of lesions. Primarily a histopathological examination is mandatory to confirm the diagnosis and provide information that could be used to predict the biological behaviour of the tumour. Second, it is important to make an accurate determination of the spread of the malignancy at local (primary), regional (cervical lymphadenopathy) and distant levels by clinical examination supplemented by imaging studies. This information needs to be collated to inform management decisions.

25.16.1 Imaging

The advances made in imaging technology over the last few decades have a significant impact in the management of oral cancer. The most widely used imaging modalities are computed tomography (CT) scans and magnetic resonance imaging (MRI). The improved resolution in CT and MRI scans used in contemporary practice helps in accurate dimensional measurements of primary and metastatic lesions and a higher level of sensitivity to pick up cervical lymphadenopathy that is not large enough to be detected during a clinical examination. A skilled radiologist may even predict between malignant and non-malignant lymphadenopathy based on the short-axis dimension and architectural features of imaged lymph nodes. CT scans better assess skeletal involvement, while MRIs provide better soft tissue imaging. Advanced cross-sectional imaging has significantly improved the accuracy in establishing:

- Local spread of the primary tumour
- Spread to locoregional lymph nodes
- Metastatic spread of the disease
- Detection of synchronous primary tumours

Ultrasound scans are useful when performing guided fine-needle aspiration cytology to assess cervical lymph nodes for confirming cervical lymphadenopathy for malignancy. Positron emission scanning (PET scans) is a newer addition that uses a radioisotope (18-fluorodeoxyglucose) injected intravenously to identify hypermetabolic cancerous or inflamed tissues.

The main indication for PET scanning is for the evaluation of malignant lymph nodes without clinically apparent primary tumour (occult tumour). It is also valuable in the evaluation of suspected recurrence amidst post-treatment changes on conventional imaging modalities. Combining PET with CT fuses the functional tissue metabolic map with anatomical details, providing invaluable information to the clinician. In contemporary practice, plain radiography (dental pantomography and intraoral radiographs) is used mainly to assess the patient's dental status and to plan to optimize oral health before undergoing treatment for oral cancer.

Information obtained from imaging studies should be interpreted in association with clinical findings to assess the spread of malignancy and arrive at staging. The best prognostic indicator is the TNM staging proposed by the American Joint Committee on Cancer staging (AJCC). TNM classification assigns values according to the extent of the primary (T_{1-4} and subtypes), regional metastasis (N_{0-3} and subtypes) and distant metastasis (M_{0-1}). The AJCC has recently revised (eighth edition) the staging system for lip and oral cavity cancers to include histopathological information such as depth of invasion (DOI) under the tumour size and extra-nodal extension (ENE) under nodal involvement. The latest inclusions have made the classification more comprehensive and include various subtypes within the values assigned for T and N status. By grouping the TNM values, OSCC can be staged (stages 1–4_{A-C}) to use in prognostication, treatment planning and post-treatment follow-up (Tables 25.2 and 25.3).

Table 25.2 The eighth edition AJCC staging for lip and oral cavity cancers

Tumour size (pT) staging for lip and oral cavity	Criteria
pTx	Tumour size cannot be assessed.
pT1 (lip and oral cavity)	Tumour less than or equal to 2 cm in greatest dimension and less than or equal to 5 mm depth of invasion.
pT2 (lip and oral cavity)	Tumour less than or equal to 2 cm in greatest dimension and more than 5 mm depth of invasion OR Tumour more than 2 cm but not more than 4 cm in greatest dimension and depth of invasion not more than 10 mm.
pT3 (lip and oral cavity)	Tumour more than 4 cm in greatest dimension or any tumour with depth of invasion more than 10 mm.
pT4a (lip)	Tumour invades through the cortical bone, inferior alveolar nerve, floor of the mouth or skin (chin or nose).
pT4a (oral cavity)	Tumour invades through the cortical bone of mandible or maxillary sinus, or skin of the face.
pT4b (lip and oral cavity)	Tumour invades masticatory space, pterygoid plates or skull base or encases the internal carotid artery.

Note: Superficial erosion of the bone/tooth socket by gingival primary is not sufficient to classify as pT4a.

Table 25.2 (continued)

Tumour size (pT) staging for lip and oral cavity	Criteria
Nodal metastasis (pN) staging for lip and oral cavity	Criteria
pNx	Regional lymph nodes cannot be assessed.
pN0	No regional lymph node metastasis.
pN1	Metastasis in a single ipsilateral lymph node, 3 cm or less and without extra-nodal extension.
pN2a	Metastasis in a single ipsilateral lymph node, 3 cm or less and with extra-nodal extension OR Metastasis in a single ipsilateral lymph node more than 3 cm but less than 6 cm in greatest dimension and without extra-nodal extension.
pN2b	Metastasis in multiple ipsilateral nodes more than 3 cm but less than 6 cm in greatest dimension and without extra-nodal extension.
pN2c	Metastasis in contralateral or bilateral nodes more than 3 cm but less than 6 cm in greatest dimension and without extra-nodal extension.
pN3a	Metastasis in a single lymph node more than 6 cm and without extra-nodal extension.
pN3b	Metastasis in a single ipsilateral lymph node more than 3 cm in greatest dimension and with extra-nodal extension OR Multiple ipsilateral or contralateral or bilateral lymph nodes any with extra-nodal extension.
Distant metastasis (pM) staging for lip and oral cavity	Criteria
pM0	No distant metastasis.
pM1	Distant metastasis present.

Table 25.3 Prognostic stage groupings in the eighth edition AJCC staging system for the lip and oral cavity cancers

Stage	pT	pN	pM
0	Tis	N0	M0
I	T1	N0	M0
II	T2	N0	M0
III	T3	N0	M0
	T1, T2, T3	N1	M0
IVA	T4a	N0, N1	M0
	T1, T2, T3, T4a	N2	M0
IVB	Any T	N3	M0
	T4b	Any N	M0
IVC	Any T	Any N	M1

25.17 Histopathological Examination

In most instances, the diagnosis of malignancy is made on an incision biopsy specimen from the primary lesion. The histopathological assessment should include the confirmation/exclusion of malignancy. Further, the report should, where possible, include information on the degree of differentiation, depth of invasion, advancing tumour front and the presence/absence of perivascular, lymphatic and perineural invasion.

Pre-treatment cytological assessment of a fine-needle aspiration sample obtained from a suspected enlarged cervical lymph node may be useful to confirm/provisionally exclude regional metastatic spread. Occasionally, surgeons may request a frozen section examination of a sentinel lymph node harvested at the time of surgery to guide on-the-table determination of the extent of surgery required.

25.18 Histopathological Features

The epithelial tumour cells show nuclear and cellular pleomorphism, altered nuclear:cytoplasmic ratio, hyperchromatic nuclei, increase in the number and the size of nucleoli, mitotic figures (including atypical forms), dyskeratotic cells and keratin pearls in varying degrees. The tumour cells invade the underlying connective tissue in cords, nests or islands.

25.18.1 Histopathological Grading

The grading of OSCC is based on the extent of differentiation of the epithelial cells to the normal epithelium. It also takes into consideration the histopathological features that are mentioned previously. The OSCCs are graded based on "Broder grading" into four grades: well-differentiated (◘ Fig. 25.6a), moderately differentiated (◘ Fig. 25.6b), poorly differentiated (◘ Fig. 25.6c) and undifferentiated OSCC. It was previously reported that the grades of differentiation are considered an important prognostic indicator for lymph node metastasis and survival. The poorly differentiated and undifferentiated OSCC might be difficult to recognize histologically under haematoxylin and eosin stains (◘ Fig. 25.6c). In that situation, immunostaining with pan-cytokeratin antibody helps identify the cell of origin of the tumour (◘ Fig. 25.6d).

The pattern (mode) of invasion (POI) can be broadly divided into two types (cohesive and non-cohesive). They are subdivided into four types (type I, II, III and IV). Types I and II POI fall under the cohesive type. Type I POI shows a broad pushing invasive front with bulbous rete pegs, which tend to infiltrate at the same level (◘ Fig. 25.7a). Type II POI shows infiltrating cords, strands or large islands, which are branching and continuous with the main tumour mass (◘ Fig. 25.7b). Types III and IV are the non-cohesive type. Type III POI shows small islands and cords that are separated

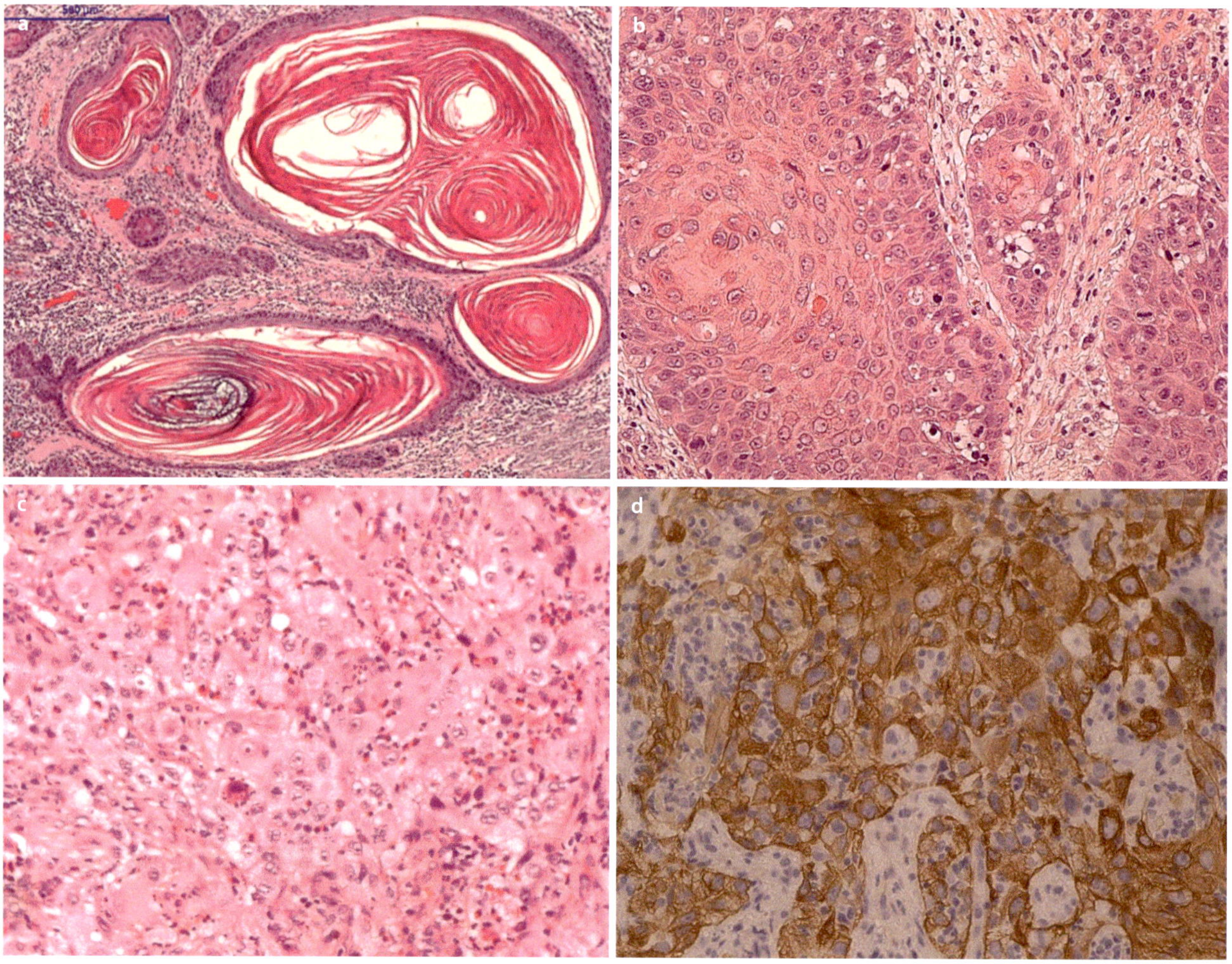

◘ **Fig. 25.6** Photomicrographs show a (**a**) well-differentiated squamous cell carcinoma, (**b**) moderately differentiated squamous cell carcinoma and (**c**) poorly differentiated squamous cell carcinoma and (**d**) strong cytokeratin (CK) immunopositive tumour cells in a poorly differentiated squamous cell carcinoma

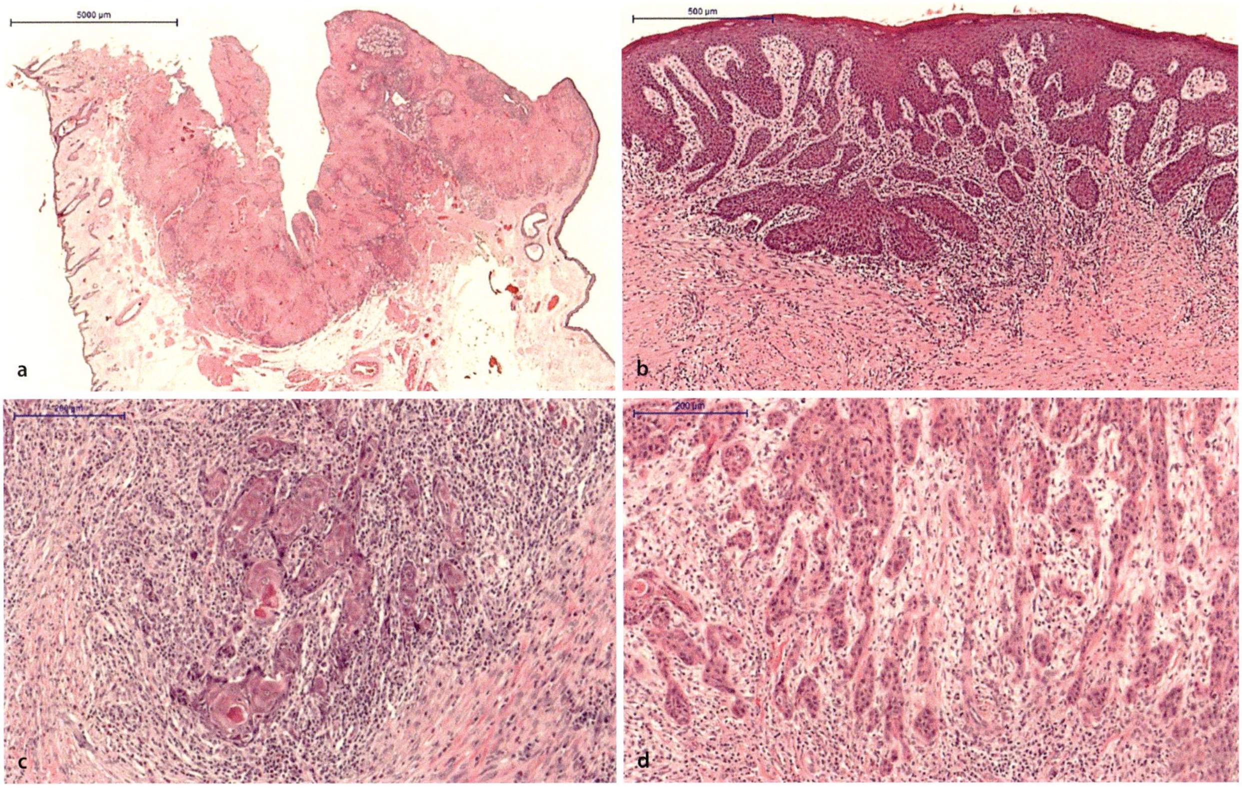

Fig. 25.7 Photomicrograph shows (**a**) type I pattern of invasion (cohesive), (**b**) type II pattern of invasion (cohesive), (**c**) type III pattern of invasion (non-cohesive) and (**d**) type IV pattern of invasion (non-cohesive)

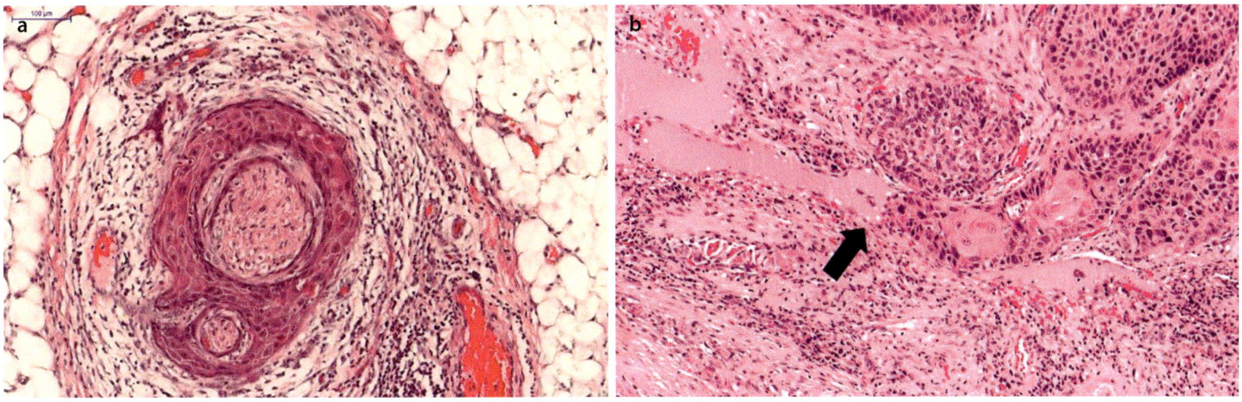

Fig. 25.8 Photomicrographs shows (**a**) perineural invasion and (**b**) lymphovascular invasion (black arrow)

from the main tumour (Fig. 25.7c), and type IV POI shows widely infiltrating small islands or individual cells of the tumour (Fig. 25.7d). Tumours with cohesive POI are said to be less aggressive when compared to tumours with non-cohesive POI. Thus, POI has been shown to be an important prognosticator in predicting the behaviour of OSCC.

Perineural invasion is defined as invasion around and through peripheral nerves by the tumour cells. Perineural invasion is seen in some OSCCs (Fig. 25.8a), and it may indicate regional nodal metastasis, higher local recurrence and decreased survival. Lymphovascular invasion (LVI) is defined as the presence of aggregates of tumour cells within endothelial lined channels or invasion of the media of a vessel with ulceration of the intima. This provides a route for the tumour cells to metastasize to distant sites in the body. Lymphovascular invasion is seen in some OSCCs (Fig. 25.8b), and it indicates higher regional nodal metastasis, recurrence and poor survival.

When treated with surgery through wide-local excision with or without cervical lymphadenectomy (neck

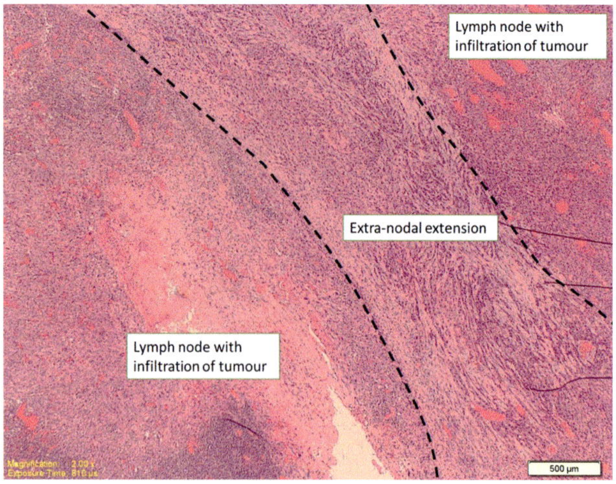

Fig. 25.9 Photomicrograph shows extra-nodal extension in a lymph node. (Courtesy: Dr Noratikah Awang Hasyim)

dissection), the excised specimen should be subjected to a detailed histopathological assessment. The post-excisional histopathological assessment, in addition to all pre-treatment markers reported, should also include an assessment of the excision margins for adequate tumour clearance at a microscopic level and the presence of lymph node involvement and, in particular, the presence/absence of extra-nodal spread. This assessment informs decisions on the possible necessity of further treatment in the line of adjuvant or salvage therapy to improve treatment outcomes.

The extra-nodal extension (ENE) also referred to as extra-capsular spread is the invasion of the nodal metastasis beyond the capsule of the lymph nodes (Fig. 25.9).

25.18.2 Treatment

The principal objective of cancer treatment is to eradicate primary and metastatic disease to achieve for disease-free survival with minimal post-treatment morbidity and good quality of life. Cure is difficult in situations of advanced disease at presentation. The aim is to achieve palliation with optimal pain control, feeding, and to secure airway in order to provide a good quality of life (QoL) until they pass away from the disease or from another cause. Diagnosis of cancer brings with it a huge psychological trauma to both the patient and his/her loved ones. Thus, the management of cancer includes providing both physical and psychological therapy to ease the disease burden. Hence, efficient cancer treatment involves a multidisciplinary approach, with each speciality contributing its expertise to achieve the best outcomes for the patient.

Surgery to completely excise the primary disease with an adequate margin where necessary coupled with a selective or a radical neck dissection to excise the draining cervical lymph nodes is regarded the most appropriate treatment for OSCC provided the patient's general health allows such treatment. Neck dissection is considered the most efficient way of controlling the regional metastatic disease. Even in the absence of clinically or radiologically evident cervical lymphadenopathy, it is often used prophylactically with the aim of eradicating potential occult lymphatic spread. The ablative surgery sometimes needs extensive reconstruction to provide structural and functional rehabilitation. Microvascular surgical techniques and the use of dental prostheses supported by osseointegrated implants have made significant advances in post-surgical rehabilitation to provide a good quality of life.

Radiotherapy (RT) is considered equally effective to surgery in managing early stage tumours. However, the most frequent use of RT is in the form of an adjuvant, delivered 6–8 weeks after surgical excision to provide control against potential recurrences from close-surgical margins and from disease deemed aggressive by observations made on the post-excision histopathology. Radiotherapy can also be used as a neoadjuvant modality to debulk a mass to facilitate surgical excision, to salvage a post-surgical recurrence or an advanced disease that is deemed inoperable. The curative doses of radiotherapy range from 60 to 70 Gy given in fractions of 1.8–2 Gy per day over 6–8 weeks. For some cancers, combining with concurrent chemotherapy (chemoradiation) provides effective control although the side-effect profiles could be higher from such protocols.

Recently, immunotherapy concurrent with radiotherapy has been offered as an alternative to chemoradiation in head and neck SCC (HNSCC). Immune check points pathways such as programmed death receptor-1 (PD-1) and its ligand (PD-L1) have been targeted therapeutically with nivolumab or pembrolizumab (anti-PD-1 monoclonal antibodies). These anti-monoclonal antibodies are given as a loading dose before RT and then followed concurrently with RT in HNSCC. However, immunotherapy remains experimental in the management of OSCC and is at various trial phases. Whatever the mode of treatment for OSCC, they come with their own set of morbidity and/or side-effects.

25.18.3 Dental Practitioners' Role

Dentists have an important role in the pre-operative/radiation preparation of a patient. Patients must have a thorough assessment of their mouth and the existing dentition. Any untreated caries should be managed either by stabilizing through restorations or, if deemed unrestorable, should be extracted. Such interventions are important to minimize the risk of osteoradionecrosis, should an extraction become necessary in the post-irradiation period. All appliances must be in good condition and should not cause trauma to the oral tissues during radiation therapy.

Patients going for radiotherapy will be advised to avoid cariogenic diets as the altered saliva in quantity and quality will make the teeth highly susceptible to caries. Radiation-induced mucositis will also make chewing and swallowing hard food difficult. Therefore, patients are advised to consume softer food and plenty of water while receiving radiation treatment. Toothbrushing is best done with a toothbrush having a small head and soft bristles. If this is not tolerated, patients can resort to using cotton tips soaked in normal saline. Oral moisturizer may help relieve the effect of dry mouth secondary to radiation. In severe xerostomia, saliva substitute is indicated. Topical fluoride application on remaining teeth should be undertaken to reduce the risk of radiation caries.

Dental health professional can also contribute immensely both in the prevention of oral cancer and in post-treatment follow-up. Prevention strategies can vary from providing health education, helping patients avoid/give up adverse health habits (smoking, alcohol, betel quid chewing) and targeted screening of high-risk populations for OPMDs and early malignancies. With their familiarity with oral anatomy and their inherent training to recognize incipient disease (early, asymptomatic caries and periodontal disease), dental practitioners should make routine dental visits an opportunity to examine for incidental oral mucosal pathology. Similarly, they should regularly review post-treatment cancer patients to maintain their oral health and use the same opportunity to maintain vigil in identifying any recurrent disease at its early stages.

25.18.4 Prognosis

Prognosis of OSCC is measured as (i) overall survival (OS) from the date of diagnosis to the date of deceased/date of the last follow-up, (ii) disease-free survival (DFS)/relapse-free survival (RFS) from the date when primary treatment ends until the date when a patient survives without any signs and symptoms of cancer, (iii) disease-specific survival (DSS) from the date of diagnosis to the date of death caused by cancer/the date of the last follow-up. The 5-year overall survival of OSCC is about 50–60%. Factors that strongly impact the prognosis of OSCC are the extent of primary and metastatic disease at presentation for treatment, depth of invasion, perineural/perivascular infiltration, tumour-positive excision margins, metastasis to cervical nodes with extra-nodal spread and the time to incur recurrence from the completion of definitive treatment.

Salient features of oral squamous cell carcinoma	
Clinical features	Present as a white lesion, red lesion, mixed red and white lesion, chronic non-healing ulcer with rolled margins and indurated base, swelling or exophytic growth.
Histopathological features	Oral squamous cell carcinoma is a malignant tumour that arise from the surface squamous epithelium of the oral mucosa and invades into the underlying epithelium with a break in the basement zone. The epithelial tumour cells show nuclear and cellular pleomorphism, altered nuclear:cytoplasmic ratio, hyperchromatic nuclei, increase in the number and the size of nucleoli, mitotic figures (including atypical forms), dyskeratotic cells and keratin pearls in varying degrees. The tumour epithelial cells invade into the underlying connective tissue in cords, nest or islands.
Treatment	Surgery, radiotherapy, chemotherapy in isolation or as combined therapy used in the form of neoadjuvant, concurrent, adjuvant or as salvage.
Prognosis	Early stage disease treated appropriately has a reasonably good prognosis. Overall, 5-year survival is 50% and has not improved significantly over the past few decades. However, modern therapeutic approaches provide good quality of post-treatment life.

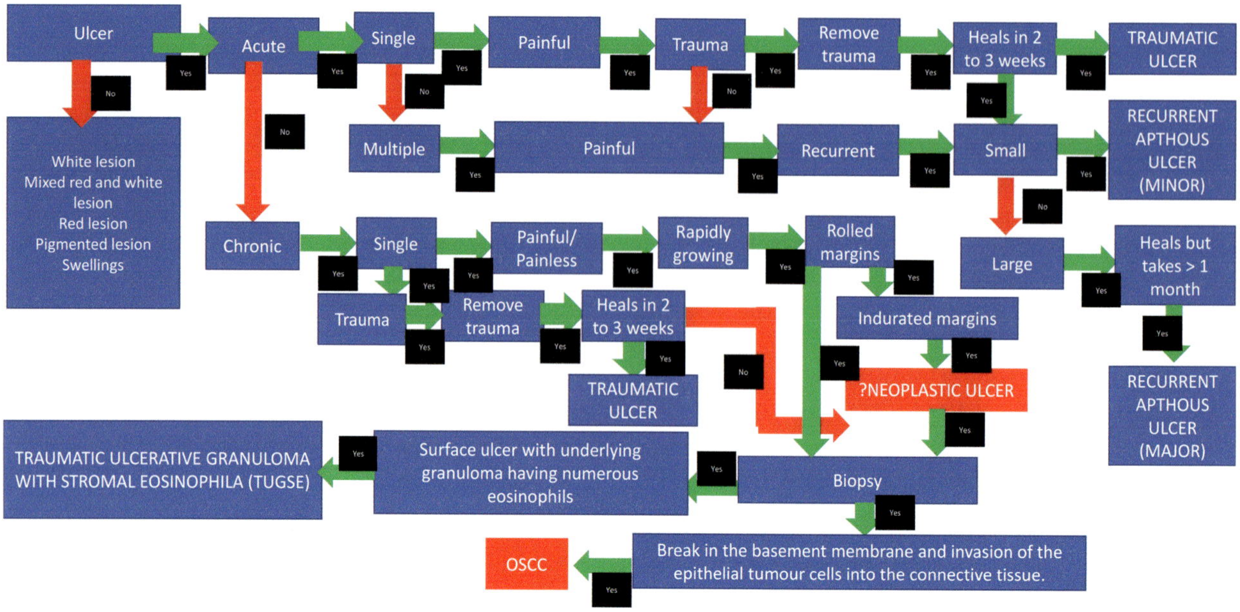

Diagnostic algorithm for an oral ulcer

Self-Assessment Questions

1. Discuss the different clinical presentations of OSCC.
2. Describe the risk factors for OSCC.
3. How would you differentiate between traumatic and neoplastic ulcers?
4. State the key histopathological features of OSCC.
5. Discuss the different modalities of treatments of OSCC.

Summary

Oral squamous cell carcinoma is a disease with significant morbidity and mortality. The affected patients need early diagnosis and aggressive treatment to achieve cure or prolonged disease-free survival. A majority of oral cancers are preceded by a potentially malignant disorder which could be a window of opportunity for therapeutic interventions to mitigate the malignant transformation risk or a chance to institute close monitoring for early diagnosis. Many histopathological features have gained attention as diagnostic and prognostic indicators. Recent advances in molecular genetics and cell cycle events appear promising towards discovering a surrogate switch that determines progression from normal epithelium to dysplasia and carcinoma. Surgery and radiotherapy are the primary treatment modalities, and chemotherapy is usually used as an adjunct. Dental practitioners have an important role in the prevention, early diagnosis and management of oral cancers. The upkeep of oral hygiene is paramount for ensuring good quality of life for oral cancer patients.

Further Reading

Bagan J, Sarrion G, Jimenez Y. Oral cancer: clinical features. Oral Oncol. 2010;46(6):414–7. https://doi.org/10.1016/j.oraloncology.2010.03.009.

Butterworth C, McCaul L, Barclay C. Restorative dentistry and oral rehabilitation: United Kingdom National Multidisciplinary Guidelines. J Laryngol Otol. 2016;130(S2):S41–4. https://doi.org/10.1017/S0022215116000414.

IARC Working Group on the Evaluation of Carcinogenic Risks to Humans. Personal habits and indoor combustions. Volume 100 E. A review of human carcinogens. IARC Monogr Eval Carcinog Risks Hum. 2012;100(Pt E):1–538.

Lewis-Jones H, Colley S, Gibson D. Imaging in head and neck cancer: United Kingdom National Multidisciplinary Guidelines. J Laryngol Otol. 2016;130(S2):S28–31. https://doi.org/10.1017/S0022215116000396.

Neville B, Damm DD, Allen C, Chi A. Oral and maxillofacial pathology. 4th ed. Elsevier; 2015.

Solan P, Gale N, Hunter K, et al. Malignant surface epithelial tumours. In: El-Naggar AK, Chan JKC, Grandis JR, Takata T, Slootweg PJ, editors. WHO classification of head and neck tumours, vol. 9. 4th ed. Lyon: IARC; 2017. p. 109–11.

Warnakulasuriya and Greenspan. Textbook of oral cancer prevention, diagnosis and management. Springer; 2020.

Warnakulasuriya S, Tilakaratne WM. Oral medicine & pathology. A guide to diagnosis and management. 1st ed. New Delhi: Jaypee.

Tumours of Odontogenic Origin

Contents

Large Swelling of the Back of the Lower Jaw: Ameloblastoma

Harsha Lal De Silva and Wanninayake M Tilakaratne

Contents

W. M Tilakaratne, T. G. Kallarakkal (eds.), *Clinicopathological Correlation of Oral Diseases*,
https://doi.org/10.1007/978-3-031-24408-7_26

Learning Goals

1. Frame appropriate questions to elicit an accurate, comprehensive clinical history.
2. Use the information from history taking to develop a preliminary differential diagnosis.
3. Follow a logical sequence to perform a comprehensive clinical examination.
4. Combine history and examination findings to formulate a working clinical differential diagnosis.
5. Judiciously select special investigations to gather appropriate additional diagnostic information.
6. Comprehend and apply clinicopathological correlations to arrive at the final diagnosis.
7. Formulate a comprehensive management plan underpinned by meaningful clinicopathological relationships.
8. Use appropriate diagnostic algorithms in clinical practice to facilitate patient management.

26.1 Main Complaint

A 38-year-old male attended the Oral and Maxillofacial surgery outpatients' clinic, referred by his family doctor for a self-noticed swelling inside his right jawline.

26.2 History of Complaint

Question: How can we help you today?

A couple of months back, I felt something unusual beneath my jawline. I was applying aftershave lotion and felt a hard "bump" inside my right jawline.

Question: Why didn't you consult a doctor immediately?

I felt puzzled, but this got forgotten with my busy work schedule. Besides, there was no pain to bother me. I am a marine engineer working for international shipping companies on a contract basis and spend 3–4 months on assignments away from home. Recently, on returning home, I casually mentioned this to my wife, and she immediately hit the panic button and insisted I see our family doctor.

Question: Did you or your wife notice any swelling in your face?

She thinks my face looks a little fuller on the right side. My doctor examined my face and neck and suggested I meet you for advice.

Question: Did you feel any pain, discomfort or anything unusual in your lower jaw or your neck at any time, apart from the "bump"?

No, I never had any pain or discomfort. Now that you asked, I do remember experiencing a funny feeling in my lip a few times. It felt like an insect crawling on my lower lip, on the right side. These episodes lasted only a few minutes and would pass away when I became involved with some other work. I thought this might be due to my teeth becoming sensitive to cold weather. I am unsure whether some of my teeth are becoming weaker and shaky.

26.3 Past Dental, Medical and Social History

Question: Do you visit a dentist regularly for check-ups?

No, I don't have a regular dentist. I haven't had many dental problems. I had crowded teeth in my teenage years, and my parents took me to an orthodontist to align my teeth with braces. At the end of this treatment, he advised I have my wisdom teeth removed. I had them taken out before I finished secondary school.

Question: Do you have any general health problems?

No, I am pretty healthy and fit. I don't take any regular medications or supplements. I am not allergic to any drugs but I do get mild seasonal hay fever that I manage well with over-the-counter medications.

Question: Do you smoke or drink alcohol?

I don't smoke now. I smoked a few cigarettes with my friends during my teenage years. I don't consume spirits but enjoy an occasional glass of beer or red wine in social gatherings.

Question: Are you married?

Yes, I am happily married for the past 12 years, and we have two school-going children.

26.4 Findings of Clinical Examination

He appeared to be an otherwise fit and healthy individual. There was mild facial asymmetry, with the lower half of his right cheek showing diffuse enlargement. The skin overlying this region was not tender or inflamed

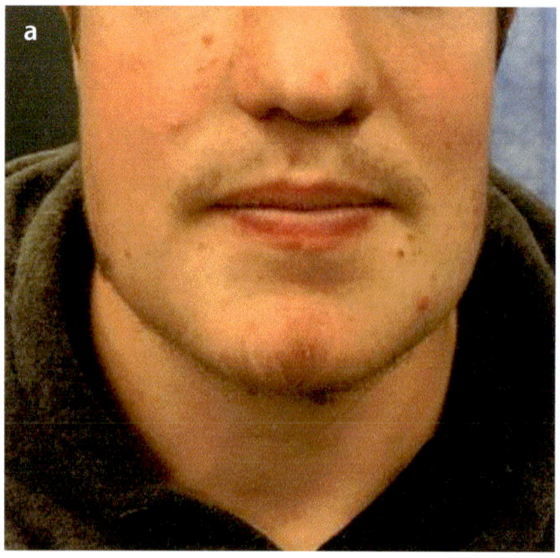

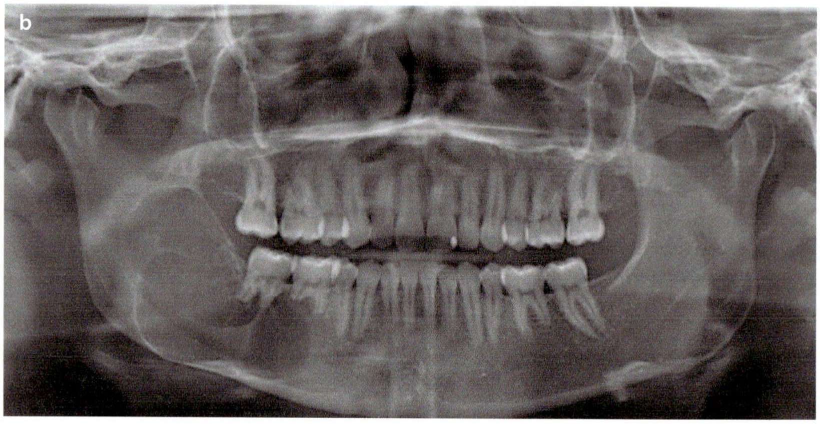

Fig. 26.1 Conventional ameloblastoma arising in the right posterior mandible. Expansion of the right mandibular buccal cortex producing mild facial asymmetry (**a**) and Dental Pantomograph (DPT) showing a large multi-locular radiolucency involving the right mandibular body and ascending ramus with evidence of root resorption in right mandibular molar teeth (**b**)

(Fig. 26.1a). His mouth opening and jaw movements were normal. No clicking or crepitation was felt over the temporomandibular joints.

On palpation, a non-tender, bony hard, expansile enlargement was felt beneath the lower border of his right mandible. There was no clinically detectable sensory deficit on the facial and neck skin, nor was there any impairment of facial nerve function. Further, no palpable cervicofacial lymphadenopathy was detected.

He had complete dentition barring third molars. There were no obvious untreated caries. None of his teeth was tender to gentle percussion. His oral hygiene appeared satisfactory, with no obvious gingival bleeding and periodontal pocketing, but the right mandibular first molar tooth (#46) had grade-1 mobility. Examination of the right mandible revealed a palpable non-tender smooth-surfaced expansion beneath the buccal vestibule extending from the right mandibular second premolar to beyond the second molar tooth. A more pronounced, irregular "bumpy" expansion was felt deep in the lingual cortex, extending from the right mandibular premolar region to the gonial angle and further superiorly on the medial aspect of the ascending ramus. There was no inflammation/ulceration of the overlying mucosa. No other clinically obvious anomalies were detected in the intra-oral examination.

26.5 What is your Differential Diagnosis with the findings from the History and Clinical Examination? Give a justification for including different entities.

1. Ameloblastoma
2. Odontogenic keratocyst (OKC)
3. Other odontogenic tumours/cyst
4. Giant cell lesion/tumour

The lack of pain/tenderness related to this expansile lesion of the mandibular bone indicates the possibility of a cyst or a tumour growing within the bone as opposed to a lesion of inflammatory origin. Although the reported history is short, the lesion may have grown over time before making its presence felt. The age group and the anatomical location favour ameloblastoma and OKC. However, the possibility of any other tumour/cyst of an odontogenic origin or giant cell lesions of bone cannot be excluded with certainty from history and clinical examination alone.

26.6 What is the most likely Clinical Diagnosis?

Ameloblastoma is the most likely clinical diagnosis. Despite OKC being more common, the cortical expansion, age, gender, tooth mobility and the reporting of occasional unusual feeling in the right lower lip make the diagnosis lean towards ameloblastoma of the right posterior mandible. In particular, mobility of the lower right first molar tooth in the absence of any inflammatory periodontal disease indicates the possibility of root resorption or resorption of supporting bone: a clinical feature more commonly seen with locally invasive neoplasms like ameloblastomas. Involvement of inferior alveolar nerve leading to anaesthesia/paraesthesia of the lip too is more common with ameloblastoma than with cysts. Furthermore, OKCs tend to grow in an anteroposterior direction rather than expanding the buccal and lingual cortices. Other tumours (odontogenic/non-odontogenic) and giant cell lesions are relatively uncommon. Despite radicular cysts and dentigerous cysts being more common, there is no obvious carious tooth or a missing tooth in the right lower quadrant to suggest the possibility of an odontogenic cyst.

26.7 What are the necessary investigations that should be performed in a logical sequence?

26.7.1 Pulp Sensibility Test

Pulp sensibility was performed in the right lower quadrant to help exclude the rare possibility of this lesion being a radicular cyst associated with a non-vital tooth. Further, it is a benchmark to monitor the vitality of any teeth which may be retained but with potentially compromised blood supply following future definitive surgical interventions.

26.7.2 Dental Pantomograph (DPT)

A dental pantomogram (DPT) revealed the presence of a multi-locular radiolucency involving the right mandible (◘ Fig. 26.1b). The radiolucency extended posteriorly from the right mandibular second premolar to involve the body of the mandible, reaching the lower border inferiorly and extending superiorly along the ascending ramus to almost the sigmoid notch and the base of the coronoid process. There were no unerupted teeth or displacement of erupted teeth associated with the radiolucency. Cortical expansion and cortical thinning were noted immediately anterior to the gonial angle, and the inferior alveolar canal appeared slightly displaced towards the lower border. No other lesions of significance were evident in the DPT.

26.7.3 Aspiration Biopsy

An aspiration under local anaesthesia performed using a syringe coupled to a 14G needle yielded straw-coloured fluid. This was performed primarily to exclude the lesion being a vascular anomaly which could complicate more invasive and diagnostic and surgical interventions.

26.7.4 Incision Biopsy

Under local anaesthesia, a mucoperiosteal flap was raised to expose the buccal bone distal in the mandibular retromolar region. A bony window was created to expose the lesion. The lesion appeared to be cystic with solid tissue masses in some areas. A sizable sample of tissue was harvested and sent in formalin for histopathological examination. Cystic cavity was irrigated with saline, and the mucoperiosteal flap was replaced using 3/0 Vicryl (Polyglactin 910) sutures.

26.8 What were the Histopathological findings?

The haematoxylin/eosin-stained sections showed an unencapsulated tumour comprised of ameloblastic follicles of varying sizes. Peripheral cells of the follicles were columnar, and nuclei exhibited hyperchromatism and reversal of polarity. Stellate reticulum-like cells were observed in the centre of the follicles. There was no evidence of cytological atypia (◘ Fig. 26.2).

26.9 Three-dimensional (3D) imaging

A computerized tomography (CT) scan was performed to accurately assess the extent of the lesion to help plan definitive treatment. Imaging showed expansion of both buccal and lingual cortices of the body of the right mandibular mandible with thinning of the expanded cortex towards the lower border on the lingual aspect and on the medial aspect of the ascending ramus. There was significant cortical thinning with an area of a potential lingual cortical breach (◘ Fig. 26.3).

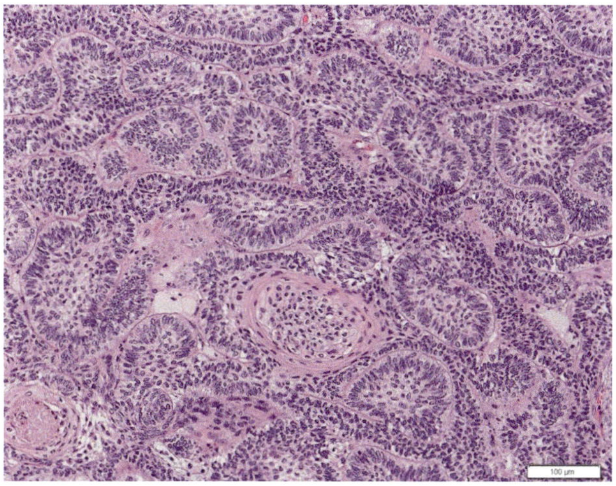

◘ **Fig. 26.2** Haematoxylin/eosin-stained section shows ameloblastic follicles with peripheral columnar cells. The cells are hyperchromatic and exhibit reverse polarity of nuclei

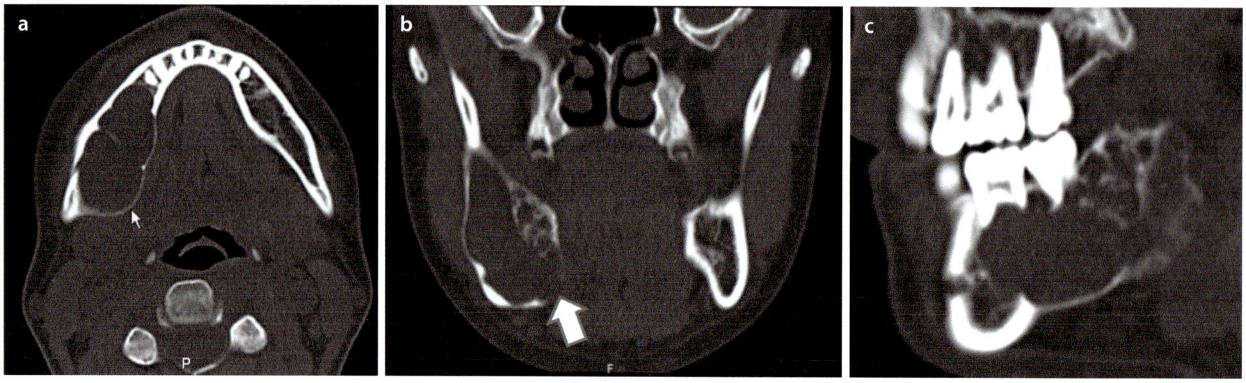

Fig. 26.3 Axial **a**, coronal **b** and sagittal **c** computerized tomographic images demonstrating multi-locularity, cortical expansion (small arrow in **a**) breached lingual cortex (large arrow in **b**) and root resorption of first and second mandibular molars (seen in **c**)

26.10 What is the definitive diagnosis?

The lesion is consistent with a conventional ameloblastoma (follicular type) involving the right mandibular body and ascending ramus, expanding both cortices with no radiographically evident extra-osseous extension.

26.11 What specific findings help you to arrive at the diagnosis?

The insidious nature of the swelling with minimal symptoms suggested a slow, potentially benign disease process. This is further endorsed by the lack of tooth displacement. The involvement of the tooth-bearing region is strongly indicative of a lesion of an odontogenic origin. Multi-locular radiolucency involving the posterior mandible in a male in his thirties, with no clinical and radiological association with an unerupted tooth or a non-vital tooth further narrows the diagnosis towards ameloblastoma or an OKC. The cortical thinning and expansion increase the likelihood of it being a tumour. Other odontogenic and non-odontogenic tumours are rare. Hence, cortical expansion and the reporting of occasional paraesthesia-like symptoms in the ipsilateral lower lip heavily favoured the diagnosis of ameloblastoma ahead of histopathological confirmation.

Like in many oral lesions, histopathology is the confirmatory diagnostic test for ameloblastoma. Despite known limitations of representativeness, an incisional biopsy is a prudent option when dealing with a large lesion. Early histopathological confirmation of the diagnosis of conventional ameloblastoma helped formulate an appropriate treatment plan to offer this patient.

26.12 What is the rationale for treatment?

Ameloblastoma is a benign yet, locally invasive tumour with a significant tendency to recur, particularly following inadequate treatment. Radiotherapy has little to no place in its treatment and should be avoided. Complete surgical removal of the lesion is the currently recommended definitive treatment. Given its known biological behaviour patterns, meticulous planning should be employed to ensure a complete cure with minimal functional and cosmetic disability from a definitive surgical intervention. Furthermore, the patient's general medical status and the ability to cope with ablative and reconstruction surgery too become determinant factors in management decisions.

It is widely accepted that conventional ameloblastoma is associated with a more invasive local growth and is best treated with wide local excision/resection incorporating a 10–15 mm wide cuff of macroscopically normal tissue where it is possible to do so without compromising vital structures. This is more critical when the tumour breaches cortical bone and extends into soft tissue. In the mandible, this involves either marginal or segmental resection of the bone together with any associated teeth, overlying soft tissues in areas of any cortical breach and in particular, the scar tissue of any previous biopsy sites. Depending on the extent and nature of the surgical defect, an appropriate reconstructive method should be employed to best restore function and aesthetics. This could be performed either immediately or preferably as a delayed procedure following confirmation of complete excision of the tumour (Fig. 26.4).

Unicystic ameloblastomas and peripheral ameloblastomas are treated more conservatively as these are believed to have a lower recurrence rate following enucleation and curettage/excision. The use of adjunctive

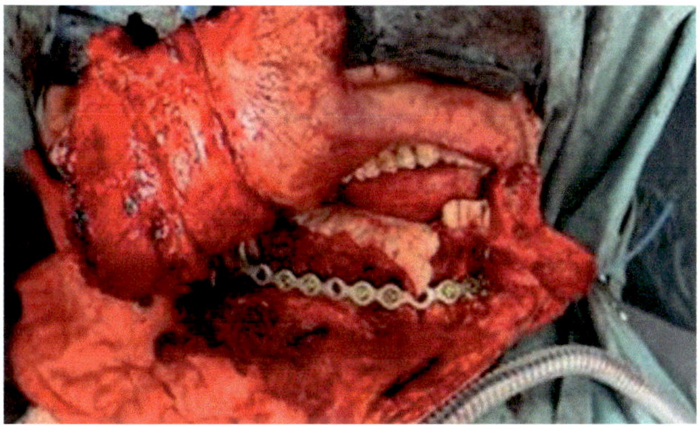

Fig. 26.4 Segmental resection of right mandible from condylar neck to the ipsilateral canine region and immediate reconstruction of the surgical defect with a fibular osteo-cutaneous flap using microvascular anastomosis. The skin paddle had been de-epithelialized to promote re-epithelialization with oral mucosal cells

methods like liquid nitrogen cryotherapy and/or the application of Carnoy's solution to destroy residual tumour cells in the surgical field was a popular practice to reduce potential recurrences. Despite its efficacy in mitigating the development of the recurrent disease, recent concerns on potential carcinogenicity have resulted in the discontinuation of Carnoy's solution in many jurisdictions. Recent reports on using a chloroform-free "Modified Carnoy's solution" have not shown the same efficacy for reducing recurrences when used in the management of OKCs.

26.13 Follow-up and Prognosis

All ameloblastoma needs vigilant follow-up following surgical excision to monitor for potential recurrent disease. A yearly clinical and radiological follow-up for a minimum of 5 years, then extending to a two-yearly review for a further 6–10 years, is considered appropriate for conventional ameloblastoma. The unicystic and peripheral variants may align with a slightly less frequent follow-up visit plan.

26.14 Ameloblastoma

26.14.1 Definition and Epidemiology

Ameloblastoma is an odontogenic tumour with benign but locally aggressive behaviour and a high tendency to recur locally following treatment. The tumour is believed to arise from the odontogenic epithelium of the enamel organ, dental lamina or such epithelial remnants located in the oral epithelium. It has an estimated annual incidence of 0.5 per million population, accounting for 1% of cysts and tumours involving jaws and 10% of all odontogenic tumours. Arguably, it is the second most common odontogenic tumour behind odontomas. More than 80% of ameloblastomas occur in the mandible with a marked predilection for the angle and body of the mandible. Ameloblastomas are more commonly seen in darker-skinned people, particularly among Africans. There is no significant gender predilection and it commonly presents in the third and fourth decades of life.

Recent literature shows that ameloblastoma is caused by dysregulated MAPK and Hedgehog signalling pathways. BRAF V600E appears to be the activating mutation in the MAPK pathway. Mutations in RAS genes (KRAS, NRAS, HRAS) and FGFR2 may also contribute to pathogenesis. Alterations in the Hedgehog signalling pathway may participate in maxillary lesions, where SMO is the most frequent mutation to co-occur with the MAPK mutation.

26.14.2 Clinical Presentation

Ameloblastoma seldom causes troublesome symptoms like pain, tenderness or ulceration and therefore is commonly picked up as an incidental finding in a radiograph taken at a routine dental check or for other reasons. Larger lesions may announce their presence by causing expansile enlargement of the alveolus/jaw, displacement of erupted teeth to cause a malocclusion, mobility of erupted teeth or sensory deficits, which could manifest as anaesthesia/paresthesia in the distribution of an involved nerve. Occasionally the tumour may obstruct a tooth from erupting into the mouth and may mimic the clinical and radiographical presentation of a dentigerous cyst or an OKC (Fig. 26.5). Rarely, large tumours may weaken the mandible to such an extent that a pathological fracture is its first presentation.

26.14.3 Radiological Appearance

Two distinct radiographical appearances (a unilocular cystic radiolucency or a multi-locular, soap-bubble-type appearance) have been described. Sometimes a close relationship to an unerupted tooth (which may or may not have been displaced into an ectopic position) is seen, more so with unilocular lesions involving the angle of the mandible or the maxillary tuberosity region. Large lesions may show cortical expansion, which may result in thinning and perforation. There can be evidence of

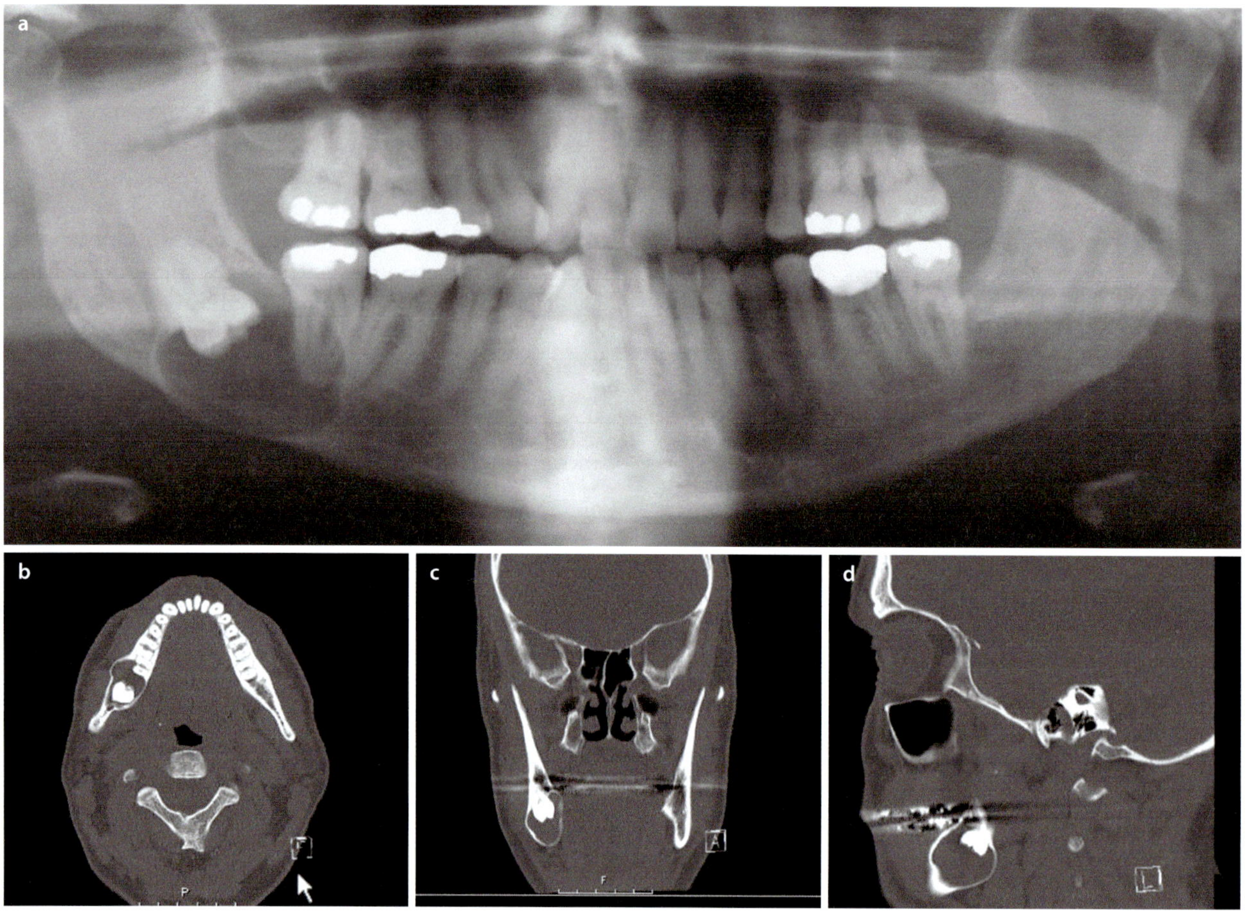

Fig. 26.5 Unicystic ameloblastoma of the right posterior mandible: presentation mimicking a dentigerous cyst. (**a**) Dental pantomograph showing unilocular radiolucency associated with unerupted tooth #48, which appears to have been displaced posteriorly into the ramus. (**b**, **c** and **d**) Computerized tomography in axial, coronal and sagittal planes showing buccal and lingual cortical expansion

displacement of erupted teeth, resorption of roots and displacement of the inferior alveolar canal. The periphery is well demarcated in the majority of unicystic lesions, and the appearance of a well-defined or an ill-defined periphery may be a reflection of the tumour's growth pattern. When a lesion presents as a multilocular radiolucency especially at the angle or body of the mandible, differential diagnoses include ameloblastoma, odontogenic keratocyst, ameloblastic fibroma, odontogenic myxoma, central giant cell granuloma, brown tumour of hyperparathyroidism and aneurysmal bone cyst. Proper clinicopathological correlation helps to arrive at a reasonable working diagnosis.

Advanced three-dimensional imaging provides accurate information on the extent of the tumour, which is invaluable when planning surgical excisions and reconstructive surgery to rehabilitate. Computerized tomography (CT) or cone-beam computerized tomography (CBCT) provides details on the extension within the bone, while magnetic resonance imaging (MRI) is best suited to assess soft tissue involvement when the tumour breaches cortical bone and extends to involve overlying soft tissues.

26.14.4 Histopathology

Ameloblastoma has different clinicopathological subtypes and histopathological variants. Recently the World Health Organization (WHO) updated its classification of head and neck tumours. The main differences between the last three classifications (2005, 2017 and 2022) on ameloblastoma are summarized in Table 26.1.

Clinicopathologically, ameloblastomas are subclassified into conventional, unicystic, peripheral (extraosseous), adenoid and metastasizing variants in the WHO's 2022 classification. The solid-multicystic subtype and the desmoplastic subtype of the 2005 classification have been amalgamated into a broad conventional ameloblastoma category while adding a new subtype called metastasizing ameloblastoma (MA) which has been separated from rare but frankly malignant ameloblastic carcinoma. MA was classified under malignant odontogenic tumours in the 2005 classification. The move to drop the term "solid-multicystic" stems from many conventional ameloblastomas having cystic degeneration with no difference in biological behaviour. The desmoplastic ameloblastoma too, despite its unique histopathological features, shows no behavioural difference. The term conventional ameloblastoma was reintroduced in the 2022 classification. The vast majority (nearly 90%) are conventional ameloblastomas, while 6–22% are unicystic ameloblastomas and the remainder are peripheral ameloblastomas and metastasizing ameloblastoma subtypes.

Table 26.1 Changes between WHO classifications of 2005, 2017 and 2022 for ameloblastoma

WHO 2005	WHO 2017	WHO 2022
Solid-multicystic ameloblastoma	Ameloblastoma	Conventional ameloblastoma
Unicystic ameloblastoma	Unicystic ameloblastoma	Unicystic ameloblastoma
Peripheral ameloblastoma	Peripheral ameloblastoma	Peripheral ameloblastoma
Desmoplastic ameloblastoma	Metastasizing ameloblastoma	Metastasizing ameloblastoma
		Adenoid ameloblastoma

26.14.5 Conventional Ameloblastoma

These tumours appear grey-white and are expansile masses consisting of either solid or a mixture of solid and cystic areas. Microscopic features include the presence of cells resembling odontogenic epithelium with hyperchromatic nuclei. Epithelial cells adjacent to the basement membrane have palisading nuclei exhibiting reverse polarity. Subluminal basal cells may show subnuclear vacuolization. The central cells of epithelial nests are loosely packed, resembling cells of the stellate reticulum. Mitotic figures are rare. The arrangement of the epithelial cells may show follicular or plexiform patterns. In the follicular pattern, tumour cells form islands that comprise tall columnar cells with reverse polarity at their periphery. Central cystic degenerations may be present. Plexiform pattern features interconnecting strands of epithelium. Some tumours may also show acanthomatous, basaloid, granular or clear cell change in the area of stellate reticulum-like cells in the centre of follicles (Fig. 26.6). It is not uncommon to observe both follicular and plexiform types in the same lesion which is sometimes referred to as mixed type. The term desmoplastic ameloblastoma is used when dense fibrous stroma is observed in conventional ameloblastoma. These different variants have no significant implications on biological behaviour or prognosis following treatment and therefore does not significantly impact clinical decisions.

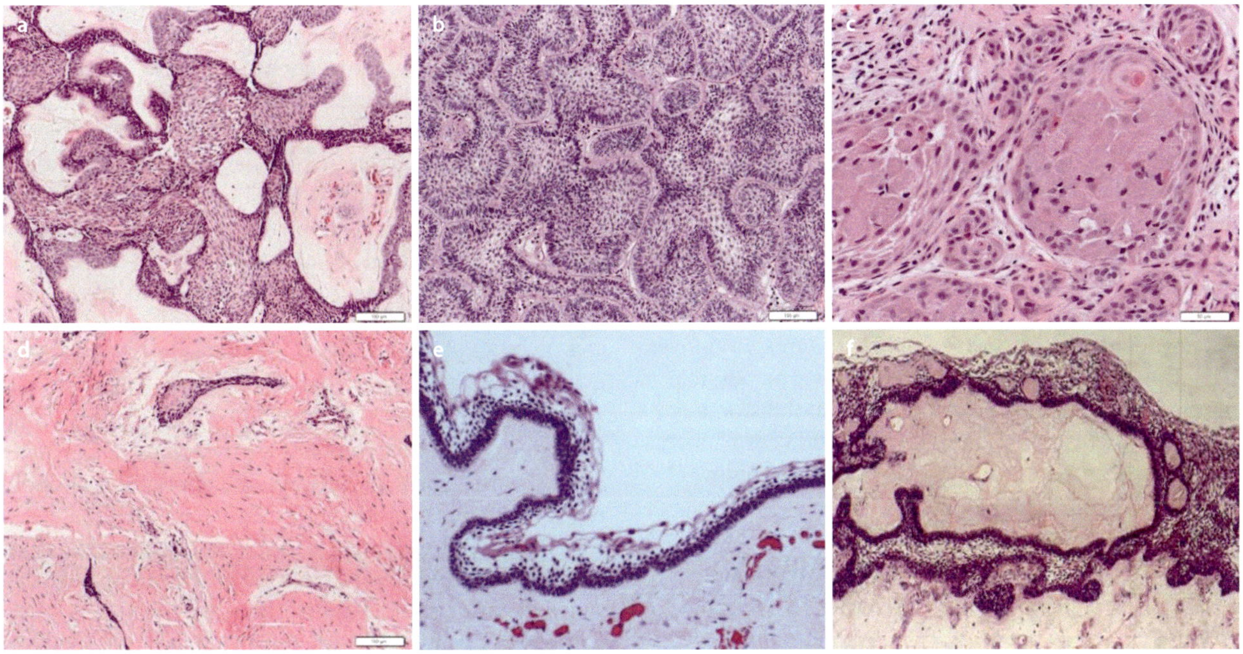

Fig. 26.6 Histological variants of ameloblastoma: plexiform (**a**), follicular (**b**), granular cell (**c**), desmoplastic (**d**), unicystic luminal (**e**) and unicystic mural (**f**) patterns

26.14.6 Unicystic Ameloblastoma

Unicystic ameloblastoma, as the name reflects, commonly shows a single cyst architecture, both radiographically as well as macro/microscopically. The entire cyst lining or some areas of the lining show ameloblastic epithelium featuring reverse polarity and the stellate reticulum-like cells with vacuolations on the surface. Occasionally a clear cell or an acanthomatous change may occur. However, differentiation of unicystic ameloblastoma from an inflamed dentigerous cyst and a radicular cyst may be difficult. Certain features such as reverse polarity and hyperchromatism of basal cells and vacuolated surface cells in unicystic ameloblastoma may help differentiate it from cysts. This combination of features is known as Vickers and Gorlin criteria for diagnosing ameloblastoma. Based on the arrangement of the neoplastic epithelium, unicystic ameloblastomas are further classified into luminal, intra-luminal and mural variants. These findings may have implications on the propensity for recurrence and prognosis.

26.14.7 Peripheral Ameloblastoma

Peripheral ameloblastoma usually presents as a gingival nodule. These tumours have ameloblastic epithelium arranged into islands with the reverse polarity of the nuclei. Most tumours show cells of basaloid morphology. The loosely arranged stellate reticulum-like cells are not a prominent feature, and the ameloblastic epithelium may fuse with the oral epithelium.

26.14.8 Metastasizing Ameloblastoma

Metastasizing ameloblastoma is a rare entity. This is now recognized as a distinct entity from ameloblastic carcinoma and is grouped as a subtype alongside ameloblastoma with metastasis to distant sites. There is no clear explanation for its metastatic behaviour despite having identical histopathological features to conventional ameloblastoma. Therefore, it is not possible to predict the metastatic potential of ameloblastoma from histological features alone. The common sites of metastasis appear to be cervical lymph nodes and lungs.

26.15 Diagnostic Challenges (Clinical/Radiological/Histopathological)

Other lesions may also present as unilocular or multilocular radiolucencies in the jaws. They may also share some clinical features with ameloblastoma. For instance, root resorption, tooth displacement and involvement of the inferior alveolar nerve leading to sensory deficit may occur with other tumours or rarely with some cysts, particularly when there is secondary infection.

Unicystic ameloblastoma may mimic an odontogenic cyst, mainly when it displaces an unerupted tooth. Characteristic histopathological features to confirm the diagnosis of ameloblastoma may not be present in all parts of the cyst lining. Thus an incision biopsy may not be adequately representative of the lesion leading to misdiagnosis or underdiagnosis and may lead to inadequate treatment and potential risk of recurrence. Therefore, the diagnosis of unicystic ameloblastoma should be confirmed only when the entire cyst lining is available for histological examination.

26.16 Treatment Strategies

Ameloblastomas have a reputation for local recurrence. Recurrence rates are highest in the first five post-treatment years, but late recurrences have been reported too. Given the locally invasive behaviour and the increased tendency to recur, ameloblastoma merits more aggressive surgery compared to the management of odontogenic cysts. Thus histopathological confirmation from an incision biopsy helps to appropriately tailor treatment. The adequacy of surgical excision to ensure complete removal of the tumour is the major determinant of successful treatment. In general, conventional ameloblastomas have a high recurrence rate if not treated aggressively with wide local resection. It can be as high as 60–80%. This is especially important for the lesions in the posterior maxilla, as recurrences with extension to the skull base have been reported. The primary objective of definitive surgery is to ensure complete excision of the tumour. Wide local excision with an adequate margin (10–15 mm) of macroscopically normal tissue is considered the gold standard for managing conventional ameloblastoma. The salient features of different ameloblastoma subtypes are summarized in ◘ Table 26.2.

Unicystic ameloblastomas are deemed to have a less aggressive biological behaviour and may respond favourably to a conservative approach. A unicystic ameloblastoma confined within the jaw bone, diagnosed on radiological appearance in conjunction with a biopsy, could be managed more conservatively by enucleation complemented with aggressive curettage and application of liquid nitrogen cryotherapy to the excision bed (◘ Fig. 26.7). However, the entire specimen should be sampled and histopathologically examined to re-confirm the initial diagnosis. In the event of some areas of the tumour showing histopathological features consistent with a mural type unicystic ameloblastoma or conventional ameloblastoma, the treatment should escalate to consider revisiting the operation site for a wider excision or at least arrange intensive clinical and radiological surveillance to monitor and deal with the potential emergence of recurrent disease.

Table 26.2 Salient features of different ameloblastoma variants

Type	Variants	Clinical presentation	Behaviour and prognosis
Conventional ameloblastoma (CA) (Follicular or plexiform patterns)	Granular cell	Usually present as multi-locular radiolucency Cortical expansion ± thinning and perforation Commonly seen in the posterior mandible	Locally invasive growth pattern Best treated with wide local resection High risk of recurrence if inadequately treated
	Basal cell		
	Acanthomatous		
	Desmoplastic	Tendency to involve anterior mandible Less radiolucent compared to other types	
Unicystic ameloblastoma (UA)	Intra-luminal	Unilocular radiolucency Cortical expansion ± thinning and perforation Could be associated with an unerupted tooth Commonly seen in the posterior mandible	Less locally invasive compared to conventional ameloblastoma May respond well to enucleation + curettage and application of cryotherapy
	Luminal		
	Mural		Behaviour is similar to conventional ameloblastoma and needs to be treated similarly
Peripheral ameloblastoma	Same as conventional ameloblastoma	Uncommon Extra-osseous location (gingiva)	Less invasive despite being histologically similar to conventional ameloblastoma Respond well for local excision
Metastasizing ameloblastoma	Same as conventional ameloblastoma	Rare May occur in the lungs, cervical lymph nodes, etc.	Needs wide local excision if appropriate The novel, targeted molecular therapies may become useful

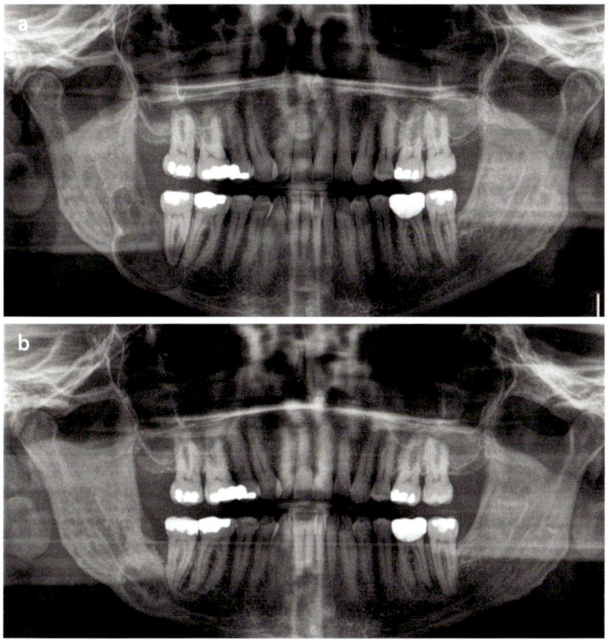

Fig. 26.7 Unicystic ameloblastoma of the right posterior mandible shown in Fig. 26.5 was managed by surgical enucleation and curettage + application of Carnoy's solution; Immediate, post-surgery (**a**) and 2 years post-surgery (**b**)

26.17 New Advances

Advanced reconstruction techniques, including the use of composite tissue transfer via microvascular anastomoses and dental implant-supported prostheses, have broadened the horizons to restore aesthetics and function following ablative surgery. Despite these improvements in post-surgical rehabilitation, the surgery remains a demanding challenge for many patients and is never free of some degree of morbidity. Recent studies have identified mutations in the mitogen-activated protein kinase (MPAK) and sonic hedgehog (SHH) signalling pathways in many ameloblastomas. BRAF V600E mutation has been reported in many tumours and is particularly common in unicystic ameloblastomas. This opens a potential avenue to explore the use of molecularly targeted therapies to treat ameloblastomas. There are a few reports on the use of single- and dual-agent therapies to treat recurrent ameloblastomas and metastasizing ameloblastomas with promising results. These agents may have potential use as neoadjuvant therapy to shrink large tumours to facilitate resection and treat recurrences that may emerge in surgically inaccessible anatomical locations.

Based on the current understanding of the biological behaviour of ameloblastomas, a decision tree for managing a large radiolucent lesion in the posterior mandible is presented in Fig. 26.8.

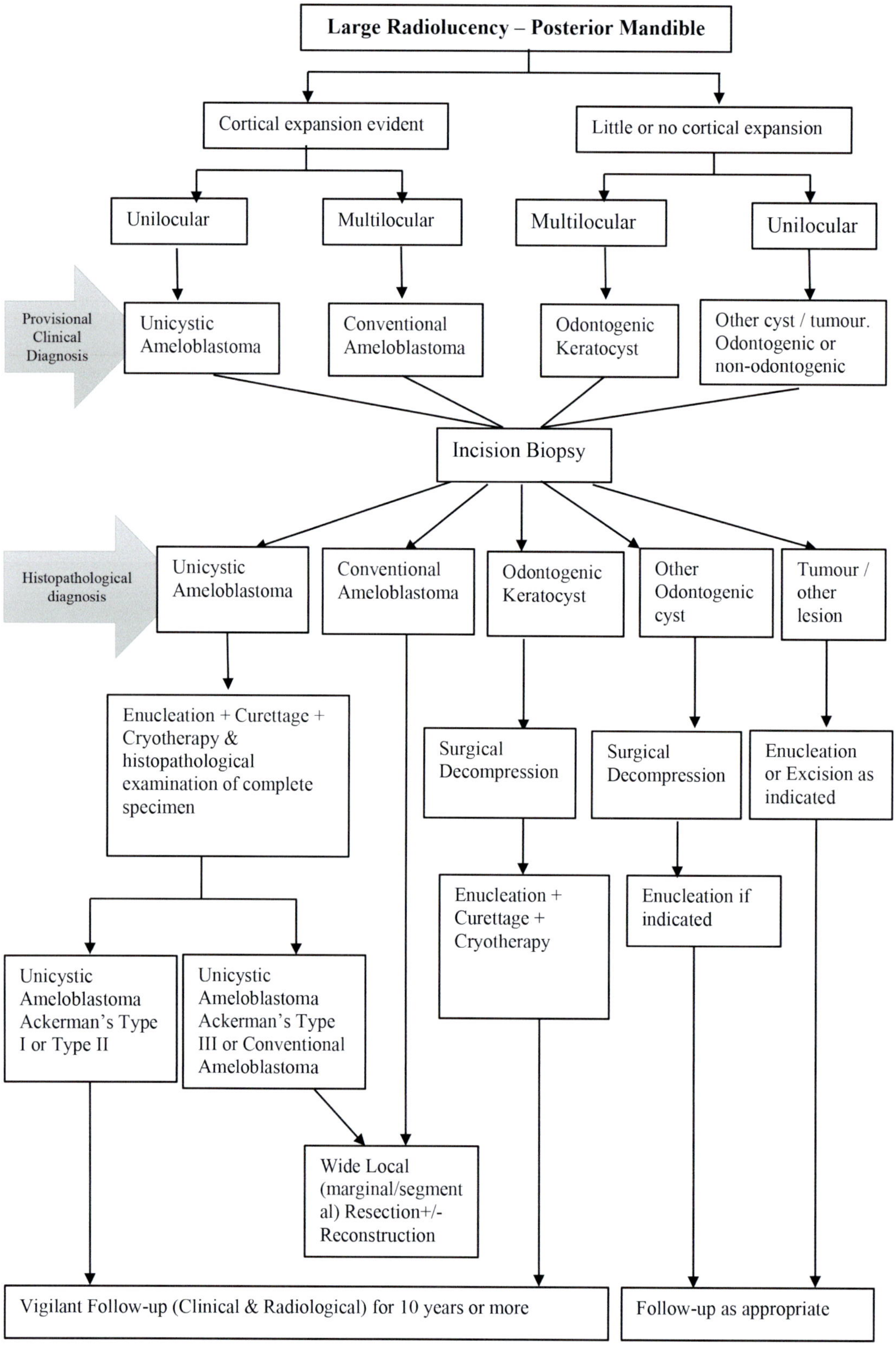

Fig. 26.8 Diagnostic and management algorithm for ameloblastoma and related lesions

Self-Assessment Questions

1. Outline the differential diagnosis of radiolucent lesions commonly occurring in the posterior mandible.
2. Describe the role of medical imaging in managing jaw cysts and tumours.
3. Discuss the rationale for using pulp sensibility testing when assessing and managing pathology affecting the jaws.
4. Describe how histopathological diagnosis will impact the management of ameloblastoma of the jaws.
5. Outline the management of ameloblastoma.

Summary

Ameloblastoma is a locally aggressive odontogenic tumour of epithelial origin. While detected as an incidental radiological finding in some instances, the tumour may also grow rapidly to infiltrate the jaw bone, expand and penetrate through cortices and involve overlying soft tissues. Histopathology remains the current gold standard in diagnosis and provides valuable information to help tailor appropriate management. Surgical excision is the mainstay in management, while a vigilant, periodic follow-up is mandatory to detect and manage the potential recurrent disease. Recent advances in molecular characterization and identification of altered gene pathways in tumorigenesis appear to show promise in developing targeted treatment to mitigate operative morbidities of current treatment options.

Further Reading

Ackermann GL, Altini M, Shear M. The unicystic ameloblastoma: a clinicopathological study of 57 cases. J Oral Pathol Med. 1988;17:541–6. https://doi.org/10.1111/j.1600-0714.1988.tb01331.x.

Bilodeau EA, Collins BM. Odontogenic cysts and neoplasms. Surg Pathol. 2017;10:177–222. https://doi.org/10.1016/j.path.2016.10.006.

Petrovic ID, Migliacci J, Ganly I, Patel S, Xu B, Ghossein R, Huryn J, Shah J. Ameloblastomas of the mandible and maxilla. Ear Nose Throat J. 2018;97(7):E26–32. https://doi.org/10.1177/014556131809700704.

Ranchod S, Titinchi F, Behardien N, Morkel J. Ameloblastoma of the mandible: analysis of radiographic and histopathological features. J Oral Med Oral Surg. 2021;27(1):6. https://doi.org/10.1051/mbcb/2020051.

Robinson RA. Diagnosing the most common odontogenic cystic and osseous lesions of the jaws for the practicing pathologist. Mod Pathol. 2017;30:S96–S103.

Shi HA, Ng CWB, Kwa CT, Sim QXC. Ameloblastoma: a succinct review of the classification, genetic understanding and novel molecular targeted therapies. Surgeon. 2021;19(4):238–43. https://doi.org/10.1016/j.surge.2020.06.009.

Siriwardena BSMS, Tennakoon TMBP, Tilakaratne WM. Relative frequency of odontogenic tumours in Sri Lanka: analysis 0f 1677 cases. Pathol Res Pract. 2012;208(4):225–30.

Zheng CY, Cao R, Hong WS, Sheng MC, Hu YJ. Marsupialisation for the treatment of unicystic ameloblastoma of the mandible: a long-term follow up of 116 cases. Br J Oral Maxillofac Surg. 2019;57(7):655–62. https://doi.org/10.1016/j.bjoms.2019.06.002.

Swelling in the Left Maxilla: Adenomatoid Odontogenic Tumour (AOT)

Kathreena Kadir, Firdaus Hariri, and Wanninayake M Tilakaratne

Contents

W. M Tilakaratne, T. G. Kallarakkal (eds.), *Clinicopathological Correlation of Oral Diseases*,
https://doi.org/10.1007/978-3-031-24408-7_27

27.1 Main Complaint

A 17-year-old female presented with a painless swelling on the left mid-face region. She was initially seen by an otolaryngologist and was referred to the oral and maxillofacial surgery clinic for an incidental radiographic finding of an impacted tooth associated with a mixed radiolucent and radiopaque lesion in the left maxilla.

27.2 History of Complaint

Question: How long have you noticed the swelling?

I noticed the swelling 6 months ago and it has been slowly enlarging since then.

Question: Is this the first time you have experienced a swelling in this region?

Yes. I have never noticed a swelling at this site before.

27.3 Additional Complaints

Question: Do you experience any other symptoms besides the swelling?

I have nasal congestion and occasional 'runny nose.' This has been worsening ever since the swelling began increasing in size.

Question: Is the swelling painful? Were there any episodes of fever concurrent with the swelling?

I do not feel any pain. I have had no history of fever prior to or during the development of the swelling.

Question: Has the swelling ever reduced in size before?

No. I have noticed that the swelling has been slowly increasing in size.

Question: Was there any history of toothache or loose tooth?

I have no history of toothache or loose tooth.

Question: Was there any previous history of trauma to the area?

I am unable to recall any previous trauma leading to the swelling.

Question: Do you have any numbness over the region of the swelling?

I do not have any numbness over the face in the region of the swelling.

Question: Do you have any difficulty in opening your mouth wide with the present swelling?

I have no difficulty to open the mouth.

Question: Did you notice any lumps elsewhere on your body?

I do not have any swelling on any other part of my body.

27.4 Past Medical/Dental and Social History

Question: Are you suffering from any other medical problems like heart disease, high blood pressure, diabetes, bleeding disorder, respiratory diseases? If yes, what kind of medications, have you been taking until now?

I am fit and healthy. I do not suffer from any medical conditions and not taking any medication.

Question: Have you undergone any dental treatment?

I visit the dentist occasionally for dental scaling. My previous dental check-ups and treatment were done in a private dental clinic.

Question: What is your social background?

I am a high school student in a local secondary school and currently living with my parents.

Question: Are you a smoker?

I am a non-smoker.

Question: Do you take alcohol?

I do not take alcohol.

27.5 With the Findings From the History, What Is Your Differential Diagnosis?

1. Odontogenic cyst
2. Odontogenic tumours and tumour-like lesions of the maxilla
3. Non-odontogenic tumours

27.6 How Do You Justify Your Differential Diagnosis After History Taking?

The patient presented with a complaint of a swelling on the left cheek. There was an incidental radiographic finding of an impacted tooth associated with a mixed radiolucent and radiopaque lesion in the underlying region. The swelling was painless and was slowly increasing in size. These features may suggest a cystic lesion or a tumour as they typically grow slowly and expansively, and are usually symptomless unless infected. Occasionally, when the swelling has expanded to a larger size, it may form a compressible and fluctuant swelling if it extends into the soft tissue. The patient also has a history of nasal decongestion on the left side, which has worsened due to the increasing size of the swelling. The swelling is likely to be benign in nature based on the slow-growing nature of the swelling.

Based on the onset of the swelling and absence of history of systemic symptoms like pyrexia, it is unlikely that the swelling is related to infection. There are no other lumps and patient does not have any risk habits associated with malignancy such as the use of tobacco and alcohol consumption, hence the findings of the history are more in favour of a cyst or a benign tumour.

27.7 Findings of Clinical Examination

Extraoral examination shows minimal swelling over the left maxilla and fullness of the nasolabial fold on the left cheek (◘ Fig. 27.1). Upon palpation, the growth is bony hard in consistency and non-tender. The overlying facial skin is normal in colour and not warm. There are no sensory deficits (hypoesthesia/paraesthesia) over the region.

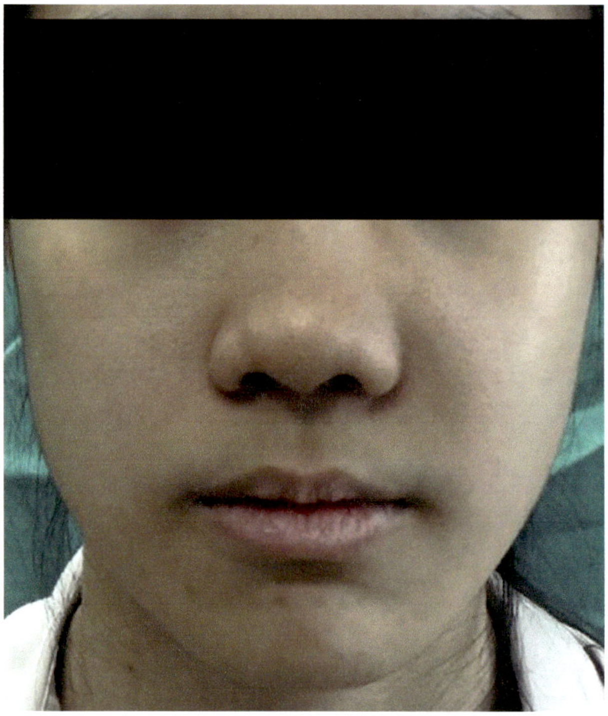

◘ **Fig. 27.1** Minimal swelling seen on left maxilla

27.8 What Other Relevant Features Are Evident?

Clinically the mouth opening is normal with no restriction of jaw movements. Eye examination also shows normal vision, without signs of epiphora. Nasal septum appeared deviated to the right side. There were no palpable lymph nodes.

Intraorally, teeth 23 and 25 are missing. Besides, there are retained deciduous teeth 63 and 65 (◘ Fig. 27.2). Otherwise, rest of the dentition is sound, with no mobility or tenderness to percussion. Electric pulp test showed all teeth to be vital. The left buccal sulcus is minimally obliterated. The swelling is bony hard and non-tender. There is a significant left palatal expansion that does not cross the midline (◘ Fig. 27.3). The palatal swelling is bony hard and non-tender on palpation. The overlying mucosa is of normal colour as compared to the surrounding soft tissue.

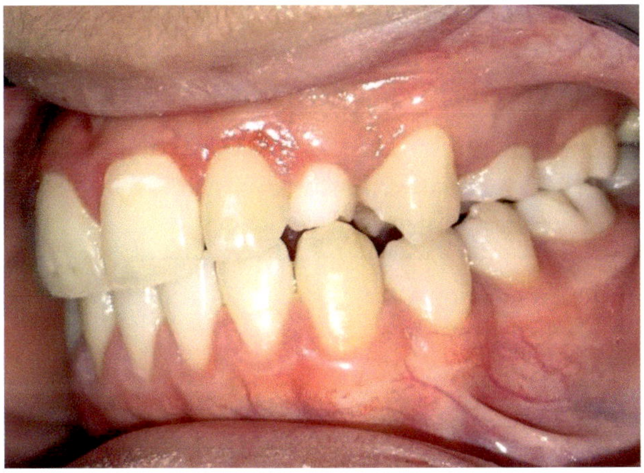

Fig. 27.2 Intraoral picture showing retained teeth 63 and 65 and missing teeth 23 and 25

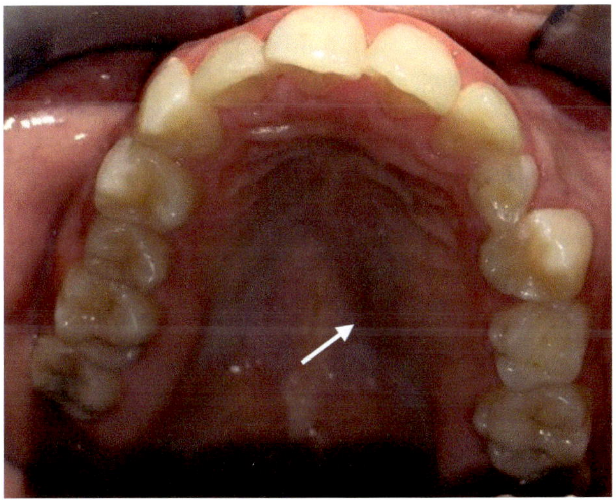

Fig. 27.3 Intraoral picture showing left palatal expansion

27.9 What Is Your Clinical Differential Diagnosis?

- Adenomatoid odontogenic tumour (AOT)
- Dentigerous cyst
- Odontogenic keratocyst (OKC)
- Other odontogenic tumours (ameloblastoma, myxoma, etc.)

27.10 What Is the Justification for Your Clinical Differential Diagnosis?

The possibility of an odontogenic cyst or tumour is highly based on the history and clinical manifestation. As there were no soft tissue abnormalities around the swelling, benign mucosal lesions could be ruled out.

Clinical examination showed expansion of the palate and obliteration of the buccal sulcus on the left side. However, the swelling was bony hard and non-tender upon palpation. The patient had retained deciduous teeth 63 and 65 and missing teeth 23 and 25 at the area of the swelling, hence this may give an indication of the possibility that the swelling could be of odontogenic origin. The history of slow-growing painless swelling in a teenager with an impacted canine suggests that it could be either an odontogenic cyst or a tumour.

27.10.1 Adenomatoid Odontogenic Tumour (AOT)

Adenomatoid odontogenic tumour (AOT) is a benign odontogenic tumour. Two-thirds of the cases are seen in females. Majority of the cases occur in the anterior maxilla and two-thirds of these cases are usually associated with an impacted tooth especially the canine thus making this the most likely differential diagnosis. It usually occurs during the second decade of life similar to the demographic background of this patient. Clinically it may present as a discrete or more obvious intra-bony swelling that is usually slow growing and asymptomatic. It does not lead to any teeth non-vitality and is bony hard and non-tender on palpation. AOT can exist in three clinico-topographic variants: (1) follicular, (2) extra-follicular or (3) peripheral. The extraosseous peripheral variant is ruled out as the swelling occurred centrally within the bone of the maxilla.

27.10.2 Dentigerous Cyst

Dentigerous cyst, also known as follicular cyst, originates by separation of follicle from around the crown of an unerupted tooth. It is the most common developmental odontogenic cyst, whereby it encloses the crown of the unerupted tooth at the cementoenamel junction. It is usually seen in the second or third decade of life with a slight male predilection. Clinically it is always associated with unerupted or impacted tooth, which often involves the mandibular third molars (75%). Other frequent sites are maxillary canines, maxillary molars and mandibular premolars. It is commonly symptomless but may also present as slow painless intra-bony expansion in the involved area, which may result in facial asymmetry if the lesion is extensively large. Infection of the cyst causes pain and causes the swelling to increase in size. These cysts are usually solitary; however, bilateral or multiple cysts may be found in association with cleidocranial dysplasia and Maroteaux–Lamy syndrome.

27.10.3 Odontogenic Keratocyst (OKC)

Odontogenic keratocyst (OKC), previously also known as keratocystic odontogenic tumour (KCOT), is a developmental odontogenic cyst, accounting for 10–20% of odontogenic cysts and is the third most common cyst of the jaws. OKC occurs over a wide age range with slight male predilection. It often affects the posterior body and ramus of the mandible. OKC may also envelop an unerupted tooth mimicking a dentigerous cyst. OKC expands preferentially along marrow spaces before causing expansion of the jaw. Hence, usually the clinical signs fail to appear until the cyst has reached a considerable size. Similar, to other jaw cysts, they are usually symptomless until the bone is expanded or infected. Root resorption is rarely seen. About 10% of patients have multiple OKCs, and half of them have naevoid basal cell carcinoma syndrome (Gorlin–Goltz syndrome) who will present with other developmental anomalies.

27.10.4 Ameloblastoma

Ameloblastoma is the most common neoplasm of the jaw, which usually presents between ages of 30 and 50 years. It often affects the mandible predominately the posterior molar region involving ramus. It is locally invasive but does not metastasize. They are typically asymptomatic unless the jaw is expanded or infected. Usually they grow in the cancellous bone of the mandible and may attain a substantial size before the outer contour of the bone is appreciably altered with buccal lingual expansion. They can reach an enormous size without either invading or ulcerating through the soft tissue.

27.10.5 Odontogenic Myxoma

Odontogenic myxoma is a benign odontogenic tumour which is a non-encapsulated, slow-growing and infiltrative tumour. It is thought to arise from the primitive mesenchymal odontogenic tissue and is often associated with unerupted, displaced or congenital missing tooth. It has slight female predilection and commonly occurs in posterior mandible.

The history and clinical findings of this patient may favour either dentigerous cyst or adenomatoid odontogenic tumour as the more likely clinical diagnosis.

27.11 How Would You Investigate the Patient?

- Incisional biopsy for histopathological examination
- Radiographic investigations

27.12 What Would Be the Best Imaging Modality to Investigate This Lesion?

Smaller cystic lesions or tumours of the jaws are investigated using dental intraoral or panoramic radiography. However, for larger lesions with significant expansion of the jaw bone that extend into neighbouring structures, advanced imaging such as CBCT, CT scan or MRI may be required because they may not be adequately diagnosed using conventional radiography. Some benign tumours may be locally aggressive and may be difficult to distinguish from malignant neoplasms, hence advanced imaging may aid in precise assessment of structures, extent and demarcation of the surrounding tissue.

27.13 What Are the Findings of Radiographic Investigations?

Dental panoramic tomography

A well-defined unilocular lesion in the left maxilla from the region of tooth 21 expanding towards tooth 27 is seen on the panoramic radiograph (◘ Fig. 27.4). The

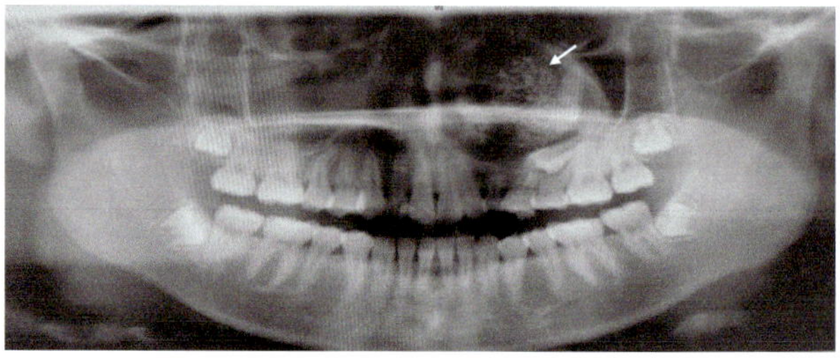

◘ **Fig. 27.4** Dental panoramic tomograph shows a well-defined unilocular lesion with mixed radiolucent–radiopaque appearance at the left maxilla. Impacted teeth 23 and 25 are seen within the lesion

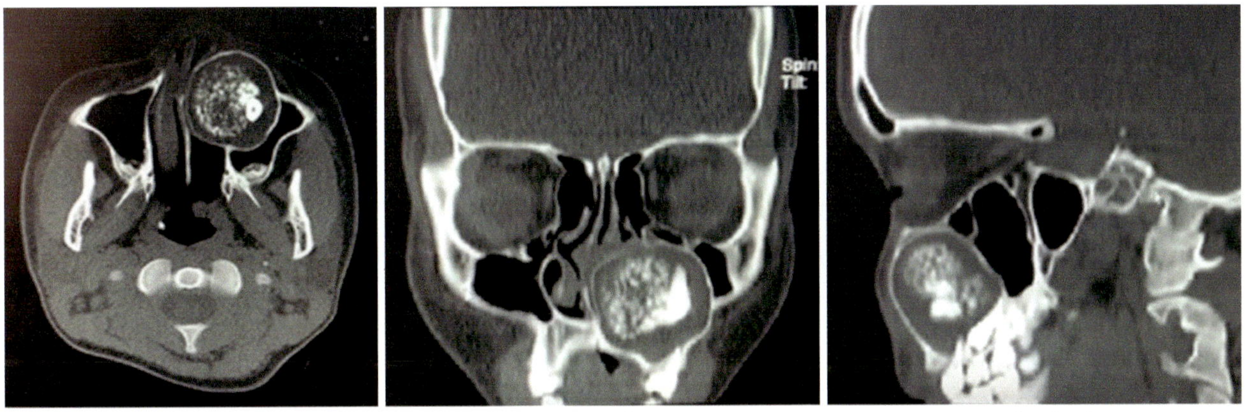

Axial Coronal Sagittal

Fig. 27.5 CT scan in different views. Axial view shows tumour expanding anterior-posteriorly and laterally involving maxillary sinus and lateral nasal wall leading to obliteration of nasal cavity and septal deviation. Coronal view shows extensive swelling with calcification and tooth structure within tumour cavity. Sagittal view shows tumour in relation to its surrounding anatomy that includes floor of left orbit, left maxillary sinus as well as teeth in the left maxillary arch

lesion consists of flecks of radiopaque calcifications together with an impacted tooth 23 within the tumour as well as a displaced and impacted tooth 25 at the inferior border of the lesion. The lesion also causes upward expansion of the left maxillary sinus floor. The permanent teeth 22 and 24 are displaced mesially and distally, respectively. Retained deciduous teeth 63 and 65 with root resorption are also evident in the dental panoramic radiograph.

27.13.1 CT Scan Findings

A well-circumscribed lytic lesion arising from left maxilla caused expansion and thinning of left maxillary cortex (Fig. 27.5). There is a tooth with adjacent amorphous calcification within the lesion. The lesion causes obliteration of the left nasal cavity and deviation of nasal septum to the right side. The lesion also bulges into the left maxillary sinus. There is splaying of the root of the incisors with no definite resorption seen.

27.14 What Is the Most Likely Working Diagnosis with the History, Clinical and Radiological Findings?

Adenomatoid odontogenic tumour.

An exploration biopsy was done via Caldwell-Luc approach and the histopathological features were consistent with an adenomatoid odontogenic tumour.

27.15 What Are the Characteristic Histopathological Features of an Adenomatoid Odontogenic Tumour?

AOT is an encapsulated lesion containing variably sized nodules of cuboidal, columnar and spindle odontogenic epithelial cells (Fig. 27.6). The stromal component is minimal. There are numerous duct-like or rosette-like structures within the nodules giving rise to a glandular appearance to the tumour. The epithelial cells are arranged into whorls in some parts of the lesion. Anastomosing strands of odontogenic epithelial cells arranged into a plexiform pattern are evident towards the periphery of the lesion. Some areas of the lesion can be prominently cystic with a lining of stratified squamous non-keratinizing epithelium or odontogenic epithelium. Eosinophilic amorphous secretory material similar to enamel matrix may present between epithelial cells and at the centre of the rosette-like structures. Foci of calcification, dentinoid-like areas and areas of haemorrhage are also present in varying amounts. AOT-like areas may present in other odontogenic tumours such as adenoid ameloblastoma, odontoma and calcifying epithelial odontogenic tumour. There is no cytological atypia and mitoses. A tooth is embedded within the lesion in the follicular variant whilst the impacted tooth is evident outside the lesion in the extra-follicular variant (Fig. 27.7).

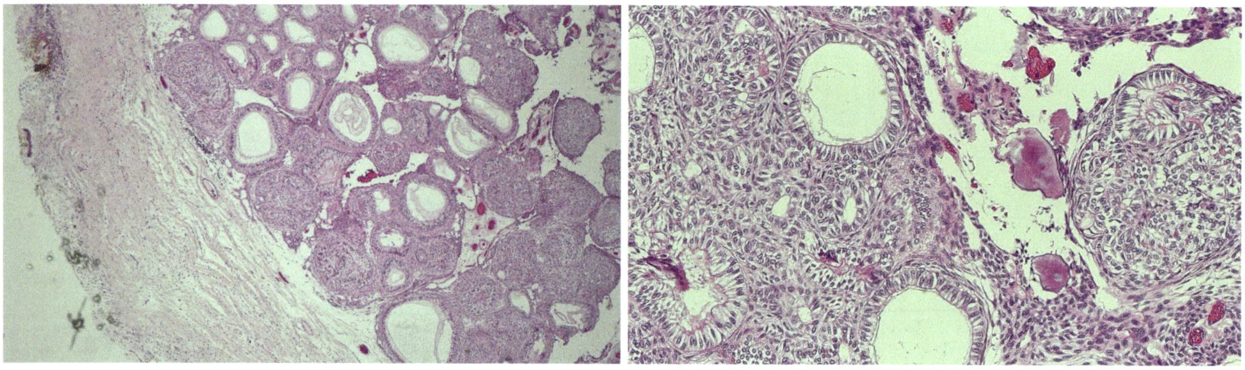

Fig. 27.6 Encapsulated tumour containing variably sized nodules of cuboidal, columnar and spindle odontogenic epithelial cells. The stromal component is minimal. There are numerous duct-like or rosette-like structures within the nodules giving rise to a glandular appearance (Left). Evidence of calcification and dentine matrix-like material (Right)

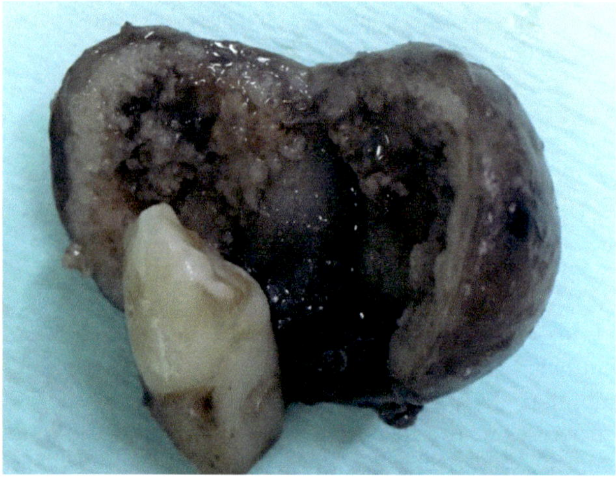

Fig. 27.7 Well-circumscribed tumour with embedded canine tooth within the lesion

27.16 How Would You Treat This Patient?

Adenomatoid odontogenic tumour is a benign lesion having some hamartomatous features. Since almost all cases are well encapsulated surgical enucleation and curettage are the treatments of choice. When the lesion is too large and in close proximity with vital structures, alternative treatment modalities such as decompression or marsupialization as initial treatment can be considered in order to reduce the damage to the adjacent anatomical structures, preventing any pathological fracture and to reduce post-operative morbidity especially in younger patients.

27.17 What Is the Prognosis for AOT?

The prognosis is excellent, and recurrence is unlikely thus justifying its conservative management. Most of the lesions are treated by enucleation. There is no difference in the prognosis between follicular, extra-follicular or peripheral variants.

27.18 Adenomatoid Odontogenic Tumour (AOT)

Adenomatoid odontogenic tumour (AOT) is an uncommon non-aggressive tumour of odontogenic epithelium. AOT comprises less than 5% of all the odontogenic tumours. The origin of the AOT may be from enamel organ epithelium. It is still debated whether AOT is a neoplastic or a hamartomatous lesion. Pathogenesis of AOT is not clear. However, KRAS mutations are reported in 70% of the AOTs together with activation of MAPK pathway. Multiple AOTs are reported in association with Schimmelpenning syndrome caused by postzygotic RAS mutations.

AOT commonly occurs in second and third decades of life, either in late adolescence or young adulthood and is predominantly seen in females. AOT can exist as an intraosseous or extraosseous lesion depending on the clinico-topographic variants. These variants are follicular, extra-follicular and peripheral. The follicular variant is associated with the crown of the embedded tooth, most frequently a permanent canine which mimics a dentigerous cyst. The extra-follicular variant may mimic either a radicular cyst if located at the apex of a tooth or totally no relationship with an embedded tooth. The peripheral type is located in the gingival mucosa and appears clinically as gingival hyperplasia or fibrous epulis. Both the follicular and extra-follicular variants are intraosseous and account for about 98% of all AOTs.

Clinically, AOT usually presents as a slow-growing, painless intra-bony swelling and is often associated with missing or delayed eruption of a permanent tooth. In some cases, mobility of the associated teeth and facial asymmetry may be present. Occasionally, the patients may manifest nasal obstruction when there is a large maxillary lesion. Occurrence of infection or pathological fracture is a rare finding in AOT. It may be found incidentally on a radiograph frequently resembling dentigerous cyst or a radicular cyst. Extraosseous or peripheral variant often presents as a gingival mass resembling gingival hyperplasia or fibrous epulis, that ranges from 1 to 1.5 cm in diameter and is more prevalent in the maxillary gingiva.

27.18.1 Investigations

About 75% of AOTs occur in the maxilla at the incisor–canine–premolar region in both jaws. Although, the tumour may have a follicular relationship with an impacted tooth mimicking dentigerous cyst radiographically, the lesion may extend apically beyond cementoenamel junction and surround a greater part of the tooth. The periphery of the lesion is well defined and well corticated or has a sclerotic border. Some lesions are completely radiolucent. However, about two-thirds of the tumours may present with flecks of calcifications within the internal structure which appear as faint radiopaque foci or dense clusters of ill-defined radiopacities. As the tumour enlarges, the teeth are frequently displaced and the tumour may inhibit the eruption of an involved tooth. Root resorption is very rarely seen. Although some expansion of the jaw may occur, the outer cortex is maintained. Extraosseous peripheral variant produces gingival swelling and may show slight erosion of alveolar bone cortex but rarely produce detectable characteristic features radiographically. AOT may be differentiated from dentigerous cyst by the presence of intra-cystic radiopaque foci. However, this feature can also be seen in calcifying odontogenic cyst. Definitive diagnosis can only be confirmed by histopathological examination.

27.18.2 Treatment and Prognosis

Almost all cases of AOT are well encapsulated. Surgical enucleation or curettage is the treatment of choice. The prognosis is excellent and recurrence is exceptionally rare. Interestingly, a few case reports show decompression or marsupialization of AOT as a possible treatment. Marsupialization combined with orthodontic treatment has been tried to assist eruption of the impacted canine. In addition, initial decompression followed by enucleation has also been tried. The rationale for the decompression first is to prevent any damage to the adjacent anatomical structures, preventing any pathological fracture and to reduce post-operative morbidity especially in younger patients. These alternatives may be an option especially when the lesion is too large and in close proximity to vital structures or, in younger patients, to allow decrease in size of the defect. However, further studies are necessary in order to assess the long-term success of these treatment modalities. The prognosis of AOT is excellent with minimum possibility of recurrence.

Salient features of adenomatoid odontogenic tumour (AOT)	
Clinical	– Slow-growing intra-bony swelling, usually in the second decade of life – Painless and often associated with a missing tooth – Two-thirds of the cases are seen in females – Two-thirds of the cases occur in the anterior maxilla – Two-thirds of the cases are usually associated with impacted tooth especially the canine
Imaging	– Well-defined radiolucency with corticated or sclerotic border – Flecks of calcifications as faint radiopaque foci or dense clusters of ill-defined radiopacities may be seen within the radiolucent lesion – Associated with impacted tooth, usually maxillary canine – Adjacent tooth may be displaced, root resorption is rare
Histopathology	– Encapsulated lesion. The epithelium is arranged into whorls and duct-like structures. Cystic areas are common. Areas mimicking enamel matrix or dentinoid-like areas are present. There is no mitotic activity or cytological atypia
Treatment	– Surgical enucleation or curettage – Marsupialization or decompression has also been tried

27

Diagnostic Algorithm

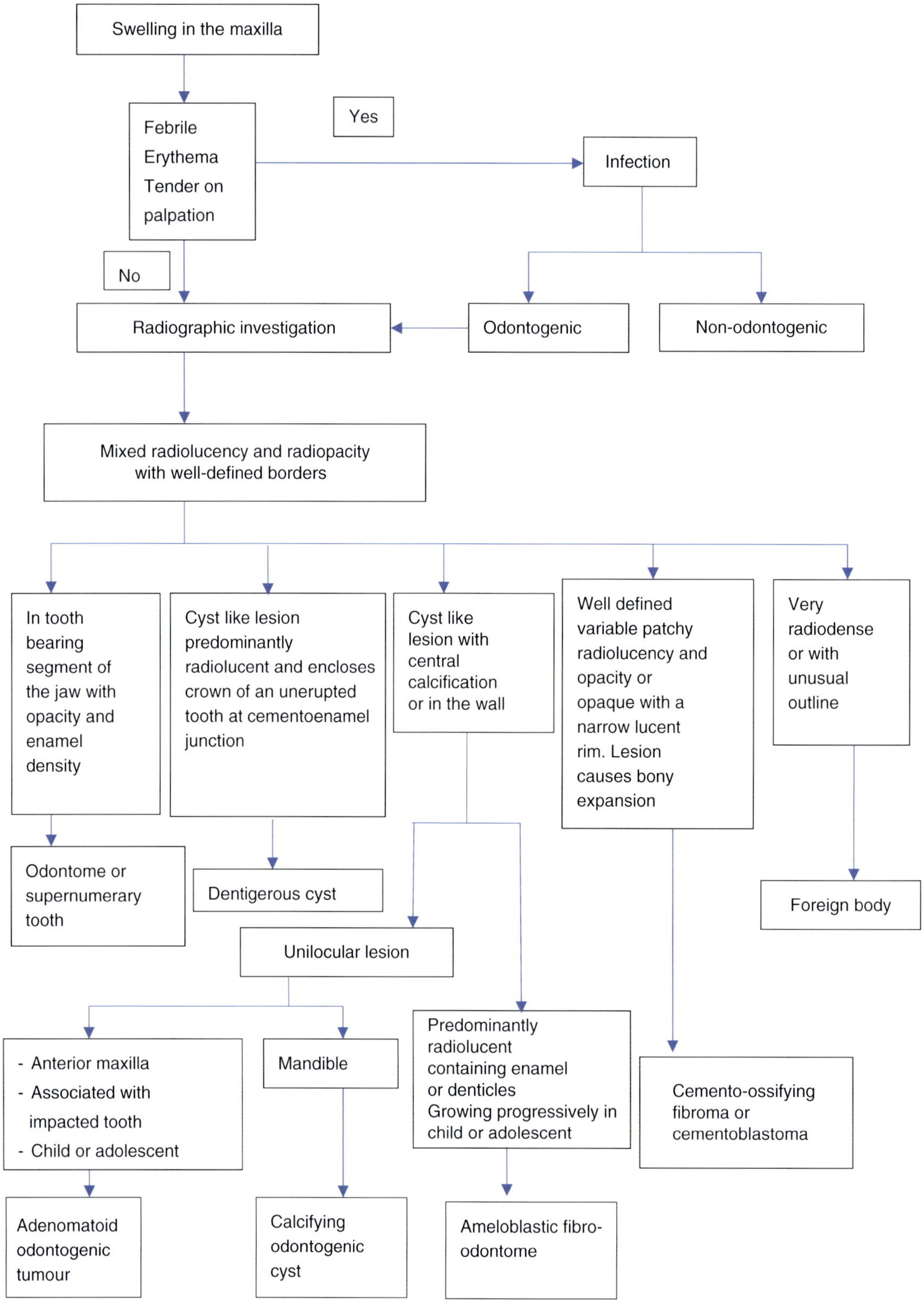

Self-Assessment Questions

1. Describe the pathognomonic clinical features of AOT.
2. List the differential diagnosis for mixed radiolucent–radiopaque jaw lesions associated with impacted teeth.
3. Describe the histopathological features of AOT.
4. Outline the management for AOT.
5. Comment on the prognosis of AOT.

Further Reading

Becker T, Buchner A, Kaffe I. Critical evaluation of the radiological and clinical features of adenomatoid odontogenic tumour. Dentomaxillofac Radiol. 2012;41(7):533–40.

Jiang M, You M, Wang H, Xu L. Characteristic features of the adenomatoid odontogenic tumour on cone beam CT. Dentomaxillofac Radiol. 2014;43(6):20140016.

Liu M, Sun G, Hu Q, Tang E. Treatment for large adenomatoid odontogenic tumors: clinical analysis of 13 cases. Int J Clin Exp Med. 2018;11:11797–803.

Philipsen HP, Reichart PA, Siar CH, Ng KH, Lau SH, Zhang X, et al. An updated clinical and epidemiological profile of the adenomatoid odontogenic tumour: a collaborative retrospective study. J Oral Pathol Med. 2007;36(7):383–93.

Wright JM, Tekkesin MS. Odontogenic tumors: where are we in 2017? J Istanbul Univ Fac Dent. 2017;51(3 Suppl 1):S10–30.

Chrcanovic BR, Gomez RS. Adenomatoid odontogenic tumor: An updated analysis of the cases reported in the literature. J Oral Pathol Med. 2019;48(1):10–6.

A Rapidly Growing Swelling in the Posterior Mandible: Clear Cell Odontogenic Carcinoma

B. S. M. S. Siriwardena and Wanninayake M Tilakaratne

Contents

W. M Tilakaratne, T. G. Kallarakkal (eds.), *Clinicopathological Correlation of Oral Diseases*,
https://doi.org/10.1007/978-3-031-24408-7_28

Learning Goals
1. Understand the clinical presentation and behaviour of intraosseous malignant tumours.
2. Recognize and classify tumours with clear cells.
3. Learn the use of immunohistochemical and molecular aids in arriving at the definitive diagnosis.

28.1 Main Complaint

A 52-year-old female presented, complaining of pain in relation to a rapidly growing lump over the left side of the body of the mandible.

28.2 History of Complaint

Question: When did you notice the lump?

It started as a hard swelling and gradually increased in size over the last 7–8 months. Initially, the swelling was painless. However, the lesion started becoming painful recently, and at present, it is moderately painful.

28.3 Additional Complaints

Question: Do you have any mobile teeth?

Recently, I experienced slight mobility of teeth on the left side posterior region.

Question: Have you noticed any ulceration inside the oral cavity?

No, I have not. However, it was difficult to chew on the affected site.

Question: Do you feel paresthesia or numbness on that side of the face or jaw?

I have mild numbness over the left lower lip.

Question: Are you suffering from any other medical conditions such as high blood pressure, heart disease, diabetes, bleeding disorder, respiratory diseases? If yes, what kind of medications have you been taking until now?

I have no other medical problems. I have been taking a few painkillers whenever I feel pain.

Question: Have you undergone any dental treatment?

I have not experienced invasive dental treatment except cleaning.

Question: What is your occupation?

I am a house wife.

Question: Do you have any specific chewing habits?

I have been chewing 3–5 betel quids per day for more than 15 years.

Question: Are you a smoker, or do you take alcohol?

I am not a smoker and do not consume alcohol.

28.4 With the Findings From the History, What Is Your Differential Diagnosis?

1. Locally aggressive intraosseous benign tumour.
2. Malignant intraosseous tumour.
3. Infection such as osteomyelitis.
4. Metastatic tumour.

28.5 How Do You Justify Your Differential Diagnosis After History Taking?

1. It started as a bony hard swelling initially that gradually enlarged within a short duration, suggesting a locally aggressive benign intraosseous tumour.
2. She experienced mobility of teeth that suggests a locally aggressive benign tumour or a malignant tumour. Mobility of teeth could be due to root resorption, bone resorption/destruction.
3. The swelling is painful. Therefore, infection leading to osteomyelitis is a possibility.
4. Although uncommon, mandible is a possible site for metastatic deposits from distant sites.

28.6 Findings of Clinical Examination

Extra-orally, the swelling appeas as diffuse measuring approximately 3 cm × 3 cm in size (Fig. 28.1). The overlying skin is normal with no inflammatory signs or draining sinuses. The swelling is firm on palpation, and the lower border of the mandible is intact. The swelling is painful on palpation. Buccal and lingual expansion of the mandible is also noted. First premolar (#34) and the first molar (#36) teeth are mobile, and second premolar

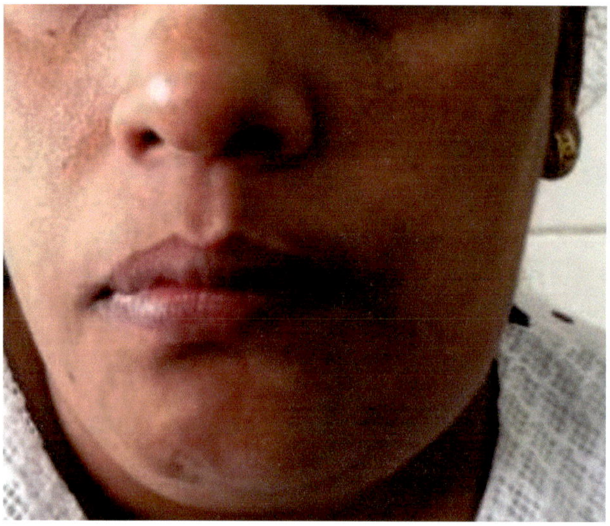

Fig. 28.1 Swelling over the left body of the mandible. (Clinical image courtesy of Dr. SAKJ Kumara)

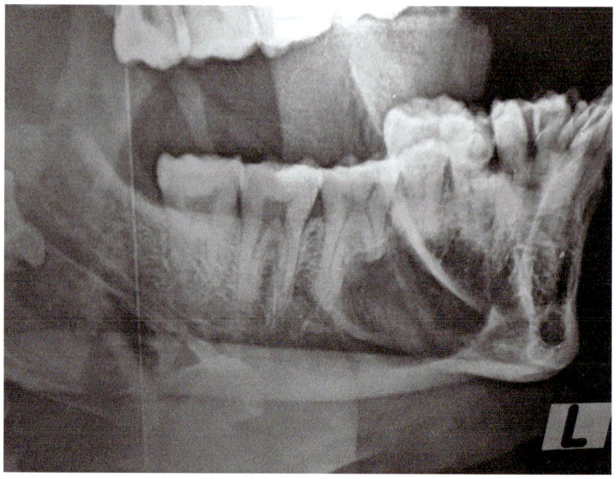

Fig. 28.2 An irregular radiolucent lesion with evidence of root resorption

tooth (#35) has grade III mobility. There is no spontaneous bleeding observed from the lesion.

28.7 What Other Relevant Features Would You Look for with the Findings You Have So Far?

There is mild numbness or paresthesia on the left side of the lower lip. There are no other swellings or ulcers in the oral cavity. Cervical lymph nodes are also not palpable.

28.8 What Is Your Clinical Differential Diagnosis?

1. Locally aggressive intraosseous benign tumour.
2. Malignant intraosseous tumour.
3. Metastatic tumour.

28.9 How Would You Justify the Inclusion of the Diseases That You Have Mentioned in the Differential Diagnosis to Arrive at a Working Diagnosis?

Clinical differential diagnoses are similar to the differential diagnoses after history taking except that the possibility of osteomyelitis can be ruled out as there are no obvious local or systemic signs and symptoms. The presence of numbness of the lower lip indicates either pressure effect on the inferior alveolar nerve or involvement of the nerve by the tumour suggestive of an aggressive lesion. Radiological investigations are necessary as it is difficult to assess the extension of the lesion and effects on adjacent structures. *Lateral oblique view* shows an irregular radiolucent lesion extending from lower left canine (#33) to first molar (#36) region with intact lower border. The tumour is destructive in nature (Fig. 28.2). Resorption of roots of first molar and premolars are evident.

28.10 What Is the Most Likely Diagnosis and Why?

Intraosseous malignant tumour. The rapid growing nature of the tumour within a short period of time, marked resorption of roots and mobility of affected teeth, paresthesia of the lower lip and osteolytic lesion are features to arrive at this working diagnosis.

28.11 How Would You Investigate This Patient?

1. Incisional biopsy.
2. Cone beam CT or a conventional CT scan to determine the extent of the lesion.

28.12 How Would You Do An Incisional Biopsy for This Patient? What Are the Important Considerations?

Biopsy must be taken from the deeper intraosseous part. A mucogingival flap should be raised followed by removal of a small piece of overlying bone, and then a representative piece should be removed from the tumour.

It is necessary to take a deep incisional biopsy including surrounding bone which facilitates to identify the infiltrative nature of the tumour.

28.13 What Specific Histopathological Features Are Helpful Leading to the Definitive Diagnosis?

H&E stained section shows cords and nests of clear cells and polygonal cells in a fibro-cellular stroma. Neoplastic clusters are entirely composed of clear cells. The peripheral cells of tumour islands show palisading. Reverse polarity is also markedly present in peripheral columnar cells. Tumour islands and strands infiltrate in between bony tissue, muscles and towards the surface epithelium. The cells reveal variable degree of nuclear pleomorphism, hyperchromatism and occasional mitotic figures (◘ Figs. 28.3 and 28.4).

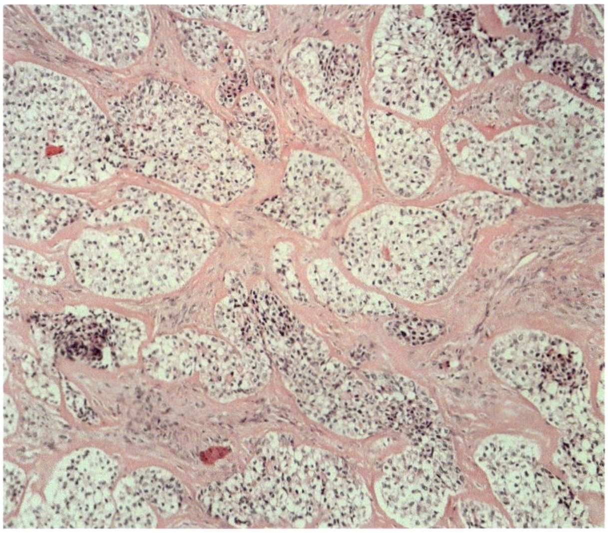

◘ **Fig. 28.3** Low-power view showing clusters of clear cells separated by thick bundles of collagen fibers

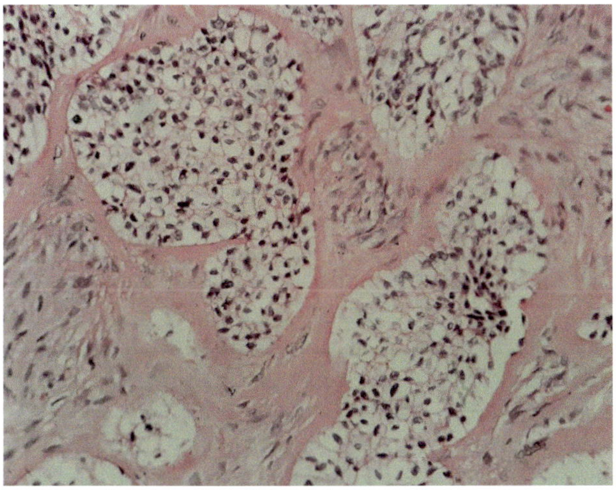

◘ **Fig. 28.4** High-power view showing reverse nuclear polarity of peripheral cells

28.14 What Is the Most Likely Diagnosis?

Clear cell odontogenic carcinoma (CCOC).

28.15 What Other Findings and Investigations Would Help You to Confirm the Diagnosis?

Findings from the history, clinical presentation, radiological features together with histopathological features confirm that it is a clear cell malignancy.

However, tumours with clear cell differentiation are not uncommon in the head and neck region. Hence, it is necessary to perform ancillary studies to confirm the diagnosis.

28.16 What Other Investigations You Would Perform in Order to Confirm the Diagnosis? Explain the Specific Reasons to Carry Out Them?

The lesion is a clear cell tumour. Therefore, it is advisable to perform other possible ancillary studies as many other entities show similar histopathological appearance. Possible differential diagnoses together with related histopathology and special investigations are given in ◘ Table 28.1. PAS-positive, diastase-sensitive granules confirmed the presence of intracellular glycogen. Mucoepidermoid carcinoma was excluded due to lack of intermediate cells, epidermoid cells and mucin (negative mucicarmine stain) within the tumour. Metastatic renal cell carcinoma was excluded as the tumour cells showed negative results with immunohistochemical stains for CK7, CD10 and renal cell carcinoma antigen. It is difficult to differentiate CCOC from hyalinizing clear cell carcinoma (HCCC) of salivary origin. However, primary intra-osseous HCCC of salivary glands is exceptionally rare. Cytokeratin 19 positivity confirmed the odontogenic origin of the tumour (◘ Fig. 28.5). In addition, demonstration of EWSR1-ATF1 fusion gene is helpful to arrive at the diagnosis of CCOC although the same is present in HCCC of salivary origin.

28

Table 28.1 Differential diagnoses for lesions with clear cells

Type	Histopathology	Special stain/ immuno marker/ molecular testing
Clear cell odontogenic carcinoma (CCOC)	Arranged in three histological patterns—biphasic pattern, monophasic pattern and clear cell nests with peripheral ameloblastoid cells with reverse polarity	PAS/DPAS+, CK19+ EWSR1-ATF1 fusion gene
Mucoepidermoid carcinoma (central) (MEC)	Epidermoid, mucous secreting and intermediate cells in a fibrous stroma. Cystic spaces may present	Mucicarmine and PAS/ DPAS+ P63+, MAML2 rearrangement
Metastatic renal cell carcinoma	Prominent vascular pattern with hemorrhagic foci within clear cells	CK7, RCCAg, CD10
Metastatic tumours from liver, prostate, and thyroid	Clear cells together with characteristic cellular features for individual tumours in non-clear cells.	Hepatocyte antigen, Prostate-specific antigen, and thyroglobulin Positivity in specific tumours
Primary intraosseous squamous cell carcinoma with clear cells (SCC)	Squamous cells, keratin pearls and high degree of cellular atypia and mitoses	Pan cytokeratin+

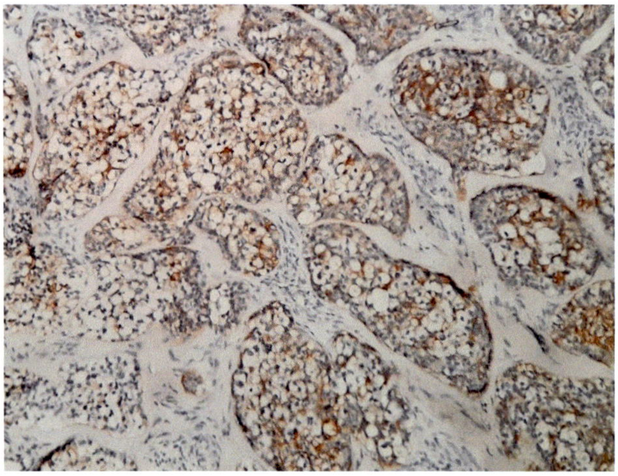

Fig. 28.5 Positive expression of CK19 confirming the odontogenic origin

28.17 What Is the Treatment for CCOC?

The treatment of CCOC is usually surgical by segmental resection of the mandible followed by appropriate reconstruction. Neck dissection and radiotherapy are recommended if there is evidence of soft tissue involvement, palpable neck lymph node or perineural invasion.

28.18 Clear Cell Odontogenic Carcinoma

Clear cell odontogenic carcinoma (CCOC) is an extremely rare odontogenic malignancy which was first described in 1981 during the International Oral Pathology meeting in Gothenburg, Sweden, by Gordon Rick, as a central clear cell tumour in the mandible with locally aggressive behaviour. Mervin Shear then defined this lesion as CCOC. In 1985, a group of people described two similar cases which they called as clear cell ameloblastoma, and in the same year, Hanson et al. described three cases introducing the term clear cell odontogenic tumour (CCOT). Later on, several cases have been published in different names with similar histology and behaviour. These findings prompted the World Health Organization (WHO) to classify this as a locally aggressive benign tumour, and the term clear cell odontogenic tumour (CCOT) was proposed in 1992. As more cases were reported with aggressive behaviour and metastasis, the name CCOC was definitively adopted by WHO in 2005 confirming it as a malignant odontogenic tumour.

The term clear cells refers to cells having a clear halo around their nuclei, which may be due to abundant glycogen or other materials which are not stained by haematoxylin and eosin. During development, the oral cavity or stomodaeum is lined by a layer of cuboidal cells, and the cytoplasm of these cells gives empty appearance due to high amount of glycogen. Histologically, this tumour shows prominent islands composed of clear cells with well-defined outline and centrally placed nuclei. Tumours with predominant clear cells are rare in the maxillofacial area and accounts for 1–2% of all tumours. Clear cells are found in many different tumours which are usually salivary, odontogenic or metastatic in origin. Although primary central clear cell carcinoma of salivary origin is extremely rare, it should be included in the differential diagnosis of central clear cell tumours of bone.

CCOC is an aggressive tumour with an infiltrative and destructive growth pattern. In some instances, it presents as a unilocular cystic lesion mimicking an odontogenic cyst. They represent the lesions of the lower end of the spectrum of malignancy. It has a 10–20% chance of metastasis particularly to lymph nodes and lungs. Clear cell odontogenic carcinomas demonstrate palisading of nuclei in peripheral cells, equal nuclear size with occasional hyperchromatic nuclei and hyalinized stroma. Perineural invasion can also be observed occasionally. There is no evidence of dentin or enamel matrix formation. Varying proportions of non-clear cells are also present. The tumour cells are positive for cytokeratins specially CK 19 but do not express myoepithelial markers such as S100 protein, GFAP, SMA and Calponin.

Molecular analysis is useful for further characterization. About 83% of CCOCs express EWSR1-ATF1 rearrangement. This rearrangement was identified in several other tumours including myoepithelial tumours of soft tissues, clear cell sarcoma, primary pulmonary myxoid sarcoma, angiomatoid fibrous histiocytoma, clear cell sarcoma–like tumour of the GI tract and salivary gland HCCC. HCCC arising in salivary glands has similar clinical behaviour to that of CCOC. They both occur in the maxillofacial region and show similar histology and immunophenotypic profiles. It has been suggested that the tumour location is a reliable distinguishing characteristic feature. Both CCOC and HCCC of salivary gland show EWSR1-ATF1 rearrangement. They can be differentiated by imaging and by demonstrating mucin in HCCC.

Wide local excision is the treatment of choice as it behaves aggressively, and there is a tendency for recurrence and metastasis. Nearly half of the patients with CCOC show recurrence. The initial mode of therapy, tumour size and extent are possible reasons for recurrence. Patients who have had conservative treatment such as curettage or enucleation experience recurrence. Conservative care and soft tissue involvement were associated with a higher recurrence rate.

CCOC is accompanied by 41% multiple recurrences and 31% metastasis. Therefore, long-term surveillance is mandatory as some cases have recurred after 20 years from the first intervention. It is mandatory to achieve clear/tumour-free surgical margins. Neck dissection and adjuvant radiation therapy may be considered in some cases. A wide local resection with 1 cm tumour free margin is recommended. Nodal excision or radiotherapy is recommended if there is evidence of soft tissue involvement, positive excision margins, palpable neck lymph nodes or perineural invasion.

Salient features of clear cell odontogenic carcinoma	
Clinical/ Radiological features	A bony hard swelling with a variable degree of pain and loosening of associated teeth. Approximately 60% of the patients show evidence of soft tissue involvement when the lesion perforates bone. Paresthesia is present occasionally. Radiologically, it is a lytic lesion with ill-defined margins. Displacement of teeth and root resorption may present
Histopathology	Solid islands and strands of cells with clear cytoplasm in most areas. Trabecular arrangement is frequent. Tumour islands show peripheral palisading with reverse polarity. Mild degree of cellular and nuclear atypia with occasional mitoses can be seen. Clear cells contain glycogen that can be demonstrated by PAS and DPAS stains. Expression of CK19 confirms odontogenic origin
Treatment	Surgical excision with or without neck dissection and radiotherapy

Self-Assessment Questions

1. List the tumours that contain prominent clear cell component in the maxillofacial region.
2. Describe how you would differentiate clear cell tumours using ancillary studies.
3. Discuss the available molecular tools to differentiate clear cell tumours in the head and neck region.
4. Describe the clinical/histopathological features of CCOC.
5. Outline the treatment options of CCOC.

28

- **Diagnostic Algorithm for Clear Cell Odontogenic Carcinoma**

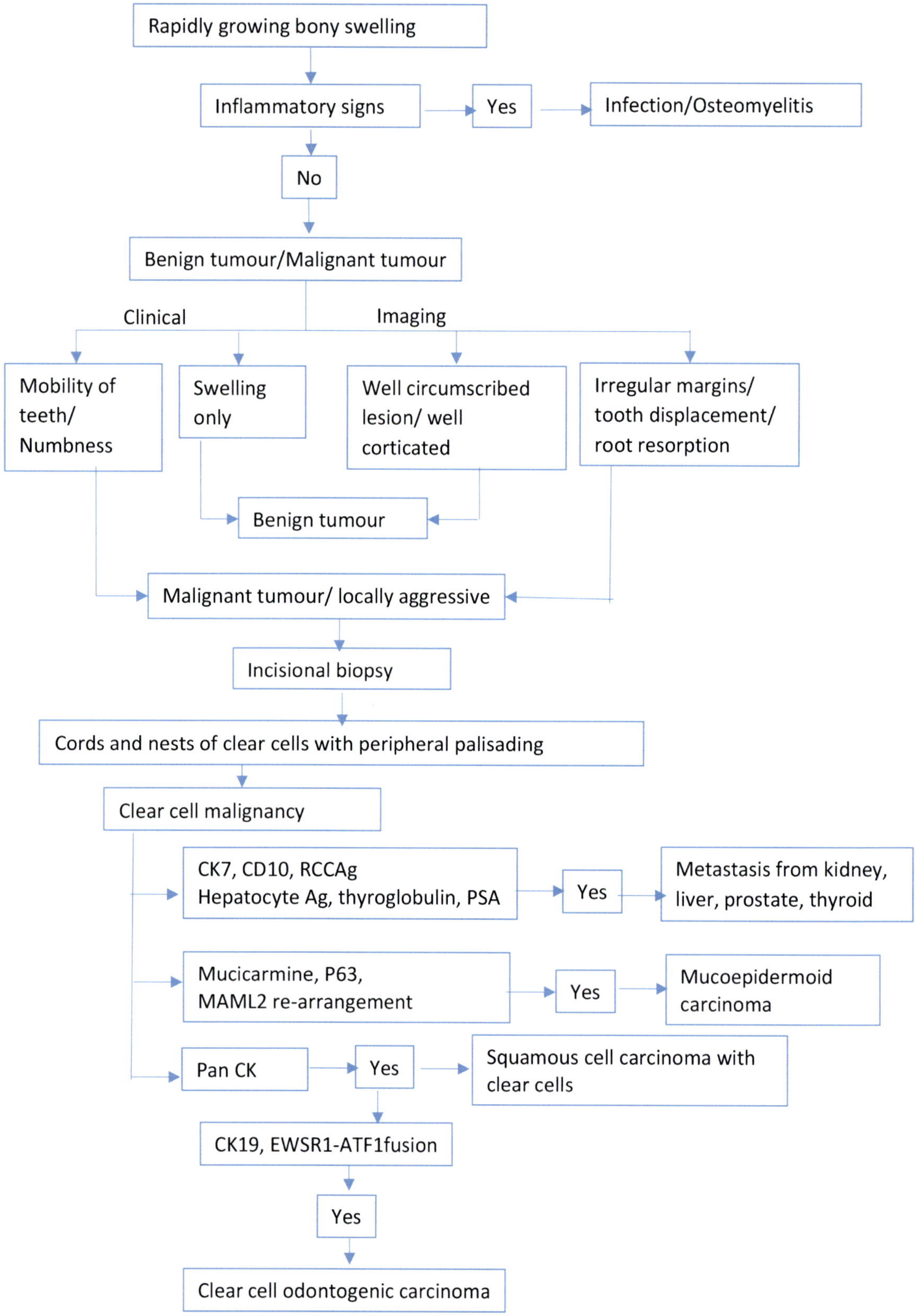

Summary

A locally aggressive central clear cell tumour recently named as clear cell odontogenic carcinoma is a rare type of malignant odontogenic tumour. Clear cell baring tumors in the head and neck region are salivary, odontogenic and metastatic tumours. Hence, it is important to arrive at a definitive diagnosis with ancillary studies. Some CCOCs may infiltrate locally whilst others may metastasize. Following surgical management, long-term surveillance is mandatory.

Further Reading

Bilodeau EA, Prasad JL, Alawi F, Seethala RR. Molecular and genetic aspects of odontogenic lesions. Head Neck Pathol. 2014;8(4):400–10. https://doi.org/10.1007/s12105-014-0588-7.

Capodiferro S, Limongelli L, Mastropasqua MG, Favia G, Lajolo C, Colella G, Tempesta A, Maiorano E. Metastatic tumors of the oro-facial tissues: clear cell renal cell carcinoma. a clinico-pathological and immunohistochemical study of seven cases. J Clin Med. 2020;9(4):1151. https://doi.org/10.3390/jcm9041151.

Hunter KD, Speight PM. The Diagnostic usefulness of immuno-histochemistry for odontogenic lesions. Head Neck Pathol. 2014;8(4):392–9. https://doi.org/10.1007/s12105-014-0582-0.

Jain A, Shetty DC, Juneja S, Narwal N. Molecular characterization of clear cell lesions of head and neck. J Clin Diagn Res. 2016;10(5):ZE18–ZE23. https://doi.org/10.7860/JCDR/2016/14394.7867.

Loyola AM, Cardoso SV, de Faria PR, et al. Clear cell odontogenic carcinoma: report of 7 new cases and systematic review of the current knowledge. Oral Surg Oral Med Oral Pathol Oral Radiol. 2015;120:483–96. https://doi.org/10.1016/j.oooo.2015.06.005. Review

Speight PM, Takata T. New tumour entities in the 4th edition of the World Health Organization Classification of Head and Neck tumours: odontogenic and maxillofacial bone tumours. Virch Arch. 2018;472(3):331–9. https://doi.org/10.1007/s00428-017-2182-3.

Developmental Alterations of the Oral Mucosa

Contents

Bilateral White Patches on the Cheek: White Sponge Naevus

Pilana Vithanage Kalani Shihanika Hettiarachchi and Wanninayake M Tilakaratne

Contents

W. M Tilakaratne, T. G. Kallarakkal (eds.), *Clinicopathological Correlation of Oral Diseases*,
https://doi.org/10.1007/978-3-031-24408-7_29

Learning Goals

1. Devise the correct way of compiling the history with appropriate questions.
2. Develop a differential diagnosis after history taking.
3. Deduce appropriate procedures in clinical examination.
4. Formulate a differential diagnosis combining findings in the history and clinical examination.
5. Justify the relevant investigations required to arrive at the diagnosis.
6. Comprehend the importance of clinicopathological correlation in arriving at the correct diagnosis.
7. Outline the management plan.
8. Recognize the importance of a diagnostic algorithm in arriving at a diagnosis.

29.1 Main Complaint

A 28-year-old male patient presented to the oral medicine clinic complaining of soft white lesions on both the cheeks and tongue.

29.2 History of Complaint

Question: When did you first notice this?

I initially noted these lesions many years ago. Since then, the lesions have remained asymptomatic with no increase in size. Therefore, I had not sought any medical advice until now.

29.3 Additional Complaints

Question: Do you have any abnormal features associated with your nails?

I did not notice any abnormality in relation to my nails.

Question: Do you have any lesions on your palms and soles or any other pigmented skin lesions?

I have no abnormalities in any other extra oral sites.

Question: Have your parents noticed these intra oral lesions since childhood?

I vaguely remember them mentioning about these lesions earlier.

Question: Do you feel any burning sensation especially on eating spicy food?

I don't specifically experience any burning sensation; however, sometimes I have a mild on and off burning sensation when eating spicy food.

Question: Does any of the other family members have similar lesions?

None of the immediate family members have similar lesions.

Question: Are you suffering from any other medical problems like asthma or diabetes or on any medications?

I am on an inhaler for asthma since the past 3 years.

Question: Have you been experiencing excessive thirst or need to urinate frequently?

I do not have any such symptoms.

Question: What is your occupation?

I am an undergraduate student.

Question: Do you have any specific habits such as chewing, smoking or taking alcohol?

I am a smoker and have been smoking about three to four cigarettes per day for the past 5 years.

29.4 With the Findings From the History, What Is Your Differential Diagnoses?

1. White sponge naevus (WSN).
2. Pseudomembranous candidosis.
3. Leukoedema.
4. Oral lichen planus (OLP).

29.5 How Do You Justify Your Differential Diagnosis After History Taking?

1. White plaque-like lesions in the oral cavity may occur due to many reasons; some of the most common reasons include leukoplakia, oral submucous fibrosis, white sponge naevus, leukoedema, oral lichen planus, pseudomembranous candidosis and dyskeratosis congenita. Since he does not have a suggestive habit history, and as the lesions were present bilater-

ally, the possibility of both leukoplakia and oral submucous fibrosis are unlikely. Although proliferative verrucous leukoplakia can present like this, the duration and no change in size may not be compatible with this condition. As there is no involvement of extra oral sites with skin pigmentation and no changes in the nails, dyskeratosis congenita can also be excluded.

2. He appears to be on long-term inhalers that may have predisposed him to develop candidosis leading to burning sensation. Further, the presence of white plaques may be due to candidal infection.
3. The presence of burning sensation to spicy food, and considering the sites of involvement, oral lichen planus can also be considered as a differential diagnosis. Leukoedema may also present as grayish, whitish discoloration of the buccal mucosa.
4. The presence of generally asymptomatic, longstanding white lesions involving multiple intra oral sites which have not increased in size over the time allows considering benign lesion-like white sponge naevus in the differential diagnosis.

29.6 Findings of Clinical Examination

Both upper and lower lips appear depigmented and scaly. Intra orally, white "sponge" plaque-like lesions present on bilateral buccal mucosae, dorsal and ventral surface of the tongue and on the floor of the mouth (◘ Fig. 29.1).

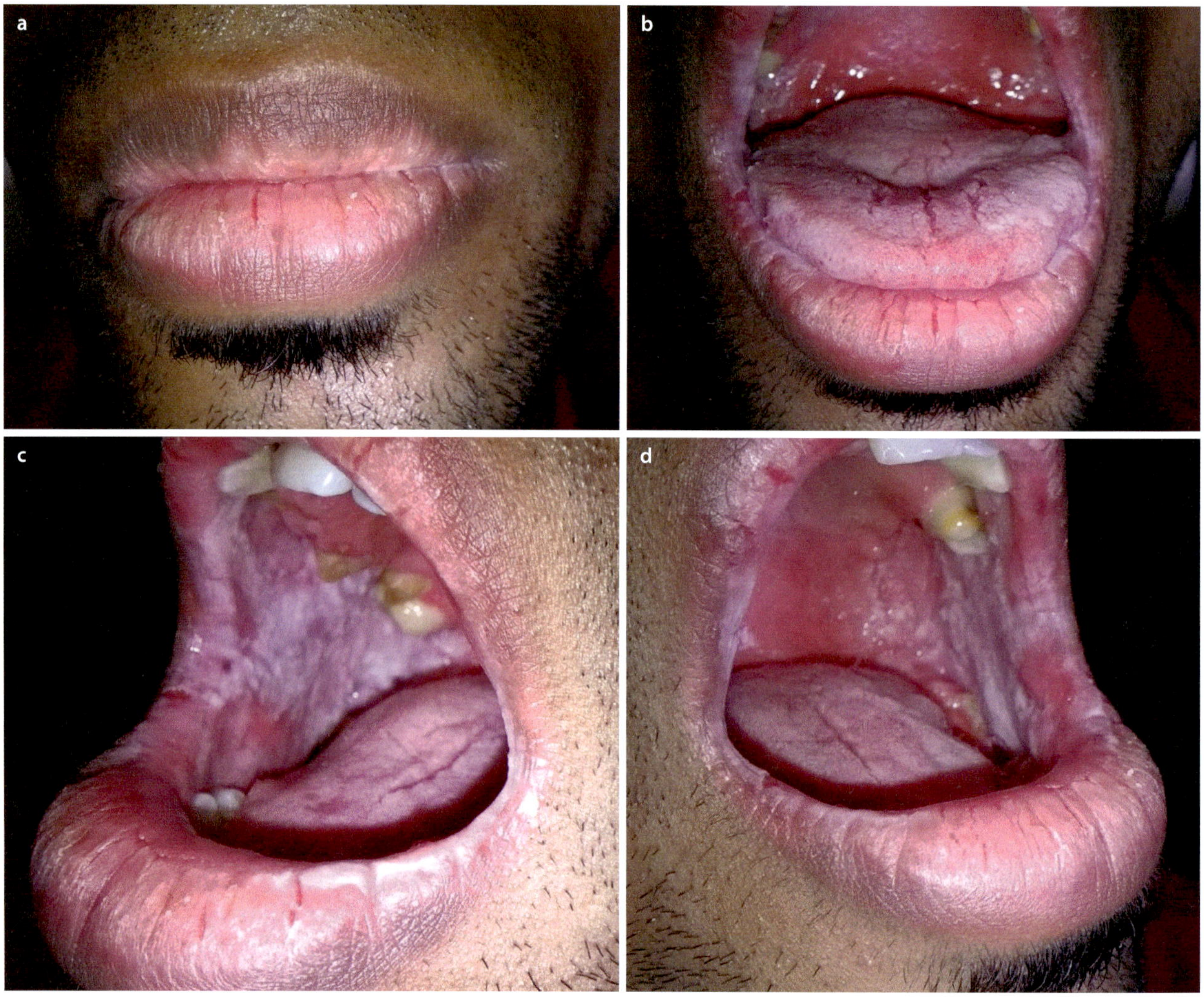

◘ **Fig. 29.1** Depigmented and scaly appearance of the lips (**a**). Intra oral white spongy plaque-like lesions present on dorsal surface of the tongue and on bilateral buccal mucosae (**b**, **c** and **d**)

29.7 What Other Relevant Features Would You Look for with the Findings You Have So Far?

The lesions did not demonstrate any reticular pattern or could not be removed by scraping off leaving an erythematous base. The lesions on the buccal mucosa did not disappear upon stretching of the mucosa.

29.8 What Is Your Clinical Diagnosis?

White sponge naevus.

29.9 How Would You Exclude Other Conditions and Justify the Inclusion of the Diseases That You Have Mentioned in the Differential Diagnosis to Arrive at a Working Diagnosis?

29.9.1 Leukoedema

This is a normal anatomical variation that usually appears as a white opalescence of the bilateral buccal mucosa (◘ Fig. 29.2a). It may present on labial mucosa or soft palate. This is commonly seen in people with dark skin and especially in smokers. Characteristically

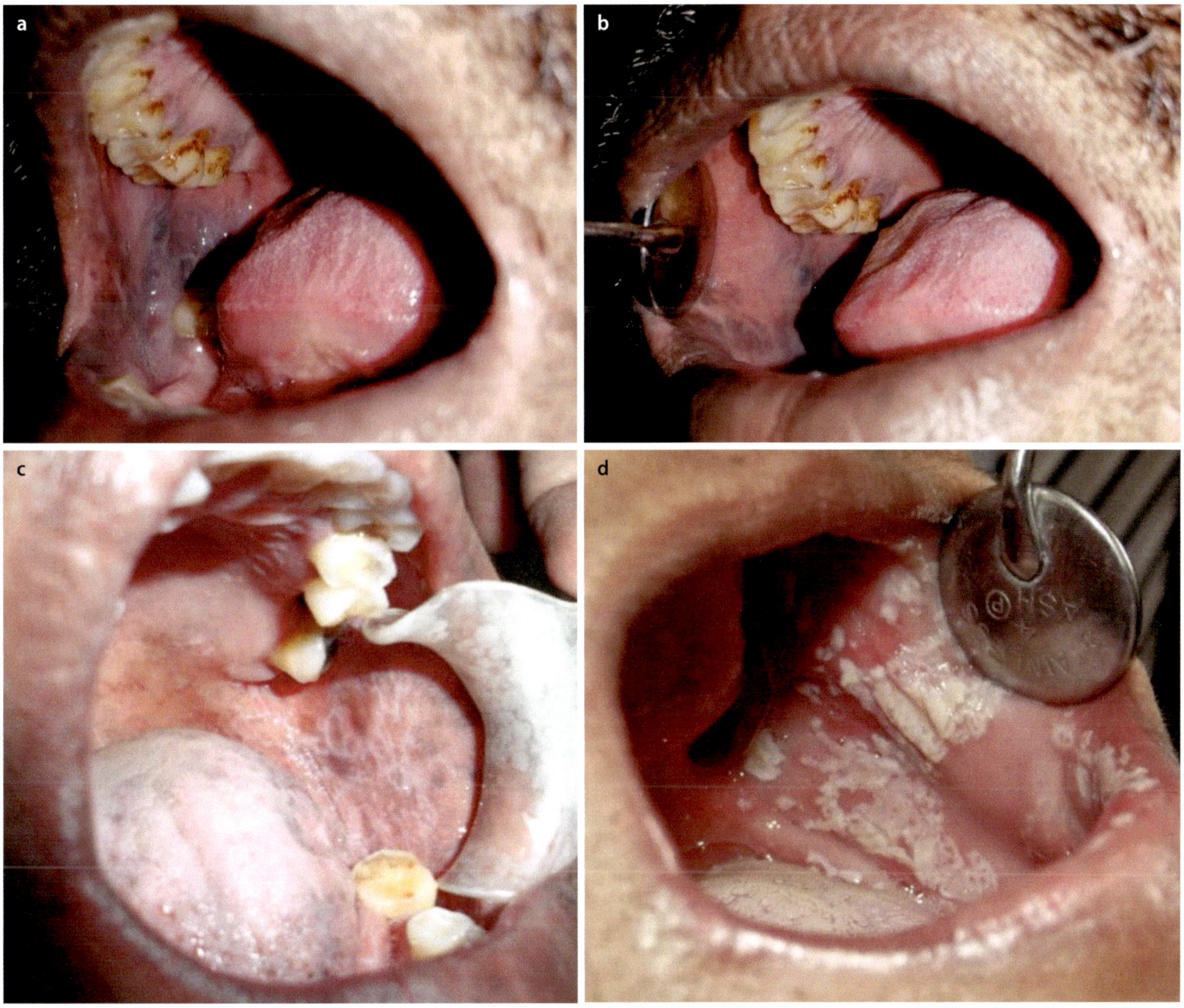

◘ **Fig. 29.2** Leukoedema of the right-side buccal mucosa with whitish/grayish discoloration (**a**); note the discoloration disappears once the mucosa is stretched (**b**); characteristic appearance of reticular lichen planus with Wickham striations on left buccal mucosa (**c**); white lesions due to acute pseudomembranous candidosis (**d**). These are characterized by leaving an erythematous region when wiped off with a piece of gauze these lesions disappear or become less prominent when the mucosa is stretched and reappears upon relaxation (◘ Fig. 29.2b). However, these lesions do not disappear upon stretching; therefore, the possibility of leukoedema is unlikely.

29.9.2 Oral Lichen Planus

Oral lichen planus (OLP) is a common chronic inflammatory mucocutaneous disorder that typically affects the skin and/or oral cavity. Oral lesions typically present as white striations (Wickham striae), white papules, white plaques, erythema, erosion or blisters (◘ Fig. 29.2c). They usually present as symmetrical and bilateral or multiple lesions. The common sites of involvement are buccal mucosa, dorsum and ventral surface of the tongue and gingivae (desquamative gingivitis). The diagnosis of OLP is initially based on the clinical presentation, which has the typical appearance of a reticular pattern which is not present in this case.

29.9.3 Pseudomembranous Candidosis

These are white, curd-like (creamy) patches or plaques, most frequently occurring on the buccal mucosa and tongue, but also seen on the palate, floor of the mouth and gingiva, usually associated with a burning sensation (◘ Fig. 29.2d). Clinically, these white plaques can be easily rubbed off with gauze, leaving a tender, red, raw area beneath, which may bleed. The ability to remove these plaques is a diagnostic feature that differentiates pseudomembranous candidosis from other forms of white lesions on the oral mucosa. In the present case, these plaques are not patchy and could not be rubbed off. Therefore, candidosis is unlikely to be the primary diagnosis for his complaints.

29.10 What Is the Most Likely Diagnosis?

White sponge naevus

29.11 How Would You Investigate This Patent?

Incisional biopsy for the confirmation of diagnosis and to plan long-term management.

29.12 How Would You Do An Incisional Biopsy for This Patient? What Are the Important Considerations?

This patient did not present with the typical family history in order to confirm the diagnosis. Hence an incisional biopsy is mandatory. Further, a white patch on the buccal mucosa may mimic oral potentially malignant disorders such as leukoplakia and oral submucous fibrosis. Therefore, an incisional biopsy will help to exclude the possible oral potentially malignant disorders. Biopsy report confirms the previous clinical diagnosis of White Sponge Naevus.

29.13 What Are the Histopathological Features That Help in the Diagnosis?

H&E sections reveal marked hyperkeratosis and acanthosis of the stratified squamous epithelium together with perinuclear eosinophilic condensation and cytoplasmic clearing in keratinocytes. The surface keratin layer is irregular due to traumatic changes. These histopathological features, taken in conjunction with the clinical findings, are consistent with the definitive diagnosis of white sponge naevus (WSN) (◘ Fig. 29.3).

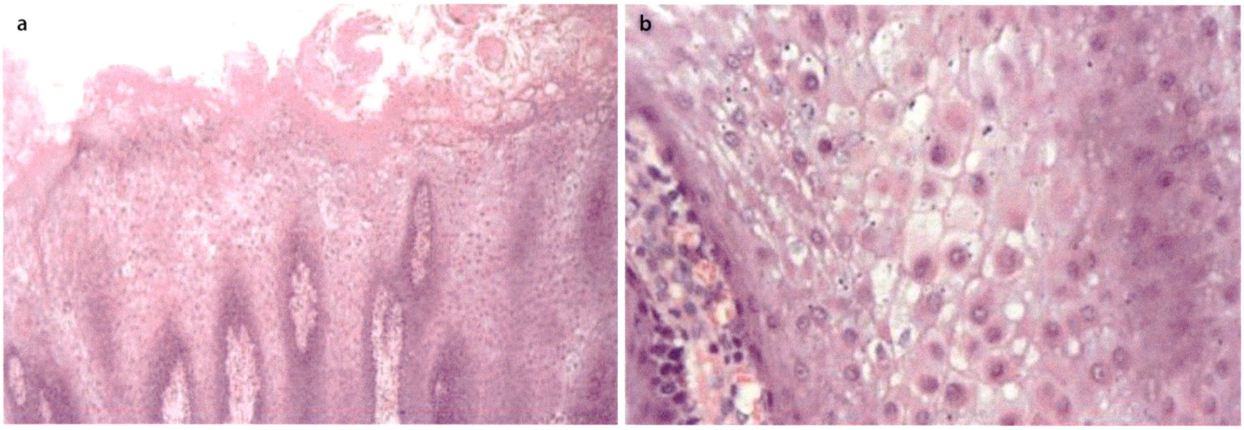

◘ **Fig. 29.3** Hyperkeratosis and spongiosis (**a**), cytoplasmic clearing and perinuclear condensation of keratin (**b**)

29.14 How Would You Manage This Patent?

The patient was reassured. Since he was asymptomatic only antiseptic mouth wash (0.2% chlorhexidine gluconate) was prescribed and planned to follow-up in 3-month intervals.

29.15 White Sponge Naevus (WSN)

WSN is a rare genetic disorder inherited as an autosomal dominant trait with wide variability of expression and penetrance and hence familial reports are not very common. This may also occur as a result of sporadic mutation. Lesions of WSN usually appear at birth or in early childhood, but sometimes the condition develops during adolescence. The reported prevalence rate is below 1 in 200,000.

Mutations in the KRT4 or KRT13 gene cause WSN. The keratin 4 protein (produced from the KRT4 gene) and the keratin 13 protein (produced from the KRT13 gene) partner together to form molecules known as intermediate filaments. These filaments assemble into networks that provide strength and resilience to different mucosae. Networks of intermediate filaments protect the mucosae from being damaged by friction or other everyday physical stresses. Keratin 4 and 13 proteins are only produced in the oral, nasal, esophageal and anogenital mucosae. Mutations in the KRT4 or KRT13 gene disrupt the structure of the keratin protein. As a result, keratin 4 and keratin 13 are mismatched and do not fit together properly, leading to the formation of irregular intermediate filaments that are easily damaged with little friction or trauma. Damage to intermediate filaments leads to inflammation and promotes the abnormal growth and division of basal cells of the epithelium, causing mucosal hyperkeratosis and acanthosis resulting in white sponge naevus.

Diagnosis of WSN is challenging in some cases and many other different types of white lesions should be considered in the differential diagnosis. There is a need for precise identification through prompt histopathological examination to differentiate this condition from more serious, potentially malignant disorders such as oral lichen planus, oral lichenoid drug reaction, lupus erythematosus, other genodermatoses such as hereditary benign epithelial dyskeratosis or Witkop disease, pachyonychia congenita, as well as cheek chewing and possibly candidosis. Pachyonychia congenita can be excluded based on the absence of extra oral skin lesions (thickened nails and hyperkeratotic palms and soles). Histopathology of Witkop disease is identical to WSN except that scattered spinous cells show premature keratinization and pyknosis of nuclei in the former. Differentiation of these two conditions is very important as Witkop disease may lead to blindness due to formation of gelatinous plaques on bulbar conjunctiva. Pseudomembranous candidosis and chronic hyperplastic candidosis can often be confused with WSN. However, inability to demonstrate fungal hyphae and characteristic histopathological features help to differentiate these. Although cheek biting, chemical burns and smoking have similar clinical features, they can be excluded by proper history taking. Leukoedema shows disappearance of its grey, pale appearance upon stretching the mucosa, which helps to differentiate it from WSN clinically. Lichen planus may look similar, but the age of onset and the presence of white reticular lesions are clinically characteristic. Further, histopathologically the two lesions can be differentiated. Biopsy is mandatory for the diagnosis and to exclude the possible potentially malignant disorders such as leukoplakia and oral submucous fibrosis.

WSN is usually asymptomatic, unless superinfection is present. The corrugated plaques of WSN easily harbor microorganisms and provide the best conditions for colonization. Maintenance of good oral hygiene and daily use of an antiseptic mouthwash are recommended for these patients to avoid such superinfections. During acute severe exacerbations, topical as well as systemic antibiotic treatment is recommended in the literature. Topical tetracycline 0.25% or 1% has been used with good symptomatic control.

Failed attempts of surgical excision of the lesions using laser are also reported in the literature. This may be due to its genetic pathogenesis. There is no definitive and standard treatment for WSN. Lesions may persist throughout the life but is completely benign in nature.

29

Salient features of oral malignant melanoma	
Clinical	White to grey, diffuse, asymptomatic, sponge and folded plaques affecting intra oral sites (mainly buccal mucosae). Lesions of WSN usually appear at birth or in early childhood, but sometimes the condition may develop during adolescence
Histopathology	– Parakeratosis, acanthosis with formation of large blunt rete ridges and spongiosis – Extensive vacuolation of suprabasal keratinocytes – Dyskeratotic cells exhibit dense peri and paranuclear eosinophilic condensations, which correspond to tonofilament aggregates
Treatment	– There is no definitive and standard treatment – Progression usually stops at puberty – There is no risk for malignant transformation

Self-Assessment Questions

1. State the important conditions that need to be included in the differential diagnosis of white lesions on the buccal mucosa.
2. List the information in the history that is important to differentiate WSN from other white lesions of the buccal mucosa.
3. Describe the important histopathological findings of WSN.
4. Explain the pathogenesis of WSN.
5. Outline the management for WSN.

Diagnostic Algorithm for White Sponge Naevus

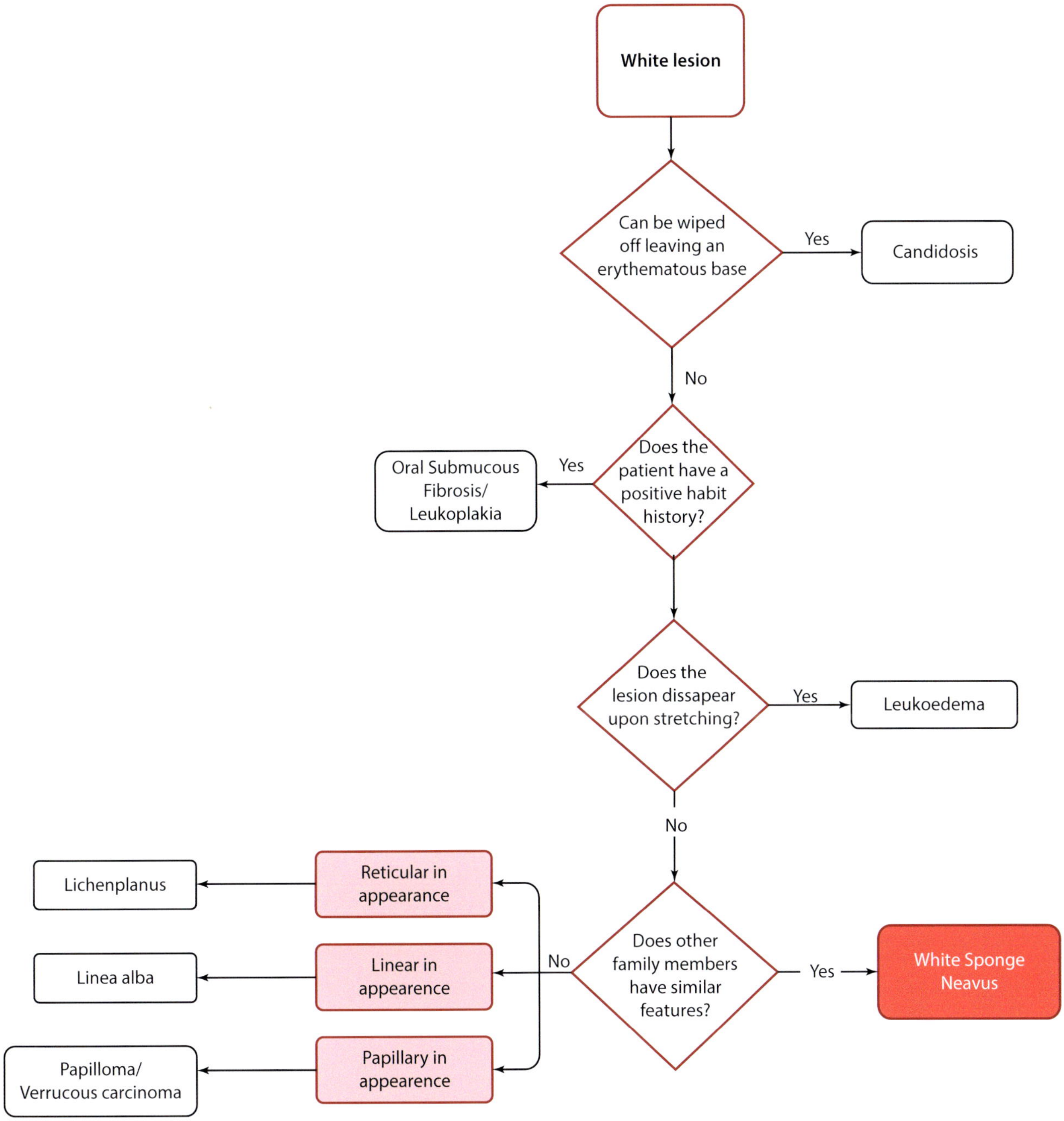

Further Reading

Hettiarachchi PVKS, Jayasinghe JCM, Siriwardena BSMS, Jayasinghe RD. White sponge nevus in the oral cavity: case report and a review of literature Sri Lanka. Dent J. 2018;48(01):41–5.

Marrelli M, Tatullo M, Dipalma G, Inchingolo F. Oral infection by Staphylococcus aureus in patients affected by white sponge nevus: a description of two cases occurred in the same family. Int J Med Sci. 2012;9(1):47–50.

Sharma S, Srivastava K, Gaur P, Gupta S. An autosomal genetic disease: white sponge nevus. Int J Contempor Med Res. 2018;5(7):G5–7.

Sobhan M, Alirezaei P, Farshchian M, Eshghi G, Ghasemi Basir HR, Khezrian L. White sponge nevus: report of a case and review of the literature. Acta Med Iran. 2017;55(8):533–5.

Songu M, Adibelli H, Diniz G. White sponge nevus: clinical suspicion and diagnosis. Pediatr Dermatol. 2012;29(4):495–7.

Bilateral Whitish Patches on the Inner Cheek: Leukoedema

Firdaus Hariri

Contents

W. M Tilakaratne, T. G. Kallarakkal (eds.), *Clinicopathological Correlation of Oral Diseases*,
https://doi.org/10.1007/978-3-031-24408-7_30

Learning Goals

1. Devise the correct way of compiling the history with appropriate questions.
2. Develop a differential diagnosis after history taking.
3. Deduce appropriate procedures in clinical examination.
4. Formulate a differential diagnosis combining findings in the history and clinical examination.
5. Justify the relevant investigations required to arrive at the diagnosis.
6. Comprehend the importance of clinicopathological correlation in arriving at the correct diagnosis.
7. Outline the management plan.
8. Recognize the importance of a diagnostic algorithm in arriving at a diagnosis

30.1 Main Complaint

A 35-year-old male patient complains of a white patch on both left and right cheek mucosa.

30.2 History of Complaint

Question: When did you first notice the white patch?

I have been noticing it for a long time but only decided to come.

Question: What is the nature of the patch?

The patch has been present for years. It remains irregular in shape, is painless and presents on both sides of the inner cheek.

Question: Has the patch progressively been changing in appearance?

The patch has remained irregular in shape and appeared whitish-grey from the time I first noticed it.

Question: Have you tried to scrape the patch off the surface?

I have tried to scrape it off occasionally while brushing my teeth, but the patch remains unscrapable.

Question: Do you have any other associated oral symptoms such as swelling and ulceration?

I do not have any other symptoms.

Question: Do you have any history of oral tissue injury such as cheek biting or trauma to the cheeks?

I do not have any history of trauma and injury to the oral tissues.

Question: Did you notice any other lesions at any part of your mouth?

I do not have any other lesions inside my mouth.

Question: Do you have general symptoms such as tiredness, loss of weight and loss of appetite?

I do not have any such symptoms.

30.3 Past Medical History

Question: Do you have any other medical problems? If yes, what kind of medications have you been taking until now?

I have not been diagnosed with any other medical problems till now.

Question: Have you been admitted to the hospital or had any surgical procedure done before?

I do not have any history of hospital admission or surgical procedure.

Question: Do you have any allergy?

I have no history of allergy.

30.4 Past Dental History

Question: How often do you visit a dentist?

I am an irregular dental attendee but have no remarkable dental treatment history.

Question: How often do you brush your teeth?

I usually brush my teeth once a day.

30.5 Social History

? Question: Is there any family history of cancer?

✓ There is no history of cancer within my family members.

? Question: Does any of your family members have similar lesions in their mouth?

✓ I am not aware of any of my family members having similar lesions in their mouth.

? Question: What is your occupation?

✓ I work as a security guard.

? Question: Do you have any high-risk habits such as smoking cigarettes, alcohol consumption or betel-quid chewing?

✓ I smoke an average of 10 cigarettes per day for the last 15 years. I do not have any other high-risk habits such as alcohol consumption and betel-quid chewing.

? Question: Tell me about your dietary habits.

✓ I rarely skip my meals. I have no food allergies and often take spicy food.

30.6 What Is Your Differential Diagnosis with the Findings From the History?

1. Linea alba
2. Leukoedema
3. Morsicatio buccarum
4. Fordyce granules (FGs)
5. White sponge naevus (WSN)
6. Oral lichen Planus (OLP)
7. Oral leukoplakia (OL)

30.7 How Do You Justify Your Differential Diagnosis?

All the lesions included in the differential diagnosis carry the similar clinical manifestation of an intra-oral white lesion. Linea alba is a relatively common condition. It usually presents as a bilateral horizontal white scalloped line. However, linea alba may be more pronounced in some individuals and appear as a thickened plaque. It occurs on the buccal mucosa at the level of the occlusal plane of the adjacent teeth extending from the commissure to the posterior teeth. Frictional irritation or sucking trauma from facial surfaces of the adjacent teeth is the causative factor. The patient's complaint of long-standing bilateral white patches on the buccal mucosa is an indicator to include lineal alba in the differential diagnosis.

Leukoedema is a relatively common oral condition which is considered to be a normal variant rather than a disease. It tends to occur more commonly in smokers and has also been found to occur with increased frequency in betel quid chewers. Clinically, it presents as a diffuse greyish-white, smooth, oedematous film bilaterally on the buccal mucosa. A history of bilateral white patches that has been present for a long period of time and chronic smoking in this patient suggests the possibility of leukoedema as a differential diagnosis.

Trauma arising from chronic biting or chewing of the non-keratinized mucosa results in white lesions. These lesions are referred to as morsicatio buccarum or morsicatio labiorum depending upon the location of the lesions on the buccal mucosa or the labial mucosa, respectively. They occur in young patients usually in their second and third decades of life and present as whitish grey papules and plaques that are usually bilateral. These lesions may resolve and recur. The patient does not have any history of cheek biting or trauma to the cheek mucosa. However, morsicatio buccarum should be considered in the differential diagnosis as the patient complains of bilateral lesions which may have arisen as result of inadvertent parafunctional habits such as chronic cheek biting.

FGs are ectopic sebaceous glands found on the genital and oral mucosa. The prevalence of FGs increases from childhood to adulthood and is slightly more common in adult males. They occur predominantly on the upper lip vermillion, retro molar area and buccal mucosa where they appear as pinhead-sized yellowish macules or papules. A bilaterally symmetrical pattern of distribution is very common. A differential diagnosis of FGs is considered as the patient complains of bilateral white lesions that have been present for a long period of time.

WSN is a rare hereditary mucocutaneous disorder that is inherited as an autosomal dominant trait with a high degree of penetrance and variable expressivity. The characteristic clinical presentation is that of diffuse, symmetrical, thickened, corrugated and white plaques on the bilateral buccal mucosae. The lesions are asymptomatic and manifest since early childhood. The patient complains of chronic white patches on the right and left buccal mucosae. However, there is no positive family history in this patient for such lesions.

OLP is a common chronic mucocutaneous disease that frequently involves the buccal mucosa, tongue and gingiva. The lesions are usually bilaterally symmetrical. The clinical variants of OLP include the reticular, papular, plaque, erosive, atrophic and bullous forms. The reticular, papular and plaque forms are usually asymptomatic but may manifest with a burning sensation and appear clinically as white keratotic lesions. WSN and OLP are considered in the list of differential diagnoses owing to the patient's complaint of bilateral white patches that have been present for a long period of time.

OL is amongst the most common oral potentially malignant disorders (OPMDs) encountered in clinical practice. It is defined as a predominantly white plaque of questionable risk having excluded other known diseases or disorders that carry no increased risk for cancer. Benign white lesions including frictional keratosis, biting of the lip/cheek/commissures (morsicatio labiorum/buccarum), alveolar ridge keratosis, leukoedema, white sponge nevus and Fordyce granules should be excluded to confirm the diagnosis of OL. It is not associated with any chemical or physical causative agents except tobacco, alcohol or betel quid. Clinically, OL can be sub-classified into homogeneous and non-homogeneous types based on distinct clinical features such as colour and surface texture. Homogeneous OLs present as a thin white plaque or a patch with a smooth surface texture and consistent topography throughout. OLs are usually solitary lesions that may vary in size from a small and circumscribed plaque to an extensive lesion involving a large area of the oral mucosa. Presence of multifocal OLs should arouse the suspicion of proliferative verrucous leukoplakia (PVL) which is a distinct, aggressive form of OL with a high risk of malignant transformation. OL is included in the differential diagnosis as the patient is a chronic smoker which may have predisposed him for OL.

30.8 What Are the Findings of Clinical Examination?

30.8.1 Extra-oral

There are no peripheral signs of systemic disease. There are no abnormalityes detected extra-orally.

30.8.2 Intra-oral

Intra-orally, the patient has moderate oral hygiene with all permanent teeth present. The lesion on each side of the buccal mucosa is whitish-grey in colour and slightly edematous. It has irregular borders and involves the buccal mucosa near the lower second molar teeth extending to the retromolar trigone area. The lesion is non-scrapable and disappears upon mucosal stretching. There is no abnormality detected at the other intra-oral sites.

30.9 What Is Your Clinical Diagnosis?

Leukoedema

30.10 How Do You Investigate the Patient to Confirm Your Diagnosis?

Leukoedema can be diagnosed clinically and easily differentiated from other lesions included in the differential diagnosis. A characteristic finding is that upon stretching or retracting the affected buccal mucosa, the lesions will disappear. In leukoedema, the affected tissue appears slightly edematous, and there is no loss of pliability of the involved tissues.

30.11 Do You Need to Do a Biopsy to Confirm the Diagnosis of Leukoedema?

Leukoedema is a clinical diagnosis. A biopsy is not warranted to confirm the diagnosis of leukoedema.

30.12 What Histological Features Would You Expect to See If a Biopsy Is Performed?

Histopathological examination reveals hyperparakeratosis (◘ Fig. 30.1) and acanthosis of the epithelium. The rete ridges appear broad and elongated (◘ Fig. 30.2). A marked intra-cellular oedema is observed within the cells of the spinous cell layer (◘ Fig. 30.3). These cells appear vacuolated and have pyknotic nuclei (◘ Fig. 30.4).

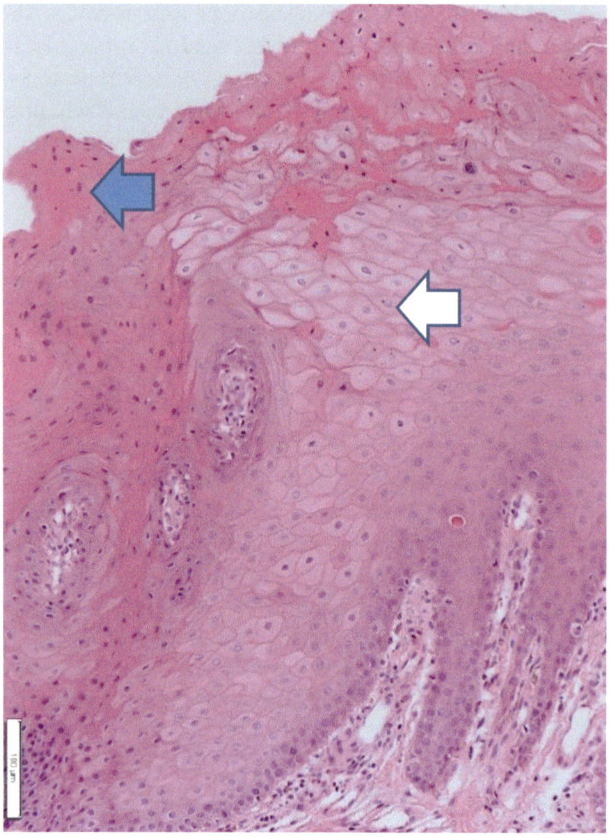

■ **Fig. 30.1** Hyperkeratosis of the epithelium (blue arrow) and marked intracellular oedema of the cells of the spinous cell layer (white arrow)

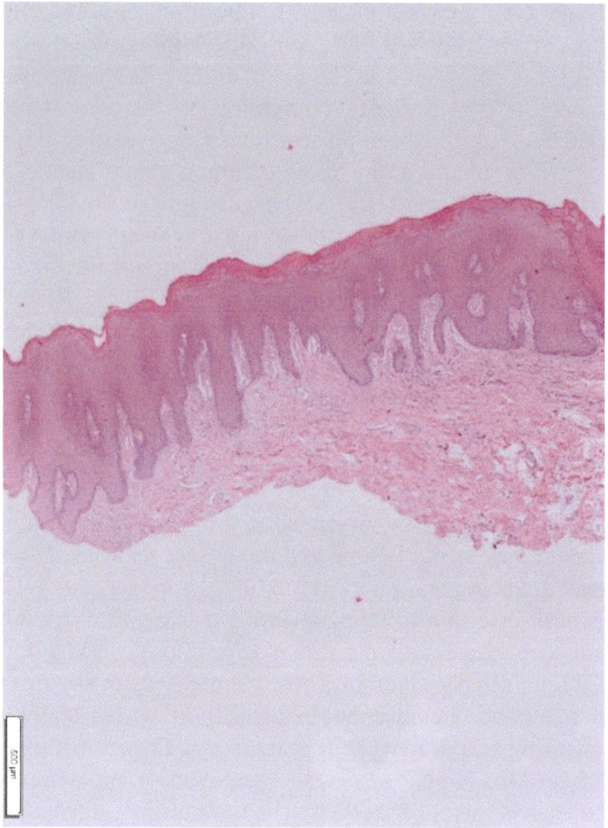

■ **Fig. 30.2** The epithelium shows broad and elongated rete ridges

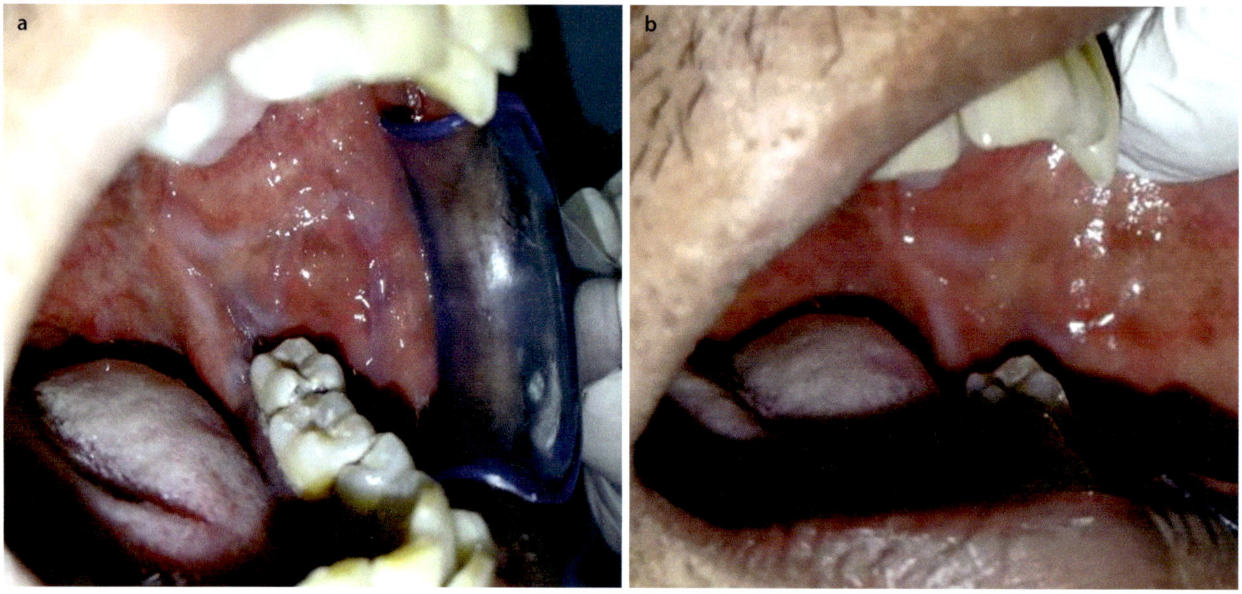

■ **Fig. 30.3** Leukoedema presenting as diffuse, greyish milky-white and opalescent film on the buccal mucosa (**a**). The lesion disappears or becomes less obvious upon mucosal stretching (**b**)

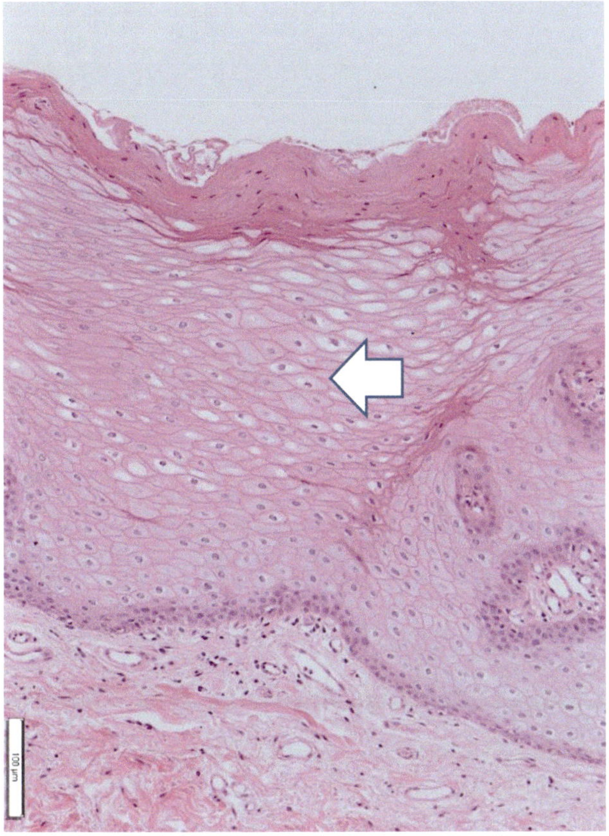

■ **Fig. 30.4** Cells in the spinous layer appear vacuolated and have a pyknotic nucleus (white arrow)

30.13 What Is the Definitive Diagnosis?

Leukoedema

30.14 How Would You Justify Your Definitive Diagnosis?

The patient presented with a long-standing history of whitish patches on both sides of his buccal mucosa. Clinically, the lesions were irregular in shape, non-scrapable and disappeared after the mucosa was stretched (■ Fig. 30.3b). The clinical diagnostic characteristics of the lesion are specific and do not necessitate histopathological examination.

30.15 How Would You Manage This Patient?

Leukoedema does not require treatment. A topical application of tretinoin gel can be considered as it has shown a promising result in symptomatic cases. The patient would require occasional periodical follow-up to assess the progress of the lesion if the patient is concerned about the lesion. Reassurance of the patient is all what is necessary for most cases. Leukoedema is harmless and is not associated with malignancy.

30.16 Leukoedema

Historically, leukoedema was once considered to be a potential precursor to leukoplakia. Recent studies show that leukoedema is a common normal variation of the oral mucosa. It may clinically resemble leukoplakia and lichen planus. Although rare, another white lesion that may have a similar presentation is white sponge nevus. The aetiology of leukoedema is not well understood and is often linked to areas exposed to local irritation, smoking habit and poor oral hygiene. Nevertheless, its association and suspicion to malignancy have been excluded. The prevalence of leukoedema varies in different ethnic groups and in different countries. It may occur in both adults and children, but the incidence of leukoedema varies globally. Studies have shown a definitive racial predilection among individuals of African origin. Leukoedema is most prevalent in adults in the 41–45-year-old age group, but there is no sex predilection. It may occur either unilaterally or bilaterally similar to other white lesions but clinically can be potentially differentiated with a detailed oral mucosal examination as listed in ■ Table 30.1.

Leukoedema is an interesting lesion as there is no consensus on its aetiology. Few studies categorize leukoedema as a congenital white lesion. The association between smoking habit and leukoedema is controversial where some studies have reported a non-significant association. Other conditions such as poor oral hygiene and daily use of spices in highly seasoned foods have been suggested as possible aetiological agents. It is also proposed that leukoedema can be considered as an acquired benign lesion that develops secondary to repeated subclinical insults to the oral mucosa by certain low-grade irritants.

Histopathological examination provides characteristic features. There is an increase in the thickness of the epithelium. The epithelial surface is frequently parakeratinized, and the rete ridges are broad and elongated. The intra-cellular edema secondary to the alteration of semipermeable cell membrane that allows the absorption of extracellular fluid is pronounced within the cells of the stratum spinosum (■ Fig. 30.5). These vacuolated cells appear large and have pyknotic nuclei.

Even though this lesion may have a similar presentation with other white lesions, leukoedema can essentially be diagnosed clinically from the specific salient manifestations, thus not necessitating a biopsy.

Table 30.1 Clinical oral examination to differentiate white lesions

Specific mucosal examination	Characteristic	Clinical diagnosis
Stretching of the mucosa	Lesion becomes less obvious or disappears	Leukoedema
	Lesion does not change significantly	White sponge nevus
	Lesion becomes more prominent	Lichen planus
Scraping of lesion	Unscrapable	Leukoedema
	Scrapable	Pseudomembranous candidiasis
Surface examination	Irregular whitish-grey Mucosal folds with wrinkles or whitish streaks	Leukoedema
	Superficial erosions with irregular white flakes	Morsicatio buccarum
	Fine, white, linear and lace-like lesions on the buccal mucosa	Reticular lichen planus
	Diffuse, thick and corrugated folded white lesions on the buccal mucosa surface	White sponge naevus
	Uniformly white and non-scrapable lesion The surface is flat or slightly wrinkled	Homogenous leukoplakia

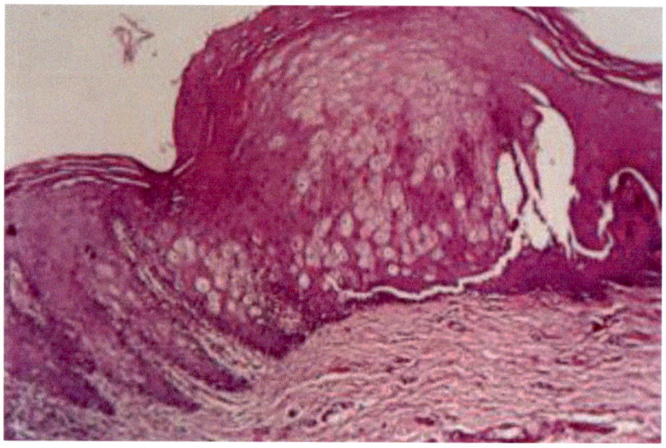

Fig. 30.5 Edematous spinous layer (Nayak et al. 2018)

Salient features of leukoedema	
Clinical features	Diffuse greyish-white, smooth, oedematous film Usually presents bilaterally on the buccal mucosa It tends to occur more commonly in smokers and has also been found to occur with increasing frequency in betel quid chewers
Histopathological features	Hyperparakeratosis and acanthosis of the epithelium. The rete ridges appear broad and elongated. A marked intra-cellular oedema is observed within the cells of the spinous cell layer. The cells appear vacuolated and have a pyknotic nucleus
Treatment	No treatment

Diagnostic Algorithm for Bilateral White Patches of Inner Cheek

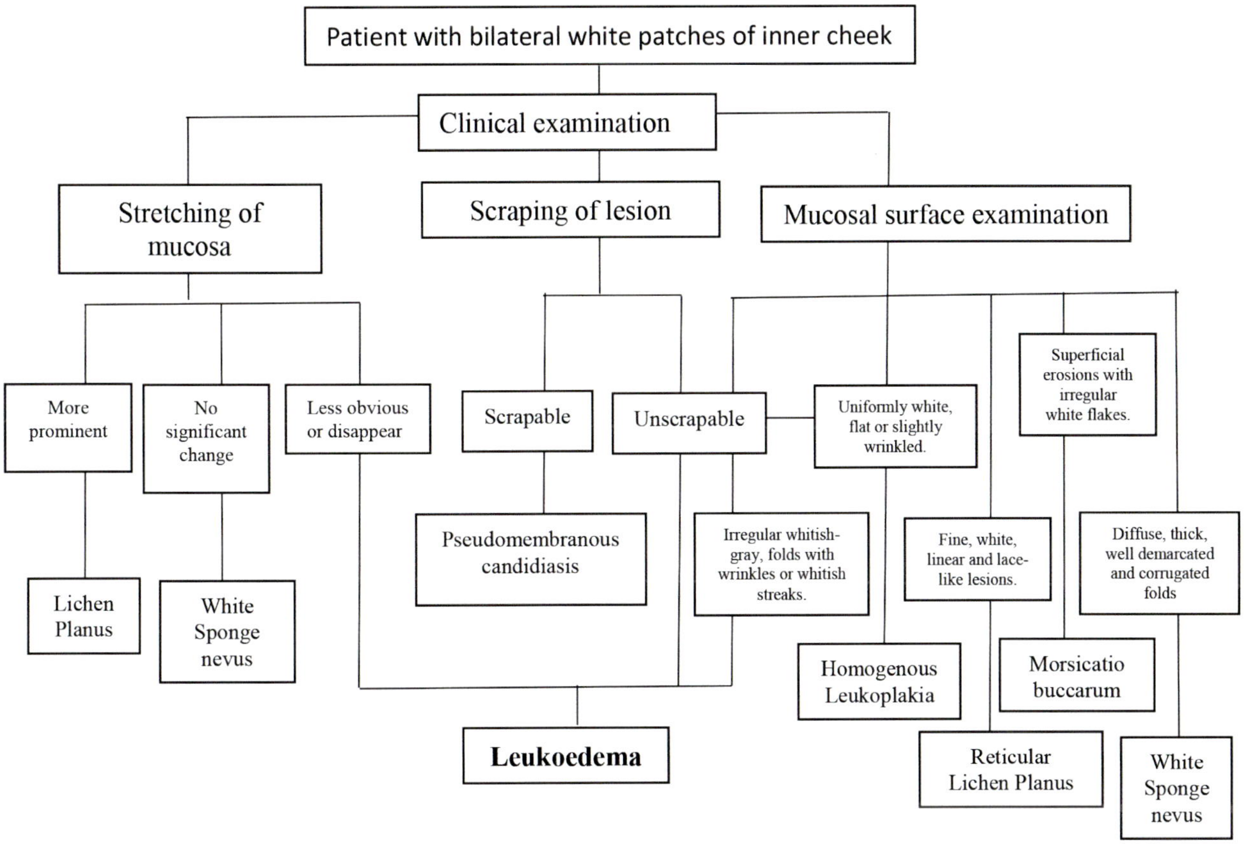

Self-Assessment Questions

1. Discuss the differential diagnosis for bilateral white patches on the buccal mucosa.
2. Describe the specific intra-oral examination findings that can be used to differentiate the different types of oral white lesions.
3. Describe the specific histopathological characteristics that differentiate leukoedema from other white lesions.
4. Outline your management plan for a patient presenting with bilateral white lesions on the buccal mucosa.

Summary

Bilateral white patches on buccal mucosa are relatively common intraoral findings among adult population. Differential diagnoses include leukoedema, lichen planus and white sponge nevus, among others. Arriving at the correct diagnosis is compulsory as different diseases in this group are diverse in terms of behaviour and treatment.

Further Reading

Anuna LM, Keerthilatha MP, Amar AS, Manoj V. The prevalence of oral mucosal lesions in patients visiting a dental school in southern India. Indian J Dent Res. 2008;19:99–103.

Hammer JE, Mehta FS, Pindborg J, Daftary DK. An epidemiologic and histopathologic study of leukoedema among 50, 915 rural Indian villagers. Oral Surg Oral Med Oral Pathol. 1971;32:58–65.

Huang BW, Lin CW, Lee YP, Chiang CP. Differential diagnosis between leukoedema and white spongy nevus. J Dent Sci. 2020;15:554–5.

Joshi M, Tailor M. Prevalence of most commonly reported tobacco-associated lesions in Central Gujarat: a hospital-based cross-sectional study. Indian J Dent Res. 2016;27:405–9.

Martin JL. Leukoedema: a review of the literature. J Natl Med Assoc. 1992;84:938–40.

Mortazavi H, Safi Y, Baharvand M, Jafari S, Anbari F, Rahmani S. Oral white lesions: an updated clinical diagnostic decision tree. Dent J (Basel). 2019;7(1):15. https://doi.org/10.3390/dj7010015.

Nayak VN, Girish HC, Murgod S, Narahari R, Kumar BNY. Leukoedema of the buccal mucosa -a case report. J Med Radiol Pathol Surg. 2018;5:16–7.

Negm SA. Unilateral leucoedema-case report. Int J Dent Clin. 2013;5:21–2.

van Wyk CW. An investigation into the association between leukoedema and smoking. J Oral Pathol. 1985;14:491–9.

Irregular Red Patches on the Dorsum of the Tongue: Benign Migratory Glossitis

Nadeena S. S. Jayasuriya and Wanninayake M Tilakaratne

Contents

W. M Tilakaratne, T. G. Kallarakkal (eds.), *Clinicopathological Correlation of Oral Diseases*,
https://doi.org/10.1007/978-3-031-24408-7_31

Learning Goals

1. Devise the correct way of compiling the history with appropriate questions.
2. Develop a differential diagnosis after history taking.
3. Deduce appropriate procedures in clinical examination.
4. Formulate a differential diagnosis combining findings in the history and clinical examination.
5. Justify the relevant investigations required to arrive at the diagnosis.
6. Comprehend the importance of clinicopathological correlation in arriving at the correct diagnosis.
7. Outline the management plan.
8. Recognize the importance of a diagnostic algorithm in arriving at a diagnosis.

31.1 Main Complaint

A 40-year-old man complained of a red area on the left side of the dorsum of his tongue.

31.2 History of Complaint

Question: When did you first notice this?

I noticed it about 6 months ago.

31.3 Additional Complaints

Question: Have you noticed similar lesions elsewhere in the mouth?

I also noticed similar lesions on the right side of the tongue. But now they have healed.

Question: During this time, did you notice any change to its shape or position?

The red area seems to have healed and appeared in a new area.

Question: Does the red area hurt or cause any irritation?

I have no symptoms and can consume normal food without any discomfort or pain.

Question: Do you have fissuring or grooves on the surface of the tongue?

I have not noticed any fissuring or any other anomalies on the surface of the tongue.

Question: Do you have a similar red area on the roof of the mouth?

I don't have red patches anywhere else in the mouth.

Question: Do you eat green vegetables and meat?

I eat a healthy meal.

Question: Did you have any abdominal pain or was diagnosed with abdominal and intestinal conditions?

I had no symptoms and was not diagnosed with any gastro-intestinal disorders.

Question: Do you have any family history of blood disorders?

There is no family history of blood disorders.

Question: Do you get tired easily?

I don't get tired after doing my daily chores. I routinely go to the gym.

Question: Have you taken anti-worm treatment as recommended?

I have taken it a long time ago.

Question: Do you have diabetes? Did you notice a recent weight loss, increased urination?

I don't have any symptoms to suggest diabetes.

Question: Do you have allergies, asthma, psoriasis or other skin conditions?

I have no known symptoms to suggest any allergic or skin conditions.

Question: Did you have joint pains, eye irritations or other red patches anywhere else in the body?

I don't have such symptoms, and I am otherwise healthy.

Question: Do your parents have such patches on their tongue?

My parents do not have any similar lesions on the tongue.

Question: Did you have any other illnesses, or have you undergone surgeries in the past?

I don't have any significant past medical or surgical history.

Question: Do you have habits such as betel chewing, smoking or excessive alcohol consumption?

31

I don't have these habits except taking a little alcohol in social gatherings.

31.4 With the Findings From the History, What Is Your Differential Diagnosis?

1. Benign migratory glossitis (BMG).
2. Anaemia.
3. Erythematous candidosis.
4. Median rhomboid glossitis (MRG).
5. Erosive lichen planus (ELP).
6. Early stage of Reiter's syndrome.
7. Atopic or allergic stomatitis.
8. Fissured tongue/ scrotal tongue.
9. Erythroplakia.

31.5 How Do You Justify Your Differential Diagnosis After History Taking?

The patient has a red patch on the dorsum of his tongue. Such depapillated red areas on the tongue may occur due to various reasons such as BMG, median rhomboid glossitis, oral lichen planus (erosive type), allergies and scrotal tongue.

BMG can appear as a reddish patch on the dorsum of the tongue which changes its position with time. BMG is mostly asymptomatic and should be the first in the list of differential diagnoses. The patient noticed the migrating nature which is suggestive of BMG.

Anaemia due to hook worms and nutritional deficiencies cause depapillation of the tongue with atrophy of filiform and fungiform papillae. As hook-worm infestation is common in South Asia, this could be considered as a possible differential diagnosis. Blood disorders such as thalassemia and haemophilia can lead to blood loss and anaemia. Though anaemia is a possibility, depapillation due to loss of both fungiform and filiform papillae may cause a more generalized atrophy of the tongue which was not the complaint in the present case. In addition, the patient is well nourished, has no family history of blood disorders and has no symptoms to suggest anaemia. He also doesn't have any abdominal symptoms to suggest chronic intestinal disease. Considering the above, depapillation due to anaemia is unlikely although it can be included in the differential diagnosis.

Erythematous candidosis is characterized by red lesions and includes acute atrophic candidosis, chronic atrophic candidosis. Acute atrophic candidosis presents as erythematous patches commonly on the palate, buccal mucosa and dorsum of the tongue. The predisposing factors include a course of broad spectrum antibiotics, HIV disease, oral corticosteroids, uncontrolled diabetes mellitus, iron and Vit-B12 deficiency anaemia. Chronic atrophic candidosis appears as erythematous areas restricted to the oral mucosa in contact with the dentures. The patient is healthy otherwise with no history of antibiotic or corticosteroid therapy. The patient is not a denture wearer. However, erythematous candidosis is included in the differential diagnosis owing to the history of red lesions on the tongue.

Median rhomboid glossitis (MRG) is a common reddish/pinkish patch on the dorsum of the tongue and should be included in the differential diagnosis. It is mostly seen in adult patients and may be symptomatic in some. Usually, a corresponding lesion may also be seen on the palate. As the patient clearly complains of red areas on the lateral side of the dorsum of the tongue together which was migratory in nature, MRG may be an unlikely differential diagnosis.

Erosive oral lichen planus (EOLP) may also present on the dorsum of the tongue as a reddish patch. EOLP is usually symptomatic involving multiple areas of the oral mucosa. As the lesion is asymptomatic and confined to the tongue, the possibility of EOLP unlikely.

Atopic or allergic stomatitis may be caused by oral hygiene products, dental materials, habits, as well as low-grade oral inflammatory conditions. The characteristic clinical manifestations include angioedema, erosions, bullous and ulcerative lesions, burning sensation, redness of the mucosa, white patches, lichenoid reactions and dysesthesia. The patient does not have any history of allergies. There are no findings in the history to suggest any source of allergies such as dental treatment or dental hygiene products such as use of a new mouth wash or a tooth paste. Atopic or allergic stomatitis is included in the differential diagnosis in view of the history of red lesions on the tongue.

Erythematous lesions of the tongue associated with Reiter's syndrome (RS), allergies and fissured tongue should also be excluded with the history. Reiter's syndrome is accompanied with arthritis, conjunctivitis and urethritis. Erythema of the tongue may be the first presentation of Reiter's syndrome and may mimic a geographic tongue. Therefore, RS should be suspected.

Fissured tongue is characterized clinically by multiple fissures and grooves on the dorsal surface of the tongue. Although fissured tongue is thought to be hereditary, published studies show that its occurrence is influenced by age. As the patient claims not to have fissuring of the tongue or burning sensations, a fissured tongue is not a favoured differential diagnosis.

Erythroplakia is a high-risk oral potentially malignant disorder presenting as a fiery red lesion. However, this is an unlikely differential diagnosis as the patient says that the lesion is migrating and some areas have healed which is not a feature of erythroplakia. In addition, the patient does not practice any risky habits.

31.6 Findings of Clinical Examination

His extra-oral examination is normal. Intra-orally, a pinkish/reddish area is noted on the left side of the dorsum of the anterior two-thirds of the tongue (Fig. 31.1).

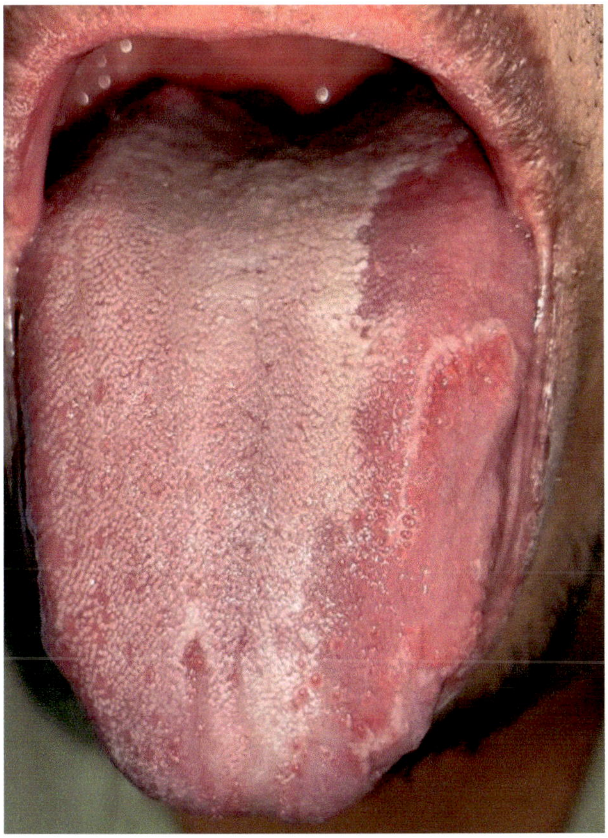

Fig. 31.1 Well-defined reddish/pinkish depapillated area is present on the left dorsum of the anterior two-thirds of the tongue. The margins are slightly elevated with a white colour

The erythematous areas are depapillated and well demarcated with clear elevated margins. The tongue is not fissured. There are no other similar lesions elsewhere in the oral cavity.

31.7 What Other Relevant Features Would You Look for with the Findings You Have So Far?

The patient has a normal body mass index with a healthy appearance. Anaemia was excluded as his palpebral conjunctivae and oral mucous membrane are of the normal pink colour. On general examination, no other skin lesions are noted.

31.8 What Is Your Clinical Differential Diagnosis?

1. BMG.
2. Anaemia.
3. Median rhomboid glossitis—candidal infection. (Although candiadal infection is a differential diagnosis, MRG is unlikely as the site is not correct)
4. Erosive lichen planus/lichenoid reaction.

31.9 How Would You Exclude Other Conditions and Justify the Inclusion of the Diseases That You Have Mentioned in the Differential Diagnosis to Arrive at a Working Diagnosis?

31.9.1 BMG

Asymptomatic well-defined depapillated areas on the dorsum of the tongue are mostly suggestive of BMG. The asymmetric location on the dorsum of the tongue is typical for BMG as it spreads to the lateral margins. In this patient, the typical elevated whitish margins around the pink areas are seen clearly. The patient noticed migration of the lesions with time. Considering the above findings, BMG is a highly suggestive diagnosis.

31

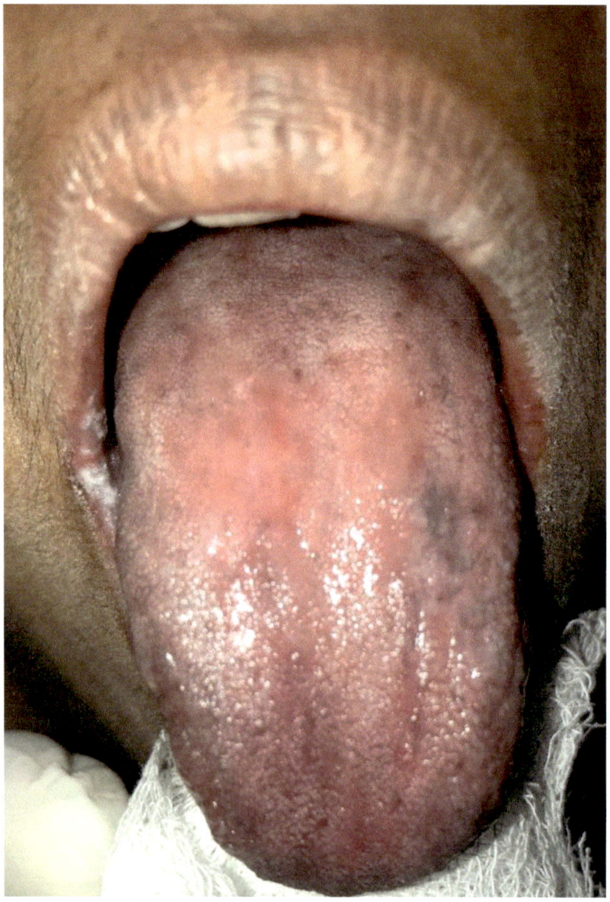

Fig. 31.2 The diagram shows the tongue of a patient with generalized depapillation associated with anaemia. Angular stomatitis can also be seen on the right commissure of the lip

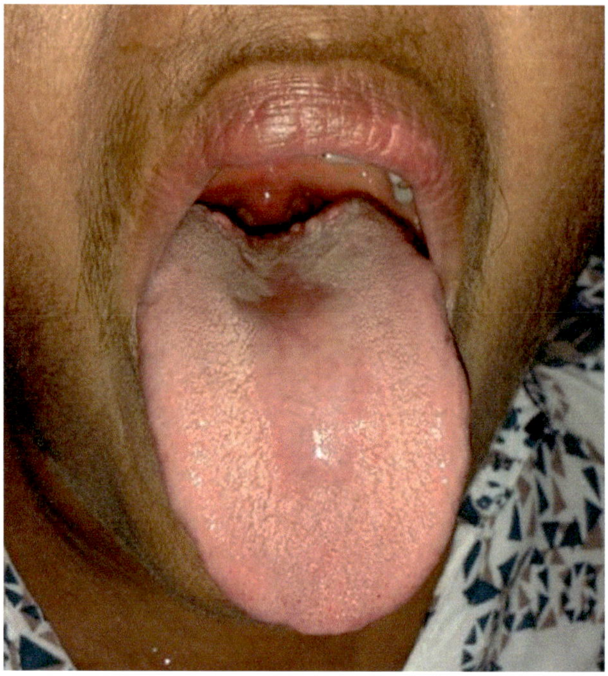

Fig. 31.3 Patient with median rhomboid glossitis of the tongue. Depapillation is seen at the central area on the dorsum of the tongue. (Courtesy of Dr. Chandira Gunasena)

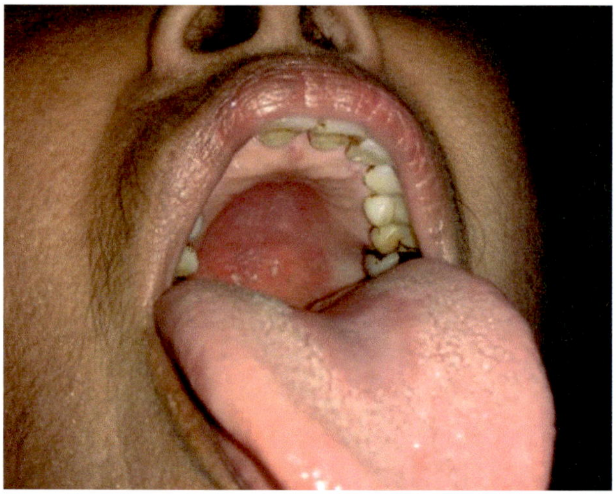

Fig. 31.4 "Kissing lesion" on the palate in a patient with median rhomboid glossitis. (Curtesy of Dr. Chandira Gunasena)

31.9.2 Anaemia

Depapillation with pinkish areas would be suspicious of glossitis due to anaemia. As his palpebral conjunctivae and oral mucous membranes are of normal colour, anaemia is unlikely. The typical feature of anaemia would be a generalized depapillation of the tongue (Fig. 31.2). Therefore, anaemia is unlikely in this patient.

31.10 Median Rhomboid Glossitis (MRG)

Median rhomboid glossitis causes a prominent reddish area on the centre of the tongue (Fig. 31.3). It is usually symptomatic and associated with a similar erythema on the palate also known as a kissing lesion due to candidate infection (Fig. 31.4). MRG is mostly a single large area on the middle part of the dorsum of the tongue. The absence of these clinical features makes MRG an unlikely differential diagnosis.

31.11 Erosive Oral Lichen Planus (EOLP)

Erosive lichen planus may appear as a red area on the dorsum of the tongue (Fig. 31.5). These lesions are symptomatic with burning sensation especially when consuming spicy food. The typical raised margins would not be seen in EOLP. Due to these reasons, EOLP is unlikely.

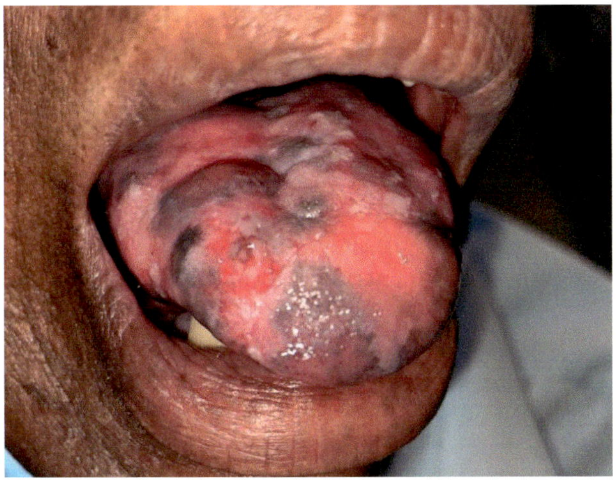

Fig. 31.5 A patient with erosive lichen planus of the dorsum of the tongue. Active lesions are seen as red areas, and the healed lesions are pigmented

31.12 What Is the Most Likely Diagnosis?

Benign Migratory Glossitis (BMG).

31.13 How Would You Investigate This Patent?

1. Full-blood count and blood picture.
2. Brush biopsy for candidal infection.

31.14 What Findings Would You Expect From the Above Investigations?

The patient's blood report is normal with good levels of haemoglobin and with normochromic normocytic cells. In case of anaemia, low haemoglobin levels with an abnormal blood picture would be expected. The brush biopsy and cytological examination did not show candidal hyphae.

31.15 How Can We Confirm the Diagnosis of BMG?

The diagnosis of BMG can be arrived at with the findings of the history and examination and by excluding other similar conditions. BMG is mostly asymptomatic. Rare forms of symptomatic BMG can be seen in some patients. In such patients, investigations to exclude the differential diagnoses are important.

31.16 What Are the Histopathological Features of BMG?

Histopathologic examination reveals hyperparakeratosis, spongiosis, acanthosis and elongation of the epithelial rete ridges. Collections of neutrophils are observed within the epithelium. The intense neutrophilic infiltrate may be responsible for the destruction of the superficial portion of the epithelium producing an atrophic and reddened mucosa (Figs. 31.6 and 31.7) The histopathological features can resemble those of psoriasis.

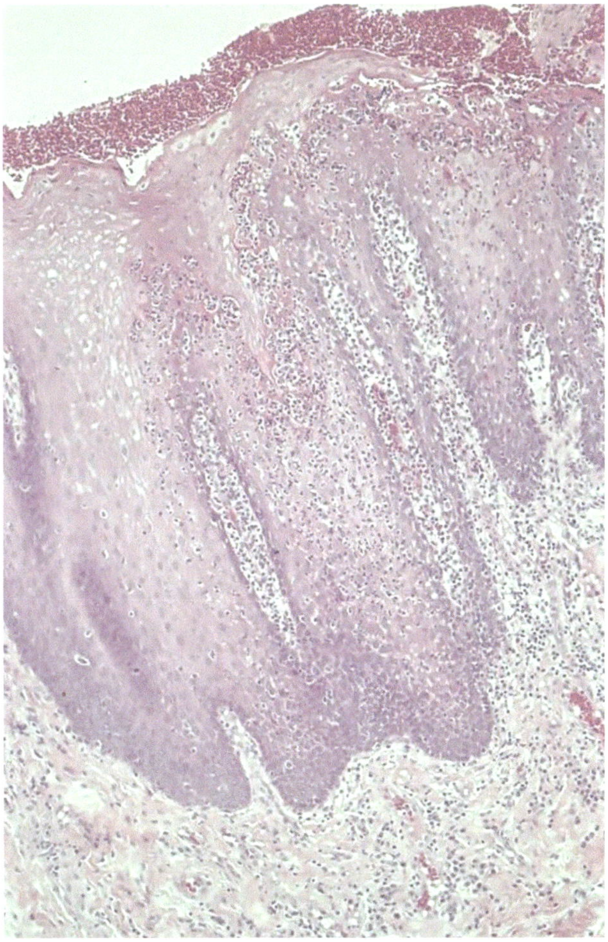

Fig. 31.6 Benign migratory glossitis: The epithelium showing hyperparakeratosis, spongiosis, acanthosis and elongation of the epithelial rete ridges

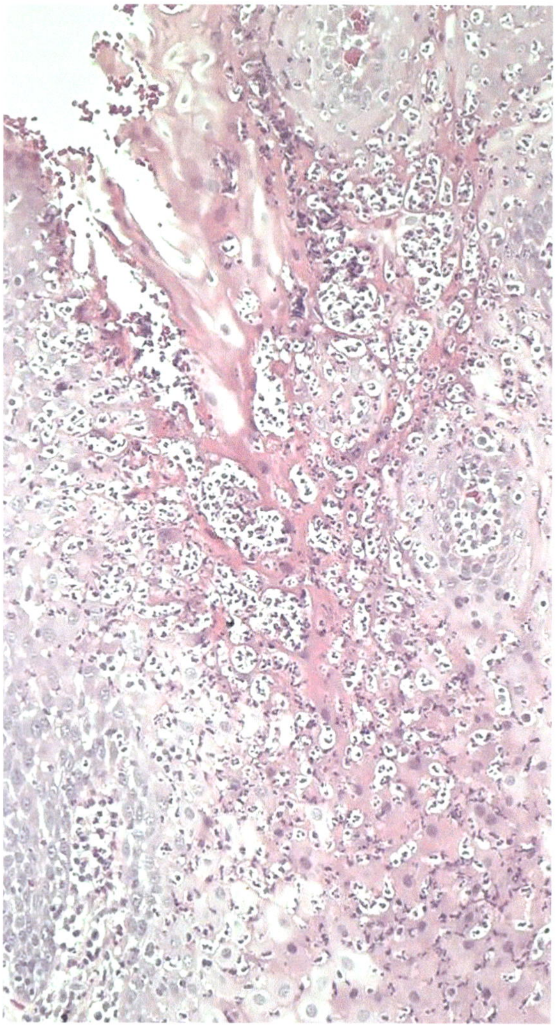

Fig. 31.7 Benign migratory glossitis: Numerous foci of collection of neutrophils are observed within the epithelium

31.17 How Would You Manage This Patent?

The patient is asymptomatic. Hence, the management should include only reassurance and education. The patient can be reviewed in the clinic if he develops symptoms.

31.18 What Is the Follow-Up Plan and Prognosis?

BMG is a benign condition and is asymptomatic. No further investigations or treatment is necessary. Patient maybe followed up in the clinic if symptoms develop. The condition has a good prognosis.

31.19 Benign Migratory Glossitis (BMG)

Benign migratory glossitis is referred to by multiple names such as geographic tongue (due to the world map-–like appearance), erythema migrans, annular migrans and wandering rash of the tongue. BMG is a harmless inflammatory condition of the dorsum of the tongue of unknown aetiology. BMG was first described by Rayer in 1831. BMG is characterized clinically by depapillation of the tongue which is non-ulcerative and bordered by a well-defined raised white/yellow margins. The lesions start to appear from a younger age and is found in 1–3% of the general population. BMG is more common in children, and the incidence reduces with age and maybe twice as common in females than males. Classically, BMG has no association with other disease conditions. Some clinicians postulate a hereditary nature to the condition.

The differential diagnoses for BMG include early changes of anaemia, median rhomboid glossitis and erosive oral lichen planus. Apart from these, BMG can have similarities with Reiter's syndrome, atopy and allergies, fissured tongue, psychological imbalances and in conditions such as diabetes. At least 50% of geographic tongue is associated with fissured tongue and has a higher frequency of occurring in parents and siblings suggesting a genetic inheritance. Psoriasis, geographic tongue and fissured tongue share a polygenic inheritance. Though, majority of the cases are asymptomatic, symptomatic lesions have also been reported in the literature. Even in asymptomatic patients, significant anxiety may develop due to fear of oral cancer. The symptoms can develop when there are extensive lesions. Burning sensation, discomfort and pain are some of the reported symptoms. As there is no specific investigation for the diagnosis of BMG, history and the clinical findings of a long-standing migratory reddish patch which changes its colour and shape in the absence of any other disease condition are confirmatory of BMG.

The management is focused on reassuring the patients of the benign and self-limiting nature of the condition. For symptomatic patients, topical steroids, anti-inflammatory agents or topical anaesthesia may be prescribed. For refractory cases, systemic antihistamines, systemic steroids or immune modulators such as tacrolimus can be used. All patients should be advised to avoid spicy food and irritants and to maintain good oral hygiene. Due to the association with more serious conditions mentioned above, even an asymptomatic patient needs to be clinically screened. Referral to a relevant specialist maybe considered when other symptoms or signs are suspected.

Management of BMG

Disease manifestation	Clinical presentation	Investigations	Management
Asymptomatic BMG	Pinkish red areas on the dorsum of the tongue that change position with time. No pain or burning sensation when consuming food.	Not needed	Reassurance
Symptomatic BMG	Pinkish red areas on the dorsum of the tongue that change position with time. Pain or burning sensation when consuming food	Smear from the surface of the tongue to exclude candidal infection	If negative for a fungal infection Topical • Steroids • Anti-inflammatory agents • Analgesics Systemic • Steroids • Antihistamines Immune modulators If positive for fungal infections Treatment with topical antifungals
Associated with other systemic conditions	Apart from the tongue lesions, the patient may develop other symptoms and signs E.g.: Psoriatic skin lesions-psoriasis Polyarthritis-Reiter's syndrome	Blood investigations C-reactive protein and ESR to assess an inflammatory disease process Incision biopsy to exclude oral lichen planus/psoriasis	Referral to a specialist

Salient features of Benign migratory glossitis	
Clinical	Reddish/pinkish asymptomatic patches on the dorsum of the tongue that are bordered by a raised white/yellow border. The areas change position from time to time. Symptomatic forms maybe present rarely. Some forms of BMG like lesions may occur with other conditions such as fissured tongue, Reiter's syndrome and psoriasis
Histopathology	Hyperparakeratosis, spongiosis, acanthosis and elongation of the epithelial rete ridges. Collections of neutrophils are observed within the epithelium
Treatment	When asymptomatic, no treatment is necessary. Symptomatic lesions can be treated with mild steroids, anti-inflammatory agents and antifungals (if positive for fungal infections)

BMG is a benign asymptomatic condition that can cause concern in patients. Management includes patient education and reassurance. When these lesions are associated with other systemic conditions, referral to a specialist is necessary.

31

Management Algorithm of BMG

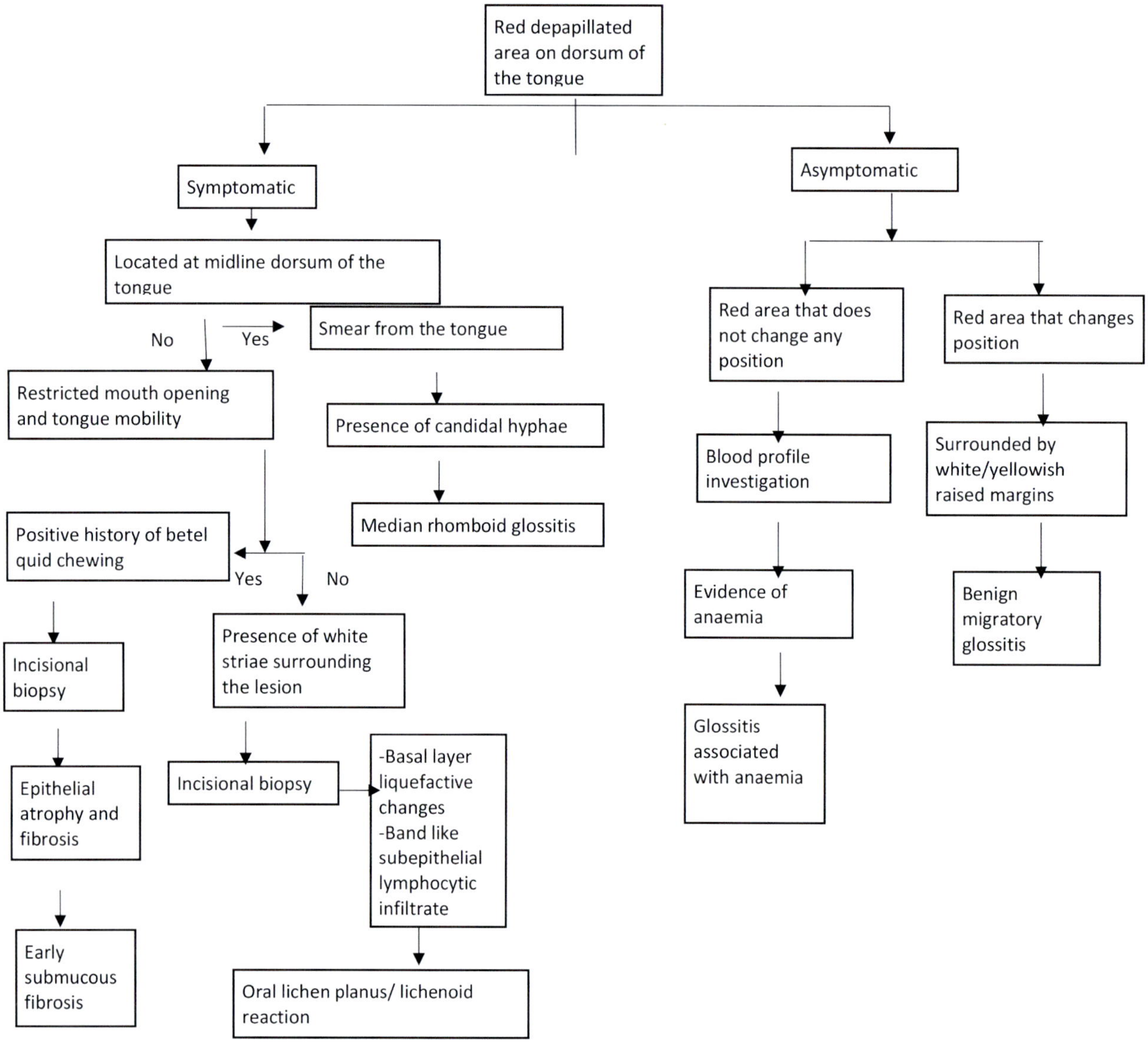

Self-Assessment Questions

1. Name the characteristic clinical features of BMG that helps in the diagnosis.
2. Discuss the differential diagnoses of BMG.
3. Describe the histopathological features of BMG.
4. Discuss the investigations for a patient with erythematous area on the dorsum of the tongue.
5. Outline the treatment for a symptomatic case of BMG.

Further Reading

Assimakopoulos D, Patrikakos G, Fotika C, Elisaf M. Benign migratory glossitis or geographic tongue: an enigmatic oral lesion. Am J Med. 2002;113(9):751–5.

Bánóczy J, Szabó L, Csiba Á. Migratory glossitis: a clinical-histologic review of seventy cases. Oral Surg Oral Med Oral Pathol. 1975;39(1):113–21.

de Campos WG, Esteves CV, Fernandes LG, Domaneschi C, Júnior CAL. Treatment of symptomatic benign migratory glossitis: a systematic review. Clin Oral Investig. 2018;22(7):2487–93.

Marks R, Czarny D. Geographic tongue: sensitivity to the environment. Oral Surg Oral Med Oral Pathol. 1984;58(2):156–9.

Nandini DB, Bhavana SB, Deepak BS, Ashwini R. Paediatric geographic tongue: a case report, review and recent updates. J Clin Diagn Res. 2016;10(2):ZE05–ZE9. https://doi.org/10.7860/JCDR/2016/16452.7191.

Wysocki GP, Daley TD. Benign migratory glossitis in patients with juvenile diabetes. Oral Surg Oral Med Oral Pathol. 1987;63(1):68–70.

Zegarelli DJ. Burning mouth: an analysis of 57 patients. Oral Surg Oral Med Oral Pathol. 1984;58(1):34–8.

Zunt SL, Tomich CE. Erythema migrans—a psoriasiform lesion of the oral mucosa. J Dermatol Surg Oncol. 1989;15(10):1067–70.

Oral Mucosal Ulcerations

Contents

Ulceration Related to New Dentures: Traumatic Ulcer

Thomas George Kallarakkal and Karthick Sekar

Contents

W. M Tilakaratne, T. G. Kallarakkal (eds.), *Clinicopathological Correlation of Oral Diseases*,
https://doi.org/10.1007/978-3-031-24408-7_32

Learning Goals

1. Devise the correct way of compiling the history with appropriate questions.
2. Develop a differential diagnosis after history taking.
3. Deduce appropriate procedures in clinical examination.
4. Formulate a differential diagnosis combining findings in the history and clinical examination.
5. Justify the relevant investigations required to arrive at the diagnosis.
6. Comprehend the importance of clinicopathological correlation in arriving at the correct diagnosis.
7. Outline the management plan.
8. Recognize the importance of a diagnostic algorithm in arriving at a diagnosis.

32.1 Chief Complaint

A 58-year-old male patient presented to the clinic with a complaint of pain and discomfort inside his mouth.

32.2 History of Complaint

Question: Where do you feel the pain?

I feel the pain inside the mouth at the back region of my lower right jaw.

Question: When did you first notice the pain?

I first felt the pain about 3 weeks ago. It initially started as mild soreness and later on increased in severity.

Question: How did the pain start?

I got a new set of upper and lower dentures a month ago. I started to feel soreness at the back region of my lower right jaw about 1 week after using the new dentures. I ignored the soreness and continued to use the dentures till the pain became very severe.

Question: How severe is the pain if you were to grade the pain on a scale of 0–10?

The pain is very severe and can be graded as 8/10. I am not able to eat with the dentures on.

Question: What is the nature of the pain?

The pain is usually burning in nature.

Question: Does the pain radiate anywhere?

The pain radiates to my neck on the right side.

Question: Does the pain follow any pattern as being present during specific times of the day?

The pain does not follow any specific pattern and is present throughout the day.

Question: Are there any aggravating or relieving factors associated with the pain?

The pain becomes more severe when eating spicy, salty and sour food. The pain also gets aggravated upon taking hard food with my dentures on and especially while biting on the right side.

Question: Did you take any medications to relieve the pain?

I took tablet Ibuprofen 400 mg three times a day for 1 week. I used to get relief from the pain on taking the medication. I stopped taking the medication as I was feeling nauseous and constipated after taking the medication.

Question: Are there any signs or symptoms associated with the pain?

I noticed an ulcer at the area where I felt the pain. I am worried about the ulcer, and so I decided to get an appointment.

Question: Do you have a history of recurrent ulcers in the past?

In the past, I occasionally used to get oral ulcers due to accidental trauma during tooth brushing or biting on the tongue or cheek during mealtimes. I haven't got any ulcers in my mouth ever since my teeth were extracted.

Question: Did you hold any medications such as aspirin or ibuprofen in the area to relieve the pain?

I did not hold any medications in the area to relieve the pain.

Question: Did you have any fever or sore throat associated with the ulcer?

I did not have any such symptoms.

Question: When did you first notice the ulcer?

- I first noticed the ulcer 3 days ago, when I removed my dentures to inspect the area of pain as it was becoming worse.

- Question: Is the ulcer painful?

- The ulcer is very tender.

- Question: Where is the ulcer located?

- The ulcer is located near my lower posterior gum on the right side adjacent to the area where the denture rests.

- Question: Did you notice a blister prior to the development of the ulcer?

- I do not remember noticing any blister in that area.

- Question: Is there any bleeding from the ulcer?

- The ulcer does not bleed.

- Question: Do you have ulcers anywhere else inside the mouth or elsewhere on the body?

- I do not have any ulcers elsewhere in my mouth or on the body.

- Question: Are you using the new pair of dentures now?

- I used to wear the new dentures regularly until 3 days ago. I have not been wearing them regularly ever since due to the pain.

- Question: Did you experience similar soreness or ulcers with your old dentures?

- I never experienced any kind of similar symptoms with my old dentures.

- Question: What was the reason to get a new pair of dentures?

- My old lower denture broke about 1 year ago after using it for almost 5 years. The dentures were similar to my new dentures. I was not able to eat well for the past 1 year as I was unable to chew without my dentures. Due to lack of time and financial constraints, I could not make a new pair immediately.

- Question: Did you come in for the follow-up appointment after the dentures were given to you?

- I could not come for the follow-up appointment as I had work commitments.

- Question: Do you have any other medical problems such as heart disease, high blood pressure, diabetes, bleeding disorder or respiratory diseases?

- I was diagnosed with hypertension 4 years ago, and I am currently on tablet Amlodipine 10 mg once a day.

- Question: Does anybody in your family have a history of similar ulcers?

- My family members are all healthy and do not have a history of similar oral ulcers.

- Question: Do you have multiple sexual partners?

- I do not have multiple sexual partners. I live with my wife and two children.

- Question: Are you allergic to any foods?

- I do not have any allergies.

- Question: Do you have any gastrointestinal symptoms such as abdominal pain, diarrhoea, constipation or blood in stools?

- I developed nausea and constipation a few days after taking tablet Ibuprofen for the pain. I do not have any such symptoms now as I stopped taking the medication.

- Question: Why did you have your teeth extracted?

- I got all my teeth removed, over time since the age of 48 years as they had become very loose gradually.

- Question: Have you undergone any surgery?

- I have not undergone any surgery in the past.

- Question: Do you have any risk habits such as smoking or drinking alcohol?

- I smoke about 5–10 cigarettes a day and drink when I meet up with my friends.

- Question: Are you employed?

- I am currently working as a supervisor at a furniture company.

32.3 With the Findings From the History, What Is Your Differential Diagnosis?

1. Traumatic ulcer
2. Drug-induced ulcer
3. Major aphthous ulcer
4. Oral squamous cell carcinoma

32.4 How Do You Justify Your Differential Diagnosis After History Taking?

The patient complains of severe burning pain over the lower back region of his right lower jaw that initially started as a soreness and eventually developed into a painful ulcer. The pain is exacerbated upon eating spicy, salty and sour food and on using the dentures to chew hard food. The symptoms coincide with the use of his new dentures. Traumatic ulcers are usually acute in onset and appear in short painful episodes.

Drug-induced ulcers generally manifest as isolated, solitary ulcers usually on the side of the tongue. They are relatively resistant to treatment and persist until the offending agent is removed. Non-steroidal anti-inflammatory agents are the drugs most likely to cause oral ulcers. Other drugs that can cause oral ulcers include antithyroid drugs, calcium channel blockers, cytotoxic drugs, bisphosphonates and beta blockers. The patient is currently on calcium antagonist, tablet Amlodipine 10 mg once a day. He has also been taking tablet Ibuprofen 400 mg three times a day until a week ago for his pain. Hence, drug-induced ulcer is included in the differential diagnosis.

Recurrent aphthous stomatitis (RAS) is an inflammatory disease of unknown origin characterized by recurrent and painful ulcers that usually affects the non-keratinized oral mucosa such as the buccal mucosa, labial mucosa, ventral surface of the tongue, floor of the mouth and soft palate. RAS usually has a multifactorial aetiology which may include stress, familial and genetic factors, autoimmune factors, hormonal changes, hypersensitivity to certain foods, drugs, B12 or folate deficiencies, zinc deficit, tobacco, local trauma, infectious agents and various systemic diseases. A diagnosis of RAS is unlikely as the patient did not give a history of recurrent episodes of oral ulceration. He also did not have any history to suggest hereditary causes or any underlying systemic disease. However, the patient has not been eating well for the past 1 year as his old denture had broken. He might have developed nutritional deficiencies that may have predisposed him to (RAS). A major aphthous ulcer is included in the differential diagnosis as the patient complains of only a single painful ulcer.

Oral squamous cell carcinoma (OSCC) is the most common malignancy in the oral cavity and is associated with risk habits such as tobacco and alcohol use. The patient is a smoker and consumes alcohol. OSCC tends to occur more commonly in elderly males with high-risk habits. OSCC can manifest as a chronic solitary ulcer that may be asymptomatic in the early stages. The patient presents with an acute painful ulcer of few days duration. It may be possible that the ulcer might have been present earlier but was left unnoticed due to its asymptomatic nature. The gender, age of the patient, history of high-risk habits and the clinic presentation of an ulcer warrant inclusion of OSCC in the differential diagnosis.

Syphilis was not considered in the differential diagnosis as the patient did not give a history of sexual promiscuity. The primary lesion in syphilis, a chancre is typically a painless, large ulcer with an indurated margin. There is often an associated painless regional lymphadenopathy. In the present case, the ulcer was painful unlike that seen in patients with syphilis. Moreover, the location of the ulcer was not a common site for chancre which tends to occur more commonly on the lips, tongue and palate. The patient did not give any history suggestive of an immunosuppressed or immunocompromised status. He did not have any symptoms such as weight loss, cough or haemoptysis consistent with systemic bacterial infections such as tuberculosis and fungal infections such as histoplasmosis. Disseminated bacterial and fungal infections can manifest as chronic painful solitary ulcers usually on the ventral or the dorsal surface of the tongue and are a severe complication secondary to HIV infection. He did not have any gastrointestinal symptoms such as abdominal pain or diarrhoea to suggest Crohn disease and ulcerative colitis. The primary oral manifestation in Crohn disease is multiple, deep, linear ulcers on the buccal mucosa and mucobuccal folds, whereas in ulcerative colitis, aphthous-like ulcers and scattered or clumped linearly oriented pustules on an erythematous base are seen.

32.5 Findings of Clinical Examination

The patient is stable, afebrile with a blood pressure of 136/82 mm of Hg and a pulse rate of 82 beats per minute. Extra-oral examination does not reveal any facial asymmetry. The range of mouth opening is normal with no signs of clicking or symptoms of pain in the temporomandibular joints. There is a palpable submandibular lymph node on the right side measuring less than 1 cm in size. The lymph node is tender and not fixed to the underlying tissue or overlying skin.

On intra-oral examination, the patient is completely edentulous. The oral mucosa appears moist with pooling of saliva in the floor of the mouth. The residual alveolar ridge is of fair height and width on the upper

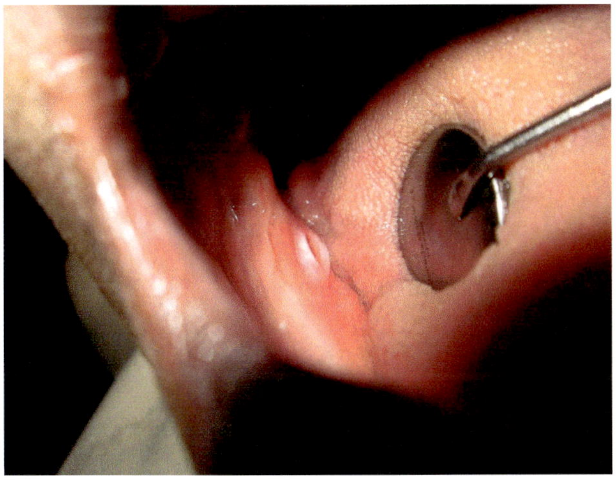

Fig. 32.1 A solitary ulcer measuring approximately 1 cm × 0.5 cm on the right lower alveolar ridge on the lingual aspect. (Picture courtesy: Prof Dr. Ruwan D Jayasinghe Faculty of Dental Sciences, University of Peradeniya, Sri Lanka)

and lower jaws. The mucosa overlying the residual alveolar ridge is of normal colour, texture and consistency. There is a solitary ulcer measuring approximately 1 cm × 0.5 cm, located on the right lower alveolar ridge on the lingual aspect (Fig. 32.1). The ulcer is oval in shape with a yellowish grey base and has well-defined keratotic margins. The margins of the ulcer are slightly everted. On palpation, the ulcer is tender and not indurated. The rest of the oral cavity is normal with no other ulcers, red or white lesions and blisters seen.

Examination of the patient's dentures shows that they are made of heat-cured acrylic and replace all teeth in the upper and lower jaws. The denture hygiene is good. They are fairly well fitting. The lower denture is slightly less stable and has an over extended lingual flange, especially on the right side.

32.6 What Is the Most Likely Clinical Differential Diagnosis?

Traumatic Ulcer

32.7 How Would You Exclude Other Conditions and Justify the Inclusion of the Diseases That You Have Mentioned in the Clinical Differential Diagnosis?

The patient has been taking tablet Amlodipine 10 mg once a day for the past 4 years. He did not have any similar episodes of oral ulceration in the past other than that caused due to trauma while brushing his teeth or eating when he was dentulous. Hence, it is highly unlikely that the patient's ulcer might have been induced by tablet Amlodipine. He also took tablet Ibuprofen 400 mg three times a day for 1 week for relief of his pain. The ulcer persisted even after stopping the medication. Drug-induced ulcers normally resolve after stopping the offending drug. Hence, it is not likely that the ulcer seen in this patient would have been induced by tablet Ibuprofen. Recurrent major aphthae present as deep painful ulcers that are usually more than 1 cm in size and have a predilection for the lips and the soft palate. They persist for several weeks and heal with scarring. The absence of any scarring on the oral mucosa and a negative history of recurrence excluded a diagnosis of recurrent aphthous major.

The patient presented with a painful ulcer. The ulcer might have been present for many days even though the patient noticed it only 3 days ago. On clinical examination, the ulcer was not indurated. The ulcer had a yellowish-grey base with well-defined keratotic margins. There was a palpable right submandibular lymph node that was tender and mobile. These features were more consistent with an inflammatory process rather than a neoplastic ulcer.

32.8 What is the Most Likely Diagnosis?

Traumatic oral ulcer.

32.9 How Would You Investigate This Patient?

1. Blood investigations including a full-blood count and film and measurement of inflammatory markers and haematinics (serum ferritin, serum B12, serum and red cell folate) to exclude nutritional deficiencies.
2. A thorough systemic examination to rule out any other causes of oral ulcers such as gastrointestinal diseases.
3. Incisional biopsy if the ulcer is persistent after the removal of the traumatic aetiology.

32.10 Should a Biopsy Be Done Immediately?

A traumatic ulcer resolves once the offending cause is removed. If the ulcer persists after the removal of the traumatic aetiology, it is advised to do an incisional biopsy of the ulcer to rule out squamous cell carcinoma or any other pathology.

32.11 If a Traumatic Ulcer Does Not Heal, A Biopsy Should Be Performed. How Would It Appear Under the Microscope?

Microscopically, there is discontinuation of the epithelium (Fig. 32.2a). The ulcer surface is covered by a fibrinopurulent exudate (Fig. 32.2b). The epithelium adjacent to the area of ulceration may show pseudoepitheliomatous hyperplasia, while the ulcer bed contains granulation tissue. Regenerating atypia may be present in the adjacent epithelium. The granulation tissue shows proliferating endothelial cells and fibroblasts. Neutrophil predominant inflammatory infiltrate is present in the ulcer bed (Fig. 32.3).

The patient's blood investigations were within the normal limits. There was no evidence of a nutritional deficiency state. A thorough systemic examination did not suggest any underlying systemic disease.

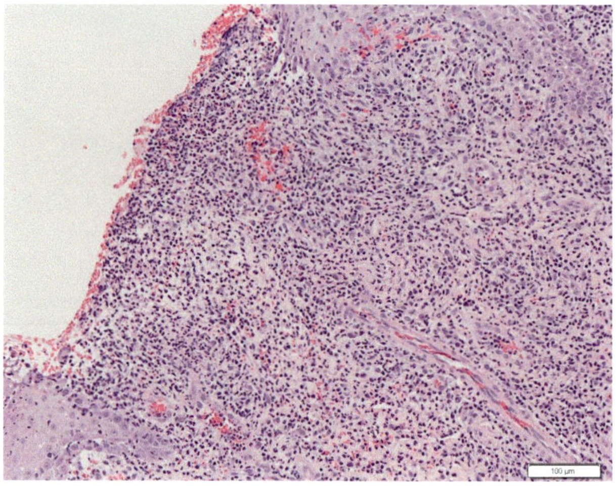

Fig. 32.3 An intense mixed inflammatory infiltrate is present in the ulcer bed

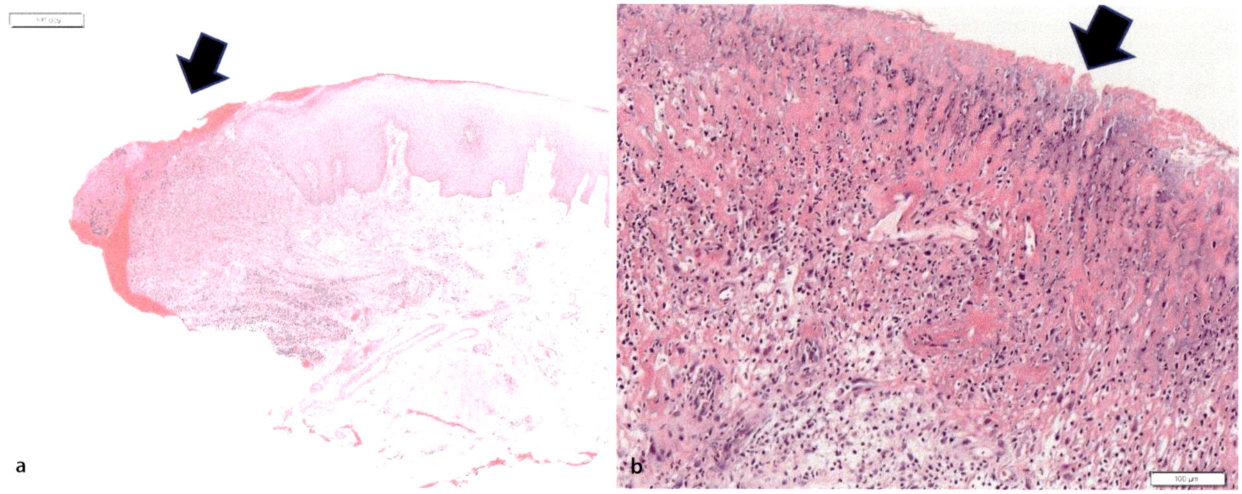

Fig. 32.2 There is a discontinuation of the surface epithelium (black arrow) (**a**). The ulcerated surface is covered by a fibrinopirulent membrane (black arrow) (**b**)

32.12 What Is the Final Diagnosis?

Traumatic ulcer.

32.13 How Would You Manage This Patient?

1. The lower denture is over-extended. An over-extended denture flange causes the denture to lose its peripheral seal, hence affecting stability and retention of the denture. The constant impingement of the denture flange on the mucosa injures the oral mucosa resulting in an ulcer. The over-extended lingual flange should be trimmed to reduce the trauma to the mucosa. This will help the denture to be more stable and improve retention.
2. The patient should be instructed not to wear the dentures for 1 week.
3. Antiseptic mouthwash such as chlorhexidine gluconate to prevent secondary infection.
4. Analgesic mouth washes such as benzydamine hydrochloride and lidocaine rinse to provide pain relief.
5. A soft and bland diet to reduce the irritation to the ulcerated area.
6. A review appointment after 7–10 days. Traumatic ulcers heal well once the source of irritation is removed.

32.14 Traumatic Oral Ulcer

Ulcers are caused due to several factors and are characterized by loss of tissue involving both the epithelium and the underlying connective tissue. Ulcers are one of the most common oral lesions to occur. Ulcers of the oral cavity can be classified into two main groups: a) acute ulcers with abrupt onset and b) chronic ulcers with slow onset and progression. An ulcer that lasts for more than 2 weeks is generally considered as a chronic ulcer. A list of acute and chronic ulcers is summarized in ◘ Table 32.1.

A traumatic oral ulcer is an open sore that can occur anywhere inside the mouth, and it is caused by trauma. The trauma can be physical, chemical or thermal. It can be acute and severe arising due to an inadvertent lip bite or cheek bite, tooth brush abrasion, accidental bite on sharp foods and lip biting due to numbness after local anesthesia. Traumatic ulcers can arise from chronic irritation like a sharp tooth or broken restoration rubbing against the cheek or tongue, and denture-induced irritation (◘ Fig. 32.4).

◘ **Table 32.1** List of acute and chronic oral ulcers

Acute oral ulcers	Chronic oral ulcers
Traumatic ulcer	Traumatic ulcer
Recurrent aphthous stomatitis	Drug-induced ulcers
Behcet disease	Erosive lichen planus
Viral infections	Pemphigus vulgaris
Bacterial infections	Mucous membrane pemphigoid
Necrotizing sialometaplasia	Lupus erythematosus
Allergic reactions	Reiter syndrome
Erythema multiforme	Tuberculosis
	Mycosis
	Other bacterial and parasitic diseases
	Eosinophilic ulcer
	Oral squamous cell carcinoma (OSCC)

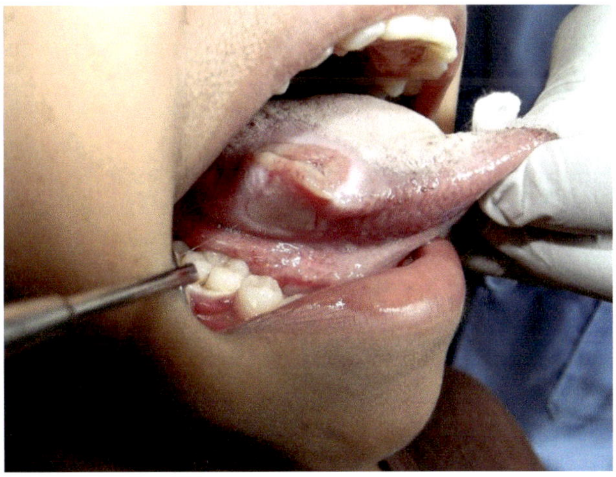

◘ **Fig. 32.4** A solitary chronic ulcer arising due to trauma from a sharp tooth on the right dorsum and extending on to the ventral surface of the tongue. (Picture courtesy: Prof Dr. Ruwan D Jayasinghe Faculty of Dental Sciences, University of Peradeniya, Sri Lanka)

Self-inflicted wounds caused by nocturnal clenching or lip biting or factitial injuries can cause traumatic ulcers as well. Consuming very hot liquids or solid foods may damage the mucosa causing an ulcer. Chemical irritation from medications such as topical acetylsalicylic acid,

pancreatic supplements, potassium tablets, bisphosphonates, trichloroacetic acid and certain oral care

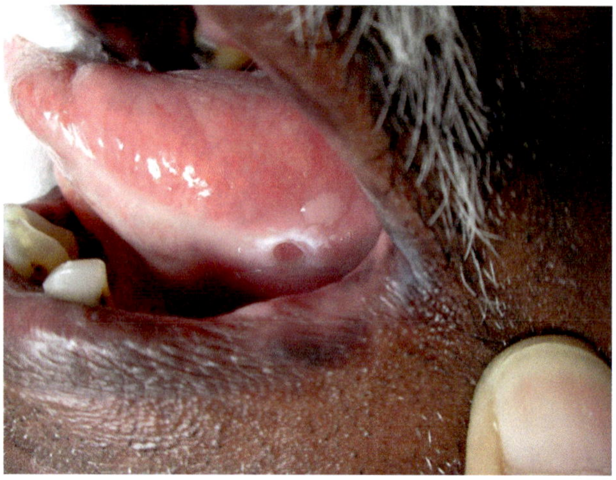

Fig. 32.5 A solitary chronic ulcer with a raised white periphery on the left ventral surface of the tongue. (Picture courtesy: Prof Dr. Ruwan D Jayasinghe Faculty of Dental Sciences, University of Peradeniya, Sri Lanka)

products can also lead to ulceration and sloughing of the oral mucosa. Oral ulcerations have also been caused due to the topical application of cocaine. Electrical burns of the oral cavity are rare but have been reported in children after biting or sucking electric cables, sockets or plugs.

Traumatic ulcers are usually painful, single and occur close to the cause of the trauma. The trauma causes a breach in the epithelium resulting in an ulcer with a yellowish greyish slough and fibrin and a reddish halo of inflammation. There might be some swelling, erythema and inflammation of varying degrees on the mucosa surrounding the ulcer, depending on the cause and duration since the trauma. They are characterized by acute pain of moderate intensity. Ulcers due to chronic irritation may present with a slightly raised white periphery (keratin builds up due to trauma) (Fig. 32.5) and may have some induration as well due to repeated trauma and healing.

Histopathological examination shows the ulcer surface covered by a fibrinopurulent exudate (Fig. 32.2b). The epithelium adjacent to the area of ulceration may show pseudoepitheliomatous hyperplasia, while the ulcer bed contains granulation tissue. The granulation tissue shows proliferating endothelial cells, fibroblasts and a mixed inflammatory infiltrate.

A thorough medical history, oral examination together with complementary diagnostic methods are essential to arrive at a specific diagnosis of oral ulcers. Traumatic ulcers with mild or moderate tissue damage are usually treated symptomatically with a topical anesthetic to relieve the pain. In instances with more severe tissue damage, non-potent topical corticosteroids such as triamcinolone in an adherent vehicle of carboxymethylcellulose, orabase (carmellose sodium) or denture adhesive paste may be helpful. Patients who are prescribed topical steroids in an adherent vehicle should be instructed to apply a small amount to the ulcerated area after meals (3–4 times per day) and not to eat or drink for at least 30 min after application. Traumatic ulcers heal spontaneously with the removal of the causative factor. However, of utmost importance is that follow-up appointments must be given to monitor the ulcer. The ulcer would need to be examined to check if it has healed. A persistent ulcer of more than 3 weeks duration warrants immediate referral to an Oral Medicine specialist. Further investigations should be carried out to rule out a malignancy or any underlying pathology such as bacterial and fungal infections or immune-mediated mucocutaneous disorders.

Salient features of traumatic ulcer	
Clinical features	Painful, single in number and occur close to the cause of the trauma. It usually manifests as an ulcer with a yellowish greyish slough and fibrin and a reddish halo of inflammation. There might be some swelling, erythema and inflammation of varying degrees on the mucosa surrounding the ulcer. They are characterized by acute pain of moderate intensity. Ulcers due to chronic irritation may present with a slightly raised white periphery (keratin builds up due to trauma) and may have some induration as well due to repeated trauma and healing.
Histopathological features	The ulcer surface is covered by a fibrinopurulent exudate. The epithelium adjacent to the area of ulceration may show pseudoepitheliomatous hyperplasia, while the ulcer bed contains granulation tissue. Regenerate atypia may be present in the adjacent epithelium.
Treatment	Symptomatic treatment with a topical anesthetic to relieve the pain. In instances with more severe tissue damage, non-potent topical corticosteroids such as triamcinolone in an adherent vehicle of carboxymethylcellulose, orabase (carmellose sodium) or denture adhesive paste may be helpful.

Self-Assessment Questions

1. Discuss the differential diagnosis for traumatic ulcers.
2. Describe the clinical features of traumatic ulcers.
3. Describe the investigations that need to be carried out to confirm the diagnosis of a traumatic ulcer.
4. Describe the histopathologic features of a traumatic ulcer.
5. Discuss the management for traumatic ulcers.

Diagnostic Algorithm

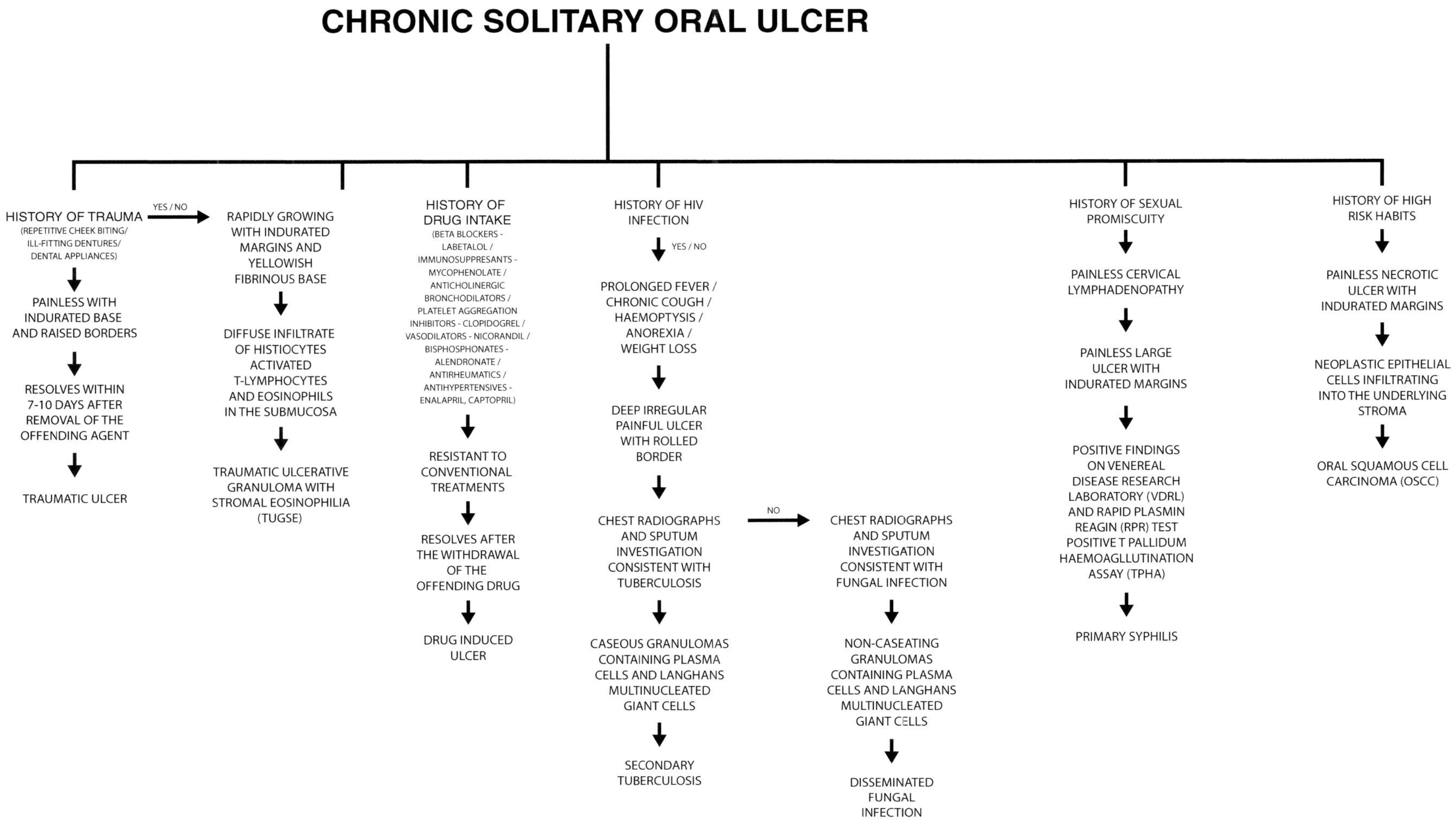

Summary

Ulcers are one of the most common oral lesions to occur. They are caused due to several factors and are characterized by loss of tissue involving both the epithelium and the underlying connective tissue. A traumatic oral ulcer is an open sore that can occur anywhere inside the mouth due to trauma. The trauma can be physical, chemical or thermal. Traumatic ulcers manifest in short painful episodes and occur close to the cause of the trauma. The trauma causes a breach in the epithelium resulting in an ulcer with a yellowish greyish slough and fibrin and a reddish halo of inflammation. Traumatic ulcers with mild or moderate tissue damage are usually treated symptomatically with a topical anesthetic to relieve the pain. In instances with more severe tissue damage, non-potent topical corticosteroids such as triamcinolone in an adherent vehicle of carboxymethylcellulose, orabase (carmellose sodium) or denture adhesive paste may be helpful.

Further Reading

Bruce AJ, Dabade TS, Burkemper NM. Diagnosing oral ulcers. J Am Acad PAs. 2015;28(2):1–10.

Cawson RA, Odell EW. Cawson's essentials of oral pathology and oral medicine e-book. Elsevier Health Sciences; 2017.

Field EA, Allan RB. Oral ulceration–aetiopathogenesis, clinical diagnosis and management in the gastrointestinal clinic. Aliment Pharmacol Ther. 2003;18(10):949–62.

Muñoz-Corcuera M, Esparza-Gómez G, González-Moles MA, Bascones-Martínez A. Oral ulcers: clinical aspects. A tool for dermatologists. Part I. Acute ulcers. Clin Exp Dermatol. 2009a;34(3):289–94.

Muñoz-Corcuera M, Esparza-Gómez G, González-Moles MA, Bascones-Martínez A. Oral ulcers: clinical aspects. A tool for dermatologists. Part II. Chronic ulcers. Clin Exp Dermatol. 2009b;34(4):456–61.

Neville BW, Damm DD, Allen C, Chi AC. Oral and maxillofacial pathology. Elsevier Health Sciences; 2015.

Sivapathasundharam B. Shafer's textbook of oral pathology-E book. Elsevier Health Sciences; 2016.

Warnakulasuriya S, Tilakaratna WM, editors. Oral medicine & pathology: a guide to diagnosis and management. JP Medical Ltd.; 2013.

A Painful Non-healing Ulcer on the Tongue: Traumatic Ulcerative Granuloma with Stromal Eosinophilia (TUGSE)

Daniel Lim

Contents

W. M Tilakaratne, T. G. Kallarakkal (eds.), *Clinicopathological Correlation of Oral Diseases*,
https://doi.org/10.1007/978-3-031-24408-7_33

33.1 Complaint

A 46-year-old gentleman is referred by a general dental practitioner for management of a painful non-healing ulcer on the left ventrolateral surface of the tongue.

33.2 History of Complaint

Question: When did you first notice the ulcer?

I noticed the ulcer about 3 weeks ago. It began as a small pin-point ulcer and progressively increased to its present size.

Question: What made you notice the ulcer?

The ulcer is painful.

Question: Is there any associated discharge or bleeding?

There is no bleeding or discharge from the ulcer.

Question: What are the symptoms of the ulcer?

The pain is worsened whenever the tongue moves. Besides that, spicy and sour food or drinks aggravate the pain. I apply the ulcer gel provided by my dentist to relieve the pain. Otherwise, the painful ulcer does not affect my daily activities much.

Question: Has the ulcer increased in size since it was first noticed?

The ulcer has progressively increased in size for the past 3 weeks. It has changed from a pinpoint to an oval-shaped ulcer. This ulcer differs from the usual ulcers that I experience as those ulcers usually resolve in less than 2 weeks.

Question: Did you have any similar ulcers in the mouth earlier?

I vaguely remember having ulcers previously.

Question: What do you think caused the ulcer?

I am not sure of the cause of the ulcer and cannot recall if there was any incident of injury to the tongue prior to the ulcer formation.

33.3 Past Dental and Medical and Social History

Question: Are you suffering from any other medical problems such as heart disease, high blood pressure, diabetes, bleeding disorder or respiratory diseases? If yes, what kind of medications have you been taking until now?

I have been diagnosed with hypertension and dyslipidemia in the last 30 years. I am on treatment with amlodipine and atorvastatin. I attend my medical check-up regularly.

Question: Have you undergone any surgery?

I have not undergone any surgery in the past.

Question: Have you undergone any dental treatment?

I go for my dental check-up annually. For this particular problem, I have visited two dental clinics and was prescribed with antibiotics and ulcer gel.

Question: What is your occupation?

I am a lorry driver.

Question: Do you have any specific chewing habits?

I used to chew betel quid for about 5 years but have stopped completely for the past 15 years ever since my mother passed away due to oral cancer.

Question: Are you a smoker?

I used to smoke 10–15 cigarettes per day for about 10 years but have stopped smoking together with my betel quid chewing habit.

Question: When did you last have a sexual encounter?

I meet up with prostitutes every month when I am outstation, but I always practice safe sex.

Question: Do you drink alcohol?

I am a social drinker.

33.4 With the Findings From the History, What Is Your Differential Diagnosis?

Major aphthous ulcer.

Traumatic ulcer.

Traumatic ulcerative granuloma with stromal eosinophilia.

Primary syphilis (syphilitic chancre).

Necrotizing sialometaplasia.

Oral squamous cell carcinoma (OSCC).

33.5 How Do You Justify Your Differential Diagnosis After History Taking?

33.5.1 Major Aphthous Ulcer

Major aphthous ulcers can present as ulcers of more than 1 cm in diameter and can last for more than 2 weeks. This variant of aphthous ulcers usually occurs on the lip, tongue, soft palate and palatal fauces. He did mention that he had history of recurrent ulcers that healed.

33.5.2 Traumatic Ulcer/Traumatic Ulcerative Granuloma with Stromal Eosinophilia

This lesion is commonly seen on the tongue, presenting as an ulcer with indurated margins. Sharp adjacent tooth surfaces may have caused trauma to the tongue without him realizing.

33.5.3 Primary Syphilis (Syphilitic Chancre)

Oral chancre may appear 3–4 weeks after infection. The ulcer may occur mainly on the lip and tongue. It usually measures around 1 cm with indurated edges. His monthly casual sexual practice may have put him at risk of contracting the infection.

33.5.4 Necrotizing Sialometaplasia

This condition is believed to be caused by ischaemia leading to the infarction of the minor salivary glands. Among the factors that may lead to ischaemia are trauma, smoking, alcohol, cocaine and local anaesthetic administration. Trauma from the adjacent teeth and history of smoking may predispose this patient to necrotizing sialometaplasia. However, this lesion is exceptionally rare on the tongue.

33.5.5 Oral Squamous Cell Carcinoma (OSCC)

Besides having a positive family history of oral cancer, his previous habit of betel quid chewing puts him at risk for oral cancer. Moreover, the ulcer has been there for more than 2 weeks.

33.6 Findings of Clinical Examination

33.6.1 Extra-oral Examination

There are no palpable lymph nodes or any other abnormalities.

33.6.2 Intra-oral Examination

There is a 1.5 cm × 1 cm solitary ulcer on the left ventral surface of the tongue which is oval in shape. The ulcer base is slightly indurated without everted margins (◘ Fig. 33.1). The ulcer base is yellowish in colour. Teeth 33 and 35 are relatively sharp as a result of attrition. Otherwise, the surrounding tissue is normal. Tongue movement and sensation are intact. There is evidence of scarring on the oral mucosa.

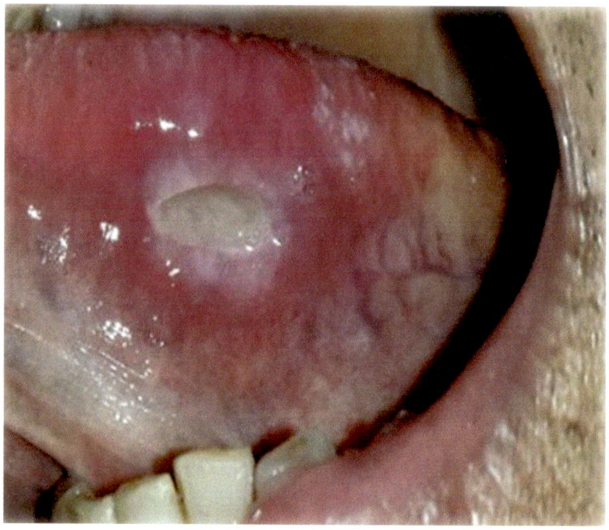

◘ **Fig. 33.1** Deep ulcer with necrotic base and regular margins. There is no evidence of rolled or everted margins

33.7 What Is Your Clinical Differential Diagnosis?

Major aphthous ulcer.

Traumatic ulcerative granuloma with stromal eosinophilia.

Primary syphilis (syphilitic chancre).

Oral squamous cell carcinoma (OSCC).

33.8 How Would You Justify the Inclusion of the Diseases That You Have Mentioned in the Differential Diagnosis to Arrive at a Working Diagnosis?

According to the history, the patient has a vague memory of previous ulceration. However, there is no evidence of scarring to suggest previous major aphthous ulceration. It suggests that the present ulcer may not be a major aphthous ulcer. However, it cannot be excluded completely. Necrotizing sialometaplasia is rarely observed on the tongue. Therefore, it is an unlikely diagnosis in this case. Syphilitic ulcers usually present on the anterior dorsal surface or at the tip of the tongue. Although it is an unusual site, the possibility of a syphilitic ulcer cannot be excluded together with the findings in the history. OSCC and traumatic ulcerative granuloma with stromal eosinophilia (TUGSE) are difficult to distinguish in some cases as they present as deep ulcers with some degree of induration. However, in this patient, there is no marked induration. In addition, the patient has stopped practicing risky habits many years ago making the possibility of OSCC less likely. This leads to the working diagnosis of this patient more towards TUGSE than OSCC.

33.9 How Would You Investigate This Patient?

Serology tests such as (Rapid Plasma Reagin (RPR) & Venereal Disease Research Laboratory (VDRL) tests.

Incisional biopsy.

33.10 How Would You Do An Incisional Biopsy for This Patient? What Are the Important Considerations?

It is important that during incisional biopsy to include part of the normal tissue together with the lesional tissue. Incision must be deep to include the base of the lesion extending to muscle.

33.11 What Are the Histopathological Features?

Histological sections from patient's biopsy show a deep ulcer extending into the muscle and characterized by a distinct eosinophilic infiltration. Variable numbers of other inflammatory cells are also present. In addition, granulation tissue formation with prominent endothelial cell proliferation is also evident in the ulcer bed. The surface epithelium at the edge of the ulcer shows hyperplastic changes (◘ Fig. 33.2).

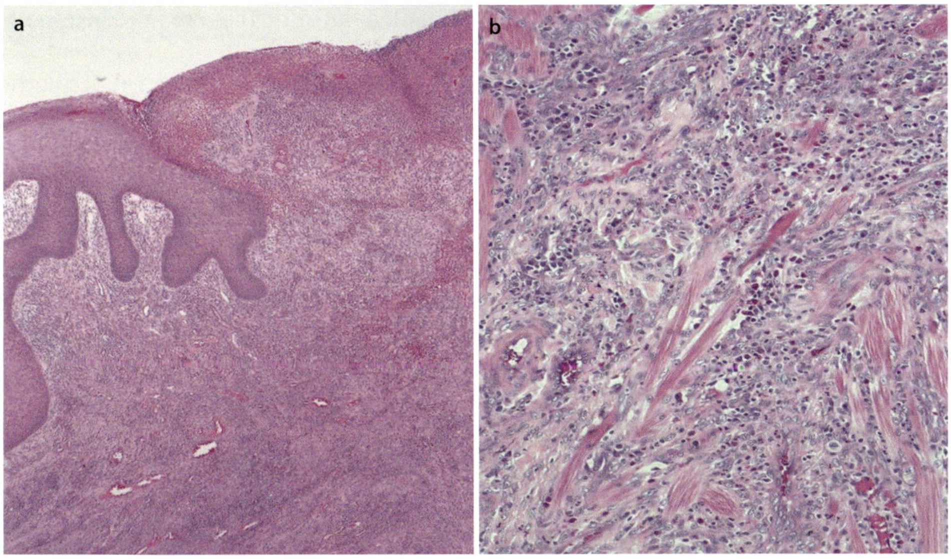

◘ **Fig. 33.2** (**a**) Discontinuity of the surface epithelium and presence of fibrinopurulent membrane indicative of ulceration. (**b**) Eosinophilic infiltration is seen extending in between the deeper muscle layer

33.12 What Specific Findings Help You to Arrive at the Diagnosis (History, Clinical and Investigations)?

Clinically, TUGSE is a single deep ulcer with some degree of induration at the base of the ulcer. It is usually of a few weeks' duration. The definitive diagnosis is mostly from histopathological examination supported by clinical features. Histology showing deep ulcer extending into muscle and characterized by a distinct eosinophilic infiltration is pathognomonic for TUGSE. Besides this, failure to detect Treponema pallidum spirochetes in the biopsy either by silver-impregnation staining techniques or immunohistochemistry in addition to serologic tests would help to rule out syphilitic chancre. A negative serological test (Rapid Plasma Reagin (RPR) & Venereal Disease Research Laboratory (VDRL) tests) ruled out syphilis. OSCC should show dysplastic features in the epithelium and evidence of invasion.

33.13 What Is Your Definitive Diagnosis?

Traumatic ulcerative granuloma with stromal eosinophilia (TUGSE).

33.14 What Is the Treatment and Prognosis?

TUGSE is generally a self-limiting disorder. It usually resolves spontaneously in a few weeks. As long as malignancy is being excluded, no specific treatment is necessary for the ulcer. In cases of persistent ulcer, excision of the ulcer has been advocated. Any possible etiology or source of trauma needs to be addressed. These include smoothening sharp tooth surfaces, restoring chipped or fractured tooth or extracting sharp retained roots. In some instances, a lower soft splint may be prescribed to protect the soft tissue from being traumatized especially during the ulcer healing period. As a symptomatic relief, topical or oral analgesics can be prescribed to help in reducing the pain.

Recurrence following excision is unlikely.

33.15 Traumatic Ulcerative Granuloma with Stromal Eosinophilia (TUGSE)

Traumatic ulcerative granuloma with stromal eosinophilia (TUGSE) is a self-limiting obscure lesion that affects oral mucosa. Ever since it was first described in 1956, various terms have been used to describe the lesion. These include eosinophilic ulcer of the oral mucosa, oral traumatic granuloma and traumatic eosinophilic granuloma.

While the aetiology of TUGSE remains unclear, trauma has been advocated as the main cause. Traumatic event introduces unidentified causes such as microorganisms, toxins or foreign proteins into connective tissue. Any of these factors is believed to cause T-cell-mediated immune response leading to activation of T lymphocytes which in turn produce lymphokines (IL-1, IL-5 and TNF). These chemicals then lead to eosinophil maturation and chemotaxis and differentiation of mast cells. The end result of these reactions is tissue destruction and delayed healing.

Clinically, TUGSE presents as a fast-growing ulcer in the oral cavity with elevated and indurated borders. The ulcer is characterized by an erythematous periphery with white or yellow base and fibrinous membrane on the surface. This lesion can affect any part of the oral mucosa but is most commonly seen on the tongue followed by the buccal mucosa. Although TUGSE is often a solitary ulcer, metachronous lesions have been reported. Similar to most oral ulcers, TUGSE is frequently associated with pain. There is a slight female predominance with a peak incidence between the sixth and seventh decades of life. This ulcer usually regresses spontaneously within 1 month, but some experience recurrence.

Since there are no pathognomonic features, clinically TUGSE shares similar presentation with some ulcerative lesions such as major aphthous ulcer, traumatic ulcer, primary syphilis (syphilitic chancre), tuberculous ulcer, necrotizing sialometaplasia and OSCC. While some of these conditions can be ruled out with tests such as the Mantoux test (to rule out tuberculosis) and serological tests (to rule out primary syphilis), most of them require histopathology to confirm the diagnosis.

A variant of TUGSE seen in paediatric patients (less than 2 years old), Riga–Fede disease, may be a presenting sign of an underlying neurological disorder. In this group, the ulcer usually presents on the ventral aspect of the tongue due to traumatic contact with the mandibular incisors during feeding.

Histologically, TUGSE is characterized by a prominent eosinophilic infiltrate. Also frequently observed are large mononuclear cells with occasional nuclear atypia intermingled with the inflammatory infiltrate.

In most occasions, no treatment is necessary for TUGSE. The clinician can adopt a wait and watch approach. The ulcer usually heals within a few weeks. However, symptomatic relief can be achieved either with topical or oral analgesics. Some clinicians advocate excision of the ulcer, if it persists for a longer period of time. No recurrence is reported following excision.

Salient features of TUGSE	
Clinical	Painful ulcer commonly seen on the tongue with no lymph node involvement.
Histopathology	Characterized by prominent eosinophilic infiltrate. These infiltrates tend to extend to deeper underlying soft tissue, muscle and salivary gland. Poorly formed granulation tissue with increased number of capillaries and prominent endothelial cells.
Treatment	This ulcer is generally self-limiting and tends to heal spontaneously within a few weeks. Removal of source of irritation or trauma is necessary (e.g. Restoration or extraction of causative tooth). Pain can be controlled by topical or oral analgesics. If the lesion persists, it can be excised

Diagnostic Algorithm

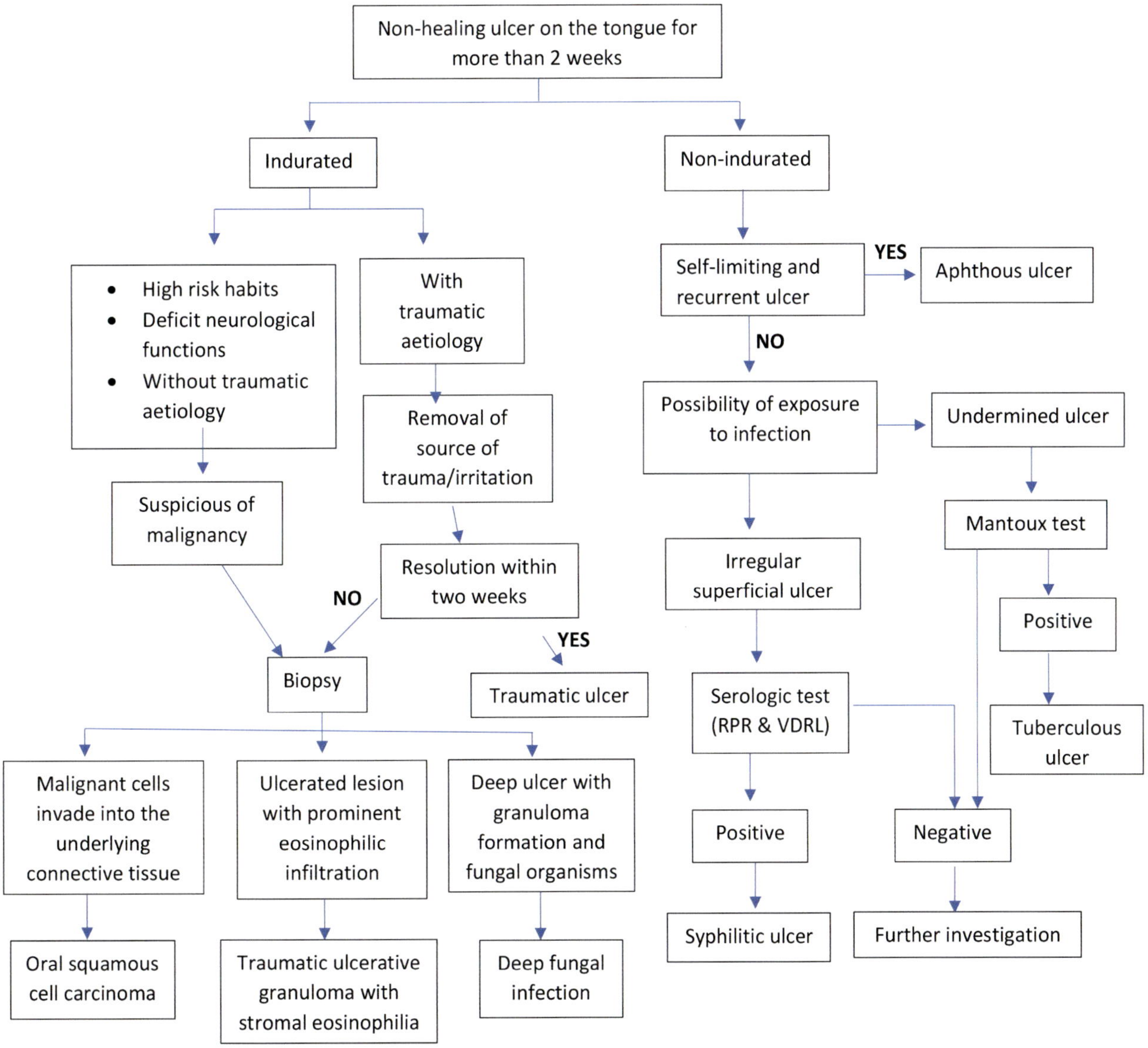

Self-Assessment Question

1. Describe the aetiopathogenesis of TUGSE.
2. Describe the histopathological features of TUGSE.
3. Discuss the differential diagnosis of TUGSE.
4. Explain the differences between TUGSE and a malignant ulcer.
5. State the management of TUGSE.

Further Reading

Cawson RA, Odell EW. Cawson's essentials of oral pathology and oral medicine. 8th ed. Edinburgh: Churchill Livingstone.

Dios PD, Scully C, de Almeida OP, Bagán JV, Taylor AM. Oral medicine and pathology at a glance. John Wiley & Sons; 2016.

Glick M. Burket's oral medicine. PMPH USA; 2015.

Scully C. Oral and maxillofacial medicine: the basis of diagnosis and treatment. Elsevier Health Sciences; 2012.

Segura S, Pujol RM. Eosinophilic ulcer of the oral mucosa: a distinct entity or a non-specific reactive pattern? Oral Dis. 2008;14:287–95.

Sharma B, Koshy G, Kapoor S. Traumatic ulcerative granuloma with stromal eosinophila: a case report and review of pathogenesis. J Clin Diagn Res. 2016;10:ZD07–9.

Warnakulasuriya S, Tilakaratna WM, editors. Oral medicine & pathology: a guide to diagnosis and management. JP Medical Ltd.; 2013.

Crusting and Ulceration of Lips: Erythema Multiforme

B. S. M. S. Siriwardena and Ruwan Jayasinghe

Contents

W. M Tilakaratne, T. G. Kallarakkal (eds.), *Clinicopathological Correlation of Oral Diseases*,
https://doi.org/10.1007/978-3-031-24408-7_34

Learning Goals

1. Understand the etiology and pathogenesis of immune-mediated conditions.
2. Differentiate erythema multiforme from other vesiculobullous disorders.
3. Classify immune-mediated vesculobullous diseases.
4. Identify histopathological differences.
5. Learn the assessment of severity and management.

34.1 Main Complaint

A 42-year-old female patient presents with ulceration, bleeding and moderate pain on the lips.

34.2 History of Complaint

Question: When did you notice these ulcers?

I noticed these ulcers 5 days ago. Initially, there were a few blisters. Subsequently, they ulcerated and started bleeding and crusting. It is painful while opening the mouth.

34.3 Additional Complaints

Question: Do you have ulcers elsewhere in the mouth?

I have ulcers on my cheeks.

Question: Do you have ulceration/irritation in the eyes?

I do not have any irritation or lesions in the eyes.

Question: Do you have any irritation in the throat?

I do not have any irritation in my throat.

Question: Have you experienced any change in your voice in the recent past?

I have not experienced any such discomfort.

Question: Do you have pain/burning sensation while passing urine? Is there any redness/ ulceration in the genital area?

I don't have any discomfort of that nature.

Question: Have you taken any medications recently?

I had fever a week before, and I consulted my family doctor. He prescribed antibiotics which I took three times a day for 5 days and a pain killer named Diclofenac Sodium twice a day for 3 days. Day, I developed blisters on my lips which later ulcerated and started bleeding.

Question: Do you have any ulcers/lesions on the skin?

I noticed reddish lesions on my palm and legs.

Question: Do you have any pain?

I find it difficult to eat and talk due to pain and discomfort.

Question: Have you experienced any similar lesions in the past?

I had similar lesions a few years ago which developed after taking medications for my fever. Small blisters developed on my lips which subsequently ulcerated. There was minimal bleeding, and the ulcers spontaneously regressed within a few days.

Question: Are you suffering from any other medical conditions such as high blood pressure, heart disease, diabetes, bleeding disorder, respiratory diseases? If yes, what kind of medications have you been taking until now?

I am not on any medications for medical conditions.

Question: Have you undergone any dental treatment?

I have undergone extractions of teeth due to dental caries.

Question: Do you have habits such as smoking, alcohol use or betel quid chewing? Are you allergic to anything?

I do not practice any of these habits. I have no known allergies.

Question: What is your occupation?

I work as an office secretary in a private company.

Question: Tell me about your family?

I am married and have two children.

Question: Does any of your family members or relatives suffer from similar lesions?

None of my family members or close relatives suffer from similar lesions.

34.4 With the Findings From the History, What Is Your Differential Diagnosis?

1. Erythema multiforme (EM).
2. Mucocutaneous autoimmune blistering disorder.
3. Oral lichenoid reaction.
4. Herpes simplex virus infection.

34.5 How Do You Justify Your Differential Diagnosis After History Taking?

34.5.1 Erythema multiforme (EM)

EM is a mucocutaneous immune mediated disorder. Drugs, microbes especially HSV are the commonest triggers, but at times it may be initiated with fever, sun exposure or even stress. Clinical spectrum of EM ranges from tender superficial erythematous or ulcerative areas confined to one mucosal surface to painful deep hemorrhagic bullae and erosions on multiple mucosal surfaces and skin. In the oral cavity, lips are the common site of involvement. EM starts as vesicles, soon ruptures giving rise to ulceration with bleeding which then crusts and covered with pseudo membrane. EM can cause morbidity including trismus, dysphonia, dysarthria and dysphagia. Skin lesions are not uncommon and characteristic target lesions are pathognomonic. This patient presented with lesions on the skin, oral ulceration and ulcers on the lips with bleeding and crusting after taking medications for fever. This suggests a high likelihood of EM.

34.5.2 Mucocutaneous Autoimmune Blistering Disorder

The patient had skin lesions. Oral ulcerations were preceded by blisters. The lesions were acute in onset and were recurrent in nature. The skin lesions and oral ulcers are suggestive of a mucocutaneous autoimmune blistering disorder. However, sudden onset and presence of bleeding are not in favour of autoimmune blistering disorder.

34.5.3 Oral Lichenoid Reaction (OLR)

Oral lichenoid reactions can be precipitated by oral medications. OLRs are common on the buccal mucosa, tongue and gingiva but rarely affect the lips. Bleeding is not a common feature of OLRs. The short duration of exposure to the medication and presence of bleeding and crusting on the lips make OLR an unlikely diagnosis.

34.5.4 Herpes Simplex Virus (HSV) Infection

Acute as well as recurrent HSV infection can cause vesicles and ulcerations on the oral mucosa. Acute infection is seen in children and characterized by gingival involvement. Recurrent infection (herpes labialis) affects the lips but is unilateral.

34.6 Findings of Clinical Examination

The patient has bloody encrustations and irregularly shaped superficial ulcerations and erosions with fresh bleeding spots on the lips (◘ Fig. 34.1). Lips are edematous. Multiple, diffuse, irregular superficial ulcerations are seen on both buccal mucosae and upper and lower labial mucosa. The ulcers are covered with slough and surrounded by diffuse erythema. Patient has halitosis. There are two target lesions on the palmar surface of the right hand (◘ Fig. 34.2). Bilateral submandibular lymph nodes are palpable and tender.

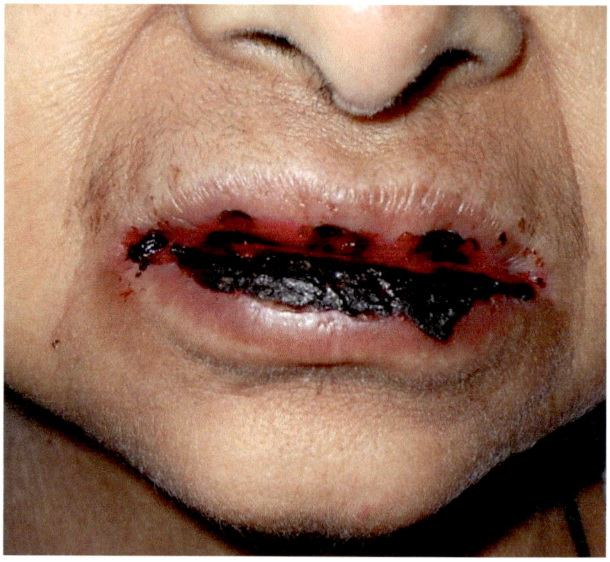

◘ **Fig. 34.1** Ulcerations with bleeding and crusting on the lips

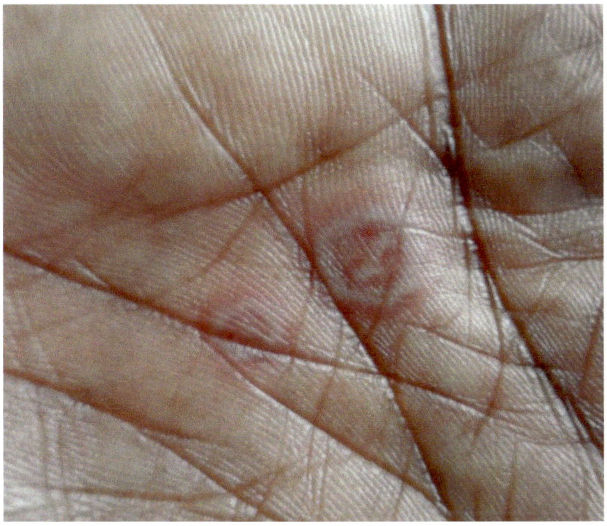

Fig. 34.2 Characteristic target lesions on the palm

34.7 What Other Relevant Features Would You Look for with the Findings You Have So Far?

The patient was referred to a dermatologist to rule out lesions involving the skin and other mucosal surfaces. There were no other blisters identified, and the dermatologist confirmed that the other mucosal sites such as the nasal, genital, conjunctival and oesophageal mucosae were free of lesions.

34.8 What Is Your Clinical Differential Diagnosis?

1. Erythema multiforme (EM).
2. Mucocutaneous autoimmune blistering disorder.

34.9 How Would You Exclude Other Conditions and Justify the Inclusion of the Diseases Mentioned in the Differential Diagnosis to Arrive at a Working Diagnosis?

Erythema Multiforme (EM) is an acute, immune-mediated condition, commonly induced by Herpes Simplex Virus (HSV) infection or by the use of certain medications and presents with cutaneous or mucosal lesions or both. EM can present only with oral lesions or associated with characteristic target lesions on the skin with concentric colour variation. It has also been reported that primary EM can be confined only to the oral mucosa, but the subsequent attacks can produce more severe forms of cutaneous EM. Considering the appearance of the lesions and a positive drug history, EM is the most likely diagnosis in this case.

Oral lesions can be the initial presentation in some patients with pemphigus and subsequent cutaneous involvement in 75% of affected patients. All mucosal surfaces may be affected, but soft palate is the most commonly involved site, followed by the buccal mucosa, tongue and gingiva causing desquamative gingivitis. Lesions start as vesicles or blisters with clear content that develop on normal or erythematous skin, but oral lesions soon rupture leaving erosions or ulcerations. Intact vesicles/bullae may be seen on the skin but rare in the mouth. Bullous pemphigoid (BP) and mucous membrane pemphigoid (MMP) are autoimmune diseases, most commonly seen in middle-aged to older females. MMP is characterized by bullous eruptions and ulceration, particularly in the oral mucosa and conjunctiva. Healing occurs with scarring giving rise to complications. The commonest site of involvement is gingiva causing desquamative gingivitis. The presence of characteristic lesions of EM on patient's palm excludes the possibility of autoimmune blistering disorders.

34.10 What Is the Most Likely Diagnosis and Why?

Drug-induced erythema multiforme (EM).

Presence of bloody encrustations and irregularly shaped superficial ulcerations and erosions on lips and characteristic target lesions on the palm with the recent drug history in arriving at the working diagnosis of drug-induced erythema multiforme.

34.11 How Would You Investigate This Patient?

There are no specific laboratory tests that are specific for the diagnosis of EM. However, when the characteristic clinical features are not present, other autoimmune blistering disorders should be excluded before arriving at the diagnosis.

1. Incisional biopsy – for routine histopathology and direct immunofluorescence (DIF).
2. Smear or swab for HSV PCR.

34.12 How Would You Do An Incisional Biopsy for This Patient? What Are the Important Considerations?

The biopsy of oral mucosa should be obtained from the lesion including perilesional area as well. Presence of epithelium is necessary in order to perform DIF. Punch biopsy can be performed for skin lesions. The sample should not be fixed in routine 10% formal saline, and it should be sent to the laboratory immediately for freezing (on a piece of gauze soaked in saline). If it is necessary to send to a distant laboratory, it should be transported in a suitable media (Michel solution). However, DIF can now be performed on formalin fixed tissues as well.

The biopsy results confirmed the diagnosis of EM.

34.13 What Histopathological Features Are Helpful to Arrive at the Definitive Diagnosis?

Mucous membrane EM and cutaneous EM have similar histopathological features. Within the epithelium, there is evidence of liquefactive degeneration of the basal cells, necrotic keratinocytes and exocytosis of lymphocytes. In some cases, subepithelial clefts and vesiculation may develop secondary to extensive basal cell degeneration. The advanced lesions show epithelial necrosis and intraepithelial vesicle formation. Mild to moderate lymphohistiocytic infiltrate in a lichenoid pattern may be observed at the epithelial connective tissue interface (◘ Figs. 34.3 and 34.4).

The purpose of direct immunofluorescence (DIF) in EM is to exclude other diseases that are considered in the differential diagnosis as histopathological features of EM can be nonspecific. There is evidence of granular deposition of C3 and immunoglobulin M (IgM) at the basement membrane zone and around superficial blood vessels. Occasional epithelial cells exhibit homogeneous C3 and IgM staining in regions of epidermal necrosis. However, overall findings of DIF can be considered as non-specific.

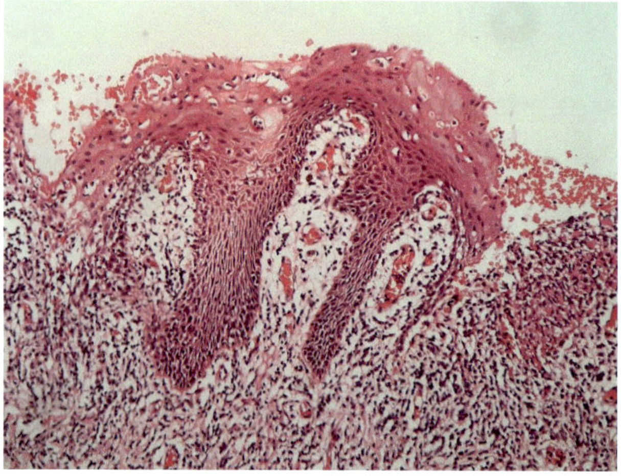

◘ Fig 34.3 Liquefactive degeneration of the basal cells and a lichenoid pattern of lymphocytic infiltrate

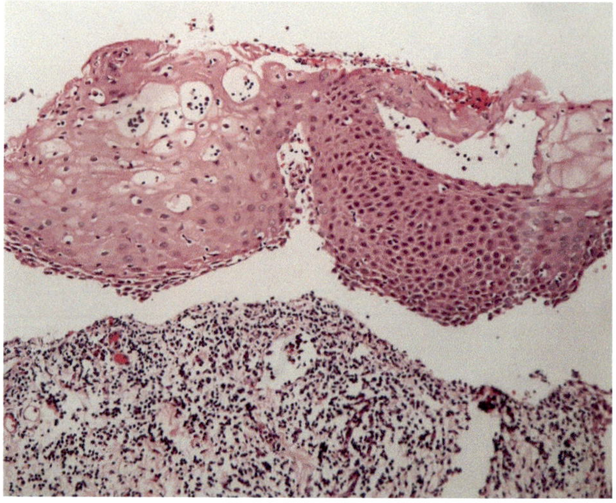

◘ Fig. 34.4 Intra and subepithelial vesciculation

34.14 What Is the Definitive Diagnosis?

Erythema multiforme (EM).

34.15 What Is the Treatment Protocol?

An important element in the treatment of EM is the discontinuation of all triggering factors. The management depends on the presence of mucosal disease, the development of recurrent disease and overall disease severity. Mucosal involvement in EM may vary in severity.

Milder forms such as painful erosions can be treated with high-potency topical corticosteroid gel, oral antiseptic washes and oral anesthetic solutions. The patients who have extensive lesions that prevent sufficient oral intake may require systemic glucocorticoids to decrease severity and disease duration. Ophthalmology consultation is imperative for patients with ocular involvement.

In patients with HSV-associated recurrent EM and idiopathic recurrent EM, the first line of treatment is antiviral prophylaxis. Treatment recommendations include acyclovir (200 mg 5 times daily) or valacyclovir (500 mg twice daily) or famciclovir (250 mg twice daily). The treatment goal is to reduce the frequency of occurrence and to induce remission. As all these drugs can induce significant side effects, careful follow-up and monitoring of the patients are essential to identify the side effects.

34.16 Erythema Multiforme (EM)

Erythema multiforme (EM) is an acute, immune-mediated, mucocutaneous condition, and the commonest triggering factor is herpes simplex virus (HSV) infection. Use of certain medications can also be a trigger. The spectrum of EM includes four clinical conditions that overlap with regard to their clinical features and suspected etiology and pathogenesis (◘ Table 34.1).

EM is characterized by distinct targetoid lesions with concentric colour variation. These lesions may be accompanied by oral, genital or ocular and mucosal erosions or a combination of these. Typical target acral lesions with involvement of a single mucosa, often the mouth, are termed as EM minor. Extensive skin lesions (not exceeding 10% of the body surface area) with severe involvement of mucosa, at least two different mucosae and having target lesions, are known as EM Major. EM usually resolves spontaneously in 3–5 weeks but has a tendency to recur. The spectrum of EM includes EM minor, major (Stevens–Johnson syndrome; SJS) and toxic epidermal necrolysis (TEN). The exact incidence is unknown, and literature indicates that infection, medication, autoimmune diseases, underlying malignancy and radiation are some of the causative factors of EM. Although there are many drugs, the most common EM precipitating drugs are NSAIDs, antibiotics and anti-epileptic drugs (◘ Table 34.1).

More than 50% of EM patients carry specific HLA alleles (e.g. HLA-DQB1*0301, HLA-B35, HLA-B62). The mechanism behind HSV-associated EM is due to cell-mediated immune reaction against the viral DNA. Once HSV infection occurs, the phagocytic cells (macrophages, CD34+ Langerhan cell progenitors) that carry the virus present in the blood are transported to the epidermis where the virus DNA is released into keratinocytes. This leads to activation of HSV-specific CD4+ T helper 1 (TH1) cells and production of cytokines (IFN-γ) leading to non- specific inflammation. Further, there is an upregulation of E-cadherin that promotes binding of virus DNA containing Langerhan cells which leads to increased vascularity with inflammation. It is

◘ **Table 34.1** Features of the spectrum of EM

Type	Course	Precipitating factor	Duration (weeks)	Mucosal involvement	Skin involvement	Systemic symptoms	Prognosis
EM minor	Acute, self-limiting, rarely recur	Infection (HSV)	1–3	Absent or mild confined to one mucosa	Typical target lesions	None	Remits, full recovery
EM major	Acute, self-limiting can be recurrent	Infection (HSV, mycoplasma)	1–6	At least 2 mucosae	Typical target lesions	Fever, arthralgia	Generally remits
SJS	Acute, progressive systemic disease	Drugs Antibiotics (penicillins, cephalosporins, sulfonamides etc.), antiepileptic (carbamazepine, phenytoin etc.), others (NSAIDs, paracetamol, ayurvedic and homeopathic medicine)	2–6	At least 2 mucosae Extensive	Dusky macular atypical target lesions <10% body surface area (BSA) detachment	Fever, lymphadenopathy, cytopenias, hepatitis	10% mortality
TEN	Prodromal mucosal Involvement acute Deterioration Widespread skin Lesions	Drugs Antibiotics (penicillins, cephalosporins, sulfonamides etc.), antiepileptic (carbamazepine, phenytoin etc.), others (NSAIDs, paracetamol, ayurvedic and homeopathic medicine)	2–6	At least 2 mucosae Severe. Respiratory and GIT involvement	Dusky macular atypical target lesions >30% body surface area (BSA) detachment	Fever, lymphadenopathy, cytopenias, hepatitis	30% mortality

reported that drug-induced erythema multiforme is associated with tumor necrosis factor-α (TNF-α) that causes epidermal destruction.

Clinical presentation may vary from patient to patient. However, early target lesions are usually round, edematous papules with erythema mimicking insect bites. Later they enlarge and form a concentric pattern which is characteristic to EM. These lesions are predominantly seen in extremities and extensor surfaces. In total, 25–60% of patients develop mucosal lesions which usually occur simultaneously with skin lesions. Some patients may present without skin involvement. The commonest mucosal site that is affected is oral mucosa. Labial and buccal mucosae, gingivae and vermillion of the lips are commonly involved sites. Lesions may range from tender superficial erythematous and hyperkeratotic plaques to painful deep hemorrhagic erosions. Laboratory tests are not useful to confirm EM. However, serum antinuclear antibody (ANA) is helpful to differentiate cutaneous lupus erythematosus.

Histopathologically, liquefactive degeneration of basal cells in the epidermis, necrotic keratinocytes and exocytosis of lymphocytes can be seen. In some cases, subepidermal/subepithelial separation may develop due to extensive degeneration of basal cells. Mild to moderate lymphohistiocytic infiltrate in a lichenoid pattern may obscure the dermo–epidermal junction. In the dermis or in the submucosa, lymphohistiocytic infiltrate is evident around blood vessels.

Direct immunofluorescence in EM is non-specific and can be helpful to differentiate from other autoimmune blistering disorders.

Stevens–Johnson syndrome is characterized by widespread erythematous or purpuric macules that are prominent on the trunk and spreads distally. Histologically, it may show more extensive epidermal necrosis with fewer inflammatory cells than minor forms of EM. Prompt recognition is essential because of the possibility of life-threatening complications and the risk for progression to toxic epidermal necrolysis.

Paraneoplastic pemphigus (PNP) is the closest differential diagnosis characterized by progressive skin and mucosal involvement with the presence of underlying malignancy. Pathologically, vacuolar or lichenoid interface dermatitis with suprabasilar acantholysis may be present similar to EM. However, PNP can be differentiated from EM by DIF. IgG and C3 deposition along cell surfaces and/or BMZ can be seen in PNP. Urticaria, Stevens–Johnson syndrome, fixed drug eruption, Sweet syndrome, Rowell syndrome, polymorphous light eruption and small-vessel vasculitis are other clinical differential diagnosis for EM.

Although symptomatic treatment may be sufficient in managing mild cases of EM, HSV-associated recurrent EM and idiopathic recurrent EM require treatment with antiviral prophylaxis.

Salient features of Erythema multiforme	
Clinical features	Initially presents as erythema with mild edema and progress to superficial erosions with pseudomembrane formation. Presence of bloody encrustations and irregular shaped superficial ulcerations and erosions on lips. Early target lesions on the skin are round, erythematous, edematous papules surrounded by areas of blanching.
Histopathology	Liquefactive degeneration of the basal cells, necrotic keratinocytes and exocytosis of lymphocytes. Subepithelial clefts and vesiculation may develop. Mild to moderate lymphohistiocytic infiltrate in a lichenoid pattern may be observed at the epithelial connective tissue interface.
Treatment	Management by a multidisciplinary team. Treatment of choice is systemic corticosteroid therapy. In patients with HSV-associated EM, the first line of treatment is antiviral prophylaxis.

Self-Assessment Questions

1. Discuss the triggering/causative factors of EM.
2. Discuss the pathogenesis of EM.
3. List the clinical differential diagnosis of EM.
4. Describe the histopathological features of EM.
5. Outline the management of EM.

▪ Diagnostic Algorithm for Erythema Multiforme

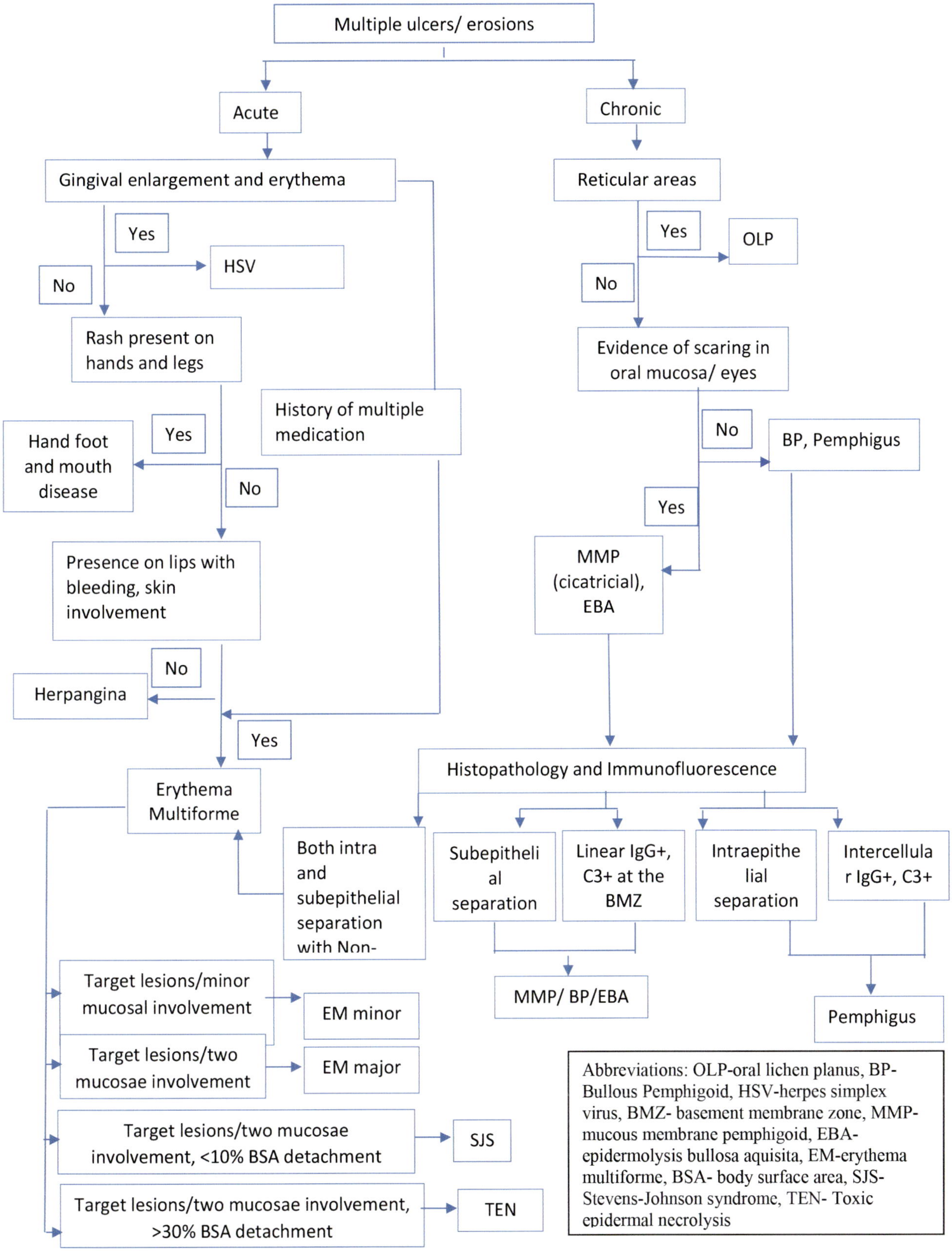

Summary

Erythema multiforme is an acute, immune-mediated, mucocutaneous condition and the commonest triggering factor is herpes simplex virus infection. Use of certain medications can also be a trigger. The spectrum of EM includes four clinical conditions, namely EM minor, EM Major, SJS and TEN. Targetoid lesions with concentric colour variation are characteristic. EM usually resolves spontaneously in 3–5 weeks but has tendency to recur. Although there are many drugs, the most common EM precipitating drugs are NSAIDs, antibiotics and anti-epileptic drugs.

Further Reading

de Risi-Pugliese T, Sbidian E, Ingen-Housz-Oro S, Le Cleach L. Interventions for erythema multiforme: a systematic review. J Eur Acad Dermatol Venereol. 2019;33(5):842–9. https://doi.org/10.1111/jdv.15447. Epub 2019 Feb 28. PMID: 30680804

Grünwald P, Mockenhaupt M, Panzer R, Emmert S. Erythema multiforme, stevens-Johnson syndrome/toxic epidermal necrolysis—diagnosis and treatment. J Dtsch Dermatol Ges. 2020;18(6):547–53. https://doi.org/10.1111/ddg.14118. Epub 2020 May 29

Samim F, Auluck A, Zed C, Williams PM. Erythema multiforme: a review of epidemiology, pathogenesis, clinical features, and treatment. Dent Clin N Am. 2013;57(4):583–96. https://doi.org/10.1016/j.cden.2013.07.001. PMID: 24034067

Soares A, Sokumbi O. Recent updates in the treatment of erythema multiforme. Medicina (Kaunas). 2021;57(9):921. https://doi.org/10.3390/medicina57090921. PMID: 34577844; PMCID: PMC8467974

Painful Recurrent Ulcers in the Mouth: Aphthous Ulcers

Karthick Sekar

Contents

W. M Tilakaratne, T. G. Kallarakkal (eds.), *Clinicopathological Correlation of Oral Diseases*,
https://doi.org/10.1007/978-3-031-24408-7_35

Learning Goals

1. Devise the correct way of compiling the history with appropriate questions.
2. Develop a differential diagnosis after history taking.
3. Deduce appropriate procedures in clinical examination.
4. Formulate a differential diagnosis combining findings in the history and clinical examination.
5. Justify the relevant investigations required to arrive at the diagnosis.
6. Comprehend the importance of clinicopathological correlation in arriving at the correct diagnosis.
7. Outline the management plan.
8. Recognize the importance of a diagnostic algorithm in arriving at a diagnosis.

35.1 Main Complaint

A 40-year-old female presented to the clinic with a complaint of a recent increase in frequency and severity of mouth ulcers.

35.2 History of Complaint

Question: How long have you been having these ulcers?

I have been having mouth ulcers for the past 10 years.

Question: How many ulcers do you get at any one time?

I usually get only one ulcer at a time.

Question: Where do you get the ulcers more commonly in the mouth?

I usually get the ulcers on the inner surface of the upper and lower lips.

Question: Do you have ulcers in other areas of the body such as genital mucosa or any history of ulcers in eyes?

I don't have ulcers elsewhere on my body.

Question: Are the ulcers painful?

The ulcers are extremely painful.

Question: How often do you get these ulcers?

Previously the frequency was less but for the past 6 months, it has been occurring more often.

Question: Do the ulcers heal spontaneously?

The ulcers usually resolve in 4–6 weeks time.

Question: Do the ulcers affect your speech and eating?

The ulcers are painful and create discomfort while eating food.

Question: Do the ulcers cause scarring once they heal?

There are some remaining scars of the previous ulcers.

Question: Are you suffering from any other medical problems, like heart disease, high blood pressure, diabetes, bleeding disorder, respiratory diseases, or gastrointestinal disorders?

I occasionally experience gastric reflux. I also have irregular menstrual cycles and excessive bleeding during menstruation. I am currently on follow-up under a gynaecologist. Besides that, I have skin allergies and I am under regular review with a dermatologist for my skin condition.

Question: How is your bowel habits?

I think my bowel habits are normal.

Question: Are you taking any medications?

I often take esomeprazole for my gastric reflux and acidity problem as advised by my physician. I also apply few topical steroid creams and anti-itch creams for my skin allergy.

Question: Are you suffering from any mental stress or anxiety disorders?

I lost my job 6 months ago and I am currently under great stress due to the uncertainty regarding my employment.

Question: Do the ulcers appear in relation to the consumption of any specific type of food products?

I have not noticed any such relation.

Question: Are you allergic to any food products?

I am not allergic to any food products.

Question: Have you undergone any dental treatment?

I visit the dentist once a year for my routine scaling.

I have had multiple fillings done. My dentist told me that I am a night grinder.

Question: Can you relate the appearance of ulcers to any episode of trauma in that region?

I can't relate anything to that effect.

Question: Do you habitually bite your lips or cheeks?

I don't have such habits.

Question: Do you have any habits like smoking or alcohol consumption?

I smoke (5–7 cigarettes per day) since past 22 years.

Question: What is your occupation?

Previously I worked as a manager at a bank for 10 years but I lost my job 6 months ago and I currently work at a call centre with back-to-back shifts.

Question: Does anyone in your family have the same condition as yours?

Both my siblings also had the problem of oral ulcers. I do not remember it being very severe like what I experience. My mother has gastric ulcers and my father is hypertensive.

With the findings from the history what are your differential diagnoses?

- Recurrent aphthous ulcer (RAU)
- Traumatic ulcers
- Behcet disease
- Crohn's disease
- Celiac disease

35.3 How Do You Justify Your Differential Diagnosis After History Taking?

A characteristic clinical feature of aphthous ulcers is its recurrent nature. Usually, RAU minor occurs as multiple shallow ulcers, whereas RAU major occurs as a single large ulcer as in this case. The RAU, depending on if it is minor or major type, heals within 2 weeks or 4–6 weeks, respectively. In this case the ulcers tend to heal in 4–6 weeks time suggesting a diagnosis of RAU major. The RAUs are extremely painful especially the RAU major as in this case. Due to extreme pain, the function of the oral cavity may be affected, such as resulting in difficulty in eating, speaking and sometime swallowing food depending on the site of the ulcers. This patient experienced difficulty in eating. Moreover, this patient is under stress and has a family history of recurrent mouth ulcers. Irregular menstrual cycles may suggest a hormonal imbalance. RAU should be considered in the differential diagnoses as emotional stress, genetic factors and hormonal imbalances have been considered to be potential predisposing factors for RAU. The patient may also be suffering from anaemia as she has a history of excessive bleeding during menstruation. The differential diagnoses for RAU are vast and range from idiopathic benign causes to inherited fever syndromes, to connective tissue disease, or even inflammatory bowel diseases, drug-induced mucocutaneous syndromes, autoimmune disorders, haematologic disorders, nutritional deficiencies, vesiculobullous diseases, and infections.

Traumatic ulcers are common on the oral mucosa. A sharp tooth or broken restoration/denture which is the cause of the trauma can be identified and should be removed. The patient should be reviewed in 2–3 weeks. If the ulcer has healed then it could be a traumatic ulcer. Usually, traumatic ulcer does not recur once the cause has been removed. However, at times patient might not able to recall any episodes of trauma. Therefore, traumatic ulcer cannot be completely excluded even though the cause of trauma is not present in this patient. However, the patient has bruxism which is a source of constant trauma. Moreover, extreme pain is a feature of both traumatic ulcer, RAU, and other ulcers.

Behcet disease shows multiple ulceration in numerous sites, including oral, genital, and ocular mucosa. In addition, cutaneous, neurological, and vascular problems may also present in some patients. Presence of only oral ulcers suggest that Behcet disease is least likely in this patient.

Inflammatory bowel diseases, such as Crohn's and Celiac disease, are known to present with oral ulceration. Therefore, those diseases can be included in the differential diagnoses. However, the absence of gastrointestinal manifestations does not make them likely differential diagnoses in this case.

35.4 What Are the Clinical Examination Findings?

Intraorally, there is an ulcer at the midline of the upper lip. It is shallow and measures approximately 8–12 mm in diameter with well-defined margins. The surrounding mucosa appears inflamed with a narrow rim of erythema around the ulcer (Fig. 35.1). The base of ulcer

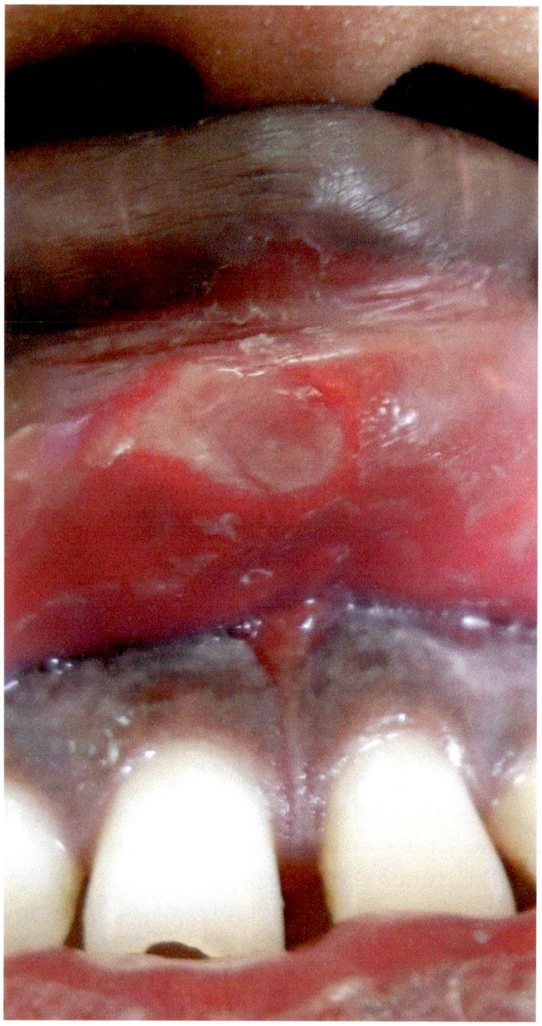

Fig. 35.1 A well-defined shallow ulcer with a whitish base and erythematous margin in the midline of the upper lip. Evidence of scarring due to previous ulcers is also noted on the adjacent mucosa. (Picture courtesy: Prof Dr. Ruwan D Jayasinghe Faculty of Dental Sciences, University of Peradeniya, Sri Lanka)

appears whitish. There is also a temporary restoration in relation to upper right canine. There are no other ulcers in the oral cavity. Multiple scars suggestive of previous ulcers are noted at the lip and buccal mucosa. Oral hygiene is fair. Mild gingivitis with multiple amalgam fillings is noticed, and a few of them seem to be fractured or defective. Traumatic cause in relation to the ulcer is not evident.

Extra oral examination does not reveal any ulcers in the ocular or genital areas. There are no significant cutaneous lesions. The conjunctiva is slightly pale in colour. The submandibular and submental lymph nodes are tender on palpation.

35.5 What Are the Clinical Differential Diagnoses?

1. Aphthous ulcer
2. Traumatic ulcer

35.6 How Would You Exclude Other Conditions and Justify the Inclusion of the Diseases That You Have Mentioned in the Differential Diagnoses to Arrive at a Working Diagnosis?

Several conditions can present with RAU, for which a thorough workup is necessary to narrow the diagnosis. A thorough intraoral examination should be performed to rule out trauma secondary to dental causes.

A complete blood count should be carried out to rule out haematologic and nutritional deficiencies. A variety of underlying disorders may predispose patients to develop RAU. They include iron deficiency anaemia, folic acid, or vitamin B12 deficiency, as well as a selective vitamin B12 reabsorption defect and neutropenia.

The history of excessive bleeding associated with menstruation in this patient suggests the possibility of iron deficiency anaemia. This, coupled with the stress and hormonal changes the patient is undergoing, might have caused the ulcers. Anaemia might not be the only cause for RAU in this patient but it might be an additional factor contributing to it.

In addition, genetic factors may be important. The family history is positive in up to 40% of patients with RAU. Gastric and hormonal abnormalities are also predisposing factors for RAS. One of the major aetiological factors of RAU is stress and gastroesophageal reflux disease (GERD). In this case the patient does have a positive family history of mouth ulcers and her mother also has history of gastric ulcers. This indicates a relationship of hereditary factors predisposing for RAU in this patient. In addition, the patient complains of irregular menstrual cycles suggesting a possible hormonal imbalance which is a known contributory factor for RAU.

The recurrent nature of ulcers with evidence of scarring are supportive for the diagnosis of major RAU. Crohn's disease can be excluded as the patient did not have any significant gastrointestinal symptoms other than the gastric reflux. Usually, gastric manifestations are preceded by oral features. Celiac disease can also be excluded from the differential diagnosis as the patient did not have any history of food allergy of gluten sensitivity.

Behcet disease is a rare disorder that causes inflammation of blood vessels throughout the body in which oral and genital ulcers are major diagnostic criteria. They can include mouth sores, eye inflammation, skin rashes and lesions, and genital sores. The patient had a history of skin allergy, but that is not sufficient enough to be diagnosed as Behcet disease.

Traumatic ulcers due to sharp tooth edges and broken fillings need to be ruled out. On clinical examination it was confirmed that there were no sharp edges in relation to the current ulcer. The patient is a night grinder which explained the sharp edges and broken fillings. However, it is difficult to exclude traumatic ulcer completely in this case.

35.7 What Is the Most Likely Diagnosis?

35.7.1 Recurrent Aphthous Major (RAU)

A diagnosis of recurrent aphthous (major) ulceration is made based on the history and clinical features. In addition, other possible diseases are excluded with the findings in the history and clinical examination. The most likely factors causing RAU in this patient are GERD, haematological, hormonal abnormalities, and stress.

35.8 How Would You Investigate This Patient?

All possible underlying systemic causes for recurrent oral ulceration must be excluded, with appropriate investigations. This includes a full blood count along with iron assay serum folic acid and vitamin B12 assay. Gastrointestinal diseases should be excluded by endoscopic retrograde cholangiopancreatography (ERCP). Blood investigation might not be useful in the diagnosis of Behcet disease. However, pathergy test is required for the diagnosis of Behcet disease. In this test, a sterile needle is inserted into skin. After one or two days the area around the inserted needle is examined for a small red bump under the skin. If a small red bump is seen under the skin, then the pathergy test is considered positive indicating that the immune system is overreacting to minor injury.

35.9 Recurrent Aphthous Ulcers

Recurrent aphthous ulcers also known as aphthae or canker sores are characterized by recurrent ulceration of the oral mucosa. The term "aphthae" is derived from the Greek word "aphthi" which means "to set on fire" or "to inflame." It was first used by the philosopher Hippocrates to describe the pain associated with a common disorder of the mouth during his time (most likely aphthous stomatitis). RAU can be classified into three different types: (i) minor aphthous ulcer, (ii) major aphthous ulcer, and (iii) herpetiform ulcers.

Aphthous ulcers present as well demarcated, oval or round recurrent oral ulcers which have a white or yellowish pseudo-membrane and an erythematous halo. Ulcers that are long standing have a greyish membrane which replaces the initial central yellow pseudo-membrane. These ulcers are associated with pain and discomfort causing difficulty in mastication and speech and may also have a prodromal burning or tingling sensation. Aphthous ulcers predominantly affect the non-keratinized and movable mucosa. In decreasing prevalence for the site, RAU occurs on the labial mucosa, buccal mucosa, ventral and lateral tongue, floor of the mouth, soft palate, and the oropharynx.

RAUs are conventionally classified, based on their size, duration, and presence or absence of scarring after healing into minor, major, and herpetiform ulcers. Minor aphthous ulcers are the commonest form of recurrent ulcers with a prevalence of around 75% to 85%. Their size ranges from 1 to 10 mm and they occur mostly as 1–5 ulcers per episode. Minor aphthous ulcers are painful and heal within 1–2 weeks. The most common site of these ulcers is labial and buccal mucosa which has non-keratinized mucosa. The key feature distinguishing minor from major aphthous ulcers is the absence of scarring after healing in minor ulcers. The occurrence of local lymphadenopathy is unlikely but may oocur based on the location, severity, and the number of the ulcers. The healing process is self-limited. In some cases, there is a simultaneous process of new ulcers forming as the old ones heal.

The major form, also known as Sutton disease, is less common than the minor RAU. It represents around 10–20% of all cases of RAU. Their size varies from more than 10 mm in diameter. They are deeper and can be associated with dysphagia and fever. The healing of major aphthous ulcers can take weeks to months, leaving scars. Major aphthous ulcers prevail on the keratinized as well as non-keratinized mucosa. Major aphthous ulcers may usually be initiated at puberty with a tendency to reappear chronically for up to 20 years or more. In comparison they are more painful and discomforting than minor form and also take longer time to heal. Scarring is more commonly appreciated. The longer prevalence of these ulcers makes them increasingly prone to superimposing bacterial and fungal infections.

The third type of RAU is the herpetiform ulcers which are rare and presents as clusters of pinpoint ulcers. They vary in size from 1 to 3 mm in diameter and manifests in large numbers of around 5 to 100 ulcers simultaneously. A large and irregular lesion can be formed as these small ulcers merge and become confluent. They may persist for about 7–14 days. Healing occurs in 1–2 weeks. These lesions persist for 1–3 years with short remissions. The age of onset of these ulcers is generally late unlike the major and minor forms. The salient features of different type of aphthous ulcers is given in ◘ Table 35.1.

Numerous aetiological and predisposing factors have been implicated for RAU. They range from local to systemic factors. The local factors include trauma, tobacco use, chemical irritants, sodium lauryl sulphate in tooth paste, and infections. Systemic factors include nutritional deficiencies, gluten sensitivity, hormonal changes, systemic disease (systemic lupus erythematosus, celiac disease, and Crohn's disease) drugs, alcohol, physical or psychological stress, and genetics.

Local trauma has been implicated as one of the local factors that may paly role in initiation of the mucosal injury resulting in ulcer formation in RAU patients. However, experimental biopsies have failed to show any histopathological difference between mechanically induced ulcers and spontaneous ulcers.

Individuals who smoke or chew tobacco tend to have fewer RAUs than non-smokers or non-chewers. The reason being, these habits tend to increase the keratinization of the oral mucosa. This keratinization may protect the oral mucosa against the penetration of the possible aetiological agent of RAU. Nicotine in tobacco tends to increase anti-inflammatory cytokines such as IL-10 and decreases pro-inflammatory cytokines, such as IL-1β and TNFα. This results in immunosuppression and a reduced inflammatory response in smokers. However, since smoking or chewing tobacco is harmful and these risk habits have been implicated in oral and lung cancer, the recommendation to use these habits as a protective factor in RAU is not viable and should be avoided.

Previously *viridian streptococci* were implicated in the destruction of oral mucosa in RAU but has been disproved. The heat shock protein (HSP) of L-form of *Streptococcus sanguis* has been implicated in the aetiology of RAU. HSP is said to cross-react with a common antigen of oral epithelium resulting in the tissue destruction. Patients with RAU show significant increase in serum antibodies to HSP. Another microorganism that has been implicated in RAU is *Helicobacter pylori* which has been detected in the oral ulcers. However, the frequency of serum IgG to *Helicobacter pylori* is not increased in RAU and the microorganism is not proven to cause RAU.

Certain chemical irritants have been suggested as aetiological agents in some patients with RAU. One such chemical irritant is sodium lauryl sulphate, a detergent that is found in most of the tooth pastes.

Many foods, such as chocolate, coffee, peanuts, cereals, almonds, strawberries, cheese, tomatoes, and wheat flour containing gluten, have been implicated in some patients with RAU. RAU patients diagnosed to be reactive to benzoic acid show clinical improvement when certain food substances are avoided.

Nutritional deficiencies are one of the systemic causes or predisposing factors for RAU. About 20% of patients with RAU tend to have either deficiency of iron or folic acid or vitaminB12. Folate or vitaminB12 deficiency occurs in these RAU patients due to lower dietary intake. Hormonal changes in women have also been suggested as a predisposing factor for RAU.

Psychological stress may play a role as trigger or a modifying factor in RAU. However, no studies have conclusively proven stress as a causative or precipitating factor for RAU.

Genetics may play an important role in RAU. Single nucleotide genetic polymorphisms (SNP) in genes related to the functioning of immune system, such as TLR4, MMP9, E-selectin, IL-1β, and TNFα, are said to

◘ Table 35.1 Salient features of different types of aphthous ulcers

Features	Minor RAU	Major RAU	Herpetiform RAU
Gender predilection	Equal	Equal	Female
Morphology	Round or oval shallow ulcers with greyish-white pseudomembrane and erythematous halo	Round or oval deep ulcers with greyish-white pseudomembrane and erythematous halo	Small, deep ulcers that commonly converge with irregular contour
Distribution	Lips, cheeks, tongue, and floor of mouth	Lips, soft palate and pharynx	Lips, cheeks, tongue, floor of mouth, and gingiva
Number of ulcers	1–5	10–20	10–100
Size of ulcers	<10 mm	>10 mm	2–3 mm
Prognosis	Lesions resolve in 4–14 days. No scarring	Lesions persist for >6 weeks. High risk of scarring	Lesions resolve in <30 days. Scarring is uncommon

be risk factors for RAU. The probability for the development of RAU in patients with SNP ranges from two to eleven times. It is said that persons carrying the SNP are in the state of "sensitization." Therefore, they tend to have a disproportionate tissue response after a minor trigger. This tissue response is characterized by the dysregulation of the local cell-mediated response resulting in an inappropriate focal accumulation of cytotoxic T-lymphocytes. These cytotoxic T-lymphocytes cause tissue damage which clinically manifest, such as oral ulceration.

Behcet disease, is, an inflammatory disease characterized by vasculitis and is associated with significant oral, ocular, and genital ulcerations. In almost 80% of cases mucosal aphthous ulcers are the presenting sign. Additionally, there can be ocular involvement as uveitis, skin lesions, such as erythema nodosum, and less commonly, central nervous system deficits. Vascular lesions may appear in small and large vessels and can cause coronary arteritis, arterial, or venous thrombosis. There are no specific tests that can confirm the diagnosis of Behcet disease although a positive pathergy test can be useful.

General dentists should be vigilant to the variant clinical presentation of this condition as they are most likely to encounter patients with RAU. Every clinical case has to be individualized and treated according to the character and severity of the disease. Treatment is usually palliative and not curative. The essential objective of the treatment along with relieving the pain symptoms is the identification of the factors that aggravate the pain and the risk of recurrence. The treatment of RAU includes anti-inflammatory agents, such as 5% amlexanox, or topical corticosteroids, such as 0.1% triamcinolone acetonide, which are used in patients who develop early symptoms to prevent the progression of any kind of lesions. In cases of already established aphthae, the former medications can be used to reduce the inflammatory effects. Additionally, a combination of these drugs with antiseptics, such as chlorhexidine and triclosan, and antibiotics, such as tetracyclines, hyaluronic acid, or pomades containing organic substances, such as myrtle or quercetin, can accelerate ulcer healing along with providing sufficient pain relief. A systemic drug treatment is more appropriate when the outbreak is constant and severe. In instances of major aphthous ulcers, when the intensity of pain is higher and topical treatment is insufficient to provide comfort, different drugs can be used to control the symptoms, such as colchicine 1.5 mg/day, dapsone 50 mg/day, clofazimine 100 mg/day, or pentoxifylline 400 mg 3 times a day. However, the most universally accepted treatment modality is systemic corticosteroids, such as prednisone 25 mg/day, and immune modulators, such as thalidomide 50–100 mg/day. These drugs almost completely cause remission of the disease, but the adverse effects of such heavy medication should be kept under consideration. Tetracycline syrup and capsule have also been used to treat RAU by inhibition of protein synthesis of bacterial cell wall and hence giving anti-bacterial effects. Triamcinolone 0.1% in Orabase (Kenalog in Orabase) and lidocaine 2% has been used topically by applying directly on dry ulcers to reduce pain and give numbing effect. Colchicine and corticosteroids are anti-inflammatory drugs. Colchicine prevents microtubule assembly and thereby disrupts inflammasome activation, microtubule-based inflammatory cell chemotaxis, generation of leukotrienes and cytokines, and phagocytosis. Corticosteroids are used for decreasing swellings and inflammations. Prednisone decreases inflammation via suppression of the migration of polymorphonuclear leukocytes and reversing increased capillary permeability. Thalidomide is an immunomodulatory medication and works by a number of mechanisms, including stimulating T cells and decreasing TNF-α production. However, its use is limited as thalidomide is teratogenic and is known to produce other adverse effects, such as irreversible polyneuropathy. As an antimicrobial agent, dapsone and clofazimine have bacteriostatic action. It inhibits the synthesis of dihydrofolic acid thereby inhibiting nucleic acid synthesis. Dapsone reduces tissue damage during inflammation. Clofazimine works by binding to the guanine bases of bacterial DNA, thereby blocking the template function of the DNA and inhibiting bacterial proliferation. *Pentoxifylline* has two major clinical effects: increasing microvascular blood flow, thereby enhancing oxygenation of ischemic tissue. It is a competitive non-selective phosphodiesterase inhibitor which raises intracellular cAMP, activates PKA, inhibits TNF and leukotriene synthesis, and reduces inflammation and innate immunity.

Avoidance of food triggers, especially alcohol, carbonated beverages, spicy foods, such as pepper, and spicy curry food is recommended. Patients should be instructed to avoid oral hygiene products that contain sodium lauryl sulphate. Oral hygiene is essential and needs to be stressed because poor oral hygiene might introduce a microbial and infectious component leading to recurrence or persistence of RAU.

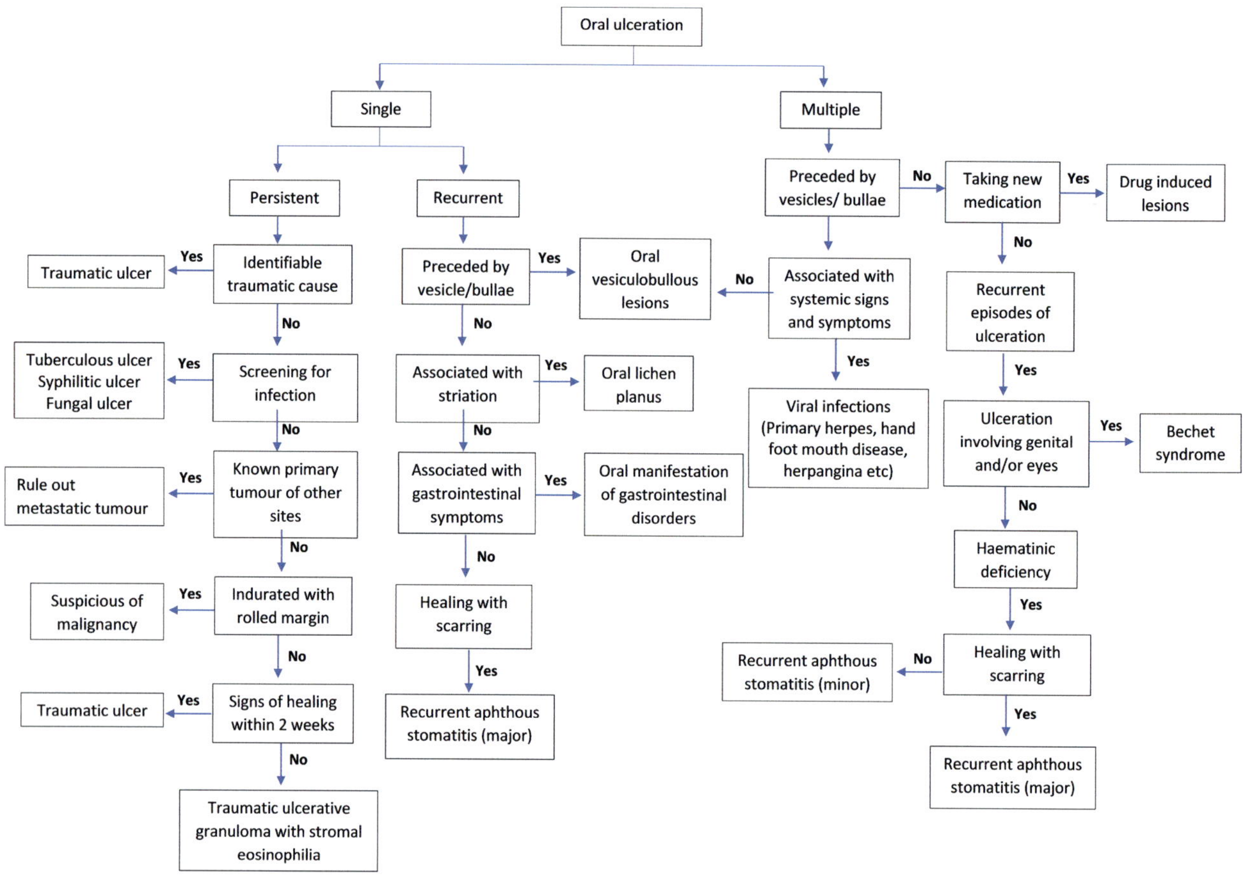

Self-Assessment Questions

1. Discuss the differential diagnoses for aphthous ulcers.
2. Describe the causes and predisposing factors of aphthous ulcers.
3. Describe the different types of aphthous ulcers and their clinical features.
4. Discuss the commonly associated systemic illness with aphthous ulcers.
5. Describe the management of patients with RAU.

Summary

Recurrent aphthous ulcers (RAUs) also known as aphthae or canker sores present as well demarcated, oval or round recurrent oral ulcers. Numerous aetiological and predisposing factors ranging from local to systemic factors have been implicated for RAU. The local factors include trauma, tobacco use, chemical irritants, sodium lauryl sulphate in tooth paste, and infections. Systemic factors include nutritional deficiencies, gluten sensitivity, hormonal changes, systemic disease, drugs, alcohol, physical or psychological stress, and genetics. RAU predominantly affects the labial mucosa, buccal mucosa, ventral and lateral tongue, floor of the mouth, soft palate, and the oropharynx. General dentists should be vigilant to the variant clinical presentation of this condition as they are most likely to encounter patients with RAU. Every clinical case has to be individualized and treated according to the character and severity of the disease. The essential objective of the treatment along with relieving the pain symptoms is the identification of the factors that aggravate the pain and the risk of recurrence.

Further Reading

Arun Kumar M, Ananthakrishnan V, Goturu J. Aetiology and pathophysiology of recurrent aphthous stomatitis: a review. IJCRR. 2014;06(10):16.

Belenguer-Guallar I, Jiménez-Soriano Y, Claramunt-Lozano A. Treatment of recurrent aphthous stomatitis; a literature review. J Clin Exp Dent. 2014;6(2):e168–74.

Compilato D, Carroccio A, Calvino F, Di Fede G, Campisi G. Haematological deficiencies in patients with recurrent aphthosis. J Eur Acad Dermatol Venereol. 2010;24(6):667–73.

Edgar NR, Saleh D, Miller RA. Recurrent aphthous stomatitis; a review. Journal of clinical aesthetics. Dermatology. 2017;10(3):26–36.

Femanio F, Lanz A, Buonaiuto A, et al. Guidelines for diagnosis and management of aphthous stomatitis. Paediatric Infect Dis J. 2007;26(8):728–32.

Oral and Maxillofacial Medicine. The basis of diagnosis and treatment. 3rd ed. Crispian Scully; 2012. ISBN: 9780702049484

Oral and Maxillofacial Pathology. Neville BW, Damm DD, Allen CM, Angela C 4th Edition.

Oral Medicine and Pathology. Guide to diagnosis and management. 2014, 1st Edition: Saman Warnakulasuriya, WM Tilakaratne. Jaypee ISBN: 9789350252215.

Rivera C, Muñoz A, Puentes C, Aguayo. Risk factors for recurrent aphthous stomatitis: a systematic review. Int J Morphol. 2021;39(4):1102–8.

Infections of the Oral Cavity

Contents

Multiple White Lesions of Recent Onset: Candidosis

Ruwan Jayasinghe and Wanninayake M Tilakaratne

Contents

W. M Tilakaratne, T. G. Kallarakkal (eds.), *Clinicopathological Correlation of Oral Diseases*,
https://doi.org/10.1007/978-3-031-24408-7_36

Learning Goals

1. Devise the correct way of compiling the history with appropriate questions.
2. Develop a differential diagnosis after history taking.
3. Deduce appropriate procedures in clinical examination.
4. Formulate a differential diagnosis combining findings in the history and clinical examination.
5. Justify the relevant investigations required to arrive at the diagnosis.
6. Comprehend the importance of clinicopathological correlation in arriving at the correct diagnosis.
7. Outline the management plan.
8. Recognize the importance of a diagnostic algorithm in arriving at a diagnosis.

36.1 Main Complaint

A 65-year-old female patient presents to the clinic with the complaint of multiple whitish lesions in the mouth.

36.2 History of Complaint

Question: How long have you been having these whitish lesions?

It has been there for more than a month. Initially it started at the back of the mouth but with time lesions started to appear all over the mouth.

Question: Is there any pain associated with the white lesions?

There is no pain or burning sensation associated with them. Sometimes I feel that the whitish lesions get peeled off specially during brushing.

36.3 Additional Complaints

Question: Have you noticed or felt any other changes or difficulties in the mouth?

I also have dryness in the mouth and altered taste, difficulty in swallowing, and bad breath.

Question: Did you have any previous episodes of similar whitish lesions in the mouth?

I do not have any previous history of similar lesions.

Question: Do you have any lesions elsewhere in the body?

I don't have any lesions other than the difficulties present in the mouth.

Question: Are you suffering from any other medical problems, like heart disease, high blood pressure, diabetes, bleeding disorder, and respiratory diseases? If yes, what kind of medications have you been taking until now?

I was diagnosed with diabetes mellitus more than 15 years ago. I am currently on oral medication. I don't take my medicines regularly and my blood sugar control is not satisfactory at the moment.

Question: Have you undergone any surgery?

I have not undergone any surgery in the past.

Question: Have you undergone any dental treatment?

I have undergone restorations and multiple dental extractions in the past without any complications. I have been edentulous for the last 10 years.

Question: What is your occupation?

I used to work as a management assistant in a private company and retired 12 years ago. Currently I am not employed.

Question: Do you have any specific chewing habits?

I am not a betel quid chewer.

Question Are you a smoker?

I am not a smoker.

Question: Do you take alcohol?

I don't consume alcohol.

36.4 With the Findings From the History, What is Your Differential Diagnosis?

1. Candidosis
2. Leukoplakia

3. Oral lichen planus or oral lichenoid reaction
4. Chemical burns

36.5 How Do You Justify Your Differential Diagnosis After History Taking?

1. She has whitish lesions all over the mouth that has been there for more than a month. They appear to be scrapable. She is a known diabetic patient. The features that she describes are suggestive of pseudomembranous candidosis considering that the patient is a diabetic with poor immune status. She has dryness in the mouth and has difficulty in swallowing suggestive of xerostomia consequent to her diabetic state. The xerostomia could have contributed to pseudomembranous candidosis due to the alteration in the normal oral microflora.
2. Leukoplakia presents as an asymptomatic white plaque mostly in people with risk habits. Even though very rarely it can be seen in multiple sites, it is generally confined to one location. Leukoplakia is not scrapable. Presence in multiple sites, recent onset, lack of risk habits, and scrapable nature of the lesions reduce the possibility of leukoplakia as a differential diagnosis.
3. Oral lichen planus (OLP) is a common immune-mediated mucocutaneous condition with unknown etiology that is commonly seen in females. Oral lichenoid reaction (OLR) has a similar clinical presentation but its etiology can be identified. OLR is commonly associated with dental materials especially amalgam or drugs, such as antihypertensive and antidiabetic medications. OLP/OLR has multiple clinical presentations, including plaque and reticular forms which are usually asymptomatic but at times can cause burning sensation especially with spicy foods. Plaques in OLP/OLR are not scrapable by activities, such as brushing. The plaque type OLP is commonly seen on the tongue and can be associated with genital or skin lesions. As this patient has been on antidiabetic drugs for some time OLP/OLR is a possibility but the scrapable nature of the white lesions makes OLP/OLR an unlikely differential diagnosis.
4. Chemical burns can cause white plaque like lesions in the mouth. However, these lesions are short lived, and patient can usually recall the incident of using a chemical. In most instances, these lesions are painful.

36

36.6 Findings of Examination

The patient is totally edentulous. Whitish plaques are observed all over the mouth. These plaques can be wiped off with a piece of gauze and a reddish base is observed in the areas where the plaques have been removed. Slight bleeding is observed from these areas. No reticular lesions are observed. The patient does not show any abnormalities on extra oral examination. There is no evidence of cervical lymphadenopathy.

36.7 What Other Relevant Features Would You Look for with the Findings You Have So Far?

Generalized dryness is observed in the mouth with lack of salivary pooling in the floor of the mouth. Whitish plaques are observed on the dorsal surface of the tongue (Fig. 36.1). Multiple white homogeneous plaques are observed on both sides of the buccal mucosae extending from the commissure to the retro-molar areas (Fig. 36.2).

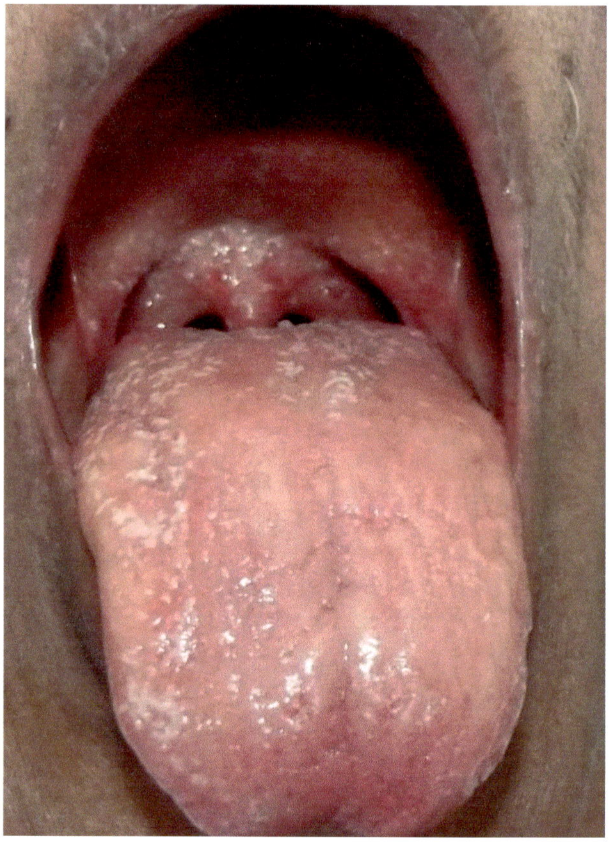

Fig. 36.1 Whitish plaques on the soft palate and tongue retained in some areas after wiping off

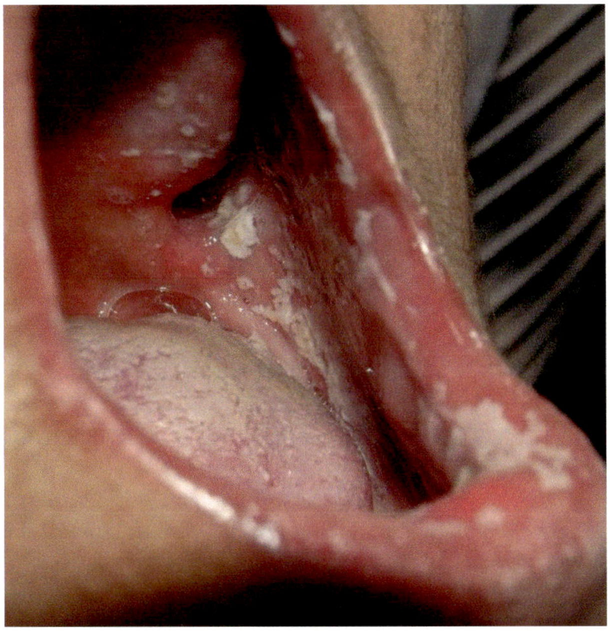

Fig. 36.2 Diffusely distributed whitish plaques on the left side buccal mucosa

36.8 What Is Your Clinical Diagnosis?

1. Pseudomembranous candidosis (Oral Thrush)

36.9 How Would You Arrive At This Working Diagnosis?

Oral thrush is usually present in people who have predisposing factors for opportunistic infections, especially in immune compromised patients. This patient has a history of diabetes which is not under control. Lesions present as white plaques which can be wiped off without causing pain or burning sensation but leaving a bleeding/reddish base. These features are diagnostic for oral thrush as any other whitish lesion present in the mouth cannot be wiped off.

36.10 How Would You Confirm Your Clinical Diagnosis?

Diagnosis of oral thrush is essentially clinical but can be confirmed microbiologically by either taking a swab for culture to identify the presence of pathological forms of candida or by staining a smear from the affected area to demonstrate fungal hyphae. The periodic acid–Schiff (PAS) stained smears obtained from the dorsum of the tongue and buccal mucosa show tangled masses of fungal hyphae along with numerous yeast forms. The background shows numerous normal squamous epithelial cells (Fig. 36.3). Presence of neutrophils is also a common finding.

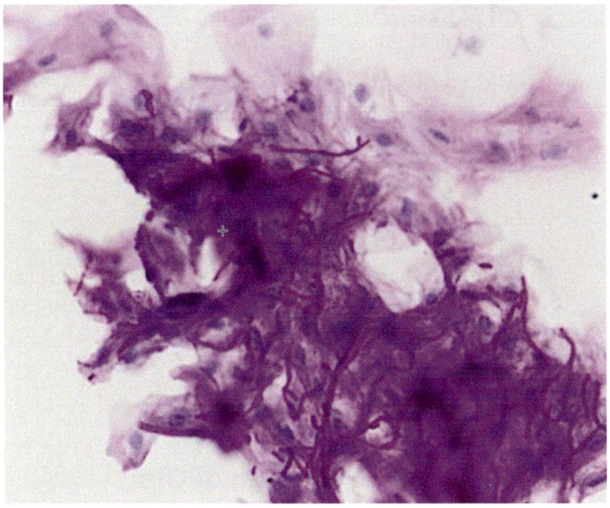

Fig. 36.3 PAS stained smear showing nucleate squamous epithelial cells and numerous fungal hyphae

36.11 How Would You Manage This Patent?

It is very essential to identify the predisposing factors for oral candidosis. In this patient, the most likely predisposing factor would be the poorly controlled diabetic status which has to be managed properly by a physician or an endocrinologist. In addition, basic investigations, such as full blood count, liver function tests, and renal function tests, have to be carried out to identify any other coexisting comorbidities that can result in poor immune status of the patient. Her dry mouth can also predispose to oral candidosis. Dry mouth is most likely due to diabetes and may improve once the disease is under control. Until such time, it is essential to improve salivary secretion by local measures and if needed systemic sialagogues. Improvement of oral hygiene and denture hygiene is essential.

Oral candidosis is managed by antifungal agents. Topical antifungals are preferred considering the side effects of systemic antifungals. Nystatin is the drug of choice. Nystatin is available as an oral rinse, pastille, and suspension. It has a poor availability in the oral cavity. Hence, the recommended dosage is four times a day for at least 2 weeks. Its taste is not tolerable by some patients resulting in poor compliance at times. Other side effects of Nystatin include nausea, vomiting, and diarrhea. Clotrimazole can be used as an alternative.

Culture and sensitivity testing should be undertaken if initial therapy with topical antifungals is unsuccessful. If the patient does not respond to topical antifungal treatment, systemic antifungals have to be considered. The drug of choice is Fluconazole as it has relatively lesser side effects.

36.12 Oral Candidosis

Oral candidosis may be classified as follows:

1. Type I—oral candidosis
   (a) Pseudomembranous
   (b) Erythematous
   (c) Hyperplastic
   (d) Candida-associated lesions–*Candida*-associated denture stomatitis, angular cheilitis, median rhomboid glossitis, and linear gingival erythema.
2. Type II—mucocutaneous candidosis with or without oral involvement.

36.13 Clinical Presentation of Oral Candidosis

Oral candidosis is not a single clinical entity. It occurs in four distinct primary forms. There are two transient types, namely, pseudomembranous candidosis and acute erythematous candidosis. Chronic erythematous candidosis and chronic hyperplastic candidosis (CHC) are the two persistent forms. Candida is also implicated in angular cheilitis, liner gingival erythema (Red band gingivitis), and median rhomboid glossitis. Each type of infection is associated with characteristic clinical signs and symptoms that are influenced by a range of predisposing factors that include the following:

Local and systemic host factors

- Local host factors
  - Wearing dentures
  - Use of steroid inhaler
  - Reduced salivary flow
  - Poor nutritional status
- Systemic host factors
  - Extremes of age
  - Endocrine disorders such as diabetes
  - Immunosuppression
  - Use of broad-spectrum antibiotics

36.14 Pseudomembranous Candidosis/Oral Thrush

Oral thrush is reported in 5–10% of neonates and elderly. It is characterized by the presence of superficial white plaques that can be easily removed by gentle rubbing. Ability to remove these plaques is a diagnostic feature that differentiates pseudomembranous candidosis from other white lesions of the oral mucosa. Cytological examination reveals fungal elements in the form of yeast and filamentous forms, together with epithelial cells.

36.15 Acute Erythematous Candidosis

This condition is also referred to as antibiotic sore mouth, as it tends to develop following a reduction in levels of bacterial component in the oral microflora after receiving broad-spectrum antibiotics. A decrease in bacterial flora results in reduced microbial competition for candida in terms of nutrition and adherence sites. This leads to an ecological shift in normal homeostatic balance of the microbial community.

This form of candidosis presents as a painful red lesion. Although the palate and buccal mucosa may be involved, the most common site of infection is dorsum of the tongue (Fig. 36.4). Cessation of antibiotic therapy results in normal levels of bacteria, which subsequently resolves candidosis without any intervention. Concomitant use of steroid therapy, particularly in inhaler form, is an additional contributing factor, as this can create a localized area of immune suppression within the mucosa that permits overgrowth of candida.

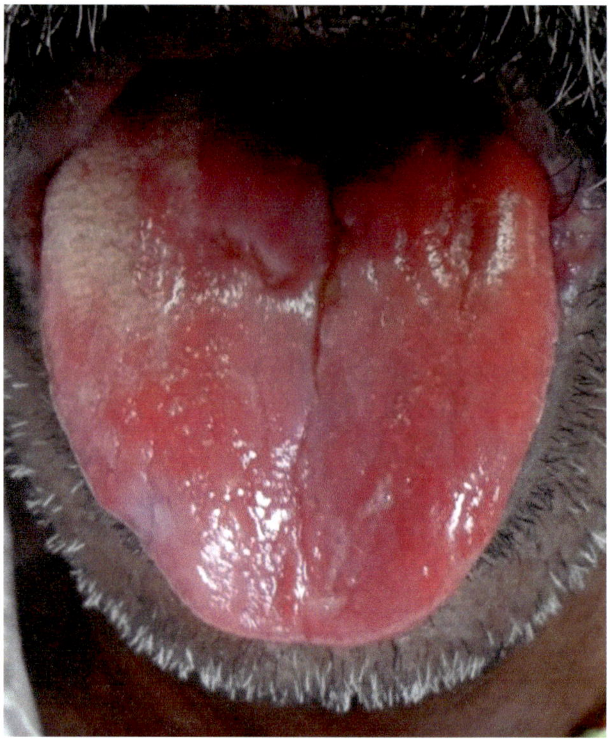

Fig. 36.4 Glossitis in acute erythematous candidosis

36.16 Chronic Hyperplastic Candidosis

Chronic hyperplastic candidosis characteristically presents as a thickened white plaque, most frequently at the commissure of the mouth (◘ Fig. 36.5) or on the dorsum of the tongue. It has questionable potential for the development of squamous cell carcinoma.

Two clinical types are recognized, including homogeneous (smooth white lesions) and non-homogeneous (areas of erythema resulting in a nodular, speckled appearance). CHC can be diagnosed by a smear or by histopathological examination of lesional tissue. The latter allows for evaluation of any epithelial dysplasia in the lesion. Microscopically, the sections reveal candidal hyphae invading the epithelium with the underlying corium containing a chronic inflammatory cell infiltrate (◘ Fig. 36.6). However, dysplasia grading should be carried out only after antifungal treatment as candida can exaggerate dysplastic features.

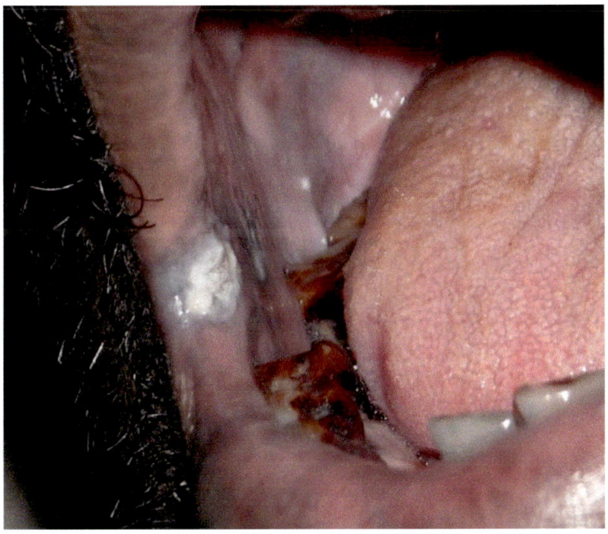

◘ Fig. 36.5 Chronic hyperplastic candidosis presenting as a thick white non-scrapable plaque at the commissure

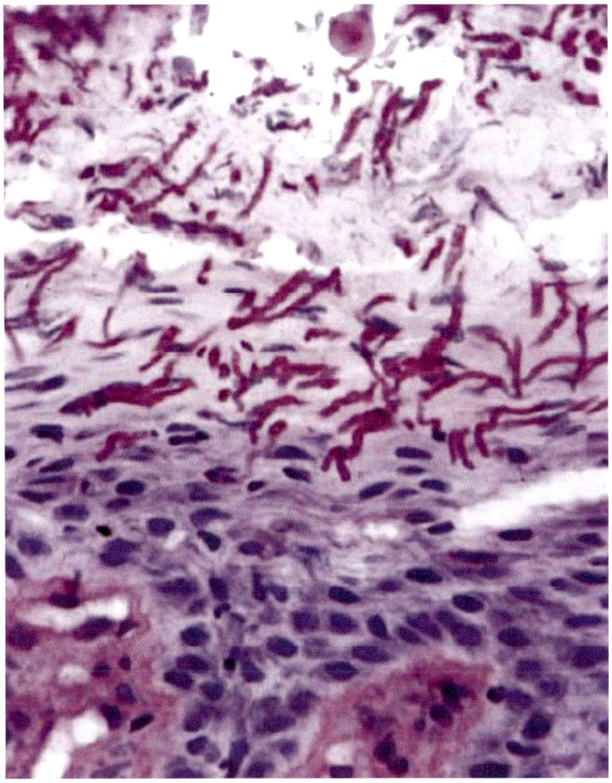

◘ Fig. 36.6 PAS staining shows numerous fungal hyphae invading into surface layers of the epithelium in CHC

36.17 Candida-Associated Denture Stomatitis/Chronic Atrophic Candidosis/Chronic Erythematous Candidosis

This condition is characterized by reddening of mucosa beneath the fitting surface of the denture. This may develop under any acrylic denture/intra-oral appliance, and is common on palatal tissues. Principle host factors associated are inadequate oral hygiene, failure to remove dentures whilst sleeping, or ill-fitting dentures. This is the most prevalent form involving up to 75% of denture wearers. Depending on the severity, denture stomatitis can be classified into three groups: type I (pinpoint erythema; ◘ Fig. 36.7); type II (diffuse erythema; ◘ Fig. 36.8); and type III (granular/papillary lesions; ◘ Fig. 36.9).

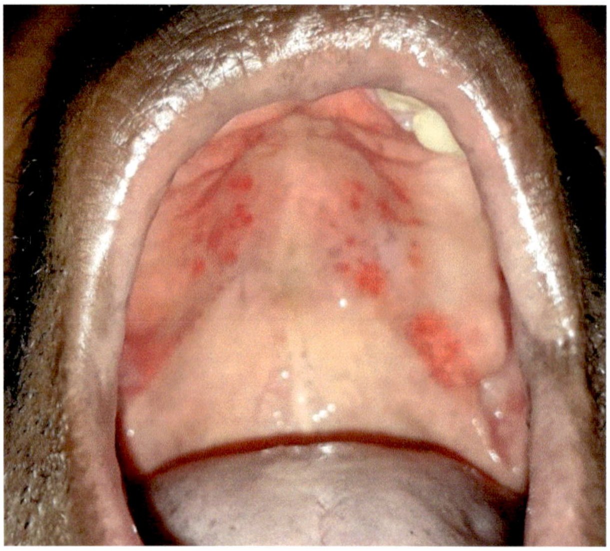

◘ Fig. 36.7 Pinpoint erythema on the palate

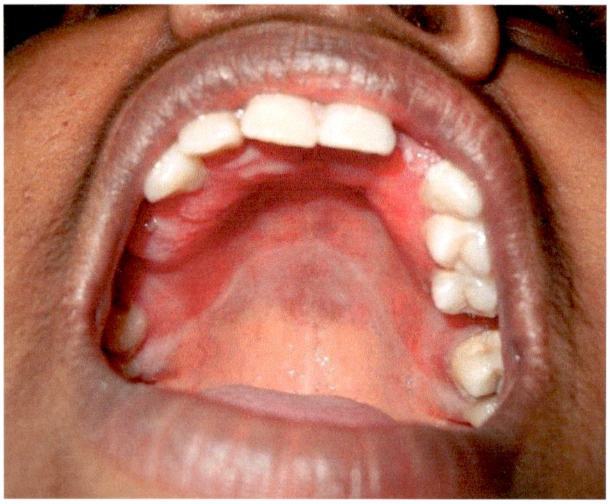

◘ Fig. 36.8 Diffuse erythema on the palate

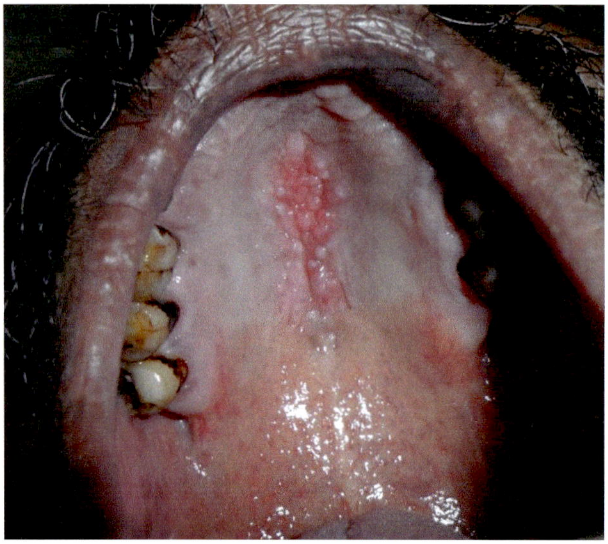

◘ Fig. 36.9 Papillary hyperplasia of the palate

36.18 Angular Cheilitis

Angular cheilitis is characterized by erythematous lesions on one side, or usually both angles of the mouth (◘ Fig. 36.10). In addition to candida, a spectrum of microorganisms recovered from these lesions include staphylococcus aureus and streptococcal species, either alone or in combination.

The exact role of candida in angular cheilitis remains unclear. It often occurs in patients with a pre-existing primary form of oral candidosis, most frequently chronic erythematous candidosis. Increased levels of candida within the mouth of such patients is most likely to be a major contributing factor.

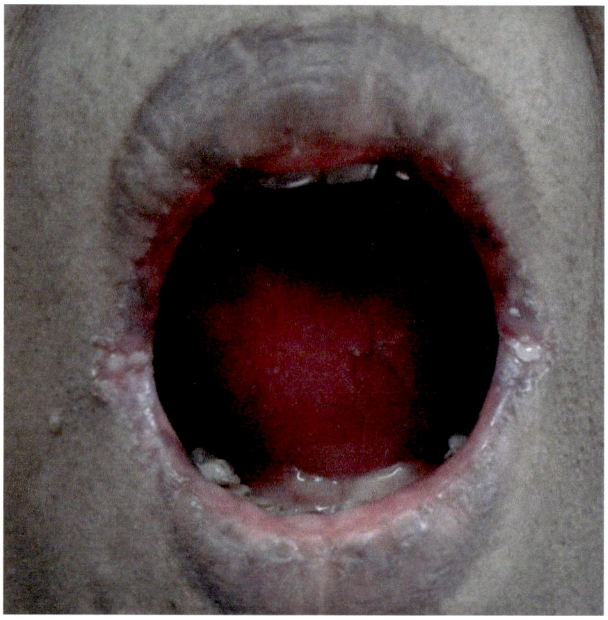

◘ Fig. 36.10 Angular cheilitis showing bilateral lesions

36.19 Median Rhomboid Glossitis (MRG)

Median rhomboid glossitis appears on the dorsal surface of the tongue as a depapillated area (Fig. 36.11). It is usually present in the midline of the tongue at the junction between anterior two-thirds and posterior one-third. Even though the name suggests a rhomboid morphology, it may take many shapes ranging from round, oval to irregular. It is well demarcated, smooth, and depapillated, but at times it can present as a lobulated area (Fig. 36.12). There can be associated lesions on the palate (kissing lesions) suggesting the infective nature of the lesion.

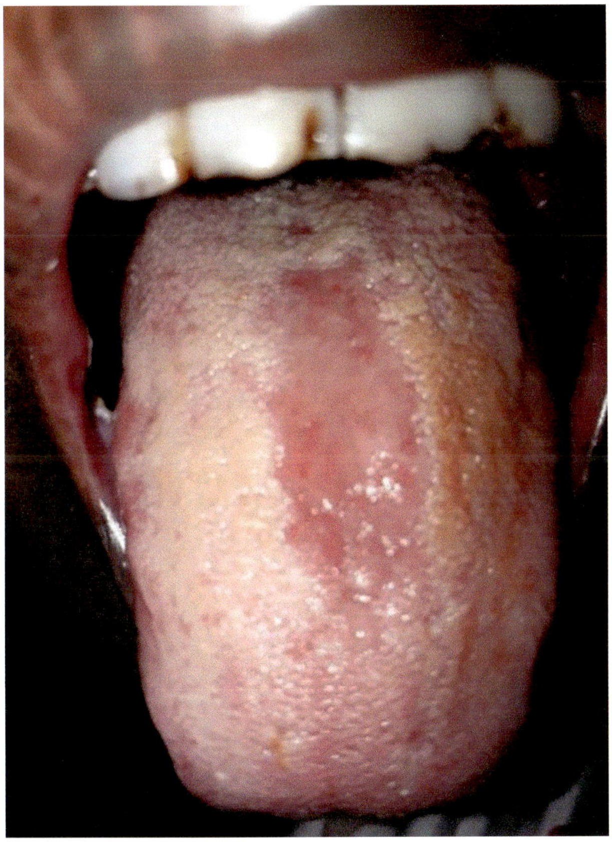

Fig. 36.11 Median Rhomboid Glossitis (MRG); Atrophic area on the dorsum of tongue

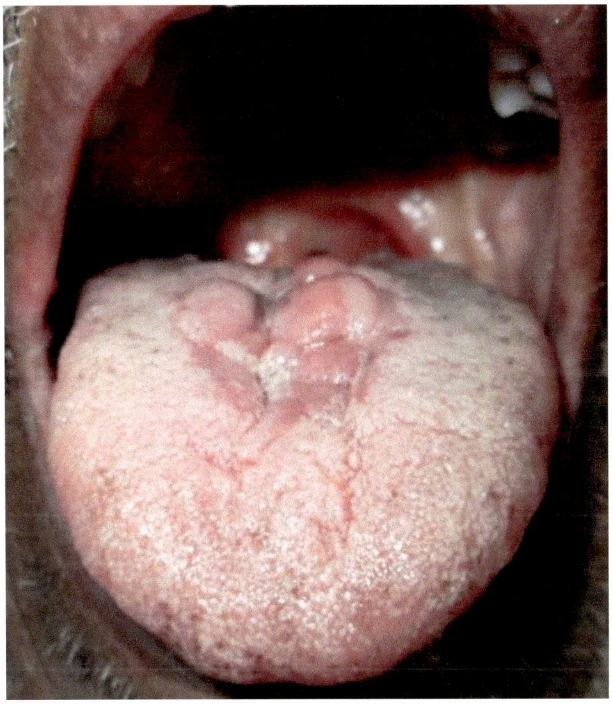

Fig. 36.12 Median Rhomboid Glossitis (MRG); lobulated appearance

36.20 Management of Oral Candidosis

Diagnosis of oral candidosis is by combination of history, clinical features, and microbiological investigations. In the case of CHC, histopathological investigations may be useful.

An effective management of oral candidosis can be achieved by the following simple guidelines:

1. Correction of local and systemic predisposing factors whenever possible.
2. Maintenance of proper oral hygiene and denture hygiene if the patient is wearing dentures.
3. Use of antifungal agents based on the severity of the infection and susceptibility of the candida species prevalent in that patient (Table 36.1).

Table 36.1 Antifungals agents for the management of oral candidosis

Antifungal agent	Mode of application	Dosage	Duration	Remarks
Nystatin suspension (100,000 U/mL)	Topical	4–6 mL four times a day	7–14 days	Bad taste, possibility of vomiting, nausea and diarrhea
Nystatin pastilles (200,000 U each)	Topical	1–2 pastilles four times a day	7–14 days	Bad taste, possibility of vomiting, nausea and diarrhea
Clotrimazole troches	Topical	10 mg five times a day	7–14 days	
Miconazole gel	Topical	3–4 times a day	14–28 days	For treating uncomplicated infections in healthy patients. Drug of choice for angular cheilitis
Fluconazole	Systemic	100–200 mg daily	7–14 days	Need to monitor liver function, possibility of development of resistant strains
Itraconazole	Systemic	200 mg daily	28 days	Need to monitor liver function, possibility of development of resistant strains

Self-Assessment Questions

1. List the pathognomonic clinical features of oral thrush.
2. Discuss the predisposing factors for oral candidosis.
3. State the different types of oral candidal infections.
4. Discuss the investigations for oral candidosis.
5. Outline the management plan according to the type of infection.

Diagnostic Algorithm

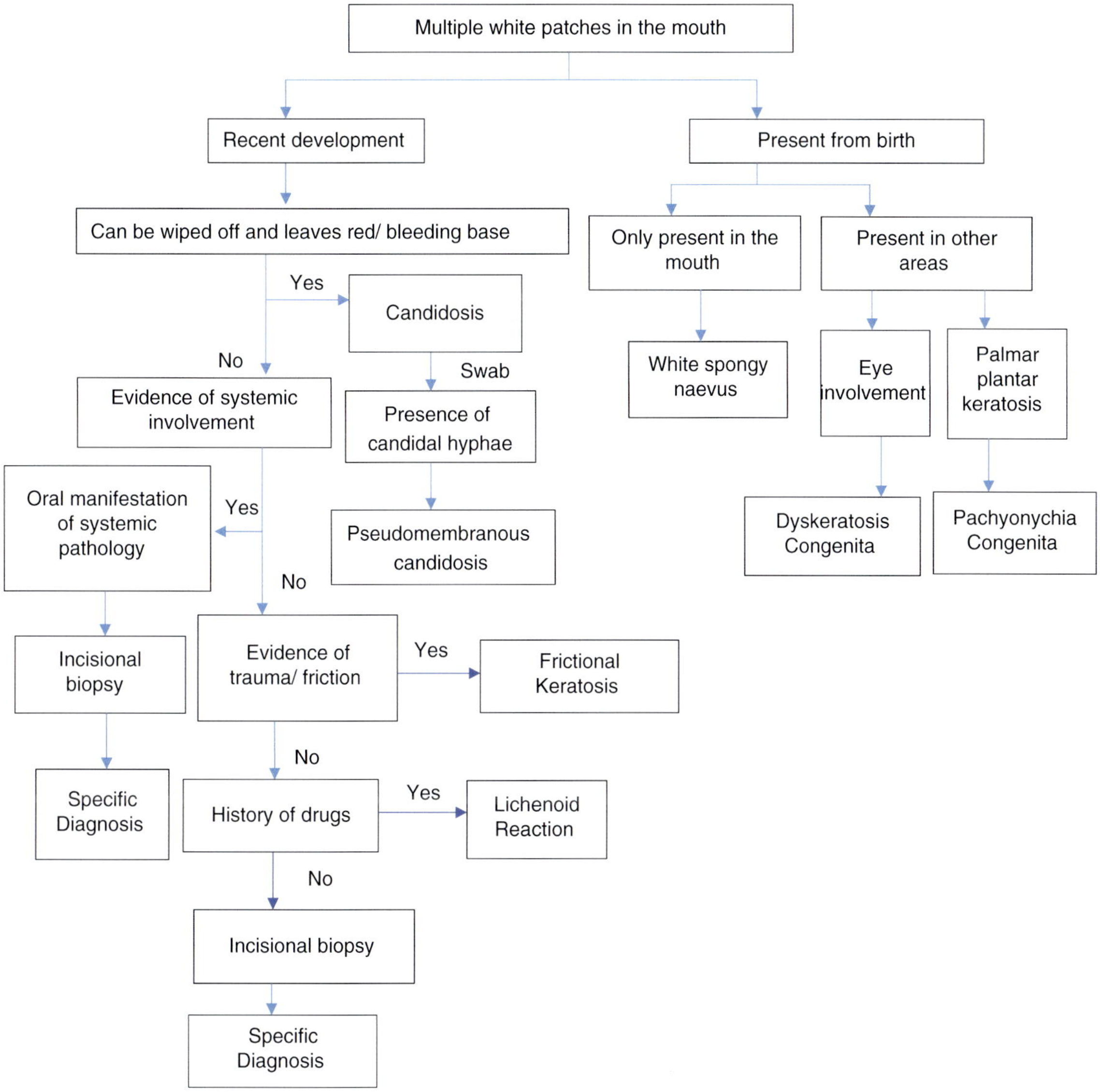

Summary

Oral candidosis has multiple clinical presentations causing a challenge in the management. Diagnosis of oral candidosis needs combination of history, clinical features, and microbiological and at times histopathological investigations. Management of oral candidosis is by correcting predisposing factors, maintenance of proper oral/denture hygiene, and use of antifungal agents which can be topical or systemic.

Further Reading

Akpan A, Morgan R. Oral candidosis. Postgrad Med J. 2002;78:455–9.

Bandara HMHN, Samaranayake LP. Viral, bacterial, and fungal infections of the oral mucosa: types, incidence, predisposing factors, diagnostic algorithms, and management. Periodontology. 2000;2019(80):148–76.

Patil S, Rao RS, Majumdar B, Anil S. Clinical appearance of oral candida infection and therapeutic strategies. Front Microbiol. 2015;6:1391. https://doi.org/10.3389/fmicb.2015.01391.

Samaranayake L. Essential microbiology for dentistry. 5th ed; 2018. ISBN: 9780702074356

Vila T, Sultan AS, Montelongo-Jauregui D, Jabra-Rizk MA. Oral candidosis: a disease of opportunity. J Fungi. 2020;6:15. https://doi.org/10.3390/jof6010015.

Williams D, Lewis M. Pathogenesis and treatment of oral candidosis. J Oral Microbiol. 2011;3:5771. https://doi.org/10.3402/jom.v3i0.5771.

Slow Growing Lump on the Labial Mucosa: HPV Infection (Squamous Cell Papilloma/ Condyloma/ Viral Wart)

Ruwan Jayasinghe and Wanninayake M Tilakaratne

Contents

W. M Tilakaratne, T. G. Kallarakkal (eds.), *Clinicopathological Correlation of Oral Diseases*,
https://doi.org/10.1007/978-3-031-24408-7_37

Learning Goals

1. Devise the correct way of compiling the history with appropriate questions.
2. Develop a differential diagnosis after history taking.
3. Deduce appropriate procedures in clinical examination.
4. Formulate a differential diagnosis combining findings in the history and clinical examination.
5. Justify the relevant investigations required to arrive at the diagnosis.
6. Comprehend the importance of clinicopathological correlation in arriving at the correct diagnosis.
7. Outline the management plan.
8. Recognize the importance of a diagnostic algorithm in arriving at a diagnosis.

37.1 Main Complaint

A 55-year-old male patient presents to the clinic with the complaint of a lump on the lower lip.

37.2 History of Complaint

Question: How long have you been having this lump?

It has been there for over 6 months. Initially it appeared as a very small white thickening and grew slowly for about 6 months. It has not enlarged in size after that.

37.3 Additional Complaints

Question: Do you have any pain or irritation in relation to the lump?

I don't have any difficulty with it. There is no pain or burning sensation. It does not interfere with my normal activities, such as eating or talking.

Question: Did you have any trauma to the lower lip or do you have habitual lip biting/sucking habit?

I can't recollect any trauma to the area. I don't have any habit of lip biting or sucking.

Question: Has this lump ruptured earlier?

It has been there as a firm lump from the day I noticed it and has been enlarging very slowly. I don't think it ruptured at any moment.

Question: Have you noticed any bleeding from it.

There was no bleeding from it at all.

Question: Do you have any similar lesions elsewhere on the body?

There are no other similar lesions on my body other than this lump.

Question: Do you have any specific chewing habits?

I have been chewing around two–three betel quids a day for a few years but stopped it about 6 months ago.

Question: Are you a smoker?

I used to smoke about ten cigarettes a day for 5 years in the past.

Question: Do you take alcohol?

I don't use alcohol.

Question: Are you married?

I am married and live with my wife and two children.

Question: Did you have multiple sexual partners during the last few years?

I did not have any such relationships.

37.4 With the Findings From the History, What is Your Differential Diagnosis?

1. Mucocele
2. Minor salivary gland tumor
3. Varix
4. Fibro-epithelial polyp
5. Pyogenic granuloma
6. Papilloma
7. Verruca vulgaris (Viral wart)

37.5 How Do You Justify Your Differential Diagnosis After History Taking?

1. He has a slow growing, painless lesion on the lower lip. Mucocele is one of the commonest lesions to occur on the lower lip, but it is usually seen in children and adolescents who have a history of trauma to the lip. It has a bluish tint. It enlarges slowly and ruptures often only to recur in few days. However, a long-standing mucocele can give rise to a firm lump similar to this patient's lesion.
2. Minor salivary gland tumors can rarely occur on the lower lip. Majority of the minor salivary gland tumors occur on the upper lip. Therefore, a minor salivary gland tumor cannot be ruled out completely.
3. A pathological dilatation of vessels (Varix) is common on the low lip in middle aged or elderly. It has a bluish/purple color. Its growth potential is limited.
4. Fibro-epithelial polyps are not common on the lower lip. It has a pale color and is associated with chronic irritation. However, it should be considered in the differential diagnosis as it is the most common reactive lesion to occur in the oral cavity.
5. Pyogenic granuloma is relatively common on the lower lip. It has a reddish color and is associated with chronic irritation. It bleeds very easily. Although it is a possibility in this case, the findings in the history do not make it a lesion which should be considered highly.
6. Papilloma is a common benign tumor caused by the human papilloma virus (HPV). It is usually a single lesion and enlarges slowly. Lip and tongue are the common oral sites. It is usually white in color. It does not cause any pain or episodes of ulceration and bleeding. Therefore, papilloma is included in the differential diagnosis.
7. Verruca vulgaris (Viral wart) is not very common in the oral cavity. When it occurs, lip is a common site of involvement. It is also a lesion caused by HPV. It tends to spread to other intra oral and extra oral sites and enlarges slowly. Most of the attributes are similar to papilloma and should be considered in the differential diagnosis for this patient.

37.6 Findings of Examination

He has a whitish exophytic lesion with finger-like surface projections (Fig. 37.1). The lesion is attached to the mucosa with a narrow base (pedunculated). The surrounding labial mucosa appears to be normal in color and texture. The surface of the lump contains small projections mimicking a cauliflower-like appearance. The lump is approximately 1 cm in diameter.

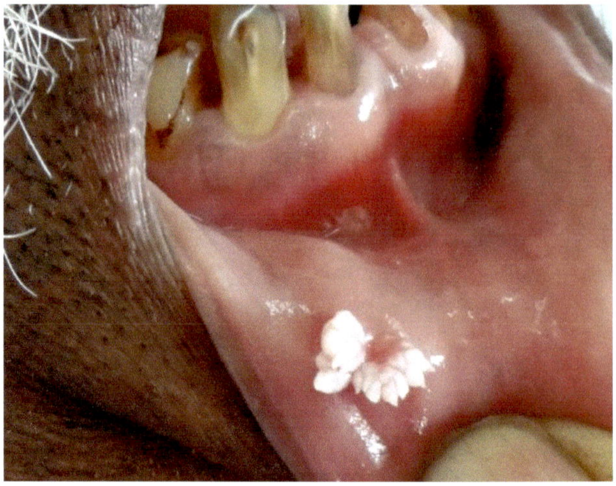

Fig. 37.1 Right labial mucosa showing a whitish exophytic lesion with finger-like projections

37.7 What are the Other Relevant Features That You Will Look For?

Palpation demonstrates it as a firm lesion without any tenderness. There is no clinical evidence of trauma. He does not have any similar lesions elsewhere in the mouth or on the visible areas of the body. Oral hygiene appears to be satisfactory.

37.8 What is Your Clinical Differential Diagnosis?

1. Squamous cell papilloma
2. Condyloma acuminatum
3. Verruca Vulgaris (Viral wart)

37.9 How Would You Justify the Inclusion of the Diseases That You Have Mentioned in the Differential Diagnosis to Arrive at a Working Diagnosis?

37.9.1 Squamous Cell Papilloma

Squamous cell papilloma is the commonest benign epithelial tumor of the oral cavity. Clinically, it presents as a whitish, exophytic growth with a papillary surface exhibiting finger-like projections. Clinically, significant number of papillomas have a "P"-shaped appearance. A papilloma has a relatively rapid growth and within the first few months, it reaches to a maximum diameter of 1 cm in most cases. The present case fulfills most of these clinical criteria and is also supported by findings in the history.

37.9.2 Condyloma Acuminatum

Condylomata is considered as a sexually transmitted disease caused by HPV. Lesions are commonly seen on the genital area and oral sex is considered as route of transmission to oral cavity. Oral lesions in the condylomata are rare. Lesions of condylomata typically appear as soft, pink/white nodules that can coalesce together to form cauliflower-like masses. Lip and tongue are the common sites of occurrence. They can present as single or multiple lesions. Most cases have an inverted "C"-shaped appearance clinically. They can grow to a larger size than papilloma or verruca vulgaris. They are mostly sessile lesions and are rarely pedunculated.

37.9.3 Verruca Vulgaris (Viral Wart)

Verruca vulgaris (VV) or common wart or viral wart is a virus-induced lesion of the oral mucosa or skin caused by HPV. Vermilion border of the lip, labial mucosa, and tongue are the common oral sites for VV. Clinically, VV appears as a painless, slow growing whitish papule, or nodule with papillary projections and can be pedunculated or sessile. The projections usually have a sharp point mimicking an inverted "V"-shaped appearance.

37.10 What is the Most Likely Diagnosis?

Squamous cell papilloma.

37.11 How Would You Investigate This Patient?

A definitive diagnosis of squamous cell papilloma is established by histopathology. Excision of the lesion followed by histopathological examination is recommended.

37.12 What are the Risk Factors for Oral HPV?

Risk factors for oral HPV infection include oral sex, multiple sexual partners, smoking, drinking alcohol, and open mouth kissing.

37.13 How Would You Manage This Patient?

Surgical excision and histopathological examination is the treatment of choice. It is an invasive procedure. Cryotherapy or liquid nitrogen therapy is a simple, painless procedure but may need multiple cycles of treatment, and there will be no tissue available for histopathological examination. Laser therapy is also an effective method.

37.14 What are the Histopathological Features of Squamous Cell Papilloma?

Hematoxylin and Eosin (H&E) sections show a mucosal nodule covered by both ortho and parakeratinized stratified squamous epithelium containing many finger-like epithelial projections (◘ Fig. 37.2). These epithelial projections are composed of a fibrovascular connective tissue core. The epithelium does not show any evidence of cytological atypia. Virally damaged epithelial cells (koilocytes) are evident in the superficial layers of the epithelium in most cases.

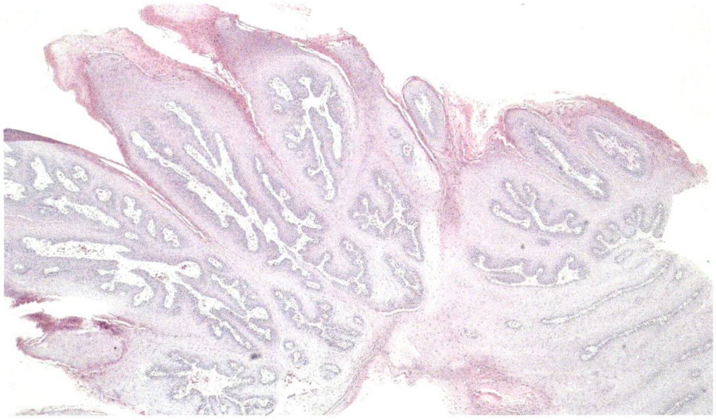

◘ **Fig. 37.2** A mucosal nodule surfaced by both ortho and parakeratinized stratified squamous epithelium showing numerous finger-like projections

37.15 What are the Important Histopathological Differential Diagnosis of Squamous Cell Papilloma?

1. Verruca vulgaris
2. Condyloma acuminatum
3. Verrucous hyperplasia (smaller lesions)
4. Multifocal epithelial hyperplasia
5. Seborrheic keratosis

37.16 Oral Manifestations of HPV Infections

Human papillomavirus has been implicated in a variety of papillomatous and malignant squamous proliferations in the head and neck area, such as squamous cell papilloma, verruca vulgaris (common warts), condyloma acuminatum, multifocal epithelial hyperplasia (Heck's disease), sinonasal papillomas, laryngeal papillomas, and oropharyngeal squamous cell carcinoma. There are over 200 different HPV genotypes but not all are associated with malignancy. Some HPV types are of low risk (e.g., HPV 6 and 11), whereas some are considered as high risk types (e.g., HPV 16 and 18). Common oral non-malignant lesions caused by the HPV are verruca vulgaris (Viral wart) squamous cell papilloma condylomata and multifocal epithelial hyperplasia.

37.16.1 Oral Squamous Cell Papilloma

Oral squamous cell papilloma is a common benign epithelial tumor. Clinically, it presents as a whitish, exophytic proliferation with a papillary surface containing finger-like projections. It is commonly seen in children and in people in the third and fourth decades of life. Although it commonly occurs as a single lesion, multiple lesions are associated with some rare syndromes, such as focal dermal hypoplasia syndrome, acrodermatitis enteropathica, Cowden syndrome, Costello syndrome, and Down syndrome. Squamous cell papilloma is usually asymptomatic. Palate and tongue are the common sites of involvement. Clinically, it is characterized by a verrucous or cauliflower-like appearance. It can be sessile or pedunculated. Most lesions are whitish in appearance, but it can be pink in color as well. Usually it appears as a single lesion with a rapid growth phase enlarging to its maximum size of 1 cm in diameter within a few months.

37.16.2 Condyloma Acuminatum

Condyloma acuminatum (CA) lesions are commonly seen on the anogenital skin and mucosa. Involvement of oral mucosa is rare. When present, upper and lower labial and buccal mucosa, soft palate, and the dorsum of the tongue are the common sites (▫ Fig. 37.3). CA is caused by HPV genotypes 6 and 11. Transmission is through sexual or skin-to-skin contact. Viral particles are shed from the lesions and can cause infections if there is mucosal to skin contact and therefore clinicians should take appropriate protection when examining an infected patient. CA lesions are usually asymptomatic. They appear as pedunculated or sessile, soft papules measuring about 2–3 mm in diameter. Exact mode of transmission of oral CA is not clear, but there is evidence of transmission via oral sex. These lesions tend to recur irrespective of the type of treatment; hence, regular follow-up of the patient is recommended.

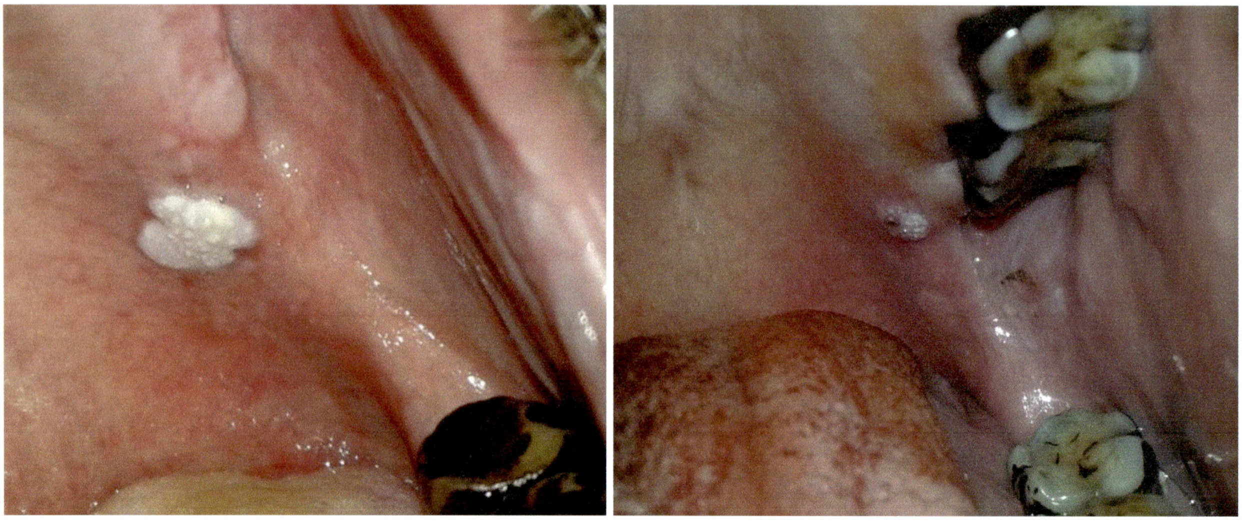

▫ **Fig. 37.3** Condyloma acuminatum on the palate

Histological features of CA are similar to squamous cell papilloma. It includes hyperplasia of the epithelium with papillary projections, slight parakeratosis, and the presence of numerous virally damaged epithelial cells (koilocytes). This feature is more frequently observed in CA compared to papilloma.

37.16.3 Verruca Vulgaris/Viral Wart

Verruca vulgaris (VV), common wart or viral wart, is a virus-induced lesion of the skin and mucosa caused by HPV. Several types of HPV are associated with VV, but HPV types 2 and 4 are the most common. Oral lesions are less common than the skin lesions and both lesions show similar clinical appearance. VV can occur at any age but is much commoner in children. Clinically, they present as whitish, sessile, circumscribed, exophytic lesions with a papillomatous surface. Oral lesions are commonly found on the vermilion border of the lip, labial mucosa, or on the tongue (◘ Fig. 37.4). Histopathologically, VVs are characterized by a proliferation of hyperkeratotic stratified squamous oral epithelium showing finger-like projections with connective tissue cores. Rete ridges are elongated and tend to converge toward the center of the lesion. A prominent granular cell layer is visible. Chronic inflammatory cell infiltrate in the underlying connective tissue is present. Koilocytes, virally damaged epithelial cells are often seen in the superficial spinous layer of the epithelium. These cells demonstrate perinuclear clear spaces and small, dark nuclei (pyknosis) with eosinophilic intra nuclear viral inclusions.

37.16.4 Multifocal Epithelial Hyperplasia (Heck's Disease)

Mutifocal epithelial hyperplasia (MFEH) is a benign rare condition associated with HPV types 13 and 32 infection with a genetic predisposition. Both genders are equally affected. Even though it can be seen at any age, it is much more common in children. Clinically, lesions of MFEH present as whitish, multiple, soft nodular elevations. Common oral sites of involvement are lower lip, buccal mucosa, and tongue (◘ Fig. 37.5). Rarely lesions can be seen on the upper lip, gingiva, and palate. They can disappear even without any treatment followed by recurrence. Important conditions that have to be included in the differential diagnosis include inflammatory fibrous hyperplasia, inflammatory papillary hyperplasia, verruciform xanthoma, verrucous carcinoma, verrucous hyperplasia, Cowden disease, and condyloma acuminatum. The diagnosis is usually made with typical clinical presentation. Histopathological features help in confirming the diagnosis. Histopathologically, characteristic features of other HPV-induced oral lesions are evident. However, the typical papillary projections seen in papilloma, VV, and CA are not observed in MFEH. In addition, presence of structures that resemble mitotic figures known as mitosoid bodies are characteristic in MFEH. As this is a self-limiting condition spontaneous healing occurs in some patients. Surgical removal of lesions can also be carried out when the lesions are traumatized or aesthetically unacceptable.

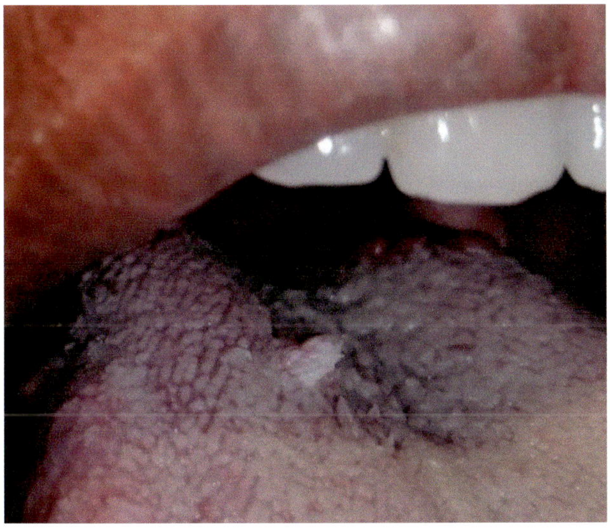

◘ **Fig. 37.4** Verruca vulgaris/viral wart on the tongue

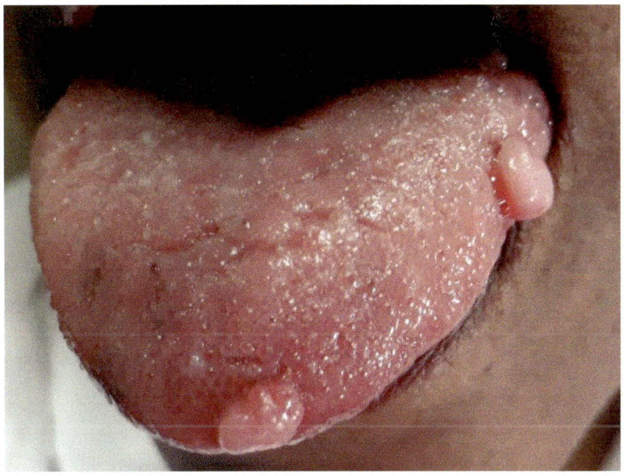

◘ **Fig. 37.5** MFEH characterized by multiple lesions on the tongue

37.16.5 Management of Common Oral HPV Lesions

Single oral lesions are treated surgically. Most of the skin lesions can be managed with topical antiviral application, but it is difficult in the oral cavity. Surgery, cryotherapy or liquid nitrogen therapy and laser therapy are the common modes of management. Other treatment modalities include drugs such as cimetidine and levamisole, retinoids, topical immunotherapy, and salicylic acid (Table 37.1).

Table 37.1 Summary of features of common oral HPV lesions

	Verruca vulgaris (common wart)	**Squamous cell papilloma**	**Condyloma acuminatum (venereal warts)**
Sexual transmission	No	No	Yes
Increased cancer risk	No	No	Yes
Clinical appearance	Sessile hairy-looking white lesion/s, elevated with discrete borders and a pointed verrucous top	Common benign pedunculated lesion, cauliflower-like surface but often indistinguishable from verruca vulgaris	Papillary proliferations with a cauliflower-like shape, small and sessile to large, larger than papillomas, often multiple
Types	HPV types 2, 4, and 40	HPV 6 and 11	HPV 6 and 11
Treatment	Surgery, cryotherapy or liquid nitrogen therapy and laser therapy	Surgery, cryotherapy or liquid nitrogen therapy and laser therapy	Surgery, cryotherapy or liquid nitrogen therapy and laser therapy

Diagnostic Algorithm

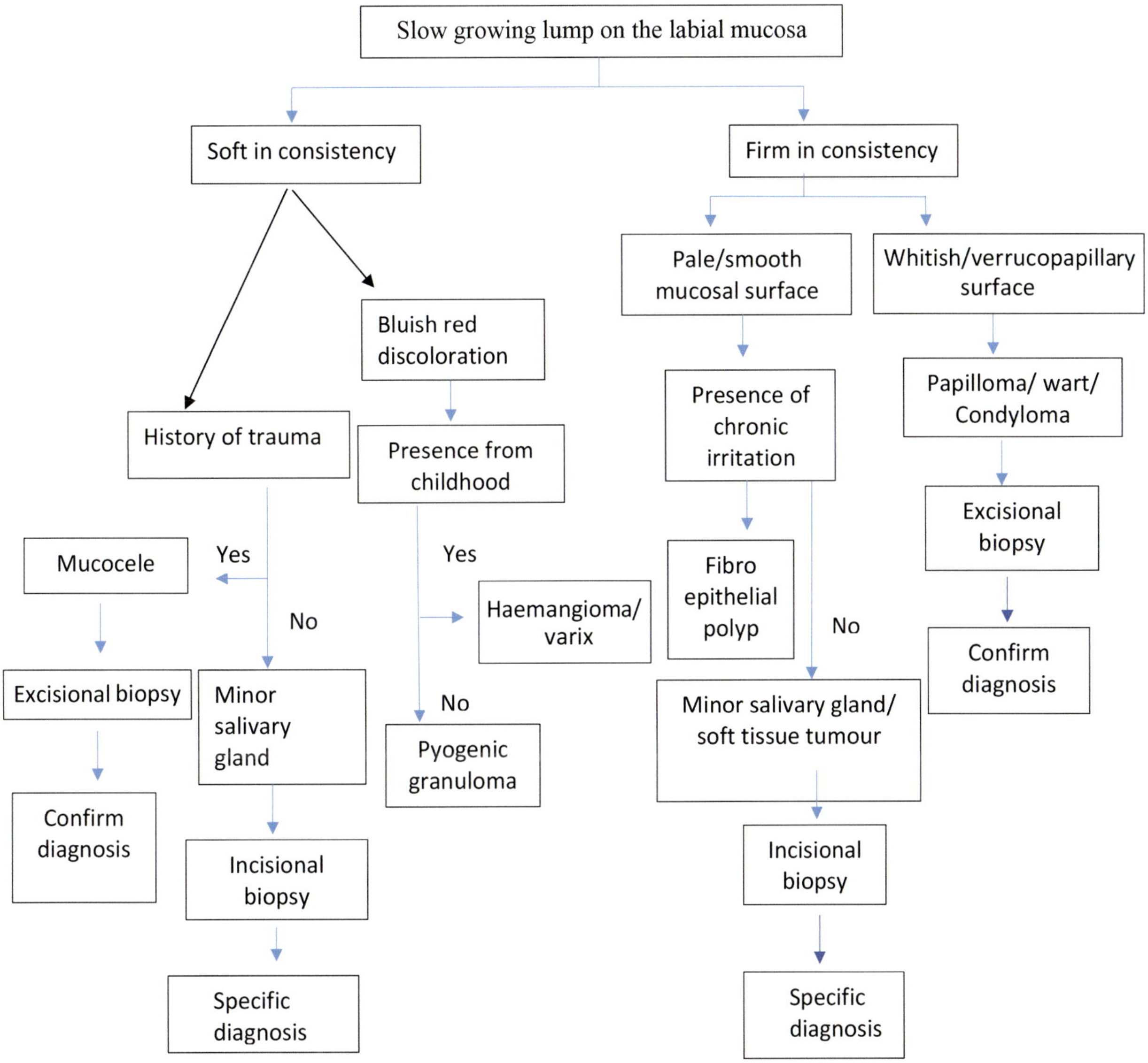

Self-Assessment Questions

1. List the common oral lesions caused by HPV.
2. Explain the clinical features of lesions caused due to HPV infection.
3. Discuss the differential diagnosis for a swelling on the lower lip.
4. Describe the histopathological features of HPV-induced lesions.
5. Outline the management plan for a patient with oral squamous papilloma.

Summary

Human papillomavirus (HPV) causes variety of lesions including squamous cell papilloma, verruca vulgaris (common warts), condyloma acuminatum, and multifocal epithelial hyperplasia (Heck's disease). They have many similarities but some features are helpful in differentiating one another. Surgery, cryotherapy, or liquid nitrogen therapy and laser therapy are the common methods used in the management.

Further Reading

Bharti AH, Chotaliya K, Marfatia YS. An update on oral human papillomavirus infection. Indian J Sex Transm Dis AIDS. 2013;34(2):77–82. https://doi.org/10.4103/0253-7184.120533. PMID: 24339456; PMCID: PMC3841675

Jayasooriya PR, Tilakaratne WM, Abeyratne S. Ranasinghe AW focal epithelial hyperplasia (Heck's disease). Oral Dis. 2004; 10:1–4.

Syrjaanen S. Oral manifestations of human papillomavirus infections. Eur J Oral Sci. 2018;126(Suppl. 1):49–66.

Toledano-Serrabona J, López-Ramírez M, Sánchez-Torres A, España-Tost A, Gay-Escoda C. Recurrence rate of oral squamous cell papilloma after excision with surgical scalpel or laser therapy: a retrospective cohort study. Med Oral Patol Oral Cir Bucal. 2019;24(4):e433–7.

Pustules on One Side of the Face: Herpes Zoster

Ruwan Jayasinghe and Wanninayake M Tilakaratne

Contents

W. M Tilakaratne, T. G. Kallarakkal (eds.), *Clinicopathological Correlation of Oral Diseases*,
https://doi.org/10.1007/978-3-031-24408-7_38

Learning Goals

1. Devise the correct way of compiling the history with appropriate questions.
2. Develop a differential diagnosis after history taking.
3. Deduce appropriate procedures in clinical examination.
4. Formulate a differential diagnosis combining findings in the history and clinical examination.
5. Justify the relevant investigations required to arrive at the diagnosis.
6. Comprehend the importance of clinicopathological correlation in arriving at the correct diagnosis.
7. Outline the management plan.
8. Recognize the importance of a diagnostic algorithm in arriving at a diagnosis

38.1 Main Complaint

A 56-year-old female patient presents to the clinic with vesicles on the right side of the face.

38.2 History of Complaint

Question: How long have you been having these lesions and what is the nature of it?

I have been having these lesions on the right side of the face since 3 days. They started as very small blisters containing fluid but increased in size over the last few days.

38.3 Additional Complaints

Question: Do you have similar blisters elsewhere on the body?

I have similar blisters inside the mouth but there are no lesions on the rest of the body.

Question: Have you noticed or felt any other changes or difficulties on the face/in the mouth?

I have a burning sensation on my face and in my mouth associated with the blisters. I find it difficult to eat or clean the mouth as the blisters cause pain during such activity.

Question: Did you have any other symptoms prior to the appearance of the blisters?

I had fever for 2 days before the appearance of blisters. I also had body aches, weakness and loss of appetite for 2–3 days. There was a burning sensation on the right side of the face and in the mouth before the appearance of the blisters and the burning sensation is still there.

Question: Are you suffering from any other medical problems like heart disease, high blood pressure, diabetes, bleeding disorder or respiratory diseases? If yes, what kind of medications, have you been taking until now?

I was diagnosed with diabetes mellitus several years ago and I am on oral hypoglycemic drugs. My sugar control appears to be unsatisfactory at the moment.

Question: Have you suffered from any similar disease that was associated with blisters in the past?

I had chickenpox when I was 48 years old.

Question: Have you undergone any surgery?

I have not undergone any surgery in the past.

Question: Have you undergone any dental treatment?

I have undergone extractions and restorations in the past. I had a bad tooth ache for few weeks and had a dental extraction 5 days before. My problems started immediately after the dental extraction.

Question: What is your occupation?

I am a daily paid manual laborer working in a tea estate.

Question: Tell me about your family.

I am married and have two children.

38.4 With the Findings from the History, What is Your Differential Diagnosis?

1. Herpes Zoster (HZ)
2. Recurrent herpes simplex infection
3. Erysipelas
4. Bullous pemphigoid
5. Pemphigus vulgaris

38.5 How Do You Justify Your Differential Diagnosis After History Taking?

1. She has multiple vesicles on the right mid face and inside the mouth since few days. There is a history of burning sensation in the same area and also prodromal symptoms like fever, body aches and loss of appetite. She is a diabetic with poor glycemic control. In addition, she has a history of a toothache followed by a dental extraction which could have triggered the reactivation of latent virus. Unilateral nature of the vesicles, presence of burning sensation and prodromal features in a patient with immunosuppression suggests a strong possibility of HZ. History of chickenpox in the past is more indicative of the diagnosis.
2. Recurrent herpes simplex virus infection (Herpes labialis) is usually seen on the lips and is not associated with prominent prodromal features. Intraoral lesions are rare in recurrent disease.
3. Erysipelas is a bacterial infection of the skin involving the upper dermis. It extends into the superficial cutaneous lymphatics. Clinically it presents as a tender, reddish, indurated plaque with clearly defined borders. Vesicles are not a feature and involvement of oral mucosa is very rare. Therefore, it can be eliminated from the differential diagnosis.
4. Bullous pemphigoid (BP) is an autoimmune disease commonly involving the skin but involvement of the mucosae can be seen in around 20% of the cases. Lesions in BP can be seen in any part of the skin and is usually multifocal. Lesions are not painful unless ulcerated or infected. Unilateral presentation restricted to mid face is not typical for BP.
5. Pemphigus vulgaris (PV) is a mucocutaneous autoimmune disease. Lesions in PV can be seen in any part of the skin or mucous membrane and is usually widespread in distribution. Lesions are not painful unless ulcerated or infected. However, unilateral occurrence restricted to mid face is not typical for PV.

38.6 Findings on Examination

She has multiple small vesicles on the right side mid face restricted to a demarcated area (◘ Fig. 38.1). There are vesicles on the oral mucosae mainly on the palate with few ulcerations (◘ Fig. 38.2). The lesions are unilateral and not crossing the midline.

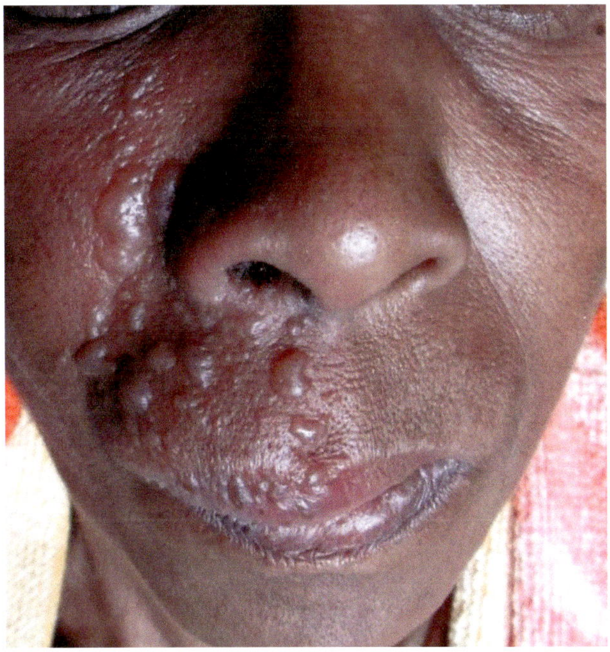

◘ **Fig. 38.1** Unilateral vesicles on the right face

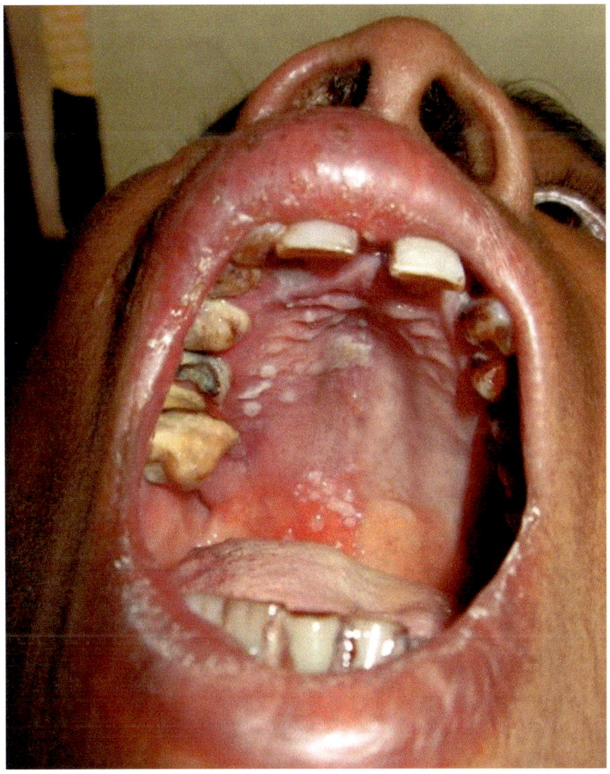

◘ **Fig. 38.2** Unilateral vesicles and ulcers on the palate on the right side

38.7 What Other Relevant Features Would You Look for with the Findings You Have So Far?

It is necessary to look for lesions in other areas such as the eye and the ear. Further, any evidence of nerve palsy should be checked. There are no lesions in the eyes or external ear. There is no evidence of facial nerve palsy.

38.8 What is Your Clinical Diagnosis?

Herpes zoster

38.9 How Would You Justify Your Clinical Diagnosis?

Diagnosis of HZ is usually done clinically by the presence of typical features of prodromal pain, characteristic vesicles and/or rash together with distinctive unilateral distribution of the lesions. The vesicles follow the distribution of a sensory nerve, usually the trigeminal nerve in the case of facial involvement. It may be confined to one or more branches of the trigeminal nerve. Lesions are always unilateral and do not cross the midline. However, diagnosis of HZ is difficult in the absence of vesicles. If the patient comes to the clinic before the appearance of rash, with the clinical symptoms of only pain and burning sensation, it may result in an incorrect diagnosis of a dental pathology or a neuralgia. Rarely HZ can occur without a rash. Diagnosis of HZ may be very difficult in children, younger adults and in immune-compromised patients due to their atypical presentations.

38

38.10 How Would You Manage This Patient?

The main aim of treatment for HZ is the reduction of pain and prevention of development of post-herpetic neuralgia. If the ophthalmic branch of trigeminal nerve is involved, urgent referral to an ophthalmologist is mandatory to prevent eye complications. Identification of the trigger or immune status is important. Patients should be educated to maintain the area clean and dry in order to reduce the risk of secondary bacterial superinfection, to avoid use of topical applications or dressings that can irritate the rash and surrounding skin or mucosa. This will help in minimizing secondary infections. They have to be educated regarding the spread of virus to others, resulting in chickenpox in non-infected individuals.

Antiviral therapy is indicated to minimize the complications and improve the healing of the lesions. Acyclovir is the drug of choice and 800 mg of Acyclovir 5 times daily for 7–10 days has to be administered. Other antiviral drugs include Famciclovir (250–500 mg 3 times daily for 7 days) and Valacyclovir (1000 mg 3 times daily for 7 days). Topical antiviral therapy is not recommended. Systemic antiviral therapy is strongly recommended. All patients with compromised immune status have to be prescribed with systemic antiviral therapy. It is also strongly recommended for immunocompetent patients who are more than 50 years of age, with moderate or severe pain and rash and with pain at night. Antiviral therapy is very helpful in reducing the chronic pain associated with HZ but not in all patients. Therefore, additional treatment may be indicated. Oral corticosteroids are helpful in reducing the acute pain but not the chronic pain. Tricyclic antidepressants are very effective in the management of chronic pain associated with HZ and post-herpetic neuralgia. Amitriptyline (25 mg once daily for three months starting immediately with the rash is the drug of choice. Opioid analgesics combined with nonsteroidal anti-inflammatory drugs (NSAIDs) are used but their effectiveness in managing chronic pain is not well established. Gabapentin and pregabalin are also effective in chronic pain management associated with HZ.

38.11 What are the Complications of This Condition?

Encephalitis: Acute varicella zoster virus (VZV) encephalitis is a very rare complication of HZ.

Varicella zoster virus retinitis: This is a complication mostly seen in immunocompromised patients. It mostly involves one eye but progression to involve both eyes occurs in some patients.

Post-herpetic Neuralgia (PHN): This is the most important, common and troublesome complication of HZ. Chronic pain can present for months or years after healing of the primary skin and oral mucosal lesions. Persisting pain for 3 months after the onset of the lesion is defined as PHN. Character of pain can vary from continuous burning or throbbing type of pain to intermittent sharp or electric shock–like pain to allodynia. Patients with HZ who are older, have a painful prodromal stage before the rash. Severe rash and severe acute pain with HZ are thought to be the important risk factors for the development of PHN.

38.12 Herpes Zoster (Shingles) and Post-herpetic Neuralgia

HZ or shingles is the result of reactivation of varicella zoster infection. A primary infection with VZV results in chickenpox. After the primary infection, VZV can travel along the sensory nerves and remain dormant in the nerve root ganglion. The reactivation of VZV in ganglia may happen frequently but remains subclinical most of the time. In patients with immunosuppression or age-related immunosenescence, it can result in the clinical disease of HZ. Involvement of trigeminal nerve is common. Any branch of the trigeminal nerve can be affected and at times, more than one branch can be involved. Involvement of ophthalmic branch is serious due to the involvement of the eye and may result in blindness unless early treatment is carried out. Rarely, HZ may involve the sensory branch of the facial nerve. When the facial nerve is involved, it is called as Ramsay Hunt syndrome. Clinically there is an erythematous vesicular rash on the external ear (zoster oticus) or in the posterior mouth together with facial nerve palsy.

Clinical presentation of HZ can be divided into three stages:

1. Prodromal (early symptoms) stage
2. Infectious rash (acute stage)
3. Resolution (healing stage)—two to four weeks duration

38.12.1 Prodrome

Prodrome is due to the infection and accompanying inflammatory response. It is seen in about 70%–80% of patients with HZ and occurs one to four days prior to the appearance of the rash. Patients experience it as a localized tingling, itching or burning sensation with constant or intermittent stabbing pain. Pain may or may not interfere with sleep. The type and intensity of pain can vary but the pain usually persists throughout. Prodrome usually lasts only 2–3 days but may persist for up to 1 week. At times this can mimic dental pain or sinusitis leading to unwarranted treatment such as tooth extraction. Other prodromal features such as malaise, fever, loss of appetite and headache may be present.

38.12.2 Rash

HZ rash typically affects a single dermatome with a unilateral band-like pattern. Even though it does not cross the midline in most cases, it may cross the midline in rare situations. The rash is commonly seen on the trunk but can occur on other sites including the face (◘ Figs. 38.3 and 38.4). Pruritus can be present and at times may be more prominent than the pain. Secondary infections over the vesicles or ulcers can occur. Virus can be transmitted from the vesicles or ulcers by direct contact to people, resulting in chicken pox. Together with the facial lesions, intraoral lesions can appear mainly on the buccal mucosa (◘ Fig. 38.5), palate (◘ Fig. 38.6) and tongue (◘ Fig. 38.7). Pain is almost always present with the vesicles/rash. Initially, rash has an erythematous and macular appearance and is difficult to identify it as HZ rash.

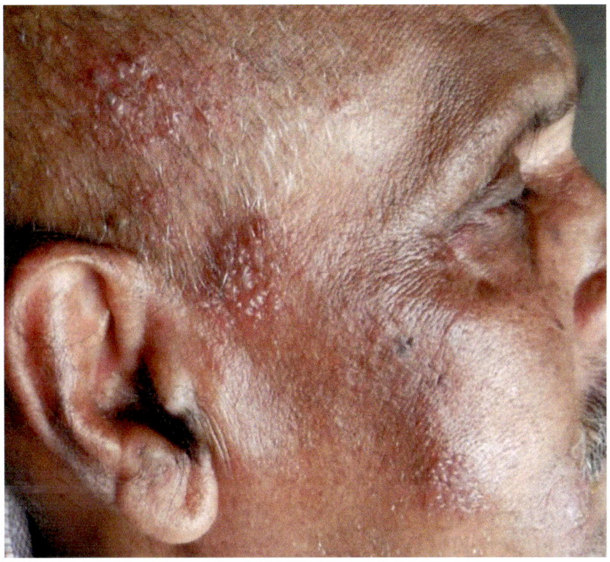

◘ **Fig. 38.3** Early vesicles/rash on the face

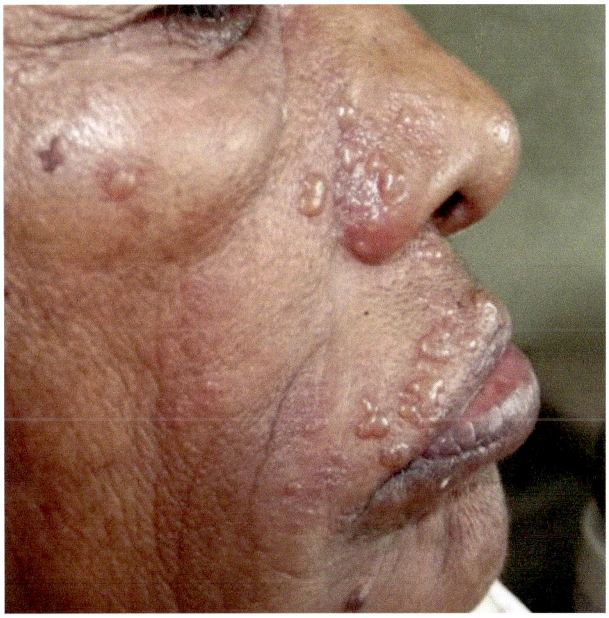

◘ **Fig. 38.4** Adavanced vesicles affecting the mid face

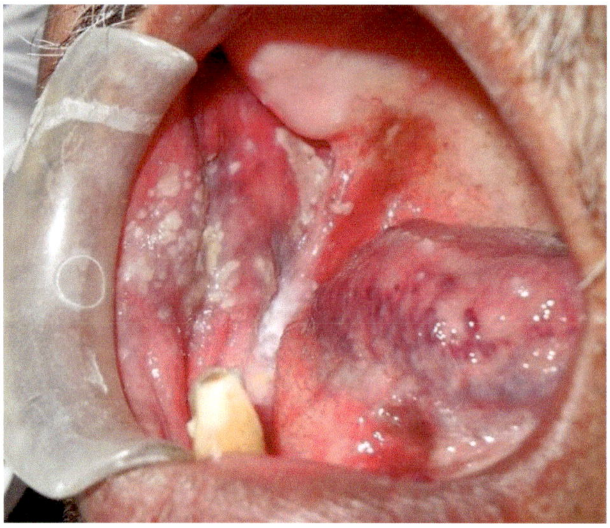

Fig. 38.5 Ulcerated lesions on the buccal mucosa

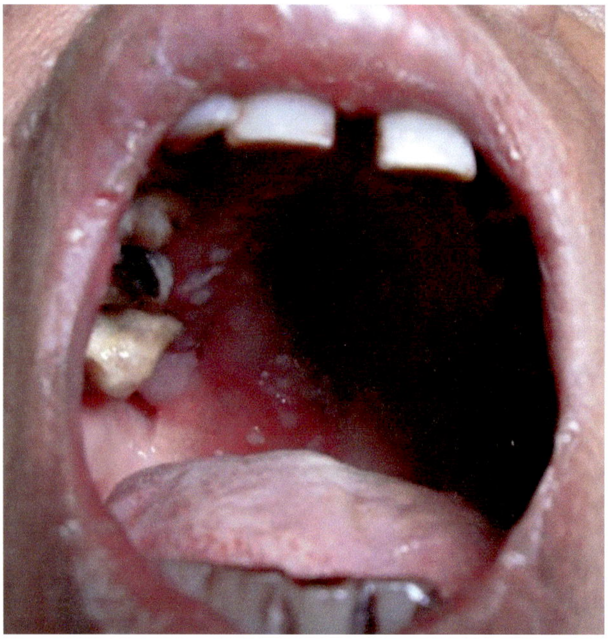

Fig. 38.6 Ulcerated lesions on the palate

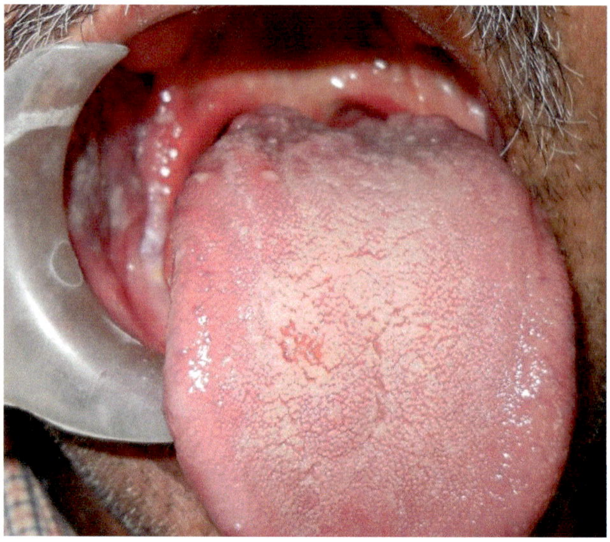

Fig. 38.7 Ulcerations on the posterior tongue

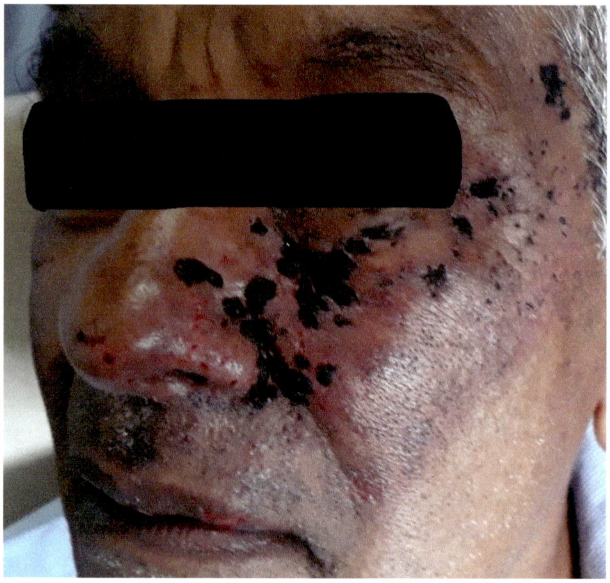

Fig. 38.8 Scarring and pigmentation involving the maxillary branch of trigeminal nerve dermatome

Over the next 3–4 days, papules appear and develop into vesicles. The vesicles pustulate within a week, followed by ulceration, crusting and scarring (Figs. 38.8, 38.9 and 38.10).

38.12.2.1 Resolution

Crusted lesions may persist for 2–4 weeks. Once the crusts are formed, the patient is no longer infectious. If new vesicles appear after 10 weeks, underlying immunodeficiency status should be investigated. Healing is delayed in immunocompromised patients and in elderly. Skin discoloration may persist for weeks or even months. Rarely reactivation of VZV in sensory nerve root ganglia can cause viremia. In patients with severe immunodeficiency, viremia can result in vesicles at a distance from the affected dermatome and can be life-threatening.

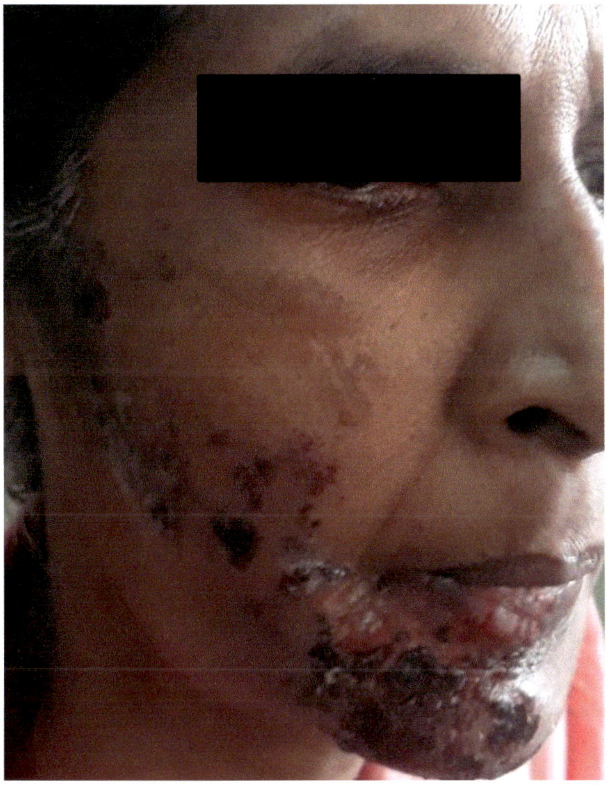

Fig. 38.9 Scaring invoving the mandibular branch of the trigeminal nerve dermatome

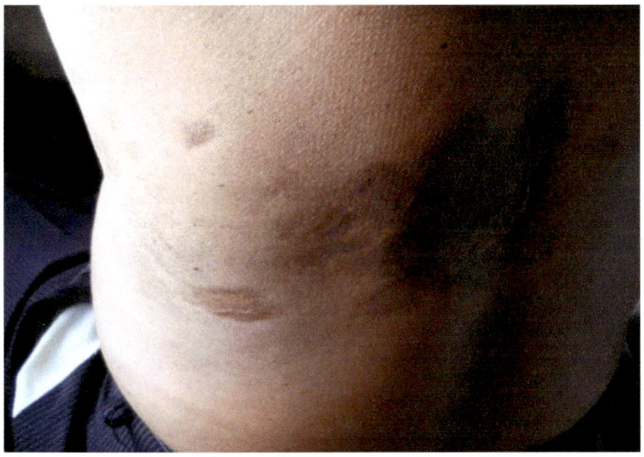

Fig. 38.10 Scarring involving the thoracic dermatome

Salient features of HZ	
Clinical	Classic features of HZ include prodromal pain, rash that evolve into pustules and distribution of the rash. It may be confined to one or more branches of the trigeminal nerve. Lesions are always unilateral and usually does not cross the midline. Lesions are localized to a single dermatome of a single sensory ganglion. Diagnosis of HZ is difficult in the absence of a rash. Diagnosis of herpes zoster may be very difficult in children, younger adults and immune-compromised patients due to their atypical presentations.
Investigations	Herpes zoster is usually diagnosed clinically. Detection of viral DNA by polymerase chain reaction (PCR) is a useful test
Treatment	Antiviral therapy is indicated in HZ to minimize the complications and improve the healing of the rash. Acyclovir is the drug of choice and 800 mg of Acyclovir 5 times daily for 7–10 days is recommended. Additional treatment may be indicated to control the pain. Oral corticosteroids are helpful in reducing the acute pain. Amitriptyline, Gabapentin and pregabalin are effective in the management of chronic pain associated with HZ.
Complications	**Post-herpetic neuralgia (PHN)** is the most important, common and troublesome complication of HZ. Prevention of PHN is very important in the management of HZ.

- Virus can be transmitted from the vesicles or ulcers by direct contact to people, resulting in chicken pox.
- In patients with severe immunodeficiency, viremia can result in vesicles at a distance from the affected dermatome and can be life-threatening.

Diagnostic features

Features	Diagnosis
In an immunocompetent individual • Prodromal symptoms • Unilateral vesicles/ blisters for few days • Limited to one dermatome • Lesions evolve from erythematous macules and papules to vesicles and pustules • Associated with burning sensation, pain or abnormal sensations • Crusting after 5–7 days • Complete healing after 2–4 weeks but pain and scaring may persist	• Clinical features alone are diagnostic • Investigations are not necessary
In an immunodeficient individual • No typical prodromal phase • Involvement of more than one dermatome • Lesions cross the midline • Previous history of herpes zoster • History of receiving VZV vaccine • Uncontrolled pain	• Clinical features alone are not diagnostic • Supportive investigations are necessary • Full blood count: Viral picture may be seen • Cytology: Testing of cells from the base of a vesicle for the presence of VZV by immunofluorescent microscopy • Real-time polymerase chain reaction (RT- PCR): Rapidly detect VZV DNA • Serology: To identify the antibodies against VZV

Self-Assessment Questions

1. Describe the etiopathogenesis herpes zoster.
2. List the clinical features of herpes zoster.
3. List the clinical features of Ramsay Hunt syndrome.
4. Outline the management of HZ.
5. State the most important complication of HZ and discuss its management.

Diagnostic Algorithm

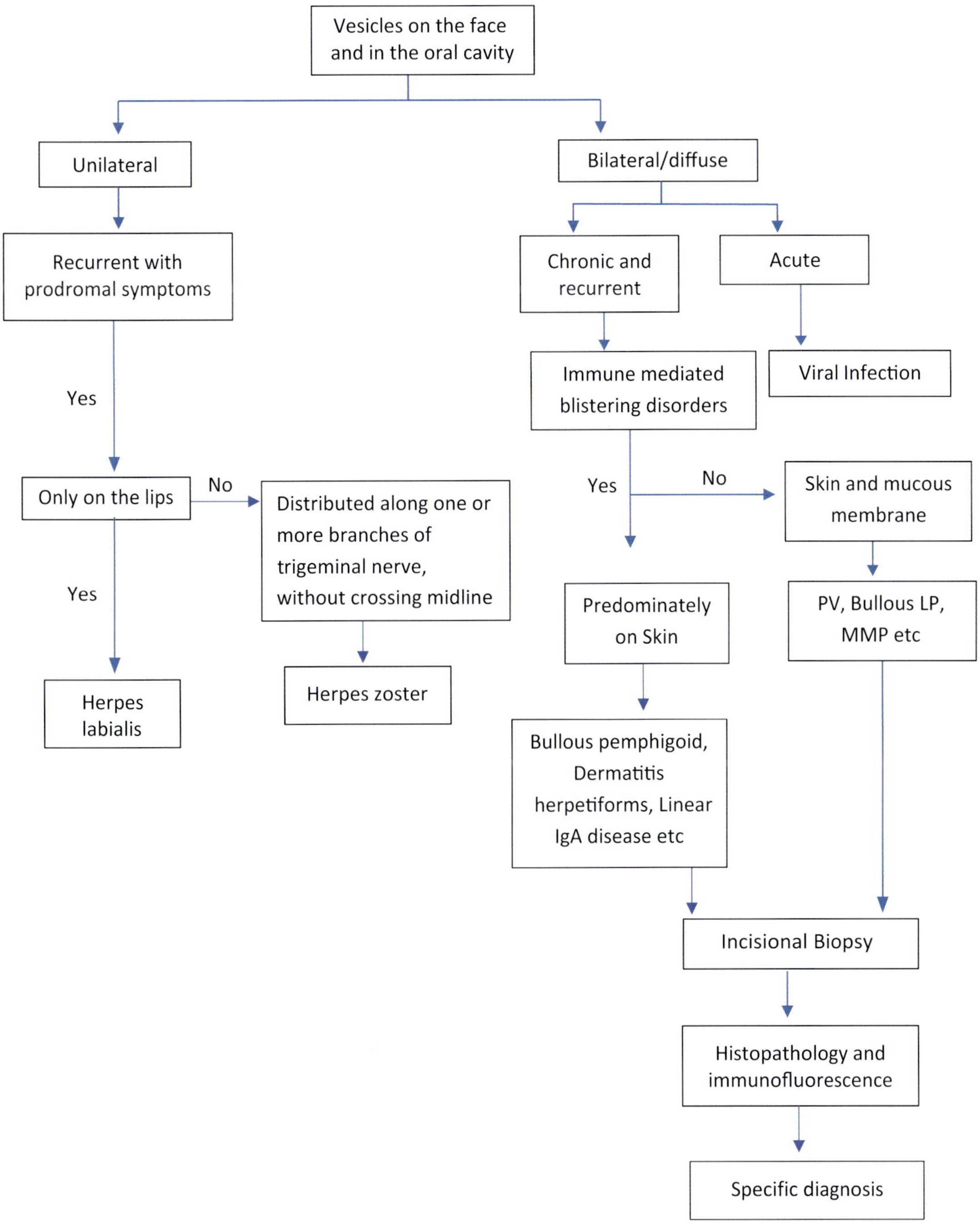

Summary

HZ/shingles is the result of reactivation of varicella zoster infection. Latent virus in the sensory ganglion can get activated causing rash along the distribution of the nerve. The trigeminal nerve is the commonly affected nerve. Antiviral therapy is indicated to minimize the complications. Postherpetic neuralgia (PHN) is the most important, common and troublesome complication of HZ.

Further Reading

Saguil A, Kane S, Mercado M. Herpes zoster and postherpetic neuralgia: prevention and management. Am Fam Phys. 2017;96(10):656–63.

Dworkin RH, Johnson RW, Breuer J, Gnann JW, Levin MJ, Backonja M, Betts RF, Gershon AA, Haanpaa ML, McKendrick MW, Nurmikko TJ, Oaklander AL, Oxman MN, Pavan-Langston D, Petersen KL, Rowbotham MC, Schmader KE, Stacey BR, Tyring SK, van Wijck AJ, Wallace MS, Wassilew SW, Whitley RJ. Recommendations for the management of herpes zoster. Clin Infect Dis. 2007;44(Suppl 1):S1–26. https://doi.org/10.1086/510206.

Klasser GD, Ahmed AS. How to manage acute herpes zoster affecting trigeminal nerves. J Can Dent Assoc. 2014;80:e42.

Sampathkumar P, Drage LA, Martin DP. Herpes zoster (shingles) and postherpetic neuralgia. Mayo Clin Proc. 2009;84(3):274–80.

Jeon Y, Lee H. Ramsay Hunt syndrome. J Dent Anesth Pain Med. 2018;18(6):333–7. https://doi.org/10.17245/jdapm.2018.18.6.333.

Non-healing Ulcer on the Palate in a Long-Term Diabetic Patient: Deep Fungal Infection

Thomas George Kallarakkal

Contents

W. M Tilakaratne, T. G. Kallarakkal (eds.), *Clinicopathological Correlation of Oral Diseases*,
https://doi.org/10.1007/978-3-031-24408-7_39

39.1 Main Complaint

A 55-year-old male patient presented to the clinic complaining of an ulcer on his palate.

39.2 History of Complaint

Question: How long have you been having this ulcer?

I noticed the ulcer a few days after I had undergone extraction of my upper left molar teeth about two months ago. I started to develop a swelling over my left face since three weeks and it has been slowly increasing in size.

Question: Why did you have your teeth extracted?

I had swollen gums, with pus discharge on the back part of my left upper jaw. My left upper molar teeth were mobile. My dentist diagnosed my condition as severe gum disease and suggested to extract the affected teeth.

Question: Were there any complications associated with the dental procedure?

The procedure was uneventful.

Question: Were you prescribed any medications after the dental procedure?

I was prescribed Tab Paracetamol and Tab Amoxicillin 250 mg, three times daily for five days. I completed my medication as prescribed.

39.3 Additional Complaints

Question: Is the ulcer painful?

I have pain on the palate in the region of the ulcer and over the left side of the face since five days. It was insidious in onset. I also have a headache since the last three days.

Question: What is the nature of the pain?

It is a gnawing persistent type of pain.

Question: Are there any factors that make the pain better or worse?

There are no aggravating factors for the pain. The pain is relieved slightly when I take a paracetamol tablet.

Question: Does the pain affect your sleep?

I find it difficult to sleep because of the pain.

Question: Is the pain radiating in nature?

The pain radiates to the left side of my head and neck.

Question: Is there any abnormal sensation or feeling of numbness over the affected area?

I do not have any abnormal sensation or numbness on my palate or over the face.

Question: Is there any pus discharge from the site of the ulcer?

I have noticed a whitish discharge from the ulcerated area. I also have a bad taste in my mouth.

Question: Do you have any difficulty in opening your mouth?

I have difficulty in opening my mouth due to the pain.

Question: Do you have any nasal congestion?

My nose is blocked on the left side.

Question: Do you have any difficulty in breathing?

I do not have any difficulty in breathing.

Question: Do you have any difficulty to swallow foods and liquids?

I do not have any difficulty in swallowing food and liquids.

Question: Do you have any other symptoms?

I have an extremely foul odor inside my mouth. My vision is blurred in the left eye.

Question: Do you have any other medical problems like heart disease, high blood pressure, diabetes, bleeding disorder or respiratory diseases?

I was diagnosed with type 2 diabetes a few years ago. I have not been taking my medications regularly for the past six months as I was advised by my friend to try alternative traditional medications.

Question: When was the last time you checked your blood sugar levels?

I did my blood tests last month and my HbA1c level was 8.5%.

Question: Are you on any other medications such as bisphosphonates?

I am currently not taking any other medications other than that prescribed for my diabetes.

Question: Do you have any history of radiotherapy in the head and neck region?

I have not undergone any radiotherapy in the past.

Question: Does anybody in your family have a history of medical illness?

My parents and my elder brother are also type 2 diabetics.

Question: Have you undergone any surgery?

I have not undergone any surgery in the past.

Question: Have you undergone any dental treatment apart from the recent dental extractions?

I have had multiple teeth extracted in the past due to gum disease.

Question: Do you have any risk habits such as smoking or drinking alcohol?

I smoke about 5–6 cigarettes a day.

Question: Do you drink alcohol?

I am a social drinker.

Question: Are you employed?

I am currently working as a senior sales manager in a local firm.

39.4 With the Findings from the History, What Is Your Differential Diagnosis?

1. Dry socket
2. Dento-alveolar abscess
3. Chronic suppurative osteomyelitis
4. Facial cellulitis
5. Deep-seated fungal infections including mucormycosis
6. Oral squamous cell carcinoma (OSCC)

39.5 How Do You Justify Your Differential Diagnosis After History Taking?

He complains of a non-healing painful ulcer on the palate that developed following extraction of his upper left molar teeth. The pain is radiating in nature. The patient also complains of bad breath and a swelling over the left side of his face since three weeks. He is a smoker and a known diabetic with a poorly controlled diabetic state. The clinical symptoms are highly suggestive of an infection probably arising as a sequelae to dental extraction. The presence of comorbidities like uncontrolled diabetes, severe periodontal disease and risk habits such as smoking may have predisposed the patient to an increased risk of infection.

1. Dry socket is the most common complication that arises 2–4 days postoperatively after tooth extraction. It is also synonymously referred to as alveolar osteitis, alveolitis sicca dolorosa, localized osteomyelitis and fibrinolytic alveolitis among others. The affected patients are usually above 40 years old. The most characteristic symptom associated with dry socket is intense pain that radiates to the ear and the neck. The affected patients are generally unwell and also complain of headache, dizziness and inability to sleep. Dry socket is an acute inflammation of the alveolar bone around the extracted tooth and normally arises as a result of breakdown of the intraalveolar blood clot whereby the socket becomes empty. The surrounding bone becomes denuded and covered by a yellow-gray necrotic tissue and the adjacent mucosa becomes erythematous. Several etiologies have been suggested to be associated with dry socket. These include traumatic, difficult and prolonged extractions, poor oral hygiene, pre-existing local infections such as pericoronitis and severe periodontal disease, bone pathologies such as Paget disease, osteopetrosis, fibrous dysplasia and irradiation that may compromise the vasculature, smoking, oral contraceptives and systemic diseases like diabetes. The patient's chief complaint is an ulcer on the palate that developed subsequently to dental extraction. It is not apparent at this stage whether the patient's chief complaint refers to the unhealed extraction socket or an ulcer that is discrete from the extraction site. Dry socket is included in the differential diagnosis owing to the positive dental history, clinical symptoms of intense radiating pain, bad breath and associated predisposing factors.

2. A dento-alveolar abscess may arise from apical periodontitis or severe chronic periodontitis. The symptoms vary from a localized swelling to a more pronounced swelling, with a risk of infection spreading to adjacent sites. Infection may spread to the maxillary sinus, the sublingual, submandibular and infraorbital regions, orbit and brain, and the parapharyngeal space, eventually resulting in mediastinitis. A dento-alveolar abscess is included in the differential diagnosis due to the positive history of dental extraction, severe periodontal disease and a clinical presentation of pain and swelling in this patient.
3. Osteomyelitis of the jaw bones is an inflammatory process that affects the medullary portion of the bone. The early phase of the disease is classified as acute osteomyelitis which is usually associated with suppuration. Chronic osteomyelitis is defined as a disease process lasting for at least 1 month. The causative factors include an odontogenic focus of infection that may be either a periapical or periodontal disease. Osteomyelitis of the jaws primarily affects the mandible while the maxilla is less commonly affected due to its good vascular supply and thinner cortical plates. It tends to occur more commonly in men over a wide age range. The characteristic clinical symptoms include intense pain, suppuration and swelling. Comorbidities such as malnutrition, alcoholism, smoking, immunosuppression, diabetes mellitus, steroid use and bone pathologies such as fibrous dysplasia, Paget disease and osteopetrosis may predispose the individuals to osteomyelitis. The patient presented with a history of advanced periodontal disease and dental extraction. His symptoms included a painful ulcer on the palate and swelling over the left face of 3–5 weeks duration. Moreover, the patient is an uncontrolled diabetic that may have predisposed him to acute suppurative osteomyelitis.
4. Facial cellulitis refers to acute inflammation and infection of the facial subcutaneous tissues caused by the spread of infection through tissue spaces and fascial planes in the head and neck region. The etiology is polymicrobial caused by highly virulent bacteria in odontogenic infections. The patient has a swelling involving the left side of his face that developed following a dental extraction which suggests the possibility of cellulitis. He is unable to open his mouth widely suggesting an inflammation of the muscles of mastication caused by the spread of infection into the masticator space. However, the patient does not have any difficulty in breathing and swallowing foods and liquids which is an indication that the infection has not spread into the retropharyngeal and lateral pharyngeal spaces.
5. Oral fungal infections (oral mycoses) are opportunistic infections. Deep fungal infections rarely affect the oral cavity and most commonly affect immunocompromised patients. Oral mucormycosis is a rare and life-threatening deep fungal infection that progresses very rapidly. The etiologic agents are filamentous, saprophytic fungi of the order Mucorales and family of Mucoraceae in fungi kingdom such as Rhizopus spp., Mucor spp. and Lichtheimia spp. These organisms frequently colonize the oral mucosa, nasal mucosa, paranasal sinuses and pharyngeal mucosa of asymptomatic patients. It generally occurs as opportunistic infections in immunocompromised hosts particularly in poorly controlled diabetics with or without ketoacidosis and severely malnourished individuals. The causative agents enter into the host tissues when the immunity is compromised or through an invasive portal, such as a dental extraction socket. Rhinocerebral mucormycosis is one of the most severe forms of mucormycosis seen in diabetic patients. It begins in the nose and paranasal sinuses and clinically manifests as severe pain, palatal ulceration, facial edema, headache and nasal congestion. The patient presents with clinical symptoms of palatal ulceration, left facial swelling, nasal congestion and headache that developed following the dental extraction. His uncontrolled diabetic state also makes him a prime candidate for mucormycosis justifying its inclusion in the list of differential diagnoses.
6. Oral squamous cell carcinoma (OSCC) can manifest clinically as a non-healing ulcer. OSCC is a chronic lesion and is painless in its initial stages. The symptoms of OSCC manifest only after the lesion has grown to a large size and has infiltrated into the adjacent tissues. The patient is a smoker which is an etiologic agent for OSCC.

39.6 Findings of Clinical Examination

The patient is stable, afebrile with a blood pressure of 140/82 mm of Hg and a pulse rate of 84 beats per minute. Extraoral examination reveals a diffuse swelling measuring approximately 5 × 5 cm involving the left mid and lower face. Periorbital swelling and ptosis is seen on the left side (Fig. 39.1). Chemosis (edema of conjunctiva) and epiphora (excessive watering of eye) are noted in the left eye. The patient also complains of diplopia (double/blurred vision) in the left eye and has restricted movement of the left eyeball, denoting paralysis of eye muscles. The overlying skin appears normal. The swelling is mildly tender, soft and slightly warm to touch. Mouth opening is restricted to 20 mm. There

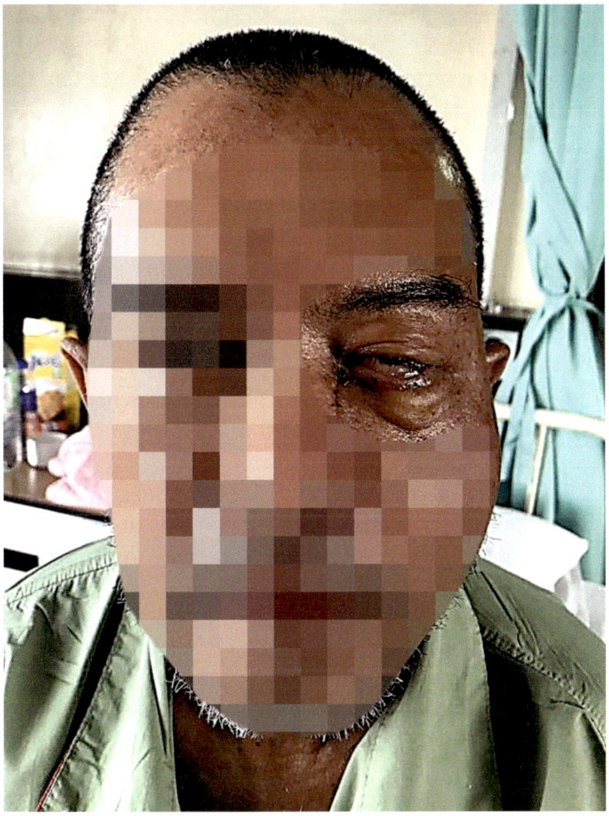

Fig. 39.1 A diffuse swelling involving the left mid and lower face. The patient also manifested periorbital swelling and ptosis involving the left eye. (Picture courtesy: Dr. Thomas Abraham, Sentosa Specialist Hospital, Selangor, Malaysia)

are multiple, enlarged submandibular lymph nodes bilaterally. The enlarged lymph nodes are tender and mobile.

The patient is fully edentulous on the upper arch. Intraorally a foul smelling necrotic ulcer is seen over the left hard palate and maxillary alveolar ridge (Fig. 39.2). The ulcer is covered by brownish yellow slough. It measures around 5 × 3 cm in size and has denuded bone in its floor, irregular margins and sloping edges. The slough is scrapable with evidence of bleeding and the surrounding mucosa is indurated.

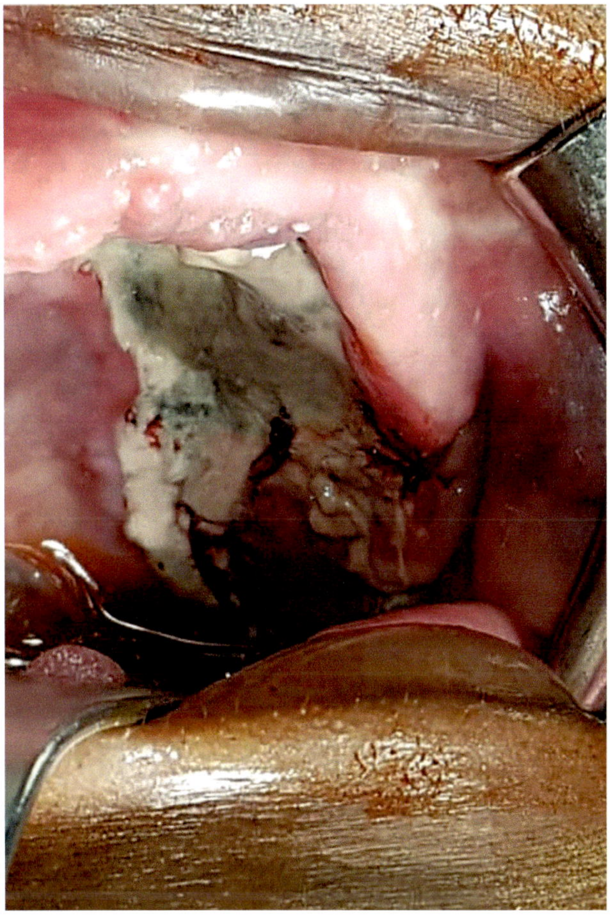

Fig. 39.2 An ulcer with denuded bone and covered with necrotic slough over the hard palate and maxillary alveolar ridge on the left side. (Picture courtesy: Dr. Thomas Abraham, Sentosa Specialist Hospital, Selangor, Malaysia)

39.7 What Is Your Clinical Differential Diagnosis?

1. Chronic suppurative osteomyelitis
2. Facial cellulitis
3. Deep-seated fungal infections including mucormycosis
4. OSCC

39.8 How Would You Exclude Other Conditions and Justify the Inclusion of the Diseases That You Have Mentioned in the Differential Diagnosis to Arrive at a Working Diagnosis?

The patient presented with a large necrotic ulcer involving the left hard palate and maxillary alveolar ridge. Dry socket was excluded from the differential diagnosis, as the intraoral findings were not consistent with a dry socket. In a dry socket, only the alveolar osseous walls of the socket are exposed due to complete or partial loss of blood clot in the interior of the socket and the perialveolar mucosa appears inflamed. A dento-alveolar abscess manifests as a localized accumulation of purulent material resulting in a fluctuant buccal or palatal swelling, with or without a draining fistula. The presence of a large necrotic ulcer with suppuration and a diffuse swelling involving the surrounding soft tissues as seen in this patient is an indication that the inflammation and or the infection has spread beyond the local confines into the fascial planes of the head and neck. Hence, a dento-alveolar abscess is excluded from the differential diagnosis.

Chronic suppurative osteomyelitis is included in the clinical differential diagnosis as the patient complained of pain, suppuration and swelling following dental extraction about 2 months ago. The intraoral finding of a necrotic ulcer and denuded bone supports the differential diagnosis of chronic osteomyelitis. Osteomyelitis could have been precipitated by an opportunistic infection owing to the patient's predisposing factors such as severe periodontal disease and uncontrolled diabetic state. Osteoradionecrosis (ORN) and medication-related osteonecrosis of the jaws (MRONJ) were not considered in the differential diagnoses at any juncture as the patient did not give any history of treatment with bisphosphonates or radiotherapy to the head and neck region.

39

Cellulitis is characterized by a hard, extremely tender, rapidly enlarging swelling that appears erythematous and warm to touch. In this patient, the mucosa surrounding the ulcerated area appeared to be indurated while the extraoral swelling was mildly tender and soft on palpation. The presence of a tender, slightly warm and diffuse swelling of the soft tissues surrounding the ulcerated area is a clinical sign that the patient is progressing to cellulitis.

Oral mucormycosis (OM) usually develops as an extension of rhinocerebral mucormycosis or direct contamination of an open oral wound. The fungal spores which are generally found in the natural environment, including soil, air, food and animal excreta, may be either inhaled or ingested. They may also exit as normal commensals in the oral cavity, nasal passage and pharynx of healthy individuals. OM has been reported to develop following extraction of maxillary posterior teeth owing to its proximity to the maxillary sinus wherein the inhaled fungal spores within the maxillary sinus cause OM in predisposed individuals. The reported clinical features of OM following extraction of maxillary teeth include edema of face, alveolar bone necrosis with palatal ulcer, nasal discharge/blockage, facial paresthesia, trismus and headache. Orbital involvement may result in chemosis, epiphora, diplopia (double/blurred vision), ptosis (drooping of upper eyelid), proptosis (protrusion of eye ball), ophthalmoplegia (paralysis of eye muscles) and loss of vision. The history and the presenting clinical features in this patient are highly suggestive of a deep-seated fungal infection such as OM.

OSCC most commonly involves the buccal mucosa, tongue and floor of the mouth. Clinically, it can manifest as a white or red patch, a proliferative growth or an ulcerated lesion. The ulcer in OSCC is a solitary lesion with rolled and indurated borders. In the present case, the ulcer did not have rolled or everted margins. The relatively acute onset of pain and swelling is more consistent with an inflammatory/infective process. However the clinical symptoms of a chronic non-healing ulcer of almost 2 months duration necessitate further investigations to rule out OSCC.

39.9 How Would You Investigate This Patient?

1. Skull radiographs (occipitomental/Waters view) to assess the involvement of the maxillary sinus and adjacent anatomic structures.
2. Cone beam computed tomography (CBCT) to determine the location, extent of the disease into the maxillary sinus and the orbit and proximity of the lesion to other vital structures in the vicinity.
3. Hematological investigations including a complete blood count (CBC) and erythrocyte sedimentation rate (ESR) to assess the severity of infection, any underlying immune deficiency status and systemic disorders such as anemia.
4. Blood biochemical investigations such as fasting blood sugar and glycated hemoglobin test (HBA1c) to assess the diabetic state.
5. Culture and sensitivity test to identify and determine the susceptibility of causative organisms to antibiotics.
6. Molecular confirmation by detection of fungal DNA in tissue samples by polymerase chain reaction (PCR) with sequencing of the 18S ribosomal DNA.
7. Incisional biopsy from the palatal ulcer and denuded bone to determine the underlying pathology.

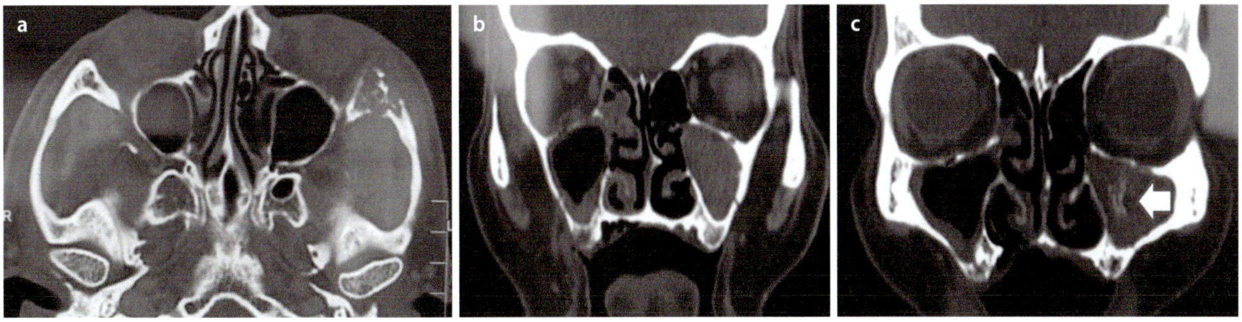

Fig. 39.3 (a) Erosion of the anterior wall of the maxillary antrum, (b) opacification of the maxillary sinus and (c) bony sequestrum within the antrum (white arrow). (Picture courtesy: Dr. Thomas Abraham, Sentosa Specialist Hospital, Selangor, Malaysia)

A computed tomography (CT) scan (Fig. 39.3) of the patient shows erosion of the anterior wall of the left maxillary antrum (Fig. 39.3a), opacification of the left maxillary antrum (Fig. 39.3b) and area of loose bone within the left maxillary antrum suggestive of bony sequestrum (Fig. 39.3c).

39.10 How Would You Do an Incisional Biopsy for This Patient? What Are the Important Considerations?

The biopsy should be deep enough and include the margins of the palatal ulcer. A biopsy from the ulcerated area alone will yield only necrotic tissue and will not be of any diagnostic significance. Sequestrum (necrotic bone fragments) obtained from the biopsy should be sent for decalcification prior to tissue processing. The tissue sections should be stained with routine hematoxylin and eosin stains and special stains such as Grocott-Gomori's methenamine silver (GMS) stain to identify the causative fungal microorganisms.

39.11 Biopsy Report Confirms the Previous Clinical Diagnosis of Mucormycosis. What Are the Histopathological Features That Help in the Diagnosis?

The hematoxylin and eosin (H & E) stained sections show densely collagenous connective tissue which is intensely inflamed with chronic inflammatory cells composed of lymphocytes, plasma cells and multinucleated giant cells (Fig. 39.4a). The decalcified sections from the bone specimen show trabeculae of necrotic bone and marrow tissue infiltrated by foamy macrophages, lymphocytes and plasma cells (Fig. 39.4b). Periodic acid Schiff (PAS) stain highlights the broad aseptate fungal hyphal forms that branch at right angles (Fig. 39.4c).

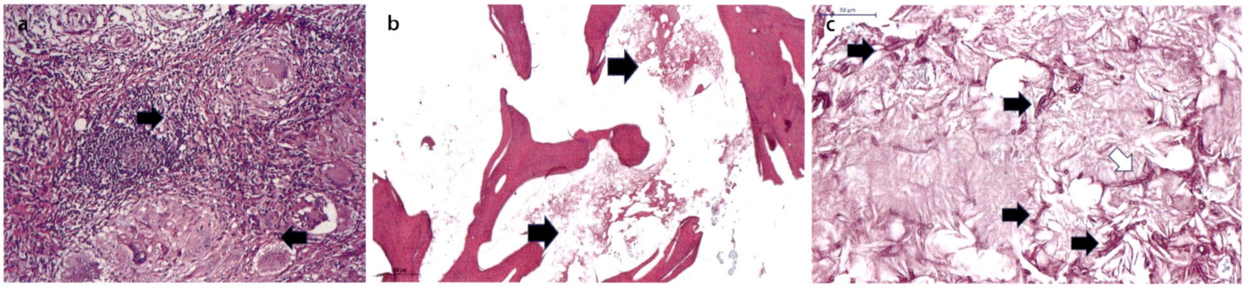

Fig. 39.4 (a) The H&E section shows granulomas (black arrows) composed of epithelioid macrophages, multinucleated giant cells and lymphocytes. (b) The decalcified section from the bone specimen shows trabeculae of necrotic bone. The intervening marrow is infiltrated by chronic inflammatory cells (black arrows). (c) PAS stained section shows broad aseptate fungal hyphal forms (black arrows) which branch at right angles (white arrow)

39.12 What Is the Final Diagnosis?

Deep-seated fungal infection consistent with mucormycosis

39.13 How Would You Manage This Patient?

The patient's biochemical examination showed high blood sugar levels with fasting blood sugar of 196 (normal range; 70–105 mg/dL) and 2 h postprandial blood sugar level of 315 (normal range; 100–180 mg/dL). The patient was admitted in the hospital as he required multidisciplinary treatment. He was administered a single daily dose of liposomal amphotericin B, 1 mg/kg body weight as an infusion in 100 mL of 5% dextrose over 1–2 h for a period of 15 days. The blood glucose level was controlled using insulin drip. The blood urea and creatinine levels were monitored for nephrotoxicity. Local surgical debridement was carried out under local anesthesia. The patient was instructed to maintain good oral hygiene and rinse his mouth three times a day after meals for 15 days.

39.14 Mucormycosis

Mucormycosis was previously termed zygomycosis as it referred to infections caused by fungi of the former phylum Zygomycota. The latter terminology is now obsolete with the phylogenetic reanalysis of the kingdom fungi. The most common pathogens are Rhizopus, which can be found in fruits, soil, dust, and manure. They are also commensals and can be cultured from the nasal mucosa of normal persons. The infection is usually acquired after inhalation of the sporangiospores through the nose or mouth. Skin lacerations can also act as a portal of entry for the pathogenic microorganisms. The infection primarily affects immunocompromised patients who are undergoing cancer chemotherapy, patients with hematologic malignancies, organ transplantation and uncontrolled diabetes with ketoacidosis. Patients with trauma are also susceptible due to the contamination of wounds with Mucorales. Mucormycosis rarely manifests in immunocompetent individuals and is an indicator of a serious underlying medical condition. It is an acute and rapidly progressing infection with a high mortality rate unless identified and treated promptly.

Mucormycosis can be classified into seven main types. They are rhinocerebral, pulmonary, cutaneous, gastrointestinal, central nervous system (CNS), disseminated and miscellaneous (e.g., bone or kidney). Rhinocerebral mucormycosis is the most common type and is characterized by involvement of the orbit, paranasal sinuses and brain. The infection tends to disseminate rapidly across tissue planes causing extensive tissue destruction. Mucormycosis often invades blood vessels, resulting in infarction, necrosis and thrombosis. Cavernous sinus thrombosis (CST) is a potential complication associated with rhinocerebral mucormycosis. Besides the hematogenous spread, rhinocerebral mucormycosis also spreads by perineural invasion. Rhinocerebral and pulmonary mucormycoses are more common in patients with hematologic malignancies.

Rhinocerebral mucormycosis develops after inhalation of fungal sporangiospores into the paranasal sinuses. Oral involvement in mucormycosis usually occurs as a transpalatal extension of rhinocerebral mucormycosis. Pain and swelling precede oral ulceration and the resulting tissue necrosis can result in palatal perforation. The palatal ulcers are well delineated, with well-defined borders. They may either develop

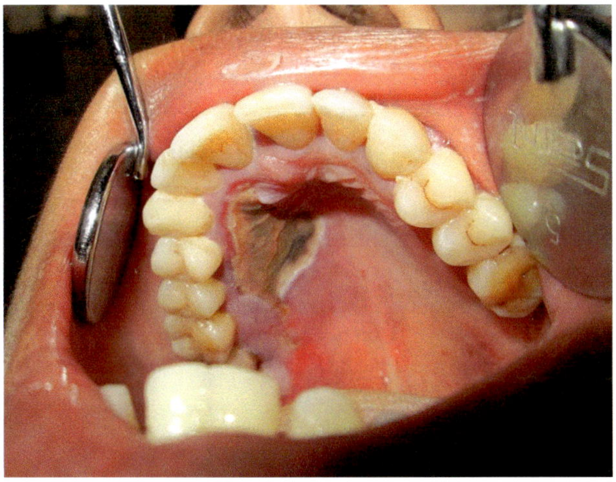

Fig. 39.5 An ulcer on the hard palate with a black necrotic eschar. (Picture courtesy: Dr. Mahima V Guledgud, JSS Dental College & Hospital, Mysuru, India)

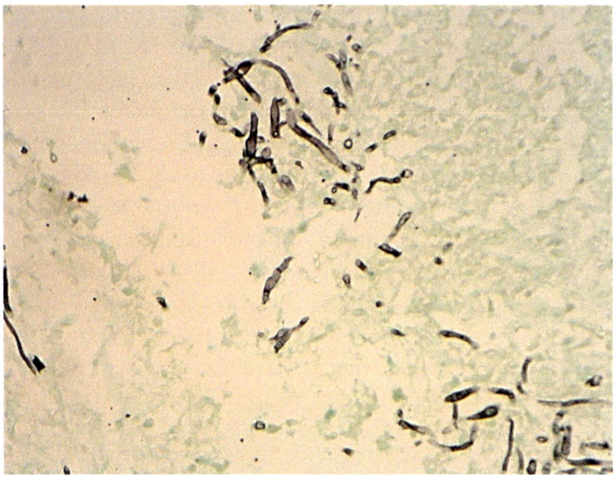

Fig. 39.6 GMS stain shows numerous, large, thin-walled, non-septate fungal hyphae having a ribbon-like appearance

slowly or very rapidly particularly when they are associated with diabetic ketoacidosis or with neutropenia. The infection may spread posteriorly to invade the sphenoid sinus, laterally into the cavernous sinus to involve the orbits, or cranially to invade the brain. The initial symptoms of rhinocerebral mucormycosis vary from sinusitis and periorbital cellulitis to facial numbness and blurring of vision. The characteristic signs and symptoms that are suggestive of mucormycosis in susceptible individuals include multiple cranial nerve palsies, unilateral periorbital facial pain, orbital inflammation, eyelid edema, acute ocular motility changes, internal or external ophthalmoplegia, headache and acute vision loss. The infected tissue which may appear normal during the earlier stages of infection progresses through an erythematous phase, with or without edema. A violaceous appearance then ensues and finally a black, necrotic eschar develops, which is a hallmark of mucormycosis (Fig. 39.5). The necrotic eschar is a result of thrombosed blood vessels and tissue infarction.

Mucormycosis may pose a challenge to diagnosis particularly in cases following a dental extraction. The reviewing clinician must be alert to symptoms of non-healing of extraction socket and associated tissue necrosis as well as symptoms that are less localized, such as disturbed vision and facial paresthesia. A cranial CT or magnetic resonance imaging (MRI) and endoscopy are highly recommended in diabetic patients with suggestive clinical features such as facial pain, sinusitis, proptosis and ophthalmoplegia. MRI is more sensitive than a CT scan to rule out spread of infection to the eye or the brain. Periodic CT scans are strongly recommended if there is a rapid spread of mucormycosis. In patients with rhinocerebral mucormycosis, CT typically shows opacification of the paranasal sinuses and thickening of the sinus mucosa and bone destruction, without an air-fluid level. Additional features such as show soft tissue swelling, proptosis and swelling of the extraocular muscles will also be evident on the CT.

Biopsy is mandatory if mucormycosis is a potential diagnosis. Histologically it may be difficult to distinguish hyphae of Mucorales from hyphae of Aspergillus or morphologically related fungi. This in turn may lead to delay in appropriate therapy. A definitive diagnosis of mucormycosis is usually established through histopathological examination of a tissue section stained with H & E, PAS or GMS stains that reveal extensive tissue necrosis and the presence of numerous, large, thin-walled, non-septate fungal hyphae branched at right angles and have a ribbon-like appearance (Fig. 39.6) invading into the tissues. The hyphae of Mucorales have a variable width of 6–16 μm, but may usually be up to 25 μm. Polymerase chain reaction (PCR) can help in diagnosis and distinguish it from other fungal infections as Mucorales are rarely separated from biologic cultures. Histologically, mucormycosis closely resembles aspergillosis. Aspergillosis differs from mucormycosis in that it has septate branching hyphae. Mucormycosis is also diagnosed by direct examination with fluorescence microscopy using fluorescent dyes such as Calcofluor, Fungifluor or Blankofluor. However, the availability of fluorescence microscopy precludes the use of this analysis in daily practice. There are no standardized tests available for detecting Mucorales-specific antigens.

The management of mucormycosis has to begin with aggressive treatment of any underlying predisposing medical conditions such as diabetes, neutropenia and graft-versus-host disease. Surgical intervention should be initiated early in the course of the treatment and should involve active debridement of all infected tissues. Aggressive cases of mucormycosis involving the oral cavity will have to be treated by radical resection, which can include partial or total maxillectomy, mandibulectomy and orbital exenteration. Amphotericin B is a widely accepted treatment in mucormycosis, with a survival rate of up to 72%. Majority of the patients who survive the disease will end up with a functional deficit such as blindness or cranial nerve palsy despite combined surgery and pharmacotherapy. Hyperbaric oxygen (HBO) that has a fungistatic activity and reduces tissue hypoxia has been used in the treatment of rhinocerebral mucormycosis. However, there is still not enough evidence regarding the effectiveness of HBO therapy.

Salient features of mucormycosis	
Clinical features	Rhinocerebral mucormycosis is the most common form Commonly affects debilitated patients with conditions such as diabetic ketoacidosis, neutropenia, immunosuppressive therapy, desferoxamine use associated with dialysis, malnutrition, leukemia, lymphoma and renal failure. Affected patients present with facial pain, headache and fever. Infection can extend to the orbit or the CNS. Involvement of the oral cavity results in a black necrotic eschar usually on the palate.
Radiological features	Opacification of the paranasal sinuses with thickening of the sinus mucosa and bone destruction. In rapidly spreading infection the CT scan also shows soft tissue swelling, proptosis and swelling of the extraocular muscles.
Histopathological features	Extensive tissue necrosis and the presence of numerous large fungal hyphae, which are non-septate and have a ribbon-like appearance, with budding and dichotomous branching.
Treatment	Treatment should be multidisciplinary. Surgical debridement, treatment of predisposing disorders and antifungal therapy using liposomal Amphotericin B. Supportive therapy includes fluid balance, nutritional supplements and correction of underlying immune deficiency. Treatment with new triazole derivative Posaconazole has also been recommended.

Self-Assessment Questions

1. Classify mucormycosis.
2. Describe the pathognomonic clinical and radiological features of mucormycosis.
3. Discuss the differential diagnoses for mucormycosis.
4. Describe the histopathological features of mucormycosis.
5. Discuss the management of mucormycosis.

■ Diagnostic Algorithm

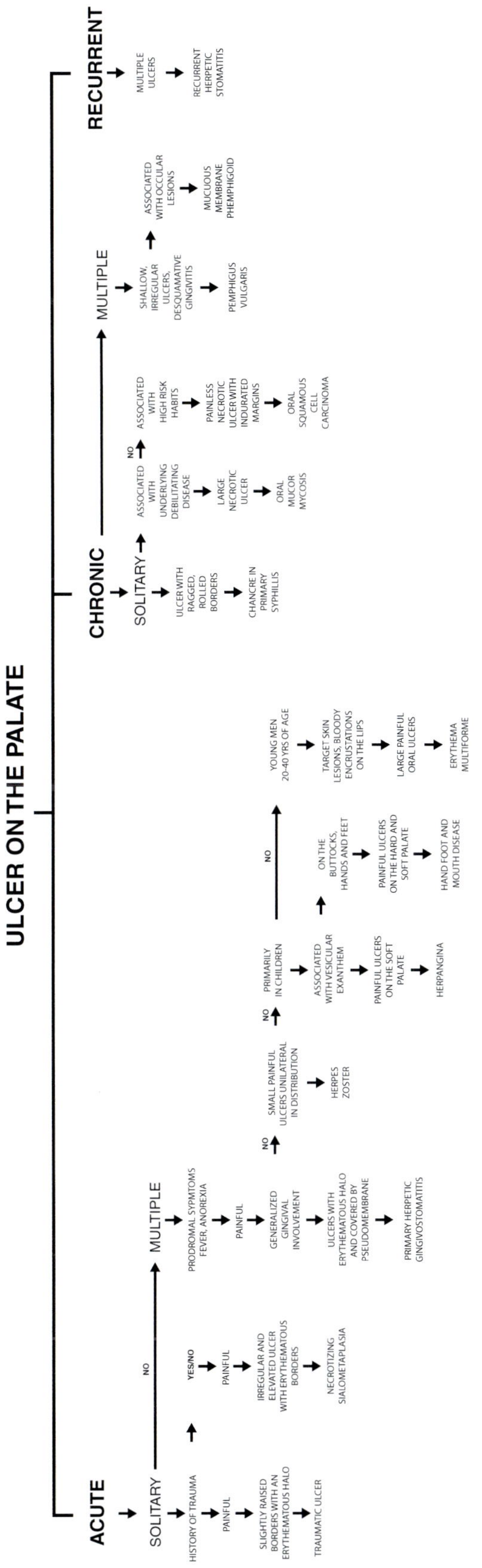

Summary

Mucormycosis was previously termed zygomycosis as it referred to infections caused by fungi of the former phylum Zygomycota. The most common pathogens are Rhizopus which can be found in fruits, soil, dust, and manure. They are also commensals and can be cultured from the nasal mucosa of normal persons. The infection is usually acquired after inhalation of the sporangiospores through the nose or mouth. Skin lacerations can also act as a portal of entry for the pathogenic microorganisms. The infection primarily affects immunocompromised patients who are undergoing cancer chemotherapy, patients with haematologic malignancies, organ transplantation and uncontrolled diabetes with ketoacidosis. Patients with trauma are also susceptible due to the contamination of wounds with Mucorales. Mucormycosis rarely manifests in immunocompetent individuals and is an indicator to a serious underlying medical condition. It is an acute and rapidly progressing infection with a high mortality rate unless identified and treated promptly.

Further Reading

Bonifaz A, Macias B, Paredes-Farrera F, Arias P, Ponce RM, Araiza J. Palatal zygomycosis: experience of 21 cases. Oral Dis. 2008;14(6):569–74.

Bonifaz A, Tirado-Sánchez A, Paredes-Farrera F, Moreno-Moreno J, Araiza J, González GM. Oral involvement in mucormycosis. A retrospective study of 55 cases. Enfermedadesinfecciosas y microbiologiaclinica (English ed.). 2021;39(10):506–9.

Cawson RA, Odell EW. Cawson's essentials of oral pathology and oral medicine e-book. Elsevier Health Sciences; 2017.

Cornely OA, Alastruey-Izquierdo A, Arenz D, Chen SC, Dannaoui E, Hochhegger B, et al. Global guideline for the diagnosis and management of mucormycosis: an initiative of the European Confederation of Medical Mycology in cooperation with the Mycoses Study Group Education and Research Consortium. Lancet Infect Dis. 2019;19(12):e405–21.

Emodi O, Ohayon C, Bilder A, Capucha T, Wolff A, Racmiel A. Post extraction mucormycosis in immunocompromised patient management and review of literature. J Oral Maxillofac Surg. 2021;

Kim J, Fortson JK, Cook HE. A fatal outcome from rhinocerebral mucormycosis after dental extractions: a case report. J Oral Maxillofac Surg. 2001;59(6):693–7.

Neville BW, Damm DD, Allen C, Chi AC. Oral and maxillofacial pathology. Elsevier Health Sciences; 2015.

Sivapathasundharam B. Shafer's textbook of oral pathology-e book. Elsevier Health Sciences; 2016.

Warnakulasuriya S, Tilakaratna WM, editors. Oral medicine & pathology: a guide to diagnosis and management. JP Medical Ltd.; 2013.

Deep-Seated Lump in the Buccal Mucosa: Dirofilariasis

Ruwan Jayasinghe and Wanninayake M Tilakaratne

Contents

W. M Tilakaratne, T. G. Kallarakkal (eds.), *Clinicopathological Correlation of Oral Diseases*,
https://doi.org/10.1007/978-3-031-24408-7_40

Learning Goals

1. Devise the correct way of compiling the history with appropriate questions.
2. Develop a differential diagnosis after history taking.
3. Deduce appropriate procedures in clinical examination.
4. Formulate a differential diagnosis combining findings in the history and clinical examination.
5. Justify the relevant investigations required to arrive at the diagnosis.
6. Comprehend the importance of clinicopathological correlation in arriving at the correct diagnosis.
7. Outline the management plan.
8. Recognize the importance of a diagnostic algorithm in arriving at a diagnosis

40.1 Main Complaint

A 57-year-old female patient presents with a complaint of a firm area on the left side cheek of 3 months duration.

40.2 History of Complaint

Question: What other features were noticed in relation to this area?

The size of the lesion has remained the same from the day it was noticed. I feel that it has become firm with time from its soft consistency. I do not feel any pain associated with it. It is more palpable over the skin than from inside the oral cavity. It is not clearly visible but I can palpate it well and I did not notice any color change on my cheek over the area. However, I remember having a slight red color on my skin of the left cheek about 2 months ago.

40.3 Additional Complaints

Question: Are you allergic to insect bites?

I have not noticed any such allergies.

Question: Have you had similar lesions in the past?

I have not experienced any lesions of this nature in the past.

Question: Have you noticed or felt any other changes or difficulties in the mouth?

It has not affected my day-to-day activities and there is no difficulty in opening my mouth, eating or talking.

Question: Do you have any lesions elsewhere on the body?

I do not have any other lesions on the body.

Question: Are you suffering from any other medical problems like heart disease, high blood pressure, diabetes, bleeding disorder, respiratory diseases? If yes, what kind of medications have you been taking until now?

I do not have any other medical problems.

Question: Have you undergone any surgery especially in the mouth?

I have not undergone any surgery in the past.

Question: Have you undergone any dental treatment?

I had a few restorations and scaling in the past without any complications.

Question: What is your occupation?

I am a retired technical officer.

Question: Do you have any specific habits such as cheek biting?

I do not have any such habits.

Question: Tell me about your family details and place of residence.

I am married and have four children. I am currently residing in an urban area closer to a water canal.

Question: Are there any mosquitoes in the area?

Yes, it is a common problem.

40.4 With the Findings from the History, What is Your Differential Diagnosis?

1. Reactive lymph node
2. Lipoma or other benign tumor
3. Epidermoid cyst
4. Salivary gland tumor
5. Parasitic nodule

40.5 How Do You Justify Your Differential Diagnosis After History Taking?

1. Reactive lymph node

   Nodules in the head and neck area commonly arise as a result of reactive lymphadenopathy. Most of the reactive lymph nodes are tender but long-standing nodes can be non-tender as well. As facial lymph nodes are in close relationship to the area of the complaint, it could be a differential diagnosis.
2. Lipomas are soft lumps usually seen in the buccal mucosa. They are painless, slow-growing lesions. It can become firm with time due to various pathological changes, although it is usually a soft lump.
3. Epidermoid/Sebaceous cyst

   Epidermoid cyst presents as a small lump beneath the skin. It is a slow-growing, painless lesion, not uncommonly seen on the face and neck. Sebaceous cysts arising from sebaceous glands have similar features to epidermoid cysts but are rare.
4. Salivary gland tumor

   Minor salivary gland tumors can occur in the buccal mucosa. Both benign and malignant minor salivary gland tumors of buccal mucosa have a significant growth potential. Over the time they become enlarged. Pain is usually not a frequent feature. Malignant salivary gland or other soft tissue tumors grow much faster. As this lesion has not changed in size, it indicates a benign process or other non-neoplastic pathology.
5. Parasitic nodule usually presents as a single non-tender subcutaneous nodule. Most lesions are asymptomatic. These lesions may show features of inflammation initially and subsequently undergo fibrosis and calcification. As time progresses, softer lesions become more firm in consistency. It is possible to suggest that the lesion could be a parasitic nodule because the lesion started as a soft area and gradually became firm. The location of the lesion is more towards the skin surface than intra-oral. Furthermore, most parasitic infections are transmitted by vectors such as mosquitoes. The patient resides in an area known for increased presence of mosquitoes. Hence, a differential diagnosis of a parasitic infection needs to be included in the differential diagnosis. Insect bites can also present in a similar manner.

40.6 Findings of Clinical Examination

The patient has a firm, movable, non-tender, localized swelling over the left cheek, which is attached to the overlying skin measuring approximately 2 cm × 1 cm in size (Fig. 40.1). The margins are not well demarcated and overlying skin and the buccal mucosa appear normal. The lesion does not show any polypoid appearance within the oral cavity. Other mucosal sites including tongue, gingiva palate and lips are normal in color and texture. Oral hygiene of the patient is satisfactory. There is no cervical lymphadenopathy.

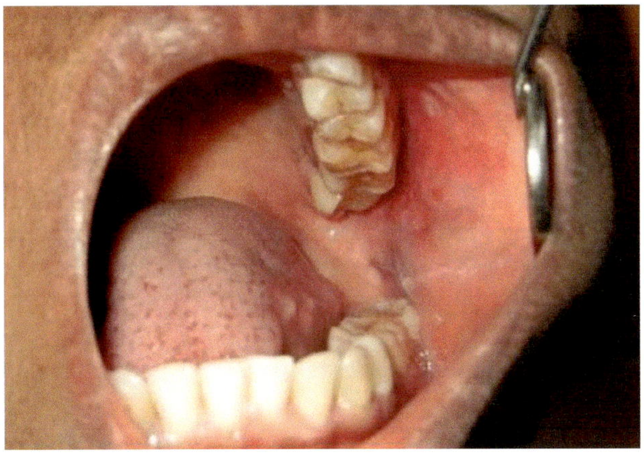

Fig. 40.1 A slightly visible lump in the buccal mucosa on the left side

40.7 What is Your Clinical Differential Diagnosis?

1. Reactive lymph node
2. Salivary gland tumor/benign soft tissue tumor
3. Epidermoid cyst
4. Healed lesion of an insect bite
5. Parasitic nodule

40.8 How Would You Justify the Inclusion of the Diseases Mentioned in the Differential Diagnosis to Arrive at a Working Diagnosis?

Justification of including those disease entities are described above. It is not possible to arrive at a single working diagnosis with the clinical presentation of the lesion until further investigations are carried out.

40.9 How Would You Investigate This Patient?

1. Full blood count (FBC)
2. Fine-needle aspiration biopsy
3. Surgical biopsy (excision)

Her full blood count was normal and fine-needle aspiration biopsy showed evidence of a chronic inflammatory process containing mixed inflammatory cells with prominent eosinophils.

40.10 What is the Next Step in the Management of this Patient?

The lesion was excised under local anesthesia and sent for histopathological examination (Fig. 40.2).

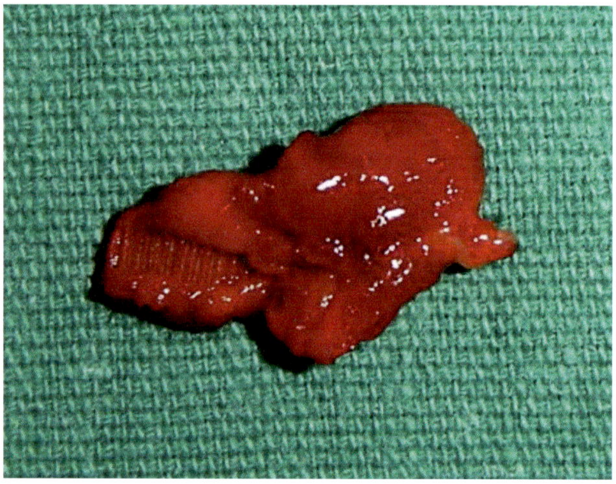

Fig. 40.2 The resected lesion comprised of a fleshy soft tissue masss measuring approximately 2 cm × 1 cm

40.11 What are the Histopathological Features Helpful to Arrive at the Definitive Diagnosis?

Excisional biopsy shows a peripheral layer of granulation tissue with an intense inflammatory cell infiltrate and conspicuous eosinophils. The center of the lesion shows a parasite exhibiting a thick cuticle with fine external longitudinal ridges and a prominent circumferential muscle layer showing transverse striations (Fig. 40.3). Sometimes dead or even live parasite can be found in early lesions (Fig. 40.4).

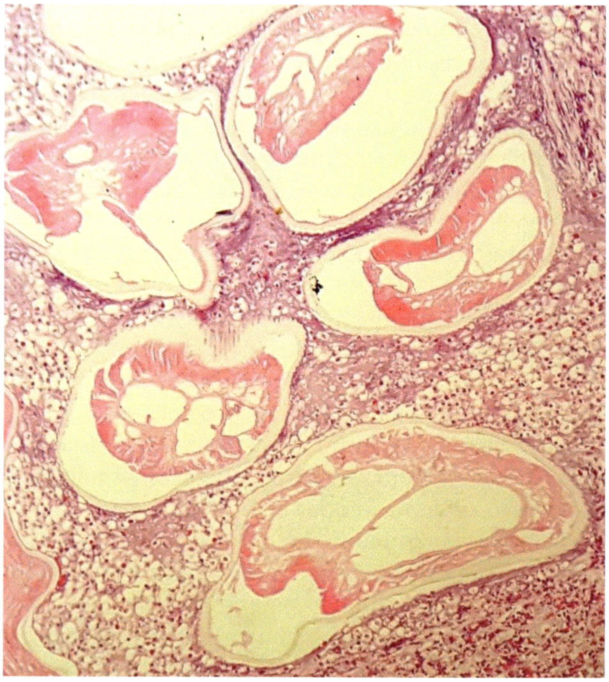

Fig. 40.3 Dead parasite with accompanying inflammatory reaction

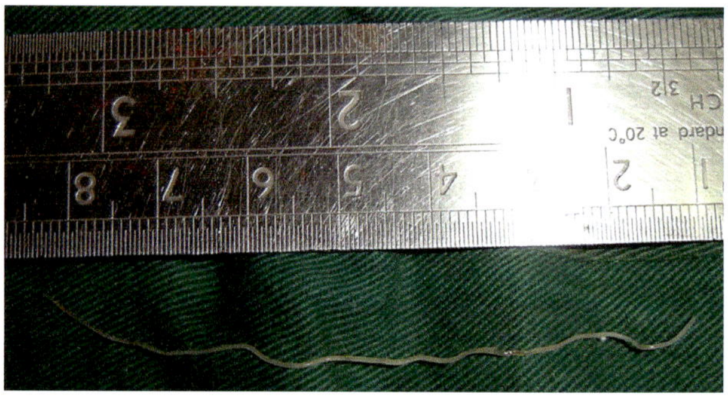

Fig. 40.4 The live *Dirofilaria* parasite removed from the lesion

40.12 What is the Most Likely Diagnosis?

Parasitic infection, consistent with dirofilariasis

40.13 What are the Specific Histopathological Features of *Dirofilaria*?

The parasite *Dirofilaria* is composed of a thick external cuticle with longitudinal ridges (micro-ruffling of the surface), leading to a cogwheel-like appearance in a transverse section, large lateral chords with tall, slender coelomian muscle layer, a single gut tube and genital tubules. The characteristic histopathological features include a dense inflammatory infiltrate composed of numerous eosinophils, neutrophils, lymphocytes, plasma cells and macrophages (◘ Fig. 40.3). Occasionally eosinophils and neutrophils partly with pyknotic nuclei can be seen on the surface of the parasite. The histopathological features may vary depending on the duration of the lesion. If the lesion is of recent onset, live parasites may be present. With time the lesion tends to get fibrosed or even calcified.

40.14 How Would You Manage This Patient?

The lesion can be easily removed surgically if the nodule is small and superficial. This provides the advantage of having the parasite for the confirmation of diagnosis by parasitological or histopathological examination. Antifilarial medicines are also effective in some cases. A single dose of ivermectin followed by three doses of diethylcarbamyzine can be used, but these must not be administered prior to surgical resection. Prevention of the disease is important. As the vector for the transmission of the disease is mosquito, this can be achieved by avoiding mosquito bites during peak biting times of the day in the areas known to be endemic for parasites. Dogs are the main host of the parasite; hence, controlling stray dogs is also helpful in controlling the spread of the disease.

40.15 Oral Dirofilariasis

Dirofilariasis is a zoonotic parasitic infection caused by a parasite nematode of the genus *Dirofilaria*, mostly living in animals, especially canines. The parasite can rarely cause infections in human beings. It is a vector-borne disease and transmission to man occurs through a bite of potential mosquito vectors. The exposed part of the body including the head and neck region and the lower extremities forms the common subcutaneous sites of involvement, with the majority of cases occurring in the ocular and periocular regions. Human dirofilarial infections are commonly seen in pulmonary, peritoneal, ocular or subcutaneous areas. There are more than 40 species that cause human dirofilariasis. *Dirofilaria repens*, *Dirofilaria ursi*, *Dirofilaria tenuis* and *Dirofilaria striata* mainly cause infections in the subcutaneous tissues, while *Dirofilaria immitis* and *Dirofilaria spectrum* are found in the heart and blood vessels.

In humans, two types of diseases occur due to dirofilarial infection. Pulmonary dirofilariasis is primarily caused by *Dirofilaria immitis*. Subcutaneous dirofilariasis is primarily caused by *Dirofilaria tenuis* and *Dirofilaria repens*. Although this infection is rare, prevalence of the disease is increasing and emerging as a significant health problem in different parts of the world. Subcutaneous dirofilariasis is commonly seen the in fourth to fifth decades of life.

Nodules may occur in any part of the body in subcutaneous dirofilariasis. Common sites are the ones that are exposed to mosquito bites. Humans are a dead-end host and therefore the parasite does not reach sexual maturity in humans. Chronic inflammatory cell infiltration is present around the living or dead parasite forming a parasitic granuloma. It commonly presents as a single non-tender subcutaneous nodule. The patients are mostly asymptomatic. The nodules become suppurative after a period of 2–12 months. Involvement of the eye is more commonly diagnosed as it causes more symptoms than subcutaneous nodules. Sub-conjunctival dirofilariasis can cause detached retina, opacity, glaucoma, uveitis and limited loss of vision. The parasitic nodule with time may undergo fibrosis or even calcification.

Hematological investigations such as full blood count (FBC) are helpful in excluding bacterial infection. FBC shows elevated levels of eosinophils as seen in any parasitic infection. Radiological investigations such as ultrasonography, computed tomography and magnetic resonance imaging may be useful. Ultrasonographic imaging is helpful in identifying the movement of the parasite inside the nodule. Detection of anti-*Dirofilaria repens* antibody level is helpful in monitoring the treatment response in cases treated with drugs.

Microscopic examination of the removed parasite or its fragments remains the most reliable method to confirm the diagnosis. Sometimes dead or even live parasite can be found in early lesions (■ Fig. 40.4).

There are multiple treatment options available for the management of subcutaneous dirofilariasis. The best treatment method is the surgical removal of the parasite. Live worm moves within the nodule giving a difficulty in locating it. In such a situation, either the nodule can be removed completely, or the parasite can be immobilized using a cryoprobe. Medical treatment is also effective in some cases. Most commonly used drugs include diethylcarbamazine (DEC), ivermectin and albendazole. DEC is very effective. It alters the membrane of the parasite by facilitating phagocytosis of the parasite by monocytes. Ivermectin is a broad-spectrum antiparasitic drug that is effective as a treatment as well as a preventive drug. Tetracycline and doxycycline have also been used with some success. The best way of minimizing the infection is by preventive measures. Proper methods to control mosquitoes and stray dogs are essential.

Salient features of subcutaneous dirofilariasis	
Clinical	• Single non-tender subcutaneous nodule. • Most patients are asymptomatic. • No particular sensation attributable to the insect bite. • Most lesions undergo fibrosis followed by calcification. • Subsequent formation of subcutaneous or subconjunctival suppurative nodules after 2–12 months. • Rarely, satellite lymphadenopathy with hyperpyrexia.
Investigations	• Hematological: FBC shows peripheral eosinophilia. • Serology: Level of anti-*Dirofilaria repens* antibodies • Radiological: Ultrasonographic imaging • Histopathological Excisional biopsy: Peripheral layer of granulation tissue with an intense inflammatory cell infiltrate. Center of the lesion shows a nematode parasite exhibiting a thick cuticle with fine external longitudinal ridges and a prominent circumferential muscle layer showing transverse striations. • Parasitological investigations
Treatment	• Surgical removal of the parasite • Medical treatment with diethylcarbamazine (DEC), ivermectin and albendazole or tetracycline and doxycycline • Preventive management: vector control

Diagnostic Algorithm

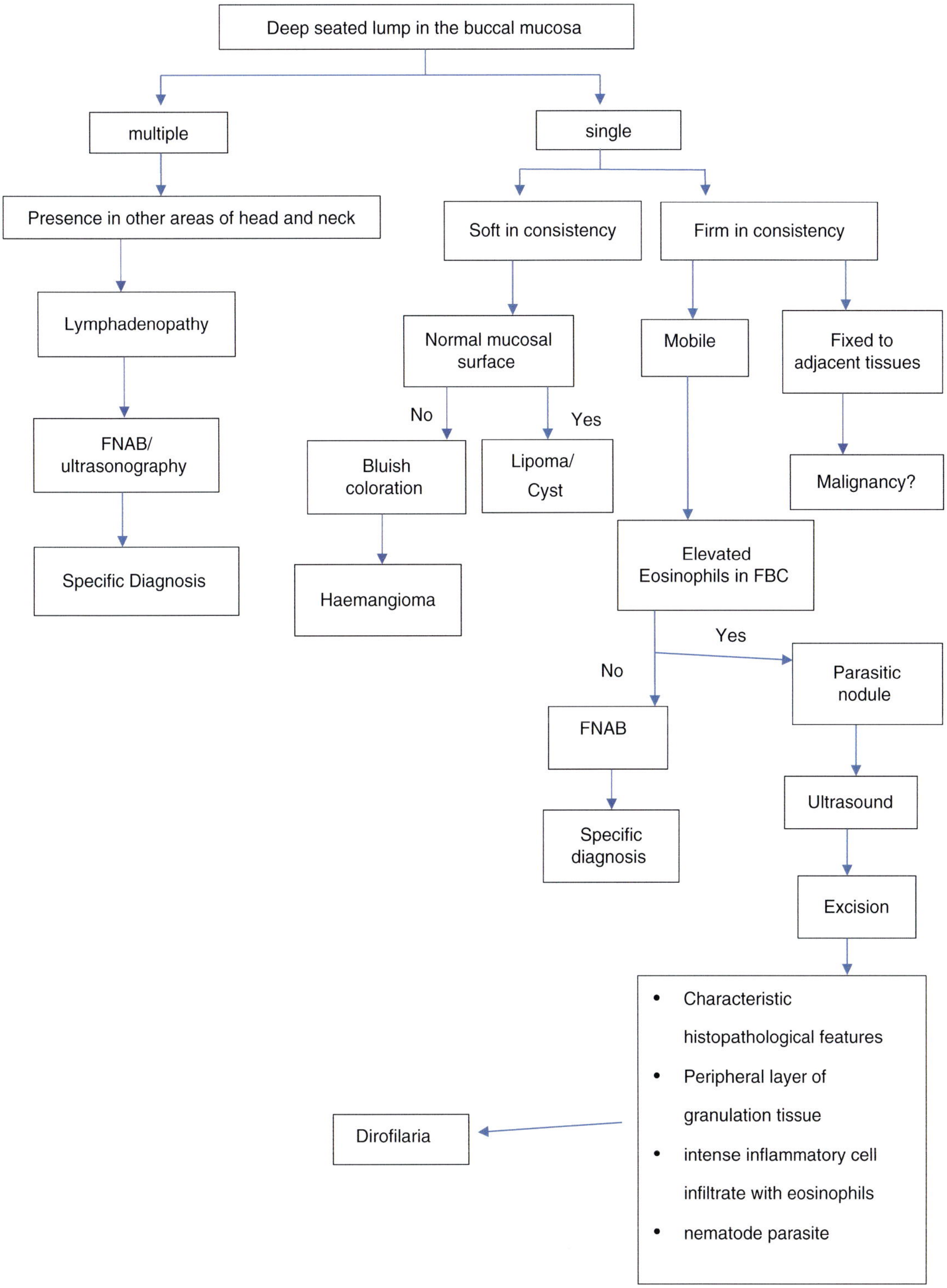

Self-Assessment Questions

1. Discuss the etiopathogenesis of subcutaneous dirofilariasis.
2. List the clinical features of dirofilariasis.
3. List the histopathological features of dirofilariasis.
4. Discuss the investigations and their findings that can be used to diagnose dirofilariasis.
5. Outline the management of subcutaneous dirofilariasis.

Summary

Dirofilariasis is a zoonotic disease caused by the parasite *Dirofilaria*, commonly *Dirofilaria repens*. It presents as a nodule commonly seen in the head and neck area. Chronic inflammatory infiltration around the parasite evokes a granulomatous reaction. It rarely causes symptoms. Hematological, radiological and immunological investigations are useful in the diagnosis. Best treatment method is surgical but medical treatment can also be used in some cases. Preventive measures are essential.

Further Reading

Genchi C, Kramer L. Subcutaneous dirofilariosis (*Dirofilaria repens*): an infection spreading throughout the old world. Parasites Vectors. 2017;10:517. https://doi.org/10.1186/s13071-017-2434-8.

Jayasinghe RD, Gunawardane SR, Sitheeque MA, Wickramasinghe S. A case report on oral subcutaneous dirofilariasis. Case Rep Infect Dis. 2015;2015:648278. https://doi.org/10.1155/2015/648278.

Riebenbauer K, Weber PB, Walochnik J, et al. Human dirofilariosis in Austria: the past, the present, the future. Parasites Vectors. 2021;14:227. https://doi.org/10.1186/s13071-021-04696-4.

Tilakaratne WM, Pitakotuwage TN. Intra-oral *Dirofilaria repens* infection: report of seven cases. J Oral Med Pathol. 2003;32(8):502–5.

Inabilty to Wear Dentures: Denture-Induced Stomatitis

Jacob John and P. L. Ranganayaki Devi S. Palaniappan

Contents

W. M Tilakaratne, T. G. Kallarakkal (eds.), *Clinicopathological Correlation of Oral Diseases*,
https://doi.org/10.1007/978-3-031-24408-7_41

Learning Goals

1. Understand the presentation and pathogenesis of denture induced stomatitis.
2. Clinically recognise and differentiate denture induced stomatitis.
3. Classify denture induced stomatitis lesions to help plan their management.
4. Recognise and appreciate the clinical challenges in their management.
5. Learn the diagnosis and assessment of denture induced stomatitis.

41.1 Main Complaint

A 78-year-old Chinese woman came to the clinic accompanied by her daughter, complaining of her ill-fitting upper denture for the last one week.

41.2 History of Complaint

Question: When did you first notice this?

My mother has been complaining about swollen palatal surface under her upper denture to her caretaker at the nursing home for the last 3 months. She is otherwise asymptomatic. However, the caretaker did not take the matter seriously until it was noticed that the patient could not use her upper denture comfortably during eating.

41.3 Additional Complaints

Question: Do you have any pain associated with the swelling?

I don't have any pain associated with the swelling.

Question: Are there any other associated signs and symptoms?

I notice pin-point areas of bleeding on the area.

Question: Is there any other lesion in and around the mouth?

I have redness at the corner of my mouth.

Question: Did you notice any swelling under your lower dentures?

The swelling is only present on my palate.

Question: Do you experience any taste alterations?

I experience a metallic taste in my mouth. I also have bad breath.

Question: Do you experience any symptoms of dry mouth or lack of saliva?

I experience dry mouth symptoms. I try to drink more water to reduce this problem.

Question: Is your present denture retentive during function? If not, do you take any steps to increase the retention?

My present denture is not fitting well nor is it retentive. I use denture adhesives to help me while eating with the denture.

Question: What is your main diet?

I usually take porridge and soft starchy food.

Question: Do you have any habits of smoking or alcohol consumption?

I do not have any such habits.

Question: Have you undergone any dental treatment?

✓ I have been edentulous since I was 65 years old. I am currently wearing my second set of dentures, constructed six years ago. Till recently, I had been having the habit of wearing my dentures throughout the day, even at night. I have been residing in a nursing home for the last 10 years, and for over a year now, I have not been able to maintain good denture hygiene by myself.

? Question: Are you suffering from any other medical problems like heart disease, high blood pressure, diabetes, bleeding disorder, or respiratory diseases? If yes, what kind of medications have you been taking until now?

✓ I have a few medical problems. I am a diabetic on medication and taking steroids for allergy. In addition, I have bronchitis and use an inhaler. I am also on antibiotics for a recent infection.

41.4 With the Findings from the History, What Is Your Differential Diagnosis?

1. Allergic contact stomatitis
2. Denture-induced stomatitis (chronic atrophic candidiasis)

41.5 Findings on Clinical Examination

The patient has a completely edentulous maxillary arch. The palatal mucosa appears erythematous with a slightly granular surface, exhibiting a cluster of multiple papules or nodules, measuring about 2 mm or less. On palpation, the palatal surface is not tender. The oral mucosa appears dry with the absence of the pooling of saliva in the floor of the mouth. The denture hygiene is poor. There is plaque and debris, both on the fitting and on the polished surface of the denture. The intraoral presentation of the patient is as seen in ◘ Fig. 41.1.

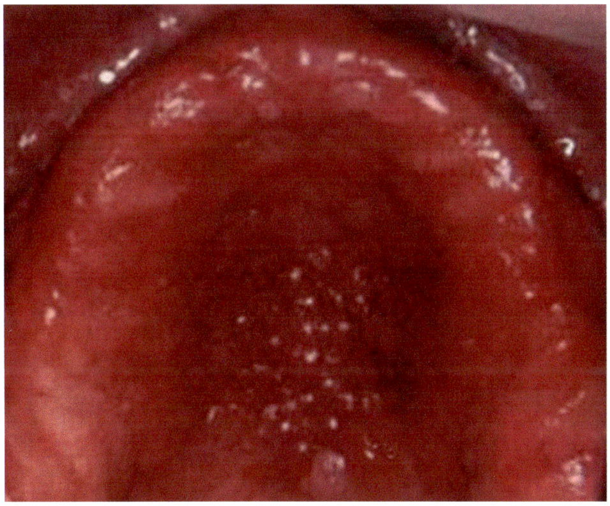

◘ **Fig. 41.1** Intraoral clinical presentation of patient

41.6 How Would You Identify Poor Denture Hygiene If Deposits Are Not Visible Clinically?

Disclosing solution can be applied on denture surfaces to reveal the deposits on the surfaces of the prosthesis. ◘ Fig. 41.2 shows marked staining deposits on the fitting surfaces and denture teeth area. This is usually due to stagnation, pooling of saliva, and the absence of contact with the tongue on the fitting surfaces.

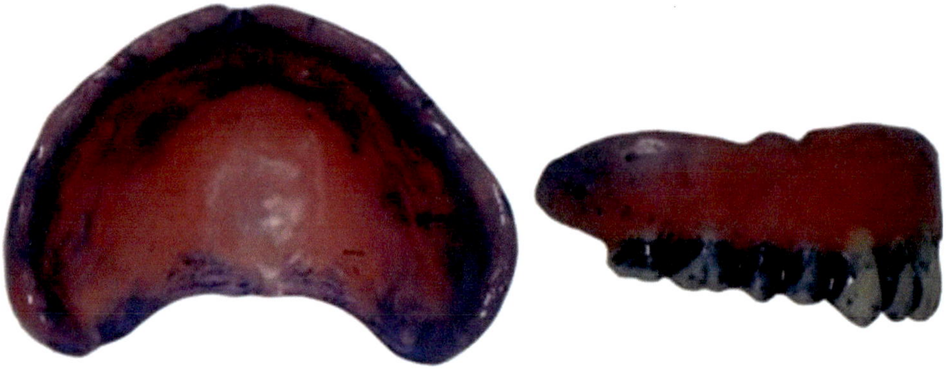

Fig. 41.2 Disclosed plaque deposition on maxillary complete denture (photos courtesy of Ikeya K et. al, 2018)

41.7 With the History and Clinical Findings, What Is Your Differential Diagnosis?

1. Allergic contact stomatitis.
2. Denture-induced stomatitis (chronic atrophic candidiasis).

41.8 How Do You Justify Your Differential Diagnosis?

Oral candidiasis is a fungal infection caused by candida species. In denture-induced stomatitis, only the denture-bearing mucosa is affected. Stomatitis rarely develops under a lower denture. Localized chronic erythema of tissues covered by dentures is the classical presentation of such a clinical scenario. Thus, some may also call this presentation erythematous candidiasis. Angular cheilitis, which is inflammation of the corners of the mouth, can coexist. This is also often associated with Candida albicans.

Inflammatory reactions of the mucosa beneath a denture can also result from irritation or allergy caused by the materials in the denture itself (acrylic, cobalt, chromium), or response to substances within denture adhesives as in allergic contact stomatitis. Incomplete curing of the acrylic resin (the prosthetic material) may also be an involved factor. For allergic reactions to occur due to the denture base material, the denture must be a new prosthesis. This patient has been using this denture for more than 6 years and hence may be an unlikely cause of allergy. The clinical presentation of denture stomatitis is erythema and oedema on the palatal mucosa restricted to the area covered by the denture base.

41.9 What Is the Most Likely Clinical Diagnosis and Your Justification?

Denture-induced stomatitis, type 3 (chronic atrophic candidiasis/chronic erythematous candidiasis)

Denture stomatitis usually does not cause any symptoms. On examination, the mucosal surface in contact with the denture is red and swollen sometimes with small red dots (petechial haemorrhages). Type 3 denture-induced stomatitis (granular type) usually involves the central part of the hard palate or the alveolar ridge. This commonly occurs due to microbial plaque accumulation, which is restricted to the denture-bearing area, often with a sharply defined edge. Patients usually do not complain of any pain.

This patient gives a history of wearing her maxillary complete denture throughout the night and this is a major risk factor for the development of this condition. Wearing dental appliances such as dentures alters the oral microbiota. A microbial plaque composed of bacteria or yeast forms on the fitting surface of the denture and on the mucosa, which is covered. Over time, this plaque may be colonized by Candida species. The local environment under a denture is more acidic and less exposed to the cleansing action of saliva, which favours high candidal enzymatic activity and may cause inflammation of the mucosa.

The patient is a diabetic and is on medication. Besides, she also uses an inhaler and is on long-term antibiotics. These factors also contribute to the development of denture-induced stomatitis. Antibiotics may destroy the bacteria that prevent Candida from growing out of control, especially if taken over a long period.

41.10 How Would You Investigate This Patient?

The diagnosis is usually made based on the clinical appearance, blood investigations to rule out systemic diseases, and swabs taken from the surface of the denture and mucosa. A clinical appearance based on the pattern of redness and swelling following the shape of the area of denture contact is the classical clinical presentation.

Investigations include basic blood tests, smears, and culture. Diabetic status should be assessed using relevant investigations. A smear of the mucosa should be performed and stained with periodic acid–Schiff stain to detect the presence of fungal organisms.

A biopsy is not indicated unless other pathologies are suspected.

41.11 How Would You Manage This Patient?

1. Good oral hygiene is mandatory. The mouth must be kept as clean as possible and a thorough rinse after meals should be performed.
2. Local factors which promote the growth of yeasts, such as smoking or wearing the dentures throughout the night, must be discouraged.
3. Dentures should be removed for as long as possible and overnight.
4. Dentures should be brushed in warm, soapy water and soaked overnight in an antiseptic solution such as bleach (10 drops of household bleach in a denture cup), chlorhexidine (not when the denture has metal components), or in any solution suitable for sterilizing baby's feeding bottles. Benzoic acid-containing products should be avoided as they induce changes in the composition of acrylic materials.
5. Denture fitting and occlusal balance should be checked to avoid trauma. A new prosthesis should be made, if necessary.
6. Tissue conditioning agents are porous materials easier to colonize than acrylic, so they are not recommended for these patients. If there is no other choice, an antifungal agent, like nystatin, miconazole or ketoconazole, may be incorporated into the tissue conditioning agent.
7. Dentures must be adequately polished and glazed, as pores increase denture contamination by oral microorganisms.
8. Treatment with low-energy lasers to reduce inflammation of the supporting mucosa is advocated.
9. Clinically inflammatory papillary hyperplasia of the palate or the granular type of denture stomatitis is a reactive tissue overgrowth, characterized by a hyperaemic mucosa with a nodular or papillary appearance, mostly covering the central part of the palate. This may need to be surgically removed (by scalpel, cryosurgery, electrosurgery, or with a laser beam) before the denture is placed but it was not indicated in this patient as the papillary lesions were not very large.
10. Mild cases may respond to antifungal treatment. Antifungal medications are recommended when yeasts have been isolated, or when lesions do not resolve with hygiene instructions.
    (a) The first-choice treatment is the topical application of nystatin or miconazole. Resistance to nystatin is rare and the drug is administered as an oral suspension. Nystatin has an unpleasant taste and can induce gastrointestinal problems and hypersensitivity.
    (b) Miconazole is available as a gel, varnish, lacquer, and chewing gum. It also provokes gastrointestinal alterations and hypersensitivity, but it tastes better. Miconazole also enhances the warfarin effect.
    (c) Systemic antifungal drugs (fluconazole, itraconazole, ketoconazole) are almost exclusively reserved for patients with systemic factors that promote the development and persistence of candidiasis, such as immunosuppression or uncontrolled diabetes.

41.12 Denture-Induced Stomatitis

The condition was described as 'denture sore mouth' by Cahn (1936), but this term was later replaced by 'denture stomatitis' as discomfort is not always present. Denture-induced stomatitis indicates an inflammatory process of the mucosa that bears a complete or partial removable dental appliance, typically a denture. It may also be called chronic atrophic or chronic erythematous candidiasis.

Denture stomatitis is a common condition. Findings from several studies suggest that it can affect as many as 35–50% of persons who wear complete dentures. The prevalence of denture stomatitis among those wearing partial dentures is markedly lower than among complete denture wearers.

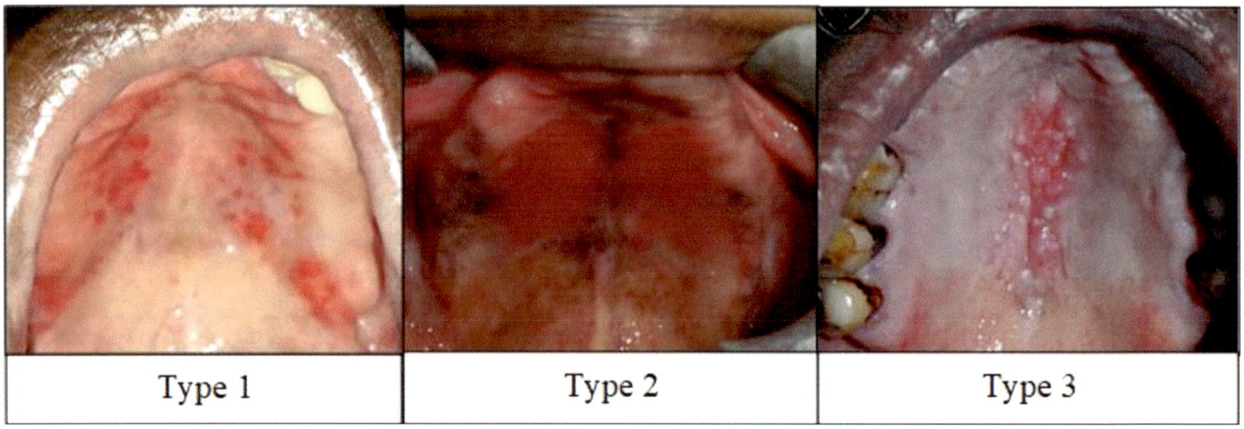

Fig. 41.3 Newton classification for denture stomatitis. Photographs courtesy of Prof. Ruwan D. Jayasinghe

There is no definite racial or sex predilection, although some authors have described a higher prevalence among women. This disorder is more frequently seen among elderly people, as they are more likely to wear removable dentures. It has been reported mostly in aged people, especially those living in nursing facilities.

Denture stomatitis may show different clinical patterns and is more frequently found in the upper jaw, especially on the palate. The absence of denture stomatitis in the lower jaw is probably due to the washing action of saliva. Even though denture stomatitis is frequently asymptomatic, patients may complain of halitosis, slight bleeding, and swelling in the involved area, burning sensation, xerostomia, or taste alterations (dysgeusia). These symptoms occur, with variable intensity.

Denture stomatitis can be classified based on the Newton Classification, 1962 (based exclusively on clinical criteria). Type 1: Localized, simple inflammation or pin-point erythema; Type 2: More diffuse generalized erythema involving part or the entire denture covering mucosa; Type 3: Granular type, usually involving the central part of the hard palate and the alveolar ridges.

Fig. 41.3 shows the clinical presentation of types 1, 2, and 3 of the Newton Classification for denture stomatitis.

The aetiology of denture stomatitis is best considered multifactorial, but denture wearing, especially when worn during the night, represents the major causative factor. There are several aetiological/predisposing factors responsible for denture stomatitis. They can be divided into prosthetic and infective factors.

41.12.1 Prosthetic Factors

Denture stomatitis cannot exist without a prosthesis. Ill-fitting, traumatic, badly maintained dentures have been considered the most frequent causes of denture stomatitis. Prosthetic traumatism is associated with functional deficiencies of the denture such as occlusal alterations, incorrect vertical dimension, retention alterations, and unstable prosthesis.

The type of material employed for construction is also a contributing factor for the development of denture stomatitis. Newton-type III is five fold more frequently associated with acrylic dentures than with metallic ones. The tissue surface of the dentures sometimes shows micropits and microporosities. Microorganisms harbouring in these areas are difficult to remove mechanically or by chemical cleansing. The microbial contamination of denture acrylic resin occurs very quickly, and yeasts seem to adhere well to denture base materials. Surface roughness may facilitate microbial retention and infection. Dentures with a fine texture and absence of porosity do not allow attachment of plaque by penetration of surface defects or by mechanical fixation to surface irregularities.

41.12.2 Infectious Factors

The denture can produce several ecological changes that facilitate the accumulation of bacteria and yeasts.

Certain bacterial species, like Staphylococcus species, Streptococcus species, Neisseria species, Fusobacterium species, or Bacteroides species, have been identified in patients with denture stomatitis, although no direct relationship between bacteria and the aetiology of denture stomatitis could be proved.

Candida species, particularly Candida albicans, have been identified in almost all patients. Patients with denture stomatitis show higher intraoral concentrations of fungi than individuals without this disorder and the lesions objectively improve after antifungal drug administration. However, the role of this organism as the sole etiologic factor remains unclear.

There are numerous predisposing factors for oral candidiasis.

1. Systemic factors
   (a) Physiological (advanced age)
   (b) Endocrine dysfunctions
   (c) Nutritional deficiencies
   (d) Neoplasia
   (e) Immunosuppression
   (f) Broad-spectrum antibiotics
2. Local factors
   (a) Antimicrobials and topical or inhaled corticosteroids
   (b) Carbohydrate-rich diet
   (c) Tobacco and alcohol consumption
   (d) Hyposalivation
   (e) Poor oral hygiene
   (f) Wearing dentures (especially through the night)

Fig. 41.4 from Jacob S. A et. al, 2013 describes the events which take place in the causation of denture stomatitis that is triggered by the prosthesis and plaque leading to alteration of the pH. Colonization of organisms also contributes to lower pH levels which result in mucosal irritation.

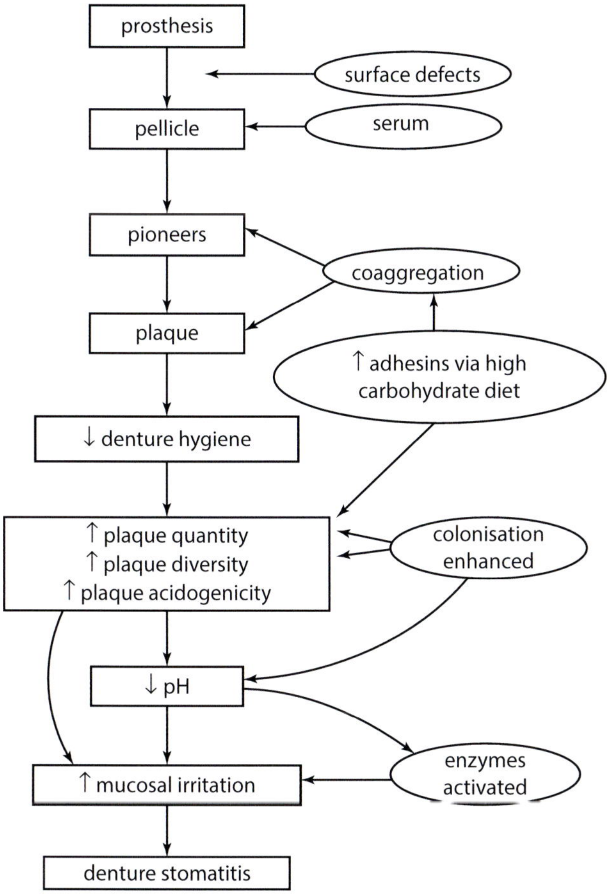

Fig. 41.4 Events in the aetiopathogenesis of denture-induced stomatitis

The clinical presentation of erythema and oedema on the palatal mucosa covered by the denture base (but not beyond) is a diagnostic feature. A smear of the palate stained with periodic acid–Schiff demonstrates the presence of Candida species. Other techniques for identifying fungal isolates such as imprint cultures may also be applied. Exfoliative cytology should be performed on mucosal surfaces to examine for the presence or absence of Candida albicans infection as determined by periodic acid–Schiff (PAS) (Fig. 41.5).

BBL culture swab (Becton, Dickinson and Company) is used to swab the denture and the mucosal surface. Samples obtained from swabbing are cultured on Sabouraud dextrose agar containing quercetin succinate. Samples are spiral plated to Sabouraud's dextrose plates to obtain a quantitative value of colony-forming units per millilitre (CFU/mL). Candida colonies are counted after 48 h, and the patients classified according to the number of CFU as follows: negative (CFU/mL = 0), carrier (CFU/mL <400), and positive (CFU/mL >400).

If untreated, denture-induced stomatitis can cause soreness and palatal inflammatory papillary hyperplasia and may lead to poorly fitting dentures in the future. The administration of topical antifungal therapy, removal of mechanical trauma caused by the denture, and reinforcement of hygienic measures ease the disappearance of the lesions.

However, local recurrences are frequent if aetiopathological factors persist. The prognosis of this

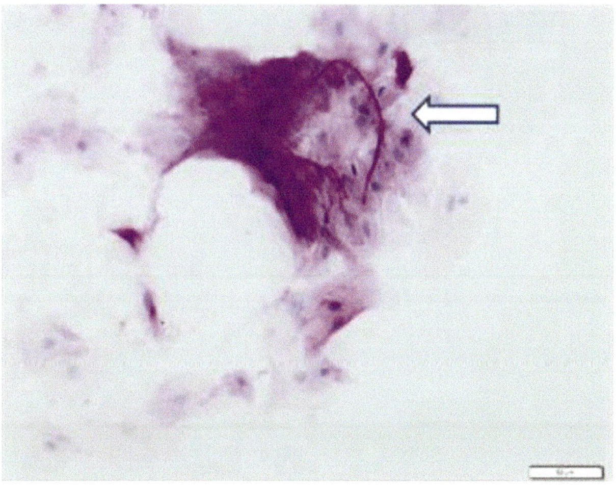

Fig. 41.5 PAS-stained smear shows candidal hyphae (white arrow)

disorder is good, as there is no risk of malignant transformation. Continuous aspiration and swallowing of Candida species may rarely have potentially fatal consequences in severely immunocompromised patients.

It is mandatory to include prevention of denture-induced stomatitis in oral healthcare programmes. Dental professionals working with geriatric patients must promote this preventive programme among all healthcare workers, home caregivers, members of the patient's family, and the patients themselves.

A preventive programme should include:

- A routine basic inspection of the oral cavity for screening for this disorder, even when the lesions are asymptomatic.
- Proper denture sanitization and good oral hygiene.
- Appropriate denture-wearing habits, instructing the patient to take his/her denture out of the mouth for 6–8 h each day.
- Patients with partial dentures should undergo periodic professional plaque control.

Salient Features of Denture-Induced Stomatitis	
Clinical Presentation	Frequently restricted to the maxillary denture-bearing area. Denture stomatitis is frequently asymptomatic. However, patients may complain of halitosis, slight bleeding and swelling in the involved area, burning sensation, xerostomia, or taste alterations.
Investigations	Swab taken from the mucosa covering the denture surface is the most ideal form of investigation. Results may reveal the presence of Candida albicans.
Treatment	1. Newton's type I and II denture stomatitis can be successfully treated with low-energy lasers to reduce inflammation of the supporting mucosa. Inflammatory papillary hyperplasia usually needs to be surgically removed (by scalpel, cryosurgery, electrosurgery, or with a laser beam) before the denture is placed. 2. Mild cases may respond to antifungal treatment. Antifungal medications are recommended when yeasts have been isolated, or when lesions do not resolve with hygiene instructions.

Diagnostic Algorithm for Denture-Induced Stomatitis

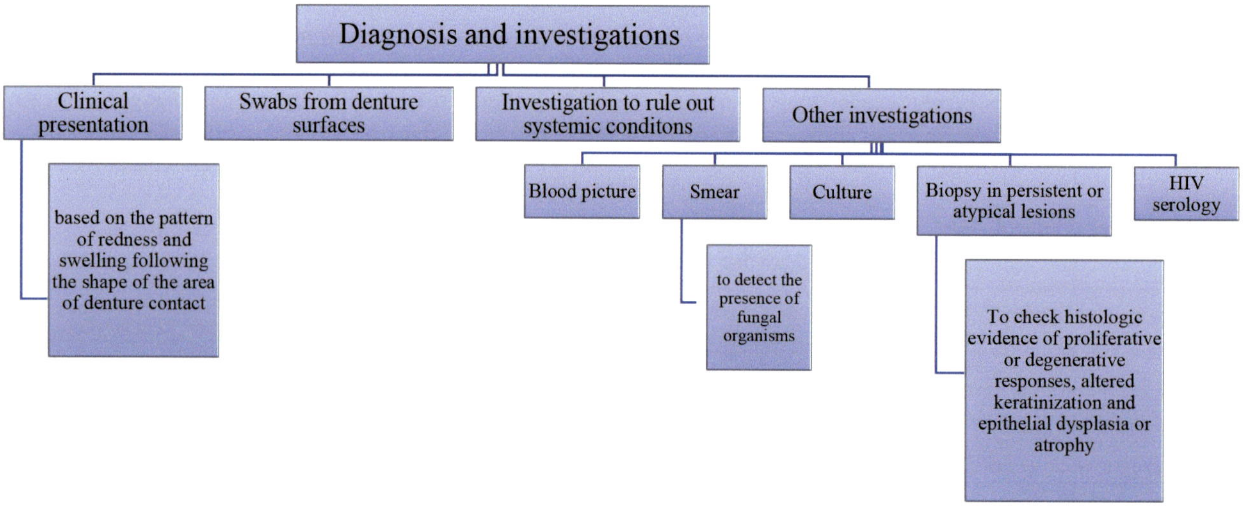

Self-Assessment Questions

1. Describe the clinical features of denture-induced stomatitis.
2. Explain the aetiology of denture-induced stomatitis.
3. Describe the investigations required to diagnose denture-induced stomatitis.
4. Explain a management plan for a patient with denture-induced stomatitis
5. Describe the steps to prevent denture-induced stomatitis.

Summary

Denture induced stomatitis is frequently seen on the maxillary denture bearing area. Denture lining materials which include tissue conditioners and soft denture liners may colonize Candida within. Fungal growth is known to destroy the surface properties of the liner and this may lead to irritation of the oral tissues. This is due to a combination of increased surface roughness and high concentrations of exotoxins and metabolic products produced by the fungal colonies. Other factors that contribute to the occurrence of denture induced stomatitis include denture cleanliness and some systemic diseases. Swabs taken from the denture surfaces are the most ideal form of investigation.

Further Reading

Altarawneh S, Bencharit S, Mendoza L, Curran A, Barrow D, Barros S, Preisser J, Loewy ZG, Gendreau L, Offenbacher S. Clinical and histological findings of denture stomatitis as related to intraoral colonization patterns of Candida albicans, salivary flow, and dry mouth. J Prosthodontics Implant Aesthetic Reconstr Dentistry. 2013 Jan;22(1):13–22.

Cawson RA, Odell EW. Cawson's essentials of oral pathology and oral medicine e-book. Elsevier Health Sciences; 2017.

Ikeya K, Iwasa F, Inoue Y, Fukunishi M, Takahashi N, Ishihara K, Baba K. Inhibition of denture plaque deposition on complete dentures by 2-methacryloyloxyethyl phosphorylcholine polymer coating: a clinical study. J Prosthetic Dent. 2018;119(1):67–74.

Jacob SA, Gopalakrishnan A. Saliva in prosthodontic therapy-all you need to know. J Dent Sci. 2013;1(1):13–25.

Pattanaik S, Vikas BV, Pattanaik B, Sahu S, Lodam S. Denture stomatitis: a literature review. J Indian Acad Oral Med Radiol. 2010;22(3):136.

Neville BW, Damm DD, Allen C, Chi AC. Oral and maxillofacial pathology. Elsevier Health Sciences; 2015.

Sivapathasundharam B. Shafer's textbook of oral pathology-e book. Elsevier Health Sciences; 2016.

Warnakulasuriya S, Tilakaratna WM, editors. Oral medicine and pathology: a guide to diagnosis and management. JP Medical Ltd.; 2013.

Fever with Ulcers in the Mouth: Herpes Simplex Infection

Ruwan Jayasinghe and Wanninayake M Tilakaratne

Contents

W. M Tilakaratne, T. G. Kallarakkal (eds.), *Clinicopathological Correlation of Oral Diseases*,
https://doi.org/10.1007/978-3-031-24408-7_42

Learning Goals

1. Devise the correct way of compiling the history with appropriate questions.
2. Develop a differential diagnosis after history taking.
3. Deduce appropriate procedures in clinical examination.
4. Formulate a differential diagnosis combining findings in the history and clinical examination.
5. Justify the relevant investigations required to arrive at the diagnosis.
6. Comprehend the importance of clinicopathological correlation in arriving at the correct diagnosis.
7. Outline the management plan.
8. Recognize the importance of a diagnostic algorithm in arriving at a diagnosis

42.1 Main Complaint

A 6-year-old girl, who complains of multiple ulcers in the mouth, was brought to the clinic by her parents. She had fever with body aches, loss of appetite, and headache few days ago but the fever had settled just before the ulcers appeared.

42.2 History of Complaint

Question: How long have you been having these ulcerations and have you had any similar ulcers in the past?

The ulcers have been there for a few days.

Question: Are they painful and disturb your normal functions?

The ulcers are painful and I am having difficulties in eating and brushing my teeth.

Question: Did you have similar ulcers in the past?

She had not had any oral ulcerations in the past and this is the first time that she developed oral ulcers according to her parents.

42.3 Additional Complaints

Question: Have you noticed or felt any other changes or difficulties in the mouth?

She has reddish swollen gums which bleed when brushing her teeth. Her mother had felt glands in the neck and the child is complaining difficulty in swallowing.

Question: Do you have any lesions elsewhere in the body?

The child does not have any ulcers or lesions elsewhere in the body.

Question: Do you get a bad breath from the mouth?

Neither the child nor the mother complains of any bad breath from the mouth.

Question: Does she get recurrent episodes of fever?

She gets fever once in a while but not frequently.

Question: Is she suffering from any other medical problems like asthma, heart disease, bleeding disorder, respiratory diseases, or taking any medication?

She does not have any other medical problems and she is not on any medication.

Question: Has she undergone any surgery?

She has not undergone any surgery in the past.

Question: Has she undergone any dental treatment?

She has not undergone any dental treatment in the past.

Question: Were there any other children in her class with fever and/or oral ulceration recently?

Her best friend had fever about a week ago and there were few other girls who missed the classes due to fever during the last few weeks.

42.4 With the Findings from the History, What is Your Differential Diagnosis?

1. Primary herpetic gingivostomatitis
2. Herpangina
3. Hand foot and mouth disease
4. Aphthous ulceration

42.5 How Do You Justify Your Differential Diagnosis After History Taking?

1. This patient is a child with multiple oral ulcers in the mouth. In addition, she had fever with body aches, loss of appetite, and headache few days ago but the fever settled just before the ulcers appeared which is consistent with the prodromal stage of a viral infection. A few girls in her class had fever during the last few weeks indicating a possible viral infection. Together with the age, oral ulceration, fever, and reddish swollen gingiva are indicative of primary herpetic gingivostomatitis.
2. Herpangina is also another common viral infection seen in children. It is clinically similar to primary herpetic gingivostomatitis but it is a milder disease with smaller and fewer ulcers than in primary herpetic gingivostomatitis. Ulcers in herpangina are mostly seen in the posterior mouth and gingival involvement is minimal.
3. Hand foot and mouth disease also presents with similar clinical features as primary herpetic gingivostomatitis but it has characteristic involvement of hands and feet. Infection is milder and ulcers are smaller, fewer and mostly seen in the posterior mouth. This is not the most likely differential diagnosis unless it is a very early stage of the disease before the development of ulcers on hands and feet.
4. Aphthous ulceration can present with similar ulcers but it is not common in this age. Even though lymphadenopathy can be present due to secondary infection, other features seen in this child are not characteristic for aphthous ulceration. Therefore, this is an unlikely differential diagnosis.

42.6 Findings of Examination

The patient is ill looking with dry lips. There are multiple small roundish ulcers on both buccal mucosae, tongue (◘ Fig. 42.1a), and lower labial mucosa (◘ Fig. 42.1b). Gingiva is reddish and swollen (◘ Fig. 42.2). There are multiple mobile, tender palpable lymph nodes in the submandibular region.

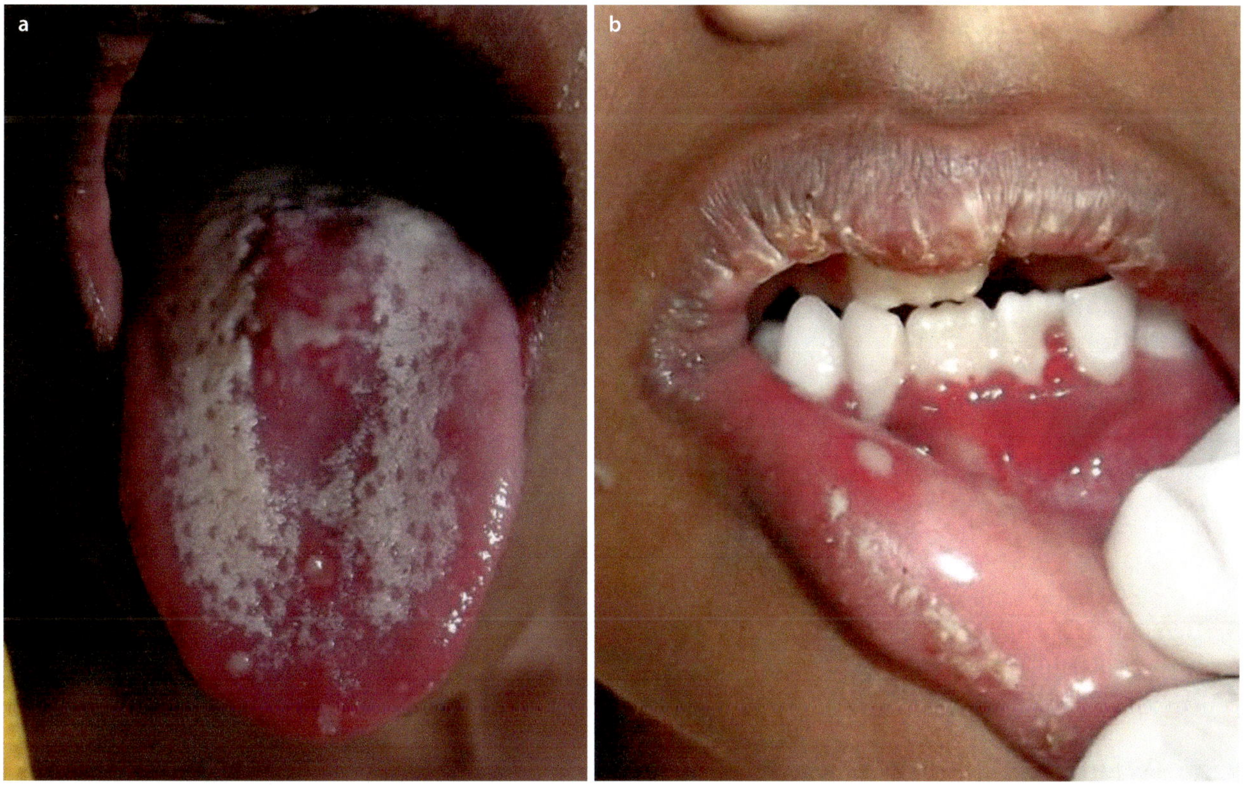

◘ **Fig. 42.1** (**a**) Ulcers on the tongue and buccal mucosa. (**b**) Multiple ulcers on the labial mucosa

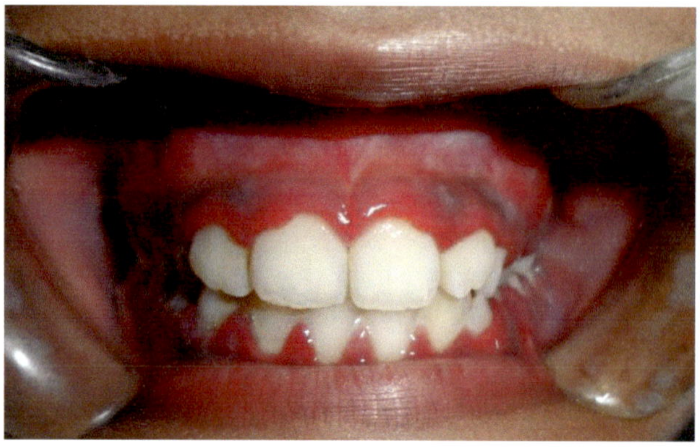

Fig. 42.2 Reddish and swollen gingivae

42.7 What Other Relevant Features Would You Look for with the Findings You Have So Far?

There is no evidence of pale colour in the oral mucosa or conjunctiva suggestive of anaemia. It is important to look for evidence of spontaneous bleeding or bleeding with minor provocation to exclude thrombocytopenia.

42.8 What is Your Working Diagnosis After History Taking and Clinical Examination?

Primary herpetic gingivostomatitis

42.9 How Would You Investigate This Patient?

Typical clinical features are helpful in the diagnosis of primary herpetic gingivostomatitis and the following investigations may be necessary in atypical cases and especially in immuno-compromised patients.

1. Full blood count (FBC) to exclude haematological disorders
2. Cytology smear from a vesicle or ulcer
3. Immunological and serological tests to identify anti-herpes virus antibodies
4. Virus culture and PCR

42.10 What is the Significance of Immune Status of the Patient?

Herpes virus infection is a mild viral infection with spontaneous recovery within a few days. Patients with compromised immune status can have a prolonged disease with atypical clinical presentation complicating the clinical diagnosis. Even though most of the cases can be diagnosed only with the clinical presentation, investigations may be necessary for the diagnosis in immuno-compromised patient. The management is also different in these patients.

42.11 How Would You Manage This Patient?

The treatment for primary herpetic gingivostomatitis is usually symptomatic. Mild cases of HSV type 1 infection are treated by pain and fever management with simple analgesics and antipyretics, topical analgesics/anaesthetics, adequate hydration, and maintenance of good oral hygiene. Antiviral therapy is not usually indicated and limited for patients with prolonged disease or immuno-compromised patients. Drug of choice is acyclovir 200 mg 5 times a day for 5 days. Valacyclovir and famciclovir are the other alternatives.

42.12 What is the Possible Complication of this Condition?

Herpes virus can travel along the sensory nerves and remain dormant in the nerve root ganglion. Later, they can get reactivated and cause recurrent infections called herpes labialis which is characterized by unilateral vesicles and ulcerations on the lip (Fig. 42.3).

Herpetic whitlow is a painful infection on a finger caused by the herpes simplex virus. It can be caused by infection due to HSV-1 or HSV-2. HSV-1 whitlow is often seen in healthcare workers especially in dental healthcare workers who come in contact with infected individuals.

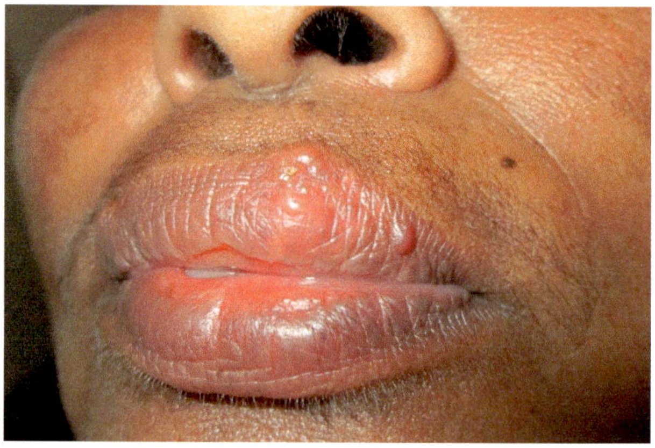

Fig. 42.3 Herpes Labialis affecting the left side upper lip in another patient

42

42.13 Primary Herpetic Gingivostomatitis

This is the most common manifestation of primary herpes simplex virus type 1 (HSV-1) infection in young children. The virus is transmitted by saliva from an infected adult or child, and the incubation period varies from days to weeks. The child then develops a prodromal stage which is characterized clinically by high fever, irritability, and inability to eat or drink. After a day or two, the child develops vesicles on the oral mucosa followed by ulceration. The disease is characterized by severe gingivitis and vesicular lesions on the tongue, buccal mucosa, and palate with extension to the lips and face. Reactive cervical lymphadenopathy may be evident. The disease lasts between 3 days to 3 weeks, and patients may still remain infectious for days to weeks after symptoms have disappeared. Diagnosis of the disease is mainly on clinical grounds but FBC and scraping from a vesicle for cytology may be helpful. Special investigations (◘ Table 42.1) may be helpful when the disease is prolonged, atypical or present in an immuno-compromised patient. The patient can be managed with symptomatic treatment including analgesics and antipyretics. Improvement of oral hygiene and hydration prevents complications. Antiviral therapy is only indicated in immuno-compromised patients. Once HSV infection occurs, the virus often travels along sensory nerves to nerve root ganglion and enters into a latent state. Reactivation of HSV-1 results in herpes labialis (◘ Fig. 42.3). Reactivation may be associated with other illnesses, trauma, or even sun exposure. Patients have vesicles involving mouth and lips often with a prodrome of pain, tingling, burning, and itching. Recurrent lesions frequently appear on the same site.

Self-Assessment Questions

1. List the pathognomonic clinical features of primary herpetic gingivostomatitis.
2. State the important conditions that need to be included in the deferential diagnosis.
3. List the different investigations that may help in the diagnosis of HSV infection in a patient with immunosuppression.
4. Outline the management of the disease.
5. State the most important complication of HSV infection and describe the clinical features.

◘ **Table 42.1** Investigations for HSV infection

Investigation	Specimen	Findings	Comment
Full Blood count	Blood	Normal or reduced total white cell count with prominent lymphocytosis	Nonspecific finding only indicates that the patient is having a viral infection
Cytology	Swab/ scraping from a vesicle or an ulcer	Ballooning degeneration (enlarged cells with intranuclear inclusions) and multinucleate keratinocytes	Nonspecific findings. Helpful when urgent results are needed
Virus isolation	Virus culture and PCR		100% sensitivity
Antibody detection	Serum	Multiple modalities Western blot is the gold standard.	Useful in identifying asymptomatic carriers. Not much useful in clinical practice as development of antibodies takes time

Salient Features of Primary Herpetic Gingivostomatitis	
Clinical	In most cases of primary herpetic gingivostomatitis, patients experience a prodromal stage with fever, myalgia, nausea, vomiting, burning, itching, or tingling sensations of the skin or mucosa for a day or two. HSV infection may be subclinical or may cause pharyngitis. Oral lesions start as vesicles/blisters and soon become ulcerated, are common on the lips and less frequent on the tongue, palatal, and buccal mucosae. Ulcers are painful and present as small, shallow ulcers with a red base. There is swollen, intensely erythematous gingiva with possible bleeding. Cervical lymphadenopathy is a common feature.
Investigations	Clinical features are helpful in the diagnosis and investigations are usually for atypical or prolonged cases or to exclude other related diseases. Full blood count and cytology are helpful. Virus culture and antibody levels can also be helpful.
Treatment	Patients are managed with symptomatic treatment including analgesics and antipyretics, improvement in oral hygiene and hydration. Antiviral therapy is only indicated in immuno-compromised patients.
HSV often travels along sensory nerves to nerve root ganglion and enters a latent state. Reactivation of HSV-1 results in herpes labialis.	

Diagnostic Algorithm

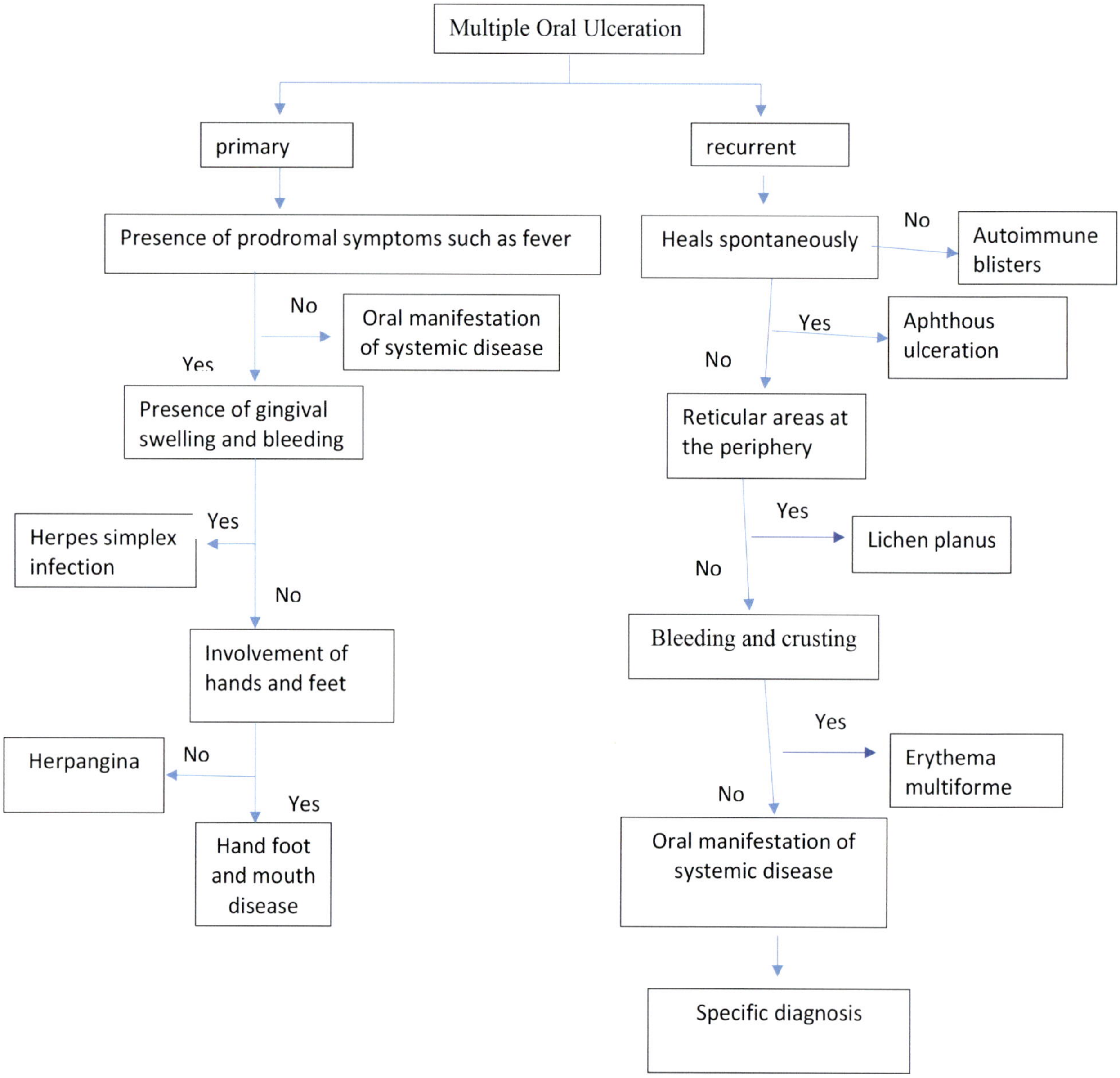

42

Summary

Primary herpetic gingivostomatitis is a manifestation of primary HSV-1 infection. It has a prodromal stage followed by vesicles and ulceration of oral mucosa. Severe gingivitis is a characteristic feature. Diagnosis is mainly on clinical features. Management is mostly symptomatic. Healing takes place in 5–7 days' time. Reactivation results in herpes labialis.

Further Reading

Aslanova M, Ali R, Zito PM. Herpetic Gingivostomatitis. 2021 Jun 25. In: StatPearls [Internet]. Treasure Island (FL): StatPearls Publishing; 2021 Jan.

Bandara HMHN, Samaranayake LP. Viral, bacterial, and fungal infections of the oral mucosa: Types, incidence, predisposing factors, diagnostic algorithms, and management. Periodontology. 2000;2019(80):148–76.

Huang CW, Hsieh CH, Lin MR, et al. Clinical features of gingivostomatitis due to primary infection of herpes simplex virus in children. BMC Infect Dis. 2020;20:782. https://doi.org/10.1186/s12879-020-05509-2.

Petti S, Lodi G. The controversial natural history of oral herpes simplex virus type 1 infection. Oral Dis. 2019;25(8):1850–65. https://doi.org/10.1111/odi.13234. Epub 2019 Nov 27

Persistent Ulcer on the Tongue with Cough: Tuberculosis

Ruwan Jayasinghe and Wanninayake M Tilakaratne

Contents

W. M Tilakaratne, T. G. Kallarakkal (eds.), *Clinicopathological Correlation of Oral Diseases*,
https://doi.org/10.1007/978-3-031-24408-7_43

Learning Goals

1. Devise the correct way of compiling the history with appropriate questions.
2. Develop a differential diagnosis after history taking.
3. Deduce appropriate procedures in clinical examination.
4. Formulate a differential diagnosis combining findings in the history and clinical examination.
5. Justify the relevant investigations required to arrive at the diagnosis.
6. Comprehend the importance of clinicopathological correlation in arriving at the correct diagnosis.
7. Outline the management plan.
8. Recognize the importance of a diagnostic algorithm in arriving at a diagnosis

43.1 Main Complaint

A 35-year-old male patient presented to the clinic complaining of an ulcer on the tongue.

43.2 History of Complaint

Question: How long you have been having this ulcer?

The ulcer has been there for a few months. It started small and then increased to the present size in recent weeks.

Question: Do you have any other problems such as pain, bleeding or pus discharge associated with the ulcer?

I don't have any pain, bleeding or pus discharge from the ulcer.

Question: Do you have any difficulty in speaking, swallowing or moving your tongue?

I don't have any difficulty in moving my tongue. I find it a little difficult to eat and speak.

Question: Can you relate any particular incidence such as a traumatic injury to tongue with the onset of ulcer.

I can't remember having any such incidents.

43.3 Additional Complaints

Question: Have you had similar ulcers in the mouth in the past?

I have had few small ulcers in the mouth from time to time but they were much smaller than the present ulcer and it usually healed within few days.

Question: Have you noticed or felt any other changes or difficulties in the mouth?

I don't have any other problem in the mouth.

Question: Do you have any difficulty in opening your mouth?

I don't have any difficulty in opening my mouth.

Question: Do you have any loss of appetite?

I have developed loss of appetite since two to three weeks.

Question: Do you have any lesions elsewhere in the body?

I don't have any other ulcers anywhere in the body.

Question: Do you have any other problems?

I have been having low grade fever for few weeks. I have lost some weight. I feel weak and have occasional night coughs.

Question: Are you suffering from any other medical problems like heart disease, high blood pressure, diabetes, bleeding disorder, respiratory diseases, and recurrent infections? If yes, what kind of medications, have you been taking until now?

I don't have any other medical problems.

Question: Have you undergone any surgery?

I have not undergone any surgery in the past.

Question: Have you undergone any dental treatment?

I have not undergone any dental treatment in the past.

Question: What is your occupation?

I am a daily paid manual laborer working in a poultry farm.

Question: Do you have any specific chewing habits?

I am not a betel chewer.

Question: Are you a smoker?

I am a smoker and have been smoking about 20 cigarettes a day for more than 15 years.

Question: Do you take alcohol?

I do take alcohol occasionally.

Question: Tell me about your family and place of residence.

I am married and have four children. I stay with my in-laws in a small two room house in the middle of the town. Altogether there are eight people living in that house.

43.4 With the Findings from the History, What Is Your Differential Diagnosis?

1. Oral cancer
2. Tuberculous ulcer
3. Deep fungal infection
4. Major aphthous ulcer

43.5 How Do You Justify Your Differential Diagnosis after History Taking?

43

1. He has been having a chronic ulcer on the tongue for a few months. There is no pain bleeding or discharge from the ulcer. He is a heavy smoker and occasionally takes alcohol. He is from a low socio-economical background. Oral cancer is common especially in people with risk habits. Hence, it has to be considered in the differential diagnosis.
2. The incidence of tuberculosis is increasing and may present as pulmonary or extrapulmonary tuberculosis. He is a heavy smoker with a low socio-economical background. He has additional symptoms like fever for few weeks, loss of appetite, cough, and weight loss. He lives in a crowded house without proper facilities. All these clinical features and living conditions are strongly supportive to include tuberculosis as a differential diagnosis. Tongue is the commonest intraoral site for oral tuberculosis and usually presents as a non-healing ulcer on the dorsal surface.
3. He works in a poultry farm where the chances of getting a deep-seated fungal infection like histoplasmosis are high. Tongue is a common site for deep fungal infections and it can present with or without pain depending on the type of fungal organism involved.
4. He gives a history of recurrent oral ulceration lasting only for few days which is suggestive of minor aphthous ulceration. Patients with minor aphthous ulceration can get major aphthous ulcer (MAU) from time to time. It presents as a non-healing ulcer which can last up to 6 weeks or more. Usually, MAU involves the non-keratinized mucosa and it causes pain, discomfort, and difficulty in moving the tongue. Although this can be considered as a differential diagnosis, presentation is not highly supportive for a MAU.

43.6 Findings of Clinical Examination

He has a pale single ulcer with sharp margins on the dorsal surface of the posterior tongue. The margins appear undermined. There is a necrotic slough on the ulcer and the base is soft (Fig. 43.1).

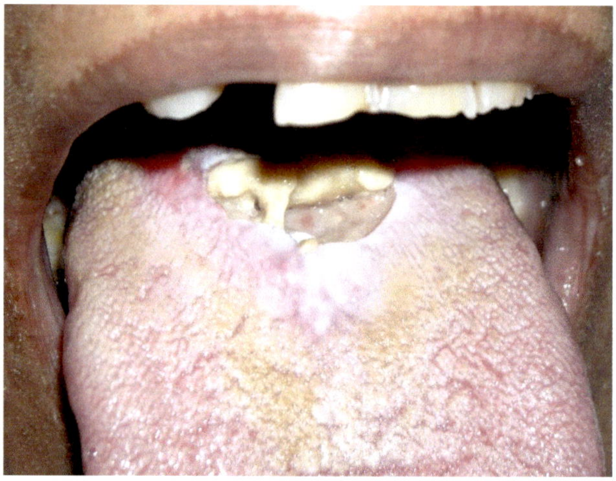

Fig. 43.1 Ulcer on the dorsal surface of the tongue with undermined margins

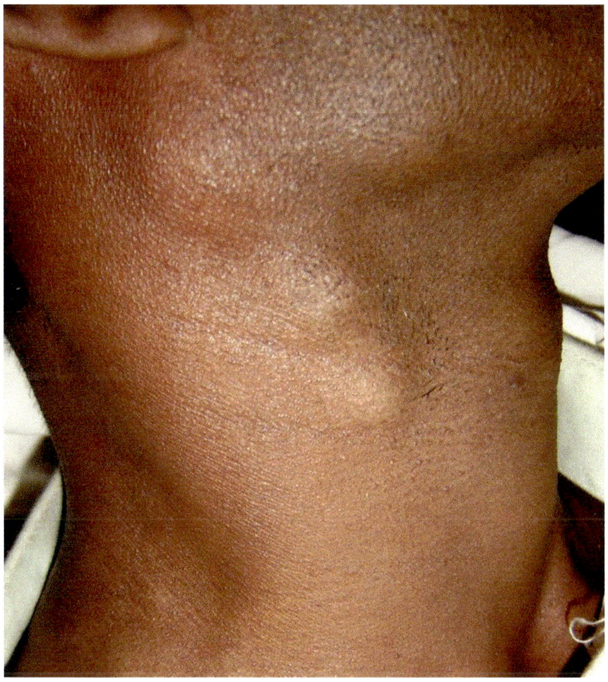

Fig. 43.2 Cervical lymphadenopathy affecting levels I, II, and III

43.7 What Other Relevant Features Would You Look for with the Findings You Have So Far?

There is no induration of the ulcer base or rolled and everted margins. Multiple enlarged lymph nodes are present but not fixed (Fig. 43.2).

43.8 What Is Your Clinical Differential Diagnosis?

1. Tuberculous ulcer
2. Deep fungal infection
3. Oral cancer

43.9 How Would You Justify the Inclusion of the Diseases That You Have Mentioned in the Differential Diagnosis to Arrive at a Working Diagnosis?

43.9.1 Tuberculous Ulcer

Tuberculosis (TB) can present as pulmonary tuberculosis or extrapulmonary tuberculosis. Oral cavity is a site for extrapulmonary manifestations. Oral tuberculosis may occur as an isolated lesion or in combination with pulmonary tuberculosis. Tongue is the commonest oral site and usually it presents as a non-healing ulcer on the dorsal surface of the tongue. TB causes lymphadenopathy especially in the neck. TB is common among people with poor socio-economical background and with other medical comorbidities such as AIDS. The patient has systemic features such as weight loss, fever, and chronic cough highly supportive of the diagnosis of pulmonary TB. This patient is a heavy smoker who belongs to a low socio-economical background having fever, loss of appetite, chronic cough, and weight loss. In addition, cervical lymph node involvement is a common head and neck manifestation of TB. Therefore, TB needs to be considered as a likely possibility in the differential diagnosis.

43.9.2 Deep Fungal Infection

Deep fungal infections are rare infections mostly seen in immunocompromised patients. Most of them are seen in the respiratory tract and may present in the oral cavity occasionally. Posterior mouth including soft palate, faucial region, and posterior tongue are the common sites. Clinically, it presents as a nodule or an ulcer. As the patient appears to be immunocompetent, the possibility of a deep fungal infection is less. However, this should be excluded with relevant investigations.

43.9.3 Oral Cancer

Oral cancers present as non-healing, painless ulcers commonly on the buccal mucosa, retromolar area, lateral border of the tongue, and floor of the mouth. Dorsal surface of the tongue is not a common site for oral cancer. Oral cancers show loco-regional spread to the cervical lymph nodes. He has a non-healing ulcer without pain, bleeding, and discharge on the tongue since few months. He is a heavy smoker and belongs to a low socio-economical background. He also consumes alcohol occasionally. Oral cancer has to be considered in the differential diagnosis as it is associated with high-risk habits. However, presence of an ulcer on the dorsal surface of the tongue without an indurated base and everted edges is not in favor of oral cancer. As it can have unusual presentations in some patients, oral cancer has to be excluded with investigations.

43.10 How Would You Investigate This Patient?

1. Incisional biopsy for the confirmation of diagnosis
2. Radiograph of the chest
3. Microbiological culture of sputum and/or material taken from the oral ulcer
4. Mantoux test
5. Polymerase chain reaction (PCR) from sputum.

43.11 His Biopsy Report Confirms the Clinical Diagnosis of TB. What Are the Histopathological Features that Help in the Diagnosis?

The hematoxylin and eosin (H & E) stained sections reveal epithelioid granulomas with occasional Langhan-type giant cells and lymphocytes at the periphery (◘ Fig. 43.3). There are foci of caseous necrosis. Ziehl-Neelsen (acid fast) stain demonstrates the presence of Mycobacterium tuberculosis (◘ Fig. 43.4).

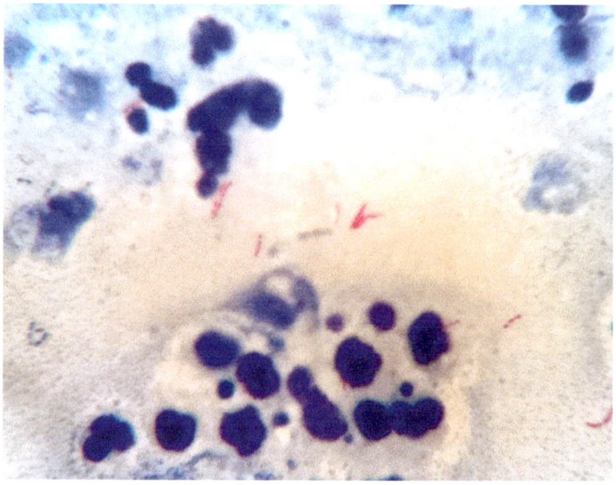

◘ **Fig. 43.4** Ziehl–Neelsen (Acid fast) stain reveals presence of frequent Mycobacterium tuberculosis organisms stained in pink color (courtesy of Professor Sumedha Jayathilake)

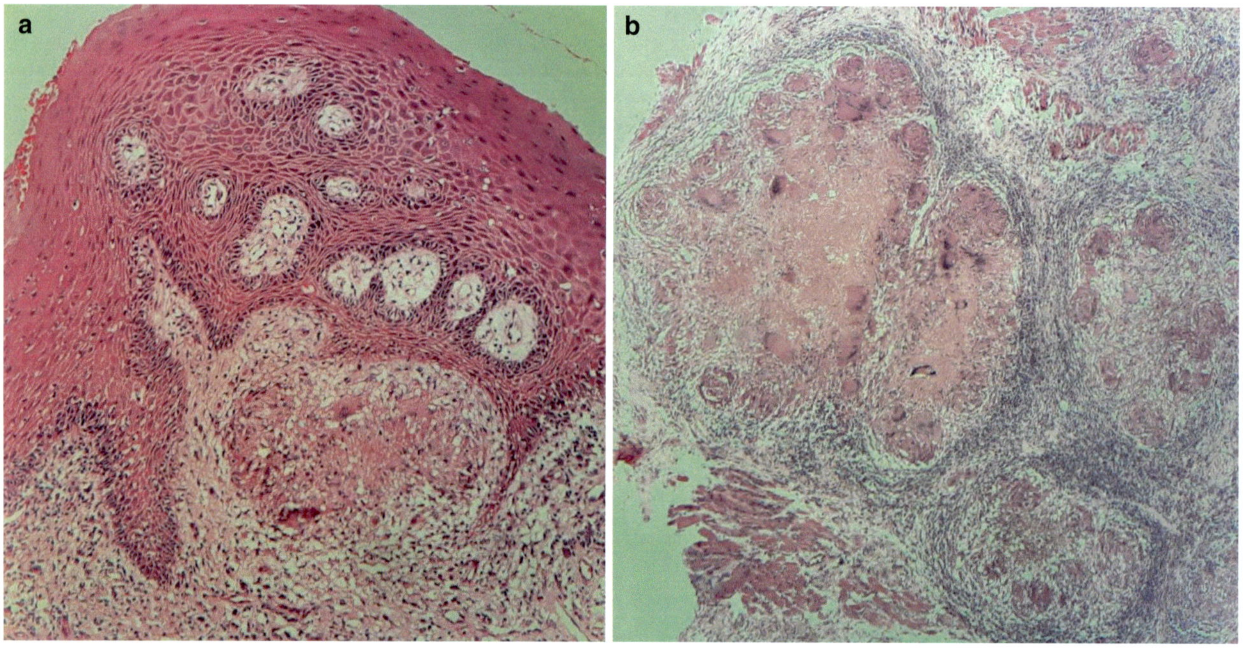

◘ **Fig. 43.3** (**a**) H & E section showing oral mucosa containing an epithelioid granuloma below the surface epithelium and (**b**) well-formed granulomas in the deeper tissues with frequent Langhan-type giant cells and foci of caseous necrosis (right)

43.12 What Are the Findings Expected to be Seen in Other Investigations?

Posterior-anterior (PA) and lateral view chest radiographs show disseminated infiltrations, nodules, fibrotic scars, cavities in the lungs, hilar, or mediastinal lymphadenopathy. Pleural effusion may also be visible.

Mantoux (tuberculin) skin test is positive in patients with TB. A positive result does not always mean active TB as it can be positive in patients with past infection or administration of BCG vaccine.

PCR investigation confirms the presence of Mycobacterium tuberculosis.

43.13 How Would You Manage This Patient?

Management of a patient with TB in the oral cavity is carried out with systemic anti-tuberculosis therapy. Therefore, the patient should be referred to a chest physician. Pulmonary TB and other extrapulmonary manifestations need to be identified. Management of TB is comprised of two stages and extends to 6 months. A patient who is receiving proper treatment is not infective and can go back to the society. The first line of treatment includes 3 or 4 antibiotics to prevent drug resistance as the development of multidrug resistance in TB is a serious concern. The usual choice for the first phase which lasts for 2 months includes isoniazid, rifampicin, pyrazinamide, and ethambutol. The second phase over the next 4 months is usually with isoniazid and rifampicin. Topical application of anti-inflammatory ointments and protective agents is useful for the symptomatic management of the ulcer. Improvement of oral hygiene and elimination of possible traumatic causes are also important.

43.14 Tuberculosis

Tuberculosis (TB) is usually caused by *Mycobacterium tuberculosis* in humans. Rarely, it can be due to atypical strains of mycobacteria. It is very much prevalent in countries of the developing world but gradual increase in the number of TB cases has been seen in the developed countries and is mostly associated with AIDS. Unsatisfactory living conditions without proper ventilation in the house, poor general health and hygiene, poor socio-economic status, drug abuse, HIV infection/AIDS, and immunosuppression are the most important predisposing factors for the development of TB. Oral TB may be associated with poor oral hygiene, local trauma, and chronic irritation.

Most often, it affects the lungs, giving rise to pulmonary TB although some patients may develop the disease in other organs and systems known as extrapulmonary TB which accounts for about 25% of the cases. Manifestation in the head and neck region is common with 10–35% extrapulmonary cases presenting in this region. Oral lesions due to TB are extremely rare. Oral TB presents as ulcers or nodules (Tuberculomas). Although any oral mucosal surface can be affected the commonest site for oral TB is the dorsal surface of the tongue. In addition, it may be seen on the palate, lips, buccal mucosa, gingiva, palatine tonsil, soft palate, floor of the mouth, and in salivary glands. Most of the time oral TB is a secondary manifestation of pulmonary TB but rarely it may present as a primary manifestation usually in young adults. Usual presentation of oral TB is as a pale, single painless ulcer covered by inflammatory exudate and slough. Clinically, it mimics the appearance of a malignant ulcer. Cervical lymphadenopathy is a common finding especially in secondary oral TB. Important conditions which have to be considered in the differential diagnosis include oral cancer, traumatic ulcer, major aphthous ulcer, syphilitic ulcer, median rhomboid glossitis, and deep fungal infection specially histoplasmosis (Table 43.1).

Median rhomboid glossitis (MRG) / central papillary atrophy of the tongue affects 0.01%–1.0% of the population. MRG is typically located around the midline of the dorsum of the tongue anterior to the circumvallate papillae. It presents as a well-demarcated, symmetrical, depapillated area. The surface of the lesion can be smooth (Fig. 43.5) or lobulated (Fig. 43.6). Usually, it is asymptomatic but rarely it can cause pain, irritation, or pruritus. MRG can have a concomitant lesion on the palate referred to as *kissing* lesion. MRG may be associated with smoking, denture wearing, diabetes mellitus, and candida infection.

Oral squamous cell carcinoma mimics oral TB ulcer. Oral cancer (Fig. 43.7) usually presents as a non-healing, painless ulcer with indurated base and everted margins. Common sites include buccal mucosa, retromolar area, lateral border of the tongue, and floor of the mouth. It is very rare to see oral cancer involving dorsal surface of the tongue. Oral cancers exhibit loco-regional metastasis; hence, involvement of cervical lymph nodes is common. Presence of risk habits, anatomical site, and induration help in differentiating oral cancer from TB. In addition, ulcers due to oral cancer show rolled and everted margins whilst tuberculous ulcers have undermined margins. However, histopathological investigation after an incisional biopsy is mandatory for the definitive diagnosis.

Table 43.1 Differential diagnosis for oral TB ulcer

Condition	Number of ulcers	Pain/ tenderness	Duration	Clinical presentation
Oral TB	Single	No	More than 3 weeks	Pale, irregular ulcer covered with slough
Syphilis	Single	No	2–6 weeks, heals spontaneously	Smooth, maybe indurated base
Deep fungal infection	Single	Yes	More than 3 weeks	Irregular, maybe indurated base
Major aphthous ulcer	Single/ Multiple	Yes	4–6 weeks, heals spontaneously	Shallow ulcer with erythematous halo
Traumatic ulcer	Single/ Multiple	Sometimes painful	Lasts until the trauma is present, heals spontaneously once the cause is eliminated	Shallow or deep ulcer with slightly elevated margins
Oral cancer	Single	Pain only in late stage	Long duration	Ulcer with irregular and everted margins, indurated base

Salient Features of Oral TB

Clinical	Single ulcer is the commonest manifestation of Oral TB but rarely it can present as a nodule (tuberculoma). Commonest site for oral TB is the dorsal surface of the tongue but it may involve the palate, lips, buccal mucosa, gingiva, palatine tonsil, soft palate, floor of the mouth, and salivary glands. Oral TB ulcer presents as a pale, single, painless ulcer covered with slough. Differential diagnosis includes oral cancer, traumatic ulcer, major aphthous ulcer, syphilitic ulcer, and deep fungal infection.
Investigations	Diagnosis of oral TB has to be done by investigations together with history and clinical examination. Histopathology, Chest X-ray, Mantoux test, sputum cultures, and PCR help in the diagnosis.
Treatment	Treatment for oral TB has to be done by a respiratory physician using anti-TB drugs. Anti-inflammatory ointments and protective agents can be applied topically to reduce symptoms of the oral ulcer. Oral hygiene needs to be improved and possible traumatic causes should be eliminated.

Deep fungal infections (Fig. 43. 8) are rare infections caused by different fungal species. It is mostly seen in immunocompromised patients but may rarely be seen in immunocompetent people as well. Most of the deep fungal infections are seen in the respiratory tract and involvement of oral cavity is rare. When it is present in the oral cavity, posterior mouth including soft palate, faucial region, and posterior tongue are the common sites. Involvement of paranasal sinuses is common. Clinically, it presents as a nodule or an ulcer. Histopathology and mycological investigations help in differentiating it from other pathologies.

Diagnosis of oral TB with history and clinical examination alone is not easy as it mimics oral cancer. Any ulcer lasting more than 3 weeks needs an incisional biopsy for correct diagnosis. Chest X-ray, Mantoux test, sputum cultures, and PCR helps in arriving at the definitive diagnosis. Treatment for a patient with oral TB has to be multidisciplinary and should include a respiratory physician. Pulmonary TB and other extrapulmonary manifestations need to be identified. The management of TB should be carried out in two stages as described above. Development of multidrug resistance in TB is a serious global concern.

Topical application of anti-inflammatory ointments and protective agents is useful for the symptomatic management of the ulcer. Improvement of oral hygiene and elimination of possible traumatic causes are important. Routine barrier protection with standard infection control protocols should strictly be followed as there is a risk of disease transmission in the dental clinic to dental health care professionals. Dental treatment must be confined only to essential treatment procedures in patients with active oral TB.

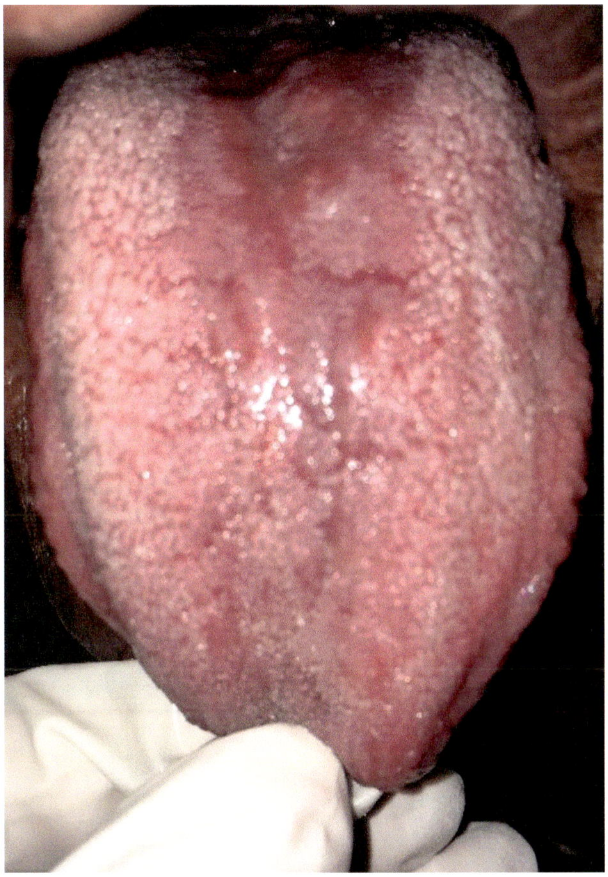

Fig. 43.5 Atrophic Median Rhomboid Glossitis

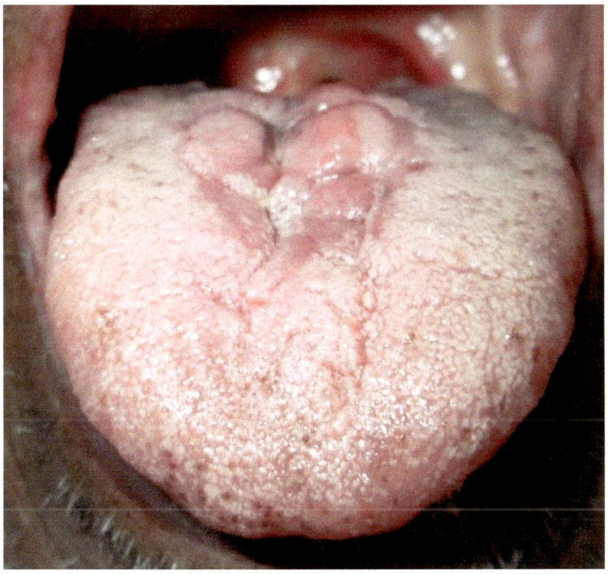

Fig. 43.6 Nodular Median Rhomboid Glossitis

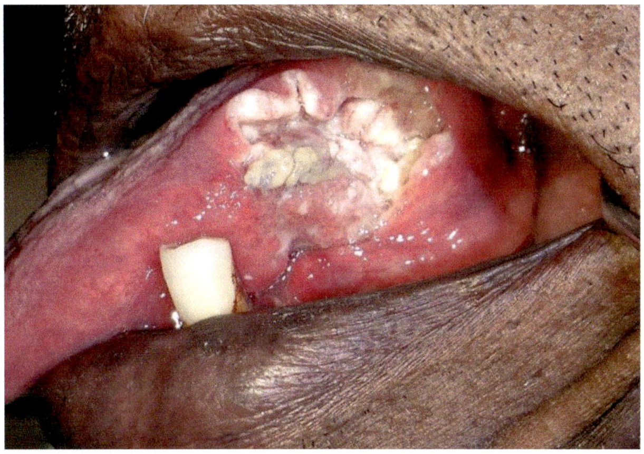

Fig. 43.7 Squamous cell carcinoma of the lateral border of tongue presenting as an ulcer with everted margins

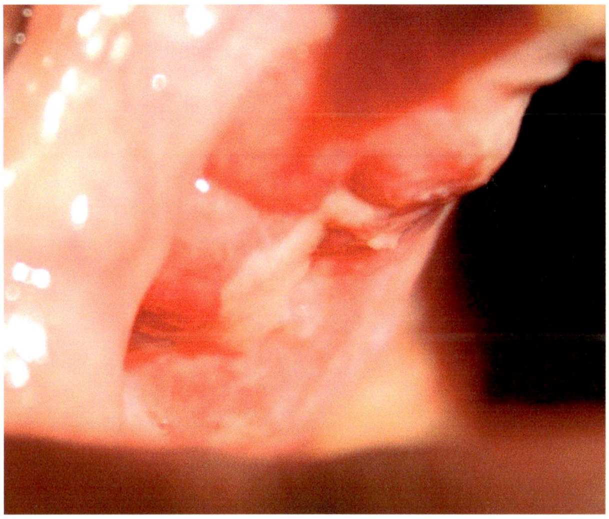

Fig. 43.8 Deep fungal infection (histoplasmosis) presenting as an ulcer

Self-Assessment Questions

1. Discuss the clinical features of oral TB.
2. State the important conditions that need to be included in the differential diagnosis.
3. List the different investigations that may help in the diagnosis of oral TB.
4. Outline the management of oral TB.
5. In order to minimize transmission of Tuberculosis in the dental clinic, what precautions should be followed by the dentist when managing a patient with oral TB.

Diagnostic Algorithm

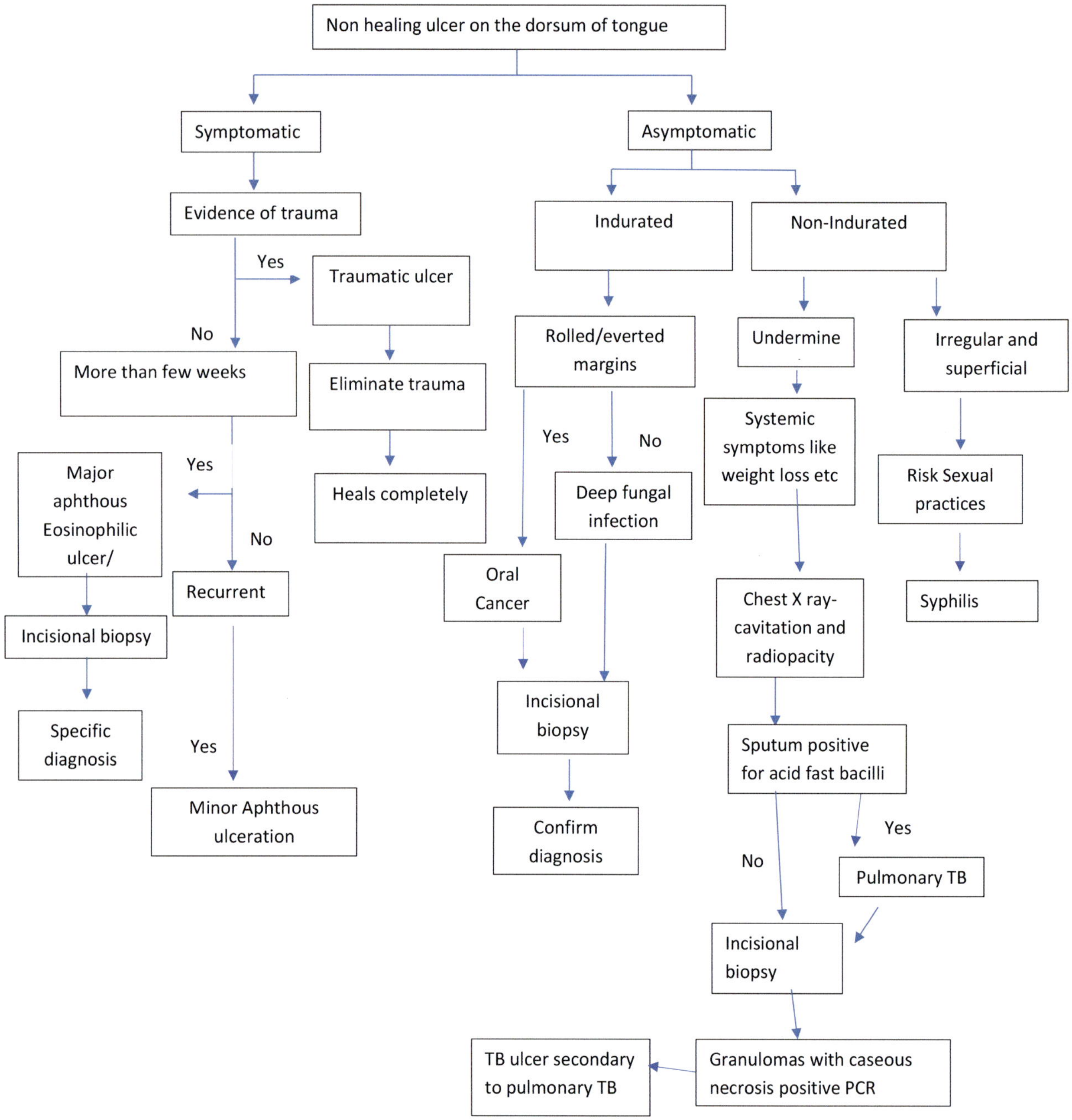

Summary

Oral TB presents as ulcers mimicking a malignancy or as nodules (tuberculomas). It may involve any oral mucosal site, but dorsal surface of the tongue is the commonest site. Mostly, it is a secondary manifestation to pulmonary TB. Diagnosis of oral TB is challenging and may need radiological, microbiological, molecular, and histopathological investigations. Treatment is multidisciplinary. Risk of disease transmission in the dental clinic need to be considered.

Further Reading

Bandara HMHN, Samaranayake LP. Viral, bacterial, and fungal infections of the oral mucosa: Types, incidence, predisposing factors, diagnostic algorithms, and management. Periodontology. 2000;2019(80):148–76.

Bansal R, Jain A, Mitta S. Orofacial tuberculosis: clinical manifestations, diagnosis and management. J Fam Med Primary Care. 2015;4(3):335–41.

Ju WT, Fu Y, Liu Y, Tan YR, Dong MJ, Wang LZ, Li J, Zhong LP. Clinical and pathologic analyses of tuberculosis in the oral cavity: report of 11 cases. Oral Surg Oral Med Oral Pathol Oral Radiol. 2018;125(1):44–51. https://doi.org/10.1016/j.oooo.2017.09.015. Epub 2017 Sep 28. Erratum in: Oral Surg Oral Med Oral Pathol Oral Radiol. 2018 Apr 23.

Krawiecka E, Szponar E. Tuberculosis of the oral cavity: an uncommon but still a live issue. Postepy Dermatol Alergol. 2015;32(4):302–6. https://doi.org/10.5114/pdia.2014.43284.

Painful Swelling in the Face and Neck: Odontogenic Infection

Ajith Manjula Attygalla and Harsha Lal De Silva

Contents

W. M Tilakaratne, T. G. Kallarakkal (eds.), *Clinicopathological Correlation of Oral Diseases*,
https://doi.org/10.1007/978-3-031-24408-7_44

Learning Goals

1. Frame appropriate questions to elicit an accurate, comprehensive clinical history.
2. Use the information from history taking to develop a preliminary differential diagnosis
3. Follow a logical sequence to perform a comprehensive clinical examination
4. Combine history and examination findings to formulate a working clinical differential diagnosis
5. Judiciously select special investigations to gather appropriate additional diagnostic information.
6. Comprehend and apply clinicopathological correlations to arrive at the final diagnosis
7. Formulate a comprehensive management plan underpinned by meaningful clinicopathological relationships.
8. Use appropriate diagnostic algorithms in clinical practice to facilitate patient management

44.1 Main Complaint

A 42-year-old man attended the emergency department complaining of pain and swelling of the right side of his face.

Question: How can we help you today?

My face is swollen, and I am in severe pain. I couldn't eat and sleep properly for the past two days. I went to see my doctor today, and he suggested I come to the hospital.

44.2 History of Complaint

Question: When did the pain and swelling start?

I have had toothache like pain on and off for the past 4–5 weeks. The swelling started the day before yesterday.

Question: Why didn't you consult a dentist when you had a toothache?

I thought the toothache will gradually disappear. I have had toothaches in the past, and they usually settled with time.

Question: Can you describe the toothache like pain in more detail, please?

Initially, I couldn't take anything cold or hot as it would trigger sharp pain in the right side of my face. It settled in a few days, but one of the 'back teeth' continued to be sore to bite on.

Question: What made you go to your doctor on this occasion?

The pain became severe about five days back and wouldn't settle even with paracetamol tablets. Also, my face became a little 'puffy' on the right side. I consulted a doctor who practices closer to my home. He prescribed an antibiotic and some painkillers the day before yesterday. Still, my pain didn't improve, and the swelling got bigger. Now, I can't open my mouth fully, and the swollen area of my face feels tight and is painful to touch.

Question: Do you feel feverish?

Yes, I feel run-down and unwell. The doctor measured my temperature and told me it was higher than it should be.

Question: Do you find it difficult to breathe?

Not really. But I find it easier to breathe when I am standing or seated.

Question: Can you comfortably eat and drink?

I have been living on liquids for the past two days. It hurts when I swallow.

44.3 Past Dental, Medical, and Social History

Question: Do you visit a dentist regularly for check-ups?

No, I don't. I am busy at work and travel a lot, so my teeth are somewhat neglected.

Question: Do you have any general health issues?

My blood sugar was a little high on a few occasions and my family doctor recommended that I do regular exercise to lose weight. He also prescribed some medicine to help lower my blood sugar but I never got down to take it.

Question: Do you take any regular medications?

No, I don't.

Question: Do you have any allergies?

I don't recall being allergic to any tablets or injections.

Question: Do you smoke or drink alcohol?

I used to smoke 5–6 cigarettes a day but quit four years back when my father suffered a heart attack. I don't take alcohol regularly but may enjoy a couple of drinks at social gatherings.

Question: Are you married?

Yes, I am married for the past eleven years and we have two school-aged children.

44.4 Clinical Examination

The patient appeared somewhat unwell and was noted using a handkerchief regularly to wipe-off saliva drooling from the corner of his mouth. His body temperature measured 38.4 °C. Pulse oximetry recorded an oxygen saturation at 93% on room air and a pulse rate of 104 per minute. His blood pressure was 126/80 mmHg, and his respiratory rate was 16 per minute.

He had an obvious swelling involving the right side of his face. The swelling extended from the right masseteric region to the ipsilateral corner of the mouth and from the zygomatic arch downwards, transgressing the lower border of the mandible to involve the right submandibular region. A soft, non-tender swelling stretched across the midline to the opposite side of his upper neck. The brawny swelling felt firm to gentle palpation over the right cheek, masseteric, and submandibular region. However, it was of softer consistency in the submental region and on the opposite side of the upper neck. The lower border of the mandible could be demarcated by palpation except in the right posterior region (Fig. 44.1).

His maximum mouth opening was limited to about 10 mm (inter-incisal distance). The limited intraoral examination possible, showed an amalgam restoration on the occlusal surface of the right mandibular first molar tooth. The right mandibular first and second molars were tender to palpation. He could move his tongue but with some degree of difficulty. The anterior floor of the mouth appeared slightly oedematous but felt soft and non-tender to palpation. The lingual sulcus in the posterior mandible could not be examined due to the limited mouth opening.

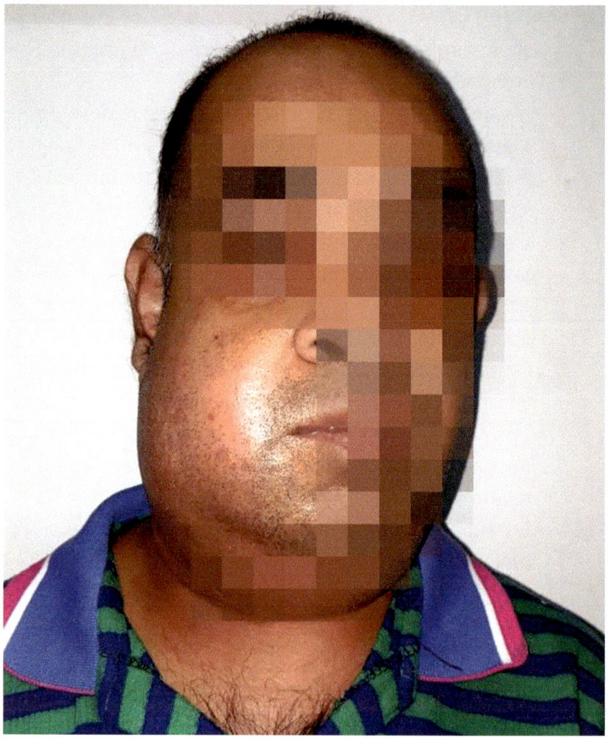

Fig. 44.1 Patient presenting with a rapidly progressing right-sided facial swelling

44.5 What Is Your Differential Diagnosis with the Findings from the History and Clinical Examination? Justify the Inclusion of Different Entities

1. A spreading infection, arising from an apical abscess (possibly from a carious right mandibular molar) and extending to involve the right submandibular and buccal spaces:

   This is the most likely scenario based on the sequence of events. Pain triggered initially by hot and cold beverages suggests the presence of untreated or secondary caries involving dentine and possibly the pulp. The subsequent change, pain triggered by biting suggests the tooth becoming non-vital and the infection reaching periapical tissues.
2. Acute pericoronitis from an impacted mandibular third molar extending to involve the right submandibular and buccal spaces:

   The mandibular third molar is the most common to become involved in pericoronitis. Although pericoronitis usually present in the late teens and early twenties, it can occur in older age groups. This patient did not give a history of pericoronitis nor a surgical removal of an impacted tooth in the right posterior mandible.

44

3. Acute right submandibular sialadenitis:
   Acute suppurative infections of the submandibular salivary gland may develop secondary to sialolithiasis, dehydration and reduced salivary flow. Usually, pain and swelling from obstruction to salivary flow occur associated with meals. Yet, an infection may sometimes cause persistent pain and swelling extending beyond the gland into the surrounding fascial spaces. Further, submandibular sialadenitis is likely to cause inflammation of the ipsilateral floor of the mouth and a purulent discharge from the orifice of the Wharton's duct.
4. Secondary infection in an odontogenic or a non-odontogenic cyst/tumour in the jaw.

44.6 What Is the Most Likely Clinical Diagnosis?

The patient appears to have developed an odontogenic infection arising from a carious tooth in the right mandibular premolar/molar region. The history of the changing nature in his pain indicates a carious lesion gradually extending deep to involve the pulp, subsequent loss of pulp-vitality leading to the development of periapical periodontitis. The two mandibular molar teeth in the right posterior quadrant were found to be extremely tender to digital pressure on their occlusal surfaces during the limited intraoral examination. The current episode, therefore, appeared to be an acute exacerbation of the pre-existing apical periodontitis, now extending beyond the periapical region to involve adjacent fascial spaces in the face and upper neck.

44.7 How Would You Manage This Patient?

The patient was admitted to the hospital for further investigation and management. The decision to offer in-patient care was based on the systemic response to the current infection as evidenced by the mild tachycardia and the elevated body temperature. On admission, venous blood samples were taken for laboratory investigations. An intravenous infusion of normal saline was started to improve his hydration. He was also given oral analgesics (paracetamol and ibuprofen) to help control his pain along with an intravenous administration of Co-amoxiclav 1.2 g as an empirically decided antibiotic therapy to combat the infection. Informed consent was obtained from the patient to examine under general anaesthesia, incise, drain and decompress any tissue space infection found, and to remove any carious teeth deemed to be the focus of the current infection, or are potential candidates for future infection episodes.

44.8 What are the Necessary Investigations that Should Be Performed Out in a Logical Sequence?

44.8.1 Laboratory Findings (On Admission to Hospital):

- Full blood count (FBC) showed leucocytosis with a markedly elevated neutrophil cell count
- C-reactive protein (CRP) was elevated and recorded 146 mg/L
- Blood urea and serum electrolytes were within normal limits
- Elevated random blood sugar—15 moles/L
- Glycated haemoglobin (Hb1Ac) was elevated and recorded a value of 76 mmol/L

44.8.2 Pulp Sensibility Test

Pulp sensibility testing is very useful to determine whether a non-vital tooth is associated with the infection. This could be performed as a cold-sensibility test or by using an electric pulp tester. This was not attempted in the patient due to the limited mouth opening.

44.8.3 Dental Pantomography (DPT)

A DPT is very useful in identifying a potential nidus of odontogenic infection, particularly when there is trismus preventing accurate positioning of a radiographic film for intraoral radiography. The DPT provides an overview of the entire dentition and the supporting jawbones to determine the presence of impacted teeth, teeth with apical pathology, jaw cysts/ tumours, and other pathologies that may cause radiographically evident changes in the jaws. Also, it may reveal radiopaque sialoliths located in major salivary glands and their main secretary ducts.

The DPT for this patient (◘ Fig. 44.2) revealed deep interproximal caries extending to involve the pulp chambers in his right mandibular first and second molar teeth. A periapical rarefaction was evident in the second molar. Furthermore, carious lesions were noted in his right posterior maxilla and the left posterior mandible along with a partially erupted, impacted left mandibular third molar tooth.

44.8.4 Aspiration

Aspiration of a sample of pus from a clinically obvious collection will help decompress the abscess as well as provide a sample for microbiological examination to identify the organism/s and their in-vitro sensitivity and resistance to different antibiotics. Given there was no clinically elicited fluctuation in this patient's face and the upper neck, indicating a deep-seated location of the infection, it was decided not to attempt an aspiration of pus from the awake patient.

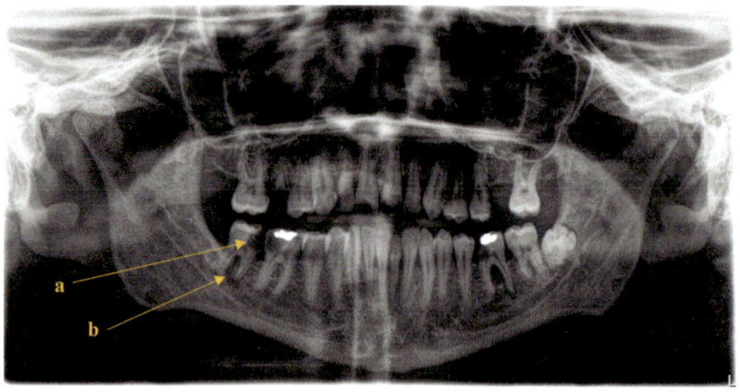

Fig. 44.2 The dental pantomogram (DPT) showing deep caries involving the pulp chambers in teeth #46 & 47 (Arrow 'a') along with periapical rarefaction in tooth #47(Arrow 'b')

44.8.5 Computerised Tomography Scanning (CT)

Three-dimensional imaging (3D) is very useful to assess the extent of soft-tissue swelling and to confirm the location and the extent of a collection of fluid/ purulent material in tissues. The infection involving the fascial spaces of the upper neck prompted the request for 3D imaging. A contrast-enhanced computerised tomography (CECT) scan confirmed the presence of a fluid collection located inferior and medial to the right posterior mandible (Fig. 44.3) suggesting an abscess involving the right submandibular fascial space. The swelling in

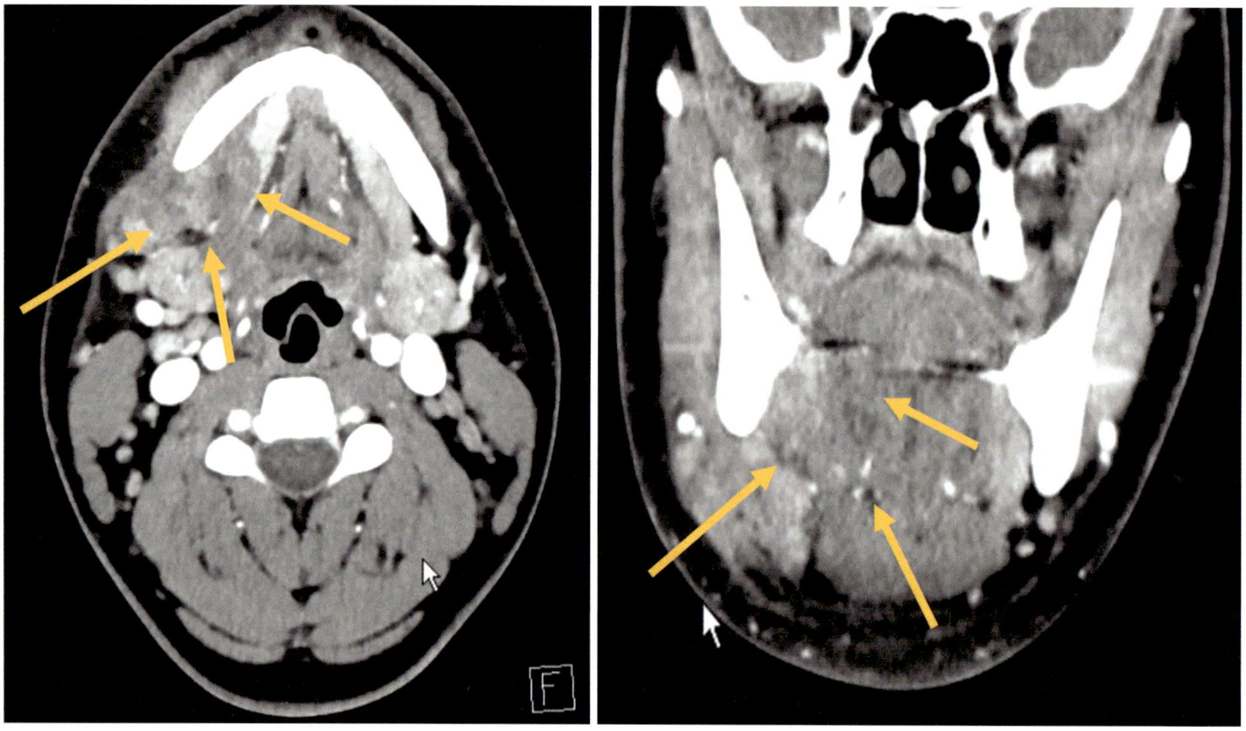

Fig. 44.3 Contrast-enhanced computerised tomograms show evidence of a collection (periphery, demarcated by arrowheads show slight 'rim-enhancement') located medial and inferior to the right posterior mandible

the buccal space was consistent with cellulitis and that in the submental and contralateral upper neck was deemed to be 'collateral oedema'.

44.9 What Is the Definitive Diagnosis?

An odontogenic infection arising possibly from the right mandibular second molar tooth extending to the right submandibular fascial space to form an abscess and cause cellulitis of the right buccal space. There is an imminent threat of infection spreading across the midline to involve the fascial spaces of the contralateral upper neck.

44.10 What Specific Findings Help You to Arrive at the Definitive Diagnosis?

Clinical examination and the DPT confirm the presence of two right mandibular molar teeth with caries involving the pulp chambers. Periapical radiolucency in the right mandibular second molar appears the likely primary source of infection. There is no impacted wisdom tooth in the ipsilateral mandible, other jaw pathology, or evidence of sialolithiasis in the major salivary glands and their main secretory ducts. The CECT scan confirms the presence of a collection of fluid infero-medial to the right posterior body of the mandible suggestive of an abscess formation in the right submandibular fascial space.

44.11 How Would You Treat This Patient?

The patient was kept fasting from admission in preparation for surgery under general anaesthesia. An intravenous infusion consisting of dextrose–insulin–potassium chloride was started to titrate and maintain his blood glucose between 4–8 mmol/L during the perioperative period. In the operating theatre, the anaesthetist performed an awake fibre-optic assisted naso-endotracheal intubation to secure the airway, induce, and maintain general anaesthesia. Following skin disinfection using a povidone–iodine solution, an incision was made 2–3 cm inferior to the lower border of the right mandible. Blunt dissection with sinus forceps through the subcutaneous tissue, platysma, and the deep fascia helped enter the right submandibular space. On reaching the abscess, the beaks of the sinus forceps were opened to initiate drainage of a copious amount of purulent material. A sample was taken and was immediately dispatched to the laboratory for microbiological culture and sensitivity testing. The abscess cavity was thoroughly irrigated with sterile saline and two corrugated rubber drains were inserted and secured to the submandibular skin with sutures to facilitate continued drainage (◘ Fig. 44.4). The muscle relaxants used for anaesthesia helped open the mouth. There was no swelling on the buccal sulcus but compressing the lingual alveolar mucosa on the right posterior mandible resulted in pus extruding from the gingival margin of the second mandibular molar. Right mandibular first and second molars showed significant mobility and were extracted along with the retained root of the right maxillary first molar and the left mandibular first molar. All tooth sockets were debrided and irrigated with saline before achieving haemostasis. The patient was recovered from general anaesthesia in the theatre but was kept moderately sedated to be nursed overnight in the intensive care unit with the naso-endotracheal tube in place. He was extubated on the second postoperative day and the corrugated rubber drains were removed on the following day.

He received regular intravenous antibiotics, oral analgesics, and antiseptic mouth rinses while recovering in the ward for the next three days. The perioperative glycaemic control achieved was maintained in the ward, gradually titrating and transferring to oral hypoglycaemics as advised by the hospital physicians. His pain, swelling, and trismus subsided rapidly and he was discharged home with instructions to maintain good oral hygiene, and appropriate glycaemic control to aim at avoiding similar catastrophic events in the future. The perioperative antibiotics, analgesics, and antiseptic mouthwashes were continued for a further 7 days. Also prescribed were the oral hypoglycaemic agents started in the postoperative phase, for continuation monitored by his family physician.

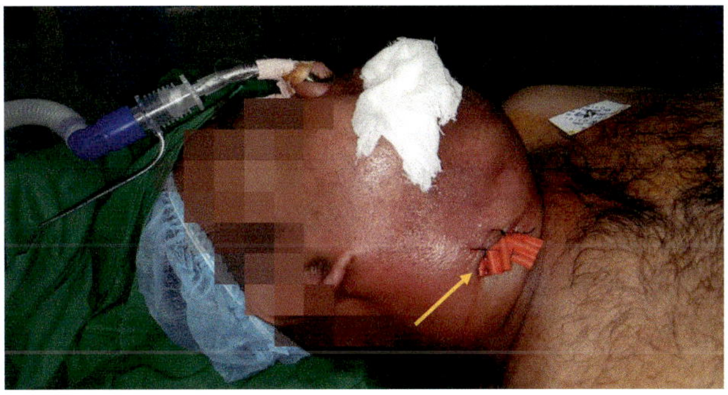

◘ **Fig. 44.4** Incision and drainage of the submandibular fascial space infection via an extraoral skin incision. Note the corrugated rubber drains (indicated by the arrow) inserted through the submandibular skin to facilitate continued drainage

44.12 What Is the Rationale for Treatment Provided?

This patient presented with an acute infection showing signs of spreading to involve adjacent tissue spaces in the face and neck. There was evidence of systemic involvement (raised body temperature and tachycardia), significant trismus, and swelling starting to cross the midline of the neck to the contralateral side. The reported difficulty in swallowing could be a forerunner for impending involvement of the tissues surrounding the airway. Moreover, neglected glycaemic control may cause diminished host resistance and facilitate a further rapid spread of infection to involve 'high-danger spaces' that could have catastrophic outcomes. Hence, the decision to admit the patient to the hospital, investigate, and treat aggressively.

The collection in the submandibular space mandates incision and drainage and is best performed under general anaesthesia. Obtaining adequate depth of local anaesthesia amidst spreading infection could be difficult. Further, a general anaesthetic administered by a skilled anaesthetist is safer, help secure the airway, and provide muscle relaxation to overcome the trismus to extract the offending tooth/teeth to remove the source of infection.

A diligent glycaemic control in the perioperative period is required for mitigating the risk of potential acute hypoglycaemia and maintaining normoglycaemic status through the postoperative recovery, healing, and beyond.

44.13 Follow-up and Prognosis

The patient was reviewed in the outpatient clinic a week from discharge. The incision sites and extraction wounds showed good healing. There was only minimal, non-tender, residual oedema in the face and the upper neck with no clinical signs of acute inflammation. He was discharged from the clinic with advice on the need to maintain good oral health and optimal glycaemic control.

44.14 Odontogenic Infections

44

44.14.1 Definition and Epidemiology

Odontogenic infections originate in teeth and/or their supporting structures. They form the bulk of the infections arising in the head and neck and are the commonest to be referred to oral and maxillofacial surgical services. A vast majority of odontogenic infections result from dental caries and their sequelae. The next common are infections arising from pericoronal and periodontal tissues. Furthermore, infections may occur in a tooth extraction socket or any other oral wound or as a secondary infection of a pathological lesion.

Most odontogenic infections are caused by a mixed flora of microorganisms, dominated by both obligatory and facultative anaerobes. Commonly isolated species include *Peptostreptococci, Bacteroides, Prevotella,* and *Fusobacterium nucleatum*. Alpha haemolytic *Streptococci* are common aerobes isolated. Organisms may act as a multispecies biofilm. The initial colonisation may be by aerobic bacteria that consume oxygen to facilitate the growth and proliferation of anaerobic species, which predominate in established infections.

A non-vital tooth resulting from caries or trauma may develop apical periodontitis. It usually remains localised and dormant for years. However, in some instances, it may develop acute exacerbations. The clinical course of infection is determined by the balance between the virulence of the organisms versus the integrity of host defences. The common medical conditions that facilitate acute exacerbation and spread of odontogenic infections include brittle diabetes, systemic autoimmune disorders, immunosuppressive therapy, antiresorptive/ antiangiogenic medications, osteoradionecrosis, and excessive mental stress. While the majority are trivial and easily managed, few odontogenic infections can spread rapidly and escalate to life-threatening situations (Fig. 44.5).

44.14.2 Clinical Presentation

Increasing levels of pain, inability to bite on the affected tooth, some inflammatory oedema of the surrounding gingiva, and the alveolar mucosa with palpable tender lymphadenopathy in the upper neck are the early signs and symptoms of an acute exacerbation. This can happen without forewarning or could result from compromised immunity from concurrent medical comorbidities.

An abscess resulting from an acute exacerbation of periapical periodontitis may remain localised in the periapical region bone. Alternatively, the pus may track buccally or lingually (taking the path of least resistance) to perforate the cortical bone and extend to overlying soft tissues. The majority will burst through to the buccal or lingual vestibule to form a fluctuant swelling or may discharge itself, forming a draining sinus in the alveolar mucosa. In the maxilla, periapical abscesses from lateral incisors, less commonly from the first premolar and first molar, may track palatally to form a palatal abscess.

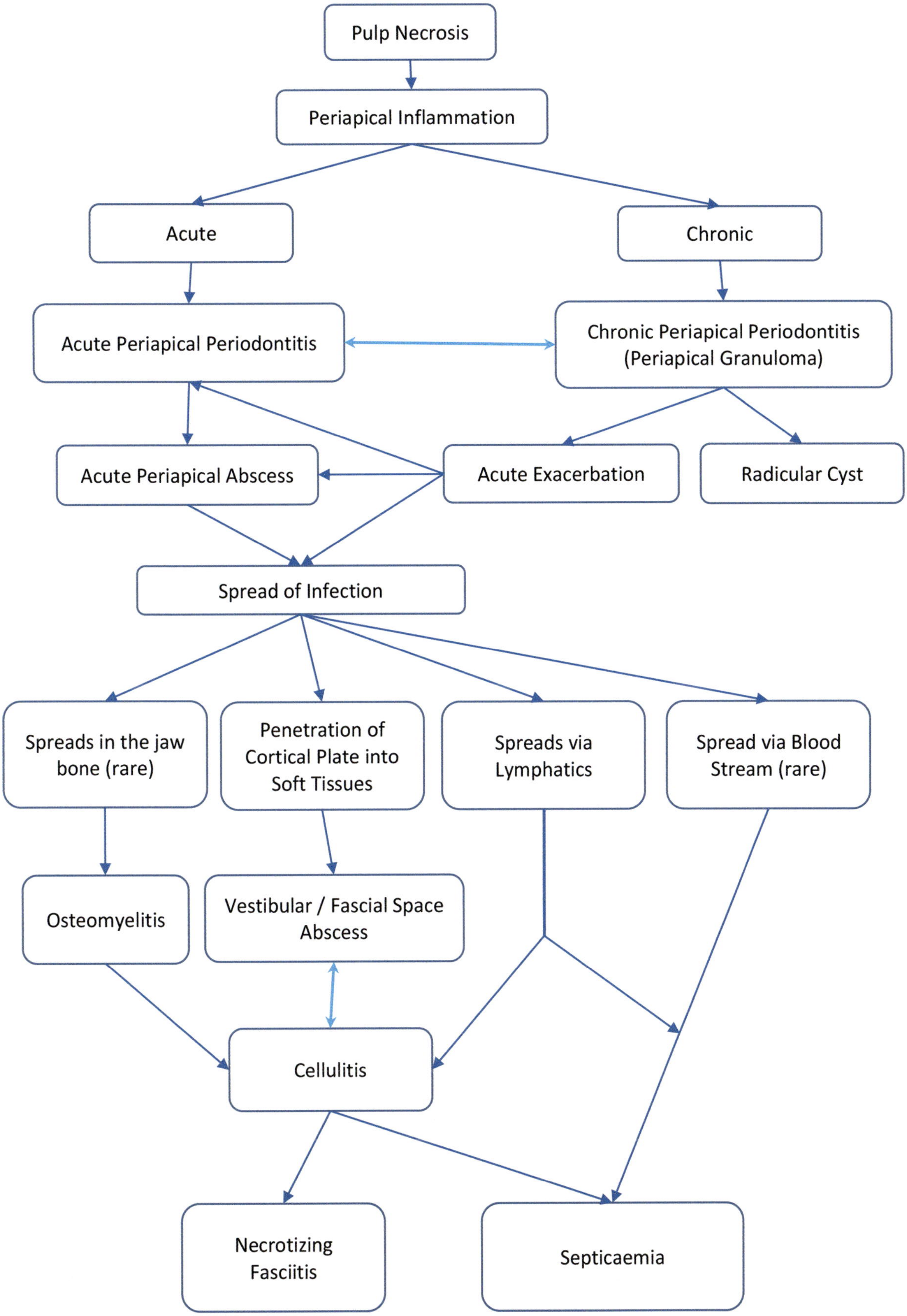

Fig. 44.5 Potential sequelae of pulpal necrosis

Table 44.1 Primary and secondary fascial spaces associated with odontogenic infections

Danger level	Fascial Spaces		
	Primary Spaces		Secondary Spaces
	Maxilla	Mandible	
Low	Vestibule Buccal Palatal	Vestibule Buccal Submental	
Medium	Infratemporal	Sublingual Submandibular Submasseteric Pterygomandibular	Superficial-temporal Deep-temporal Infratemporal
High	Canine fossa		Lateral-pharyngeal Retropharyngeal Alar Prevertebral

If the cortical bone is penetrated superiorly (in the maxilla) and inferiorly (in the mandible) to muscle attachments (buccinator, levator labii group, mentalis, and mylohyoid), the infection could enter deep primary fascial spaces of the face and neck (Table 44.1). Pericoronitis is primarily a soft-tissue infection and if arising in the mandibular third molar region may spread to involve the buccal, pterygo-mandibular, submandibular, and sublingual tissue spaces.

Once in the soft tissues, further spread of infection to involve secondary fascial spaces and beyond is determined by the attachment of muscles and fascia. Yet, highly virulent infections may disregard these anatomical barriers and spread widely and haphazardly. An inadequately treated infection may spread rapidly and extensively to involve distant anatomical sites with drastic consequences (Fig. 44.6).

Clinical presentation of spreading infection into tissue spaces may include increased pain and swelling, trismus due to involvement of masticatory muscles, and systemic signs of fever, malaise, dehydration, and tachycardia. If not treated urgently, the symptoms may escalate to difficulty in swallowing shown as drooling of saliva. Further progression may compromise the airway evidenced by the patient adopting a 'seated, sniffing position' to breathe. The deterioration is rapid in immunocompromised patients but may occur in others too.

44

44.14.3 Principles of Management

The vast majority of infections remain dormant and may show minimal clinical signs of their existence. They are easily treated by eliminating the cause. If a non-vital tooth is identified as the source of infection it needs to be treated either with a pulpectomy or if deemed unrestorable, should be extracted at the first available opportunity. On the contrary, impacted teeth with clinical evidence of involvement in pericoronitis are best removed as an elective surgical procedure, after using antibiotics to control any acute infection. Pathological lesions like cysts and tumours too should be managed similarly.

Increased awareness among clinicians, development of targeted investigations, and management strategies in contemporary clinical practice have made a paradigm shift in the way we treat odontogenic infections and their consequences. The contemporary approach could be summarised as 'treat surgically and manage medically'. The steps outlined below should move forward in a seamless continuum.

1. Assess the severity and decide the setting of care
2. Determine the level of integrity of host defences
3. Determine and eliminate the source of infection
4. Establish and maintain drainage
5. Administer appropriate antibiotics as necessary
6. Support and monitor general health and regularly review clinical progress
7. Follow-up focused on prevention

44.14.4 Assess the Severity and Decide the Setting of Care

Odontogenic infections which show signs of spread or systemic involvement are best referred to an oral and maxillofacial surgeon for specialised care. A quick but thorough assessment of the severity of the infection and the level of systemic response will help decide between managing as an outpatient or admitting to a hospital.

Fig. 44.6 The potential routes of spread for odontogenic infections

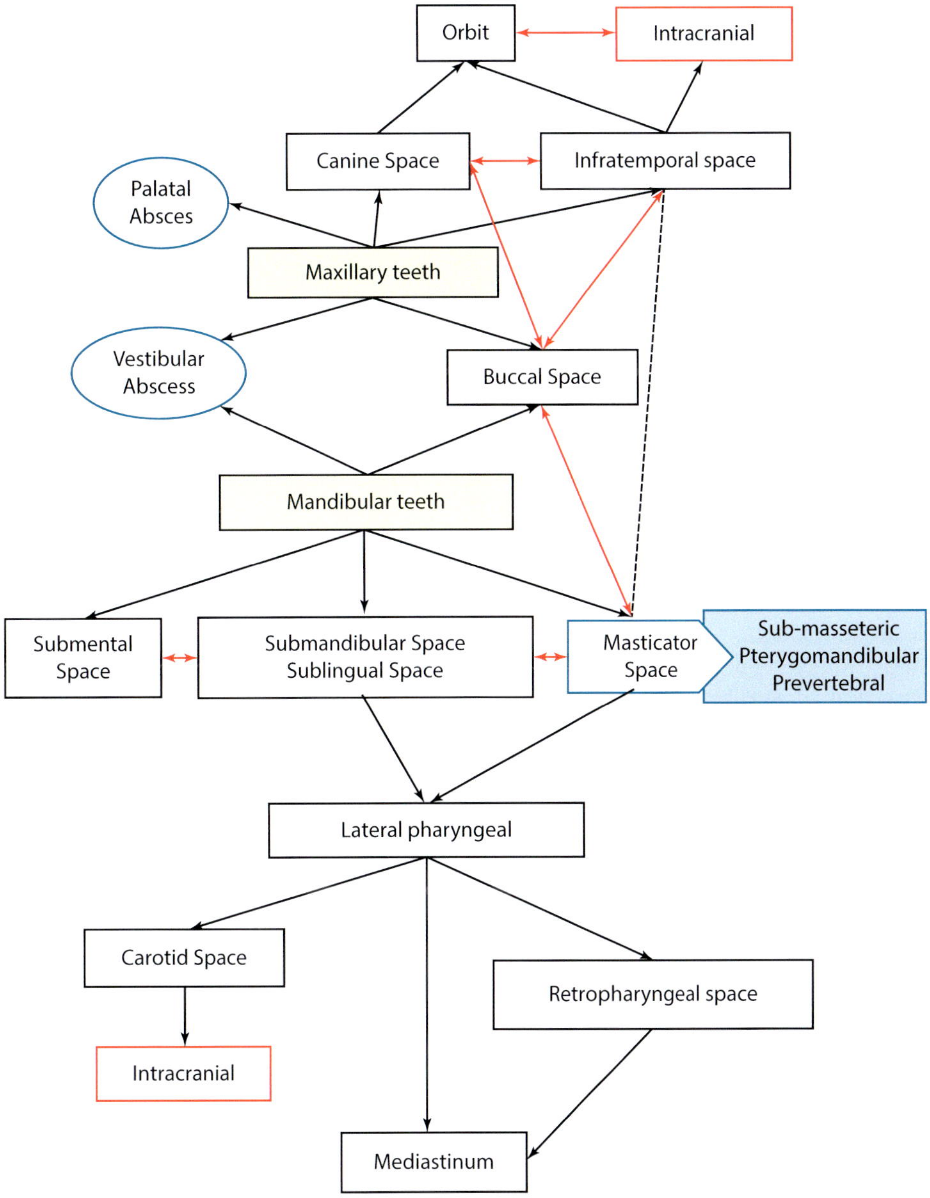

Hospital admission should be considered for,

1. Inability to maintain airway without sitting and leaning forward
2. Inability to maintain oxygen saturation of 92% or more on room air
3. Infections involving moderate or high-danger fascial spaces
4. Rapidly progressive swelling
5. Drooling from an inability to swallow
6. Severe trismus
7. An apparent need for in-patient control of systemic diseases
8. An apparent need for general anaesthesia for incision and drainage
9. Pyrexia of 38 °C or higher
10. Evidence of dehydration

Clinical examination complemented by imaging studies and laboratory indices will help decision making. The threshold for admission should be lower for patients with compromised immunity.

44.14.5 Determine the Level of Integrity of Host Defences

Past medical history should be reviewed to identify medical comorbidities or drug therapy that may lower host immunity. Poorly controlled diabetes mellitus is a common culprit. Even in those who are not known diabetics, it is prudent to check the glycaemic status which may unravel an undiagnosed disease.

44.14.6 Determine and Eliminate the Source of Infection

Eliminating the source of infection will help expedite clinical improvement and prevent a recurrence. Clinical examination, pulp sensibility testing, and radiography will help identify the primary source. Retaining or extraction of an offending tooth is made on clinical judgement, the strategic value of the tooth in the dental arch, and on the patient's preference.

44.14.7 Establish and Maintain Drainage

Any identified collection of pus should be drained as soon as possible. When limited to the periapical region, drainage could be established through a pulpectomy and lavage or by extraction of the tooth. Usually, abscesses in the vestibule or the palate can be incised and drained with topical local anaesthesia. Deep-seated abscesses are best incised and drained under general anaesthesia and may need insertion of a rubber drain to maintain drainage over 24–48 h. Extraction of the offending tooth can be done concurrently when it is difficult to obtain an adequate depth of anaesthesia in the presence of local infection.

44.14.8 Administer Appropriate Antibiotics as Necessary

Antibiotics should never be used as an alternative to incision and drainage of pus and the elimination of the source of infection. Yet, the judicious use of an appropriately selected antibiotic therapy can complement surgical management to expedite clinical improvement. Acute infections showing signs of rapid spread through fascial spaces, and for those occurring in patients with compromised immunity, antibiotic therapy should be started early. It is common practice to start a beta-lactam antibiotic (penicillin or co-amoxiclav) chosen empirically while waiting on the results of a culture and sensitivity test. Empirically started antibiotics should be changed only if the in-vitro sensitivity test recommends otherwise <u>and</u>

1. there is no tangible improvement in 48 h <u>or</u>
2. there is a rapid clinical deterioration of patients' general condition.

44.14.9 Support and Monitor General Health and Regularly Review Clinical Progress

It is very important to maintain adequate hydration, nutrition, provide pain relief, and control pyrexia as appropriate. A close cooperation with medical practitioners will help manage any underlying medical comorbidities that may impact the outcome of the infection. The patient's progress should be closely monitored, both with clinical observations and laboratory indices where appropriate. A downward trend in the CRP and white blood cell count are useful confirmatory evidence of general improvement.

44.14.10 Follow-up Focused on Prevention

Any medical conditions that may have an impact on infections need to be treated and monitored with the help of the patient's physician. If the offending tooth is to be retained, then endodontics and coronal restoration should be completed and oral hygiene optimised. If the source of infection was pericoronitis associated with an impacted tooth, it is best treated as an elective surgical procedure.

44.14.11 Complications

Severe complications are rare but projected increases in elderly populations living with multiple medical comorbidities and being managed on therapeutic interventions that may compromise host immunity make it important to manage odontogenic infections aggressively and efficiently. Ludwig's angina is a rapidly spreading infection involving bilateral sublingual and submandibular spaces, commonly resulting from odontogenic infections originating from the mandibular premolar/molar region. The oedema of the floor of the mouth raises and displaces the tongue against the pharynx to produce severe dysphagia and difficulty to breathe. Importantly, the infection can rapidly spread to involve 'danger spaces' to cause acute airway obstruction. Moreover, infections entering parapharyngeal spaces can track inferiorly to the chest to cause mediastinitis. Occasionally odontogenic infections may cause necrotising fasciitis or may spread intracranially to cause cavernous sinus thrombosis. The latter is caused mainly by infections involving the canine space and the infratemporal space, which may potentially spread intracranially in a retrograde manner via orbital veins and/or pterygoid plexus of veins. Furthermore, severe infections, especially in patients with compromised immunity, may progress to toxaemia and septic shock syndrome with fatal consequences.

? Self-Assessment Questions

1. List the common sources for odontogenic infections.
2. Describe the investigations that help in identifying the source of an odontogenic infection.
3. How will you decide whether an odontogenic infection could be managed in your practice or would need a referral to a hospital/specialist.
4. Explain the relevance of fascial spaces in head and neck infections.
5. Discuss the complications that may arise from inappropriate management of odontogenic infections (◘ Fig. 44.7).

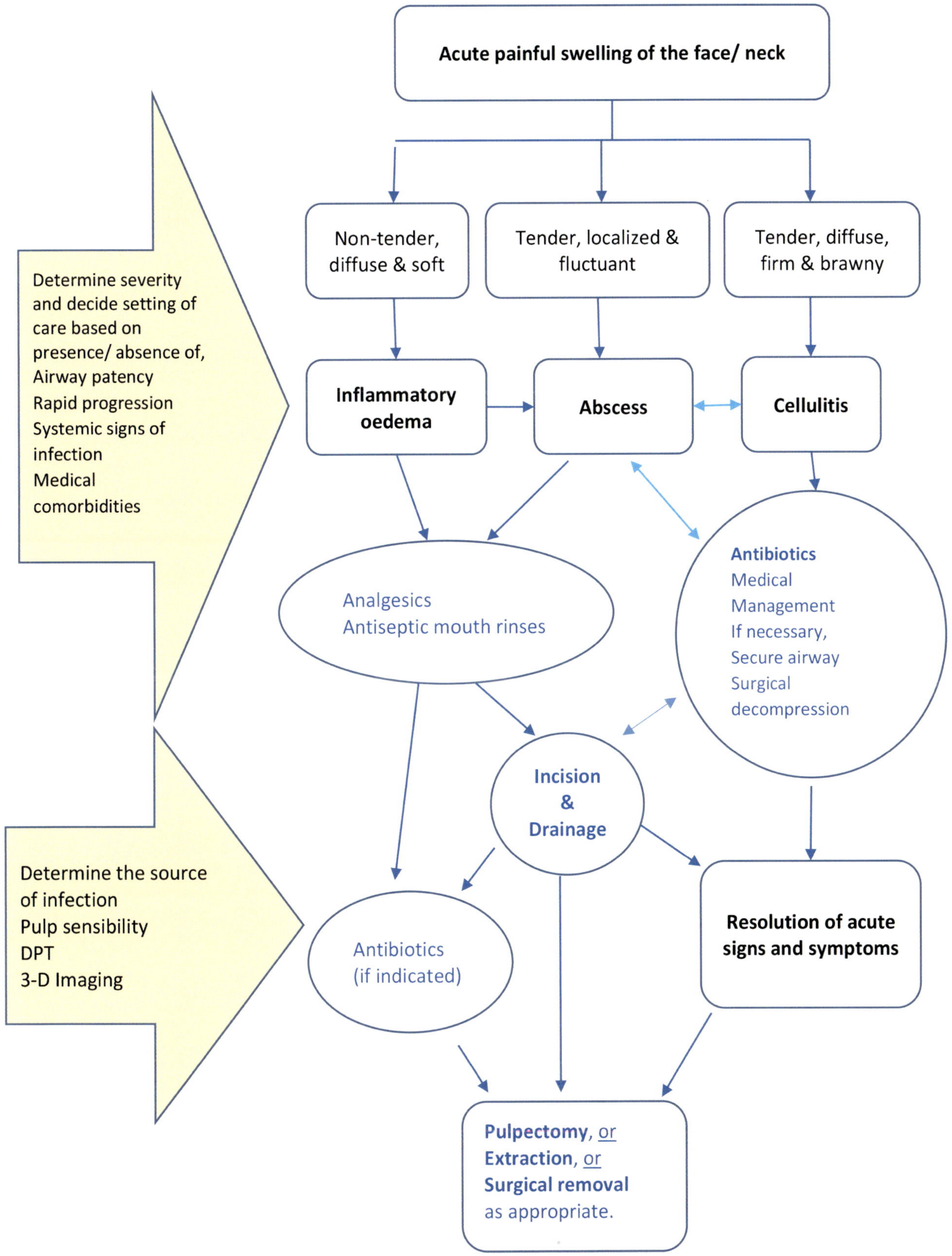

Fig. 44.7 Diagnostic and management protocol for acute, painful jaw/ facial swellings

Summary

Odontogenic infections are a common clinical presentation. The severity of these infections may vary from mild to moderate or life-threatening. Virulence of the organisms and the level of host resistance is pivotal in determining the course of infection. Prompt recognition of the severity of the infection, and initiation of targeted treatment in an appropriate clinical setting are important requisites to avoid escalating into potentially life-threatening situations. Surgical interventions aiming to remove the source of infection and drainage of pus alongside medical management focusing on supportive therapy help achieve optimal clinical outcomes.

Further Reading

Bahl R, Sandhu S, Singh K, Sahai N, Gupta M. Odontogenic infections: microbiology and management. Contemp Clin Dent. 2014;5(3):307.

Chang J-S, Yoo K-H, Yoon SH, Ha J, Jung S, Kook M-S, et al. Odontogenic infection involving the secondary fascial space in diabetic and non-diabetic patients: a clinical comparative study. J Korean Assoc Oral Maxillofac Surg. 2013;39(4):175–81.

Chi T-H, Tsao Y-H, Yuan C-H. Influences of patient age on deep neck infection: clinical etiology and treatment outcome. Otolaryngol--Head Neck Surg Off J Am Acad Otolaryngol-Head Neck Surg. 2014 Oct;151(4):586–90.

Gonçalves L, Lauriti L, Yamamoto MK, Luz JGC. Characteristics and management of patients requiring hospitalisation for treatment of odontogenic infections. J Craniofac Surg. 2013;24(5):e458–62.

Holmes CJ, Pellecchia R. Antimicrobial therapy in management of odontogenic infections in general dentistry. Dent Clin. 2016;60(2):497–507.

Hupp JR, Ellis E, Tucker MR. Contemporary oral and maxillofacial surgery. 7th ed. St. Louis: Elsevier; 2019.

Jevon P, Abdelrahman A, Pigadas N. Management of odontogenic infections and sepsis: an update. Br Dent J. 2020;229(6):363–70.

Ogle OE. Odontogenic infections. Dent Clin. 2017;61(2):235–52.

Opitz D, Camerer C, Camerer DM, Raguse JD, Menneking H, Hoffmeister B, Adolphs N. Incidence and management of severe odontogenic infections—A retrospective analysis from 2004 to 2011. J Cranio-Maxillofac Surg. 2015;43(2):285–9.

Vytla S, Gebauer D. Clinical guideline for the management of odontogenic infections in the tertiary setting. Austr Dent Js. 2017;62(4):464–70.

Pain in the Lower Jaw with Numbness of the Lip: Osteomyelitis of the Mandible

Parakrama Wijekoon and Wanninayake M Tilakaratne

Contents

W. M Tilakaratne, T. G. Kallarakkal (eds.), *Clinicopathological Correlation of Oral Diseases*,
https://doi.org/10.1007/978-3-031-24408-7_45

Learning Goals

1. Understand the presentation and pathogenesis of osteomyelitis in the head and neck region
2. Clinically and radiologically recognize and differentiate different types of osteomyelitis.
3. Classify osteomyelitis of jaw bones to help plan their management
4. Understand the treatment of osteomyelitis.

45.1 Main Complaint

A 71-year-old lady presented to the Oral and Maxillofacial surgery clinic with a painful swelling of the lower left side of the face and unbearable pain originating from the lower left side of the jaw.

45.2 History of Complaint

Question: How long have you been having the pain and swelling?

I have been having the symptoms for the last three months.

Question: What is the type of pain and how did it start?

It is a sharp and continuous pain, which started suddenly.

Question: Where did it start?

I felt that it originated from the lower left back teeth.

Question: Does it radiate to any other areas?

It radiates towards the left ear region.

Question: Have you taken any medicine for the pain?

I took paracetamol for pain but there is no relief.

Question: Have you noticed any other features?

I had a bad smell in the mouth and a salty taste. It was extremely difficult for me to open my mouth or chew food. In addition, I noticed a swelling of the lower left side of the face extending towards the lower lip. I also had fever. My pain and swelling have been getting worse with time.

Question: Do you have any abnormal sensation in the area?

I do feel some numbness in the lower lip and chin area on the same side.

Question: Have you had similar episodes in the past?

I had a similar problem in 2019 and underwent surgery under general anaesthesia for the same. I did not have any problem after surgery until the current episode.

45.3 Past Medical History

Question: Are you suffering from any medical problems such as heart disease, high blood pressure, diabetes, bleeding disorder, or respiratory diseases? If so are you on any treatment?

I am under treatment for hypertension and hyperlipidaemia.

At the last follow-up visit, my BP was 130/80 mm/Hg, and I was asked to continue the same drugs with the same dosage. I also had a mild heart attack and was admitted to the hospital for a few days.

45.4 Past Dental History

Question: Have you undergone any dental treatment?

I have been to my dentist on several occasions with toothache. He filled several teeth and removed some under local anaesthesia. The wounds healed without any complications except the last time.

Question: What happened during the last extraction?

The last extraction was followed by pain and swelling for a long time. I had fever on and off.

Question: Do you notice any pus coming out from the site?

I feel that there is a discharge with salty taste. I also feel mobility of surrounding teeth.

Question: Have you ever had bleeding from gums?

I have not had any bleeding from the gums.

Question: Are you wearing any dentures?

I never had dentures.

45.5 Social History and Family History

Question: Are you employed and if so, what is your occupation?

I am a housewife and now I stay with my children who are married.

Question: Is there anyone in your family affected with similar problems in the mouth?

I am not aware of any family members with a similar problem.

Question: Are you a betel chewer?

I chew betel very occasionally (one quid per day and I do not take tobacco or lime with it).

Question: Are you a smoker?

I am not a smoker.

Question: Do you take alcohol?

I have never taken alcohol.

45.6 With the Information From the History, What Is Your Differential Diagnosis?

1. Chronic suppurative osteomyelitis
2. Chronic periapical abscess
3. Infected periapical cyst
4. Chronic periodontal infection

45.7 How Would You Justify your Differential Diagnosis after Taking the History?

1. She has a history of complicated extraction followed by pain and purulent discharge for a long time for which she underwent surgical intervention. She also has a soft tissue swelling of the same area with a few episodes of fever and numbness on the affected side supporting a possible differential diagnosis of chronic suppurative osteomyelitis.
2. A chronic periapical abscess can present with pain, soft tissue swelling, discharge, bad smell and salty taste, and limitation of mouth opening. Some of the features found in this patient make chronic periapical abscess also a possible differential diagnosis.
3. A periapical cyst could have been present at the time of initial extraction. If the dental surgeon did not notice it at the time of extraction, it could get infected and present with symptoms described by the patient.
4. Bad smell and salty taste, pain, and soft tissue swelling are the main complaints of chronic periodontal infection. The presence of these symptoms in this patient justifies including chronic periodontal infection in the differential diagnosis.

45.8 Findings of Clinical Examination

On extra-oral examination, she looks ill, exhausted, and febrile. She has a core temperature of 39 degrees centigrade while all other vital signs are within normal range. There is a facial asymmetry with a diffuse tender swelling on the left side of the lower lip, cheek, and submandibular region (Fig. 45.1a). Features of inflammation are seen over the swelling with a slightly increased temperature and right submandibular lymphadenopathy. The lymph nodes are tender and not fixed.

She has a slight loss of sensation over the right mental nerve area. Her motor nerve function (facial nerve) is normal. Mouth opening is restricted to 11 mm with limitation in chewing leading to difficulty in taking food. The general oral hygiene of this lady is poor with the presence of plaque and calculi. Her alveolar ridge of the lower left quadrant is slightly swollen but there is no septic root, or ulceration of the mucosa. Severe pain over the left alveolar ridge is elicited on palpation. There is a discharging sinus present in the left buccal sulcus over the alveolar ridge and the teeth adjacent to the area show grade 1 mobility and tenderness on percussion (Fig. 45.1b). There is no bleeding from the gums.

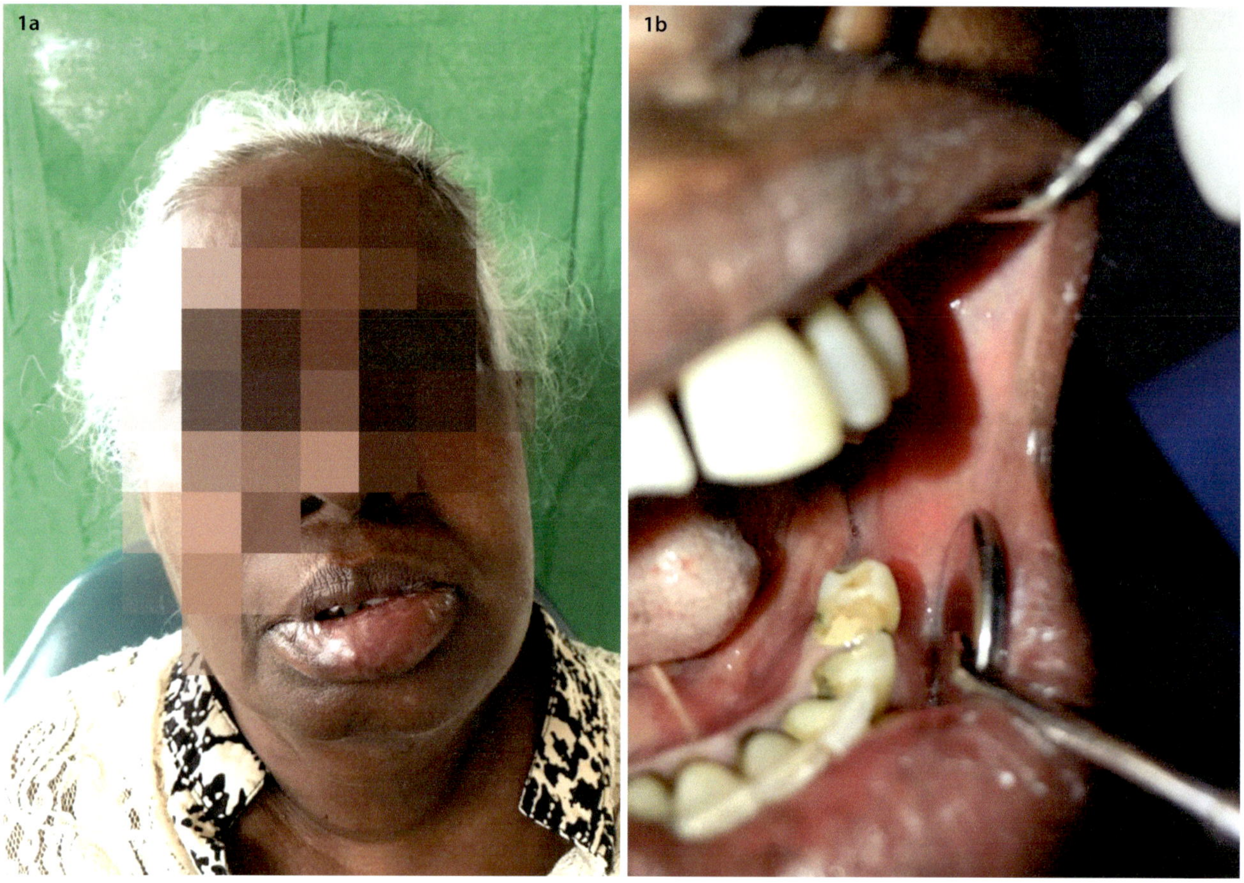

Fig. 45.1 Swelling of the left side of the face extending from the angle of the mandible to the lower lip (**a**). Slight swelling in the buccal gingivae and sulcus with evidence of pus discharge (**b**) (courtesy of Dr Thanuja Pathiraja)

45.9 What Is Your Clinical Differential Diagnosis?

1. Chronic suppurative osteomyelitis
2. Chronic periapical abscess
3. Infected periapical cyst

45.10 Explain the Justification for Your Clinical Differential Diagnosis

1. Clinical examination findings such as fever, limited mouth opening, loss of sensation over mental nerve area, mobility and tenderness of adjacent teeth, intraoral discharging sinus, swelling of the lower lip and cheek are pointers towards the clinical diagnosis of chronic suppurative osteomyelitis.
2. A chronic periapical abscess can cause tenderness of adjacent teeth, discharging sinuses, local soft tissue swelling, and inflammatory signs around the area. Although this can be included in the clinical differential diagnosis, it is an unlikely diagnosis with the presenting features.
3. The clinical presentation of an infected cyst is similar to a chronic periapical abscess which makes it one of the clinical differential diagnoses.

45.11 What Is the Working Diagnosis?

After considering the history, symptoms, duration, presentation, and physical signs, chronic suppurative osteomyelitis is considered as the working diagnosis.

45.12 How Would You Investigate This Patient?

1. Haematological assessment
2. Imaging—dental panoramic tomography (DPT)

Her haemoglobin level was normal with a value of 11.1 g/dL. Her full blood count showed neutrophilic leucocytosis (WBC 19.38 × 10^9/L) and elevated levels of CRP (38 mg/dL) and ESR (80 mm/hr).

The DPT (Fig. 45.2) showed a diffuse irregular radiolucency in relation to the region of teeth 35, 36, 37

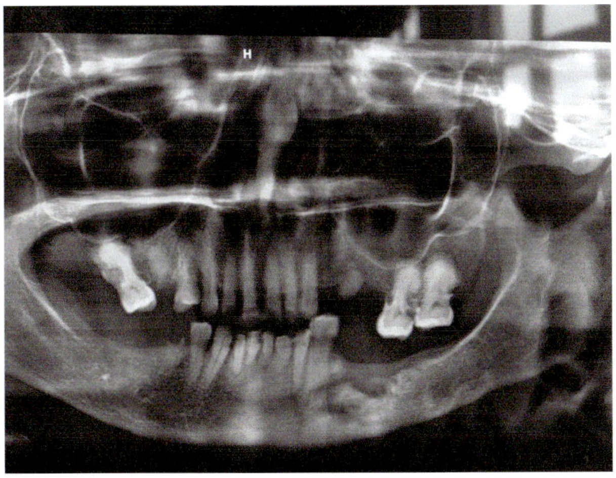

Fig. 45.2 DPT shows an irregular mixed radiopaque to radiolucent lesion in the body of the mandible on the left side

with a moth-eaten appearance. A mixture of osteolytic and sclerotic areas were seen in the DPT representing radiopaque involucrum and radiolucent sequestrum in the left mandibular body region, suggestive of chronic osteomyelitis.

45.13 What Is the Most Likely Diagnosis?

Based on history, clinical examination, and findings of the investigations, the most likely diagnosis is chronic suppurative osteomyelitis

45.14 How Would You Manage This Patient?

The treatment of chronic suppurative osteomyelitis involves thorough surgical debridement and prolonged antimicrobial therapy along with symptomatic, supportive management, and long-term treatment. Based on the findings, it was decided to carry out local curettage and saucerization of the infected bone along with a course of antibiotics.

All aspects of management were explained to the patient, and written consent was obtained for the procedure. As the patient had suffered from mild heart attack in 2019, medical clearance for surgery was obtained.

The procedure was carried out under general anaesthesia with nasal intubation. The area was infiltrated with 2% lignocaine containing 1/80,000 adrenaline. An incision was made parallel to the alveolar ridge, and the mucoperiosteal flap was raised buccally. Necrotic bone fragments with suppuration were seen on the buccal side of the mandible (Fig. 45.3).

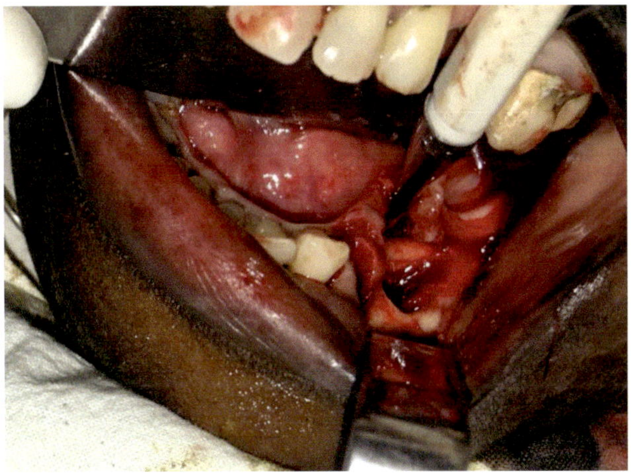

Fig. 45.3 Intraoperative view of the mandible showing necrotic bone which was removed up to bleeding bone

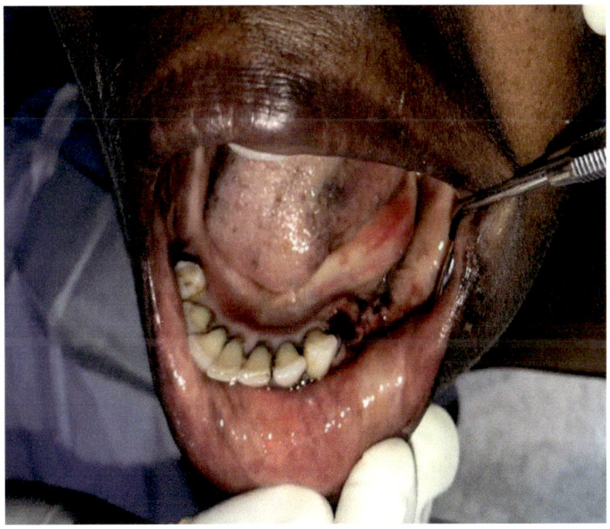

Fig. 45.4 Postoperative intraoral view after one month showing healed surgical site

All necrotic material was removed with a rose head bur, and bone was removed till the healthy bone was identified (bleeding). The sample was collected for culture and antibiotic sensitivity test (ABST). The removed tissue was sent for histological examination and the wound was irrigated profusely with normal saline. The wound was closed with 3/0 vicryl simple interrupted sutures. The postoperative period was uneventful.

Postoperatively, the patient was kept on amoxycillin with clavulanic acid (Augmentin) 1.2 g 12 hourly, infusion of metronidazole 500 mg 8 hourly, and gentamycin 80 mg intravenously 12 hourly for 7 days followed by oral Augmentin 675 mg and metronidazole 400 mg three times a day for two weeks. Postoperative pain was controlled by diclofenac sodium 50 mg twice a day.

The postoperative course of the patient was uneventful with satisfactory intraoral healing (Fig. 45.4).

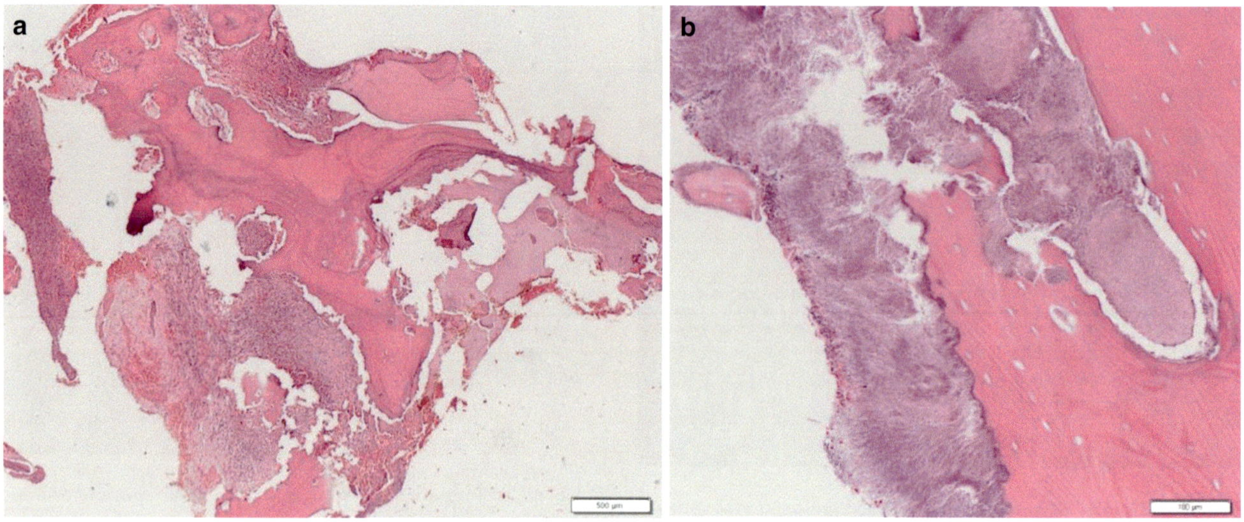

Fig. 45.5 (a) H & E stained decalcified sections show bone and soft tissue containing a dense mixed inflammatory infiltrate and evidence of granulation tissue formation. (b) Numerous bacterial colonies and bone with empty lacunae suggesting nonvital bone

45.15 What Are the Histopathological Findings of the Surgically Removed Lesional Tissue?

The haematoxylin and eosin (H&E)-stained decalcified sections showed bone and soft tissue containing a dense mixed inflammatory infiltrate and evidence of granulation tissue formation. Bacterial colonies were scattered throughout the lesion. Some areas revealed bone with empty lacunae suggesting nonvital bone (sequestrum) (Fig. 45.5). In most cases of chronic osteomyelitis, the periphery contains newly formed bone (Involucrum).

The histopathological features together with clinical and radiological findings confirm the diagnosis of chronic suppurative osteomyelitis

45.16 Osteomyelitis

In the past 20 years, the clinical presentation of osteomyelitis has changed significantly. Currently, there are an increased number of patients with osteomyelitis despite all the benefits associated with the advances in medicine and dentistry. There are several factors responsible for this trend including, development of microorganism resistance to commonly used antibiotics, increased number of immunocompromised patients such as patients with diabetes, HIV, organ transplants, patients who undergo radiation therapy and patients treated with bisphosphonates.

Chronic suppurative osteomyelitis is characterized by an inflammatory process resulting in necrosis of mineralized bone and marrow tissue, suppuration, resorption, and sclerosis. The primary cause of chronic osteomyelitis is usually microbiologic, and it results from odontogenic infection, postextraction complications, inadequate removal of necrotic bone, early termination of antibiotic therapy, inappropriate selection of antibiotics, diagnostic failure, trauma, inadequate treatment for a fracture, or irradiation to the mandible.

Many classification systems exist for osteomyelitis based on a variety of features such as clinical course, pathological–anatomical or radiological features, aetiology, and pathogenesis. This leads to difficulties in diagnosis and also comparing the results of different studies. A simple classification system based on the aetiology and pathogenesis of the disease known as Zurich classification is used by many due to its simplicity and clarity.

Three main types of osteomyelitis are described in the Zurich classification.

1. Acute osteomyelitis,
2. Secondary chronic osteomyelitis,
3. Primary chronic osteomyelitis.

Acute and secondary chronic osteomyelitis is the same disease, the only difference it being separated by an arbitrary time limit of one month after onset of the disease. The clinical presentation and course may vary significantly depending on the intensity of the infection and the host response.

45.16.1 The Zurich Classification of Osteomyelitis of the Jaws

Acute Osteomyelitis (<1-Month Duration) → Secondary Chronic Osteomyelitis

1. Neonatal, tooth germ–associated
2. Trauma-/fracture-related (e.g. open fracture)

3. Odontogenic
4. Periodontal
5. Pulpal
6. Paranasal sinus related
7. Extraction wound related
8. Chronic neck infection (actinomycosis, tuberculosis)
9. Implant-associated (dental implant or internal fixation device)
10. Graft-associated (bone grafts for reconstruction)
11. Associated with bone pathology and/or systemic disease (Albers–Schönberg disease, Paget disease)
12. Not classifiable

Primary Chronic Osteomyelitis
1. Early onset (juvenile chronic osteomyelitis)
2. Adult onset
3. Radiation-induced avascular bone necrosis
4. Osteo-chemonecrosis (corticosteroids, antineoplastic drugs, bisphosphonate therapy)
5. Syndrome-associated (e.g. chronic recurrent multifocal osteomyelitis)
6. Garre's sclerosing osteomyelitis,
7. SAPHO (synovitis, acne, pustulosis, hyperostosis, and osteitis)

Osteomyelitis of the jaws is predominantly seen in the mandible due it its limited vascularity. In the upper jaw, it accounts for only 1–6% of patients. Acute and secondary chronic osteomyelitis of the jaws is caused mostly by a bacterial focus (odontogenic disease, pulpal, and periodontal infection, extraction wounds, foreign bodies, and infected fractures). Primary chronic osteomyelitis of the jaw is rare and usually non-suppurative.

Early diagnosis of osteomyelitis is very important to carry out appropriate treatment which will help to minimize severe functional and aesthetic deformity. Clinical diagnosis, imaging, and pathological diagnosis remain the main modality for diagnosis. The clinical findings of chronic suppurative osteomyelitis include local pain, fever, swelling, purulent discharge, intraoral and skin fistula, unhealed soft tissue lesions in the oral cavity, paraesthesia in the involved area, pathologic fracture, and trismus.

Imaging is a very important diagnostic tool in the assessment of acute and chronic osteomyelitis of the jaws. To confirm and assess osteomyelitis of the jaws, a range of radiological techniques is available. Conventional radiographs still serve as the first line of investigation. Among conventional radiographs, the DPT is of primary importance as it shows the status of the dentition, reveals the osseous confines and internal osseous structure of the jaws, and provides adequate basis for a follow-up examination. The DPT may be occasionally supplemented by intraoral radiographs. Computed tomography (CT) or cone-beam CT (CBCT) and magnetic resonance imaging (MRI) are well-established high-resolution cross-sectional imaging techniques that provide precise morphological information regarding bone (CT) and soft tissue (MRI) involvement.

Scintigraphy is a well-recognized tool in the early diagnosis of osteomyelitis of jaw bones. Due to the sensitivity of this investigation, the extent of the infectious lesion can be determined accurately thus providing important information before surgical therapy. An additional useful feature of bone scans is their ability to monitor activity during the course of the disease and hence determine the effectiveness of therapy as well as detecting relapse.

Positron emission tomography (PET) is a relatively new non-invasive technique to investigate various bone and soft tissue pathologies. The development of fused PET/CT images is particularly promising since it combines the advantages of detailed imaging of the anatomy combined with detection of local metabolic activity patterns. High costs and limited availability are the major drawbacks for PET and fused PET/CT investigation.

Histopathology has always been regarded as valuable in the diagnostic process of osteomyelitis, especially distinguishing it from other diseases of bone. Histopathology of osteomyelitis varies according to the nature of the disease including acute, chronic, specific types such as sclerosing type or Garre's osteomyelitis (proliferative periostitis). In addition, specific features are present if it arises in the background of other bone diseases such as Paget disease or osteopetrosis. In acute forms of osteomyelitis, the lesional tissue is characterized by dense infiltrate of inflammatory cells, predominantly neutrophils. In addition, numerous bacterial colonies are present. Chronic forms are dominated by granulation tissue formation with a dense infiltrate of mixed inflammatory cells, dead bone (sequestrum), and new bone formation (involucrum). Sclerosing forms and proliferative periostitis show evidence of new bone formation either with minimal inflammatory infiltrate or without inflammatory features and bacterial colonies. Culture and antibiotic sensitivity test (ABST) has its own value in selecting appropriate antibiotics for the ongoing infection.

The objective of treatment for acute and secondary chronic osteomyelitis of the jaws is to increase the host defences, reduce causative microorganisms, and to allow the body to overcome the infection. Reduction of pathogens is achieved by surgical removal of infected and necrotic tissue as well as by antibiotic therapy.

Treatment depends on the type of osteomyelitis. Acute suppurative osteomyelitis usually responds to antibiotic therapy alone but in the case of chronic suppurative osteomyelitis, in addition to antibiotic therapy, it is necessary to combine surgery that aims to remove all necrotic soft and hard tissue. In acute suppurative osteomyelitis, persistent infections not responding to treatment are seen in some patients. It may indicate inadequate antimicrobial therapy either due to wrong or missing microbiological data (superficial swab instead of deep biopsy) or due to antimicrobial treatment with an insufficient drug (low bioavailability, unexpected resistance, emergence of resistance during therapy, or superinfection).

Chronic suppurative osteomyelitis is managed by surgery and antimicrobial therapy. Surgery is a form of surgical decortication which exceeds conventional surgical debridement in order to remove all necrotic tissue and to bring well-vascularized tissue to the affected area. This facilitates healing and allows antibiotics to reach the target area. Therefore, surgery and antibiotics are considered as major arrays of treatment in osteomyelitis of the jaws. Empirical broad-spectrum antibiotics should be started after surgery and appropriate antibiotic should be prescribed as soon as the results of ABST are available.

The surgical management of acute and secondary chronic osteomyelitis varies depending on the extent of the infected bone, from incision and drainage to local resection (◘ Fig. 45.6).

Hyperbaric oxygen (HBO), which is considered as an adjunctive therapeutic modality in the treatment of acute and secondary chronic osteomyelitis, supports host-defensive mechanisms and promotes tissue vascularization as well as has direct toxic effects on microorganisms causing the infection.

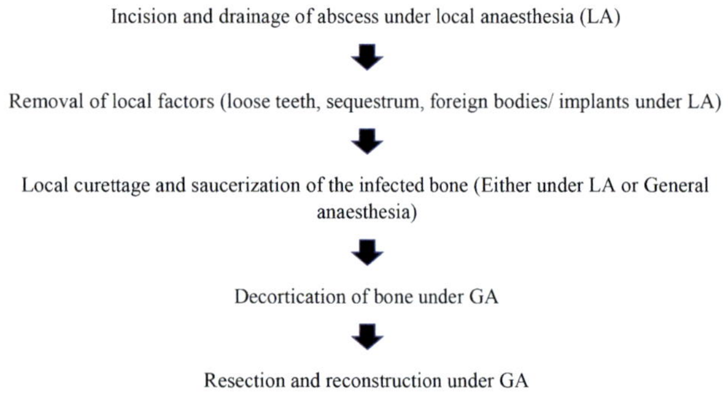

◘ **Fig. 45.6** Surgical management of acute and secondary chronic osteomyelitis

Due to the nature of the disease, patients with osteomyelitis of the jaws need careful and regular clinical and radiological follow-up visits for at least 2 years to rule out relapse of the disease and to evaluate the effectiveness of therapy. Patient education plays a key role in long-term management. During the initial phase, clinical signs (local signs of inflammation, fever) and laboratory (C-reactive protein, leucocyte counts) indicators of infection should be closely monitored.

Salient Features of Osteomyelitis	
Clinical	• Local intense pain, • Tenderness, • Fever, • Painful or painless swelling, • Purulent discharge, • Intraoral fistula, • Skin fistula, • Trismus, • Hypoesthesia of the inferior dental nerve, • Pathologic fracture
Radiological	• Areas of radio-opacity with loss of bony trabeculae • Areas of radiolucency with interruption of cortical bone • Sequestrum formation • Pathological fracture • New bone formation (involucrum)
Histopathology	• Mixed inflammatory infiltrate (more neutrophils in acute form) • Granulation tissue formation • Bacterial colonies • Dead bone (sequestrum) and new bone (involucrum)
Treatment	• Antibiotic therapy • Surgical intervention • Hyperbaric oxygen as adjuvant therapy
Necrotic tissue removed during the surgery should be sent for histopathological diagnosis and culture and antibiotic sensitivity test to determine the antibiotic of choice.	

Management Algorithm

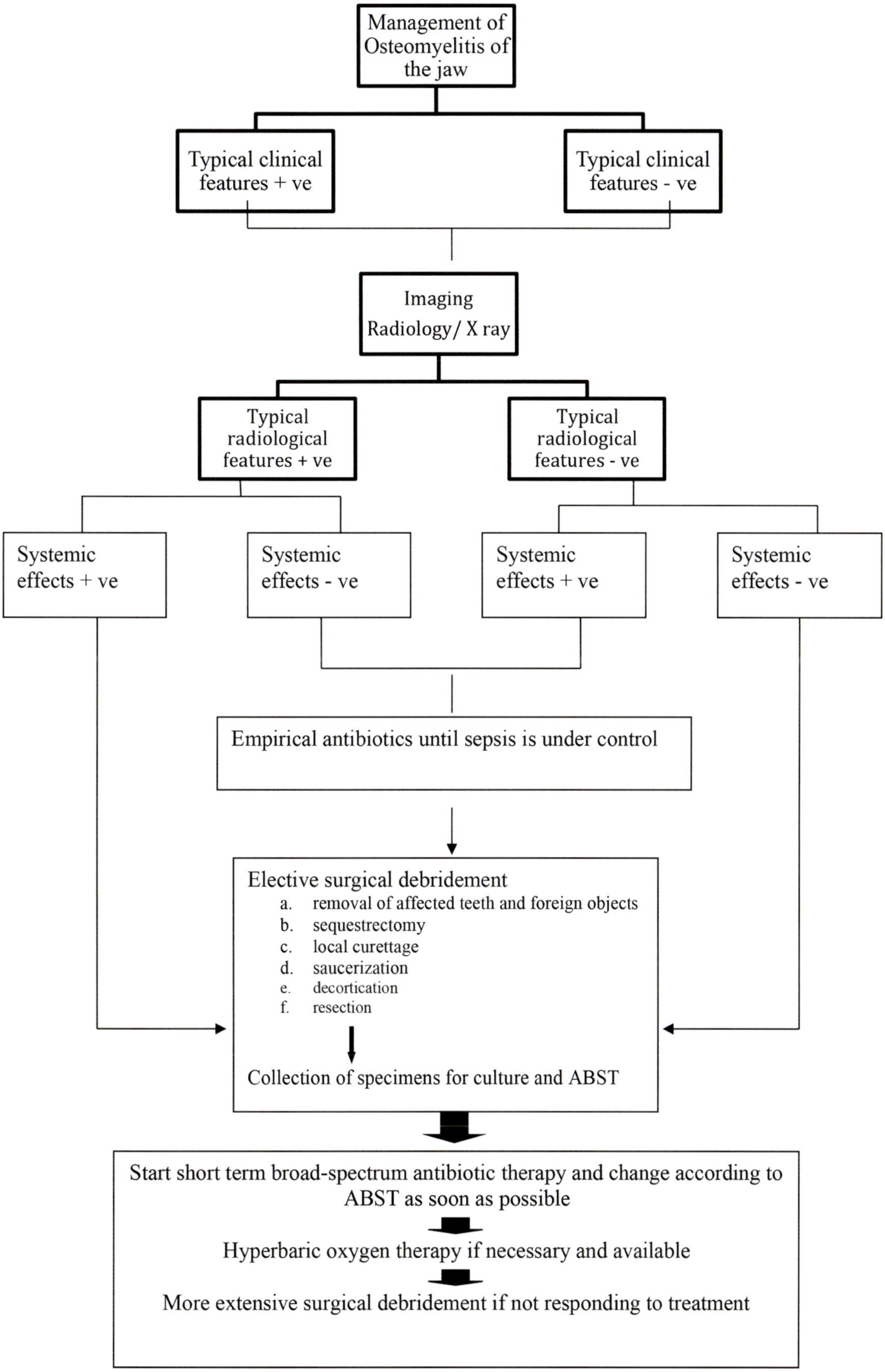

- **Diagnostic Algorithm of Osteomyelitis**

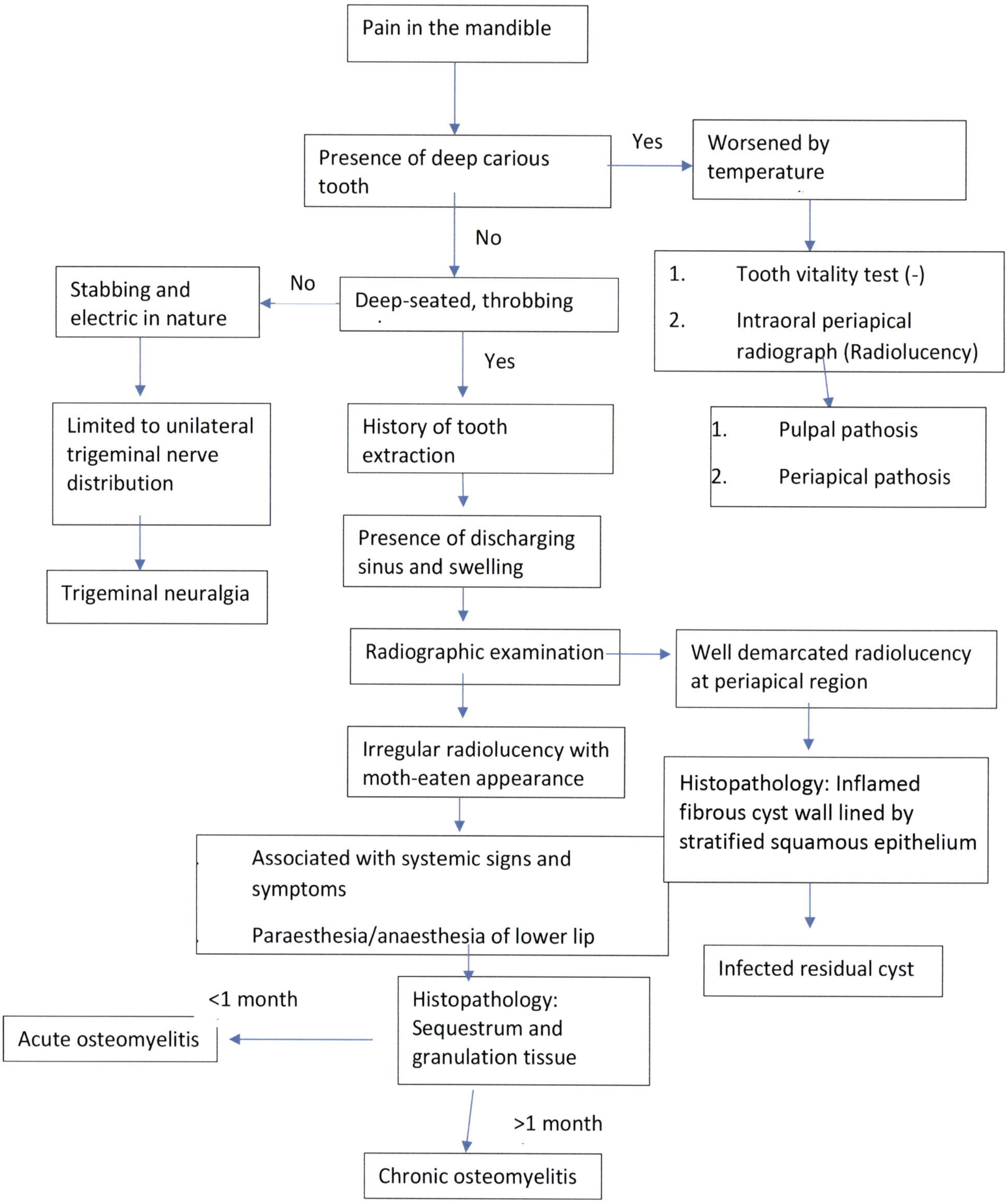

Self-Assessment Questions

1. Give a classification for osteomyelitis of jaw bones.
2. Describe the aetiological and predisposing factors of osteomyelitis.
3. Describe the clinical features of osteomyelitis.
4. Describe the radiological features of different forms of osteomyelitis.
5. Describe the treatment of osteomyelitis.

Summary

Osteomyelitis of the jaws has become a rare disease with the introduction of antibiotics and meticulous surgical techniques. It is commonly seen in the mandible. The primary cause of chronic osteomyelitis is usually microbiologic infection, and it results from odontogenic infections, inadequate treatment and inappropriate selection of antibiotics, and diagnostic failure. Diagnosis of osteomyelitis is carried out with the help of patient history, clinical examinations, radiographic findings, and the surgical presentation. Histopathologic examinations can confirm the diagnosis. The main treatment of localized osteomyelitis in a patient without any systemic conditions is to remove the aetiology of the disease as well as antibiotic therapy to prevent post-surgical infection.

Further Reading

Agarwal A, Kumar N, Tyagi A, De N. Primary chronic osteomyelitis in the mandible: a conservative approach. BMJ Case Rep. 2014;2014:bcr2013202448. Published 2014 Apr 3. https://doi.org/10.1136/bcr-2013-202448.

Baltensperger M. A retrospective analysis of 290 osteomyelitis cases treated in the past 30 years at the Department of Cranio-Maxillofacial Surgery Zurich with special recognition of the classification. Med Dissertation,. Zurich; 2003.

Baltensperger M, Eyrich GK. Osteomyelitis of the Jaws. 1st ed. Berlin Heidelberg: Springer-Verlag; 2009. https://doi.org/10.1007/978-3-540-28766-7.

Berglund C, Ekströmer K, Abtahi J. Primary chronic osteomyelitis of the jaws in children: an update on pathophysiology, radiological findings, treatment strategies, and prospective analysis of two cases. Case Rep Dent. 2015;2015:152717. https://doi.org/10.1155/2015/152717.

Daramola JO, Ajagbe HA. Chronic osteomyelitis of the mandible in adults: a clinical study of 34 cases. Br J Oral Surg. 1982;20:58–62.

Mallikarjun K, Kohli A, Kumar A, Tanwar A. Chronic suppurative osteomyelitis of the mandible. J Indian Soc Pedod Prev Dent. 2011;29(2):176–9.

Park MS, Eo MY, Myoung H, Kim SM, Lee JH. Early diagnosis of jaw osteomyelitis by easy digitalized panoramic analysis. Maxillofac Plast Reconstr Surg. 2019;41(1):6. Published 2019 Feb 1. https://doi.org/10.1186/s40902-019-0188-2.

Painless and Exposed Bone in the Maxilla: Medication-Related Osteonecrosis of the Jaw (MRONJ)

Firdaus Hariri, Muhammad Kamil Hassan, and Thomas George Kallarakkal

Contents

W. M Tilakaratne, T. G. Kallarakkal (eds.), *Clinicopathological Correlation of Oral Diseases*,
https://doi.org/10.1007/978-3-031-24408-7_46

Learning Goals

1. Devise the correct way of compiling the history with appropriate questions.
2. Develop a differential diagnosis after history taking.
3. Deduce appropriate procedures in clinical examination.
4. Formulate a differential diagnosis combining findings in the history and clinical examination.
5. Justify the relevant investigations required to arrive at the diagnosis.
6. Comprehend the importance of clinicopathological correlation in arriving at the correct diagnosis.
7. Outline the management plan.
8. Recognize the importance of a diagnostic algorithm in arriving at a diagnosis

46.1 Main Complaint

A 75-year-old female patient presented to the dental clinic complaining of a hard white-yellowish lesion on her front upper jaw.

46.2 History of Complaint

Question: How long have you noticed this lesion?

I have been noticing this lesion for about 3 months now. It occurred spontaneously. Initially, it was only a small lesion. Gradually, my gums started to grow away from the lesion. I feel that the bone of my jaw in the region is exposed. It has not been painful nor giving any other symptoms.

46.3 Additional Complaints

Question: Have you noticed or felt any other changes or difficulties in the mouth?

Since the occurrence of the lesion, I could not fit my upper partial denture well and decided not to wear it. Otherwise, I have no problem in eating or speaking.

Question: Are you suffering from any medical problems such as heart disease, high blood pressure, diabetes, bleeding disorder, respiratory diseases? If yes, what kind of medications have you been taking until now?

I have high blood pressure which is managed with 5 mg amlodipine. I have no other problems. However, I am taking a certain medication to strengthen my bones, which was prescribed by my oncologist.

Question: Can you elaborate the details of your treatment under the oncologist?

I am currently receiving treatment for my breast cancer. I completed chemo-radiation therapy one year ago. Subsequently, six months later, my oncologist diagnosed lytic lesions in my vertebrae and pelvic region which was later confirmed as bone metastasis of breast cancer. I was immediately started on IV Zometa (bisphosphonate) 4 mg every four weeks.

Question: Have you undergone any surgery?

I have undergone right mastectomy for breast cancer.

Question: Have you undergone any dental treatment?

I had an extraction 5 months ago (1 month after starting IV Zometa regime) of my upper left central and lateral incisors which were grossly carious. I also have upper and lower acrylic partial dentures which are more than 5 years old.

Question: What is your occupation?

I am a pensioner but previously worked as a teacher.

Question: Are you a smoker?

I used to smoke 10 cigarettes per day for the past 30 years. I stopped smoking after being diagnosed with the breast cancer.

Question: Do you take alcohol?

I do not use alcohol.

46.4 With the Findings From the History, What Is Your Differential Diagnosis?

1. Medication-related osteonecrosis of the jaws (MRONJ)
2. Metastatic lesion from breast cancer
3. Osteoradionecrosis (ORN)
4. Osteomyelitis

46.5 How Do You Justify Your Differential Diagnosis After History Taking?

1. The patient presents with a lesion suggestive of an area of exposed bone in the anterior maxilla for more than eight weeks' duration. It occurred spontaneously. The patient had undergone treatment for breast cancer which involved surgery and adjuvant chemo-radiation therapy to eradicate the disease. However, she developed bone metastasis and was started on IV Zometa (zoledronic acid) which is a bisphosphonate type medication to prevent bone resorption from metastatic lesions. MRONJ is a known condition and complication in patients taking bisphosphonate medications.
2. The patient received radiation therapy as an adjunct following her breast cancer surgery. The radiotherapy is commonly localized to the breast and axillary lymph node region. It is very unlikely for the radiotherapy to involve the head and neck region, resulting in osteoradionecrosis (ORN). However, both MRONJ and ORN do present in a very similar way clinically.
3. The patient is likely to be immunosuppressed following chemotherapy. Immunosuppression is one of the risk factors for developing osteomyelitis of the jaw, although it is more common in the mandible compared to the maxilla.
4. Any lesions that look abnormal in the oral cavity in a patient with a history of cancer elsewhere should always be suspicious for metastatic lesions.

46.6 Findings of Clinical Examination

She has normal extraoral findings with no cervical lymphadenopathy and normal mouth opening.

Intra-orally, there is a 5 cm × 2 cm area of exposed necrotic bone in the upper left anterior maxilla which is firm (Fig. 46.1). The mucosa looks erythematous on the labial surface with slough covering the superior portion of the exposed bone. There is evidence of pus formation. She also does not claim of any nasal discharges or epistaxis. There are no signs of ulceration, induration, or neurosensory disturbances.

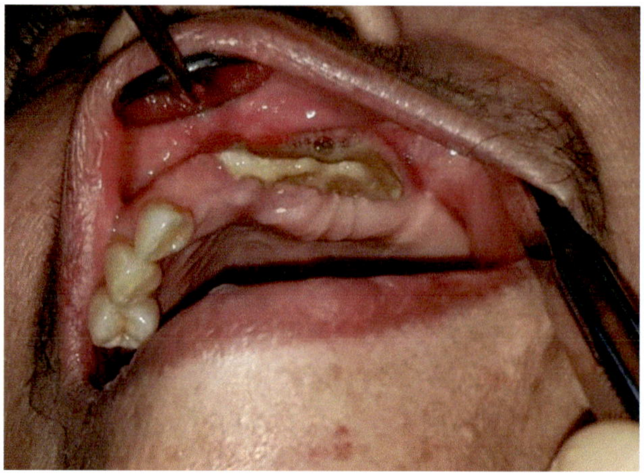

Fig. 46.1 An area of exposed necrotic bone in the upper left anterior maxilla

46.7 What Other Relevant Features Do You Look for with the Findings You Have So Far?

There are no signs of nasal blockage or discharge suggestive of any growing pathological lesions or chronic inflammatory conditions. There are no ulcerations, bleeding, and/or neurosensory disturbances that raise a suspicion of malignancy.

46.8 What Is Your Clinical Differential Diagnosis?

1. Medication-related osteonecrosis of the jaws (MRONJ)
2. Metastatic lesion from breast cancer

46.9 How Would You Exclude Other Conditions and Justify the Inclusion of the Diseases That You Have Mentioned in the Differential Diagnosis to Arrive at a Working Diagnosis?

46.9.1 Medication-Related Osteonecrosis of the Jaws (MRONJ)

The patient presents with a history of exposed bone for more than eight weeks duration. Her medical history which indicates that she is currently receiving bisphosphonate (antiresorptive medication) for treatment of metastatic bone lesions with no history of radiation to the head and neck region correlates with the classic definition of MRONJ. It can occur spontaneously without any external causes such as odontogenic infections or trauma. The patient is receiving intravenous bisphosphonates which carries a tenfold increase in risk of developing MRONJ compared to oral bisphosphonates. Therefore, the most likely working diagnosis is MRONJ.

46.9.2 Osteoradionecrosis (ORN)

Osteoradionecrosis of the jaws is a condition that presents with exposed or non-exposed necrotic bone following radiotherapy to the head and neck region. The clinical presentation of ORN and BRONJ is very similar and not clinically distinguishable. However, without radiotherapy to the head and neck region, the diagnosis of ORN should not be considered.

46.9.3 Osteomyelitis

Osteomyelitis, an inflammatory condition of the bone marrow, may or may not be precipitated by infection. Immunosuppression is a known risk factor for developing osteomyelitis; however, the incidence has greatly reduced with the advances in antibiotic treatments. It often presents with the classical signs of inflammation such as pain, redness, heat, and loss of function. It occurs most often in the mandible compared to the maxilla. Hence, osteomyelitis is an unlikely working diagnosis.

46.9.4 Metastatic Lesion

Any abnormal presentation in the oral cavity in a patient with a history of cancer should be suspicious of metastatic lesion. This includes lesions with non-healing ulcers, swellings, indurated areas, and neurosensory disturbances. Metastatic lesions in the oral cavity may present without cervical lymph node involvement. Thus, the possibility of a metastatic lesion should not be ruled out completely until proven with a biopsy although findings in the history and clinical examination are more towards MRONJ.

46.9.5 What Is the Most Likely Diagnosis?

Medication-related osteonecrosis of the jaws (MRONJ)

46.9.6 How Would You Investigate This Patient?

1. History with clinical correlation
2. Imaging: Dental panoramic tomograph (DPT)/Computed tomography (CT)/Cone beam computed tomography (CBCT)
3. Biopsy of necrotic bone and surrounding tissues

46.9.7 A DPT Was Taken for This Patient. What Features Do You See in This DPT?

In the upper left anterior maxilla, there is thickening of lamina dura of the socket of tooth 11 (◘ Fig. 46.2). The tooth was extracted 5 months ago, and remnants of the lamina dura may indicate little or no remodelling of the alveolar bone post-extraction. The edges of the bone also look ragged and rough. In the right mandible, there are areas of diffuse osteosclerosis with osteolysis. In the left mandible, there are tooth sockets with remnants of lamina dura. These features may indicate osteonecrosis in the mandible although not yet exposed through the soft tissues.

46.9.8 Is Biopsy Always Necessary in All Cases?

Biopsy is not always indicated for all MRONJ cases. An exception is for cases of MRONJ that develop after therapy for hypercalcaemia or bone metastasis in cancer patients. It is necessary to do a biopsy to rule out metastatic lesions in the jaw region, which may influence the overall management of the patient.

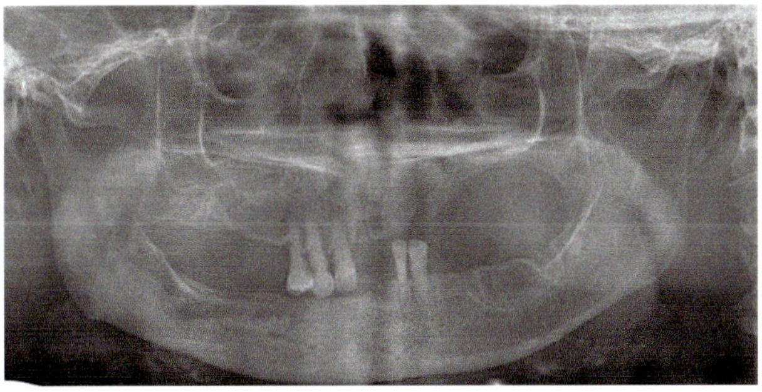

◘ **Fig. 46.2** The socket of tooth 11 showing thickened lamina dura and rough and ragged bone edges

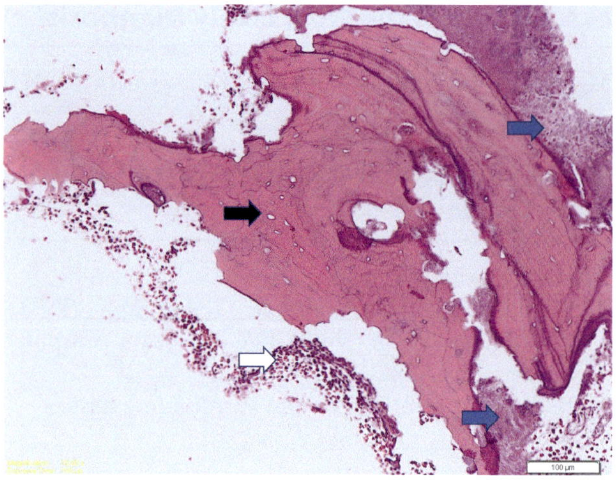

Fig. 46.3 Necrotic bony trabeculae with empty lacunae (black arrow). An abundant inflammatory infiltrate is associated with the necrotic bone (white arrow). A plethora of microorganisms is present within the marrow spaces and the surface of the necrotic bone (blue arrows)

46.9.9 What Do You Expect to See If Biopsy Is Performed?

The lesional tissue in MRONJ exhibits necrotic bony trabeculae with empty lacunae (Fig. 46.3). Osteoclasts are rare and present only focally. A significant inflammatory infiltrate is always present. An abundance of microorganisms consisting of gram-positive and gram-negative cocci, rods, and filamentous forms are present within the marrow spaces and on the surface. A consistent histological finding in MRONJ is the presence of Actinomyces species within the specimens.

46.9.10 How Would You Manage This Patient?

Management of MRONJ remains a difficult task. Various surgical and non-surgical modalities have been published in the literature with mixed results and success. The important part of management includes obtaining a proper working diagnosis for MRONJ. The information for type of bisphosphonate medication, dosage, and route of administration is crucial to assess the risk of developing MRONJ. Nitrogen containing bisphosphonates, higher doses, and intravenous administration increases the risk for MRONJ. In symptomatic cases, clinicians must address them prior to a definitive surgical or non-surgical management. MRONJ may be asymptomatic but could also present with common inflammatory signs and symptoms and also infection. Pain should be managed with analgesia appropriate to the severity, whereas infection is treated with incision and drainage (when an abscess is present) or antibiotics (where spread of infection is evident).

Following symptomatic relief, radiographic investigation should be performed to assess the extent of necrotic bone and affected teeth, tissues, or other anatomical structures/spaces. A CT or CBCT imaging is ideal to allow assessment in all planes. In the present case, the extent of necrotic bone involved the nasal floor.

The staging of the MRONJ can influence the overall management. A discussion with the oncologist is important to ensure that the surgical management does not contradict the current oncologic management and that the patient is fit for surgical intervention.

In this case, the patient did not consent for any surgical intervention and only agreed for symptomatic relief. Eventually, she returned with an oro-nasal fistula and nasal regurgitation following exfoliation of the necrotic bone in the anterior maxilla. An upper acrylic denture with obturator for the oro-nasal fistula was constructed for the patient.

46.10 Medication-Related Osteonecrosis of the Jaws (MRONJ)

Medication-related osteonecrosis of the jaw (MRONJ) is defined as a severe adverse drug reaction, consisting of progressive bone destruction in the maxillofacial region. Due to the growing number of osteonecrosis cases related to both antiresorptive and antiangiogenic therapy reported globally, the old nomenclature bisphosphonate-related osteonecrosis of the jaw (BRONJ) was changed to MRONJ.

Other medications have been added to the list of causative drugs for MRONJ as shown in Table 46.1.

Even though the pathophysiology of MRONJ is not completely elucidated, several hypotheses have been described. They include multi-aetiological factors associated with inflammation or infection, microtrauma, altered bone remodelling or oversuppression of bone resorption, angiogenesis inhibition, soft tissue bisphosphonates toxicity, biofilm of the oral cavity, terminal vascularization of the mandible, suppression of immunity, and vitamin D deficiency.

Bisphosphonates have high affinity to bone, particularly at active sites of bone remodelling. Excess bisphosphonates that are not retained in bone are excreted renally. On a biochemical level, bisphosphonates incorporate into adenosine triphosphate (ATP) molecules which cause it to be cytotoxic to osteoclasts, leading to cellular apoptosis. This activity of bisphosphonate drugs then limits the disease progression in bones. However, devastating side effect occurs in the jaws where bone remodelling is high due to the masticatory process. Inhibition of bone remodelling in the bone due to bisphosphonates leads to osteonecrosis of the jaws.

In RANK-ligand inhibitor therapy for osteoporosis or metastatic bone diseases, the antiresorptive medication inhibits osteoclast function, decreases bone resorption, and increases bone density. In antiangiogenic medications, the development of novel blood vessels is impaired thus blocking the angiogenesis-signalling cascade.

Table 46.1 List of medications related to osteonecrosis of the jaws

Category	Molecule	Indication
Bisphosphonate	Alendronate Ibandronate Risedronate Neridronate Tiludronate Pamidronate Zoledronate	Osteoporosis Paget's disease, osteogenesis imperfecta Bone metastases
Tyrosine kinase inhibitors	Sorafenib Sunitib	Hepatocellular carcinoma Renal cell carcinoma
Humanized monoclonal antibody	Bevacizumab	Metastatic colorectal cancer Non-squamous non-small cell lung carcinoma Metastatic renal cell carcinoma
Receptor activator of nuclear factor kappa-B-ligand inhibitors	Denosumab	Bone metastases Osteoporosis
Mammalian target of rapamycin pathway	Sirolimus	Organ rejection in renal transplant

Patients with MRONJ commonly present with a non-healing area of exposed jawbone which may appear necrotic. The surrounding mucosa may also be inflamed, and in an infected condition, the lesions appear erythematous, sloughy, and may present with pus.

Other findings are often associated with the site of the lesion. MRONJ in the maxillary region may lead to signs of nasal blockage or presence of discharge whereas neurosensory disturbance within the distribution of inferior alveolar nerve may occur in severe conditions of the mandible.

Radiographically, the most common features of MRONJ include thickening of lamina dura, diffuse osteosclerosis with or without osteolysis, and bony sequestra. These features are not specific to MRONJ alone and must be correlated with history and clinical findings.

A common finding in suppurative osteomyelitis of jaws (SOJ), MRONJ, and osteoradionecrosis of jaws (ORNJ) is necrotic bone with empty osteocyte lacunae, empty Haversian systems, and Volkmann canals (Fig. 46.4a). Similarly, inflammation within the marrow spaces (Fig. 46.4b), the presence of bacteria (Fig. 46.4b), and reactive bone formation is a feature seen in all the three conditions. Osteoclasts are generally scarce in MRONJ and osteomyelitis, while it is completely absent in ORN (Fig. 46.4c). The empty lacunae at the periphery of the bone depicts apoptosis of osteoclasts (Fig. 46.4c). There are no distinctive histopathological features that can differentiate SOJ, MRONJ, and ORNJ from one another. The role of histopathological analysis is to serve as an adjunct to diagnosis and it must be supported by the patient's history and imaging findings. The American Association of Oral and Maxillofacial Surgeons (AAOMS) in their position paper on the definition, staging, and the management of patients with MRONJ states that histological analysis and radiographic features are not a

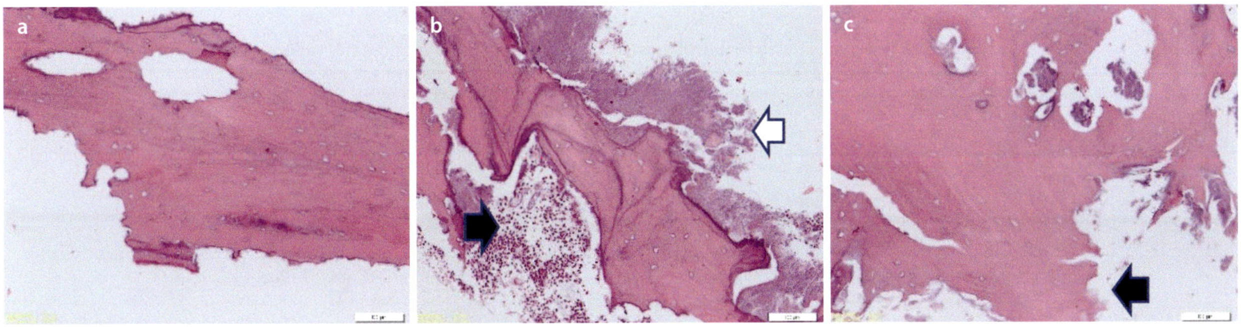

Fig. 46.4 (a) Necrotic bone with empty osteocyte lacunae, (**b**) inflammation (black arrow) and non-specific bacteria (white arrow), (**c**) and empty Howship's lacunae without osteoclasts (black arrow)

prerequisite for its diagnosis. The diagnosis is primarily based on clinical features alone and most patients do not undergo a biopsy from the exposed necrotic bone.

To aid in treatment planning and disease progression, a classification for MRONJ has been proposed. In this classification, 5 stages have been defined together with their proposed management. This is summarized in ◘ Table 46.2 below:

Conservative management for MRONJ includes oral hygiene instructions, dental restorations, endodontics and periodontal treatments, application of topical and antibacterial mouth rinses such as chlorhexidine and local and systemic antibiotics for infections.

Surgical treatment is indicated when conservative management is deemed ineffective or unlikely to respond due to the staging of the disease. Surgical treatment includes removal of teeth in affected necrotic sites, debridement of necrotic bone, and resection of affected sites (◘ Fig. 46.5). On principle, a full-thickness mucoperiosteal flap is raised to assess the whole area of necrotic bone, followed by removal of necrotic bone until "healthy" bone is seen (through bleeding). The sharp edges of bone are smoothened and rounded to prevent trauma to overlying tissues which may cause wound dehiscence.

The difficulty of surgical debridement or resection is that there are no "clear margins" for MRONJ, unlike in cases involved by tumours. This is because the medications diffuse systemically and any bone in the body could be affected. Bisphosphonate medications are retained in bones for many years.

Adjuvant therapies include laser therapy, ozone therapy, and application of platelet-rich plasma/fibrin. All the adjuncts aim to minimize surgical trauma, increase oxygen tension in tissues, and aid healing of the surgical wound. However, the results of these adjuvant therapies remain conflicting.

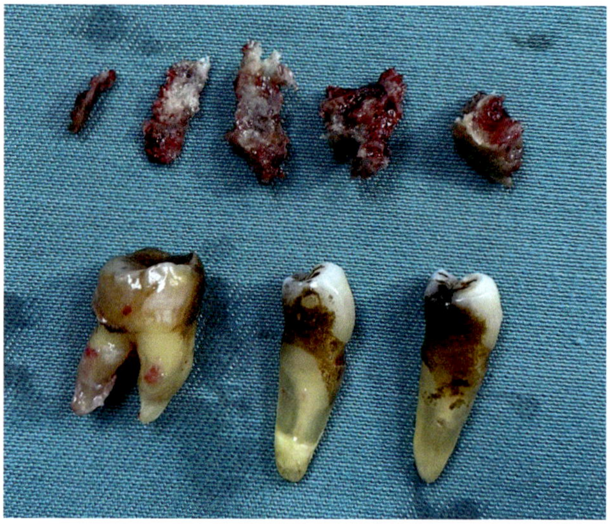

◘ **Fig. 46.5** Removal of affected teeth and necrotic bone in MRONJ stage 2

◘ **Table 46.2** Staging of MRONJ according to AAOMS position paper published in 2014

Stage	Clinical and radiological features	Treatment/management
At risk	No apparent necrotic bone in patients who have been treated with either oral or IV bisphosphonates.	• No treatment indicated. • Patient education.
0	No clinical evidence of necrotic bone, but non-specific clinical findings, radiographic changes, and symptoms.	• Systemic management, including the use of pain medication and antibiotics.
1	Exposed and necrotic bone, or fistulae that probes to bone, in patients who are asymptomatic and have no evidence of infection.	• Antibacterial mouth rinse. • Clinical follow-up on a quarterly basis. • Patient education and review of indications for continued bisphosphonate therapy.
2	Exposed and necrotic bone, or fistulae that probes to bone, associated with infection as evidenced by pain and erythema in the region of the exposed bone with or without purulent drainage.	• Symptomatic treatment with oral antibiotics. • Oral antibacterial mouth rinse. • Pain control. • Debridement to relieve soft tissue irritation and infection control.
3	Exposed and necrotic bone or a fistula that probes to bone in patients with pain, infection, and one or more of the following: exposed and necrotic bone extending beyond the region of alveolar bone, (inferior border and ramus in the mandible, maxillary sinus and zygoma in the maxilla) resulting in pathologic fracture, extraoral fistula, oral antral/oral nasal communication, or osteolysis extending to the inferior border of the mandible of sinus floor.	• Antibacterial mouth rinse. • Antibiotic therapy and pain control. • Surgical debridement/resection for longer term palliation of infection and pain.

Diagnostic and Management Algorithm

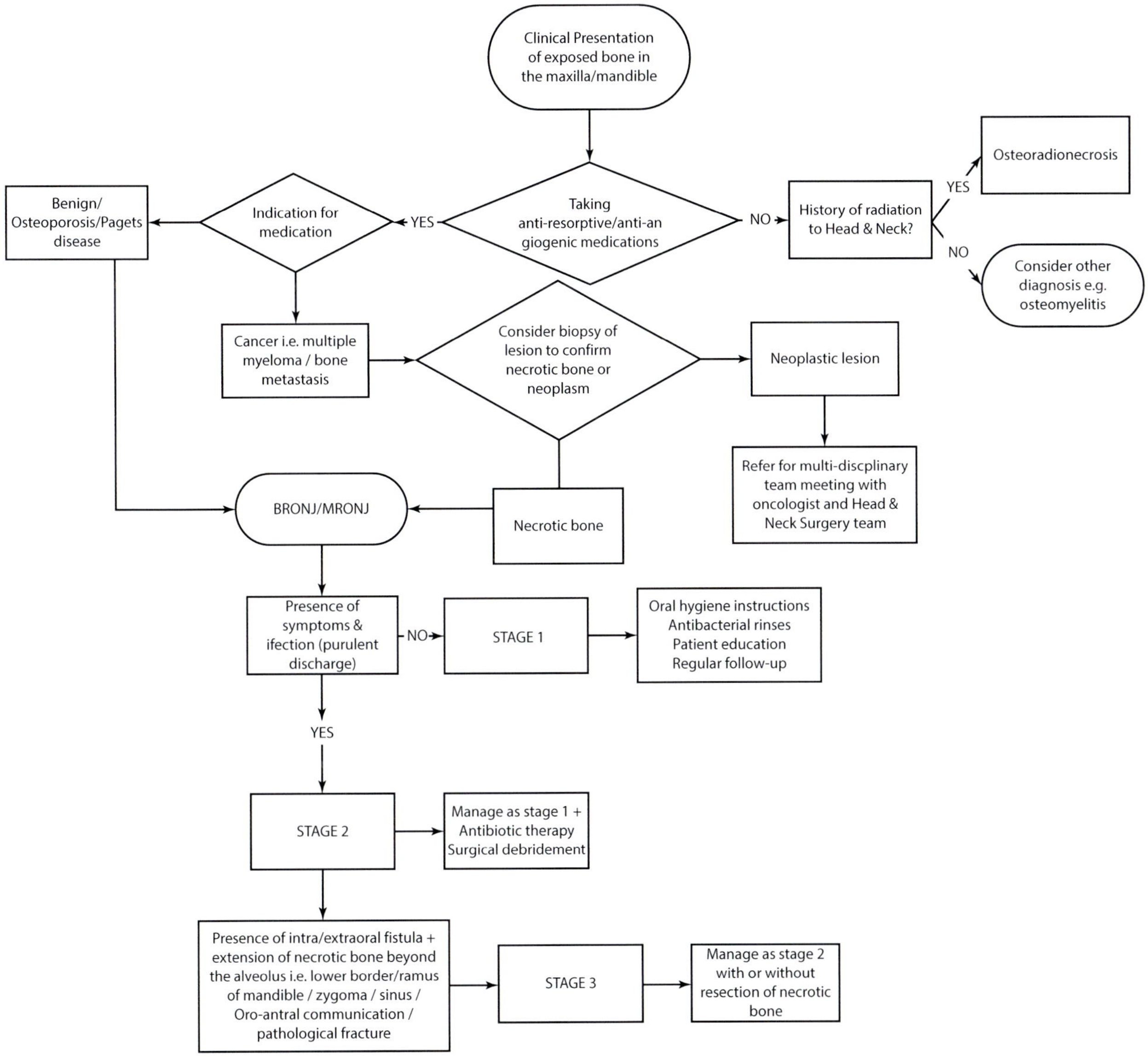

Salient features of BRONJ/MRONJ	
Clinical	Exposed bone, or unexposed bone that can be probed through a fistula. Exposed and necrotic bone are yellowish-grey in colour and not painful to touch. Surrounding soft tissues may appear normal or erythematous. Infection and purulent discharge may be associated with the lesion. May present with or without symptoms. Symptoms may correlate with extent of osteonecrosis (mobile teeth, paraesthesia of mandibular nerve, trismus due to chronic infection or pathological fracture, oro-antral communication).
Histopathology	Necrotic bony trabeculae with empty osteocyte lacunae. The empty lacunae at the periphery of the bone depict apoptosis of osteoclasts. Presence of bacteria especially Actinomyces species.
Treatment	Depending on the stage of disease. Pre-medication dental treatment is vital to prevent future dental problems and risk of developing BRONJ/MRONJ. Patient education is important to ensure they are aware of the risk of developing the condition which may also occur spontaneously. Symptomatic relief is required when the condition causes pain or discomfort. Antibiotics is indicated in infection cases. Surgery is reserved when patients do not or unlikely to respond to conservative management. Surgical treatment involves removal of teeth in affected sites, bone debridement, or resection of bone in advanced cases.

Self-Assessment Questions

1. Define BRONJ.
2. Describe the clinical features of BRONJ.
3. Discuss the differential diagnosis for BRONJ.
4. Describe the classification and stages in BRONJ
5. Discuss the pathophysiology of BRONJ and MRONJ.
6. Describe the histopathological features of BRONJ.

Summary

In the past twenty years, the clinical presentation of osteomyelitis has changed significantly. Currently, there are an increased number of patients with osteomyelitis despite all the benefits associated with the advances in medicine and dentistry. There are several factors responsible for this trend including development of microorganism resistance to commonly used antibiotics, increased number of immunocompromised patients such as patients with diabetes, HIV, organ transplants, patients who undergo radiation therapy, and patients treated with bisphosphonates.

Osteomyelitis of the jaws is predominantly seen in the mandible due to its limited vascularity. In the upper jaw, it accounts for only 1–6% of patients. Acute and secondary chronic osteomyelitis of the jaws is caused mostly by a bacterial focus (odontogenic disease, pulpal, and periodontal infection, extraction wounds, foreign bodies, and infected fractures). Primary chronic osteomyelitis of the jaw is rare and usually non-suppurative. Imaging is a very important diagnostic tool in the assessment of acute and chronic osteomyelitis of the jaws. To confirm and assess osteomyelitis of the jaws, a range of radiological techniques is available.

Histopathology has always been regarded as valuable in the diagnostic process of osteomyelitis, especially distinguishing it from other diseases of bone. Histopathology of osteomyelitis varies according to the nature of the disease including acute, chronic, specific types such as sclerosing type or Garre's osteomyelitis (proliferative periostitis).

Treatment depends on the type of osteomyelitis. Acute suppurative osteomyelitis usually responds to antibiotic therapy alone but in the case of chronic suppurative osteomyelitis, in addition to antibiotic therapy, it is necessary to combine surgery that aims to remove all necrotic soft and hard tissue.

Suggested Readings

Drake MT, Clarke BL, Khosla S. Bisphosphonates: mechanism of action and role in clinical practice. Mayo Clin Proc. 2008;83(9):1032–45. https://doi.org/10.4065/83.9.1032.

Rosella D, Papi P, Giardino R, Cicalini E, Piccoli L, Pompa G. Medication-related osteonecrosis of the jaw: clinical and practical guidelines. J Int Soc Prev Community Dent. 2016;6(2):97–104.

Ruggiero SL, Dodson TB, Fantasia J, et al. American Association of Oral and Maxillofacial Surgeons position paper on medication-related osteonecrosis of the jaw—2014 update. J Oral Maxillofac Surg. 2014;72:1938–56.

Shuster A, Reiser V, Trejo L, Ianculovici C, Kleinman S, Kaplan I. Comparison of the histopathological characteristics of osteomyelitis, medication-related osteonecrosis of the jaw, and osteoradionecrosis. Int J Oral Maxillofac Surg. 2018; https://doi.org/10.1016/j.ijom.2018.07.002.

Oral Manifestations of Autoimmune Disorders

Contents

Blisters and Ulcers on the Soft Palate: Pemphigus

B. S. M. S. Siriwardena and Ruwan Jayasinghe

Contents

W. M Tilakaratne, T. G. Kallarakkal (eds.), *Clinicopathological Correlation of Oral Diseases*,
https://doi.org/10.1007/978-3-031-24408-7_47

Learning Goals

1. Understand the pathogenesis of autoimmune blistering disorders
2. Learn different clinical manifestations of blistering disorders
3. Clinically differentiate PV from other vesiculo-bullous disorders
4. Identify histopathological differences
5. Learn different management strategies

47.1 Main Complaint

A 47-year-old male patient presents to the clinic complaining of non-healing multiple painful ulcers on the posterior palate.

47.2 History of Complaint

Question: When did you feel the pain and notice these ulcers?

These ulcers started to appear two months ago. Initially, they appeared as fluid-filled blisters which then ruptured soon leaving reddish patches. It took few weeks to heal. In the meantime, new blisters erupted.

47.3 Additional Complaints

Question: Do you have ulcers elsewhere in the mouth.

I don't have any, but it is difficult to brush my teeth due to reddish and sore gums.

Question: Did you have any similar ulcers in the past?

I have had similar ulcers at multiple times in the past.

Question: How frequently do these lesions appear and have you had any disease-free intervals?

I have been suffering for almost one year. These lesions appear frequently, and I have had about 6–7 recurrent attacks from the onset.

Question: Have you had any treatment for ulcers, or did they heal spontaneously?

I used a topical oral gel that was prescribed by my dentist. Although the ulcers disappeared for 1–2 months, it recurred from time to time.

Question: Do you have any whitish striations on the buccal mucosa or the tongue?

No, I haven't noticed any such lesions.

Question: Do you have ulceration/ irritation in the eyes?

I do not have any ulceration or irritation in my eyes.

Question: Do you have any irritation in the throat?

I do not have any irritation in my throat.

Question: Have you noticed any change in your voice in the recent past?

I have not experienced any such discomfort.

Question: Have you noticed any changes in your nails such as longitudinal ridging and grooving or splitting?

I do not have such changes.

Question: Do you have pain/burning sensation while passing urine? Is there any redness/ ulceration in the genital area?

I haven't had any discomfort while passing urine and no visible redness or ulcerations in the genital area.

Question: Do you have ulcers/lesions on the skin?

I have had scaly areas on the skin on my upper chest area from time to time, during last year. They initially presented as fluid-filled blisters then ruptured leaving erosions.

Question: Are you suffering from any other medical conditions such as high blood pressure, heart disease, diabetes, bleeding disorder, respiratory diseases? If yes, what kind of medications, have you been taking until now?

I am suffering from asthma and I am on Salbutamol inhaler.

Question: Have you undergone any dental treatment?

✓ I have undergone extraction of teeth due to dental caries.

? Question: Do you have any specific chewing habits?

✓ I used to chew betel quid with all ingredients (betel leaf, areca nut, lime and chewing tobacco), about 8–10 quids per day for more than 20 years.

? Question: Are you a smoker, or do you take alcohol?

✓ I do not smoke but take alcohol occasionally

? Question: What is your occupation?

✓ I am a farmer

? Question: Tell me about your family?

✓ I am married and have two children.

? Question: Does any of your family member or relative suffer from similar lesions?

✓ None of my family members or close relatives are suffering from similar lesions.

47.4 With the Findings from the History, What Is Your Differential Diagnosis?

1. Lichen planus
2. Mucocutaneous autoimmune blistering disorder
3. Recurrent aphthous ulceration (RAU)
4. Behcet disease
5. Erythema multiforme (EM)

47.5 How Do You Justify Your Differential Diagnosis after History Taking?

There are scaly skin lesions on the upper chest area that have been present for about a year. Ulcerations in the oral cavity are preceded by blisters. A diagnosis of a mucocutaneous skin disorder like lichen planus has to be included in the differential diagnosis. In lichen planus, there may be skin lesions that present typically as flat-topped violaceous papules usually affecting the wrists, ankles, and genitalia.

However, the ulcers are recurrent in nature; hence, a mucocutaneous autoimmune blistering disorder is also a possible differential diagnosis.

The most common recurrent ulcerations are aphthous stomatitis that consists of multiple shallow painful ulcers which recur at intervals of a few days to few months. Although the palatal mucosa is a rare site, oral lesions of this patient could be aphthous ulcers.

In Behcet disease (BD), appearance of aphthae on the oral mucosa with recurrent genital and ocular ulcers is characteristic. Genital ulcers are seen in approximately 75% of BD patients. Skin lesions in BD initially appear as red and raised, or pus-filled bumps that leave faint scars or discolourations. With the clinical description, BD could be a possible differential diagnosis.

Erythema multiforme has distinctive mucosal and skin lesions. The initial skin lesions of EM are usually round, erythematous, edematous papules surrounded by areas of blanching that may resemble insect bites or papular urticaria. Typical target lesions of the skin begins with raised center that later coalesce with indistinct borders. Oral lesions initially present as erythema with some edema and progress to superficial erosions. Although the commonly affected sites of the oral cavity are labial and buccal mucosae, palatal mucosa can rarely be affected.

47.6 Findings of Clinical Examination

He has several red-based superficial erosions on the mucosa close to tuberosity area. In the soft palate region, there are multiple, irregular, fibrin-covered erosions (◘ Fig. 47.1). There are no visible blisters. Anterior hard palate, buccal mucosa, lips, and tongue are uninvolved. There is no evidence of scarring in the oral mucosa.

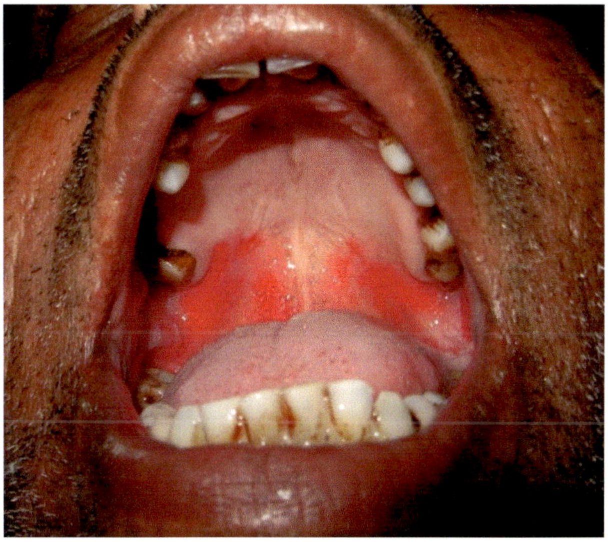

◘ **Fig. 47.1** Diffuse erosive lesions at the posterior hard palate and soft palate

Both upper and lower gingivae are reddish with mild swelling. Erosions are noted in focal areas. There is generalized plaque accumulation with the presence of calculi in a few places. Appearance is consistent with desquamative gingivitis.

47.7 What Other Relevant Features Would You Look for with the Findings You Have So Far?

Scaly lesions were noticed on the skin with evidence of healing (Fig. 47.2). The patient was referred to a dermatologist for review and management of skin lesions. There were no blisters on the skin and the dermatologist confirmed that the other mucosal sites such as the nasal, genital, conjunctival, and esophageal mucosae were free of lesions.

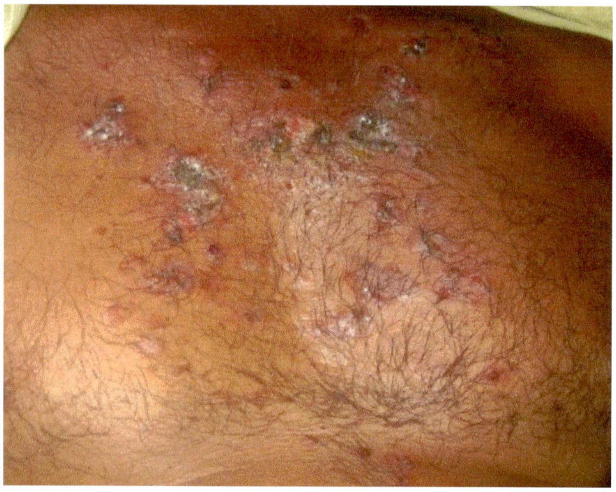

Fig. 47.2 Scaly skin lesions on the upper chest area

47.8 What Is Your Clinical Differential Diagnosis?

1. Bullous/ulcerative oral lichen planus
2. Pemphigus
3. Pemphigoid
4. Linear IgA disease
5. Dermatitis herpetiformis
6. Epidermolysis bullosa acquisita

47.9 How Would You Justify the Inclusion of the Diseases That You Have Mentioned in the Differential Diagnosis to Arrive at a Working Diagnosis?

Oral lichen planus (OLP) is a chronic mucocutaneous inflammatory condition which can present as ulcerative, atrophic, or bullous forms. Commonest sites of involvement are buccal mucosa followed by tongue and gingiva. It is very rare to see the involvement of palate. Skin lesions in OLP are commonly seen on the flexor surfaces of the hands and legs and back of the body. Lesions on the skin cause itching and are self-limiting. In most patients with bullous or ulcerative OLP, white striations can be seen in the mouth. Absence of characteristic striations and involvement of the soft palate may not be supportive of OLP.

Presence of oral lesions is the initial presentation in some patients with pemphigus. Progression to cutaneous involvement is seen in 75% of affected patients. All mucosal surfaces may be affected but soft palate is the most commonly involved oral site, followed by the buccal mucosa, tongue, and gingiva causing desquamative gingivitis. Lesions start as vesicles or blisters with a clear content that develop on normal or erythematous skin. Oral lesions rupture soon leaving erosions or ulcerations. Intact vesicles/bullae may be seen on the skin but not in the mouth. Considering the site and appearance of the lesion, pemphigus vulgaris is a very likely diagnosis in this case.

Mucous membrane pemphigoid (MMP) is an autoimmune disease, most seen in middle-aged to older females. It is characterized by bullous eruptions and ulceration, particularly in the oral mucosa and conjunctiva. Healing occurs with scaring giving rise to complications. 80% of the affected patients have oral ulcerations. The commonest site of involvement is the gingiva causing desquamative gingivitis. 70% of the affected patients may have conjunctival lesions. Laryngeal mucosa may also get involved causing changes in voice. About 20% of the patients develop skin lesions as well. Although the patient had multiple episodes of ulceration, there is no evidence of scarring in the oral cavity. This finding is not supportive of MMP.

Linear IgA disease is a rare condition mainly involving the skin of children and older adults. Patients present with itchy rash with small blisters arranged as clusters or rings. Blisters may be limited to one area of the skin or can be seen all over the body. The blisters may be arranged lying around the rim of wheal-like red patches ("string of pearls sign"). Up to 80% of affected adults can have blisters or ulcers in the mouth, eyes, or the genital region. Hard palate, soft palate, and the buccal mucosa are the common oral sites. Lesions are usually symmetrical. Absence of characteristic skin lesions may not support the diagnosis of linear IgA disease.

Dermatitis herpetiformis is an uncommon chronic skin disease that rarely affects the oral mucosa. Erythematous areas about 1–3 cm in size may appear on the palate and buccal mucosa. Aphthae can be seen on labial mucosa. Oral lesions appear months or years after the skin lesions.

Epidermolysis bullosa acquisita manifests with blistering and erosions of the skin and mucous membranes. Tense vesicles and scarred skin may see in some patients while nail dystrophy and scarring alopecia have been observed in some others. Desquamative gingivitis could be a possible clinical presentation. However, lesions appear in trauma-prone areas particularly tongue and lips. Oral manifestations are extremely rare.

47.10 What Is the Most Likely Diagnosis and Why?

The patient has recurrent ulcers that started as blisters followed by erosions. Most lesions are confined to the soft palate region and gingiva leading to desquamative gingivitis. There is no evidence of scarring in the oral mucosa. Skin lesions in PV appear as thin-walled flaccid blisters that easily rupture causing itchy and painful erosions followed by crusting. They are often arise on the upper chest, back, scalp, and face. These features are supportive to arrive at the diagnosis of pemphigus vulgaris as the working diagnosis.

47.11 How Would You Investigate This Patient?

1. Nikolsky sign: This is a supportive clinical sign for pemphigus and is produced by applying lateral pressure to the mucosa or skin in the peri-lesional area resulting in separation of the epidermis in the normal areas. However, this is not a reliable test to arrive at the diagnosis as some other lesions may show the same.
2. Incisional biopsy for routine histopathology and direct immunofluorescence (DIF) test.
3. Immunoserology: Indirect immunofluorescence (IIF) assists to detect circulating autoantibodies using normal skin or other mucosae as a substrate. Anti-desmoglein (DSG) 1 and 3 are useful in the diagnosis of pemphigus vulgaris. Evaluation of autoantibodies is very useful in assessing the treatment response in the management.

47.12 How Would You Do an Incisional Biopsy for This Patient? What Are the Important Considerations?

The biopsy should include perilesional tissue that has the epithelium for DIF. The specimen should not be fixed in routine 10% formal saline, and it should be sent to the laboratory immediately for freezing (on a piece of gauze soaked with saline). Transportation to a distant laboratory should be in a suitable transport media (Michel solution). The lesional tissue should be included for routine hematoxylin and eosin sections.

47.13 What Specific Histopathological Features Are Helpful to Arrive at the Definitive Diagnosis?

Intraepithelial separation is evident just above the basal layer (◘ Figs. 47.3 and 47.4). Acantholytic cells (Tzanck cells) can be observed within the intraepithelial blisters. Intact basal cell layer shows characteristic tomb stone appearance. A mixed inflammatory infiltrate predominantly consisting of eosinophils is seen within the underlying connective tissue. These histo-

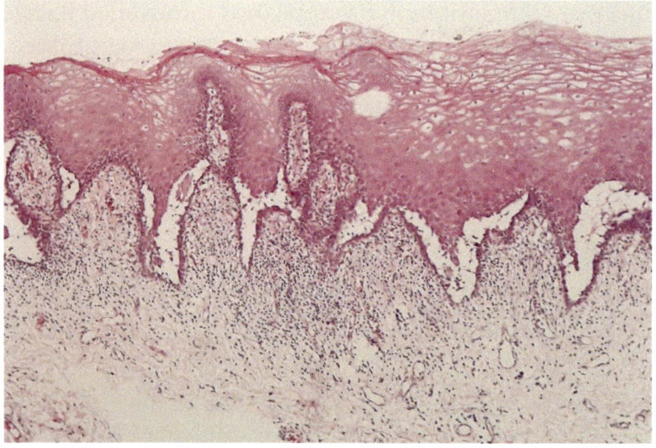

Fig. 47.3 Intraepithelial separation just above the basal layer

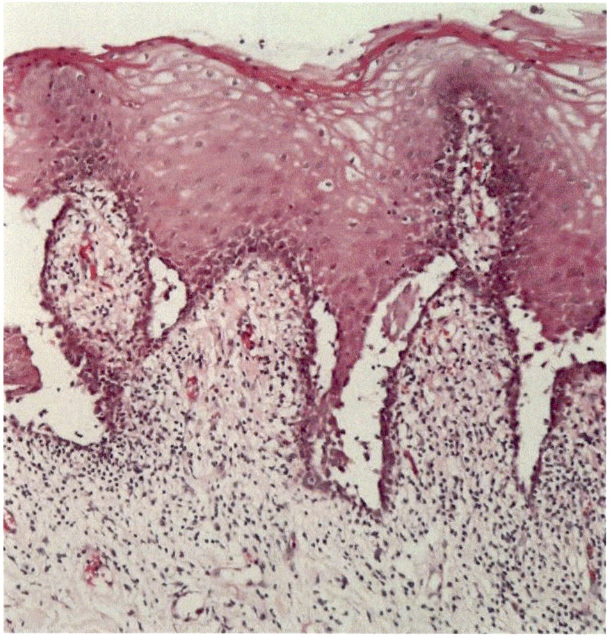

Fig. 47.4 Intact basal layer showing tomb stone appearance and Tzanck cells are present within intraepithelial blisters

pathological features are supportive for the diagnosis of pemphigus vulgaris.

A confirmatory diagnosis can be established with DIF test. In pemphigus, intercellular binding of IgG and/or C3 is found in the epidermis/epithelium (Fig. 47.5) while in pemphigoid, linear band of IgG and/or C3 is seen at the basement membrane zone.

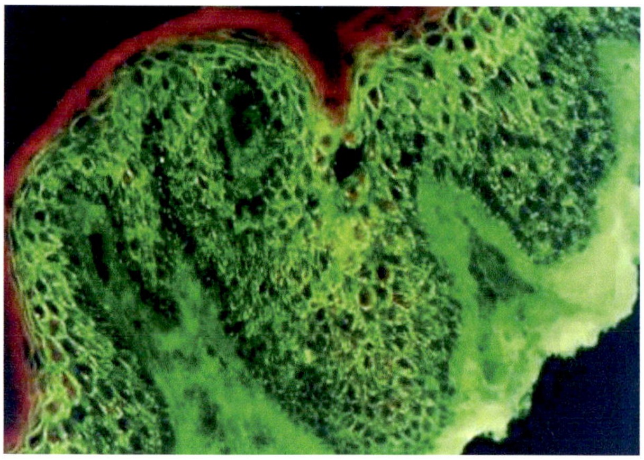

Fig. 47.5 Direct immunofluorescence showing strong intercellular binding of IgG

47.14 What Is the Definitive Diagnosis?

Pemphigus vulgaris

47.15 What Is the Treatment Protocol?

Pemphigus is a life-threatening disease in the absence of proper management due to loss of body fluids and secondary bacterial infection. Management of pemphigus has to be always carried out by specialists and within a multidisciplinary team. Treatment of choice is systemic corticosteroid therapy. Immunosuppressants and immunomodulating drugs like azathioprine, dapsone, methotrexate, cyclophosphamide, and cyclosporine are useful adjuvants or alternatives. Topical corticosteroids are useful in the remission period or only when localized oral lesions are present. Majority of cases of pemphigus vulgaris will eventually end up having skin lesions hence requiring systemic therapy at some point. Improvement of oral hygiene and minimizing irritation of the oral lesions is essential.

All these drugs used in the management of pemphigus vulgaris can induce significant side effects. Careful follow-up and monitoring of the patients are essential to identify the side effects. All patients require basic investigations such as full blood count, serum electrolytes test, blood sugar levels, renal and liver function tests prior to the treatment and should be repeated regularly during follow-up. Osteoporosis prevention guidelines have to be followed.

47.16 Pemphigus Vulgaris

Autoimmune blistering dermatoses comprise a heterogeneous group of diseases that are characterized by autoantibodies to structural components of the skin and adjacent mucous membranes. In pemphigus, autoantibodies are directed against desmosomal proteins that connect neighboring keratinocytes. The first author to describe pemphigus vulgaris in a patient was MacBride in 1777. The incidence of pemphigus is approximately 1 in 100,000 people. Pemphigus vulgaris is the most common variant of pemphigus with an incidence of 0.1 to 0.5 per 100,000 populations and is higher among Jewish patients. Various environmental and pharmacologic etiological factors have been reported in pemphigus. These factors include medications, pesticides, malignancy, ultraviolet radiation, and stress.

The diagnosis is made from the clinical picture and histopathologic studies. However, confirmatory diagnosis requires detection of autoantibodies in tissues by direct immunofluorescence (DIF) or in the circulation by indirect immunofluorescence (IIF). In addition, specific target antigen by enzyme-linked immunosorbent assay (ELISA) or Western blot can also be performed. The classification of bullous dermatoses still relies on histologic criteria, primarily according to the localization of bullae. Accordingly, blistering diseases are classified as intraepidermal/intraepithelial and subepidermal/subepithelial disorders.

The presence of acantholytic keratinocytes is considered a key element for the histologic diagnosis of pemphigus. Acantholytic cells themselves, however, are neither pathognomonic for a particular disease nor an exclusive feature of intraepithelial bullous diseases. Pemphigus is an intraepithelial bullous disorder that can present alone in the skin or mucosa or in both. Pemphigus family is comprised of different subtypes such as pemphigus vulgaris, pemphigus foliaceus, pemphigus vegetans, pemphigus erythematosus, IgA pemphigus, and paraneoplastic pemphigus (PNP). PV is the commonest type which occurs in the oral mucosa. The fully developed PV lesions are characterized by the occurrence of intraepithelial vesicles mostly located immediately above the basal layer of the epithelium.

Pemphigus vulgaris is slightly more common in women and occurs primarily in adults during the 5th or 6th decade of life. There is a strong genetic background to pemphigus with linkage to HLA class II alleles and ethnic groups such as Ashkenazi Jews and those of Mediterranean and Indian origin. The primary feature of pemphigus vulgaris is that it typically runs a chronic course, almost invariably causing blisters, erosions, and ulcers on the oral mucosa and skin. These lesions may occur on the mucosae of pharynx, larynx, esophagus, nose, conjunctiva as well as genital regions. On the oral mucosa, lesions can occur anywhere, but the soft palate and buccal mucosa are the most commonly affected sites followed by involvement of the palatal, lingual, and labial mucosa. Gingiva is the least commonly affected site and desquamative gingivitis is the commonest manifestation of the disease when gingiva is involved. Pemphigus vulgaris often begins with blister formation in the mouth. The blisters are soft and fragile. Skin lesions present as flaccid fluid-filled blisters on sites exposed to trauma. The blisters break to form large, denuded areas of skin which can prove fatal if extensive areas are involved.

In case of mucosal involvement of pemphigus vulgaris, the lesions are histologically identical to skin lesions. Any mucous membrane can be involved. Oral lesions are almost always present and can be the first manifestation of the disease. Examination of patients with exclusively oral lesions may frequently be hampered because intact bullae are difficult to find clinically due to rupture as a result of trauma or mastication and mucosal tags might lie over the ruptured bullae. Therefore, the histology of biopsy specimens might only show erosions or ulcerations. Therefore, biopsy specimens should preferably be obtained from the margin of a denuded area, where specific histological alterations can be detected. In patients with only oral lesions, the specimen should be obtained from intact oral mucosa for DIF assay, which is more sensitive than routine light microscopic study. Histological examination alone is not sufficient to make a precise diagnosis of pemphigus vulgaris. The diagnosis should be confirmed by DIF, IIF assay, or ELISA using Dsg1 and Dsg3 recombinant fusion proteins. The bullae in pemphigus rupture easily. Therefore, it is important to obtain a biopsy specimen from an early lesion to make an accurate diagnosis. A biopsy specimen should also be obtained from a very small lesion (a bulla as a whole) so that the epidermis/epithelium remains attached to the dermis/submucosa. Punch biopsy should not be performed due to the shear moment and possible epidermis detachment from the dermis. Previous application of a cooling spray is recommended if a punch technique is used. A bulla can be excised with a scalpel.

Mortality from PV before the development of effective therapies was as high as 90% and was often fatal mainly from dehydration or secondary systemic infection. It has reduced to approximately 5–15% with the advent of effective therapies.

The etiology of pemphigus vulgaris is uncertain. A strong association with certain HLA Class II alleles (DRBI*0402 and DQBI*0503) has been demonstrated in pemphigus vulgaris. Other initiating factors reported include certain foods (garlic), infections, neoplasms, and drugs (thiol group, rifampicin).

In oral pemphigus vulgaris, autoantibodies are produced against desmosomes, especially desmoglein 3 (Dsg 3). Another important component of desmosome is desmoglein 1 (Dsg1). The latter is the target of autoantibody formation in pemphigus foliaceous that affects cutaneous sites only. Dsg 3 is predominantly expressed in oral epithelium while both Dsg 1 and Dsg 3 are expressed in skin. Dsg1 is expressed more intensely in the superficial layers and Dsg 3 is found more abundantly in the basal and suprabasal layers. Dsg 1 and 3 are components of desmosomal cadherins which hold the epithelial cells together. The loss of adhesive function results in bulla formation. If the autoantibodies are directed against Dsg 3, the vesicle forms immediately suprabasally, and if it is directed against Dsg 1, the vesicle is more superficial.

Histopathological characteristics, immunofluorescence analysis, and further immunologic laboratory testing must be integrated with the clinical findings in order to establish an accurate diagnosis. Histopathologically, pemphigus vulgaris displays acantholysis, suprabasal separation of the epithelium, and sparse inflammatory infiltrate. These findings occur due to IgG autoantibodies targeting the desmosomal protein desmoglein 3, which serves an important role in intercellular adhesion of the epidermis and epithelium. DIF on a perilesional mucocutaneous biopsy displays intercellular deposition of IgG antibody and/or C3 complement along the epithelial cell surfaces. IIF shows the presence of circulating serum IgG autoantibodies through intercellular deposition on substrates such as human skin or monkey esophagus. Enzyme-linked immunosorbent assay (ELISA) allows for further specificity. Antibody levels of Dsg 1 and Dsg 3, detected by ELISA, correlates well with disease severity at cutaneous and oral sites, respectively. In future, the diagnosis and long-term follow-up of patients with pemphigus would rely on detecting and quantifying antibodies against desmoglein proteins using ELISA.

The treatment for pemphigus vulgaris is by systemic corticosteroids even if confined to oral mucosa. Oral lesions may partially respond to topical steroid applications, but it is necessary to treat systemically if the disease is widespread with involvement of the skin and other mucosal surfaces. Before the advent of steroids, the mortality rate was 30% and currently it is about 6% due to the effects of immunosuppressive therapy. The initial dose of corticosteroids is typically about 0.75–1 mg/kg/day, and it can be increased depending on the responsiveness by 25%–50% in every 5–7 days. If more than 1 mg/kg/day of prednisolone is needed, adjuvant immunosuppressants are added such as azathioprine, cyclophosphamide, and mycophenolate for their "steroid-sparing" effect. Tapering of steroids should be done by 25% every 2 weeks. When the patient reaches a dose <20 mg, taper more slowly. 5 mg reduction every 4 weeks could be suitable for most of the patients. The duration of corticosteroid therapy is variable.

The histopathological diagnosis along with DIF is necessary to confirm the diagnosis. ELISA is helpful to determine the severity of the disease and can measure the response level after systemic therapy of corticosteroids. As it is a life-threatening disease, it is important that the dental professionals are able to recognize oral manifestations of pemphigus vulgaris and refer appropriately.

Salient features of pemphigus vulgaris	
Clinical features	Presence of erosions on the soft palate and other oral sites together with desquamative gingivitis and blisters on the skin.
Histopathology	Intraepithelial cleft just above the basal layer with acantholytic cells (Tzanck cells) and intact basal layer (Tomb stone appearance). A mixed inflammatory infiltrate with eosinophils. Direct immunofluorescence on a perilesional biopsy displays intercellular deposition of IgG antibody and/or C3 complement along the cell surfaces.
Treatment	Management by a multidisciplinary team. Treatment of choice is corticosteroid therapy.

Self-Assessment Questions

1. Discuss the clinical differential diagnoses when a patient presents, with blisters and erosions on the oral mucosa.
2. Describe different types of pemphigus.
3. Describe the histological features of pemphigus.
4. Explain the advanced molecular techniques used to confirm the diagnosis of pemphigus.

Diagnostic Algorithm for Pemphigus

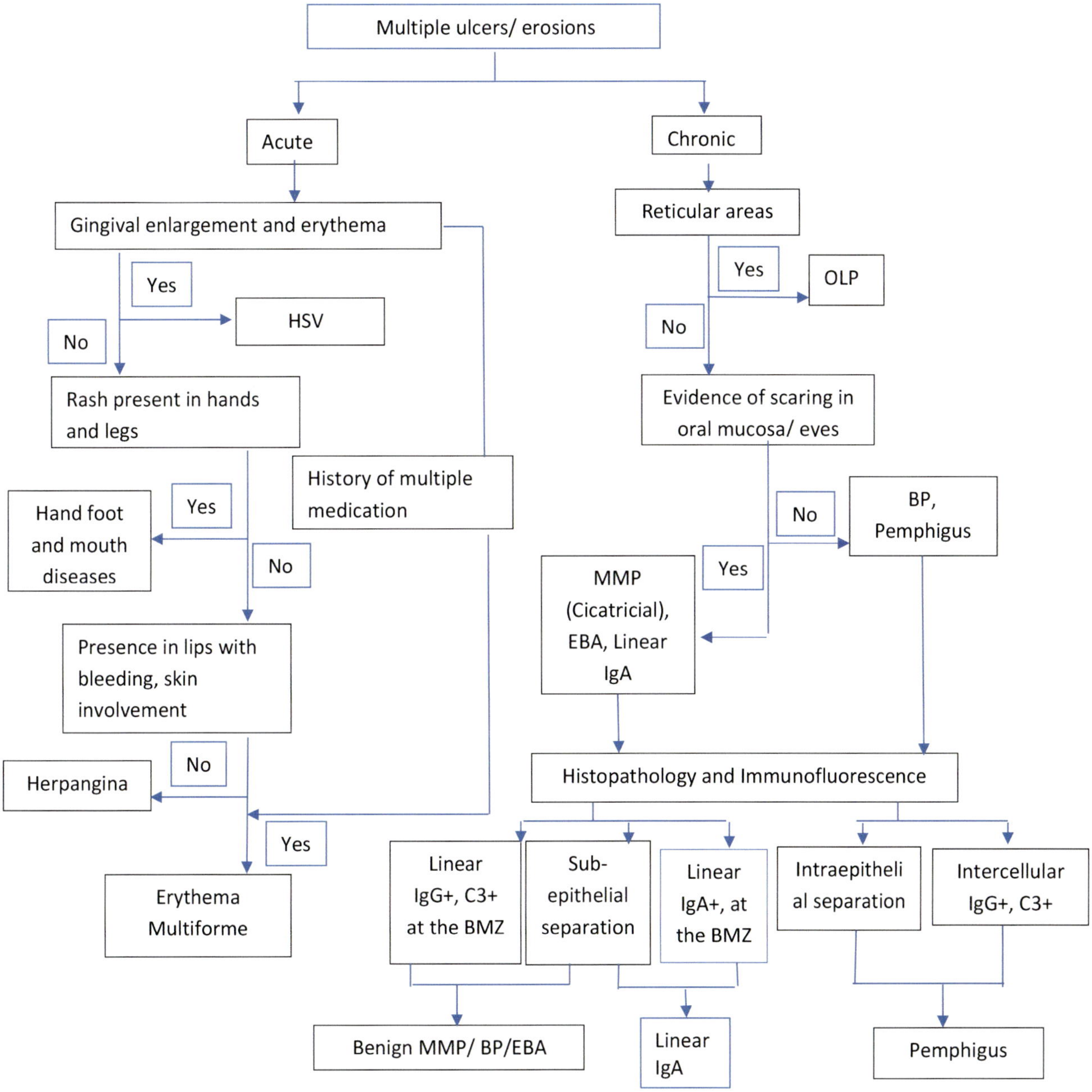

HSV- herpes simplex virus, OLP-oral lichen planus, BP- bullous pemphigoid, MMP- mucous membrane pemphigoid, BMZ- basement membrane zone, EBA- epidermolysis bullosa aquisita.

Summary

Pemphigus is defined as a group of life-threatening blistering disorder of skin and mucous membrane characterized by intraepithelial blistering induced by circulatory autoantibodies to intercellular adhesion molecules. Definitive diagnosis of pemphigus vulgaris can be achieved by histopathology and direct immunofluorescence. Pemphigus vulgaris is generally managed with local and systemic corticosteroid therapy.

Suggested Readings

Eduardo Calonje J, Brenn T, Lazar A, Billings S. McKee's pathology of the skin. 5th ed. Elsevier; n.d. 2019.

Hannah R, Ramani P, Tilakaratne WM, Sukumaran G, Ramasubramanian A, Krishnan RP. Critical appraisal of different triggering pathways for the pathobiology of pemphigus vulgaris: a review. Oral Dis. 2021; https://doi.org/10.1111/odi.13937.

Kasperkiewicz M, Ellebrecht C, Takahashi H, et al. Pemphigus. Nat Rev Dis Primers. 2017;3:17,026. https://doi.org/10.1038/nrdp.2017.26.

Manocha A, Tirumalae R. Histopathology of pemphigus vulgaris revisited. Am J Dermatopathol. 2020; https://doi.org/10.1097/DAD.0000000000001838.

Sanders WJ. A brief review of pemphigus vulgaris. Biomed Dermatol. 2017;1:7. https://doi.org/10.1186/s41702-017-0008-1.

Saschenbrecker S, Karl I, Komorowski L, Probst C, Dähnrich C, Fechner K, Stöcker W, Schlumberger W. Serological diagnosis of autoimmune bullous skin diseases. Front Immunol. 2019;10:1974. https://doi.org/10.3389/fimmu.2019.01974.

A Patient Presenting with Desquamative Gingivitis: Mucous Membrane Pemphigoid

B. S. M. S. Siriwardena and Ruwan Jayasinghe

Contents

W. M Tilakaratne, T. G. Kallarakkal (eds.), *Clinicopathological Correlation of Oral Diseases*,
https://doi.org/10.1007/978-3-031-24408-7_48

- **Learning Goals**
  1. Understand the pathogenesis of autoimmune blistering disorders
  2. Learn the oral manifestation of subepithelial blistering disorders
  3. Clinically differentiate from other vesiculo-bullous type disorders
  4. Identify histopathological differences
  5. Learn the management

48.1 Main Complaint

A 55-year-old woman presents to the clinic with painful, reddish, and ulcerated gingivae.

48.2 History of Complaint

Question: When did you notice these changes?

I noticed these changes three to four months ago. It shows different appearances from time to time.

Question: Can you explain those changes?

It starts as reddish areas on the gums followed by occasional blisters which subsequently rupture and become ulcers. They are painful and take several weeks to heal.

48.3 Additional Complaints

Question: Do you have ulcers elsewhere in the mouth?

I do not have any at the moment but previously there were occasional blisters and similar ulcers in the mouth on the right side of the cheek. I also notice that the mucosa is peeling off while eating or brushing my teeth.

Question: Do you feel any roughness or scarring inside the mouth on the right cheek?

I do feel roughness inside the mouth on the right cheek.

Question: Do you have ulceration/irritation in the eyes?

I do not experience such difficulty.

Question: Do you have any irritation in the throat?

I do not have any discomfort of that nature.

Question: Did you notice any change in your voice in the recent past?

I haven't noticed any such change.

Question: Do you have any nasal bleeding?

I do not have any nasal bleeding.

Question: Do you have pain or burning sensation while passing urine? Have you noticed redness or ulceration in the genital area?

I have not had any discomfort while passing urine. I have not noticed any visible redness or ulcerations in the genital area.

Question: Do you have any ulcers or blisters on the skin?

I do not have any ulcers or blisters on my skin

Question: Are you suffering from any other medical conditions such as high blood pressure, heart disease, diabetes, bleeding disorder, and respiratory diseases? If yes, what kind of medications, have you been taking until now?

I am not suffering from any other medical problems. I am not taking any medications other than the analgesics prescribed by my family doctor for pain.

Question: Have you undergone any dental treatment?

I have undergone dental treatment for two teeth due to caries.

Question: Do you smoke or take alcohol?

I do not smoke or consume alcohol.

Question: What is your occupation?

I am a housewife.

Question: Tell me about your family?

I am married and have three children.

? Question: Does any of your family members or relatives suffer from similar lesions?

✓ None of my family members or close relatives suffer from similar lesions.

48.4 With the Findings from the History, What is Your Differential Diagnosis?

1. Mucus membrane (Cicatricial) pemphigoid
2. Oral lichen planus
3. Pemphigus vulgaris
4. Epidermolysis bullosa acquisita
5. Contact stomatitis

48.5 How Do You Justify Your Differential Diagnosis After History Taking?

Mucous membrane pemphigoid (MMP) or cicatricial pemphigoid is a chronic autoimmune, mucocutaneous disorder commonly seen in elderly females. Lesions appear as vesicles that soon rupture leaving erosions or ulcerations. The commonest site of involvement is the gingiva affecting more than 70% of patients. MMP is one of the conditions in which desquamative gingivitis may be the only oral manifestation. Ulcers in MMP heal by scaring resulting in high morbidity. It can involve other mucous membranes like nasal, genital, and ocular mucosae. Skin involvement occurs in around 25% of the patients. The age of the patient, possible history of recurrence, clinical presentation of blisters that ulcerate and gingival involvement are strongly suggestive of MMP.

Oral lichen planus (OLP) is a chronic immune-mediated, mucocutaneous disorder commonly seen in females. OLP has multiple clinical presentations such as plaque and reticular forms, which are usually asymptomatic, and symptomatic forms include erosive, ulcerative, and bullous types. When erosive lesions of OLP involve the gingivae, the term desquamative gingivitis is used. Although OLP is a possible differential diagnosis, isolated desquamative gingivitis in OLP is rare.

Bullous pemphigoid (BP) is a chronic autoimmune blistering disorder primarily affecting the skin, with occasional mild mucosal lesions. Lesions in the oral mucosa may show erosions, bullae, and desquamative gingivitis. In the absence of skin lesions, oral involvement is exceptionally rare in BP.

Pemphigus (PV) is a life-threatening blistering disorder commonly seen in middle-age females. Oral lesions may be the initial presentation in many patients and lesions can proceed to cutaneous involvement in 75% of affected patients. All mucosal surfaces may be affected but soft palate is the commonest site, followed by the buccal mucosa, tongue, and gingiva causing desquamative gingivitis. Isolated desquamative gingivitis is rare in PV.

Epidermolysis bullosa acquisita (EBA) is a rare, autoimmune disorder, which can have involvement of mucosae. In EBA, clinical presentation may change over time. Desquamative gingivitis could be a possible clinical presentation. The lesions usually appear in trauma-prone areas particularly tongue and lips.

Contact stomatitis is a rare condition affecting the oral mucosae and is due to inflammation of the oral mucosa caused by external substances. It can be caused by a variety of substances including dental materials, drugs, or oral hygiene products. Even though oral mucosa is exposed to large number of allergenic substances, contact allergic reactions are less common in oral mucosa than in the skin. It usually presents as acute oral ulcerations which can involve any oral mucosal surface. Involvement of gingiva may cause desquamative gingivitis but involvement of gingiva alone is exceptionally uncommon.

48.6 Findings of Clinical Examination

The patient has ulcers with a creamy/whitish slough and erythema on the gingiva (◻ Fig. 48.1). The ulcers are painful. Both upper and lower gingivae are affected. Most ulcers are coalesced to form larger erythematous areas. There are no ulcers on the labial mucosa and no evidence of visible intact blisters. Her whole gingiva is reddish and swollen in most areas. Few areas of the right-side buccal mucosa are erythematous and firm on palpation. The buccal mucosa on the left side appears normal. There is evidence of scarring on the right-side buccal mucosa towards commissure. The tongue appears to be normal. Oral hygiene is acceptable with evidence of some gingival recession. The appearance of the gingivae is compatible with desquamative gingivitis.

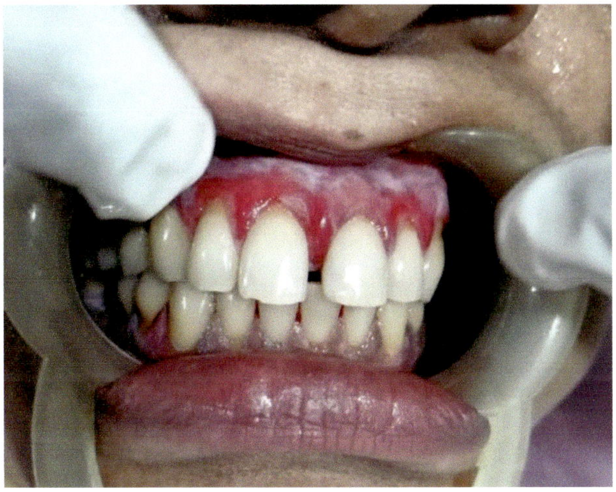

Fig. 48.1 Erythematous and swollen gingiva with focal areas showing whitish/creamy slough

48.7 What Other Relevant Features Would You Look for with the Findings You Have So Far?

The skin should be examined for any visible blisters or evidence of healed lesions. The patient should be referred to relevant specialists to confirm the presence or absence of other mucosal lesions involving nasal, genital, conjunctival, and oesophageal mucosae.

48.8 What is Your Clinical Differential Diagnosis?

1. Mucous membrane pemphigoid (MMP)
2. Pemphigus vulgaris (PV)
3. Oral lichen planus (bullous/ ulcerative)
4. Epidermolysis bullosa acquisita (EBA)

48.9 How Would You Justify the Inclusion of the Diseases That You Have Mentioned in the Differential Diagnosis?

MMP is characterized by bullous eruptions followed by ulceration, particularly of the oral mucosa and conjunctiva. Healing occurs with scaring leading to its complications. Oral ulcerations occur in 80% of the affected patients. The clinical presentation of blisters followed by ulceration, desquamative gingivitis, and evidence of scarring in this patient suggests the possibility of MMP.

OLP is a chronic mucocutaneous inflammatory condition which presents in many clinical forms. The symptomatic forms include ulcerative, atrophic, and bullous types. The common sites of involvement are the buccal mucosa followed by the tongue and the gingiva. The patients with most forms of OLP show typical features of lichen planus such as white striations elsewhere in the mouth. However, there were no such features in this patient.

Oral lesions in PV are the initial presentation in some patients and affect all mucosal surfaces with blisters followed by ulceration. Although desquamative gingivitis is one of the oral presentations, scarring is not a feature of pemphigus.

Epidermolysis bullosa manifests with blistering and erosions of the skin and mucous membranes. It occurs either as an acquired or inherited form and oral manifestations are very rare. Although EBA should be in the differential diagnosis, it is an unlikely diagnosis in this case as there are no skin lesions.

48.10 What is the Most Likely Diagnosis and Why?

MMP is the most likely diagnosis. Presence of desquamative gingivitis, ulcerations preceded by blisters on the buccal mucosa, and scarring in an elderly female patient is helpful in arriving MMP as the working diagnosis.

48.11 How Would You Investigate This Patient?

1. Nikolsky sign is a phenomenon characterized by epithelial desquamation as a result of slight pressure or rubbing the mucosa or skin. The sign is present when slight rubbing of the skin results in separation of the outermost layer, forming a blister within minutes. In the dental clinic, the presence of Nikolsky sign can be evaluated by the application of a firm sliding or rubbing force to the mucosal surface using a dental instrument. When the blister appears in the vicinity of an existing blister, it is called marginal Nikolsky sign and if it is elicited away from the blister, it is called direct Nikolsky sign. This sign is positive in both pemphigus and MMP. However, it is not a suitable method to differentiate these two lesions. Nikolsky sign on the oral mucosa may cause unnecessary injury to the tissue and pain to the patient. Therefore, it may not be ethical to perform it unless it is very essential in the diagnosis.
2. Incisional biopsy: This can be used for both routine histopathology and direct immunofluorescence.
3. Immunoserology:

Several immunoserologic tests are available to detect circulating autoantibodies. Circulating autoantibodies in serum in PV is high and therefore very useful in the diagnosis and monitoring the disease progression. However, in MMP, antibody titers are usually low and may not be helpful. Indirect immunofluorescence (IIF) is very useful in assessing the treatment response in the management of MMP.

48.12 How Would You Do an Incisional Biopsy for This Patient? What are the Important Considerations?

The biopsy should be obtained from the lesion extending to perilesional area including clinically normal epithelium. Entire biopsy from the ulcerated area may hinder diagnosis. The sample should not be fixed in 10% formal saline and it should be sent to the laboratory immediately for freezing (on a piece of gauze soaked in saline). If it is necessary to send the sample to a distant laboratory, it should be transported in a suitable media (Michel solution).

48.13 The Haematoxylin & Eosin Stained Sections from the Biopsy Showed a Subepithelial Blister. What Specific Histopathological Features and Immunofluorescence Findings are Helpful to Arrive at the Definitive Diagnosis?

MMP typically demonstrates a subepithelial blister with an eosinophil and/or neutrophil-rich leukocytic infiltrate within the superficial lamina propria and along the basement membrane zone (◘ Figs. 48.2 and 48.3). If there is a history of recurrent lesions, fibrosis may be observed. It is necessary to perform direct immunofluorescence test (DIF) for the definitive diagnosis as other subepithelial blistering disorders share similar histopathology.

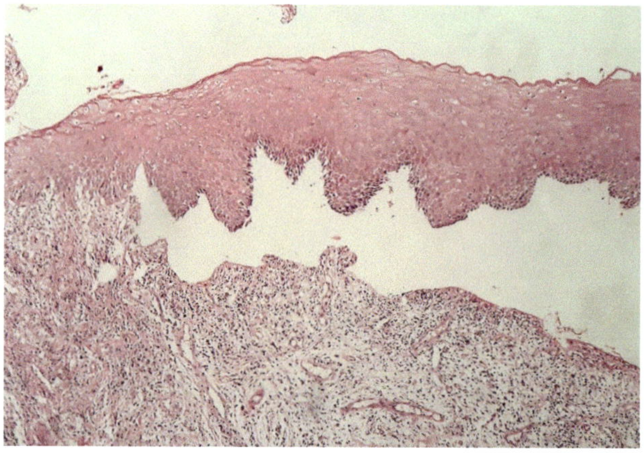

◘ **Fig. 48.2** Subepithelial separation lifting the full thickness of the epithelium creating a blister

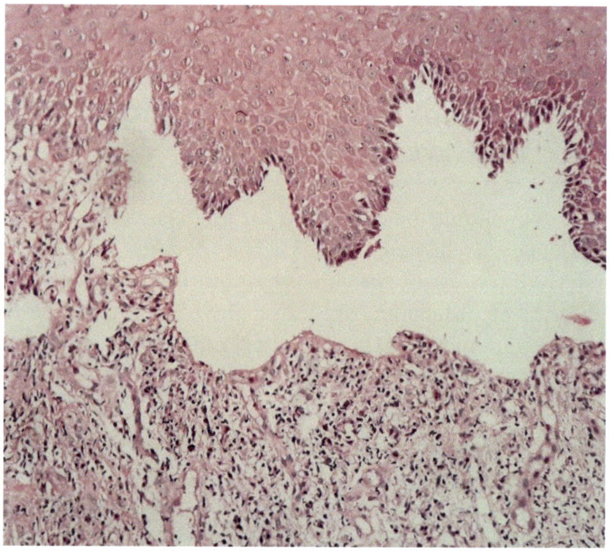

◘ **Fig. 48.3** A subepithelial blister and a moderate chronic inflammatory infiltrate is present in the superficial lamina propria

A DIF typically shows linear deposits of immunoglobulin G (IgG) and complement 3 (C3) along epithelial basement membrane zone (◘ Fig. 48.4). A minority of cases may show IgM and IgA deposits. In contrast to MMP, PV demonstrates intercellular deposits of IgG, IgM, and C3.

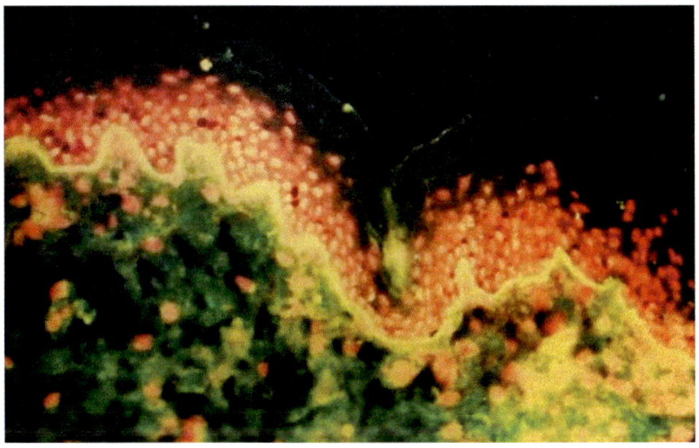

Fig. 48.4 Deposition of C3 along the basement membrane zone (immunofluorescence image courtesy of Dr Ramesh Kumar and Dr Pratibha Ramani)

48.14 What is the Definitive Diagnosis?

Mucous membrane pemphigoid

48.15 How Do You Manage This Patient?

A multidisciplinary approach is essential in the management of MMP. The first international consensus report on MMP in 2002 recommended to divide patients into low-risk and high-risk groups based upon the site of involvement. The low-risk patients were defined as having only oral mucosal or oral and skin involvement while high-risk patients should have involvement of the ocular, genital, nasopharyngeal, oesophageal, and/or laryngeal mucosae. High-risk patients require more aggressive treatment. This patient can be categorized as a low-risk patient based on the clinical presentation of having only oral lesions.

Multiple treatment modalities are available for the management of MMP. Non-specific immunosuppression, especially with corticosteroids, remains the main treatment modality. A short course of systemic steroids followed by topical application is adequate in majority of patients, but effectiveness of topical treatment can be influenced by the severity of the ulceration and site of involvement. Severe side effects of steroids and contraindications limit the use of steroids in some patients. Dapsone is a good alternative and can be started at 25–50 mg per day and increasing monthly by 25–50 mg until clinical remission is achieved or until the maximum tolerable dose is reached (usually 200 mg per day). A failure to obtain any improvement within approximately 3 months should prompt consideration of another agent such as azathioprine, methotrexate, cyclophosphamide, or hydroxychloroquine particularly if the disease affects high-risk sites such as the ocular surface.

All the above-mentioned drugs can induce significant side effects. Careful follow-up and monitoring of the patient is essential to identify the side effects such as monitoring the level of glucose-6-phosphate dehydrogenase due to the risk of haemolysis. Monitoring during therapy is required to assess for adverse effects including dose-related haemolytic anaemia and methemoglobinaemia, and other idiosyncratic side effects such as agranulocytosis and hepatitis. Furthermore, fatal hypersensitivity syndrome has been reported with the use of dapsone (dapsone hypersensitivity syndrome; DHS). DHS is a rare dose-independent adverse effect which develops several weeks to as long as six months after initiating the treatment. Manifestations of DHS include high-grade fever, skin rash, lymphadenopathy, eosinophilia, hepatitis, acute pneumonitis, neurological, and other systemic features of multi-organ dysfunction.

48.16 Mucous Membrane Pemphigoid

MMP is a mucous membrane-dominated autoimmune subepithelial blistering disease that is caused by autoantibodies against various autoantigens in basement membrane zone (BMZ) proteins. This is generally a disease of middle-aged and elderly people and has a predilection for white populations.

The pathogenesis of MMP has been poorly understood. MMP is characterized by linear deposition of autoantibodies that bind to a range of autoantigens including collagen XVII (COL17, also called BP180), BP230, laminin 332, integrin $\alpha6/\beta4$, and collagen VII (COL7) at the basement membrane zone (BMZ). The C terminus of COL17 and laminin 332 are the major autoantigens for MMP. Integrin $\alpha6/\beta4$ is associated with the occurrence of ocular lesions. However, the exact mechanism of blister formation remains unclear.

In the majority of patients, the oral mucosa is the site of onset and is the most frequently involved (85%) site followed by ocular mucosa. Desquamative gingivitis may range from localized gingival erythema to generalized inflammation with blistering or ulceration. Gingival lesions of MMP may be indistinguishable from PV, OLP, or EBA. Further, it is more difficult to differentiate from BP if patients present with mucous membrane involvement.

Scarring may lead to potentially serious complications like adhesions including fusion of the buccal mucosa and alveolar processes, the uvula and tonsillar fossa, or the tongue with the floor of the mouth. Ocular involvement is characterized by blisters that ulcerate and eventually undergo conjunctival scarring and visual impairment. Vesicles or frank blisters are not usually clinically evident in ocular MMP. The initial stages of ocular disease are often subtle, with vague symptoms such as burning, dryness, photophobia, or foreign body sensation. Furthermore, ocular MMP may lead to symblepharon (adhesion of the palpebral conjunctiva to the bulbar conjunctiva), ankyloblepharon (adhesions of upper and lower eyelid), entropion (eyelid folds tend to be inward), trichiasis (eyelashes grow inwards), corneal damage, and neovascularization (new blood vessel formation).

The diagnosis of MMP is based on the clinical, histological, and immunopathological findings. Although patients manifest a predominantly mucosal disease, it is relatively difficult to diagnose clinically due to low titer of circulating autoantibodies. Histologically, subepithelial separation with a mixed inflammatory infiltrate in the superficial lamina propria is evident. Further, MMP patients tend to have fewer inflammatory findings than BP patients. This may indicate differences in blistering mechanisms between MMP and BP. Direct immunofluorescence (DIF) test for IgG, IgA, and C3 is positive at the BMZ. Serum samples are valuable for identifying isotype binding pattern, and titer of circulating anti-BMZ antibodies. Detection of both IgG and IgA is associated with more severe disease and serial IgG titres be used to monitor disease severity and management.

DIF is often helpful for diagnosis of MMP, but it does not distinguish MMP from other subepithelial blistering disorders such as BP and EBA. MMP is usually differentiated from other mucocutaneous diseases such as OLP, erythema multiforme, and PV by routine histopathology.

Distinction should be made by combining the clinical findings with other sophisticated immunopathologic tests, which are not routinely requested in clinical practice. It is difficult to distinguish MMP from BP solely by DIF and IIF since most patients with MMP and BP have bullous pemphigoid antigen 2 (BPAG2). More specific immunological procedures have demonstrated that autoantibodies produced by MMP patients bind to the C-terminal portion of the BPAG2 antigen, whereas antibodies produced by patients with BP bind to the NC16A domain of the same autoantigen. EBA is distinguished from MMP by salt-split method where EBA-related antibodies are present at the dermal side of the artificial split. However, it is a challenge to differentiate EBA from anti-p200 pemphigoid, and anti-laminin 332 MMP, because in all of these diseases, autoantibodies deposit on the floor of the artificial blister when IIF microscopy is performed on salt-split human skin.

The main goals of the management of MMP are to halt the progression, reduce symptoms, and prevent chronic inflammation that leads to scarring. Treatment should be multidisciplinary as it is a debilitating disease. Collaboration with dermatologists, ophthalmologists, dentists, otolaryngologists, urologists, and gastroenterologists leads to better management and reduced morbidity.

Moderate-to-high potent topical corticosteroids are the first line of treatment for those who have the disease limited to the oral mucosa with or without cutaneous involvement (low-risk patients). If the patient does not respond, intralesional (more superficial) injections of triamcinolone hexacetonide at 5–10 mg/mL every 2–4 weeks are recommended. Good oral hygiene should be maintained to prevent plaque build-up. Regular dental examination is crucial.

Salient features of mucous membrane pemphigoid	
Clinical features	Presence of painful, erosive/blistering lesions. More common on gingiva, buccal mucosa, and palate. Although scarring is its clinical hallmark, this may not always be obvious.
Histopathology	Subepithelial separation at the basement membrane zone (BMZ) and a lympho-histiocytic infiltrate admixed with some granulocytes and plasma cells in early lesions in the superficial lamina propria and along the BMZ. Direct immunofluorescence on a perilesional mucosal biopsy displays a linear deposition of IgG antibody and/or C3 complement along the BMZ.
Treatment	Management by a multidisciplinary team. Treatment of choice is corticosteroid therapy.

Self-Assessment Questions

1. Discuss the clinical differential diagnoses of a patient presenting with erosions on the gingivae.
2. Discuss the differential diagnoses for subepithelial blistering disorders affecting oral mucosa.
3. Describe the steps to confirm the diagnosis of MMP.
4. Discuss the management of MMP.

- **Diagnostic Algorithm for MMP**

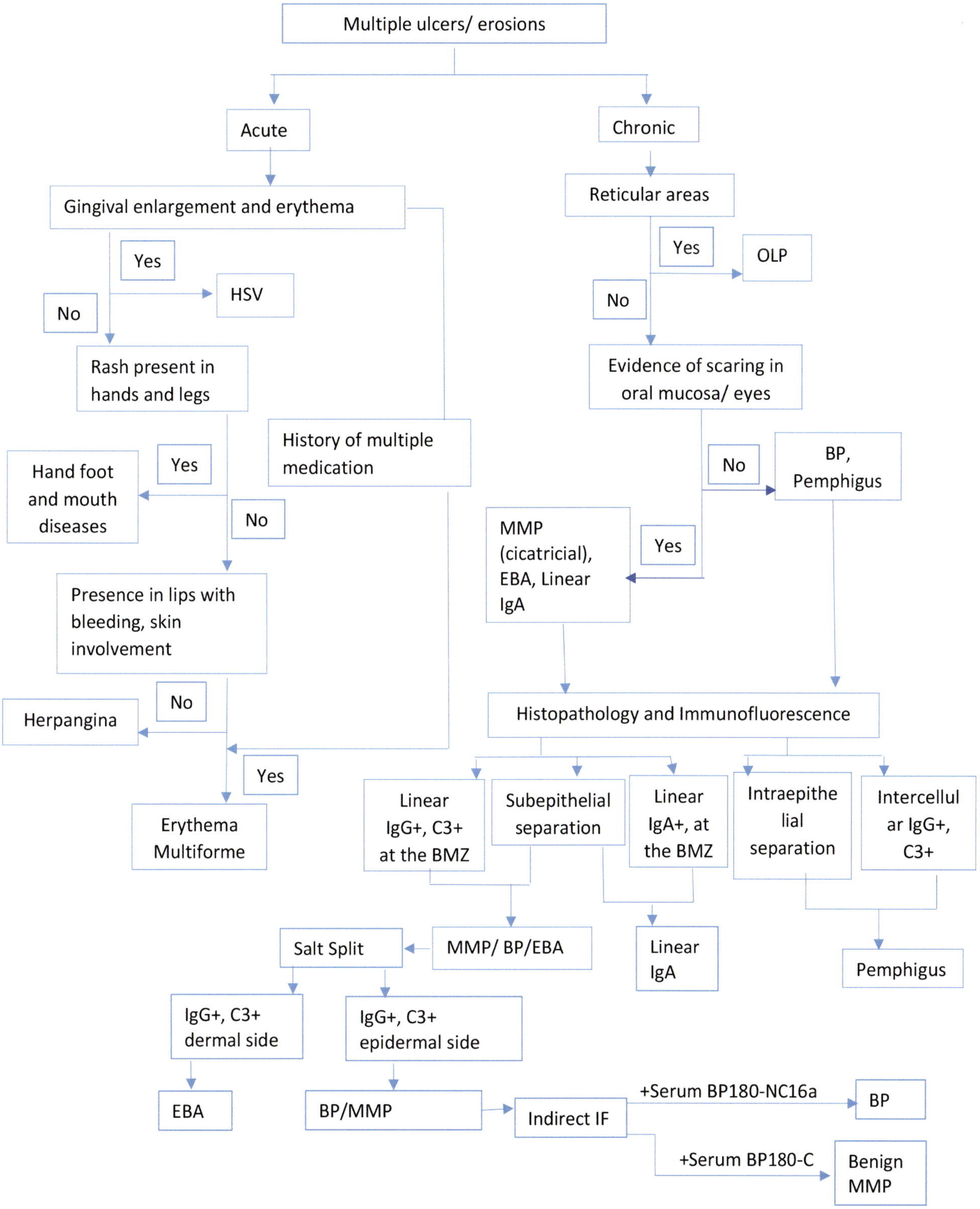

OLP- Oral Lichen Palnus
HSV- Herpes Simplex Virus infection
BP- Bullous Pemphigoid
MMP- Muocus Membrane Pemphigoid
EBA- Epidermolysis Bullosa Acquisita

Summary

The diagnosis of MMP is based on the clinical, histological, and immunopathological findings. Distinction from other subepithelial blistering disorders should be made by combining the clinical findings with other immunopathologic tests. The main goals of the management of MMP are to halt the progression, reduce symptoms, and prevent chronic inflammation that leads to scarring. Treatment should be multidisciplinary as it is a debilitating disease.

Suggested Readings

Bernard P, Antonicelli F. Bullous pemphigoid: a review of its diagnosis, associations and treatment. Am J Clin Dermatol. 2017;18(4):513–28. https://doi.org/10.1007/s40257-017-0264-2.

Daniel BS, Murrell DF. Review of autoimmune blistering diseases: the Pemphigoid diseases. J Eur Acad Dermatol Venereol. 2019;33(9):1685–94. https://doi.org/10.1111/jdv.15679. Epub 2019 Jul 11.

Eduardo Calonje J, Brenn T, Lazar A, Billings S. McKee's pathology of the skin. 5th ed. Elsevier. 2018.

Schmidt E, Rashid H, Marzano A, Lamberts A, Di Zenzo G, Diercks GFH, Alberti-Violetti S, Barry RJ, Borradori L, Caproni M, Carey B, Carrozzo M, Cianchini G, Corra A, Dikkers FG, Feliciani C, Geerling G, Genovese G, Hertl M, et al. European guidelines (S3) on diagnosis and management of mucous membrane pemphigoid, initiated by the European Academy of Dermatology and Venereology—Part II. J Eur Acad Dermatol Venereol. 2021;35(10):1926–48. https://doi.org/10.1111/jdv.17395.

Yancey KB. Cicatricial pemphigoid. In: Wolff K, Goldsmith LA, Katz SI, et al., editors. Dermatology in general medicine. 7th ed. New York: McGraw-Hill Inc; 2008. p. 481–5.

Oral Manifestations of Hematological Disorders

Contents

Multiple Reddish Swellings on the Gum: Leukemia

Wei Cheong Ngeow, Thomas George Kallarakkal, and Harsha Lal De Silva

Contents

W. M Tilakaratne, T. G. Kallarakkal (eds.), *Clinicopathological Correlation of Oral Diseases*,
https://doi.org/10.1007/978-3-031-24408-7_49

Learning Goals

1. Frame appropriate questions to elicit an accurate, comprehensive clinical history.
2. Use the information from history taking to develop a preliminary differential diagnosis
3. Follow a logical sequence to a comprehensive clinical examination
4. Recognize the importance of thinking beyond what is clinically apparent.
5. Combine history and examination findings to formulate a working clinical differential diagnosis
6. Judiciously select special investigations to gather appropriate additional diagnostic information.
7. Comprehend and apply clinicopathological correlations to arrive at the final diagnosis
8. Formulate a comprehensive management plan underpinned by meaningful clinicopathological relationships.
9. Use appropriate diagnostic algorithms in clinical practice to facilitate patient management

49.1 Main Complaint

A 40-year-old woman attended the outpatient clinic, referred by her family doctor to investigate and manage multiple swellings appearing on her gingiva of the upper front teeth.

49.2 History of Complaint

Question: How long have you had these swellings?

They have been there for several months.

Question: How did you first notice them?

I saw them while brushing my teeth. They were small initially and didn't cause me discomfort, except they occasionally bled during tooth brushing. They grew rapidly for the past six months and started bleeding spontaneously.

Question: How were your gums before this swelling appeared?

I don't remember having any swellings or gum boils before this.

Question: Do you have any other problems associated with these swellings?

I have difficulty chewing because of these swellings. I am scared that they might get traumatized and bleed if I am not careful when eating. I consciously try hard to avoid chewing on the swellings. I occasionally feel a foul odour from my mouth and wonder whether it is coming from these swellings.

Question: Have you noticed any other changes in your mouth?

Occasionally, I have had bleeding gums before. The teeth close to the swellings feel slightly loose.

Question: Have you noticed any swellings, lumps, or bumps anywhere else in your body?

I felt a few swellings on both sides of my neck and my armpits. They aren't painful.

Question: Did you feel generally unwell in the past few months?

I was frequently feeling tired and rundown. I don't have much appetite for food and recently lost a fair amount of weight.

Question: Do you become short of breath when you walk or climb stairs?

I manage my daily routines but forced to take breaks more often than I used to. I become tired very fast.

Question: Do you get fever?

Yes. I had fever, on and off, during the past six months. I had COVID-19 tests twice, but they both returned negative.

Question: Are you suffering from any other medical problems like heart disease, high blood pressure, diabetes, bleeding disorder, respiratory diseases, etc.?

I have had high blood pressure for the past four years. I visit my doctor regularly for treatment and he is happy with the blood pressure control.

Question: What medications do you take for high blood pressure?

I have been taking nifedipine (40 mg/day) and cilazapril (5 mg/day) for the past two years. I was on different pills earlier, but I cannot remember their names.

Question: Have you had any surgery in the past?

I haven't undergone any surgery in the past.

Question: Have you had any dental treatment?

I had a few decayed teeth extracted many years ago. I don't recall having any fillings or scaling within the past 10 years. I only visit a dentist if I have tooth pain.

Question: Have you had any bleeding issues when you had dental extractions?

No, there were no issues of note. The wounds healed well.

Question: What is your occupation?

I am an office clerk.

Question: Have you been exposed to chemicals or radiation?

I do not recall having exposure to any industrial chemicals or radiation

Question: Do you smoke or take alcohol?

I am a non-smoker. I enjoy an occasional glass of wine or beer at social gatherings.

49.3 Based on the Findings From the Patient's History, What Is Your Differential Diagnosis?

1. Gingival hyperplasia
2. Drug-induced gingival hyperplasia
3. Lymphoma
4. Kaposi sarcoma
5. Leukemic infiltrate

49.4 How Do You Justify Your Differential Diagnosis Based on the History?

Gingival swellings may result from local disease or systemic causes, including oral manifestations of systemic malignancies. The patient's presenting symptoms are painless multiple gingival swellings that tend to bleed spontaneously and from toothbrush trauma. Gingivitis is the commonest cause of gingival bleeding and swelling. Gingival swellings may become persistent through a hyperplastic response. The patient's medical history reveals the use of calcium channel blockers (nifedipine) which is known to be associated with gingival hyperplasia. However, the reported systemic symptoms like recurrent bouts of fever, lethargy, unintentional loss of weight, and multiple enlarged lymph nodes suggest the possibility of an underlying systemic cause. The involvement of gingiva in Kaposi sarcoma, lymphoma, and leukemia is well recognized and merits further consideration in the diagnostic process.

49.5 What Are the Findings of the Clinical Examination?

The extraoral examination is unremarkable except for multiple, discrete, non-tender, firm, movable lumps on both sides of her neck, suggestive of bilateral cervical lymphadenopathy.

Intraorally, she has multiple dark blue/purple painless exophytic gingival lesions around the upper right and left anterior teeth (Fig. 49.1). They feel soft to palpation, and the gingiva appears to have lost the stippling surface texture. Oral hygiene around anterior teeth seems compromised, possibly due to the large gingival swellings interfering with tooth brushing. The gingiva shows evidence of spontaneous bleeding and also bled significantly on gentle periodontal probing, even in areas not involved with visible gingival swellings. Despite being swollen in places and having a tendency to bleed, the gingiva generally did not appear reddish or inflamed. There is an offensive odour from the patient's mouth, and the adjacent teeth show grade 1 mobility. The buccal mucosa, the floor of the mouth, tongue, palate, and pharynx appear clinically normal.

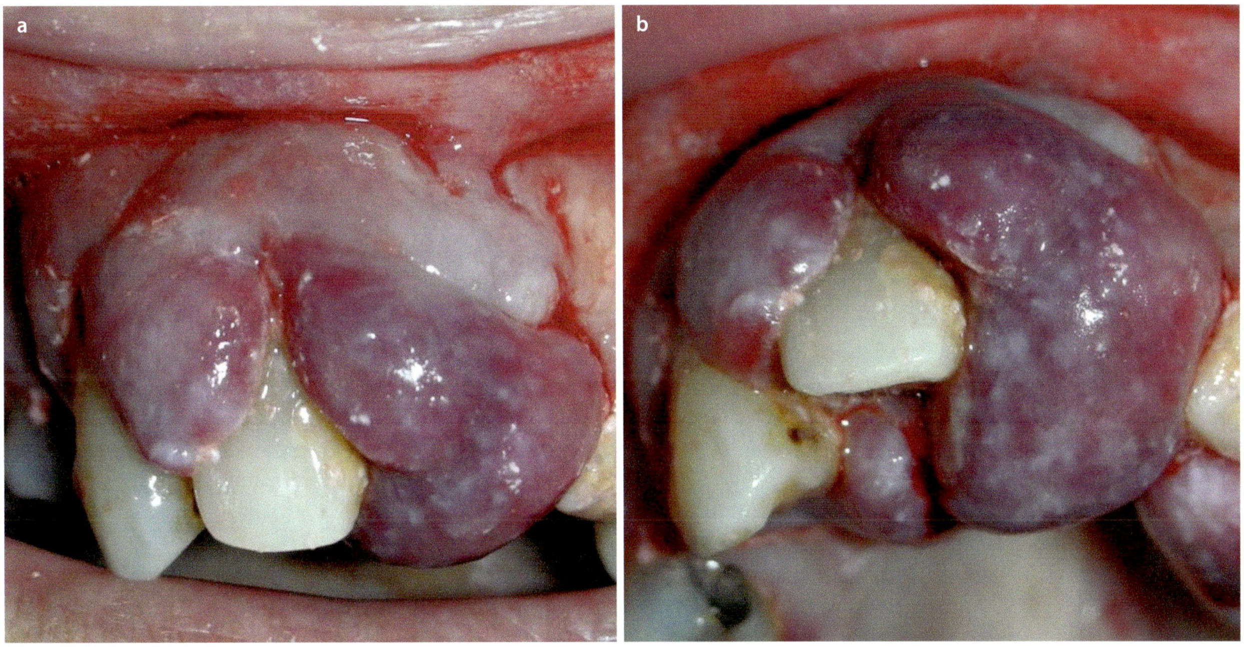

Fig. 49.1 Large bluish-purple colored swellings covering most of the labial and palatal aspects of the right upper lateral incisor and the canine (**a**) and (**b**)

49.6 What Is Your Clinical Differential Diagnosis?

1. Leukemic infiltrate of the gingiva
2. Kaposi sarcoma
3. Lymphoma

49.7 How Would You Exclude Other Conditions and Justify the Inclusion of the Diseases That You Have Mentioned in the Differential Diagnosis to Arrive at a Working Diagnosis?

Calcium channel blockers can cause gingival hyperplasia, which can become amplified with poor oral hygiene and plaque accumulation. Despite being an on-demand dental attendee, the patient's oral hygiene was satisfactory except in areas affected by exophytic gingival swellings. Gingival hyperplasia secondary to drug therapy is usually more generalized and does not cause spontaneous bleeding in the absence of inflammation. Further, it is uncommon to be associated with marked cervical lymphadenopathy or systemic signs and symptoms.

The reported systemic signs and symptoms strongly suggest the presence of an underlying systemic cause for the presenting gingival lesions. The involvement of gingiva has been reported in lymphomas, but the lesions tend to be more localized and unlikely to have a bleeding tendency. Kaposi sarcoma is a malignancy seen mostly in association with immunodeficient conditions such as HIV-AIDS.

Leukemia has many oral manifestations. The commonest reported is the bluish/ purple swellings that tend to occur in gingivae. They usually appear as multiple spongy masses which tend to bleed easily. Their appearance commonly accompanies lymph node enlargement in the neck and other sites like the axilla and inguinal regions. This patient also reported a recent, unintentional loss of weight, lethargy, and frequent bouts of fever, all characteristic of leukemia.

49.8 What is the Most Likely Diagnosis?

Leukemic infiltrate of the gingiva

49.9 What Special Investigations Are Needed to Confirm Your Diagnosis?

1. Complete blood count
2. Microscopic examination of a peripheral blood film
3. Gingival biopsy

This patient's peripheral blood showed a significantly elevated white cell count (leucocytosis). Peripheral blood smear showed marked leukocytosis with abundant blasts and monocytoid population. Both platelets and red blood cells appeared depleted.

The above changes in the peripheral blood helped confirm leukemia and exclude both lymphoma and Kaposi sarcoma.

49.10 How Would You Do an Incisional Biopsy for This Patient? What Are the Important Considerations?

The gingival incisional biopsy was performed with extreme care. Appropriate measures were taken to achieve adequate haemostasis as leukemia may increase perioperative bleeding due to depleted platelets (thrombocytopenia). The harvested tissue was sent for histopathological examination.

The hematoxylin and eosin (H & E) stained slides showed diffuse infiltration and destruction of the host tissue architecture by sheets of immature lymphoid cells with myelomonocytic features suggesting either lymphoma or leukaemic deposits as the cause for gingival enlargement (◘ Figs. 49.2 and 49.3). The gingival biopsy helps further exclude other conditions associated with gingival swelling, as they have their characteristic histopathological appearances.

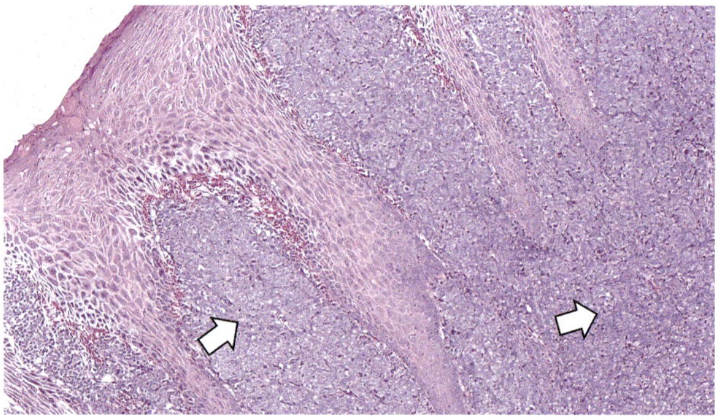

◘ **Fig. 49.2** Infiltration of small- to medium-sized atypical lymphoid cells (white arrows) with mild-to-moderate nuclear atypia in the lamina propria

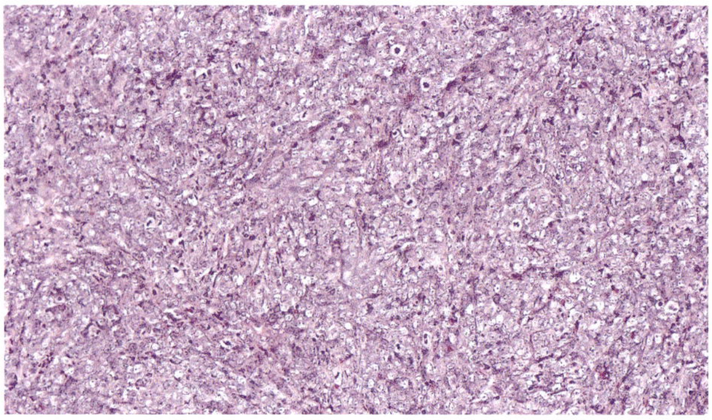

◘ **Fig. 49.3** Diffuse infiltrate of medium-sized to large atypical immature lymphoid cells throughout the lamina propria

49.11 What Other Relevant Features Would You Look for with Your Findings So Far?

A complete medical history workup and a detailed general clinical examination are crucial to arriving at the correct diagnosis and staging of the disease to formulate appropriate treatment planning. The examination should include other lymph node sites (axilla and inguinal regions) and the abdomen, focusing on potential hepatosplenomegaly. The clinical examination should be followed by targeted special investigations that may include

1. Biochemical assessment of renal and liver function
2. Serum protein electrophoresis, quantification of immunoglobulins, and immunoelectrophoresis
3. Fine-needle aspiration biopsy of an enlarged lymph node
4. Bone marrow biopsy
5. Urine analysis which includes immunofixation electrophoresis (IFE)
6. HIV, HBsAg, VDRL, and Mantoux test
7. Cytogenetic studies

The bone marrow film obtained by bone marrow biopsy confirmed the diagnosis of acute myeloid leukemia (AML). The bone marrow film showed that more than 30% of all nucleated cells were blast cells. Erythroid hyperplasia was noted, with more than 50% of all the nucleated cells being erythroblasts. More than 3% of the blast cells were positive for myeloperoxidase (MPO). Immunophenotyping with monoclonal antibodies to CD13 and CD33 confirmed myeloid-associated antigens on the cells, while the cells were negative to lymphoid antigens CD7, CD10, and CD19.

49.12 What Is the Definitive Diagnosis?

Acute myeloid leukemia (AML)

49.13 How Would You Manage This Patient?

The patient is best managed by referring to a hemato-oncologist, a medical doctor specializing in managing hematological malignancies. The medical management of leukemia includes different chemotherapeutic regimes to achieve cure or long-term remission. The treatment regime may start with induction chemotherapy followed by consolidation chemotherapy and maintenance chemotherapy if deemed necessary. Induction chemotherapy aims to return the blood counts to normal by destroying leukemic cells, while the consolidation phase targets destroying the remaining hidden leukemic cells.

Also, some patients may require maintenance chemotherapy to minimize potential recurrences following initial treatment. In some cases, complete remission and cure are not achievable with chemotherapy alone, and such patients may have to be considered for an allogeneic stem-cell transplant.

The collaborative management of this patient included a complete dental check-up and optimizing her oral hygiene to the best possible state in advance of the chemotherapy. She was prescribed alcohol-free chlorhexidine gluconate 0.12% solution and a soft toothbrush. Dental reviews were arranged in between chemotherapy cycles to encourage oral hygiene maintenance. She was provided with 2% viscous lignocaine to help soothe the oral mucositis resulting from cytotoxic drugs. The patient will attend periodic follow-up visits with the haemato-oncology department for long-term surveillance against potential relapses.

49.14 Leukemia

Leukemia, the most common malignancy of the hemopoietic system, is a disease featuring an uncontrolled proliferation of myeloid or lymphoid cells. The myeloid precursor cells in bone marrow differentiate to form erythrocytes, platelets, polymorphonuclear leukocytes, macrophages/monocytes, eosinophils, and basophils. In contrast, the lymphoid precursor cells of the bone marrow develop and mature into B-lymphocytes, T-lymphocytes, or natural killer (NK) cells. There is a maturation failure in leukemia resulting in immature blast cell accumulation and suppression of normal hematopoietic stem cells. Thus, a deficiency of mature leukocytes, erythrocytes, and platelets leads to clinical manifestation of immunodeficiency, anemia, and thrombocytopenia.

The etiology of leukemia is not well understood. Genetic disorders (chromosomal abnormalities), chemical exposures (pesticides), radiation exposure, and viral infections are some of the associated risk factors. Familial predisposition to myelodysplastic syndromes (MDS) and AML are recognized. Predisposing mutations in multiple genes, including RUNX1, CEBPA, GATA2, ANKRD26, SRP72, DDX41, ETV6, ATGB2/GSKIP (duplication) and possibly HYDIN, MUC16, NMUR2, RNF213, and ACD (TPP1) have been identified by cytogenetic studies.

Leukemia is an aggressive disease accounting for up to 4% of all deaths from malignancies. Leukemic patients may often become sick and drift quickly into an acute leukemic crisis resulting in rapid clinical deterioration. Neutropenia during acute exacerbations may lead to the development of fulminant infections with fatal outcomes. However, some leukemic patients may remain asymptomatic, in remission for long periods, and are only diagnosed following routine blood investigations. Leukemic cells may invade body tissues, such as the spleen, liver, lymph nodes, and peripheral blood. Less commonly, they may accumulate in the brain, skin, or gingiva.

There are four major types, classified first on the histogenesis and then further divided according to the onset and progression of the disease. They are, namely, acute lymphocytic leukemia (ALL), acute myeloid leukemia (AML), chronic lymphocytic leukemia (CLL), and chronic myeloid leukemia (CML).

49.14.1 Acute Lymphocytic Leukemia (ALL)

It is the most common childhood cancer, frequently affecting children between two and five years of age. Clinical manifestations include fever, fatigue, pallor, mucosal bleeding, petechiae, bone pain, hepatosplenomegaly, lymphadenopathy, and local infections. Down's syndrome is recognized as a risk factor for developing ALL.

Investigations for ALL include imaging for enlarged nodes, blood investigation, bone marrow aspiration biopsy, and nodal biopsy. Histopathological examination shows neoplastic proliferation of clonal precursor B cells or T cells. The prognosis for ALL is considered good when it occurs in children and is appropriately managed with multi-agent chemotherapy protocols. Bone marrow transplantation and Chimeric antigen receptor (CAR) T cell immunotherapy may be required to manage cases that relapse following treatment with chemotherapeutic agents.

49.14.2 Chronic Lymphocytic Leukaemia (CLL)

CLL is frequently seen among individuals in their 8th and 9th decades of life and is regarded as the commonest form of leukemia in adults. It has a similar origin to ALL, but the progression is much slower and gradual, remaining asymptomatic for several years. Lymphadenopathy and splenomegaly are common in CLL, which also tend to infiltrate into tonsils and other lymphoid bearing oral mucosal tissues. Treatment is tailored to clinical progression, provision of chemotherapy, monoclonal antibodies, or kinase inhibitors when indicated. Many patients with CLL survive for more than ten years from diagnosis.

49.14.3 Acute Myeloid Leukemia (AML)

AML is a relatively rare disease, mainly affecting blood and bone marrow. It is frequently seen in males aged >65 years, and it accounts for approximately 25% of all adult leukemias. Symptoms of AML and ALL are similar, except that the former is less likely to involve the central nervous system. AML is diagnosed from a combination of bone marrow aspirate smear morphology, cytochemistry, flow cytometry, and cytogenetics. Histologically, hypercellular bone marrow with immature cells and increased eosinophilic cells may be evident. Treatment is by multi-agent chemotherapy with or without monoclonal antibodies. AML has a variable prognosis, with one in eight developing myeloid sarcomas.

49.14.4 Chronic Myeloid Leukemia (CML)

With a similar origin to AML but with an abundance of well-differentiated cells in the bone marrow, peripheral blood, and tissues for a prolonged clinical course due to its slow growth rate, CML accounts for 20% of all cases of leukemia. It commonly affects men in their 4th and 5th decades of life. Hepatosplenomegaly and leukocytosis are typical presenting features. Sustained remission has been reported in >90% of patients treated with BCR-ABL inhibitors. Chemotherapy is given for blast crises, while stem cell transplants are curative in three-quarters of younger patients.

49.14.5 Oral Manifestations of Leukemia

Oral involvement may occur in all types of leukemia but is more frequently reported in acute leukemias. The oral manifestations can occur due to direct infiltration of leukemic cells or are secondary to underlying thrombocytopenia, neutropenia, or impaired granulocyte function. Of the four types of leukemia, AML is most often associated with oral manifestations, the prevalence being 3% to 5%. Reportedly, dentists have been responsible for initiating the diagnosis in up to 33% of AML.

The signs and symptoms of oral manifestations include toothache, gingival hyperplasia, gingival bleeding and/or gingivitis, oral ulceration, petechiae and ecchymoses of the oral mucosa, and mucosal pallor secondary to anemia. Less common symptoms reported include pericoronitis and trismus as the primary manifestations. Due to immunosuppression, recurrent herpetic gingivostomatitis, diffuse chronic mucocutaneous candidiasis, and other viral bacterial and opportunistic fungal infections can occur in leukemia.

Gingival hyperplasia has been observed with all four types of leukemia. It is mostly seen in association with AML. Gingiva enlarges due to infiltration with leukaemic cells. It is characterized by progressive enlargement of the interdental papillae and the marginal and attached gingivae. The crowns of adjacent teeth may become covered if left to enlarge. Despite being more common in patients with raised white cell counts, the development of gingival infiltration is unpredictable, being reported in people with 'aleukemia' or 'subleukemic' forms of leukemia too. Adults are more commonly affected, and there is no observed gender predilection. Pre-existing periodontal disease may aggravate leukemic infiltration and the resulting gingival enlargement. This type of gingival swelling has not been observed in edentulous sites. Often the gingival hyperplasia resolves with effective chemotherapy. Surgical intervention may be needed if it persists and disturbs the patient's ability to chew food.

49.15 Dentist's Role in Management

Dentists may be the first clinicians to become alerted to an oral manifestation that could lead to the diagnosis of otherwise asymptomatic leukemia. Hence, the dentists' vigilance to think beyond the immediately apparent clinical presentation could become lifesaving. Further, leukemic patients undergoing chemotherapy and other treatment modalities frequently develop troublesome oral mucositis. It is well recognized that improvement in oral hygiene in advance could help minimize the oral adverse effects of aggressive chemotherapy.

Algorithm for diagnosis and management of reddish-purple gingival enlargements

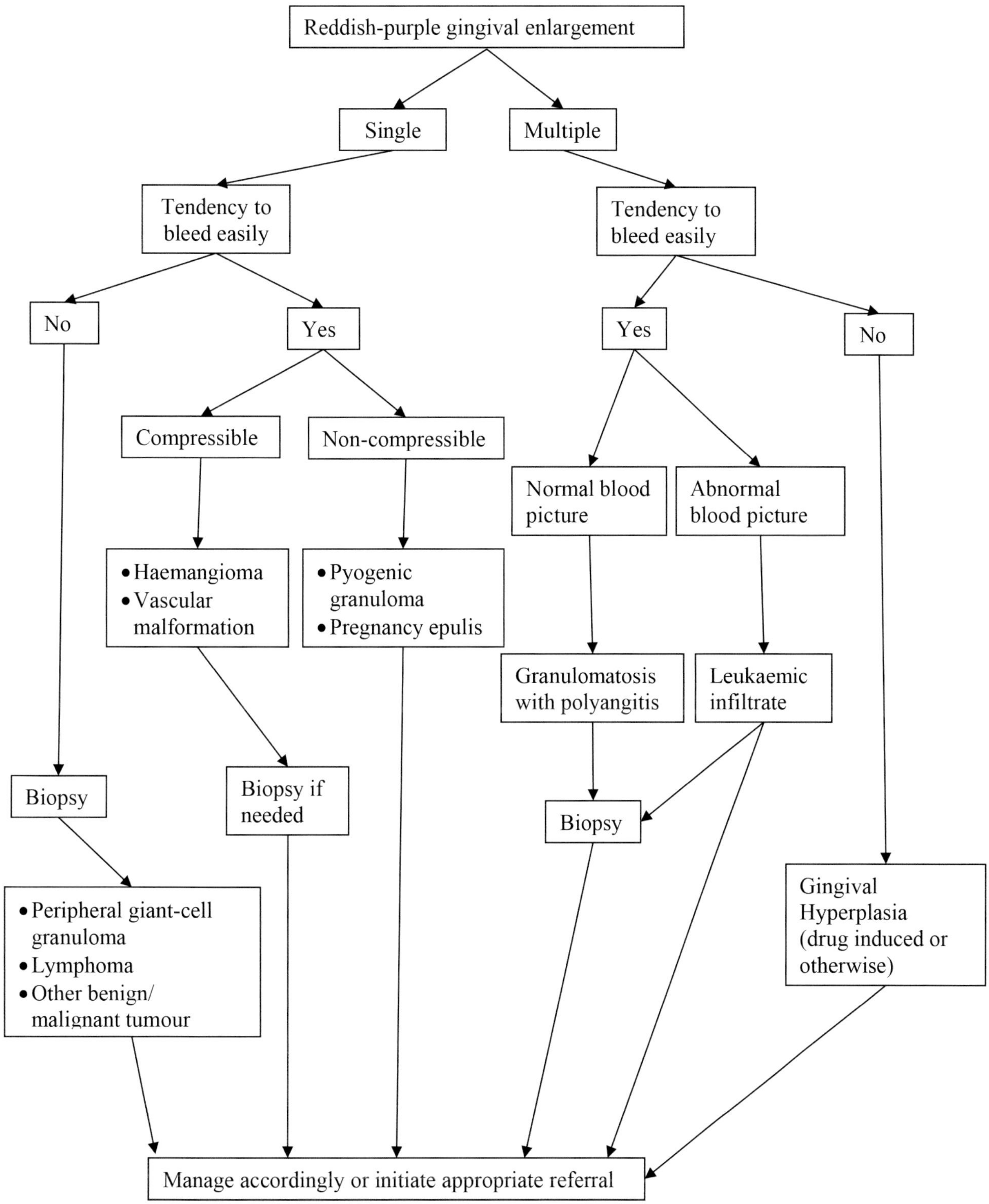
Reddish-purple gingival enlargement
Single
Multiple
Tendency to bleed easily
Tendency to bleed easily
No
Yes
Yes
No
Compressible
Non-compressible
Normal blood picture
Abnormal blood picture
• Haemangioma
• Vascular malformation
• Pyogenic granuloma
• Pregnancy epulis
Granulomatosis with polyangitis
Leukaemic infiltrate
Biopsy
Biopsy if needed
Biopsy
Gingival Hyperplasia (drug induced or otherwise)
• Peripheral giant-cell granuloma
• Lymphoma
• Other benign/ malignant tumour
Manage accordingly or initiate appropriate referral

49

Self-Assessment Questions

1. List the risk factors for leukemia.
2. List the pathognomonic clinical features of acute and chronic leukemias
3. Describe the oral manifestations of leukemia.
4. List other conditions that may clinically mimic leukemia?
5. Outline the importance of early diagnosis in the management of leukemia.
6. Describe the histopathological features of oral leukemic manifestations.
7. Describe the role of a dental practitioner in the diagnosis and management of leukemia?

Summary

Leukemia is the commonest malignancy of the hematopoietic system. While it could affect any age group, different subtypes of leukemia tend to have a predilection for distinct age groups. Presenting clinical features could be diverse and the disease could easily be missed by an unsuspecting clinician. Oral manifestations are common in acute myeloid leukemia, but other subtypes are not exempt. A vigilant dentist could be the first clinician to notice an oral manifestation that may lead to an early diagnosis and a favourable outcome for this otherwise deadly disease. Moreover, the dentist has an important role to play in the muti-disciplinary management of leukemia by optimizing oral health to mitigate troublesome oral side effects of anti-leukemic chemotherapy.

Further Reading

Anonymous. https://www.pathologyoutlines.com. Accessed October 17th, 2021; n.d.

Arber DA, Orazi A, Hasserjian R, et al. The 2016 revision to the World Health Organization classification of myeloid neoplasms and acute leukemia. Blood. 2016;127(20):2391–405.

Eyer-Silva WA, Soares PEMA, Azevedo MCVM, Silva GARD, Signorini DJHP, Neves-Motta R, Pinto JFDC, Moura LM, Basílio-de-Oliveira RP, Araujo LF, Favacho ARM, Lemos ERS. An unusual case of bacillary angiomatosis in the oral cavity of an AIDS patient who had no concomitant tegumentary lesions—case report and review. Rev Inst Med Trop Sao Paulo. 2017;59:e59. https://doi.org/10.1590/S1678-9946201759059.

Hunasgi S, Koneru A, Vanishree M, Manvikar V. Angiosarcoma of anterior mandibular gingiva showing recurrence—a case report with immunohistochemistry. J Clin Diagn Res. 2016;10(7): ZD01–4.

McCord C, Johnson L. Oral manifestations of hematologic disease. Atlas Oral Maxillofac Surg Clin North Am. 2017;25(2):149–62. https://doi.org/10.1016/j.cxom.2017.04.007.

Stern JK, Stern I, De Rossi SS, Zemse SM, Abdelsayed R. Kaposi sarcoma presenting as "diffuse gingival enlargement": report of three cases. HIV & AIDS Review. 2016;15(2):80–7. https://doi.org/10.1016/j.hivar.2016.04.001.

Generalized Weakness and Recurrent Ulcers on the Tongue: Anemia

Firdaus Hariri

Contents

W. M Tilakaratne, T. G. Kallarakkal (eds.), *Clinicopathological Correlation of Oral Diseases*,
https://doi.org/10.1007/978-3-031-24408-7_50

Learning Goals

1. Understand the pathogenesis of recurrent aphthous ulcers of the tongue.
2. Clinically recognise the characteristics of oral aphthous ulcer.
3. Appreciate the importance of comprehensive haematological investigations to diagnose different types of anaemia.
4. Recognise and appreciate the different management approaches in oral ulcer treatment and other associated medical conditions leading to anaemia.

50.1 Main Complaint

A 40-year-old female patient presented to the clinic with a complaint of recurrent ulcers on her tongue.

50.2 History of Complaint

Question: When did you first notice the ulcerations?

I noticed the ulcerations approximately 6 months ago.

Question: How often does it occur?

It occurs every 3–4 weeks.

Question: What is the nature of the ulcerations?

The ulcers are spontaneous, multiple, and occur at different sites in the mouth. They heal on their own after a few days.

Question: Do you have any other associated oral symptoms?

I have been experiencing occasional burning sensation in the mouth and dryness of the lips especially at the angle of the mouth.

Question: Do you feel tired lately?

I generally feel tired all the time.

Question: Do you have any episodes of heart racing or pounding?

I have occasional palpitations which lasts for a few minutes during each episode.

Question: Do you have any history of vomiting?

I don't have any history of vomiting.

Question: Do you experience any loss of appetite?

I have normal appetite.

Question: Did you notice any loss of weight?

I have not noticed any weight loss. My weight has remained unchanged.

Question: Have you had any episodes of shortness of breath, chest pain or dizziness?

I have been experiencing occasional periods of shortness of breath but I have not experienced other symptoms such as chest pain and dizziness.

Question: Have you been experiencing heavy menstruation? Is your menstruation cycle normal?

I have normal menstruation cycles. I don't have any history of prolonged or heavy menstruation.

Question: Do you have any history of injury such as tongue biting or trauma to the mouth?

I have no history of trauma and injury to the oral tissues.

Question: Do you have any history of fever or any other lesions on any part of your body?

I don't have any history of fever or occurrence of lesions on any part of my body other than the ulcerations of the oral tissue.

50.3 Past Medical History

Question: Do you have any systemic diseases?

I was diagnosed of having peptic ulcers a year ago and I am currently under follow-up. I have no other medical problems.

Question: Have you been admitted to the hospital or had any surgical procedure done before?

I was admitted once for an endoscopic procedure for examination of my digestive tract but have no history of any surgical procedure.

50.4 Past Dental History

Question: How often do you visit a dentist?

I visit my dentist only very rarely.

50.5 Social History

Question: Do you have any family history of cancer?

None of my family members have a history of cancer.

Question: What is your occupation?

I work as a sales executive.

Question: Do you have any high risks habits such as smoking cigarettes, alcohol consumption, or betel-quid chewing?

I don't have any such high-risk habits.

Question: Tell about your dietary habits?

I rarely skip the main three meals (breakfast, lunch and dinner). I rarely take meat due to preference for other dietary options.

50.6 What Is Your Differential Diagnosis with the Findings from the History?

Recurrent aphthous stomatitis associated with:

1. Iron deficiency anemia
2. Anemia of chronic disease
3. Aplastic anemia

50.7 How Do You Justify Your Differential Diagnosis?

Recurrent aphthous ulceration is considered as a common oral manifestation of the above anemic conditions. The patient has a history of general anemic symptoms such as shortness of breath, tiredness, and occasional palpitations. Her medical history revealed the diagnosis of peptic ulcer disease which is a known condition to cause iron deficiency anemia. Patient also manifests other oral signs and symptoms such as angular cheilitis and burning mouth sensation, respectively.

50.8 What Are the Findings of Clinical Examination?

50.8.1 Extra Oral

On extra oral examination, there is marked conjunctival pallor (Fig. 50.1a). Mild degree of angular cheilitis is observed (Fig. 50.1b). Nails of both hands show ver-

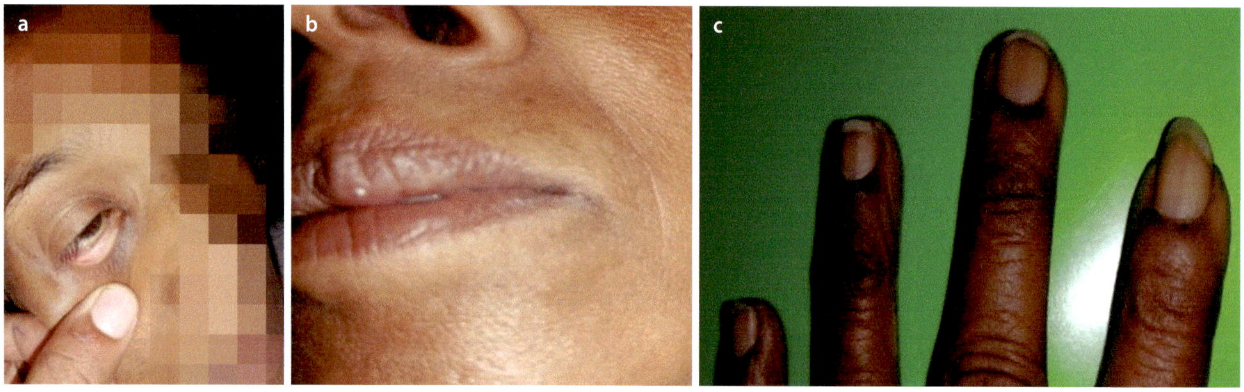

Fig. 50.1 (**a**) Marked pallor of the conjunctiva, (**b**) angular cheilitis, (**c**) and early vertical ridging of nails (Courtesy of Prof Ruwan Jayasinghe)

tical ridging (◘ Fig. 50.1c). There are no other peripheral signs of systemic disease.

50.8.2 Intraoral

Intraorally, there is erosion noticed at the left angle of the mouth. There are erosive areas and ulcers on the left lateral border and ventral surface of her tongue (◘ Fig. 50.2). All ulcers are round and superficial, sized approximately around 4 mm in diameter. The ulcers have a yellowish base and are surrounded by an erythematous halo. The tongue and surrounding oral mucosa appear pale. There is no other abnormality of intraoral tissues.

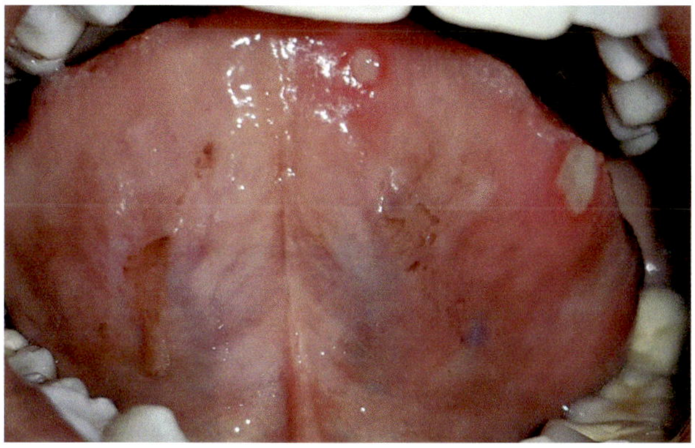

◘ **Fig. 50.2** Multiple ulcers on the lateral border and ventral surface of the tongue. The ulcers have a yellowish base and are surrounded by an erythematous halo

50.9 What Is Your Clinical Diagnosis?

Recurrent aphthous stomatitis most probably secondary to iron deficiency anemia.

50.10 How Would You Exclude Other Conditions Leading to Oral Ulceration from Your Differential Diagnosis and Justify Your Clinical Diagnosis?

Oral ulceration is a manifestation of local causes such as trauma due to various reasons and a large number of systemic diseases. However, presence of significant clinical features such as shortness of breath, tiredness, and occasional palpitations and presence of other oral signs and symptoms like angular cheilitis and burning mouth sensation are highly suggestive of anemia. In addition, she also has nail changes and pallor of the conjunctiva suggestive of anemia. Therefore, other conditions leading to oral ulceration can be excluded. Her medical history revealed the diagnosis of peptic ulcer disease which is a known condition to cause iron deficiency anemia.

50.11 How Do You Investigate the Patient to Confirm Your Diagnosis?

Full blood count must first be analysed to confirm the haemoglobin level. The Hb level will indicate whether the patient is anemic or normal. The mean corpuscular volume (MCV) can then be assessed to determine the morphological classification of the anemia and in this case, would be microcytic and hypochromic.

Specific tests to identify substance deficiency can be performed when a specific disorder is suspected as in iron deficiency anemia. These tests include serum iron, serum ferritin, and total iron-binding capacity (TIBC), among others.

Medically, the cause of iron deficiency anemia was identified as due to the history of peptic ulcers and confirmed via the haematological investigation which revealed microcytic and hypochromic red blood cells (Table 50.1).

50.12 What Is Your Definitive Diagnosis?

Recurrent aphthous stomatitis secondary to iron deficiency anemia.

50.13 What Are the Specific Findings That Help You to Confirm Your Definitive Diagnosis?

The patient presented with common oral manifestations of iron deficiency anemia such as recurrent aphthous ulcerations, burning mouth sensation, and angular cheilitis as well as other anemic symptoms such as shortness of breath, tiredness, and palpitations. Clinically, there were general manifestations of anemia such as conjunctival pallor, nail changes, and pale intraoral mucosa. In addition, all haematological parameters were consistent with iron deficiency anemia.

Table 50.1 Blood parameters indicating microcytic and hypochromic anemia

	Parameters	Patient's value		Normal value
1.	Haemoglobin (Hb)	Decreased	9 g/dL	12–13 g/dL
2.	Mean corpuscular volume (MCV)	Decreased	75 μm^3	80–100 μm^3
3.	Serum ferritin	Decreased	8 ng/mL	10–120 ng/mL
4.	Serum iron	Decreased	45 mcg/dL	60–170 mcg/dL
5.	Transferrin	Increased	450 mg/dL	204–360 mg/dL
6.	Total iron-binding capacity (TIBC)	Increased	480 mcg/dL	240–450 mcg/dL

50.14 How Would You Manage This Patient?

The primary aim of the treatment is to treat the underlying cause leading to iron deficiency anemia which is the peptic ulcer disease. Following comprehensive examinations and investigations by the gastroenterologist to confirm the peptic ulcer disease, a combination of medications was prescribed to eliminate the H. pylori bacteria and to reduce acidity in the stomach. These medications include proton pump inhibitors and antibiotics. The iron deficiency can be treated via replacement therapy using supplements or by the improvement of dietary habits which consist of iron-rich foods such as meat, eggs, and green vegetables. Most aphthous ulcers are self-limiting. Nevertheless, topical medication can be used to relieve ulcer symptoms.

50.15 Follow-up and Prognosis

The patient would require periodical follow-up to assess the underlying peptic ulcer disease as the progress and its treatment determines the prognosis of her oral health condition.

50.16 Oral Manifestations of Anemia

Anemia is defined as decreased haemoglobin (Hb) concentration for age and gender of patient. The World Health Organization (WHO) defines anemia as Hb <13 g/dL in men above 15 years, <11 g/dL in pregnant women, and <12 g/dL in non-pregnant women above 15 years of age. In general, the etiological factors of anemia are categorised based on three conditions: (1) decreased red cell production, (2) excess red cell breakdown, or (3) loss of red cells. Marrow failure is an example of decreased red cell production whereas haemolytic anemia is a condition where there is an excess of red cell breakdown. On the other hand, red cell loss may occur in any bleeding conditions such as in gastrointestinal bleeding. These underlying aetiological factors can either be acquired or hereditary in origin.

When reviewing a patient suspected of having anemia, it is important to thoroughly assess the patient for the presence of any general signs and symptoms of anemia as they can be non-specific. These signs and symptoms include pallor, tachypnoea, palpitations, tachycardia, angina, postural hypotension, claudication, and tiredness, among others. The presence of these signs and symptoms should be well documented as it may indicate the overall picture and well-being of the patient.

The investigations to determine the type of anemia require laboratory blood analysis of certain hematological parameters as discussed earlier. Among the important parameters is the analysis of red cell indices as it provides a valuable parameter for morphological classification of anemias (microcytic, normocytic, and macrocytic). In macrocytic anemia, further bone marrow analysis allows classification into megaloblastic or non-megaloblastic types. Specific tests to identify nutritional deficiency can be performed as in iron deficiency anemia.

50.16.1 Specific Oral Manifestations

The identification of specific oral manifestations of anemia allows dental or medical practitioners to provide a better and comprehensive management of an anemic patient. At the same time, the manifestation may provide important clues towards the identification of specific type of anemia when there is a high index of suspicion. For the purpose of systematic description of these manifestations, anemia is further aetiologically categorised into:

1. *Anemia due to decreased red cell production*

   An example of a condition due to decreased production of red cells is pernicious anemia, which is an autoimmune atrophic gastritis that subsequently leads to vitamin B12 deficiency. Patients with pernicious anemia suffer from malabsorption due to deficiency of intrinsic factor important for the absorption of vitamin B12 which is a vital component in the formation of RBC. Among the common manifestations in this group of patients are burning sensation of the oral tissues such as the lips, mucosa, and tongue. The mucosa may appear smooth due to papillary atrophy of the tongue surface or present with an erythematous patch. Other manifestations include aphthous-like ulcers (◘ Fig. 50.3a, b), alteration in taste, and dysphagia.

   Another serious blood disorder is aplastic anemia characterised by hypoplastic bone marrow and peripheral pancytopenia. This condition is caused by the destruction of pluripotent stem cells in bone marrow. The patient may present with the general anemic signs and symptoms as well as other investigative findings of thrombocytopenia and neutropenia. Both thrombocytopenia and neutropenia are associated with bleeding tendency and impairment of resistance towards infection, respectively. Platelet deficiency in pancytopenia may lead to bleeding manifestations such as haemorrhagic gingival spots and mucosal hematoma at any site as well as gingival hemorrhage. Ulcerative lesions are common as a result of neutropenia.

2. *Anemia due to excess red cell breakdown*

   Sickle cell anemia is characterised by mutation in the HBB (haemoglobin subunit beta) gene, which leads to replacement of amino acid glutamic acid by

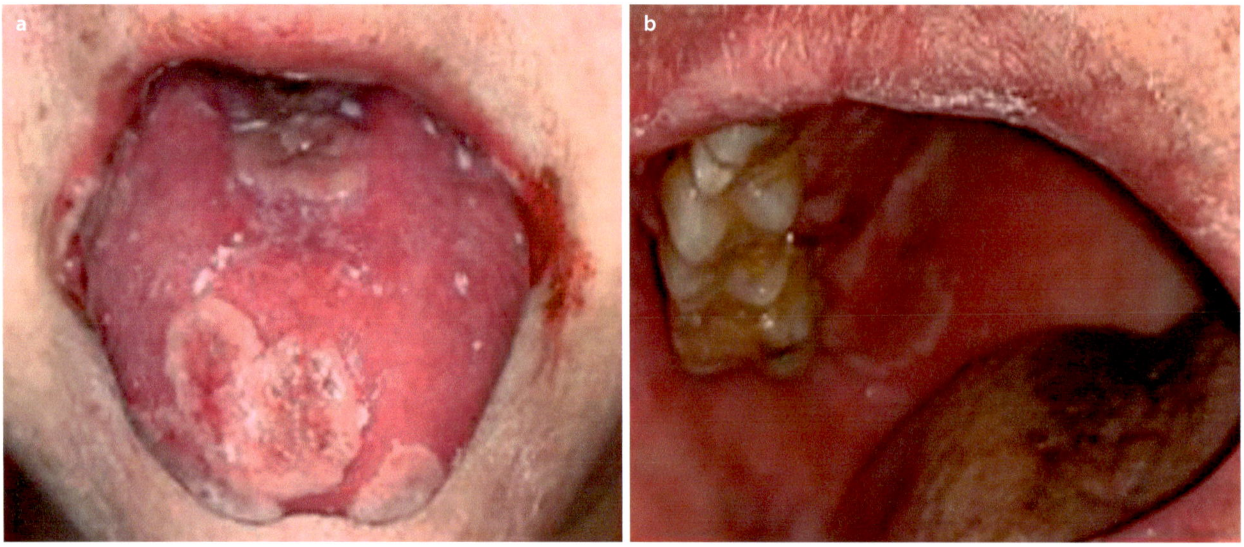

Fig. 50.3 Oral manifestation in anemic patient; (**a**) ulcerations on the tongue and angular cheilitis, (**b**) ulcerations on the palatal mucosa

valine on β-hemoglobin chain. This leads to distortion of erythrocyte shape (sickle shape) and reduced normal lifetime from 120 days to 14 days. Clinically, a patient with sickle cell anemia is characterised by multiple oro-facial manifestations which include 'step-ladder' trabecular pattern of the alveolar process of the jaws, enamel hypomineralisation, calcified canals, diastema, increased overbite, increased overjet, anaesthesia or paraesthesia of the mental nerve or inferior alveolar nerve, asymptomatic pulp necrosis. Another common blood disorder which is characterised by excessive loss of red cells is thalassemia. It is an inherited condition caused by mutations resulting in decreased rate of synthesis of α or β chains, which leads to deficiency of Hb, with additional secondary red cell abnormalities caused by the relative excess of the other unaffected globin chain. Oral manifestations are closely associated with compensatory bone marrow hyperplasia. These include radiographic findings such as attenuated lamina dura, taurodontism, spiky shaped and short roots, enlarged bone marrow spaces, small maxillary sinus, and absence of inferior alveolar canal. Clinically, thalassaemic patients may present with maxillary overdevelopment secondary to bone marrow hyperplasia, thus having a facial characteristic of prominent cheekbones, sunken nose, and labially inclined maxillary incisors and incompetent lips.

3. *Anemia due to loss of red cells*

   As discussed earlier, iron deficiency anemia is a disorder characterised by incomplete Hb synthesis leading to microcytic and hypochromic RBCs. Inadequate Hb further leads to the inability of blood to deliver oxygen to cells and tissues. The common oral manifestations of this disorder are glossitis, glossodynia, angular cheilitis, erythematous mucositis, oral candidiasis, recurrent oral ulcers, and burning mouth (Fig. 50.4).

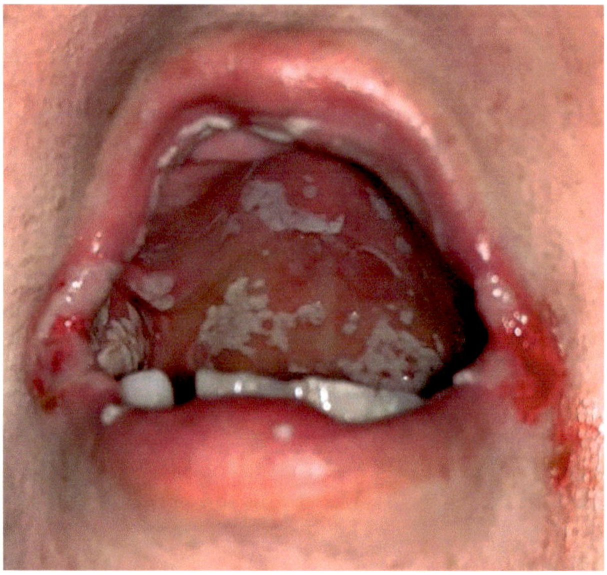

Fig. 50.4 Common oral manifestation in anemia of chronic disease. The patient manifests angular cheilitis, oral candidiasis, and ulcerations

Plummer–Vinson syndrome or Patterson–Brown–Kelly syndrome is a disorder of iron deficiency anemia characterised by atrophic glossitis or angular cheilitis and dysphagia secondary to pharyngoesophageal ulcerations and oesophageal webs. It is also associated with koilonychia or spoon-shaped nails. The salient oral features of iron deficiency anemia are summarised in Table 50.2.

■ Diagnostic Algorithm for Iron Deficiency Anemia

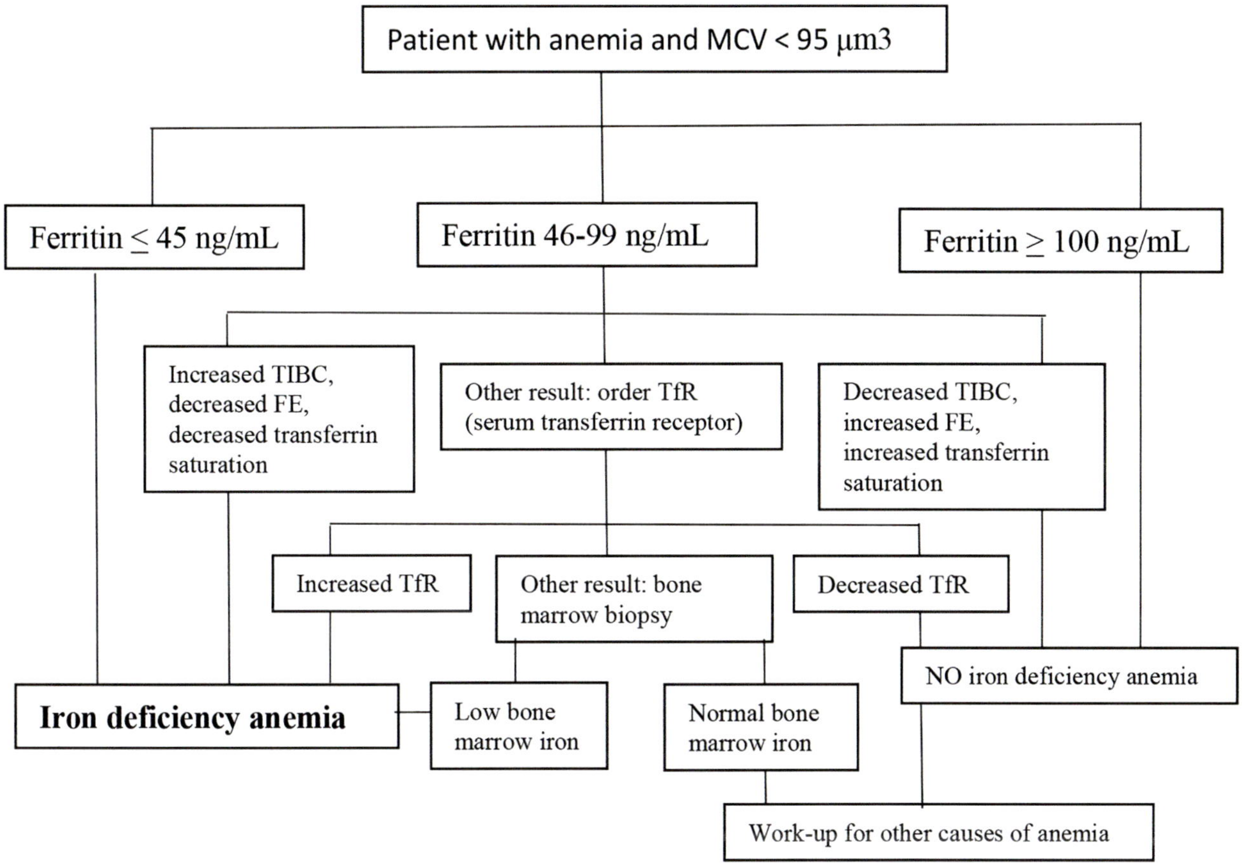

Table 50.2 Salient features of iron deficiency anemia

Salient features of oral manifestations in iron deficiency anemia
Glossitis
Glossodynia
Angular cheilitis
Erythematous mucositis
Oral candidiasis
Recurrent oral ulcers
Burning mouth

Self-Assessment Questions

1. List the common oral manifestations in an anemic patient.
2. Classify anemias.
3. Discuss the differential diagnoses of underlying hematological disorders leading to recurrent aphthous ulcers.
4. Explain the importance of hematological investigations in anemia.
5. Outline the management plan for a patient with a known hematological disorder presenting with oral manifestation.

Summary

History taking is important to determine patient's general and specific symptoms associated with anemia and recurrent oral ulcers, respectively. Medical history provides further valuable information on specific conditions such as peptic ulcer disease that could be the aetiology for anemia. Clinical characteristics of the ulcers must be recognised in order to differentiate between benign and malignant oral lesions. Comprehensive blood investigations are essential for the diagnosis of specific underlying hematological disorders such as iron deficiency anemia. Management includes symptomatic relief for oral ulcers whereas specific intervention to treat the condition leading to the anemia remains the mainstay of the treatment strategy.

50

Suggested Reading

Brennan MT, Sankar V, Baccaglini L, et al. Oral manifestations in patients with aplastic anemia. Oral Surg Oral Med Oral Pathol Oral Radiol Endod. 2001;92:503–8.

Embury SH. The not so simple process of sickle cell vaso-occlusion. Microcirculation. 2004;11:101–13.

Goddard AF, James MW, McIntyre AS, Scott BB. Guidelines for the management of iron deficiency anaemia. Gut. 2011;60:1309–16.

Greenberg MS, Glick M, Ship JA. Burket's oral medicine. 11th ed. New Delhi: CBS Publications; 2012.

Helmi N, Bashir M, Shireen A, et al. Thalassemia review: features, dental considerations and management. Electron Physician. 2017;9(3):4003–8.

Hjorting-Hansen E, Bertram U. Oral aspects of pernicious anaemia. Br Dent J. 1968;125:266–70.

Lahner E, Annibale B. Pernicious anaemia: new insights from a gastroenterological point of view. World J Gastroenterol. 2009;15(41):5121–8.

Naylor GD, Hall EH. Differential diagnosis of glossodynia. J Oral Med. 1987;42:85–8.

Taylor LB, Nowak AJ, Giller RH, et al. Sickle cell anaemia: a review of the dental concerns and a retrospective study of dental and bony changes. Spec Care Dentist. 1995;15:38–42.

Young NS. Acquired aplastic anaemia. Ann Intern Med. 2002;136:534–46.

Granulomatous Disorders

Contents

Generalized Swelling of the Lip: Orofacial Granulomatosis

Prasangi Madubhashini Peiris and Wanninayake M Tilakaratne

Contents

W. M Tilakaratne, T. G. Kallarakkal (eds.), *Clinicopathological Correlation of Oral Diseases*,
https://doi.org/10.1007/978-3-031-24408-7_51

51

Learning Goals
1. Devise the correct way of compiling the history with appropriate questions
2. Develop a differential diagnosis after history taking
3. Formulate a differential diagnosis combining findings in the history and clinical examination
4. Justify the relevant investigations required to arrive at the diagnosis
5. Comprehend the importance of clinicopathological correlation in arriving at the correct diagnosis of OFG
6. Outline the management plan
7. Recognize the importance of a diagnostic algorithm in arriving at a diagnosis

51.1 Main Complaint

A 21-year-old female patient presents to Oral Medicine clinic with a complaint of generalized upper lip swelling.

51.2 History of Complaint

Question: When did the swelling start and what is the nature of it?

The swelling started 3 months ago. Initially there was a mild swelling affecting the upper lip. The swelling increased in size slowly with time without any pain. Now I am having a rubbery feeling of my upper lip. The lower lip is not affected.

Question: Is this the first time that you are experiencing lip swelling?

During the last 6 months I had experienced two episodes of lip swelling. The swelling affected the upper lip and lasted for few days. It was painless and subsided spontaneously.

Question: Did you have any treatment for the swelling?

I didn't seek treatment as it was a mild and asymptomatic swelling and it mostly disappeared after some time.

Question: Do you have any other lesions in the mouth?

I have been suffering from recurrent oral ulcerations for several months. They are small in size but painful and heal within few days. The ulcer-free period is about 3–4 days.

Question: Are you experiencing any dryness in the mouth?

I don't have any dryness of my mouth.

Question: Are you suffering from diarrhoea and abdominal pain?

I don't have any such problems.

Question: Do you have any food or drug allergies? Can you relate taking any particular food and lip swelling?

I have experienced allergic reaction to pineapple but not to any medications. I can't relate any food habit to the lip swelling.

Question: Do you feel tired easily or find it difficult to walk a long distance or climb steps?

I do not experience any such difficulty or tiredness.

Question: Are you suffering from any medical problems? If yes, what kind of medications have you been taking up to now?

I am not suffering from any other medical problems and not on any medication.

Question: Have you undergone any surgery?

I have not undergone any surgery

Question: Have you undergone any dental treatment?

I had undergone a scaling 1 year back but did not undergo any recent dental treatments.

Question: Tell me about your meals

My diet is mostly composed of rice and curry. I use a lot of spices in my curries. I also frequently dine out on working days.

Question: Have you undergone any cosmetic procedures recently, such as injectable fillers to lips?

I have not undergone any such cosmetic procedures.

Question: Do you experience any taste disturbances?

I noticed an alteration in taste recently but without significant disturbances.

❓ Question: Do you smoke or consume alcohol?

✅ I do not smoke or consume alcohol.

❓ Question: What is your occupation?

✅ I am a clerk in a private company.

❓ Question: Tell me about your family?

✅ I am unmarried and living with my parents and brother. I have a good family support.

❓ Question: Are there any family members having a similar condition?

✅ None of my family members have similar complaints.

51.3 With the Findings from the History, What is Your Differential Diagnosis?

1. Idiopathic Orofacial granulomatosis (OFG)
2. Crohn's disease (CD)
3. Angioedema
4. Allergic reaction

51.4 How Do You Justify Your Differential Diagnosis After History Taking?

The patient is having a generalized lip swelling affecting the upper lip. It may occur due to disease conditions such as OFG, CD, angioedema and localized allergic reaction. Furthermore she is suffering from recurrent oral ulceration which is a feature of both CD and OFG. Even though CD is more prevalent than OFG, CD patients suffer from gastrointestinal symptoms such as diarrhoea and abdominal pain and features of malabsorption while this patient does not exhibit such features. However, early cases of CD may not have significant gastrointestinal symptoms. Further, very rare cases of CD can have oral features even before gastrointestinal manifestations. Therefore, at this stage both OFG and CD should be in the differential diagnosis.

According to her dietary habits, she consumes foods containing spices. Cinnamon is one of the common spices used in preparing foods. It has been suggested that cinnamon aldehyde can precipitate OFG in some individuals.

She is allergic to pineapple and according to her food habits she eats frequently from outside and it is possible to get exposed to an allergen even in minor amount causing allergic reaction or angioedema. But the duration of the lip swelling does not support these two differential diagnoses.

51.5 Findings of Examination

The patient looks fit and healthy except the main complaint. She has a generalized upper lip swelling (◘ Fig. 51.1a & b) which is rubbery in consistency without tenderness or altered sensation. There are no features of angular or median cheilitis. She does not have any palpable cervical lymph nodes or other swellings in the head and neck region. Facial nerve examination is normal without any features of nerve palsy such as Bell sign of eyes, difficulty in wind blowing, deviation of mouth to a side while smiling.

Intra orally the gingivae appear erythematous. There are three small ulcers on the upper labial mucosa (◘ Fig. 51.1c) and buccal mucosae with an erythematous halo resembling minor aphthae. The tongue appears shiny and dry without fissuring. There is no evidence of urticaria and features of anemia.

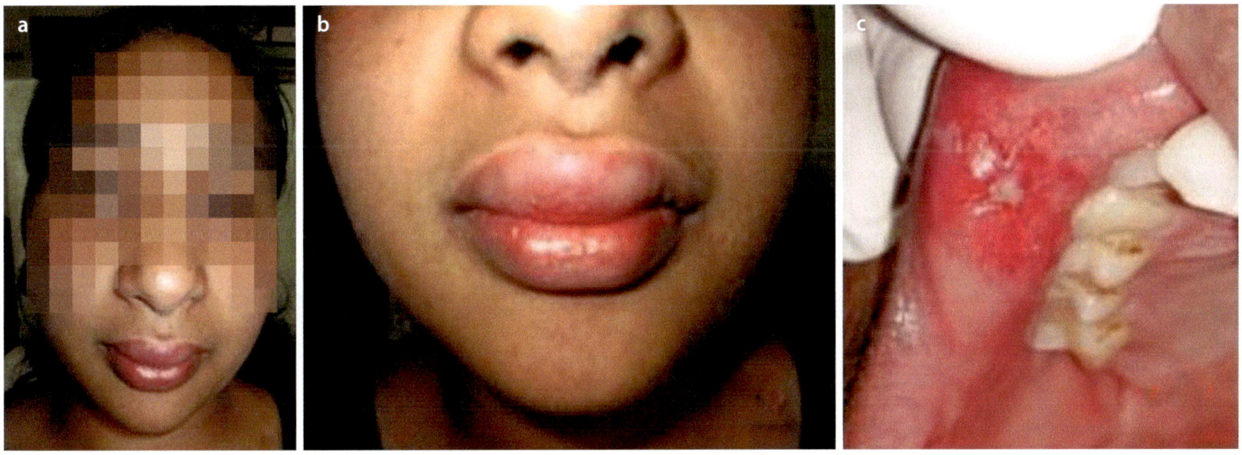

◘ **Fig. 51.1** (**a**, **b**) Generalized upper lip swelling, (**c**) aphthous-like oral ulcer on the upper labial mucosa

51.6 What is Your Clinical Differential Diagnosis?

1. Orofacial granulomatosis
2. Crohn's disease

51.7 How Would You Justify the Inclusion of the Diseases That You Have Mentioned in the Differential Diagnosis to Arrive at a Working Diagnosis?

CD is the commonest inflammatory bowel disease apart from ulcerative colitis. Abdominal pain associated with diarrhoea and features of malabsorption such as weight loss, anemia can be elicited in CD patients from history and examination. Orofacial manifestations of CD are similar to features of OFG. Rarely, oral manifestations appear before gastrointestinal features. Although unlikely, CD is a possible differential diagnosis until the gastrointestinal involvement is ruled out with colonoscopy and other related investigations.

A patient with idiopathic OFG usually presents with orofacial signs and symptoms only. In this patient, there are no features suggestive of intestinal or other system involvement. Melkersson- Rosenthal syndrome (MRS) is a clinical variant of OFG. There is a triad of features for the diagnosis of MRS which consists of lip swelling, facial nerve palsy and fissured tongue. In this case, only the lip swelling is present and facial nerve palsy and fissured tongue are absent. Although, all other recognized granulomatous disorders should be excluded to arrive at the diagnosis of OFG, history and clinical examination are supportive of OFG.

51.8 How Would You Investigate this Patient?

- Full blood count (FBC)
- Erythrocyte Sedimentation Rate (ESR) and C-reactive protein (CRP) as inflammatory markers
- Colonoscopy and bowel biopsy
- Incisional biopsy of the lip

It is important to obtain a deep biopsy for the diagnosis of OFG since in some cases granuloma formation may occur deep within the muscle layer.

51.9 What Are the Findings of the Investigations?

FBC, ESR, CRP—Values are in the normal range
Colonoscopy and bowel biopsy—Normal

51.10 What are the Histopathological Findings?

Haematoxylin and eosin-stained (H & E) sections show mucosa covered by hyperplastic non-keratinized stratified squamous epithelium. The underlying corium contains collection of macrophages forming non-caseating granulomas. The upper corium is oedematous and contains a lymphocytic infiltrate (◘ Fig. 51.2a & 51.2b). There is no evidence of any foreign bodies.

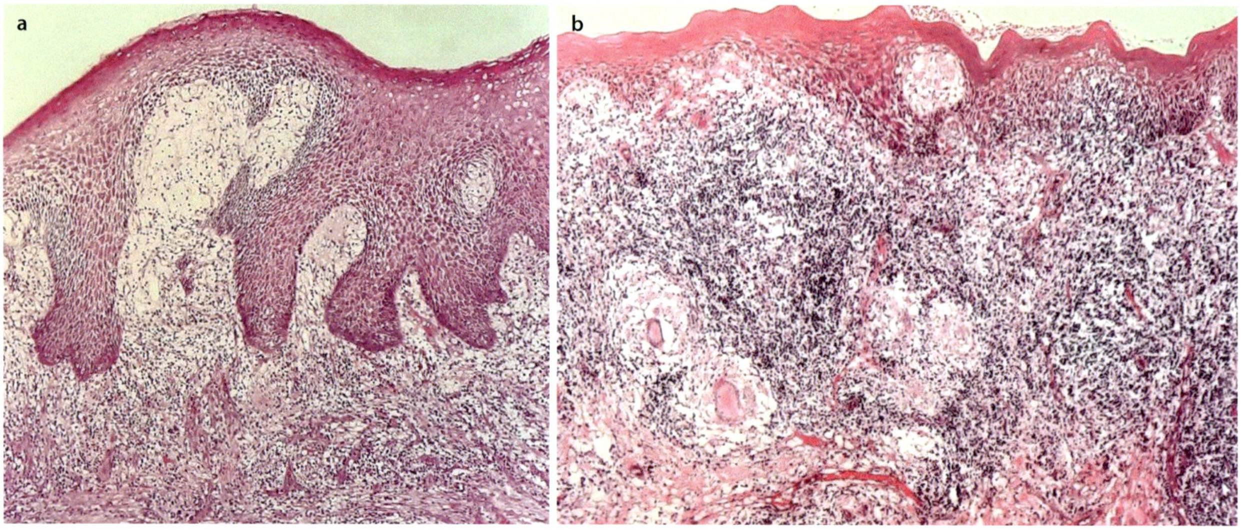

◘ **Fig. 51.2** (**a**) H&E sections showing markedly oedematous corium with spongiosis in the epithelium and (**b**) non-caseating epithelioid granulomas containing multinucleated giant cells

51.11 Do any other Investigations Need to be Performed in Order to Arrive at the Definitive Diagnosis?

It is necessary to exclude known granulomatous conditions such as sarcoidosis and tuberculosis. Polymerase chain reaction (PCR) for Mycobacterium tuberculosis is negative and serum calcium levels are normal. Chest radiograph did not reveal any abnormality.

51.12 What is the Definitive Diagnosis and Explain the Findings Which Helped You to Arrive at the Definitive Diagnosis?

Idiopathic orofacial granulomatosis.

According to the history, a recurrent lip swelling of short duration progressed to a persistent lip swelling and recurrent oral ulceration. Only orofacial features are present without systemic involvement such as abdominal pain and diarrhoea. There are no identifiable causative factors. There were no mucosal abnormalities in colonoscopy. Incisional biopsy shows granuloma formation and other known granulomatous conditions have been excluded. Therefore, the definitive diagnosis is OFG.

51.13 How Would You Manage This Patient?

There is no definitive treatment for OFG, and treatment is mostly symptomatic. Severity of the disease should be considered when deciding the treatment options. The patient can be instructed to avoid dietary allergens such as cinnamon and benzoate which are possible allergens to precipitate OFG.

Pharmacologically topical steroids can be prescribed to apply on lip swelling and intra orally for oral ulceration. Intra-lesional injection of a steroid preferably triamcinolone or methyl prednisolone can be used for lip swelling periodically. A compression device can be introduced to reduce labial swelling.

Oral hygiene instructions should be given to optimize the oral health. Chlorhexidine mouth wash supports in preventing infection of oral ulcers and maintaining periodontal health. Long-term follow-up is necessary with periodic intestinal examination, since features of CD may appear months or years after diagnosing OFG.

51.14 Orofacial Granulomatosis (OFG)

OFG is an uncommon disease which affects oral and perioral region. The first description of orofacial granuloma formation without systemic disease was by Melkerson in 1928 with a case report showing facial palsy and orofacial oedema. Later in 1932, the term Melkersson- Rosenthal syndrome (MRS) was proposed to describe the triad of persistent lip or facial swelling, facial nerve palsy and fissured tongue. Miescher's cheilitis or cheilitis granulomatosa, a monosymptomatic variant of MRS characterized by marked lip swelling was described in 1945. The term Orofacial Granulomatosis was introduced by Wiesenfield in 1985 to describe the occurrence of orofacial granulomas without any systemic involvement.

OFG is a rare condition which affects males and females equally and appears to have predilection for younger age groups. The etiology of OFG is not well understood. It has been suggested that an abnormal immune reaction triggered by an environmental insult in genetically susceptible individuals can cause granulomatous inflammation. Genetic predisposition, allergy to foods, food additives, dental materials and medications and immunological reactions have been suggested as causative factors of OFG. There is no adequate data in existing literature to suggest that OFG has a firm genetic background. However, relationship between OFG and human leucocyte antigen (HLA) has been investigated and revealed that patients with specific HLA haplotypes may be more likely to develop OFG.

The possibility of certain food substances and food additives causing or precipitating OFG by evoking a delayed type hypersensitivity reaction has been suggested. Cinnamon aldehyde, benzoates, monosodium glutamate, wheat, dairy products, eggs, chocolates, peanuts, cocoa and sun yellow dye are some of the implicated substances. Even though there are few reports of positive patch test for mercury in amalgam and cobalt chloride in OFG patients, there is no conclusive evidence to support dental materials as an etiological factor for OFG. There is an association of infection as an etiological factor for chronic granulomatous conditions such as Crohn's disease, sarcoidosis and tuberculosis. On this basis, microbial agents have been suggested for the causation of OFG. *Mycobacterium tuberculosis*, *M. paratuberculosis*, *Saccharomyces cerevisiae* and *Borrelia burgdorferi* are the most commonly suggested microbes in the etiology of OFG.

OFG shows histopathological features suggestive of delayed hypersensitivity. As a result, inflammatory/immunological factors have been suggested in the etiology of OFG. There is evidence that Th1 response in OFG patients is associated with increased IFN-gamma expression and increased levels of IL-12. Increased levels of cytokines, chemokines and chemokine receptors which are associated with Th1-mediated immune response provide further evidence to Th1 nature of the immune response in OFG patients.

The term OFG should be used when the disease is affecting only the oral and perioral region. More importantly all known granulomatous conditions should be excluded with relevant investigations before confirming the diagnosis of OFG. The most characteristic clinical feature of OFG is lip swelling. At the beginning, there can be episodes of painless, soft swelling which may affect one or both lips, more commonly the lower lip. In the absence of treatment, the condition progresses and swelling becomes persistent. Permanently enlarged lips become firm and rubbery and are prone to get median cheilitis and angular cheilitis. Similar swellings can appear in periorbital region and chin.

Intra orally OFG manifests with cobblestone appearance of the mucosa, erythematous and hyperplastic gingivae, oral ulceration and mucosal tags. Cobblestone appearance of buccal and labial mucosa is due to granuloma formation. There can be recurrent aphthous-like ulceration or long-standing deep linear ulcers in the oral mucosa (◘ Fig. 51.3). Mucosal tags may be seen in the buccal and labial sulci and retromolar region. In addition, reduced salivary flow and altered taste sensation have been reported in OFG patients.

Diagnosis of OFG should be made after the exclusion of other possible differential diagnoses. These include CD, sarcoidosis, infections such as tuberculosis and deep fungal infections, amyloidosis and foreign body reaction.

Patients with CD usually suffer from abdominal pain, diarrhoea and features of malabsorption. Haematological tests such as FBC, serum iron, serum vitamin B12 show features of anemia suggesting malabsorption. OFG and CD cannot be differentiated histopathologically. Intestinal examination with colonoscopy shows abnormalities of gut mucosa which is suggestive of CD.

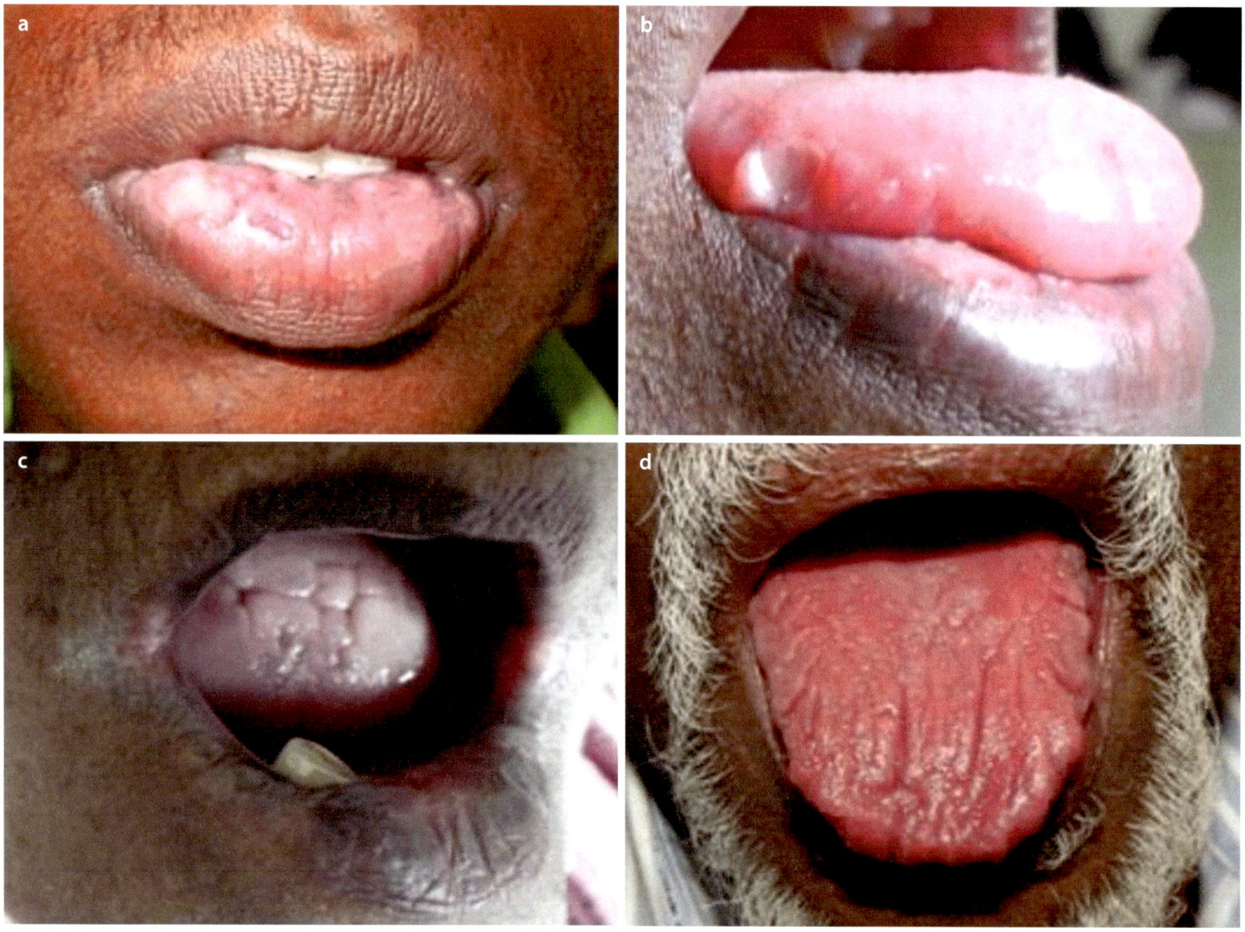

◘ **Fig. 51.3** (**a**) Lower lip swelling with mucosal ulceration, (**b**) ulcer on tongue, (**c**) angular cheilitis, (**d**) fissured tongue

Hilar lymphadenopathy in chest radiograph, increased serum calcium and raised angiotensin-converting enzyme (ACE) are findings of investigations in sarcoidosis. Tuberculosis is another differential diagnosis for OFG. Chest radiograph, tuberculin skin test, polymerase chain reaction (PCR), histopathological examination with special stains such as Ziehl-Neelsen acid-fast technique are investigations that need to be carried out in order to exclude tuberculosis. Histopathologically presence of caseating granulomas in tuberculosis is characteristic whilst there are non-caseating granulomas in OFG. Deep fungal infections can be diagnosed on histopathological examination using special stains such as Periodic acid-Schiff-diastase (D-PAS) and Grocott-Gomori's Methenamine Silver (GMS).

The histopathological features vary depending on the stage of the disease. In early disease, non-caseating granuloma formation is not clearly visible. However, oedematous corium and perivascular lymphocytic infiltration are present in early cases. Dilated lymphatics which contain macrophages causing granulomatous lymphangitis can also be visible in some cases. In advanced disease non-caseating granulomas are evident in the corium or in some cases within the muscle layer. It is common to have varying amounts of fibrosis in cases with persistent swelling. It is important to obtain a deep biopsy including muscle layer to identify deep granulomas.

Treatment of OFG is challenging since there is no cure. The treatment is mostly symptomatic with the aim of controlling the acute disease and to restore function and aesthetics. The uncertainty of the aetiology of the disease has led to a less rational therapy and response to treatment is usually slow and incomplete. When deciding the treatment for a particular patient, the severity of the disease should be considered. Elimination of possible dietary allergens such as cinnamon and benzoate can be carried out. Use of compression devices for several hours regularly may reduce the labial swelling in OFG patients. Pharmacological therapy for OFG includes corticosteroids, immune modulators and antibiotics. Corticosteroid is the first line drug. Method of administration of the drug can vary according to the severity of the disease. Topical steroids can be used for mild cases in the form of ointments, mouth washes or inhalers to control intra oral granuloma and oral ulceration. Periodic intra-lesional steroid injections to lips have shown reduction in lip swelling. In severe cases, it is necessary to use systemic corticosteroids to control the disease. Immunomodulators such as tacrolimus, azathioprine, clofazimine and thalidomide are used in treating OFG. Clofazimine is a lipophilic dye that is thought to be a scavenger of hypochloric acid reducing the chlorination of proteins by neutrophils. However, the exact mechanism in OFG remains unknown. Oral antibiotics such as metronidazole, azithromycin, lymecycline, minocycline and roxithromycin have also been used. Surgical intervention such as cheiloplasty can be carried out in recalcitrant or disfiguring cases. Disfiguring lip and orofacial swelling may affect the quality of life and psychosocial health of patients. It is important to identify the psychological aspects in patients and counselling should be carried out. Long-term follow-up with a referral to a gastroenterologist is necessary in the management of OFG patients, since it can precede gastrointestinal changes of CD.

Salient features of OFG

Clinical features	Lip swelling, median & angular cheilitis, periorbital and chin swelling, erythematous gingiva, cobblestone appearance, oral ulceration, mucosal tags, cervical lymphadenopathy.
Aetiological factors	Genetic factors, allergy, infection, immunological/inflammatory reaction.
Histopathology	Non-caseating granulomas, perivascular lymphocytic infiltration, granulomatous lymphangitis and oedematous corium.
Treatment	Elimination of possible allergens, medications (corticosteroids), physical therapy and surgery.

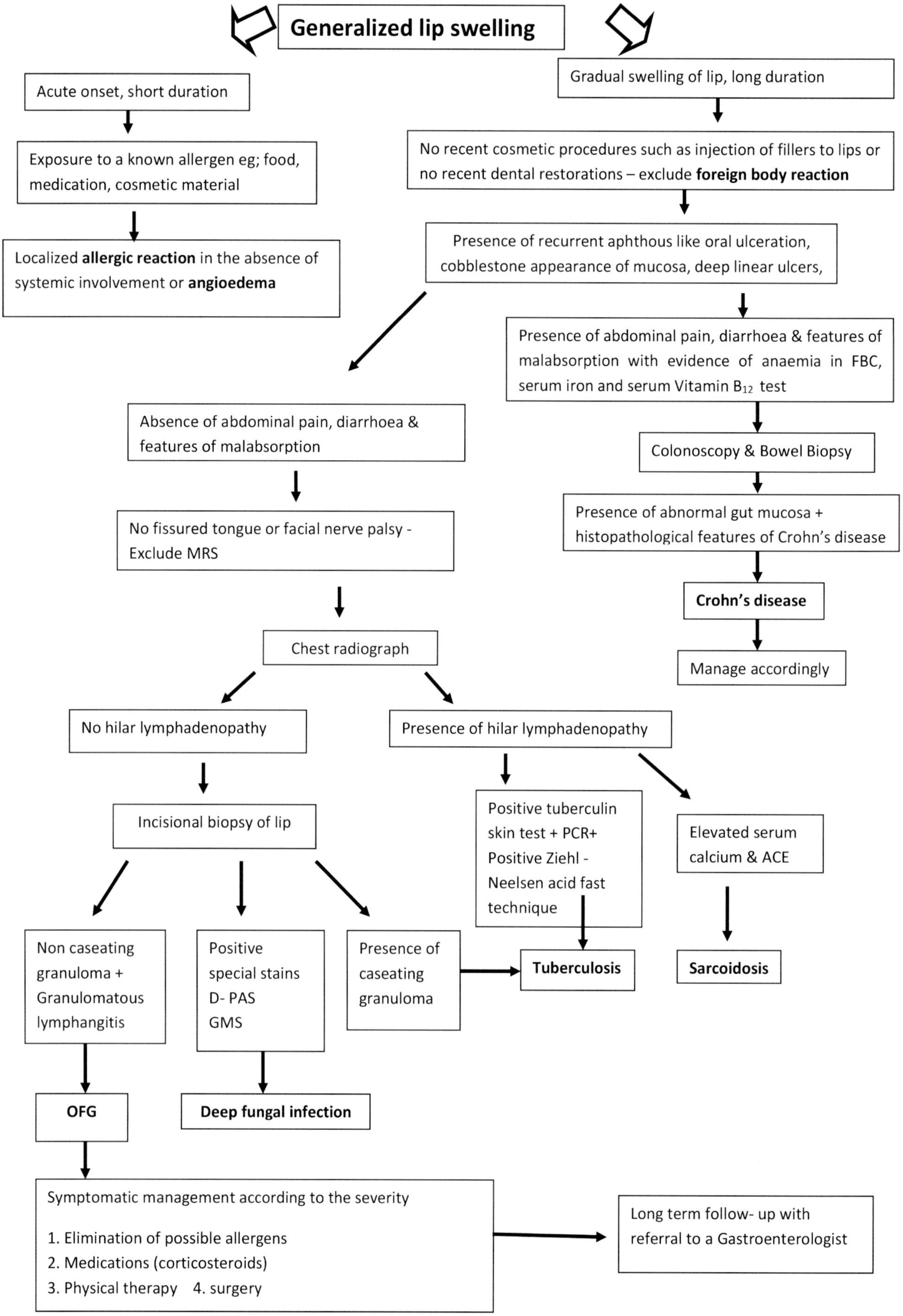
Generalized lip swelling
Acute onset, short duration
Exposure to a known allergen eg; food, medication, cosmetic material
Localized allergic reaction in the absence of systemic involvement or angioedema
Gradual swelling of lip, long duration
No recent cosmetic procedures such as injection of fillers to lips or no recent dental restorations – exclude foreign body reaction
Presence of recurrent aphthous like oral ulceration, cobblestone appearance of mucosa, deep linear ulcers,
Presence of abdominal pain, diarrhoea & features of malabsorption with evidence of anaemia in FBC, serum iron and serum Vitamin B_{12} test
Colonoscopy & Bowel Biopsy
Presence of abnormal gut mucosa + histopathological features of Crohn's disease
Crohn's disease
Manage accordingly
Absence of abdominal pain, diarrhoea & features of malabsorption
No fissured tongue or facial nerve palsy - Exclude MRS
Chest radiograph
No hilar lymphadenopathy
Presence of hilar lymphadenopathy
Incisional biopsy of lip
Positive tuberculin skin test + PCR+ Positive Ziehl - Neelsen acid fast technique
Elevated serum calcium & ACE
Non caseating granuloma + Granulomatous lymphangitis
Positive special stains D- PAS GMS
Presence of caseating granuloma
Tuberculosis
Sarcoidosis
OFG
Deep fungal infection
Symptomatic management according to the severity
1. Elimination of possible allergens
2. Medications (corticosteroids)
3. Physical therapy 4. surgery
Long term follow- up with referral to a Gastroenterologist

Self-Assessment Questions

1. Describe the clinical features of OFG.
2. List the possible aetiological factors of OFG.
3. Describe the histopathological features of OFG.
4. List the diseases that should be excluded prior to the diagnosis of OFG and state how you are going to exclude them.
5. Discuss the available treatment options for OFG.

Summary

OFG is a rare granulomatous disease which affects the oral and perioral region. The clinical features of OFG are similar to oral manifestations of systemic granulomatous diseases such as Crohn's disease. Hence a through history, clinical examination and specific investigations should be carried out to exclude other disease conditions with similar clinical presentations. Successful treatment of OFG is a challenging task for clinicians.

Suggested Reading

Grave B, McCullough M, Wiesenfeld D. Orofacial granulomatosis – a 20-year review. Oral Dis. 2009;15(1):46–51.

Miest R, Bruce A, Rogers RS. Orofacial granulomatosis. Clin Dermatol [Internet]. 2016;34(4):505–13. https://doi.org/10.1016/j.clindermatol.2016.02.024.

Müller S. Non-infectious granulomatous lesions of the orofacial region. Head Neck Pathol [Internet]. 2019;13(3):449–56. https://doi.org/10.1007/s12105-018-00997-w.

Tilakaratne WM, Freysdottir J, Fortune F. Orofacial granulomatosis: review on aetiology and pathogenesis. J Oral Pathol Med. 2008;37(4):191–5.

Wehl G, Rauchenzauner M. A systematic review of the literature of the three related disease entities cheilitis granulomatosa, orofacial granulomatosis and Melkersson–Rosenthal syndrome. Curr Pediatr Rev. 2018;14(3):196–203.

Swelling of the Lips and Shortness of Breath: Sarcoidosis

Muhammad Kamil Hassan and Wanninayake M Tilakaratne

Contents

W. M Tilakaratne, T. G. Kallarakkal (eds.), *Clinicopathological Correlation of Oral Diseases*,
https://doi.org/10.1007/978-3-031-24408-7_52

52

Learning Goals

1. Devise the correct way of compiling the history with appropriate questions
2. Develop a differential diagnosis after history taking
3. Deduce appropriate procedures in clinical examination
4. Formulate a differential diagnosis combining findings in the history and clinical examination
5. Justify the relevant investigations required to arrive at the diagnosis
6. Comprehend the importance of clinicopathological correlation in arriving at the correct diagnosis
7. Outline the management plan
8. Recognize the importance of a diagnostic algorithm in arriving at a diagnosis

52.1 Main Complaint

A 49-year-old female was referred to your dental clinic. Her main complaint is a generalized swelling of her lower lip.

52.2 History of Complaint

Question: How long have you noticed the swellings?

I have noticed it for more than 3 months. It has been there since.

Question: Do you feel that the size of the swelling is getting larger?

Yes, I feel so but I think it is only very slowly enlarging in size.

Question: Is this the first time it happened or you experienced this time to time in the past?

This is the first time I got this and it has been there through out last few months.

Question: Are you allergic to anything?

I am not aware of any.

Question: Can you relate any particular incidence such as applying a new lipstick or having a food that you didn't have in the past?

I don't remember anything like that.

Question: Is it painful, or is there any altered sensation?

I don't have any pain or altered sensation.

52.3 Additional Complaints

Question: Have you noticed or felt any other changes or difficulties in the mouth?

I feel my mouth is getting dryer and need to drink more water. I also get recurrent ulcers in my mouth. The ulcers occur every month and takes a while to heal. This causes some discomfort during eating and chewing foods. I also have a feeling that upper parts of my cheeks getting slightly swollen.

Question: Do you have any lesions anywhere else on the body? Do you have any rashes or skin conditions?

I have some skin rashes on the legs, and arms. They are tender, red and raised and vary in sizes.

Question: Do you feel dryness in your eyes?

No, I don't.

Question: Do you get tired easily? Do you experience fatigue during your daily routine?

I sometimes experience 'shortness of breath' especially when doing heavy work.

Question: Do you experience dry cough, and chest discomfort apart from the 'shortness of breath'?

Yes, I do sometimes.

Question: Do you have any joint pain?

I do, sometimes have painful joints.

Question: Have you lost weight during past few months.

I have a feeling that I have lost my weight slightly.

Question: Are you suffering from any other medical problems like heart disease, high blood pressure, diabetes, respiratory diseases, gastrointestinal problems such as abdominal pain or diarrhoea?

I do not have any medical issues and is not taking any other medications.

Question: What is your occupation?

I work as a clerk in a business company.

Question: Are you a smoker?

I am an ex-smoker. I stopped smoking since 5 years. I previously smoked about five cigarettes a day for 10 years.

Question: Do you take alcohol.

I do not drink alcohol.

52.4 With the History Findings, What Is Your Differential Diagnosis?

1. Sarcoidosis
2. Sjogren Syndrome
3. Orofacial granulomatosis
4. Crohn's disease

52.5 How Do You Justify Your Differential Diagnosis After History Taking?

1. She has swellings involving her lips. In addition, her cheek swellings are gradually becoming larger. She also experiences dryness in her mouth. Cheek swellings may arise from various tissues including the parotid glands, facial and masticatory muscles or from within the mucosa. In this case, it could be suggested that the swelling originates from the parotid gland and further suggests the possibility of Sjogren's syndrome or sarcoidosis with other associated features.
2. Skin rashes may be seen in sarcoidosis where the lesion can appear on any parts of the body. They typically appear as chronic, indurated lesions especially on the lower legs.
3. Her complaint with regards to fatigue, coughing and chest discomfort may be caused by involvement of lungs, mediastinal and paratracheal lymph nodes. This is found in 90% of the patients with sarcoidosis. Although some of these features are suggestive of tuberculosis, lip and cheek swelling with pulmonary symptoms are more suggestive of sarcoidosis.
4. Furthermore, lip swellings and oral ulceration may also suggest orofacial granulomatosis and Crohn's disease. Her weight loss may further suggest the possibility of Crohn's disease due to the effect on the gastrointestinal lining and malabsorption of nutrients.

52.6 Findings of Examination

She has an obvious, generalized swelling of the lower lip (Fig. 52.1) which is soft-rubbery in consistency and is not painful on palpation. There are erythematous mac-

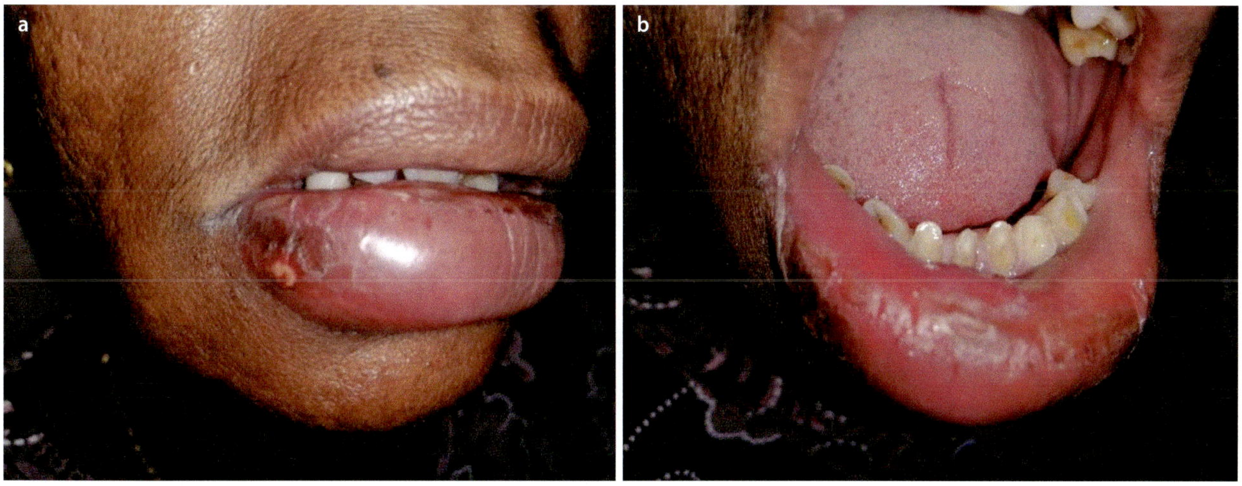

Fig. 52.1 Generalized lower lip swelling with focal ulceration. (**a**) Generalized lower lip swelling with erythematous macules. (**b**) erosive areas on the lower labial mucosa. (Courtesy of Prof Ruwan Jayasinghe)

ules with central hyperkeratosis on the lower labial mucosa. A few erosive areas are also present on the lip. The cheek swellings are mild and bilateral. The swelling feels firm and is located within the parotid gland region. Salivary duct orifices appear normal and saliva is expressed from the ducts when squeezing both the parotid and submandibular glands.

She also has red-coloured maculopapular rashes on her legs. There is no obvious dryness in her eyes. Although, the patient complains about dryness of the mouth, the oral mucosa did not appear dry except the swollen lips. There is no cervical lymphadenopathy or enlarged lymph nodes elsewhere in the body.

52.7 What Other Relevant Features Would You Look for Based on Your Current Findings?

There is thick, viscous saliva with no pooling in the floor of mouth. Oral hygiene is moderate and can be related to the dry mouth. Other oral cavity structures look normal. The buccal mucosa does not seem to be affected. Minimal saliva can be expressed from the Stensen's ducts.

52.8 What Is Your Clinical/Working Diagnosis?

Sarcoidosis

52.9 How Would You Exclude Other Conditions and Justify Your Clinical/Working Diagnosis?

52.9.1 Orofacial Granulomatosis (OFG)/Crohn's Disease

The most common site of involvement is the lips. However, the clinical presentation is highly variable. The labial tissues often present as a persistent swelling which is soft and non-tender. Other intra-oral sites may also be involved and present with various lesions such as ulcers, papules and oedema. The buccal mucosa often shows a cobblestone appearance due to submucosal enlargement. However, hyposalivation is rarely reported. Involvement of parotid gland and other skin manifestations are not features of OFG. The manifestations of Crohn's disease in the oral cavity are very similar to OFG and together with the absence of gastrointestinal features, presence of parotid and skin involvement exclude the possibility of Crohn's disease.

52.9.2 Sjogren Syndrome

Sjogren syndrome can present as a primary Sjogren syndrome or secondary with associated other autoimmune disorders such as rheumatoid arthritis. The presentation is similar to sarcoidosis especially in the head and neck region. Swelling of the parotids and other salivary glands with resulting dryness of the mouth is a typical presentation. The patient does not have significant level of dry mouth or dry eyes. In addition, the presence of skin lesions and respiratory symptoms makes it unlikely to be the working diagnosis.

52.9.3 Sarcoidosis

This disorder is a multisystem granulomatous disorder which can affect any organ, but predominantly the lungs, lymph nodes, skin, eyes and salivary glands. The presence of swollen parotid glands, skin rashes, lip swelling and respiratory symptoms highly suggest sarcoidosis as the working diagnosis. The dry mouth can be a feature as a consequence of salivary gland involvement.

52.10 How Would You Investigate This Patient?

1. Blood test including serum calcium and angiotensin-converting enzyme levels
2. Chest X-ray to show bilateral hilar lymphadenopathy (Fig. 52.2)

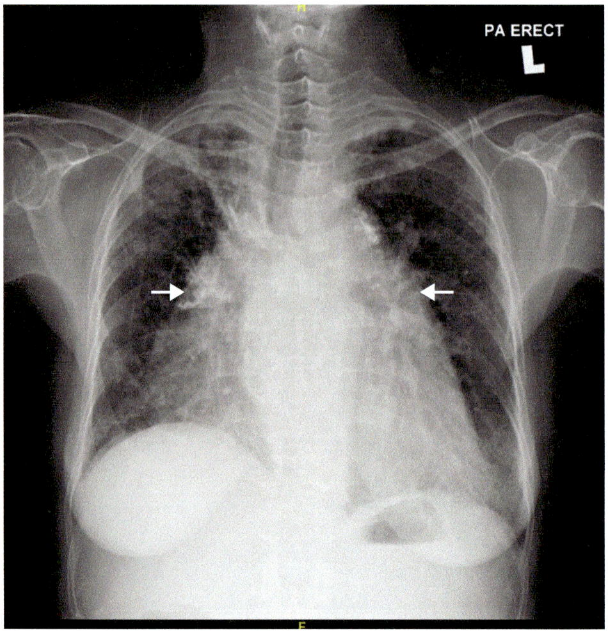

Fig. 52.2 Chest X-ray showing bilateral hilar lymphadenopathy

3. Kveim skin test (Not used much presently)
4. Minor salivary gland biopsy
5. Sialography and sialometry

52.11 How Would You Do a Lip Biopsy for This Patient?

Salivary gland biopsy can be done on both minor salivary glands and major salivary glands. Minor salivary glands are widely distributed in the labial and buccal mucosae of the oral cavity. Labial salivary glands, in particular, are easily accessible as they lie above the muscle layer, and are separated from the oral mucous membrane by a thin connective tissue layer. Minimal bleeding is anticipated as the main vessels to the lip lie deep in the muscles. There are several methods to perform a labial salivary gland biopsy. The described techniques include, horizontal, vertical, wedge-shaped and punch biopsy. Complications reported after different techniques are bleeding, external hematoma, swelling, pain and paresthesia.

Parotid gland biopsy may be avoided because of the possibility of causing a salivary fistula and damage to the facial nerve. These concerns have been reduced through the biopsy technique and incision made below the earlobe to reach the posterior superior lobe of the parotid gland. However, parotid biopsy is not indicated for this purpose.

52.12 What Are the Histopathological Features Present in Sarcoidosis?

Biopsy of the salivary glands in sarcoidosis exhibits a classic picture of granulomatous inflammation which is not specific to sarcoidosis alone. There are aggregates of epithelioid histiocytes, with a surrounding rim of lymphocytes. Multinucleated giant cells are scattered and intermixed with the histiocytes. Calcified structures namely Schaumann bodies (degenerated lysosomes) and asteroid bodies (entrapped fragments of collagen) can be seen in the granuloma. There is no evidence of necrosis which is a feature in tuberculosis (◘ Fig. 52.3).

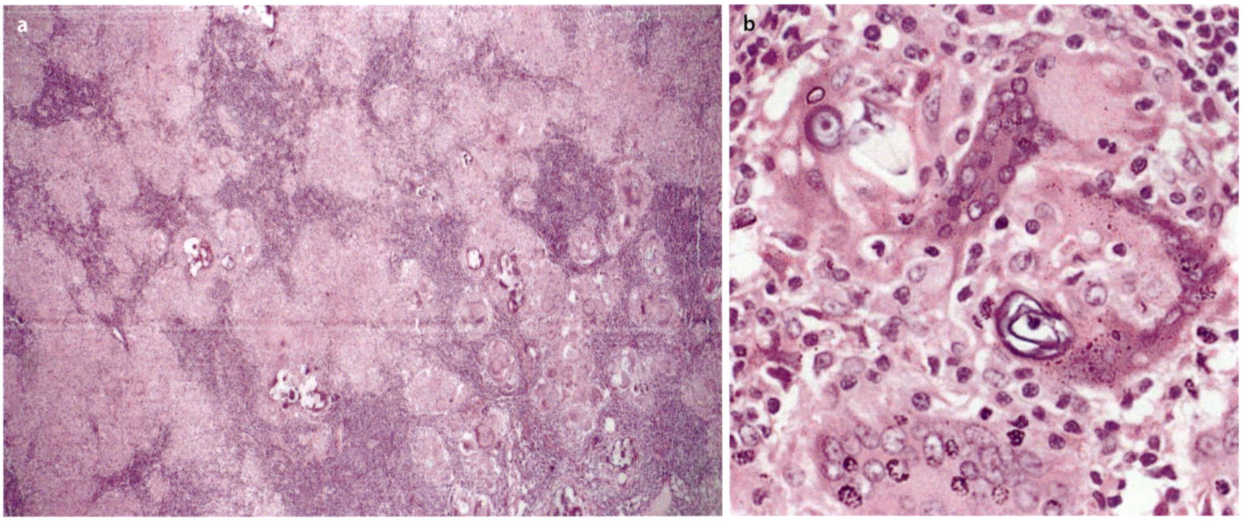

◘ **Fig. 52.3** H&E sections showing (**a**) numerous epithelioid granulomas without caseous necrosis and containing a rim of lymphocytes at the periphery. (**b**) Numerous calcified bodies and multinucleated giant cells are also present (Courtesy of Dr. Shanika Fernandopulle)

52.13 How Would You Manage This Patient?

Sarcoidosis being a multisystem granulomatous disorder, the management should involve a multi-disciplinary team comprising of Rheumatologist, Respiratory physician, Dermatologist, Ophthalmologists, Oral surgeon, Oral Pathology and Oral Medicine specialists and others.

The diagnosis of sarcoidosis should not be arrived on the biopsy alone, as histopathology is non-specific. The diagnosis should be based on the presence of non-caseating granulomas on histopathological examination, compatible clinical presentation and exclusion of other causes of granulomatous inflammation together with the findings of serological and radiological examination.

Treatment for patients with sarcoidosis is mainly reserved for those with disabling symptoms or with progressive organ damage/dysfunction. This is because approximately 60% of patients with sarcoidosis resolve spontaneously within 2 years without treatment. Medications used for treatment include corticosteroids, methotrexate, azathioprine, chlorambucil, chloroquine and cyclophosphamide.

52.14 Sarcoidosis

Sarcoidosis is a multisystem granulomatous disorder of unknown aetiology that can affect many organs. The disorder was initially described by Jonathon Hutchinson in 1875 but it was Boek in 1889 proposed the term sarcoidosis. The main features of this disorder are the non-caseating granulomas, with clusters of epithelioid macrophages and mononuclear cells in the peripheral zone. Although, the exact etiology is unknown, it is thought that both genetic predisposition, infectious agents (Epstein-Barr virus, Human Herpes virus and others) and other environmental factors play a role in the pathogenesis.

The highest incidence of the disorder is observed among African-Americans (17–35 per 100,000 population), followed by Caucasians (5–12 per 100,000 population) and then Asians and Hispanics (1–3 per 100,000 population). It is more prevalent in females with the average age at diagnosis between 35 and 50 years.

Approximately 20% of patients with the condition do not exhibit any symptoms, and the disease is discovered on routine chest radiographs. In acute cases, patients often exhibit fever, fatigue, anorexia or weight loss. These can be combined with other manifestations such as respiratory symptoms, skin lesions, polyarthritis and visual problems. The most common organs to be affected in sarcoidosis are the lungs, lymph nodes, skin, eyes and salivary glands. Over 90% of patients with sarcoidosis have affected lungs and intrathoracic lymph nodes. Pulmonary sarcoidosis can be categorized into four stages; stage I: mediastinal and hilar adenopathy without pulmonary infiltrates, stage II: mediastinal and hilar adenopathy with pulmonary infiltrates, stage III: pulmonary infiltrates without adenopathy—adenopathy regresses and stage IV: pulmonary fibrosis with volume loss and no adenopathy. The common symptoms include cough, dyspnoea and chest tightness. The prognosis for stage I is good with spontaneous regression in 80% of the patients. However, the prognosis becomes poor as the stage of the disease advances.

Skin involvement is the most common extrapulmonary manifestation of sarcoidosis and is present in one-third of the patients. Skin lesions can be specific (skin lesions with non-caseating granulomas) and non-specific (erythema nodosum). The skin lesions can present as papules/plaques or subcutaneous nodules. The plaques and papules can either be skin-coloured or hyperpigmented, erythematous and more commonly found on the extremities and head and neck region compared to the trunk and abdomen. Lupus pernio presents as chronic, violaceous indurated lesions and are frequently found on the nose, ears, lips and face. Erythema nodosum are skin lesions that are non-specific to sarcoidosis. It is typically present in the lower extremities. The presence of erythema nodosum usually indicates an acute form of sarcoidosis. Ocular involvement is noted in 25% of cases and often appears as anterior uveitis. Patients with anterior uveitis present with visual loss, eye pain and redness. When the lacrimal gland is involved, keratoconjunctivitis sicca occurs.

A combination of clinical presentations of acute sarcoidosis gives rise to two distinct syndromes. Lofgren syndrome consists of bilateral hilar lymphadenopathy, erythema nodosum and arthritis. Heerfordt syndrome patients have parotid enlargement, anterior uveitis of the eye, facial paralysis and fever. This is also referred to as uveoparotid fever.

When the head and neck region is involved, sarcoidosis manifests with the involvement of the salivary glands and oral mucosa. This can present as gland enlargement and xerostomia, mimicking Sjogren syndrome. In the oral cavity, any mucosal site can be affected. Lesions can present as ulcers, papules or submucosal masses. The mucosal lesions may present as normal mucosal colour, brown-red, violaceous or hyperkeratotic lesions. Most common site of involvement in the oral cavity is the buccal mucosa followed by gingiva, lips, tongue and palate. Crohn's disease and OFG are the closest differential diagnoses for oral manifestations of sarcoidosis.

Histopathologically, sarcoidosis exhibits the classic picture of granulomatous inflammation. There are tightly clustered aggregates of epithelioid macrophages with surrounding lymphocytes. Multinucleated giant cells are intermixed with the histiocytes. Schaumann bodies (degenerated lysosomes) or asteroid bodies (stellate inclusions) are often present in the granulomas. However, none of these features are specific to sarcoidosis.

Sarcoidosis is diagnosed by clinical and radiographical presentations, histopathological appearances and negative findings from other special stains and culture. Special blood investigations such as increase in serum Angiotensin-converting enzyme (ACE) with pulmonary involvement strongly support the diagnosis of sarcoidosis. Salivary gland biopsy complements other biopsy sites (pulmonary or intrathoracic nodes). Minor salivary gland biopsy is easily accessible but is less effective than a parotid gland biopsy. Parotid gland biopsy is associated with various complications such as salivary fistula formation and risk of injury to the facial nerve.

Approximately 60% of patients with sarcoidosis show spontaneous resolution within 2 years without treatment. Treatment of sarcoidosis is reserved for cases with progressive disease, cardiac and pulmonary involvement, skin disease and serious ocular lesions. Corticosteroids are the first-line drug therapy but it is associated with side effects and relapses.

Salient features of sarcoidosis	
Clinical	Oral cavity—ulcers, papules, submucosal mass Head and neck—salivary gland enlargement. Skin lesion on the face known as lupus pernio Eyes—anterior uveitis Skin—erythema nodosum Lungs—bilateral hilar lymphadenopathy
Histopathology	Non-caseating granulomatous inflammation; tightly clustered epithelioid macrophages with a surrounding rim of lymphocytes
Treatment	Spontaneous resolution in 60% of patients without treatment. When progressive and causes morbidity in affected organs, corticosteroid is the first-line drug therapy
Sarcoidosis is a multisystem granulomatous disorder of unknown cause. It is important to identify the disorder and differentiate it from other orofacial granulomatous diseases. Management is multi-disciplinary and often involves several medical specialties.	

- **Diagnostic Algorithm for Sarcoidosis Symptoms Presented in the Head and Neck Region**

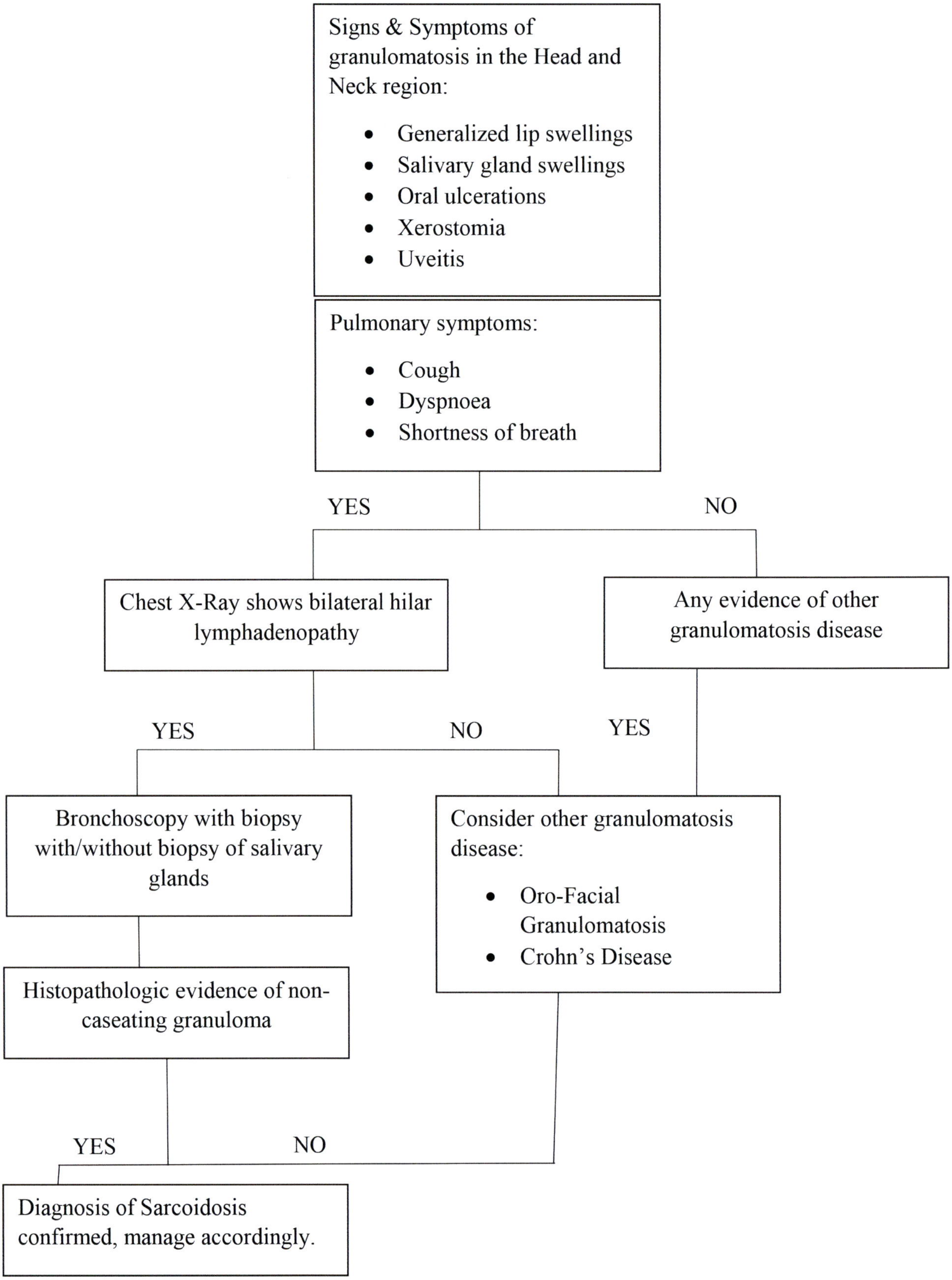

Self-Assessment Questions

1. List the pathognomonic clinical features of sarcoidosis.
2. State the important conditions that need to be included in the differential diagnosis.
3. What are the head and neck manifestations of sarcoidosis?
4. State the histopathological features of sarcoidosis.
5. Outline the management plan according to the stage of the disease.

Suggested Reading

Blinder D, Yahatom R, Taicher S. Oral manifestations of sarcoidosis. Oral Surg Oral Med Oral Pathol Oral Radiol Endod. 1997;83(4):458–61. https://doi.org/10.1016/s1079-2104(97)90145-1.

Chappity P, Kumar R, Sahoo AK. Heerfordt's syndrome presenting with recurrent facial nerve palsy: case report and 10-year literature review. Sultan Qaboos Univ Med J. 2015;15(1):e124–8.

Gupta S, Tripathi AK, Kumar V, Saimbi CS. Sarcoidosis: oral and extra-oral manifestation. J Indian Soc Periodontol. 2015;19(5):582–5. https://doi.org/10.4103/0972-124X.167167.

Llanos O, Hamzeh N. Sarcoidosis. Med Clin North Am. 2019;103(3):527–34. https://doi.org/10.1016/j.mcna.2018.12.011.

Soto-Gomez N, Peters JI, Nambiar AM. Diagnosis and management of sarcoidosis. Am Fam Physician. 2016;93(10):840–8.

Suresh L, Radfar L. Oral sarcoidosis: a review of literature. Oral Dis. 2005;11(3):138–45.https://doi.org/10.1111/j.1601-0825.2005.01014.x.

Neurological Disorders

Contents

Asymmetry of Face: Bell's Palsy

Thomas George Kallarakkal and Wei Cheong Ngeow

Contents

W. M Tilakaratne, T. G. Kallarakkal (eds.), *Clinicopathological Correlation of Oral Diseases*,
https://doi.org/10.1007/978-3-031-24408-7_53

53

53.1 Main Complaint

A 42-year-old male patient presented to the Oral & Maxillofacial Surgery clinic complaining of facial asymmetry.

? Question: How long have you been having this facial asymmetry?

✓ I noticed the facial asymmetry three days ago when I woke up in the morning and observed myself in the mirror.

? Question: Has your condition worsened over the past three days?

✓ I feel that the asymmetry has become worse. It has been slowly progressing since I first noticed it three days ago.

? Question: Have you had similar episodes in the past?

✓ I have never experienced any similar symptoms in the past.

? Question: Did you experience facial twitching prior to the onset of the facial asymmetry?

✓ I did not experience facial twitching before the onset of facial asymmetry.

? Question: Do you have weakness on one side of your body making it difficult to perform your daily activities such as walking, dressing and grabbing objects?

✓ I don't have any such difficulty.

? Question: Do you have any difficulty in comprehending/pick up words to speak?

✓ I don't have any difficulty in comprehending my speech.

? Question: Was your face exposed to a cold draught of wind prior to the development of this symptom?

✓ I don't remember my face being exposed to cold winds.

? Question: Did you splash ice cold water on your face prior to the development of the symptom?

✓ I did not splash cold water on my face. I normally wash my face only with warm water.

? Question: Do you have a history of tick bites?

✓ I do not recall any exposure to ticks.

? Question: Do you have a recent travel history to any countries that are endemic for ticks?

✓ I have not travelled beyond my state in the last six months owing to work commitments.

? Question: Do you have any rash, blisters or diffuse areas of redness on the skin of your face or body?

✓ I do not have any skin lesions

? Question: Do you feel any stiffness in your joints?

✓ I don't have any pain or stiffness in my joints.

? Question: Do you have headache, fever or feel weak and dizzy?

✓ I am perfectly fine and do not have headache and fever.

? Question: Do you have cough?

✓ I have not had any cough or running nose since many months.

? Question: Did you suffer from any trauma to your head or face?

✓ I do not recall any trauma to my head or face in the recent past.

? Question: Did you have any vaccinations recently?

✓ I had my booster vaccine (Pfizer) for covid-19, two months ago. I had a mild fever and body ache for two days after the vaccination.

53.2 Additional Complaints

? Question: Do you have any pain in or around the ear?

✓ I have been having pain in my left ear for the past 4–5 days.

? Question: Is there any pus discharge from your left ear?

✓ I have not noticed any discharge from my left ear.

❓ Question: What is the nature of the pain?

✅ It is a dull type of pain that is persistent.

❓ Question: Are there any factors that make the pain better or worse?

✅ There are no aggravating factors for the pain. I applied Neomycin ear drops that was suggested by my friend for two days. The pain did not reduce after the application of the ear drops. The pain is relieved slightly when I take Paracetamol tablets.

❓ Question: Does the pain affect your sleep?

✅ The pain doesn't affect my sleep.

❓ Question: Is the pain radiating in nature?

✅ The pain is not radiating in nature.

❓ Question: Do you have any difficulty in hearing?

✅ I do not have any difficulty in hearing. However, I feel extremely sensitive on the left side as the noises appear to be very loud.

❓ Question: Did you notice any swelling in front of the left ear or around the ear?

✅ There is no swelling in front or around my left ear.

❓ Question: Is there any abnormal sensation or feeling of numbness over the affected area?

✅ I feel numbness over the cheek on my left side.

❓ Question: Do you feel any weakness in your facial muscles?

✅ I feel that my facial muscles on the left side have become weak.

❓ Question: Do you have difficulty in eating?

✅ I cannot eat well as I find it difficult to chew my food.

❓ Question: Did you notice any alteration in your taste sensation?

✅ I feel that my food is either not sweet enough or does not contain enough salt. My food seems tasteless despite adding excess salt or sugar.

❓ Question: Do you feel that your mouth is dry?

✅ My mouth feels a little dry.

❓ Question: Do you have any difficulty to swallow food and liquids?

✅ I do not have any difficulty in swallowing food and liquids.

❓ Question: Do you have difficulty in smiling?

✅ I find it very difficult to smile properly.

❓ Question: Do you have any difficulty in closing your eyes?

✅ I cannot close my eyes fully on the left side.

❓ Question: Do you have any other medical problems like heart disease, high blood pressure, diabetes, bleeding disorder, respiratory diseases?

✅ I was diagnosed with Type 2 Diabetes a few years ago. I am currently on Tablet Metformin 200 mg twice a day. I am on regular follow-up and my HbA1c levels are within the normal range. I am also taking Tablet Amlodipine 10 mg once a day for my blood pressure.

❓ Question: Do you have a history of stroke?

✅ I don't have a history of stroke.

❓ Question: Do you have any history of surgery or radiotherapy in the head and neck region?

✅ I have not undergone any surgery or radiotherapy in the past.

❓ Question: Does anybody in your family have a history of facial paralysis?

✅ My parents and my siblings are all healthy.

❓ Question: Do you have any risk habits such as smoking or drinking alcohol?

✅ I am a smoker and smoke about 5–6 cigarettes a day.

❓ Question: Are you employed?

✅ I am currently working as a senior data analyst in a local firm.

53.3 With the Findings from the History, What Is Your Differential Diagnosis?

1. Bell's palsy
2. Ramsay Hunt syndrome
3. Stroke
4. Tumours or space occupying lesions involving the central nervous system
5. Tumours involving the parotid gland or the facial nerve
6. Acute otitis media
7. Lyme disease
8. Auto immune disorders including Gullian-Barre syndrome and multiple sclerosis
9. Lymphoreticular malignancy
10. Sarcoidosis

53.4 How Do You Justify Your Differential Diagnosis After History Taking?

He complains of facial asymmetry for the past three days. The onset was sudden and gradually progressed to the present state. He feels that the left side of his face is numb. He has facial weakness on the left side with difficulty in chewing his food. He also cannot smile properly and has difficulty in closing his eyes completely on the left side. An acute ipsilateral weakness of the facial muscles accompanied by symptoms such as facial numbness is a characteristic feature of Bell's palsy. It is suspected to arise as a result of inflammation of the facial nerve in the geniculate ganglion leading to its compression, ischaemia and demyelination. Even though the factors that give rise to this inflammation remain unclear, a probable aetiology that has been suggested is that of a reactivated herpes simplex virus type 1 (HSV-1) infection within the geniculate ganglion. HSV-1 and herpes simplex virus type 2 (HSV-2) are neurotropic viruses and the viral genome remains in a latent form within the ganglia throughout the life of the host after the primary infection. A high frequency of diabetes mellitus has been reported in patients with Bell's palsy. Diabetic patients with Bell's palsy are prone to develop a more severe injury and have a less favourable outcome. The probable aetiology for the facial palsy has been attributed to ischaemia of the facial nerve due to diabetic small vessel disease. The patient has a history of otalgia since 4–5 days which probably suggests an ear infection leading to inflammation of the facial nerve in the geniculate ganglion. Moreover his diabetic state would have also served as a predisposing factor for Bell's palsy.

Ramsay Hunt syndrome (RHS) is defined as peripheral facial nerve palsy accompanied by erythematous vesicular rash on the ear or in the mouth. RHS is a type of acute herpes zoster associated with reactivation of the varicella zoster virus (VZV) in the geniculate ganglion. Other symptoms of RHS include tinnitus, hearing loss, nausea, vomiting, vertigo and nystagmus owing to the close proximity of the geniculate ganglion to the vestibulocochlear nerve within the bony facial canal. The patient complains of a persistent dull pain in his left ear for the past 4–5 days accompanied by numbness and facial paralysis on the left side. He also has hyperacusis. There is no history of vesicular eruptions on the facial skin, around the ear and in the mouth. The patient also does not have any other symptoms suggestive of vestibulocochlear nerve involvement. A diagnosis of RHS cannot be excluded as reactivation of the VZV can manifest only as neuralgic or neuropathic pain without any vesicular eruptions on the skin. This atypical clinical presentation of HZ is known as zoster sine herpete (ZSH).

Stroke is a clinical syndrome believed to arise as a result of a focal cerebral damage which is usually sudden in onset. The characteristic features of stroke include rapid onset of clinical signs lasting for more than 24 h or leading to death. Cerebral ischaemia is the principal aetiology for stroke in majority of the patients. Cerebral haemorrhage which may be either intracerebral or subarachnoid is the causative factor in a lesser number of patients. The patient is a 42-year-old male with a history of hypertension, diabetes mellitus and smoking which are all established risk factors for stroke. He has numbness and weakness on the left side of his face. However, he does not have hemiparesis, dysphasia, dysphagia, difficulty in hearing and visual disturbances which are the clinical features of a stroke. Stroke is included in the differential diagnosis based on the history and clinical presentation of facial muscle weakness. A detailed clinical examination to determine whether the upper facial movement is preserved and evaluation of cranial nerve function, including all facial muscles will help to confirm the diagnosis.

Primary and metastatic tumours along the central cranial nerve pathways can cause cranial nerve palsy. CNS lesions above the level of the facial nucleus in the pons of the contralateral hemisphere result in unilateral weakness of the lower facial area. This is due to the fact that the cells of the facial nucleus that innervate the lower face receive corticobulbar fibres primarily from the contralateral cerebral hemisphere while cells of the facial nucleus that innervate the upper face receive corticobulbar fibres originating from both cerebral hemispheres. Besides these cortical signs such as hemiparesis, hemi sensory loss, dysarthria and self-neglect suggest a lesion of the cerebral cortex. The patient is alert and responsive with no features to suggest a cerebral cortical lesion. The patient did not give a history of facial twitch or spasm indicating continuous facial nerve irritation suggestive of a tumour. Further examination to determine whether upper facial movement as well as all cranial nerve function are preserved needs to be carried out to discriminate between cortical/central and peripheral facial nerve weakness.

Facial nerve paralysis associated with benign tumours have an insidious onset while those associated with malignant tumours have an acute onset. Malignant tumours include primary parotid tumours associated with the facial nerve and sarcomas arising from facial nerve. Benign tumours affecting the facial nerve include facial nerve schwannomas and geniculate ganglion haemangiomas. Parotid salivary gland tumours manifest as a clinically evident swelling. An estimated 70% of all salivary gland tumours occur within the parotid gland. Majority of the salivary gland tumours are benign, pleomorphic adenoma being the most common. Facial nerve paralysis or paresis is a clinical sign that a parotid mass is most likely malignant and has invaded the facial nerve. The patient did not complain of any swelling in front or around the ear suggestive of a parotid mass. However, a thorough clinical examination is mandatory to exclude the differential diagnosis of a parotid mass and intraparotid lymph node metastasis from an unknown primary tumour. Examination to evaluate the cranial nerves, lymph nodes, ears and facial skin will often elucidate the presence of a malignancy.

Facial nerve paralysis associated with acute otitis media (AOM) is relatively rare and occurs primarily in children. The characteristic clinical features include severe otalgia, fullness and conducive hearing loss involving the affected ear. In facial nerve paralysis associated with AOM, the paralysis sets in at least 1 day after AOM. The probable aetiology for nerve paralysis is direct involvement of the facial nerve by inflammation or infection from the middle ear through bony dehiscence or physiologic canaliculi in the facial canal with consequential ischaemia and infarction of the facial nerve. Facial nerve paralysis associated with chronic otitis media (COM) usually arises as a result of bony dehiscence or destruction of the facial canal by a cholesteatoma. Involvement of the temporal bone by cholesteatoma results in bone expansion and destruction with resultant hearing loss, vestibular dysfunction, facial paralysis and intracranial complications. In the present case, the patient complains of otalgia and hyperacusis without any associated pus discharge in the right ear of 4–5 days' duration. There is no history of any hearing loss. A diagnosis of otitis media is considered in the present case due to the clinical presentation of acute onset otalgia and hyperacusis.

Lyme disease is a tick-borne disease caused by the spirochete Borrelia burgdorferi. Other Borrelia species like Borrelia afzelii and Borrelia garinii have also been implicated as the causative agents. It causes infection by migration through tissues, adhesion to host cells and evasion of host immune response. The characteristic clinical manifestation in patients with Lyme disease is a skin rash referred to as erythema chronicum migrans that begins as a red macule or papule usually associated with a tick bite at the affected skin site. These lesions migrate to other skin sites owing to the haematogenous spread of the pathogenic microorganism. The affected patients may also present with severe headache, migratory musculoskeletal pain and arthralgia along with other constitutional symptoms such as, fever, chills, profound malaise and fatigue. Frank neurologic abnormalities like meningitis and cranial neuritis including bilateral facial palsy develop within a few weeks to months after the disease onset. Cardiac abnormalities like atrioventricular block, acute myopericarditis and left ventricular dysfunction ensue later. The patient is well and did not give any history of tick bites, fever, fatigue, skin lesions and musculoskeletal pain. Moreover, the facial palsy was only unilateral and acute in onset. However, a detailed examination is required to exclude early stage Lyme disease which can manifest as unilateral facial palsy.

Gullian-Barre syndrome (GBS) is characterized by a triad of progressive motor weakness, areflexia and albuminocytologic dissociation of the cerebrospinal fluid. Cranial nerve palsies are relatively common in GBS and frequently involve the facial nerve. Facial nerve involvement in GBS is frequently bilateral. GBS is usually triggered by an infection or an immune stimulus that induces an aberrant autoimmune response targeting peripheral nerves and their spinal roots. The progressive limb weakness and associated sensory and cranial nerve involvement peaks within 2–4 weeks of its onset. In the present case, the patient's clinical history did not reveal any characteristic symptoms of GBS such as progressive weakness of the limbs and peripheral neuropathy. However, GBS is included in the differential diagnosis as facial nerve palsy usually manifests in the early stage of the disease before other symptoms manifest and can be rarely unilateral. Multiple sclerosis (MS) is a progressive, chronic inflammatory disease induced by a cell-mediated immune response resulting in destruction of the myelin sheath of the central nervous system (CNS). It commonly affects young adults living in temperate climates with Canada recording the highest prevalence rates in the world. The clinical course of MS may vary from relapsing/remitting acute episodic attacks to gradually progressive deterioration of neurologic symptoms. The common presenting symptoms include monocular visual impairment with pain (optic neuritis), weakness and/or paraesthesias in one or more extremities, heat sensitivity and Lhermitte sign (electrical sensation down the spine on neck flexion) while the less common symptoms include unsteadiness of extremities, fatigue and pain and bladder urgency or retention. Trigeminal neuralgia, trigeminal sensory neuropathy and facial palsy are the most frequent orofacial manifestations in MS.

The patient did not give any history of previous episodes of facial palsy or other symptoms such as weakness of the limbs and impairment of vision. However, a detailed neurological examination is required to exclude MS from the differential diagnosis.

CNS and concomitant cranial nerve involvement can occur in the course of a lymphoreticular malignancy. Non-Hodgkin lymphomas (NHLs) account for majority of the lymphomas. However, it is very rare for any neural involvement to manifest prior to systemic symptoms. Patients with NHL present with painless lymphadenopathy, and may or may not have systemic symptoms such as fevers, drenching night sweats, weight loss, pruritus and fatigue. Cranial nerve involvement is usually characterized by recurrent or bilateral facial palsies. The patient was well with absence of any systemic symptoms and atypical features such as recurrent or bilateral facial palsies. A diagnosis of lymphoma is included in the differential diagnosis as a detailed clinical examination is needed to rule out any lymphadenopathy.

Sarcoidosis is a systemic disease of unknown aetiology with multiorgan involvement. It frequently presents with bilateral hilar lymphadenopathy, pulmonary infiltration, ocular and skin lesions. Pulmonary symptoms predominate and include dyspnoea, dry cough and chest pain while cutaneous manifestations are primarily purplish macules and plaques and erythema nodosum. Nervous system involvement is seen in a minority of cases and presents as facial palsies, hypothalamic and pituitary lesions. The patient did not present any history of pulmonary or cutaneous involvement. Nevertheless, sarcoidosis is included in the differential diagnosis owing to the clinical presentation of unilateral facial palsy. Further investigations are required to confirm the diagnosis.

53.5 Findings of Examination

The patient appears well on general examination with normal built and gait. He is afebrile with a blood pressure of 132/82 mm of Hg and a pulse rate of 84 beats per minute. On extra oral examination, his face is asymmetrical with drooping of the corner of the lips on the left side. There is absence of wrinkling of the forehead on the left side when the patient is asked to raise his eyebrows (Fig. 53.1). The patient is unable to close his left eye completely (Fig. 53.2) and demonstrates the

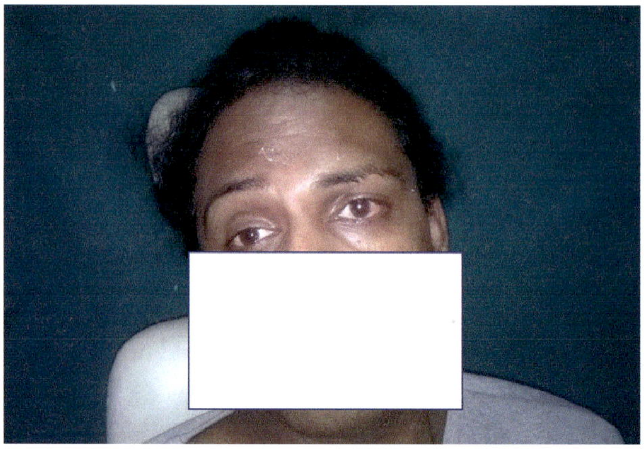

Fig. 53.1 Inability to raise his eyebrows and absence of wrinkling of the forehead on the left side when the patient is asked to do so. (Picture courtesy: Prof Dr. Ruwan D Jayasinghe Faculty of Dental Sciences, University of Peradeniya, Sri Lanka)

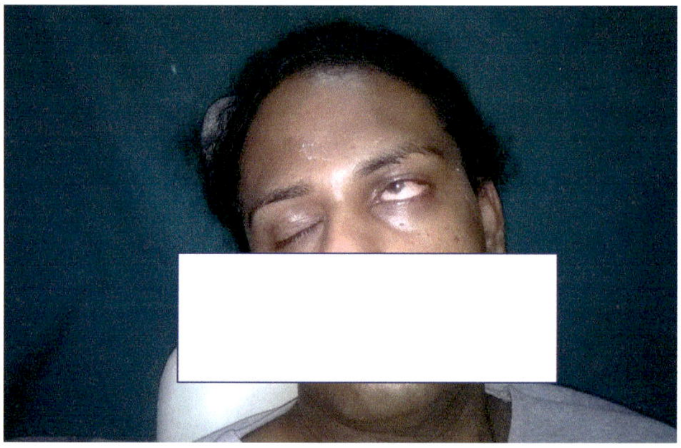

Fig. 53.2 The patient is unable to close his left eye completely. (Picture courtesy: Prof Dr. Ruwan D Jayasinghe Faculty of Dental Sciences, University of Peradeniya, Sri Lanka)

Bell's phenomenon—the eyeball moves in an upward and lateral direction when the eyelids are forcibly opened. The nasolabial fold appears flattened on the left side. When the patient is asked to puff his cheeks, his left cheek appears flattened (Fig. 53.3). He also cannot purse his lips. He cannot smile properly and show his teeth on the left side (Fig. 53.4). The face deviates to the right side upon smiling. There is no swelling associated with the parotid gland on the affected side. There is no evidence of facial muscle weakness on the right side. Examination of the trigeminal nerve function does not show any loss of sensory or motor nerve function bilaterally. The skin over the face and behind the ear appears normal. There are no other visible skin lesions elsewhere on the body. Upon intra-oral examination, the oral mucosa appears moist but there is a lack of pooling of saliva in the floor of the mouth. There are no vesicles or ulcers in the oral cavity and oropharynx.

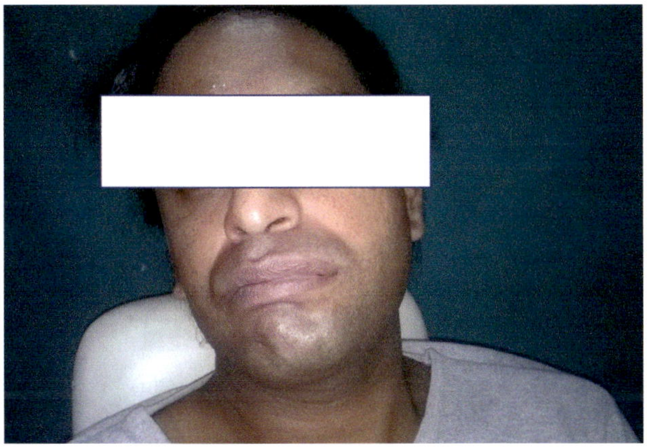

Fig. 53.3 When the patient is asked to puff his cheeks, his left cheek appears flattened. (Picture courtesy: Prof Dr. Ruwan D Jayasinghe Faculty of Dental Sciences, University of Peradeniya, Sri Lanka)

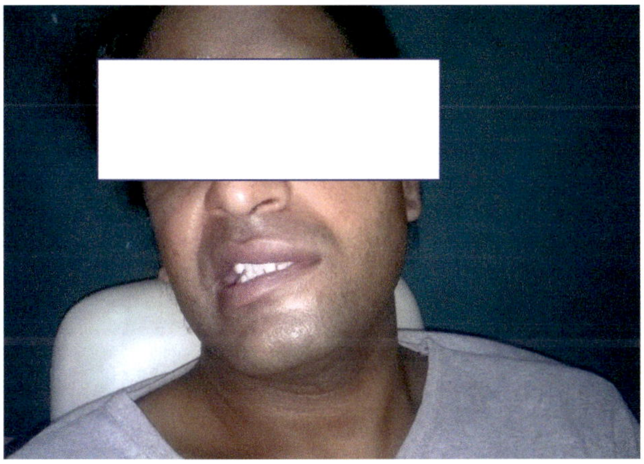

Fig. 53.4 The patient is unable to smile properly and show his teeth on the left side. (Picture courtesy: Prof Dr. Ruwan D Jayasinghe Faculty of Dental Sciences, University of Peradeniya, Sri Lanka)

53.6 What Other Relevant Features Would You Look for with the Findings You Have So Far?

Examination of the neck revealed palpable bilateral submandibular lymph nodes. There were two enlarged lymph nodes, one on each side measuring less than 1 cm in size. The enlarged nodes were mobile and mildly tender on palpation. The patient was referred to the medical physician for further examination. The physician confirmed the absence of any paresis of the limbs, dysarthria, dysphasia, visual disturbances and loss of cranial nerve function. There were also no abnormal auscultatory findings in the heart and lungs. Examination of the ear canal and the tympanic membrane did not reveal any abnormality including vesicles or otorrhoea.

53.7 What Is Your Clinical Diagnosis?

Bell's palsy

53.8 How Would You Exclude Other Conditions and Justify the Inclusion of the Disease That You Have Mentioned in the Clinical Diagnosis to Arrive at a Working Diagnosis?

Bell's palsy is a diagnosis by exclusion after having eliminated other possible causes of unilateral facial nerve paralysis. The patient presented with an acute onset of unilateral facial nerve paralysis involving the left side of his face that was of three days duration. He complained of hyperacusis, and a dull, persistent pain in his left ear that did not disturb his sleep for the past 4–5 days. He also complained of ageusia and dry mouth. Extra oral examination revealed a loss of motor function of the left facial nerve characterized by absence of wrinkling of the forehead on the left side, inability to completely close the left eye, Bell's phenomenon, drooping of the corner of the lips on the left side, difficulty in puffing out the cheeks and pursing the lips. The patient was afebrile and did not have a prodrome of pain characteristic of herpes zoster (HZ) infection. Otoscopy did not reveal any characteristic cutaneous findings of weeping vesicles and pustules in the Hunt's zone consistent with the diagnosis of RHS. The Hunt's zone includes the eardrum, the external auditory canal and the central region of the ear; the cavum conchae. There was no evidence of otorrhoea to suggest otitis media. The patient did not have any signs and symptoms of vestibulocochlear nerve involvement such as tinnitus, hearing loss, nausea, vomiting and vertigo. There were no vesicles on the skin and intraorally to suggest HZ infection. Hence RHS and acute otitis media were excluded from the differential diagnosis.

A unilateral lesion in the cortex or underlying corticobulbar fibres will produce a contralateral lower facial paralysis sparing the forehead and a contralateral hemiplegia without affecting salivary and lacrimal secretions or the sense of taste. In contrast, a unilateral paralysis of all the muscles of facial expression including the forehead is due to a nuclear or infranuclear lesion of the ipsilateral facial nerve. The patient was unable to wrinkle his forehead on the left side denoting a peripheral lesion of the facial nerve. He also complained of loss of taste and dry mouth that suggested a peripheral lesion either proximal or distal to the geniculate ganglion. A neurological examination did not reveal signs of hemiparesis, dysphasia, dysphagia, difficulty in hearing and visual disturbances suggestive of stroke and any tumours involving the CNS. The deep tendon reflexes, sensory system function and all other cranial nerve examination findings were also normal on neurological examination. Thus stroke, GBS, MS and space occupying lesions of the CNS were excluded from the differential diagnosis. There were no pathologically enlarged lymph nodes in the neck thus eliminating the possibility of a lymphoreticular malignancy.

Extra oral examination and palpation did not reveal any swelling around or in front of the left ear. The enlarged submandibular lymph nodes were consistent with inflamed nodes. Moreover facial nerve palsies consequent to tumours are insidious in onset unlike the present case where the duration of the slowly progressive symptoms was only three days. A gradual onset of more than two weeks duration is highly suggestive of a mass lesion. Symptoms due to intrinsic tumours of the facial nerve depend upon the location of the lesion and vary from gradual onset of facial weakness to hearing loss, tinnitus and vertigo. There were no such significant findings on otolaryngological examination. A diagnosis of left parotid gland and facial nerve tumours was excluded from the differential diagnosis.

The patient did not have any constitutional symptoms such as headache, fever, chills, malaise and fatigue. A specialist dermatological examination did not reveal any characteristic skin lesions consistent with Lyme disease or sarcoidosis. There were also no pulmonary signs suggestive of sarcoidosis.

The acute onset of unilateral facial paralysis together with associated symptoms like hyperacusis, otalgia, ageusia and decreased salivary secretion is highly suggestive of Bell's palsy.

53.9 What Is the Most Likely Diagnosis?

1. Bell's palsy

53.10 How Would You Investigate This Patient?

1. Fasting blood glucose levels and glycosylated haemoglobin (HbA1c).
2. A complete blood count (CBC) with differential count to exclude underlying infection or a lymphoproliferative disorder.

Imaging, serologic testing and electrodiagnostic studies are not essentially necessary when the history and physical examination are consistent with Bell's palsy. The patient should be referred to a neurologist if symptoms such as unilateral facial paralysis sparing the forehead, bilateral facial palsies, multiple cranial nerve neuropathies and paresis of the limbs are present or if the facial weakness persists without any significant improvement for more than 3 weeks. Referral to an otolaryngologist is mandatory if signs of middle ear infection and symptoms of vestibulocochlear nerve involvement such as ipsilateral deafness, manifest. The following additional investigations are mandatory in the presence of specific history and clinical findings:

1. Assessment for Lyme disease—Indicated in patients living in or who have travelled to areas endemic for Lyme disease with suggestive history and clinical presentation: Enzyme linked-immunosorbent assay (ELISA) and indirect fluorescent antibody test to detect antibodies to B. burgdorferi. If the results are positive, the diagnosis of Lyme disease should be confirmed by Western blot.
2. Serum antibody titers for herpes zoster if there is clinical evidence of herpes zoster infection.
3. Imaging—Indicated in patients with atypical findings inconsistent with Bell's palsy such as insidious onset, paresis of the limbs on the affected side, bilateral facial palsies, unilateral facial palsy sparing the forehead and symptoms that do not improve in 3 weeks: Contrast-enhanced computed tomography or gadolinium-enhanced magnetic resonance imaging of the internal auditory canal and face to image the entire course of the facial nerve.
4. Electroneurography—Indicated in patients with complete facial paralysis that persists 1 week after medical treatment to determine the extent of nerve degeneration.
5. Cerebrospinal fluid (CSF) analysis: Indicated in patients with suspected GBS and CNS infections.

The fasting blood sugar level was 90 mg/dl and the HbA1c level was 5.7%. The CBC results were not indicative of any underlying infection or haematological malignancy.

53.11 What Is the Final Diagnosis?

Bell's palsy

53.12 How Would You Manage This Patient?

The patient was started on a combination therapy of oral steroids and oral antivirals. Tablet Prednisone 50 mg was administered orally daily for five days. This was followed by tapering the dose by 10 mg each day for five days. Tablet Valacyclovir 1 g three times daily for seven days was administered in combination. Oral corticosteroids were prescribed primarily to reduce the facial nerve inflammation. Oral antivirals were prescribed as reactivation of HSV-1 has been implicated as probable aetiology for Bell's palsy. The patient was advised to use sunglasses (barrier protection), and artificial tears for eye protection and lubrication as he had a difficulty to close his right eye. The patient was also recommended to avoid dusty and windy environments. In order to prevent trauma to the left buccal mucosa during eating due to the flaccid paralysis and incontinence, the patient was asked to take a soft diet and use a straw for liquids.

53.13 Bell's Palsy

Bell's palsy, is named after the Scottish anatomist Sir Charles Bell who first described the condition along with the anatomy and the function of the facial nerve. It is an idiopathic, peripheral nerve palsy of acute onset affecting the facial nerve which supplies all the muscles of facial expression. The facial nerve also supplies parasympathetic fibres to the lacrimal and salivary glands as well as fibres of taste sensation to the anterior two-thirds of the tongue. It is the most common acute mononeuropathy and is the most common diagnosis associated with facial nerve paresis (weakness) or paralysis (complete loss of movement). The annual incidence of Bell's palsy has been reported to be about 15–30 per 100,000 persons with both men and women being affected equally. There is no specific age predilection but a peak incidence has been observed in the fourth to fifth decades of life. The right and the left facial nerves are identically prone to this condition.

The exact aetiology of Bell's palsy still remains unclear. It is primarily believed to be caused by inflammation of the facial nerve in the geniculate ganglion which leads to its compression, ischaemia and demyelination. Viral infections and auto immune diseases have been postulated as possible causative mechanisms. Diabetic patients and pregnant women are more susceptible to develop Bell's palsy. An increased incidence has also been observed in patients who have had recent influenza, common cold or other upper respiratory tract infections. Some of the affected patients also report an exposure to cold air from an air condition outlet or an open window preceding the attack. A familial occurrence has also been reported. There is increasing evidence that Bell's palsy is caused by reactivation of the latent herpes virus (HSV-1 and VZV) centred around the geniculate ganglion. Reactivation of these viruses causes inflammation of the facial nerve resulting in reversible neuropraxia and eventually Wallerian degeneration. Viral reactivation may predominantly occur in an immunocompromised host but can also occur in immunocompetent individuals. Numerous causes can produce peripheral facial nerve palsy identical to Bell's palsy. However, it is very important to differentiate Bell's palsy from facial nerve palsy arising due to secondary causes as it may significantly influence the treatment and prognosis. Secondary causes that have been implicated to cause facial nerve palsy are detailed in ◘ Table 53.1. These conditions have additional features that help to differentiate it from Bell's palsy.

A thorough history and a structured clinical approach are invaluable in establishing a diagnosis of Bell's palsy. The medical history should include history of recent rashes, arthralgias, fever and peripheral nerve palsy, exposure to influenza vaccine or new medications and exposure to ticks where Lyme disease is endemic. The pattern of facial nerve involvement (◘ Table 53.2) along with patient characteristics inconsistent with Bell's palsy (◘ Table 53.3) and a thorough physical examination will provide evidence for an alternative diagnosis and prompt appropriate investigations. Besides the above features, absence of recovery of facial tone within 4 months of onset of facial palsy rules out a diagnosis of Bell's palsy. The physical examination should include careful inspection of the ear canal, tympanic membrane and oropharynx as well as evaluation

◘ **Table 53.1** Secondary causes of unilateral facial nerve palsy

Metabolic diseases: Diabetes, preeclampsia
Stroke
Infections: Hansen disease, otitis media, mastoiditis, herpes simplex infection, varicella zoster infection, Ramsay Hunt syndrome, influenza viruses, borreliosis, cryptococcosis, neurocysticercosis, toxocarosis, tuberculous meningitis, parotitis, parotid abscess, malignant external otitis, syphilis
Surgery: Removal of cerebellopontine angle tumours
Trauma: Head trauma (crush injury), birth injury
Tumours: Facial nerve neurinoma, cerebellopontine angle tumours (neurinoma), tumours of the pons, petrosal bone, middle ear, parotid gland
Haematological malignancies: Leukemia
Lymphoreticular malignancies: Lymphomas
Immune system disorders: Guillain–Barre syndrome, Miller–Fisher syndrome, systemic lupus erythematosus, myasthenia gravis
Drugs: Interferon, linezolid
Syndromes: Moebius syndrome, Melkersson–Rosenthal syndrome

53

Table 53.2 Patterns of facial nerve involvement

Pattern	Causes
Recurrent ipsilateral facial nerve palsy	Usually associated with benign facial nerve neoplasms (Schwannoma) or benign neoplasms involving the parotid gland, temporal bone and cerebellopontine angle, Melkerrson-Rosenthal syndrome
Bilateral facial nerve palsy	Usually associated with Neurological causes: GBS Malignancies: Lymphomas, leukemias, metastatic tumours Infections: HIV, Lyme disease Autoimmune disorders: Sarcoidosis, systemic lupus erythematosus (SLE), Linezolid therapy
Slow onset of facial weakness	Usually associated with benign tumours of the facial nerve and parotid gland
Facial palsy at birth	Moebius syndrome Associated with traumatic injury at birth

Table 53.3 Symptoms inconsistent with Bell's palsy

Otovestibular symptoms: Hearing loss, vertigo, imbalance, otorrhoea
Other focal neurologic deficits: Diplopia, facial anaesthesia
Constitutional symptoms: Fever, chills, fatigue, malaise, sweats, weight loss
Lyme-specific symptoms: Recent tick bite or exposure, erythema migrans rash, arthralgia, myalgia, low back pain
Inflammatory symptoms: Orofacial swelling or parotitis, uveitis

of peripheral nerve function in the extremities and palpation of the parotid gland. Evaluation of cranial nerve function including all facial muscles should be performed to assess involvement of forehead to differentiate between central and peripheral nerve lesions.

Patients with Bell's palsy present with a partial or complete inability to voluntarily move the muscles on the affected side of the face. The characteristic symptoms include ipsilateral sagging of the eyebrow, drooping of the face, flattening of the nasolabial fold, inability to fully close the eyes, purse the lips and raise the corner of the mouth on the affected side. The eye rolls upward when the patient attempts to close the eye and is referred to as the Bell's phenomenon. Majority of the patients will have associated symptoms such as ipsilateral pain around the ear, hyperacusis and paraesthesia over the involved side of the face. The presence of associated symptoms may be explained due to the propensity of the facial nerve to form numerous connections with the adjacent cranial nerves including the trigeminal nerve (paraesthesia over the face) and vestibulocochlear nerve (hyperacusis). Patients complain of irritation in the eyes due to failure to close the eyes completely and lack of lubrication. There is pooling of food and saliva in the affected side of the mouth which may spill out from the corner. The symptoms progress to its maximum severity within three days and almost always within one week from its onset. An insidious onset or progression over more than two weeks should prompt an alternative diagnosis. Majority of the patients with Bell's palsy show at least a partial remission of their symptoms within three weeks of onset.

Table 53.4 House-Brackmann score (HBS) to grade the severity of facial nerve palsy

Grade	Description	Characteristics
I	Normal	Normal, symmetrical function in all areas
II.	Mild dysfunction	Slight weakness on close inspection, complete eye closure with minimal effort, slight asymmetry of smile with maximal effort, slight synkinesis, absent contracture or spasm
III.	Moderate dysfunction	Obvious weakness but not disfiguring, unable to lift eyebrow, complete and strong eye closure, asymmetrical mouth movement with maximal effort, obvious but not disfiguring synkinesis, mass movement or spasm
IV.	Moderately severe dysfunction	Obvious disfiguring weakness, inability to lift brow, incomplete eye closure and asymmetry of mouth with maximal effort, severe synkinesis, mass movement, spasms
V.	Severe dysfunction	Motion barely perceptible, incomplete eye closure, slight movement of corner of mouth, synkinesis, contracture, spasm usually absent
VI.	Total paralysis	No movement, loss of tone, no synkinesis, contracture, spasm

The severity of facial nerve palsy can be assessed by various scoring systems. The House-Brackmann facial nerve grading system (HBS) is the most widely used system (Table 53.4). Other available grading systems include the Yanagihara grading system, the Sunnybrook scales, the Jadad score of methodological quality and scales on computed systems. Most of the grading systems evaluate resting symmetry, degree of voluntary excursion of the skeletal muscles and the degree of synkinesis (abnormal involuntary facial movement that occurs with voluntary movement of a different facial muscle group). The degree of the nerve damage can also be assessed by nerve conduction studies. Reduction of the compound muscle action potential suggests axonal degeneration whereas increase in latency suggests demyelination of the nerve.

Further investigations are not required when the history and clinical examination findings are consistent with Bell's palsy. Serological investigations are mandatory for patients from areas endemic for Lyme disease. Imaging findings such as computed tomography of the temporal bone without contrast, and/or gadolinium-enhanced MRI of the temporal bones and parotid gland are indicated if atypical findings are present. A complete blood investigation (complete blood count, erythrocyte sedimentation rate, C-reactive protein, rheumatoid factor, antinuclear antibody, antineutrophil cytoplasmic antibody, antiphospholipid antibodies and angiotensin-converting enzyme) is indicated in cases with recurrent facial palsy or autoimmune disorders such as sarcoidosis.

Treatment of Bell's palsy should start as soon as possible after onset. Treatment may be subdivided into acute measures and measures to treat moderate or severe sequelae. The acute measures include:

- **Eye Protection:** Lubricating eye ointments or artificial tears to protect the cornea from dehydration, or abrasions due to insufficient lid closure or tearing.
- **Steroids:** Prednisone is typically prescribed in a 10-day tapering course starting at 60 mg per day. The treatment should be initiated within 72 h of the symptom onset.
- **Antivirals:** Acyclovir 400 mg is given five times per day for seven days or Valacyclovir 1 g is given three times per day for seven days. Antiviral therapy alone is not recommended as a treatment due to the lack of effectiveness of the currently available drugs and the potential for adverse drug effects.

In patients with chronic facial damage, the following treatment modalities have been found to have some effects.

Transcutaneous Electrical Nerve Stimulation (TENS): TENS has been reported to restore the function and increase the speed of recovery in patients with Bell's palsy by maintaining the tone of the facial muscles on the affected side.

Surgical Decompression (Transmastoid Decompression): This procedure is recommended in patients with complete facial paralysis and an increased likelihood of poor recovery. The potential side effects of this procedure include risk of bleeding, infection, seizures, deafness and leakage of cerebrospinal fluid.

Majority of the patients with Bell's palsy show a spontaneous and compete recovery within 3 months while a minority of the patients experience a variable degree of permanent nerve damage. The prognosticators of incomplete recovery include old age, severe facial palsy and the length of time prior to the onset of recovery. The patients should be placed on periodic follow-up. In patients, whose symptoms do not improve completely after 3 months of onset or show progression, a re-evaluation should be carried out immediately.

Salient features of Bell's palsy	
Clinical features	Partial or complete inability to voluntarily move the muscles on the affected side of the face. The characteristic symptoms include ipsilateral sagging of the eyebrow, drooping of the face, flattening of the nasolabial fold, inability to fully close the eyes, purse the lips and raise the corner of the mouth on the affected side. The eye rolls upward when the patient attempts to close the eye resulting in Bell's phenomenon.
Radiological features	NA
Histopathological features	NA
Treatment	Eye protection: To protect the cornea from dehydration, or abrasions due to insufficient lid closure or tearing. A combination therapy of steroids and antivirals should be initiated within 72 h off symptom onset. Pharmacotherapy: Prednisone 50 mg orally daily for 5 days followed by 10 mg less each day for 5 days/Prednisolone 50 mg orally daily for 10 days. Valacyclovir 1 g three times daily for 7 days/Acyclovir 400 mg five times daily for 7 days Surgical decompression is recommended in patients with poor outcome.

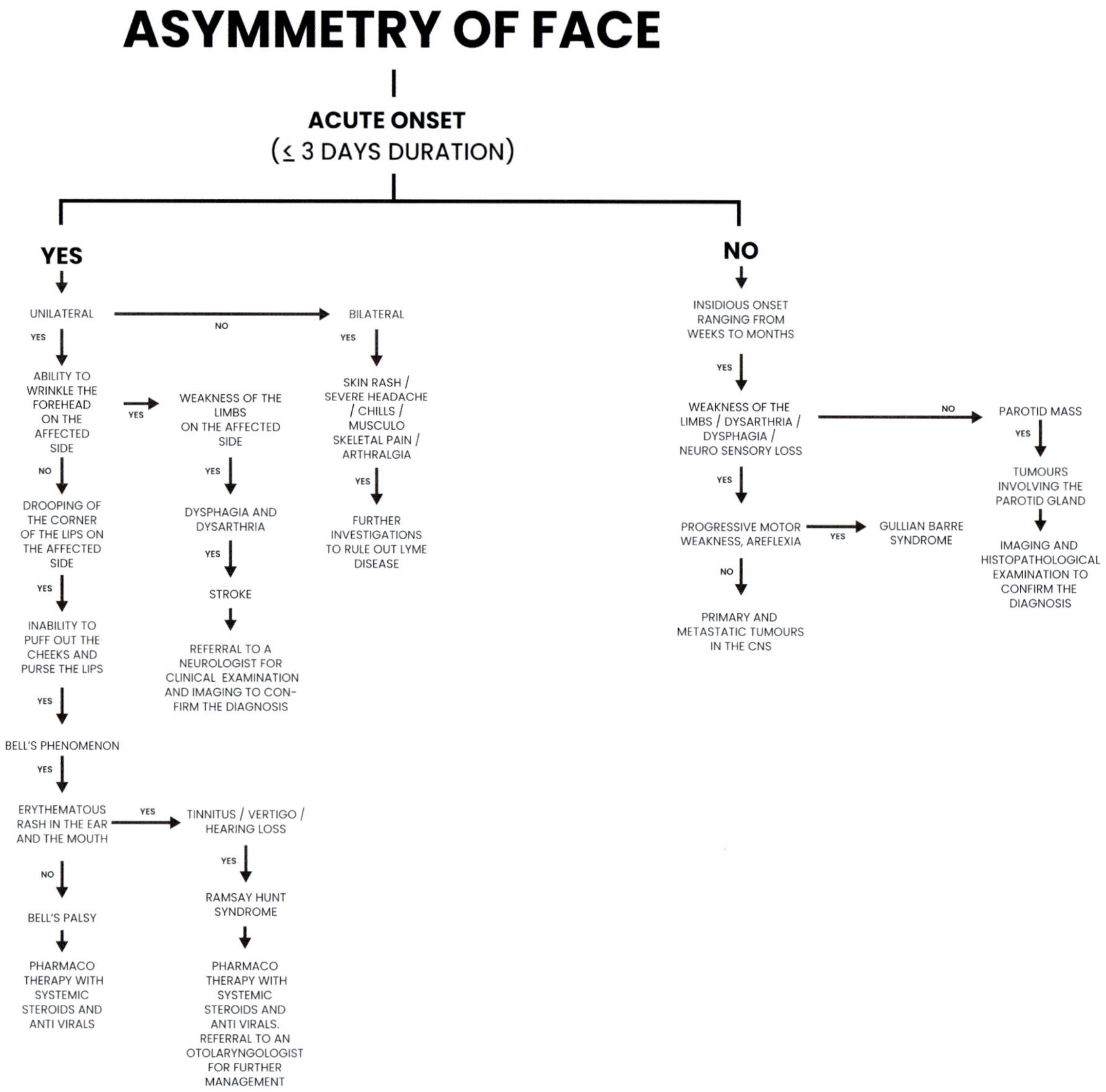

Self-Assessment Questions

1. Describe the clinical features of Bell's palsy.
2. List the various causes for unilateral facial palsy.
3. Discuss the differential diagnosis for Bell's palsy.
4. Discuss the investigations in patients with Bell's palsy.
5. Outline the treatment for Bell's palsy.

Summary

Acute ipsilateral weakness of the facial muscles accompanied by symptoms such as facial numbness is a characteristic feature of Bell's palsy. It is suspected to arise as a result of inflammation of the facial nerve in the geniculate ganglion leading to its compression, ischaemia and demyelination. Even though the factors that give rise to this inflammation remain unclear, a probable aetiology that has been suggested is that of a reactivated herpes simplex virus type 1 (HSV-1) infection within the geniculate ganglion. HSV-1 and herpes simplex virus type 2 (HSV-2) are neurotropic viruses and the viral genome remains in a latent form within the ganglia throughout the life of the host after the primary infection. A high frequency of diabetes mellitus has been reported in patients with Bell's palsy. Diabetic patients with Bell's palsy are prone to develop a more severe injury and have a less favourable outcome. The probable aetiology for the facial palsy has been attributed to ischaemia of the facial nerve due to diabetic small vessel disease. Treatment of Bell's palsy should start as soon as possible after onset. Treatment may be subdivided into acute measures and measures to treat moderate or severe sequelae. Majority of the patients with Bell's palsy show a spontaneous and compete recovery within 3 months while a minority of the patients experience a variable degree of permanent nerve damage. The prognosticators of incomplete recovery include old age, severe facial palsy and the length of time prior to the onset of recovery. The patients should be placed on periodic follow-up. In patients, whose symptoms do not improve completely after 3 months of onset or show progression, a reevaluation should be carried out immediately.

Further Reading

Baugh RF, Basura GJ, Ishii LE, Schwartz SR, Drumheller CM, Burkholder R, et al. Clinical practice guideline: Bell's palsy. Otolaryngol Head Neck Surg. 2013;149(3_suppl):S1–S27.

Cawson RA, Odell EW. Cawson's essentials of oral pathology and oral medicine e-book. Elsevier Health Sciences; 2017.

Eviston TJ, Croxson GR, Kennedy PG, Hadlock T, Krishnan AV. Bell's palsy: aetiology, clinical features and multidisciplinary care. J Neurol Neurosurg Psychiatry. 2015;86(12):1356–61.

Finsterer J. Management of peripheral facial nerve palsy. Eur Arch Otorhinolaryngol. 2008;265(7):743–52.

Gilden DH. Bell's palsy. N Engl J Med. 2004;351(13):1323–31.

Jowett N. A general approach to facial palsy. Otolaryngol Clin N Am. 2018;51(6):1019–31.

Neville BW, Damm DD, Allen C, Chi AC. Oral and maxillofacial pathology. Elsevier Health Sciences; 2015.

Sivapathasundharam B. Shafer's textbook of oral pathology-e book. Elsevier Health Sciences; 2016.

Tiemstra JD, Khatkhate N. Bell's palsy: diagnosis and management. Am Fam Physician. 2007;76(7):997–1002.

Warnakulasuriya S, Tilakaratna WM, editors. Oral medicine & pathology: a guide to diagnosis and management. JP Medical Ltd; 2013.

Unbearable Pain in the Left Lower Jaw: Trigeminal Neuralgia

Karthick Sekar

Contents

W. M Tilakaratne, T. G. Kallarakkal (eds.), *Clinicopathological Correlation of Oral Diseases*,
https://doi.org/10.1007/978-3-031-24408-7_54

54

Learning Goals

1. Devise the correct way of compiling the history with appropriate questions
2. Develop a differential diagnosis after history taking
3. Deduce appropriate procedures in clinical examination
4. Formulate a differential diagnosis combining findings in the history and clinical examination
5. Justify the relevant investigations required to arrive at the diagnosis
6. Comprehend the importance of clinicopathological correlation in arriving at the correct diagnosis
7. Outline the management plan
8. Recognize the importance of a diagnostic algorithm in arriving at a diagnosis

54.1 Main Complaint

A 55-year-old woman with a past medical history of migraine presented in the clinic with a complaint of severe and throbbing pain on the left side of her face and jaw.

54.2 History of Complaint

Question: How long have you been having this pain?

I have been having this pain since 3 weeks.

Question: Have you taken any treatment for your pain?

I took my migraine pills and analgesics that were previously prescribed by my physician, but the pain did not resolve. Additionally, I also took ibuprofen and paracetamol to reduce the pain but it was not effective. Last week, after a verbal consultation with my regular dentist, I also took a course of antibiotics for 5 days for pain relief, which did not help much.

54.3 Additional Complaints

Question: Have you had any similar episodes of pain in the past?

This is the first episode of such severe pain.

Question: What is the nature of the pain?

I feel the pain when eating, talking, brushing my teeth, washing and touching my face. The pain is sudden in onset and feels like an electric shock. I chew only on my right side currently.

Question: How long does the pain last?

The pain usually lasts for about 5–10 sec.

Question: Where do you feel the pain?

The pain is restricted mostly to the left side of my face including the middle face region near the cheeks and the lower jaw.

Question: Does the pain radiate to any other area?

The pain radiates to my left ear.

Question: Do you feel the pain deep in the ear and or back of the tongue?

I do not feel the pain deep in ear or at the back of my tongue.

Question: Does the pain become worse upon swallowing or coughing?

The pain does not increase in intensity upon coughing or swallowing.

Question: Does the pain increase in severity upon lying down or upon contact with hot or cold stimulus?

The pain is not aggravated upon lying down and on contact with hot or cold drinks.

Question: Does the pain disturb your sleep?

The pain doesnt occur or disturb during sleeping.

Question: Do you experience lacrimation, nasal congestion and facial and forehead sweating?

I do not have any such symptoms.

❓ Question: Are your eyes sensitive to bright light?

✅ My eyes are not sensitive to bright light.

❓ Question: Are you sensitive to loud sounds?

✅ I do not have any such problem.

❓ Question: Do you have any symptoms such as nausea, vomiting, visual disturbances, diplopia, malaise, fever, myalgia or weight loss?

✅ I do not have any such symptoms.

❓ Question: Are there any other symptoms associated with this pain?

✅ The pain disturbs my daily work routine. I feel tired daily after work and I have not slept well for the past four nights.

❓ Question: Do you have any history of trauma to your face?

✅ I have not suffered from any trauma involving my face or jaws.

❓ Question: Do you have a history of rash or vesicles on your face?

✅ I have not developed any rash or vesicles on my face in the past.

❓ Question: Do you have a history of stroke?

✅ I do not have a history of stroke.

❓ Question: Are you suffering from any other medical problems such as high blood pressure, diabetes, bleeding disorder, respiratory disease, etc?

✅ I have been suffering from migraine since adulthood but I have not experienced any headaches in the past couple of years. I was diagnosed with hypertension and hypercholesterolemia 10 years ago. I am under regular follow-up with my physician and my condition is well controlled as per my doctor.

❓ Question: What kind of medications have you been taking until now for your medical problems?

✅ I was prescribed sumatriptan and naproxen sodium to treat my migraine. I take atorvastatin and atenolol for my hypertension.

❓ Question: Have you undergone any surgery?

✅ I have not undergone any surgery in the past.

❓ Question: Have you undergone any dental treatment?

✅ I visit my general dentist every year for scaling. I have had multiple fillings done previously which were all uneventful. Besides that, I have no known dental illness except for a clicking noise in my jaw joint associated with opening and closing of mouth for which I have been treated. The condition has resolved since the treatment.

❓ Question: How often do you brush your teeth?

✅ I brush once a day but since the past 3 weeks, I have stopped brushing on the left side as it triggers the severe pain.

❓ Question: Does anybody in your family have a similar problem?

✅ My mother and father have no known medical illnesses but my brothers have a history of migraine.

❓ Question: Do you have any risk habits such as smoking or drinking alcohol?

✅ I do not have any risk habits.

❓ Question: What is your occupation?

✅ I work as a manager at a garment company.

54.4 With the Findings from the History, What Is Your Differential Diagnosis?

Trigeminal neuralgia (TGN)
- Acute pulpitis
- Cracked tooth syndrome
- Glossopharyngeal neuralgia
- Temporomandibular disorders (TMDs)
- Temporal arteritis
- Sinus infection
- Ear infection

54.5 How Do You Justify Your Differential Diagnosis After History Taking?

Based on the findings from the history, the patient claims to have a sharp shooting pain on the left face and lower jaw region. Hence it is likely that the patient could have TGN. A history of multiple dental fillings suggests that the pain may likely be of odontogenic origin. Acute pulpitis is associated with throbbing pain that disturbs the sleep while cracked tooth syndrome can cause symptoms of sharp pain upon biting or chewing. A differential diagnosis of glossopharyngeal neuralgia is included as the patient complains of radiating pain to the left ear even though she does not feel any pain upon swallowing and coughing. Migraine headaches usually cause facial pain, occasionally without a headache at all. The patient had previously been treated for migraine; however, she does not have any associated symptoms such as photophobia, phonophobia, nausea and vomiting during the current episode of pain. She only has unilateral pain, which is not a typical feature of migraine headaches. Additionally, upon taking medications previously prescribed for migraine, the pain did not subside. Hence a diagnosis of migraine is unlikely in the present case. A diagnosis of post-traumatic trigeminal pain is excluded as the patient does not have any history of trauma to the face or a traumatic dental procedure. A negative history of rash and vesicles on the face excludes a diagnosis of post-herpetic neuralgia. The patient also has a previous history of temporomandibular joint (TMJ) pain which, she claims to have resolved. There is a possibility that the TMD could have relapsed resulting in pain radiating to the head and neck region. Temporal arteritis is considered in the differential diagnosis as the patient presents with pain over the left side of the face including the jaw region even though there are no associated symptoms such as visual disturbances, malaise and loss of weight. It is also important to consider infections of sinus region and ear infections as an aetiology owing to the radiating nature of the pain. Trigeminal autonomic cephalalgias include cluster headaches, paroxysmal hemicrania and SUNCT (short-lasting unilateral neuralgiform headache with conjunctival injection and tearing) syndrome. Many of these conditions involve the eyes and forehead. The patient did not present with any such symptoms. Cluster headaches are excruciating attacks of pain in one side of the head, often felt around the eye. Paroxysmal hemicrania that usually begins in adulthood with symptoms like severe throbbing, claw-like, or boring pain usually unilaterally, in, around, or behind the eye; and occasionally reaching to the back of the neck. This pain may be accompanied by red and tearing eyes, a drooping or swollen eyelid, nasal congestion and attacks typically occur from 5 to 40 times per day and lasts 2–30 min. SUNCT syndrome is pain attacks resulting in unilateral headache with ipsilateral conjunctival injection, lacrimation and forehead sweating. The patient did not present with any such symptoms suggestive of trigeminal autonomic cephalalgias.

54.6 Findings of Clinical Examination

The patient is obese. She is otherwise fit and healthy with no obvious problems. She is alert, and oriented with intact cognition. Her temperature is 37 °C. Her blood pressure is 120/70 mmHg, with a heart rate of 91 beats per minute, respiratory rate of 20/min and oxygen saturation of 99% on room air. She appears to be in pain and the involved area of the face is highly sensitive to light touch. The sensory function is intact bilaterally, and the reflexes are also intact on both sides of the body. Her cranial nerve examination is also normal. There is no evident deformity on her face or eyes, and she does not have any facial muscle weakness. There is no evident clicking noise within the TMJ. Her TMJ and muscles of mastication are not tender to palpation. The patient does not have any signs and symptoms of sinusitis and ear infection.

Intra orally, the patient has a bilaterally balanced occlusion. Teeth 15, 16 and 26 have intact amalgam fillings while teeth 11, 21, 35 and 36 have intact composite fillings. Generalized gingivitis is noticed with the left upper and lower teeth having mild periodontal problems and calculus deposits as she has not been chewing on the left side or brushing her teeth on the left side for the past 3 weeks. Her teeth are not mobile and none of her teeth are tender to percussion. There is no evidence of attrition, abrasion and dental caries.

54.7 What Is Your Clinical Differential Diagnosis?

Trigeminal neuralgia

54.8 How Would You Exclude Other Conditions and Justify the Inclusion of the Diseases That You Have Mentioned in the Differential Diagnosis to Arrive at a Working Diagnosis?

Intra oral examination did not reveal any tenderness upon percussion on all her erupted teeth. There were no signs of pain from odontogenic causes. Hence acute pulpitis was not a likely differential diagnosis. None of the teeth were tender to percussion in an axial direction. Pain was not elicited using a tooth slooth. Thus, a diagnosis of cracked tooth syndrome was excluded.

Patients with glossopharyngeal neuralgia or vago-glossopharyngeal neuralgia manifest sharp, sudden, severe pain in the throat or deep in the ear. These pains may be set off by swallowing or touching the deep ear. The clinical presentation in this patient was not consistent with glossopharyngeal neuralgia as the patient did not feel any pain deep in the ear and while coughing or swallowing.

TMDs involve constant aches and pains, usually set off by talking or moving the jaw. The patient did have a history of clicking noise in the TMJ but it had been resolved. Clinical examination did not reveal any clicking noise in the joint. Her TMJ and muscles of mastication were not tender to palpation.

54.9 What Is the Most Likely Diagnosis?

TGN involving the maxillary and the mandibular divisions of the left trigeminal nerve.

54.10 How Would You Investigate This Patient?

Trigeminal nerve block provides hemifacial anaesthesia and is used predominantly in the diagnosis and treatment of neuralgia. Trigeminal nerve is responsible for sensory and motor functions which includes sensations on the face, biting, chewing and swallowing. Blocking the nerve can help stop the sensation of facial pain. An inferior alveolar nerve block was given intra orally anaesthetizing the mandibular branch of trigeminal nerve, using large bore needle and Akinosi technique for block administration as a diagnostic investigation. Pain symptoms were seen to subside temporarily after the local anaesthesia was administered.

A dental panoramic tomograph (DPT) will help to rule out any tumour or mass involving the trigeminal nerve. Additionally, neuro-imaging like MRI (magnetic resonance imaging), MRA (magnetic resonance angiogram) can also reveal the relationship of the trigeminal nerve with any other anatomical structure or mass that is impinging on the nerve causing symptoms for the patient. MRI can also rule out multiple sclerosis. MRA can also be used to inject a dye into a blood vessel to view the arteries and veins and highlight blood flow. The MRI in this patient revealed trigeminal nerve to be in close relation to the superior cerebellar artery, which was compressing the trigeminal nerve at the root entry zone hence causing pain to the patient.

TGN involving the maxillary and the mandibular divisions of the left trigeminal nerve. A diagnosis of TGN was made based on the history and exclusion of other differential diagnosis. The most likely aetiological factor in this case is the compression of the trigeminal nerve root adjacent to pons, causing demyelination of the nerve root. As an initial diagnostic step, inferior alveolar nerve block was given and there was relief of the pain temporarily. The imaging findings did not reveal any tumour involving the trigeminal nerve.

54.11 Trigeminal Neuralgia

TGN is a common facial pain disorder. The pain typically involves the lower face and jaw, although sometimes it affects the area around the nose and above the eye. This severe shooting pain usually involves one side of the face and is primarily caused by the irritation of the fifth cranial nerve, which innervates the forehead, cheek and lower jaw. The pain is typically sharp shooting and throbbing in nature. A variety of triggers may set off the pain of trigeminal neuralgia, including; shaving, touching the face, eating, drinking, brushing the teeth, talking, putting on makeup, encountering a breeze, smiling and washing the face.

TGN is also called tic douloureux (painful tic) because patients often distort the face because of severe pain. The area of pain in classical TGN will depend on which of the three branches of the trigeminal nerve is affected, though more than one branch at a time can be affected. Involvement of the ophthalmic branch affects the forehead, nose and eyes; the maxillary branch affects the lower eyelid, eyes, side of nose, cheek, upper gum, upper lip and upper teeth. Involvement of the mandibular branch has an effect on the lower jaw, teeth, gum and lip.

Trigeminal nerve compression will not always present with pain symptoms and it has been suggested that in symptomatic cases, the pressure on the nerve causes demyelination which is the wearing away of the protective outer layer referred to as the myelin sheath. This demyelination causes uncontrollable pain signals to manifest along the nerve, though this fails to adequately explain why asymptomatic remission can occur and why there is immediate pain relief post-operatively after removal of a blood vessel away from the nerve. A list of differential diagnoses that may be considered in patients presenting with severe orofacial pain is listed in ◘ Table 54.1.

TGN affects males and females of all ages. It has a prevalence of 0.1–0.2 per 1000 and an incidence ranging from 4 to 20 cases per 100,000 people per year. The female to male ratio is around 3:2. While it is common

Table 54.1 Clinical features for differential diagnoses of orofacial pain

Conditions	Location of pain	Duration of attack/pain	Shooting pain or symptoms
Cluster headache	Retrobulbar, cheek, chin	20 min–hours	Only superimposed on deep dull pain
SUNCT (short-lasting unilateral neuralgiform headache with conjunctival injection and tearing) syndrome	Forehead, retrobulbar	5s to few mins	Yes
Paroxysmal hemicranias	Forehead, retrobulbar	2–45 min	No
Cracked tooth syndrome	Upper and lower jaw	Few seconds	Yes
Post-herpetic neuralgias	Forehead, eye, cheek (rarely)	Continuous	Superimposed background pain

after 50 years of age, TGN is uncommon in young adults and rare in children. The right side of the face is reported to be more commonly involved.

TGN is usually idiopathic. However, any factor irritating the trigeminal nerve can cause it. Inflammation and compression of the trigeminal nerve are the common risk factors associated with TGN. People with multiple sclerosis (MS) are more likely to get TGN. For patients without MS, TGN is usually caused by a blood vessel pressing on the trigeminal nerve in the brain, or, rarely, a tumour. Inflammation is usually caused by an infection, and compression of trigeminal nerve results from the blood vessel or tumour. TGN also has an association with inflammatory or autoimmune conditions.

An increased risk of TGN in migraine patients has been recently recognized. The association between migraine and TGN remained significant in sensitivity analyses. Among migraine subtypes, patients with migraine and aura were at greater risk of TGN development. The condition is not dangerous, but severe persistent pain can limit daily activities.

TGN has been classified based on aetiology into two types by the international headache society (IHS)

1. Classical: It is caused by vascular compression of the nerve, the superior cerebellar artery is most commonly responsible for neurovascular compression on the trigeminal nerve, although other arteries or veins may also be responsible.
2. Symptomatic: It has the same clinical criteria but another underlying cause except vascular compression is responsible for the symptoms. Based on the symptoms, it is classified as
   (a) Typical trigeminal neuralgia (Tic douloureux) which is the most common type of TGN. It is present with minor aching or burning pain within the affected distribution of the trigeminal nerve.
   (b) Atypical trigeminal neuralgia is characterized by a unilateral, continuous and severe aching or burning pain. Both these types of pain can occur in the same patient.

The aetiological factors of TGN may be classified as follows:
1. Disease-related
2. Direct injury to the nerve
3. Poly aetiological origin

Despite the above-mentioned aetiological factors, compression of the trigeminal nerve is still considered to be the most common cause of TGN.

According to the international guidelines on TGN, anticonvulsant carbamazepine or oxcarbazepine is the drug of choice for the patients with TGN, and most of the patients respond well. Medication in the form of analgesics (paracetamol and aspirin) and anti-inflammatory tablets (ibuprofen) are ineffective for TGN pain. Common adverse effects of anticonvulsants include nausea, dizziness, confusion, drowsiness, vision problems, suicidal thoughts and allergies.

TGN is a chronic condition that requires long-term monitoring and when pharmacotherapy therapy is instituted, a full blood analysis, carbamazepine levels and liver function tests are required prior to commencement for ascertaining baseline values. On commencement of the treatment, full liver function and carbamazepine levels should be monitored closely, after the first 2 weeks and then every 3 months and whenever the dose is adjusted or adverse effects appear, and annually thereafter.

For carbamazepine, a dose of 100–200 mg should be prescribed initially for two to three times per day. Doses should be increased and titrated according to the severity of the pain up to a maximum 1200 mg per day. Serum level is a useful way of monitoring the dose of carbamazepine (6–12.5 μg/ml). If symptoms do not subside, combination therapy should be considered by adding

Table 54.2 Pharmacotherapy for management of trigeminal neuralgia

Drug	Dosage	Class	Mechanism	Adverse effects
First-line therapy				
Carbamazepine	Start: 100–200 mg Maintenance 600–800 mg Max: 1200 mg/day	Anticonvulsant	Sodium channel blockers, inhibits repetitive firing	Aplastic anaemia Fatal skin rash SIADH
Oxcarbazepine	Start 600 mg Max: 1200–1800 mg/day	Anticonvulsant	Sodium channel blocker	Less than carbamazepine Fatal skin rash
Second-line therapy				
Lamotrigine	Start: 25–50 mg Maintenance: 400 mg daily	Anticonvulsant	Sodium channel blocker, decrease glutamate release	Potentially fatal skin rash
Baclofen	Start: 15 mg/day Maintenance: 50–60 mg/day	Muscle relaxant	GABA agonist	Drowsiness, respiratory depression, rebound symptoms may occur

drugs like baclofen or phenytoin, sodium valproate, gabapentin, lamotrigine or clonazepam. For cases of TGN induced by multiple sclerosis, lamotrigine has been recently considered as a drug of choice. The choice of drugs, dosage, mechanism of action and adverse effects are listed in Table 54.2.

Management of TGN must be tailored individually, early diagnosis and prompt referral for specialized care are thus imperative. A lack of efficacy or intolerable side effects to oral medication justifies the recommendation of neurosurgical treatment to the patient. The patient must be educated of the relative efficacy of various modalities of treatments, including complications and recurrence rates.

The international guidelines further state that surgery would be a reasonable next step in the case where anticonvulsants are ineffective. Invasive treatments can be considered and implemented depending on the suitability of the patient for the procedure. Decompression of the blood vessels might cure the pain in patients with possible anatomical aetiology for TGN. A trigeminal ganglion nerve block or injections with botulinum toxin may be considered if there is no anatomical aetiology identified. There are a number of surgical options available to effectively treat TGN which include percutaneous glycerol rhizotomy (PGR), percutaneous balloon compression (PBC), percutaneous stereotactic radiofrequency thermal rhizotomy (PSRTR), gamma-knife radiosurgery (GKR), partial sensory rhizotomy (PSR) and MVD rhizotomy or gamma knife surgery to severe the nerve root may also be considered for refractory and treatment-resistant trigeminal neuralgia. However, these procedures can result in impairment of facial sensation. Surgery can provide good relief, but relapse may occur within months or years later. According to the literature, up to 95% of cases of TGN are caused by an artery or vein compressing the trigeminal nerve.

Salient features of trigeminal neuralgia	
Clinical features	Sharp shooting, lancinating, terrifying, exhausting, unbearable pain. Unilateral in distribution. Affects the midface region, along the distribution of branches of affected nerve. The pain is usually spontaneous in nature. It is aggravated by light touch, eating, talking and shaving and relieved by sleep, ID nerve block and medication. The pain lasts for seconds to minutes with periods of remission and exacerbation.
Treatment	Pharmacotherapy with anticonvulsants such as Carbamazepine and Oxcarbazepine. A dose of 100–200 mg should be prescribed initially for two to three times per day. Doses should be increased and titrated according to the severity of the pain up to maximum 1200 mg per day. For refractory cases, combination therapy should be considered by adding drugs like baclofen or phenytoin, sodium valproate, gabapentin, lamotrigine or clonazepam. Surgery is recommended in cases where anticonvulsants are ineffective.

- Diagnostic Algorithm for the diagnosis and treatment of trigeminal neuralgia

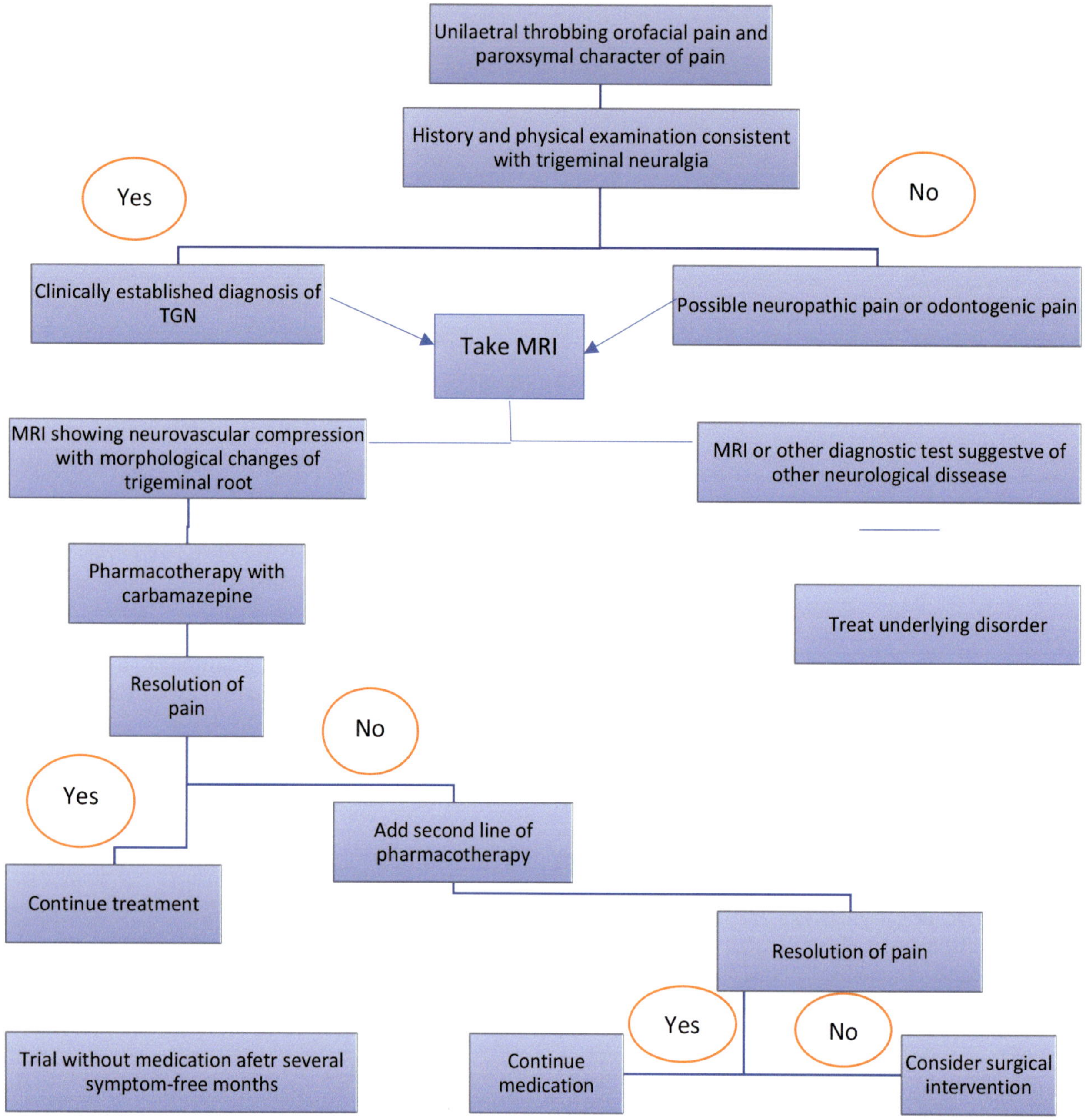

Self-Assessment Questions

1. Describe the salient clinical features of trigeminal neuralgia.
2. Describe the classification and aetiology of trigeminal neuralgia.
3. State the important conditions that need to be considered in the differential diagnosis in patients with orofacial pain.
4. Describe the important investigations required for a definitive diagnosis of trigeminal neuralgia.
5. Outline the management plan according to the aetiology of trigeminal neuralgia.

Summary

Trigeminal neuralgia (TGN) is a common facial pain disorder. The pain typically involves the lower face and jaw, although sometimes it affects the area around the nose and above the eye. It is primarily caused due to irritation of the fifth cranial nerve, which innervates the forehead, cheek and lower jaw. The pain in TGN is typically sharp shooting and throbbing in nature. A variety of triggers may set off the pain of TGN including shaving, touching the face, eating, drinking, brushing the teeth, talking, putting on makeup, encountering a breeze, smiling and washing the face. Pharmacotherapy with anticonvulsants such as carbamazepine is the treatment of choice and most of the patients respond well. A dose of 100–200 mg should be prescribed initially for two to three times per day. Doses should be increased and titrated according to the severity of the pain up to maximum of 1200 mg per day. For refractory cases, combination therapy should be considered by adding drugs like baclofen or phenytoin, sodium valproate, gabapentin, lamotrigine or clonazepam. Surgery is recommended in cases where anticonvulsants are ineffective.

Suggested Reading

Benjamin M, Zussman BS, Yaron A, Moshel. Trigeminal neuralgia, a case report.
Brisman M. Trigeminal neuralgia differential diagnosis.
Cawson RA, Odell EW. Cawson's essentials of oral pathology and oral medicine e-book. Elsevier Health Sciences; 2017.
Kashyap N, Arya A. Trigeminal neuralgia case report and treatment modalitis.
Kataria S, Ahmed Z, Ali U, et al. Trigeminal neuralgia induced headache: a case report and literature review. Cureus. 2020;12(7):e9226. https://doi.org/10.7759/cureus.9226.
Neville BW, Damm DD, Allen C, Chi AC. Oral and maxillofacial pathology. Elsevier Health Sciences; 2015.
Sivapathasundharam B. Shafer's textbook of oral pathology-e book. Elsevier Health Sciences; 2016.
Trigeminal neuralgia: case report and literature review. Stomatological Dis Sci. 2019; https://doi.org/10.20517/2573-0002.2019.08.
Turton M, Malan-Roux P. Trigeminal neuralgia: case report and literature review.
Warnakulasuriya S, TilakaraTGNa WM, editors. Oral medicine & pathology: a guide to diagnosis and management. JP Medical Ltd; 2013.
Yang X-H, Li Y, Yang L-Q, Wu B-S, Ni J-X. Nerve coblation for treatment of trigeminal neuralgia: a case report. World J Clin Cases. 2019;7(9):1060. https://doi.org/10.12998/wjcc.v7.i9.1060.

Temporomandibular Disorders

Contents

Pain During Mouth Opening: Temporomandibular Disorders (Myalgia)

Siew Wui Chan and P. Shanmuhasuntharam

Contents

W. M Tilakaratne, T. G. Kallarakkal (eds.), *Clinicopathological Correlation of Oral Diseases*,
https://doi.org/10.1007/978-3-031-24408-7_55

55

Learning Goals

1. Devise the correct way of compiling the history with appropriate questions
2. Develop a differential diagnosis after history taking
3. Deduce appropriate procedures in clinical examination
4. Formulate a differential diagnosis combining findings in the history and clinical examination
5. Justify the relevant investigations required to arrive at the diagnosis
6. Comprehend the importance of clinicopathological correlation in arriving at the correct diagnosis
7. Outline the management plan
8. Recognize the importance of a diagnostic algorithm in arriving at a diagnosis

55.1 Main Complaint

A 38-year-old lady complains of pain on the left jaw when opening her mouth wide.

55.2 History of Complaint

Question: How long have you been having this pain?

The pain started after the extraction of my upper left third molar a month ago.

Question: What is the nature of the pain?

The pain is dull and usually comes in the morning or whenever I chew hard or tough food. I have been chewing with the right side of my jaw ever since. The pain is relieved whenever I take mefenamic acid capsules.

55.3 Additional Complaints

Question: Do you have any associated pain in the temple, in the ear or in front of the ear on either side?

The pain is localized to the jaw on the left side only.

Question: Did you have any accident or trauma to the painful site recently?

I do not remember any such incident.

Question: Have you had pain or stiffness in your jaw on awakening in the morning?

I feel pain in my jaw often in the mornings.

Question: Do you have habits such as clenching, grinding or bruxism?

I do not clench or grind my teeth. However, I am unsure if I have bruxism.

Question: Have you noticed any jaw joint noise(s) when you moved your jaw recently?

I have not noticed any noises within the joint.

Question. Have you ever experienced your jaw lock or catch, even momentarily, so that it would not open all the way?

I have not had any such problems.

Question: Have you ever experienced moments when you could not close your mouth after you opened it wide?

I have not had difficulty in closing my mouth at any time.

Question: Tell me about your diet. Do you often snack on food like nuts or chewing gums?

I take a normal diet and do not have any snacking habits.

Question: Do you have any other medical problems? If yes, what kind of medications have you been taking until now?

I am medically fit and healthy. However, I take mefenamic acid capsules sometimes for the pain.

Question: Have you undergone any surgery?

I have not undergone any surgery.

Question: Have you undergone any dental treatment?

I had my left upper third molar tooth extracted 1 month ago. I have a scheduled minor oral surgery in the next 2 months for removal of my lower left third molar tooth.

Question: What is your occupation? Is your work stressful for you?

I work as a teacher. I feel stressed at work sometimes.

Question: Do you have habits of smoking, betel quid chewing or take alcohol?

I do not have any of the said habits.

55.4 From the Clinical History, What Is Your Differential Diagnosis?

1. Temporomandibular disorder (TMD)—myalgia
2. Dry socket (alveolar osteitis)
3. Pericoronitis
4. Acute periapical periodontitis
5. Cracked tooth

55.5 How Do You Justify Your Differential Diagnosis After History Taking?

1. She has pain associated with functional jaw movements such as mouth opening which is a typical presentation in TMDs. The onset of the pain suggests that she might have sustained trauma during the extraction process, leading to her present complaint. A diagnosis of myalgia is considered due to the conspicuous absence of symptoms involving her temporomandibular joints such as joint noises and locking of the jaw. The possibility of bruxism which could exacerbate her symptom in the mornings cannot be ruled out. In addition, she has work-related stress which is a psychosocial component commonly linked to the multifactorial aetiology for TMDs.
2. It is essential to rule out dental-related causes with reference to her complaint site, such as dry socket, pericoronitis, chronic periapical periodontitis or cracked tooth. Dry socket is an unpredictable complication of tooth extraction frequently associated with intense pain. Pericoronitis is a common condition affecting partially erupted teeth, but more often lower third molars. On the other end, symptoms for chronic periapical periodontitis and cracked tooth are exacerbated with biting.

55.6 Findings of Examination

Extraoral Examination

She has no facial asymmetry and no palpable lymph nodes. Her bilateral temporomandibular joints are not tender to palpation and do not present with swelling, clicking or locking. The jaw does not deviate during opening. Her left masseter muscle is tender to palpation but temporalis muscles are non-tender. Her mouth opening with pain is 29 mm. The maximum unassisted mouth opening is 40 mm, with pain felt on the left masseter. Pain is also felt with right and left lateral excursions, but not on mandibular protrusion.

Intraoral Examination

There is no mucosal lesion in the oral cavity. Extraction site of 28 is healing. Teeth in the left upper and lower quadrants are neither carious nor tender to percussion. Impacted tooth 48 is not visible clinically.

55.7 What Is the Most Likely Diagnosis?

TMD—Local myalgia of the left masseter muscle

55.8 How Do You Justify the Exclusion of the Diseases That You Have Mentioned in the Differential Diagnosis to Arrive at a Working Diagnosis?

55.8.1 Dry Socket

Dry socket or alveolar osteitis refers to localized inflammation of the alveolar bone due to premature loss of the healing blood clot after tooth extraction. In this patient, the extraction site did not exhibit signs of inflammation like erythematous and tender mucosa or empty socket with visible bone. The lymph nodes were not enlarged or tender as well.

55.8.2 Pericoronitis

Pericoronitis usually affects partially erupted teeth because maintenance of oral hygiene in these areas is difficult. The communication between the tooth follicle with the oral cavity is thought to allow bacterial infiltration which initiates infection. This diagnosis is unlikely for this patient as her impacted tooth 38 was not even clinically visible. Again, general signs of inflammation like enlarged or tender lymph nodes were absent.

55.8.3 Acute Periapical Periodontitis

Acute periapical periodontitis is often preceded by pulpal pain and usually associated with non-vital tooth. More importantly, the affected tooth can be precisely located by means of tooth percussion, which was not present for this patient.

55.8.4 Cracked Tooth

Pain from cracked tooth may be felt when chewing or biting, and especially when the bite is released. There could also be sensitivity to heat, cold or sweets. Patient's symptoms were not consistent with this condition.

55.8.5 How Would You Investigate This Patient?

A thorough clinical examination of the temporomandibular joints and the masticatory muscles should be sufficient to achieve a diagnosis for this patient. Additional investigations are mainly to rule out the dental causes. Dental panoramic tomograph is useful to show the impacted tooth 38. Intraoral periapical views may aid in identifying cracked lines on suspected tooth or demonstrate periapical changes. Pulp sensibility tests can be carried out to assess tooth vitality if indicated.

55.8.6 How Would You Manage This Patient?

Myalgia can be adequately managed via reversible and non-invasive therapy which aims to empower patient through education for self-management as well as to reduce or eliminate pain and functional limitation due to the condition. Patient would appreciate reassurance that her condition is benign and generally non-progressive even if it is somewhat fluctuating in nature. Patient should be motivated to practise self-care and adopt certain modification of habits and lifestyle. Simple generic advice regarding dietary habits is often enough to produce noticeable improvements. Patient should go on a soft diet and avoid hard and chewy food. It is also good to cut food into smaller pieces. She should avoid excessive chewing such as chewing gums and excessive mouth opening during yawning. Postures or habits that put unnecessary strain on the jaws should also be avoided. Jaw exercises and light massage can be helpful. As part of her home care, application of superficial heat and/or cold can reduce symptoms, facilitating mobilization and reducing pain thus allowing jaw exercises to be practised better. Other physical modalities such as ultrasound, low-intensity laser and pulsed diathermy can be prescribed if available. Short-term pharmacotherapy like NSAIDs can also be considered in the acute phase. If stress is a prevalent factor in patient's lifestyle, she would also benefit from relaxation techniques or just taking a break.

55.9 Temporomandibular Disorders (TMDs)

TMDs are a group of disorders comprising of myogenous and/or arthrogenous conditions (musculoskeletal disorders). It is the most common cause of chronic pain in the orofacial region with a strong predilection for females and peaks between the ages of 25 and 45.

The prevalence of masticatory muscle disorders is reported as 6–13.3%, 8.5–15.8% for disc displacement disorders and up to 8.9% for temporomandibular joint (TMJ) pain disorders in the general population. Myofascial pain with or without limitation of mouth opening is most frequently diagnosed among TMD patients whilst disc displacement with reduction is the commonest diagnosis in the general population. TMD has been acknowledged universally for its multifactorial aetiology with roles for genetics, psychological characteristics, occlusion, parafunctional habits and trauma. Psychosocial factors leading to general distress is the most striking factor for many patients with chronic TMD pain.

The TMD Research Diagnostic Criteria for Temporomandibular Disorders (RDC/TMD) or its revised version, DC-TMD, along with American Academy of Orofacial Pain are frequently referred to for their diagnostic classification for TMD. An expanded TMD taxonomy which includes less common but clinically relevant TMD was also developed through integration of both classifications (◘ Table 55.1).

The clinical presentation differs for the varying diagnoses in TMDs. Signs and symptoms of interest are pain in and around TMJ and muscles of mastication, muscle and joint tenderness on palpation, joint sounds (clicking or crepitus), limitation and incoordination of the mandibular movement, headaches, joint lock or catch and clinical indications of parafunctional habits (tooth wear facets, scalloped tongue). Masticatory muscles such as temporalis, masseter, medial and lateral pterygoids are palpated under standard examination protocols. ◘ Table 55.2 and ◘ Fig. 55.1 provide further details on the commonly diagnosed TMDs.

Investigation for TMDs is mainly by imaging especially with regard to intra-articular TMDs. However, imaging is considered adjunctive rather than definitive. It will help in excluding dental or other pathology which might mimic TMDs. Changes detected on imaging such as degeneration or erosion of the joints should not be taken at face value especially if function is not affected. Useful imaging options include conventional radiographs (mainly panoramic radiographs), computed

Table 55.1 Expanded TMD taxonomy by Peck et al. (2014)

TMJ articular disorders	Masticatory muscle disorders
1. Joint pain (a) Arthralgia (b) Arthritis **2. Joint disorders** (a) Disc disorders • Disc displacement with reduction • Disc displacement with reduction with intermittent locking • Disc displacement without reduction with limited opening • Disc displacement without reduction without limited opening (b) Hypomobility disorders other than disc disorders • Adhesions/adherence • Ankylosis (fibrous/osseous) (c) Hypermobility disorders • Dislocations (Subluxation/luxation) **3. Joint diseases** (a) Degenerative joint diseases • Osteoarthrosis • Osteoarthritis (b) Systemic arthritides (c) Condylysis/idiopathic condylar resorption (d) Osteochondritis dissecans (e) Osteonecrosis (f) Neoplasm (g) Synovial chondromatosis **4. Fracture** **5. Congenital/developmental disorders** (a) Aplasia (b) Hypoplasia (c) Hyperplasia	**1. Muscle pain** (a) Myalgia • Local myalgia • Myofascial pain • Myofascial pain with referral (b) Tendonitis (c) Myositis (d) Spasm **2. Contracture** **3. Hypertrophy** **4. Neoplasm** **5. Movement disorders** (a) Orofacial dyskinesia (b) Oromandibular dystonia **6. Masticatory muscle pain attributed to systemic/central pain disorders** (a) Fibromyalgia/widespread pain
Others	
1. **Headache attributed to TMD** 2. **Coronoid hyperplasia**	

Table 55.2 Descriptions of the most common TMDs (Schiffman et al. 2014)

Pain-related TMD	
Myalgia	Pain of muscle origin that is affected by jaw movement, function or parafunction, and replication of this pain occurs with provocation testing of the masticatory muscles.
Local myalgia	Pain of muscle origin as described for myalgia with localization of pain only at the site of palpation when using the myofascial examination protocol.
Myofascial pain with spreading	Pain of muscle origin as described for myalgia with pain spreading beyond the site of palpation but within the boundary of muscle when using the myofascial examination protocol.
Myofascial pain with referral	Pain of muscle origin as described for myalgia with referral of pain beyond the boundary of muscle being palpated using the myofascial examination protocol.
Arthralgia	Pain of joint origin that is affected by jaw movement, function or parafunction, and replication of this pain with provocation testing of the TMJ.
Headache attributed to TMD	Headache in the temple area secondary to pain-related TMD that is affected by jaw movement, function or parafunction, and replication of this headache occurs with provocation testing of the masticatory system

(continued)

Table 55.2 (continued)

Intra-articular TMD	
Disc displacement with reduction	An intracapsular biomechanical disorder involving the condyle-disc complex: in the closed mouth position, the disc is in an anterior position relative to the condyle, and the disc reduces upon opening of the mouth. Medial and lateral displacement of the disc may also be present. Clicking, popping or snapping noises may occur with disc reduction.
Disc displacement with reduction with intermittent locking	An intracapsular biomechanical disorder involving the condyle-disc complex: in the closed mouth position, the disc is in an anterior position relative to the condyle, and the disc intermittently reduces with opening of the mouth. When the disc does not reduce with opening of the mouth, intermittent limited mandibular opening occurs. When the limited opening occurs, a manoeuvre may be needed to unlock the TMJ. Medial and lateral displacement of the disc may also be present. Clicking, popping or snapping noises may occur with disc reduction.
Disc displacement without reduction with limited mouth opening	An intracapsular biomechanical disorder involving the condyle-disc complex: in the closed mouth position, the disc is in an anterior position relative to the condyle and the disc does not reduce with opening of the mouth. Medial and lateral displacement of the disc may also be present. This disorder is associated with persistent limited mandibular opening that does not reduce with the clinician or patient performing a manipulative manoeuvre. This is also referred to as closed lock.
Disc displacement without reduction without limited mouth opening	An intracapsular biomechanical disorder involving the condyle-disc complex: in the closed mouth position, the disc is anterior relative to the condyle, and the disc does not reduce with opening of the mouth. Medial and lateral displacement of the disc may also be present. This disorder is not associated with limited mandibular opening.
Degenerative joint disease	Degenerative disorders involving the joint characterized by deterioration of articular tissue with concomitant osseous changes in the condyle and/or articular eminence.
Subluxation	A hypermobility disorder involving the disc-condyle complex and the articular eminence. In the open mouth position, the disc-condyle complex is positioned anterior to the articular eminence and is unable to return to normal closed mouth position without a manipulative manoeuvre. The duration may be momentary or prolonged. When the patient can reduce the dislocation, this is referred to as subluxation. When the patient needs the assistance of the clinician to reduce the dislocation and normalize the jaw position, it is called luxation or open lock.

tomography (CT) and magnetic resonance imaging (MRI). Although imaging contributes to a definitive TMJ-related diagnosis, it should not be used routinely but rather considered when the findings will change the patient's treatment plan or prognosis. Occasionally, blood investigations may be useful for conditions like rheumatoid arthritis.

Management of TMDs can generally be divided into reversible and irreversible therapies. Reversible therapy, also considered as conservative management is the first-line intervention for TMDs. Data suggest that about 75–90% of patients respond favourably to conservative management, with early introduction yielding successful outcomes for all subtypes. This option is simple with minimal cost and mostly non-invasive. Conservative management comprises of reassurance and education, physical therapies, pharmacotherapy, occlusal splint therapy and psychological interventions. Patient should receive reassurance that TMD is a benign condition that is usually non-progressive. Patient should be motivated to encourage self-care and adopt certain modifications of habits and lifestyle. A most useful advice is a change to dietary habits like taking soft food and cutting tough food into smaller pieces. The idea is to allow the joints and muscles adequate rest to promote natural healing. Therefore, any food that requires excessive chewing should be avoided. Care should also be taken to avoid excessive mouth opening like yawning or positions subjecting the jaw to unnecessary strain.

There are a wide range of physical therapies which help to relieve pain and restore normal function of the TMJ. The simplest method is through application of superficial heat and/or cold which can be easily managed by patients themselves. Other options may require training by physiotherapist such as jaw exercises, massage and manual mobilization. Directed therapy with modalities such as ultrasound, low-intensity laser, pulsed diathermy, iontophoresis, phonophoresis and electrotherapy is dependent on the availability at the treating institution. Pharmacotherapy is usually applicable over short-term with the use of analgesics and occasionally muscle relaxants. Occlusal splint therapy with stabilization splint or anterior repositioning splint has been fairly successful in treating most common subtypes as well. Psychological interventions are to be considered when there is a strong psychosocial component in the diagnosis of TMDs.

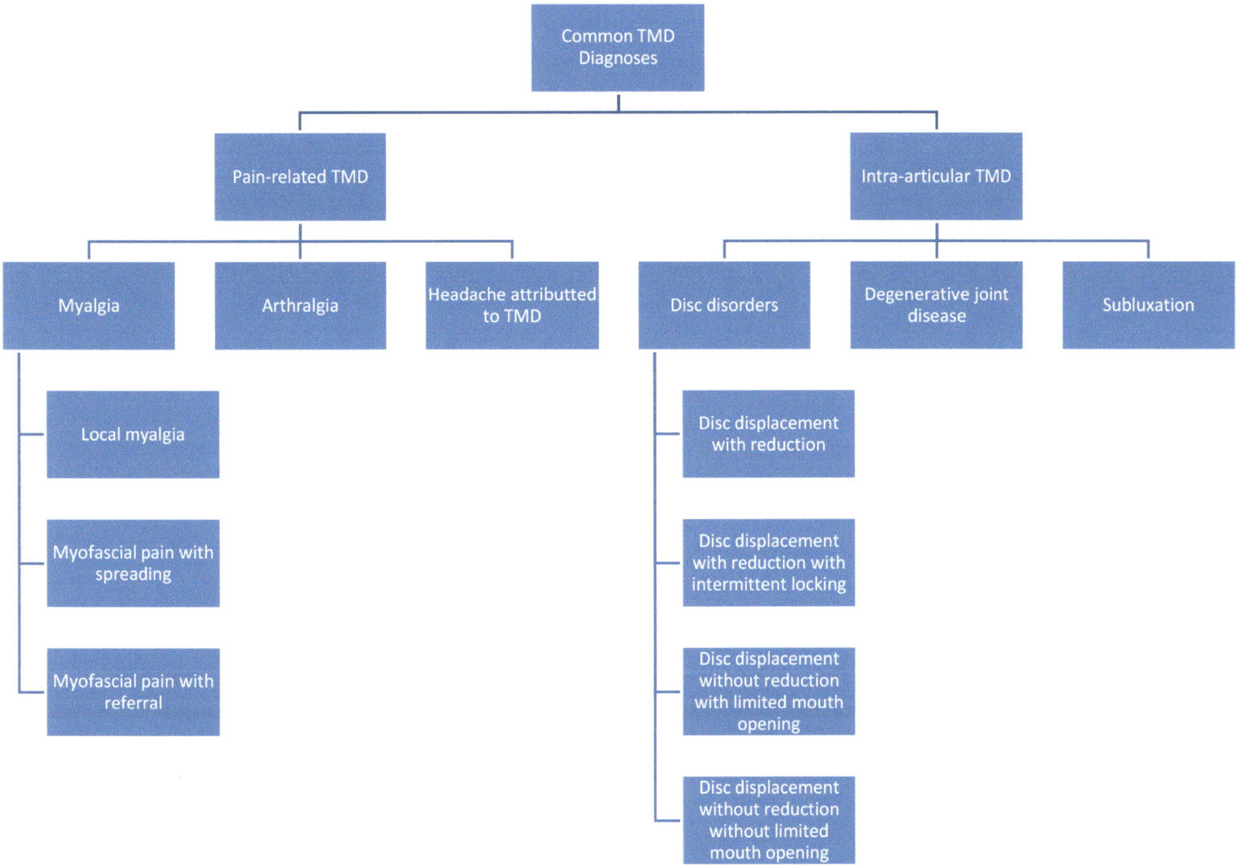

Fig. 55.1 Diagrammatic representation of common TMD diagnoses

Irreversible therapies such as orthodontics and surgery should only be considered if the severity and/or persistence of symptoms warrants it. However, the relative risk and benefits must be taken into account. Irreversible therapies should be the last resort in the treatment of TMDs. Surgical procedures from the likes of arthrocentesis, arthroscopy and joint replacement may be indicated in carefully selected cases.

Salient features of myalgia

Aetiology	• Possible aetiologic factors identified through history and examination
Clinical features	• Pain and tenderness of any of the masticatory muscles that can be directly affected by movements of the jaw • No joint signs and symptoms • Dental and other pathological causes should be excluded
Treatment	• Conservative management

Salient features of myalgia

This is chronic pain condition that requires a partnership-like effort from both patient and clinician to achieve optimum results.

Self-Assessment Questions

1. List the common types of TMD.
2. List the important signs and symptoms of TMD.
3. List different aetiological factors for TMD.
4. Explain the role of imaging in TMD.
5. Outline the management plan for TMD.

Suggested Reading

Akhter R. Epidemiology of temporomandibular disorder in the general population: a systematic review. Advances in Dentistry & Oral Health. 2019;10(3):1–13. https://doi.org/10.19080/ADOH.2019.10.555787.

de Leeuw R, Klasser GD. Chapter 8: Temporomandibular disorders. In: American Academy of Orofacial Pain, editor. Orofacial pain:

guidelines for assessment, diagnosis, and management. 6th ed. Hanover Park, IL: Quintessence Publishing; 2018.

Durham J. Summary of Royal College of Surgeons' (England) clinical guidelines on management of temporomandibular joints in primary care. Br Dent J. 2015;218(6):355–6.

Manfredini D, Guarda-Nardini L, Winocur E, Piccotti F, Ahlberg J, Lobbezoo F. Research diagnostic criteria for temporomandibular disorders: a systematic review of axis I epidemiologic findings. Oral Surg Oral Med Oral Pathol Oral Radiol Endod. 2011;112:453–62.

Peck CC, Goulet JP, Lobbezoo F, et al. Expanding the taxonomy of the diagnostic criteria for temporomandibular disorders. J Oral Rehabil. 2014;41(1):2–23. https://doi.org/10.1111/joor.12132.

Schiffman E, Ohrbach R, Truelove E, et al. Diagnostic criteria for temporomandibular disorders (DC/TMD) for clinical and research applications: recommendations of the International RDC/TMD Consortium Network and Orofacial Pain Special Interest Group. J Oral Facial Pain Headache. 2014;28(1):6–27. https://doi.org/10.11607/jop.1151.

Bilateral Pain in Front of The Ear During Mouth Opening: Temporomandibular Disorders (Disc Displacement Disorders)

Siew Wui Chan and P. Shanmuhasuntharam

Contents

W. M Tilakaratne, T. G. Kallarakkal (eds.), *Clinicopathological Correlation of Oral Diseases*,
https://doi.org/10.1007/978-3-031-24408-7_56

Learning Goals

1. Devise the correct way of compiling the history with appropriate questions.
2. Develop a differential diagnosis after history taking.
3. Deduce appropriate procedures in clinical examination.
4. Formulate a differential diagnosis combining findings in the history and clinical examination.
5. Justify the relevant investigations required to arrive at the diagnosis.
6. Comprehend the importance of clinicopathological correlation in arriving at the correct diagnosis.
7. Outline the management plan.
8. Recognize the importance of a diagnostic algorithm in arriving at a diagnosis.

56.1 Main Complaint

A 16-year-old male patient is referred for painful and clicking temporomandibular joints prior to orthodontic treatment

56.2 History of Complaint

Question: How long have you had this condition and how has it progressed?

I started to notice clicking of the left temporomandibular joint since a few years ago. It is worse during meals when I open my mouth wide or chew hard food. Recently, the clicking is more severe and frequently accompanied by pain. I also feel slight pain on the right side. The pain comes and goes.

56.3 Additional Complaints

Question: Do you have any associated pain in the temple, jaw or neck muscles on either side?

The pain is mainly in front of the ears on both the sides.

Question: Did you have any accident or trauma to the complaint site recently?

His mother relates that he had a history of fall and fracture on the left mandibular condyle when he was 2 years old but there were no such incidents in recent times.

Question: Have you had pain or stiffness in your jaw on awakening?

I don't have any pain or stiffness in the jaw on awakening.

Question: Do you have habits such as clenching, grinding or bruxism?

I don't have any such habits.

Question: Have you ever experienced your jaw lock or catch, even momentarily, so that it would not open all the way?

I have not experienced any such symptoms.

Question: Have you ever experienced moments when you could not close your mouth after you opened it wide?

I have not experienced anything like it.

Question: Are you on any special diet? Do you often snack on food like nuts or chewing gums?

I have a normal diet. I am not fond of snacking.

Question: Do you have any other medical problems? If yes, what kind of medications have you been taking until now?

I am medically fit and not taking any medication.

Question: Have you undergone any surgery?

I have not undergone any surgery.

Question: Have you undergone any dental treatment?

I have had scaling done before. Currently I am seeing an orthodontist to address my concerns of facial asymmetry and deviated teeth.

Question: Are you currently schooling? Are your studies stressing you out?

I am attending public school. I am stressed but not overly distressed.

Question: Do you have habits of smoking or take alcohol? Do you have habits such as chewing your fingers or objects like pens or pencils?

I don't have any such habits.

56.4 With the Findings from the History, What Is Your Differential Diagnosis?

Temporomandibular disorders (TMD)

1. Bilateral arthralgia
2. Disc displacement with reduction of left temporomandibular joint

How do you justify your differential diagnosis after history taking?

1. He has a typical arthrogenous TMD presentation with clicking and pain over the temporomandibular joint region, especially in association with functional jaw movements such as mouth opening and chewing. The complaint of pain and associated sites are consistent with bilateral arthralgia. The presence of clicking but absence of any limitation of mouth opening indicates that this is most likely a case of disc displacement with reduction. The history of trauma seems irrelevant even though macro trauma is a frequent cause of adhesion and ankyloses of the temporomandibular joints. The incident occurred too long ago and did not manifest as any symptom consistent with progressive loss of jaw mobility with severe limited range of motion on jaw opening.
2. Given the specificity of the symptoms, a diagnosis of TMD should be rather apparent. Nevertheless, general exclusion of dental-related causes and closely related structures should also be done. This is especially true as patient may sometimes also present with non-specific toothache or sensitivity, indicating possible pain of pulpal or periodontal origin that may radiate to the TMJ region. It is also recommended to be wary of red flag symptoms suggestive of secondary headaches, additional symptoms suggestive of pathology from the oral cavity, ear, nose or throat, as well as symptoms of temporal arteritis.

56.5 Findings of Examination

Extraoral Examination

He has facial asymmetry at rest with noticeable deviation of the chin to the left. The mandible deviates about 2 mm to the left during mouth opening. The head and neck lymph nodes are not palpable. There is tenderness on palpation over his left- and right-temporomandibular joints. There is also clicking of the left temporomandibular joint on opening and closing of the mouth. There is no evidence of jaw lock noted. The masticatory muscles are non-tender on palpation. The pain-free mouth opening is 36 mm. The maximum unassisted mouth opening is 45 mm, with pain felt over the temporomandibular region. Lateral and protrusive movements are asymptomatic.

Intraoral Examination

There is a left midline shift and dental malocclusion. There is no mucosal lesion present and the teeth are generally sound. Oral hygiene is fair.

56.6 What Is the Most Likely Diagnosis?

1. Bilateral arthralgia.
2. Disc displacement with reduction of the left temporomandibular joint

56.7 How Would You Investigate This Patient?

A combination of comprehensive history and thorough clinical examination of the temporomandibular joints and the masticatory muscles is usually enough to arrive at a provisional diagnosis for this patient. However, imaging such as MRI will further confirm the diagnosis (◘ Fig. 56.1). General examination or imaging of the dentition and closely related anatomical structures can be done to rule out other causes which may compound the original complaints (◘ Fig. 56.2).

56.8 How Would You Manage This Patient?

As with most TMD, this patient would also benefit from early conservative or non-invasive therapy. Reassurance and education of patient on the disease are helpful in improving his condition. In addition to adjusting dietary preference and modification of certain habits or lifestyle, he should be advised to avoid overloading his joints through excessive mouth opening or poor postures. Warm compression and jaw exercises will alleviate the symptoms, while physiotherapy and short-term pharmacotherapy with NSAIDS can also be considered if necessary. This patient is also suitable for splint therapy, specifically anterior repositioning splint. The splint worn over a certain period of time will reduce the symptomatic pain and clicking. It may also improve his midline shift which can be further stabilized when his orthodontic treatment is initiated. However, he will have

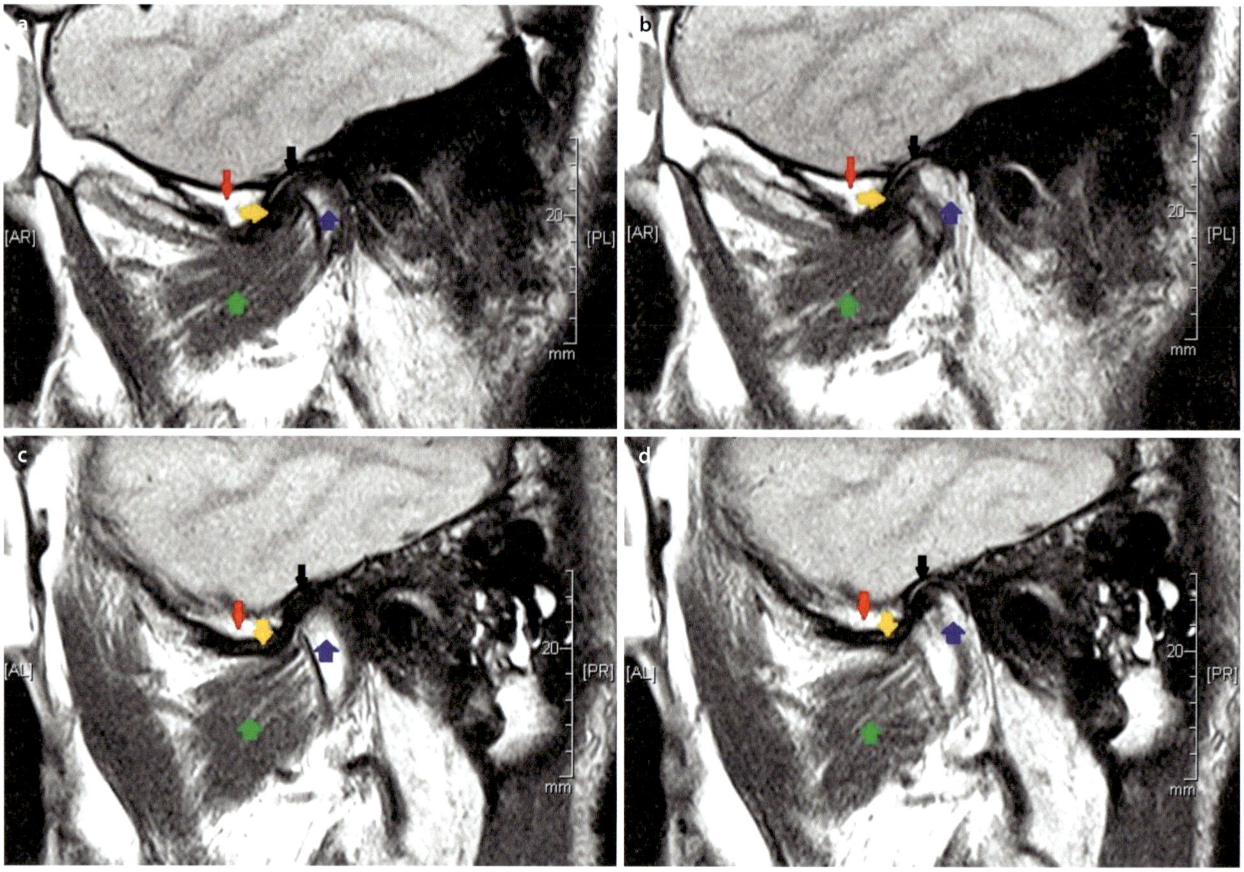

Fig. 56.1 MRI findings (T2 weighted images) for this patient exhibiting left anterior disc displacement **a** on jaw closing and jaw opening, **b** but normal TMJ relationship on the right on jaw closing **c** and jaw opening **d**. Arrows: (blue—mandibular condyle; red—articular eminence; yellow—articular disc; green—lateral pterygoid muscle; black—bilaminar zone attached to posterior margin of articular disc)

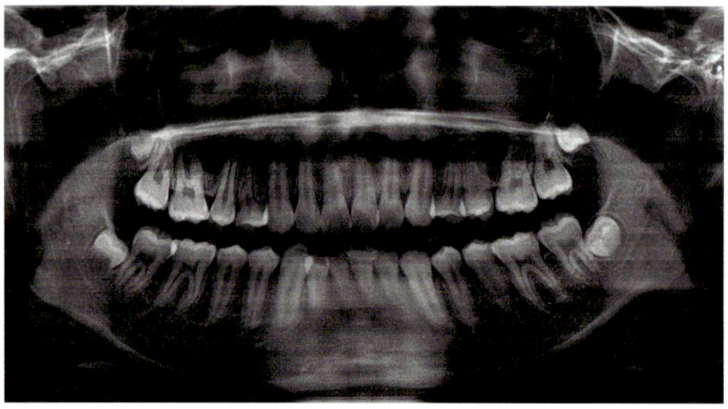

Fig. 56.2 Dental panoramic tomograph showing no underlying pathology that would explain this patient's signs and symptoms

to be closely followed up to monitor his disease progression and review the fitting as well as wear and tear of the splint. The wearing of splint can be discontinued when he is asymptomatic as prolonged wear of the splint may also result in unwanted occlusion changes. Once patient is asymptomatic, he can be referred back to his orthodontist to commence treatment.

56.9 Temporomandibular Joint Disorder (TMD): Disc Displacement Disorders

Disc displacement disorders are the most commonly diagnosed types of arthrogenous TMD, accounting for an 8.5–15.8% prevalence in the general population. According to the current Diagnostic Criteria for Temporomandibular Disorders (DC-TMD) classification, this subgroup includes disc displacement with reduction, disc displacement with reduction with intermittent locking, disc displacement without reduction with limited opening and disc displacement without reduction without limited opening. Over the years, continuous amendments to existing diagnostic classifications have led to various confusing nomenclatures in TMD-related literature. Disc displacement disorders are also known as disc derangements, internal derangements or disc-condyle complex disorders, albeit with slightly different defined subtypes.

DC-TMD has come up with several useful diagnostic algorithms for common TMDs, most of which boast acceptable sensitivity and specificity, that is recommended for clinical use or screening purpose. The diagnostic algorithms for TMJ intra-articular disorders have suboptimal diagnostic accuracy and are therefore reserved for screening of preliminary diagnoses of disk displacements or degenerative joint disease, with the only exception being disc displacement without reduction with limited opening (Table 56.1). In reference to the algorithm and the decision tree (Fig. 56.3), signs and symptoms such as temporomandibular joint noises, jaw locks, and extent of mouth opening are critical for diagnosis of disc displacement disorders. Temporomandibular joint noises refer to sounds heard by patients or heard and/or palpated by examining clinician during jaw movements, typically during opening and closing the mouth. It can be described as clicking, popping, snapping or crepitus (crunching, grinding or grating noise). However, absence of joint noises does not exclude the diagnosis of disc displacement with reduction as many MRI-confirmed cases might not present with clinically detectable joint noise or these noises are not consistently present. On a similar note, crepitus can occur without frank osseous changes and may not always be present with degenerative joint disorders.

Table 56.1 Diagnostic criterion for intra-articular TMD disorders (modified from Schiffman and Ohrbach 2016)

Disorders	Criteria	
	History	Examination findings
Disc displacement with reduction	TMJ noise(s) present.	TMJ noise present with: • opening and closing, **or,** • opening or closing, **and** lateral or protrusive movements.
Disc displacement with reduction with intermittent locking	TMJ noise(s) present **and** Jaw locks with limited opening and then unlocks.	TMJ noise present with: • opening and closing, **or,** • opening or closing, **and** lateral or protrusive movements. Note: When disorder is present in clinic, maneuver is required to open mouth (optional).
Disc displacement without reduction with limited opening	Current TMJ lock with limited opening **and** Limitation severe enough to interfere with ability to eat.	Maximum assisted opening (passive stretch) <40 mm. Note: Maximum opening includes inter-incisal opening + vertical overlap of incisors.
Disc displacement without reduction without limited opening	Prior TMJ lock with limited opening, **and** Limitation severe enough to interfere with ability to eat.	Maximum assisted opening (passive stretch) ≥40 mm. Note: Maximum opening includes inter-incisal opening + vertical overlap of incisors
Degenerative joint disease	TMJ noise(s) present.	Crepitus * present during maximum active opening, passive opening, right lateral, left lateral or protrusive movement(s).
Subluxation	TMJ locking or catching in a wide-open position that resolves with a specific maneuver (e.g., moving the jaw).	Note: When disorder is present in clinic, maneuver is required to close mouth (optional).

Jaw locks can be divided into closed locks or open locks. Closed locks refer to the inability to further open the mouth, even momentarily, from a partially opened position. Conversely, open locks refer to the inability to close the mouth, even momentarily, from a wide-open position. Both the conditions can be determined through history and/or clinical examination. In both the situations, it is also useful to note if reduction of the locks is possible, either by the patient or the clinician. On the other hand, mouth opening measurements such as pain free opening, maximum unassisted opening, and maximum assisted opening, provide a reliable objective assessment of the patient's condition. These involve measurements of the inter-incisal distance between the maxillary and mandibular reference teeth that are adjusted by taking into account the incisal overbite. Maximum assisted opening will best reflect the actual jaw mobility as the element of guarding is minimized or eliminated during the procedure. A measurement below the cut-off point of 40 mm during maximum assisted opening is regarded as limited mouth opening. Alternatively, patient's perceived limitation of mouth opening can also be taken into consideration irrespective of the measurement.

At present, there are many available diagnostic imaging modalities for the TMJ including conventional radiographs, computed tomography (CT), magnetic resonance imaging (MRI), ultrasonography (US), arthrography, and nuclear medicine studies. In addition, multidetector CT (MDCT) and cone beam CT (CBCT) are emerging new options. Conventional radiographs have limited diagnostic roles in TMD due to issues with superimposition of adjacent bony structures, low reliability and low sensitivity in detecting bony changes. Only panoramic radiography has been acknowledged for its value in screening for gross dental, periodontal, or other bony pathologies. For the most part, CT is deemed as a far superior option due to its exquisite bone details

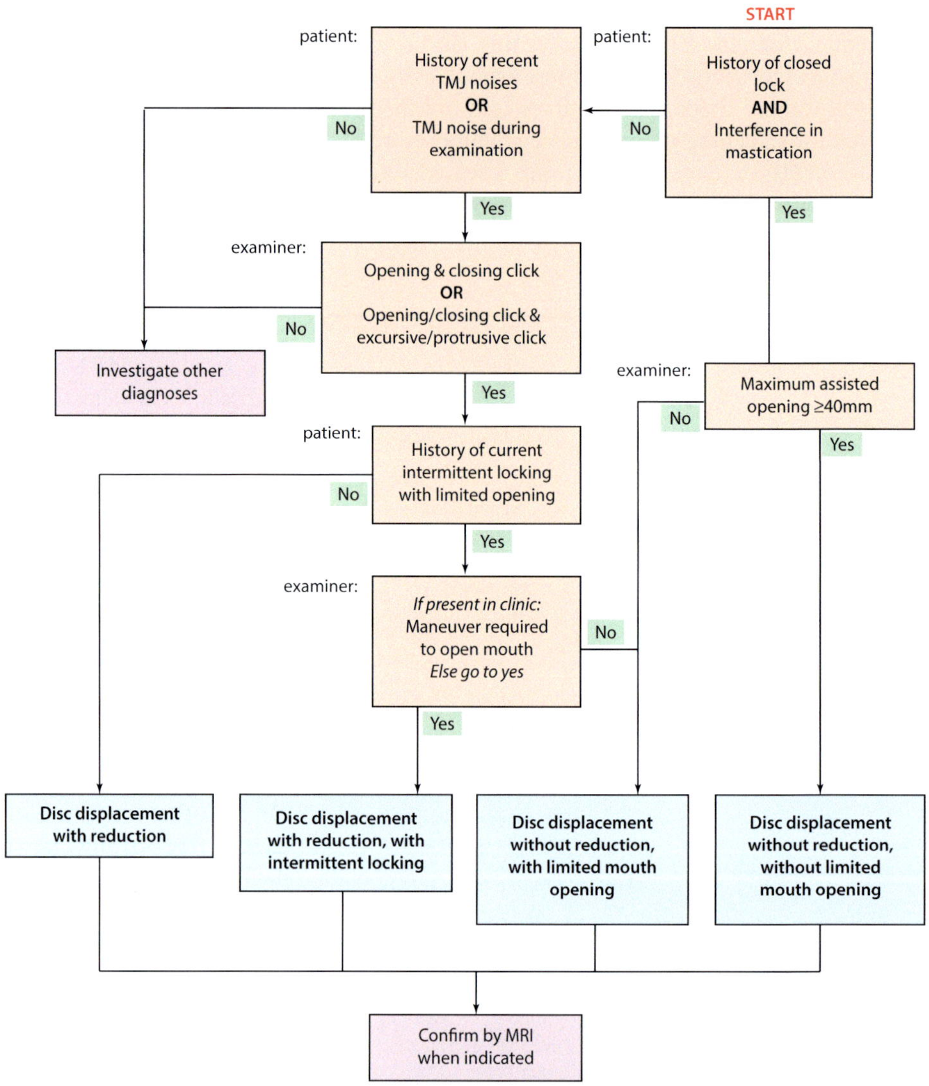

Fig. 56.3 Diagnostic decision tree for intra-articular joint disorders (modified from Diagnostic Criteria for Temporomandibular Disorders (DC/TMD): Diagnostic Decision Tree)

and three-dimensional assessments. CT is ideal to examine bony changes, fractures, bony cysts, tumor invasion, and other pathologies. CBCT is also an attractive option to detect bony abnormalities because of the lower cost and radiation dose. Meanwhile, MDCT has a slight advantage over CBCT in TMD diagnosis because it can project soft tissue details. However, MRI is still the gold standard for soft tissue evaluation. MRI is also the imaging modality of choice for the diagnosis of TMJ internal derangements. MRI provides high resolution and great tissue contrast to enable reliable assessment of disc position and detection of joint effusions. Hence, if clinically indicated, CT imaging is advocated to confirm degenerative joint disorders and MRI to confirm intra-articular joint disorders.

US is not particularly useful to diagnose intra-articular disc derangements but may be valuable in US-guided injection of medications into muscles or joint spaces. Arthrography is an invasive imaging modality that is rarely employed today as it requires injection of radiopaque contrast into the TMJ that outlines the articular disc under video fluoroscopy. Hence, MRI is a better non-invasive option without exposing patient to risk of allergic reaction to contrast, infection or radiation. Nuclear medicine studies is another invasive modality that involves the intravenous administration of a radioactive isotope which enters into tissues and is measured via either a scintillation gamma camera or single-photon emission CT (SPECT).

Most guidelines for management of TMD advocate conservative or reversible therapy as the initial intervention. For disc displacements, the primary goals remain to reduce pain and functional limitations as well as encourage self-management of the condition. In patients presenting with acute symptoms such as acute onset of pain and/or painful limitations, rest and pharmacotherapy such as non-steroidal anti-inflammatory drugs (NSAIDS) are required in short term. If disc displacement without reduction (closed lock) is present, manual reduction by the patient or attending clinician may be attempted with the aid of local anaesthesia, and if applicable oral diazepam. In addition to pharmacotherapy, non-acute or chronic cases may be complemented with any of the non-invasive reversible therapies including physical therapies, occlusal splint therapy, and psychological interventions. An example of an ideal self-care programme would contain components of cognitive behavioural therapy, relaxation techniques, simple self-administered physiotherapeutic techniques, and jaw exercises addressing muscle strength and jaw movement coordination.

Various orthopaedic appliances like hard stabilization splint, soft stabilization splint, non-occluding splint, mini-anterior splint, prefabricated splint and anterior repositioning splint have been used in the treatment of TMDs, with the most widely used being stabilization splint, anterior repositioning splint, and anterior bite splint. These appliances may theoretically alter occlusal and structural TMJ relationships, redistribute occlusal forces, prevent damage to teeth, reduce bruxism, and parafunctional habits, and treat painful myogenous and arthrogenous TMD. At the very least, these appliances may produce favourable results due to positive placebo effect or increased cognitive awareness to parafunctional habits. Current literature suggests that all occlusal splints, such as the anterior repositioning splint, hard stabilization splint, soft stabilization splint, mini-anterior splint, and prefabricated splint, are probably more effective treatments for arthrogenous and myogenous TMDs when compared to no treatment and non-occluding splints. For arthrogenous TMDs, anterior repositioning splint and counselling therapy (behaviour changes, muscle exercise, joint mobilization, self-management, professional reassurance, and relaxation sessions) in combination with a hard stabilization splint seem to be the most effective treatments in reducing TMJ pain and TMJ sounds. However, prolonged use of these appliances especially with regards to partial coverage appliance may result in major and irreversible occlusal changes.

Irreversible therapies such as orthodontics and surgery are only reserved for select cases. Surgical options ranging from minimally invasive to open joint surgery are reserved for specific articular disorders, especially cases with disabling pain or functional problems. In particular, there are suggestions to consider minimally invasive procedures such as intra-articular injections and/or arthrocentesis earlier in the management of arthrogenous TMDs. A recent network meta-analysis of randomized clinical trials has demonstrated minimally invasive procedures to be significantly more effective than conservative treatment for pain reduction and improvement of maximum mouth opening.

Salient features of disc displacement disorders	
Clinical	• Temporomandibular joint noises that could be associated with pain and/or tenderness of the TMJ • Limitation of mouth opening • Presence of jaw locks
Treatment	• Conservative management • Surgical options if clinically indicated
This is a chronic pain condition that often requires a multimodal treatment approach for effective results.	

Self-Assessment Questions

1. List the types of arthrogenous TMD.
2. Differentiate the types of jaw locks.
3. List the available imaging modalities for TMJ.
4. Explain the proposed therapeutic mechanisms of occlusal splints.
5. Discuss the components of an ideal self-care programme.

Suggested Reading

Ahmad M, Hollender L, Anderson Q, Kartha K, Ohrbach R, Truelove EL, John MT, Schiffman EL. Research diagnostic criteria for temporomandibular disorders (RDC/TMD): development of image analysis criteria and examiner reliability for image analysis. Oral Surg Oral Med Oral Pathol Oral Radiol Endod. 2009;107(6):844–60. https://doi.org/10.1016/j.tripleo.2009.02.023.

Al-Moraissi EA, Farea R, Qasem KA, Al-Wadeai MS, Al-Sabahi ME, Al-Iryani GM. Effectiveness of occlusal splint therapy in the management of temporomandibular disorders: network meta-analysis of randomized controlled trials. Int J Oral Maxillofac Surg. 2020a;49(8):1042–56. https://doi.org/10.1016/j.ijom.2020.01.004.

Al-Moraissi EA, Wolford LM, Ellis E III, Neff A. The hierarchy of different treatments for arthrogenous temporomandibular disorders: a network meta-analysis of randomized clinical trials. J Craniomaxillofac Surg. 2020b;48(1):9–23. https://doi.org/10.1016/j.jcms.2019.10.004.

de Leeuw R, Klasser GD. Chapter 8: Temporomandibular disorders. In: American Academy of Orofacial Pain, editor. Orofacial pain: guidelines for assessment, diagnosis, and management. 6th ed. Hanover Park, IL: Quintessence Publishing; 2018.

Diagnostic criteria for temporomandibular disorders (DC/TMD): diagnostic decision tree. https://buffalo.box.com/s/btzm3fzeocw5xmh3ty2x5gjtba23hai5. Accessed 8 Sept 2021.

Durham J. Summary of Royal College of Surgeons' (England) clinical guidelines on management of temporomandibular joints in primary care. Br Dent J. 2015;218(6):355–6.

Schiffman E, Ohrbach R. Executive summary of the Diagnostic Criteria for Temporomandibular Disorders for clinical and research applications. J Am Dent Assoc. 2016;147(6):438–45. https://doi.org/10.1016/j.adaj.2016.01.007.

Schiffman E, Ohrbach R, Truelove E, et al. Diagnostic criteria for temporomandibular disorders (DC/TMD) for clinical and research applications: recommendations of the International RDC/TMD Consortium Network and Orofacial Pain Special Interest Group. J Oral Facial Pain Headache. 2014;28(1):6–27. https://doi.org/10.11607/jop.1151.

Salivary Gland Disorders

Contents

Dry Mouth and Dry Eyes: Sjogren Syndrome

Anand Ramanathan, P. Shanmuhasuntharam, and Jasmin Raja

Contents

W. M Tilakaratne, T. G. Kallarakkal (eds.), *Clinicopathological Correlation of Oral Diseases*,
https://doi.org/10.1007/978-3-031-24408-7_57

Learning Goals

1. Devise the correct way of compiling the history with appropriate questions.
2. Develop a differential diagnosis after history taking.
3. Deduce appropriate procedures in clinical examination.
4. Formulate a differential diagnosis combining findings in the history and clinical examination.
5. Justify the relevant investigations required to arrive at the diagnosis.
6. Comprehend the importance of clinicopathological correlation in arriving at the correct diagnosis.
7. Outline the management plan.
8. Recognize the importance of a diagnostic algorithm in arriving at a diagnosis.

57.1 Main Complaint

A 40-year-old female patient presented to the dental clinic with a complaint of dry mouth and dry eyes.

57.2 History of Complaint

Question: Does food stick in your mouth or throat?

I notice that the food occasionally gets stuck in my mouth.

Question: Can you eat a dry cracker without water?

I cannot eat a dry cracker without sipping water.

Question: Has your taste sensation decreased?

I have altered taste sensation.

Question: Does your mouth feel dry at night and do you need to drink water?

My mouth feels dry at night and I need to wake up to sip some water.

Question: How long have you noticed the dryness of your mouth?

The dryness of mouth has been there for a year.

Question: Do you have pain or burning sensation in your mouth?

I have severe burning sensation and I am unable to eat spicy food.

Question: Do you have difficulty in speaking?

I have difficulty in speaking as my mouth feels dry.

Question: Do you have difficulty swallowing?

I have difficulty in swallowing.

Question: Do you have any other symptoms apart from dry mouth?

I sometimes feel bad odour in my mouth.

Question: Do you feel dehydrated?

I do not feel dehydrated.

Question: Do you have vomiting?

I do not have vomiting.

Question: Do your eyes itch/burn?

My eyes itch and burn occasionally.

Question: Do your eyes turn red and watery?

They sometimes turn red and watery.

Question: Do you feel something is stuck in your eyes?

Sometimes it feels like there is sand in my eyes.

Question: How long have you noticed dryness of your eyes?

I have been having dry eyes for the past 1 year.

Question: How is your eyesight?

My vision is blurred sometimes.

Question: Do you have any swelling on your face?

I sometimes notice swelling of my face near my ears.

Question: Do you have any problems in your throat?

Sometimes I feel burning sensation in my throat.

Question: Do you have hoarseness of voice?

I do not have any hoarseness of voice.

Question: Does your skin feel dry?

✔ My skin feels dry at times.

? Question: Does your vagina feel dry?

✔ It feels dry sometimes.

? Question: Do you need to wake up in the night to pass urine?

✔ I often get up at night to pass urine.

? Question: Do you feel tired?

✔ I feel extremely tired at times.

? Question: Do you have pain in your joints?

✔ I have joint pain.

? Question: How long have you been having the joint pain?

✔ I have been having the joint pain for the past 6 months.

? Question: Which of your joints are painful?

✔ The joints of both my hands which include fingers, knuckles, and wrists are painful.

? Question: Is the pain constant?

✔ The pain is not constant. Sometimes it is severe for a few days and then subsides, only to flare up again.

? Question: What is the nature of the pain?

✔ At times the pain is severe, affecting my daily activities.

? Question: Do you have any swelling of your joints?

✔ The joints are usually swollen and red when there is severe pain.

? Question: Do you feel any stiffness in your joint?

✔ I feel stiffness in the joints especially in the mornings when I wake up from sleep.

? Question: Do you have any tingling sensation of your fingers?

✔ I sometimes do have tingling sensation of my fingers.

? Question: Do you snore while sleeping?

✔ I do not snore while sleeping.

57.3 Past Medical History

? Question: Do you have any medical problems like diabetes?

✔ I do not have any other medical problems.

? Question: Are you taking any medications?

✔ I am not taking any medications.

? Question: Have you undergone any radiotherapy?

✔ I have not undergone any radiotherapy.

? Question: Have you consulted any doctor for your dry eyes?

✔ I have not consulted a doctor for my dry eyes.

? Question: What did you do for your joints?

✔ I do warm compression at home or take pain killers (bought over the counter) for the joints when the pain is severe.

? Question: Have you seen the doctor for your joint pain?

✔ I have not consulted a doctor for my joint pain.

57.4 Past Dental History

? Question: Have you got any decayed tooth?

✔ I have few decayed teeth.

? Question: Did you go to a dentist to get them fixed?

✔ I got restorations done for the decayed teeth.

? Question: Do you visit a dentist regularly?

✔ I have gone to the dentist only a few times.

? Question: Did you have any tooth extracted?

✔ I have not had any teeth extracted.

? Question: Do you have any ulcers in your mouth?

✔ I currently don't have any ulcers but I have had ulcers in my mouth a few times.

57.5 Social History

Question: Do you smoke or drink alcohol?

I do not smoke or drink alcohol.

57.6 Findings of Extraoral Examination

On extraoral examination, she has red, dry eyes (Fig. 57.1). Her joints, especially the small joints of hands and wrists, are tender, red and swollen. She has a slight swelling of the parotid salivary glands bilaterally. There is no swelling seen in her neck. Her temporomandibular joints (TMJs) are tender on palpation bilaterally. Her muscles of mastication including the masseter, temporalis, and medial pterygoid are tender upon palpation. Her mouth opening is normal but she has tenderness over her TMJs when she tries to open her mouth wide.

57

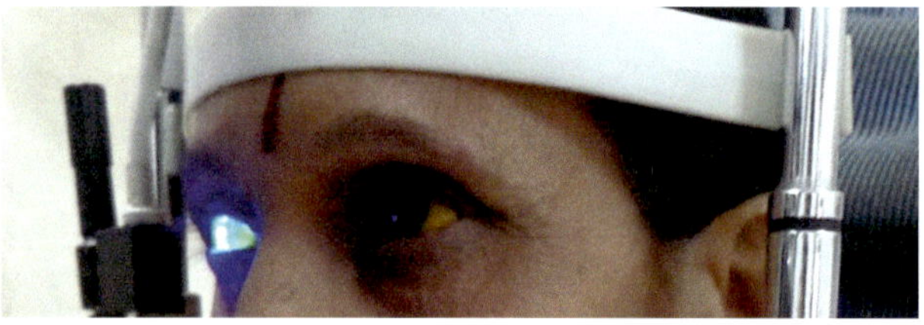

Fig. 57.1 Photograph shows red, dry eyes (Courtesy: Dr. Preeti Nair, People's College of Dental Sciences, Bhopal, India)

57.7 Findings of Intraoral Examination

The patient has poor oral hygiene. The tongue seems dry, fissured with atrophy of papillae on the dorsum (Fig. 57.2a). There are numerous teeth with cervical and root caries (Fig. 57.2b, c).

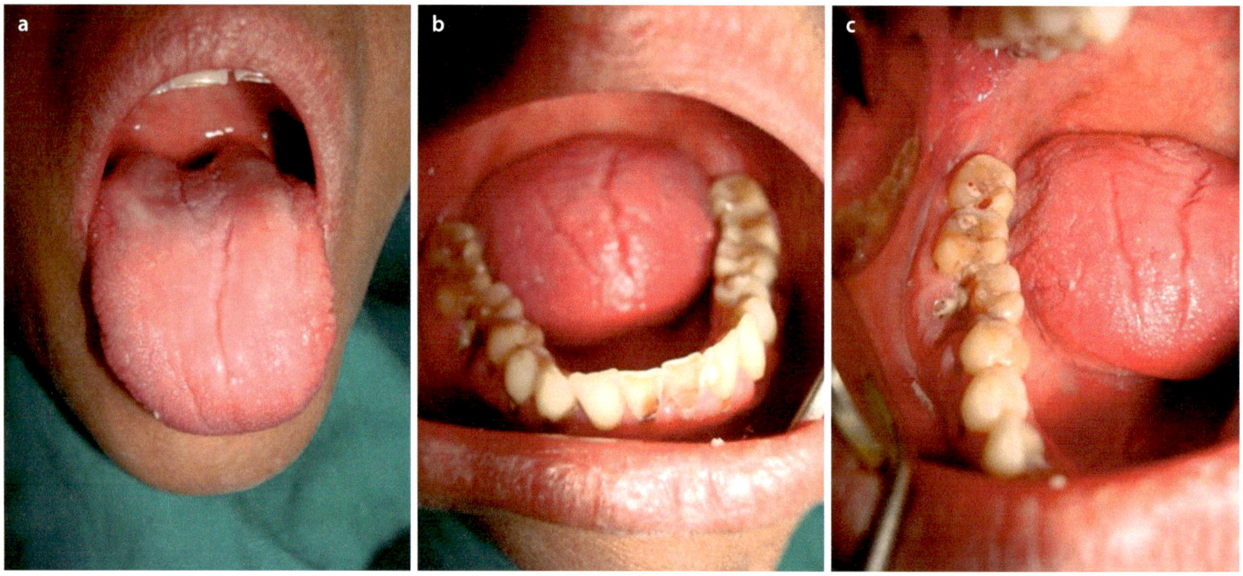

Fig. 57.2 Intraoral photographs show (**a**) dry and fissured tongue, (**b**) and (**c**) numerous cervical and root caries as well as poor oral hygiene (Courtesy: Dr. Preeti Nair, People's College of Dental Sciences, Bhopal, India)

57.8 What Is Your Provisional Diagnosis for This Patient? Give Reasons for Your Diagnosis?

Sjogren syndrome

The patient has dry mouth (xerostomia) and red, dry eyes (xerophthalmia) which are classic features of Sjogren syndrome (SS). The history and examination findings are not suggestive of any other diseases like diabetes, stroke, and HIV/AIDS. The patient does not have any history of radiotherapy in the head and neck region. She is currently not taking any medication which can cause dry mouth. She also does not have habits such as drinking alcohol, smoking, and snoring. Moreover, the patient has pain in her knee joints. Extraorally, the patient has red, dry eyes, and red, swollen knees and elbows. She also has tenderness over her TMJs and her muscles of mastication. Her parotid salivary glands are swollen. She also notices her fingers turn pale and then blue when exposed to cold, suggestive of Raynaud phenomenon. Intraorally she has dry, fissured tongue with atrophy of the papillae on the dorsum. She sometimes has ulcers in her mouth. She has multiple cervical and root caries due to xerostomia. Her oral hygiene is poor. These features are suggestive of SS.

57.9 What Investigations Need to Be Carried out for This Patient?

Sialometry
- Oral Schirmer test
- Sialochemistry
- Sialography
- Labial gland biopsy
- Schirmer test
- Serological testing

For sialometry, the unstimulated whole salivary flow rate and stimulated salivary flow rate were measured. The unstimulated salivary flow rate was <1 mL in 10 min, which when calculated per min was <0.1 mL, whereas the stimulated salivary rate was 5 mL for 10 min, which when calculated per min was 0.5 mL/min for this patient. Oral Schirmer test was carried out using Whatman number 41 filter, which was placed in the floor of the mouth for 5 min after which the length of wetness of the filter paper was measured for this patient. The length of wetness was 17 mm/5 min indicating dry mouth. Sialochemistry of the parotid saliva of this patient showed increase in total lipids. Both phospholipid and glycolipid levels were also elevated. Sodium and chloride levels were also elevated. Sailography showed snowstorm appearance in the DPT due to the leakage of contrast medium in this patient. Labial gland biopsy of the minor oral salivary gland was performed. Schirmer test was carried out for this patient (◘ Fig. 57.3). She had about 8 mm of moisture after 5 min.

Serological testing such as immunofluorescence for anti-nuclear antibodies (ANA) and extractable nuclear antigen (ENA) were carried out. ANA was positive and showed speckled pattern with a titer of 1:320 while anti-ENA antibodies, anti-Ro/SS-A and anti-La/SS-B were also positive in this patient.

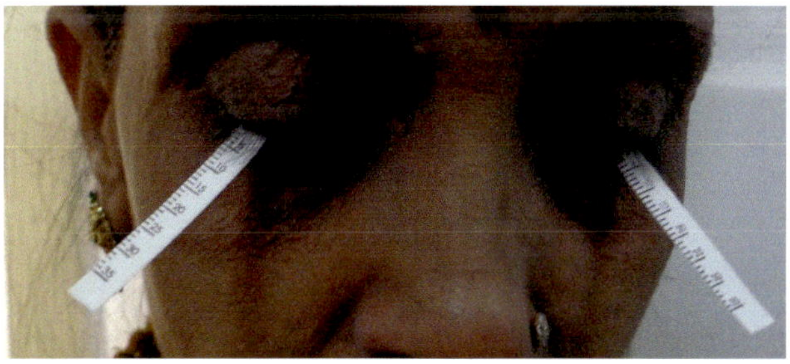

◘ **Fig. 57.3** Photograph shows a Schirmer test being carried out on this patient (Courtesy: Dr. Preeti Nair, People's College of Dental Sciences, Bhopal, India)

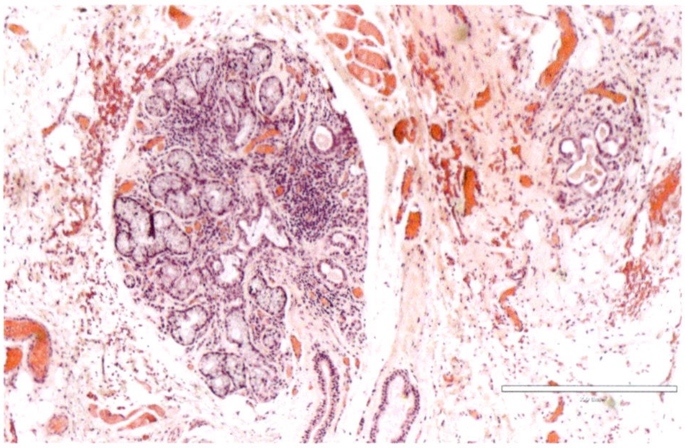

Fig. 57.4 Photomicrograph shows periductal lymphocytic clusters in the minor salivary gland

Table 57.1 2016 American College of Rheumatology/European League Against Rheumatism classification criteria for Primary SS

No.	Criteria	Score
1.	Anti-SSA/Ro antibody positivity	3
2.	Focal lymphocytic sialadenitis with a focus score of ≥1 foci/4 mm^2	3
3.	Abnormal ocular staining score of ≥5 (or van Bijsterveld score of ≥4)	1
4.	Schirmer test result of ≤5 mm/5 min	1
5.	Unstimulated salivary flow rate of ≤0.1 mL/min	1

57

57.10 What Are the Histopathological Features of the Labial Salivary Gland Biopsy?

The labial salivary gland biopsy shows periductal lymphocytic clusters (>50 lymphocytes) mostly around minor salivary gland ducts. This patient had a focus score ≥1 and some acinar destruction. Hence, it was reported as suggestive of SS (Fig. 57.4).

57.11 What Is the Definitive Diagnosis for This Patient?

Sjogren syndrome.

57.12 What Specific Findings Help You to Arrive at the Diagnosis of SS (Clinical Findings and Investigations)?

Clinical features that point towards the diagnosis are the presence of a dry mouth, red, dry eyes, and moderate burning sensation of her mouth. Extraorally, presence of joint pain, pain in the TMJs and muscles of mastication and swelling of the parotid salivary glands are features suggestive of SS. Intraorally, presence of dry tongue with atrophy of the papillae and multiple cervical and root caries are indications of severity of the xerostomia.

According to 2016 American College of Rheumatology/European League Against Rheumatism classification criteria for Primary SS (Table 57.1), the findings in this patient show that she has anti-Ro/SS-A and anti-La/SS-B antibodies giving a score of 3. Labial salivary gland biopsy shows focal lymphocytic sialadenitis with a focus score of ≥1 foci/4 mm^2 giving a score of 3. Sialometry shows reduced salivary flow which gives a score of 1. This patient has a total score of 7 which is ≥4 thus confirming that the patient is suffering from SS.

57.13 What Is the Management Plan for This Patient? Indicate the Rationale for Selecting a Particular Treatment Option If Many Available

Patients with SS have various dental and medical problems which need a multidisciplinary approach. The multidisciplinary team should include the general dentist, oral medicine specialist, ophthalmologist, and rheumatologist. The following is the management plan for this patient:

1. Oral hygiene instructions.
2. Non-surgical prophylactic treatment.
3. Extraction of non-restorable teeth.
4. Restorative treatment for dental caries.
5. Referral to oral medicine specialist for treatment of dry mouth.
6. Referral to ophthalmologist.
7. Referral to rheumatologist.
8. Review every 4 months.

In this patient, oral hygiene should be given utmost importance. She should be encouraged to brush her teeth at least two to three times a day. She should be advised to use soft-bristled toothbrush and avoid using commercial toothpaste with abrasives (whitening toothpaste) and sodium lauryl sulfate (detergent). She needs to floss at least once daily. She should be prescribed neutral sodium fluoride (0.05%) mouth rinse. This patient should be advised to take sugar-free meals and avoid taking sugar which can cause further dental caries. Alternative sweeteners such as xylitol is an option, if needed. She should be counselled on the do's and don'ts which include to keep herself hydrated by taking frequent sips of water or sucking on finely crushed ice, avoid the use of alcohol-based mouth rinse and not to drink any carbonated soft drinks which are acidic.

Gingival and periodontal status monitoring should be regularly done while required non-surgical prophylactic treatment is provided to the patients. Non-restorable teeth are indicated for extraction. Dental caries needs to be identified early and appropriate restorative treatment is important to be initiated as required. Prosthetic replacement of extracted tooth will also need to be carried out. As for the dry mouth, the patient should be referred to an Oral Medicine specialist. A multidisciplinary approach with the ophthalmologist and rheumatologist is mandatory for the management of her overall SS. Dental surveillance and management by her dentist for any caries activity is recommended every 4 months.

The ophthalmologist may advise the patient to frequently apply preservative-free artificial tears throughout the day and nightly application of lubricant ointments. Some patients may find it helpful to wear eye protection to help reduce tear evaporation. In severe cases, preservation of existing tear film can be achieved through punctal occlusion to decrease tear drainage.

The rheumatologist may prescribe non-steroidal anti-inflammatory drugs (NSAIDs) or oral steroids for flare ups and ongoing inflammation of the joints. Immunosuppressants such as hydroxychloroquine or methotrexate are used for cases of persistent inflammatory arthritis. Hydroxychloroquine may also be prescribed for patients with fatigue, which is a common manifestation of SS.

57.14 What Is the Prognosis of a Patient with SS?

The prognosis of SS patients depends on the severity of the clinical features. A critical issue in this patient is the severity of xerostomia as it affects her quality of life (QoL) with regards to chewing, eating, swallowing, speaking, and socializing. The severity of xerostomia also affects the oral hygiene of this patient. The dryness of eyes may have an impact on her vision, whereas joint pain may restrict her day-to-day activities. She also has an increased risk of lymphoma and needs to be constantly monitored for any swelling in her neck and parotid region.

57.15 Sjogren Syndrome (SS)

In 1933, a Swedish ophthalmologist Henrik Sjögren published a series of cases that were affected by dryness of eyes (keratoconjunctivitis sicca), mouth (xerostomia), and arthritis, and named it sicca syndrome. This new systemic disease was later named as Sjogren syndrome. SS is a chronic autoimmune disease of the exocrine gland characterized by infiltration of lymphocytes. It can be either primary or secondary. Primary SS consists of xerostomia and keratoconjunctivitis sicca, whereas secondary SS is diagnosed when the sicca symptoms coexist with other systemic autoimmune or connective tissue disease such as rheumatoid arthritis (RA), scleroderma or systemic lupus erythematosus (SLE). The prevalence rate of SS ranges from 0.03% in Japan to 4.8% in Europe. Women are more affected than men with a ratio of 9:1. Middle-aged women, young adults, and children can be affected. The severity of SS varies from mild dryness of the mouth and eyes to severe dryness causing pain, depression, multi-organ involvement, and development of lymphoma. Hair, skin, mucosa of the vagina, gastrointestinal tract, respiratory tract, renal, musculoskeletal, and neurological systems can be involved. The current diagnostic criteria used for SS was proposed by the Sjogren International Collaborative Clinical Alliances Cohort in 2012 and later approved by the American College of Rheumatology (ACR) and Board of Directors and the European League Against Rheumatism (EULAR) Executive Committee in 2016. The final classification criteria are based on the weighted sum of five items as described in ◘ Table 57.1.

Individuals with signs and/or symptoms suggestive of SS with a total score of ≥ 4 for the above items meet the criteria for primary SS.

Approximately, 98% of the cases of SS have presentation of dryness of mouth and eyes. Oral complications that are common are xerostomia and salivary gland hypofunction. Xerostomia is defined as the patient perception of dryness of the mouth with or without salivary gland hypofunction. If there is presence of low-salivary flow rate, then the patient is said to have salivary gland hypofunction. They often need regular sips of water to moisten their oral mucosa. Patients with SS may additionally complain of difficulty in speaking, chewing, and swallowing (dysphagia) of food due to the dry mouth. Altered taste sensation (dysgeusia), impaired phonation, and sometimes hoarseness of voice are also encountered in SS patients. Burning sensation to acidic drinks and acidic and spicy food is another frequent complaint in these patients.

Studies have shown that patients with SS tend to have temporomandibular disorders more frequently when compared to the healthy population. The symptoms include difficulty in mouth opening and pain while chewing. On extraoral examination, patients can have deviation of the jaw while opening and myofascial pain particularly in the muscles of mastication. Therefore, a thorough evaluation of the TMJ and muscles of mastication needs to be carried out in these patients. Another extraoral clinical feature that is not uncommonly seen in SS is swelling of the parotid glands (◘ Fig. 57.5a–c) with or without pain, which may be due to recurrent infection of the salivary gland causing sialadenitis. In children, recurrent sialadenitis may precede dryness of the mouth. However careful examination and investigation of the parotid salivary glands are required as patients with SS have high risk for developing lymphomas in the parotid gland. Primary SS patients have a 16-fold increased risk of developing non-Hodgkin lymphoma particularly a low-grade B-cell type extra nodal marginal zone lymphoma of the parotid gland.

The extraglandular manifestation of SS may involve various systems. Lethargy and musculoskeletal manifestations, such as arthralgia, myalgia, and non-erosive arthritis are more common. The gastrointestinal system is occasionally involved with primary biliary cirrhosis, pancreatitis, and atrophic gastritis. Renal tubular acidosis and intestinal nephritis are the manifestations seen in the renal system. Vascular involvement includes purpura, Raynaud phenomenon, cutaneous vasculitis or vasculitis causing mononeuritis multiplex or peripheral neuropathy and benign sensory trigeminal neuropathy. Interstitial lung disease or lung fibrosis can have a debilitating impact on the respiratory system. Rare occurrences in the central nervous system and endocrine alterations have also been reported.

Intraoral clinical features that can be seen in patients with SS are dryness of mouth with fissured tongue or erythematous tongue. In some cases, the tongue is depapillated and atrophic. The mucosa may be erythematous and dry. Patients with SS have the tendency to develop traumatic ulcers due to the lack of saliva which usually helps in lubricating the mucosa. On milking the Stensen ducts, there is no clear fluid seen flowing. SS patients have higher risk of developing oral candidosis when compared to healthy people. This occurs in severe xerostomia as a result of minimal salivary flow rate. Oral candidosis can cause altered taste sensation especially metallic taste. Additionally, erythematous candidosis and angular cheilitis are also more commonly seen in these patients. Erythematous candidosis presents as red areas especially on the dorsal surface of the tongue and/or palate with burning sensation. Angular cheilitis presents as painful fissures at the commissures of the mouth. The affected patients may also be troubled by dry and cracked lips with peeling of the mucosa of the lips.

The lack of flow of the saliva causes plaque accumulation on the tooth resulting in initial enamel hypocalcification or chalky enamel and gingivitis. Some patients complain of tooth sensitivity. The plaque accumulation leads to the development of cervical or root caries which may require restoration or need to be extracted due to severe caries. The DMFT scores are higher in patients with SS. Additionally, patients with SS who suffer from gastrointestinal reflux disease (GERD) are at risk of developing enamel erosion of teeth. Studies have shown that the periodontal status of patients with and without SS seem to be similar. However, if the patient has secondary SS with rheumatoid arthritis, they may suffer from periodontal disease as studies have shown strong link between rheumatoid arthritis and periodontal disease due to the presence of *Porphyromonas gingivalis*.

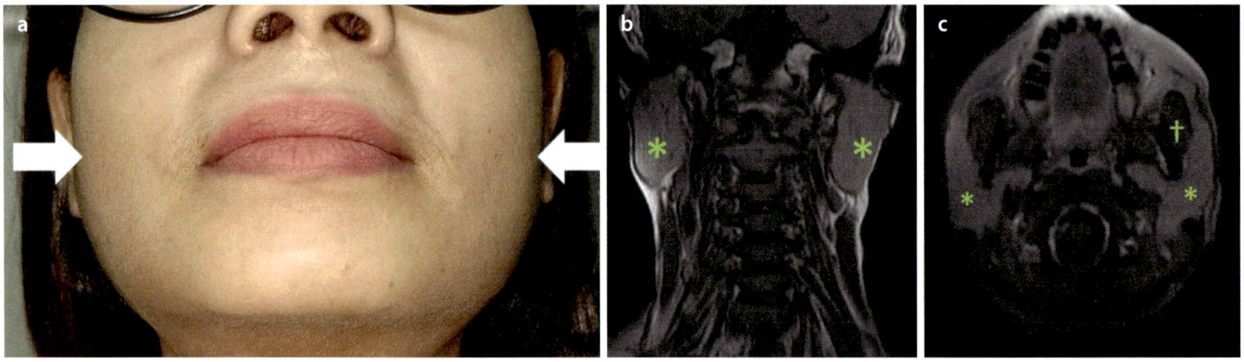

◘ **Fig. 57.5** Photographs show (**a**) bilateral diffuse swelling of both parotid glands that has been present for a few years and (**b**) MRI imaging of T1-weighted coronal window showing diffusely enlarged parotid glands and (**c**) T2-weighted axial window showing hypertrophy of the superficial and deep lobes of parotid glands (*) covering most of the masseteric muscles (†) (Courtesy: Dr. Liew Yew Toong, Faculty of Medicine, University of Malaya)

Sialometry, the measurement of salivary flow rate, is carried out for these patients to determine the hyposalivation and caries risk assessment. The unstimulated whole salivary flow rate and the stimulated salivary flow rates are measured. If the unstimulated whole salivary flow rate <0.1 mL/min or the stimulated whole salivary rate is <0.7 mL/min, it is considered as hypofunction of the salivary glands. Oral Schirmer test is used for screening. A Whatman number 41 filter placed in the floor of the mouth for 3–5 min after which the length of wetness of the filter paper is measured.

Sialochemistry in patients with SS shows that the parotid saliva has two-fold increase in total lipids with elevated phospholipids and glycolipids along with sodium and chloride levels when compared to healthy controls.

Sialography is a minimally invasive technique where water soluble low-osmolality iodine containing contrast medium is injected into the Stensen duct of the parotid gland. Two images are taken, one with the contrast medium in the salivary gland and the other at the end of the procedure to see if there is any retention of the contrast medium in the duct of the gland. Sialography shows a snowstorm appearance due to the leakage of contrast medium which occurs as a result of the sialectasis (◘ Fig. 57.6). There will be a delay in emptying of the contrast medium. Ductal atrophy may be present. Cherry blossom appearance of the obstructed ductal system can be seen in some patients. The cherry blossom appearance in the sialography is due to the presence of punctate cavitary radiocontrast-filled defects that percolate through salivary gland ducts.

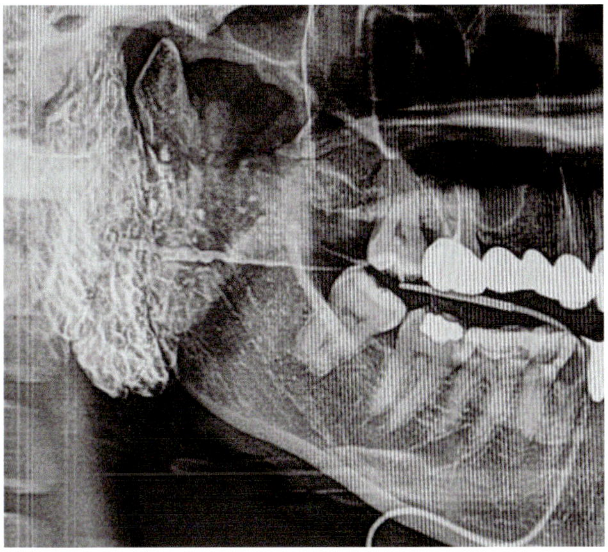

◘ **Fig. 57.6** Sialography showing snowstorm appearance of the parotid gland (Courtesy: Dr. Zakiah Mat Ripen and A/Prof. Dr. Norliza Binti Ibrahim, Faculty of Dentistry, University of Malaya)

Serological testing shows patients with SS can have raised inflammatory markers such as erythrocyte sedimentation rate (ESR) and C-reactive protein. About 50% of patients have polyclonal hypergammaglobulinemia. Rheumatoid factor (RF) is present in 50 and 90% of primary and secondary SS cases, respectively. Rheumatoid arthritis preciptin (RAP) is present in only 5% of primary SS patients, whereas it is present in 75% of secondary SS patients. Antinuclear antibody (ANA) test detects the autoantibodies which are produced against the components of nuclei of cells. If a clinician suspects the presence of an autoimmune disease, then ANA is usually ordered, either using immunofluorescence method or enzyme-linked immunosorbent assays (ELISA). ANA is non-specific since a positive result with significant titer level can be present in many other autoimmune diseases. Specific staining patterns are seen in the nucleus or cytoplasm of the reagent cells (human epithelial laryngeal carcinoma type 2 cells: HEp-2) used which may give a clue towards identification of an autoimmune condition. ANA test result is expressed as titer (it shows to what extent the blood sample can be diluted before the activity of the antibodies can no longer be detected). ANA titer of 1:40 is said to be normal, whereas 1:80 and above is said to be positive. ANA titer is significantly positive in 40–70% of SS cases. In SS, SS-A(Ro) antibodies are seen in 60–90%, whereas SS-B (La) antibodies are seen in 30–60% of cases with a fine speckled pattern present in the reagent cells. These antibodies are also seen in 10–50% of patients with lupus erythematosus.

Labial salivary gland biopsy is an important investigation to be carried out when SS is suspected in a patient. A small incision is made towards the lateral side of the lower lip to harvest the minor salivary glands (◘ Fig. 57.7) under local anesthesia. About 2–3 minor salivary glands are harvested and the incision wound is sutured with a resorbable suture to achieve hemostasis. The patient may have discomfort or pain in the biopsied area, which is relieved by analgesics. The harvested minor salivary gland tissues are sent for histopathological examination. The hematoxylin and eosin-stained (H&E) minor salivary gland tissues show periductal lymphocytic clusters (>50 lymphocytes) adjacent to normal minor salivary gland acini which is referred to as focal lymphocytic sialadenitis. The focus score is measured by counting the number of lymphocytic aggregates per 4 mm^2. If the focus score is ≥ 1, then it is considered that the patient has SS. Acinar destruction can also be seen in some areas of the minor salivary gland.

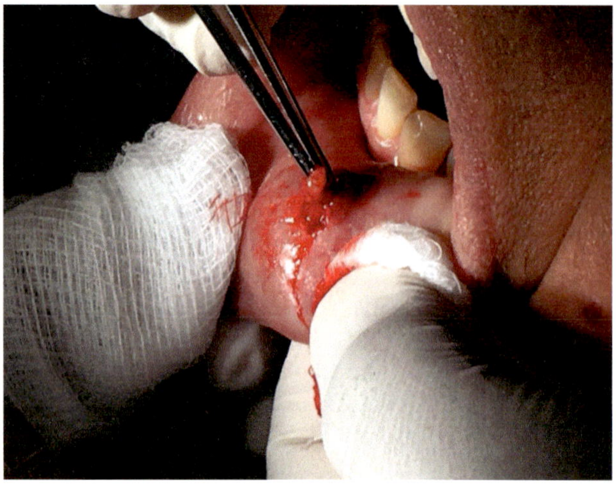

Fig. 57.7 Photograph showing the harvesting of the minor salivary gland from lower lip (Courtesy: Dr. Nadia Najwa Shuhairi)

57

SS manifests with various dental and medical problems. Therefore, it needs a multidisciplinary management approach by a team consisting of a general dentist, an oral medicine specialist, an ophthalmologist, and a rheumatologist. Other medical and dental specialists may be involved depending on the various clinical manifestations that may require their services to manage these patients.

The general dentist is mainly concerned about the oral hygiene status of these patients which is the result of the severity of dry mouth. Patients with mild xerostomia may only require proper oral hygiene education and instructions. These patients should be given oral hygiene instructions such as advise to brush their teeth 2–3 times/day after meals using soft tooth brush and tooth paste without abrasives (whitening tooth paste) and sodium lauryl sulfate (detergent). They should be advised to floss at least once daily and avoid alcohol-based mouth washes. Neutral sodium fluoride (0.05%) mouth rinse at bed time or 1.1% neutral sodium fluoride toothpaste or gel can be prescribed. Non-fluoride remineralizing agents such as amorphous calcium phosphate (ACP), casein phosphopeptide-ACP, calcium sodium phosphosilicate, and tricalcium phosphate can also be used as adjunct therapeutic agents. Patient should be advised to avoid taking sugar containing drinks or foods in order to prevent further development of dental caries and worsening of the oral hygiene. They may be advised to use sweeteners such as xylitol. They should avoid carbonated drinks, acidic drinks, acidic food, spicy food, and alcohol. Non-surgical prophylactic treatment such as scaling and polishing of the teeth should be done and the gingival and periodontal status should be monitored every 6 months.

However, in patients with moderate to severe xerostomia apart from the above-mentioned oral hygiene education and instructions, management of dental caries and periodontal disease may be required. These might range from simple to complex restorations for dental caries and from non-surgical prophylactic treatment to complex periodontal management. Teeth affected by root or cervical caries that cannot be restored should be extracted. All dental caries should be identified early and appropriate restorative treatment should be initiated as required. Cervical caries can be restored with tooth-coloured filling material such as fluoride-releasing glass-ionomer cements. Prosthetic replacement of extracted tooth should be carried out.

Patients with dry mouth should be referred to an oral medicine specialist. Management of dry mouth may vary depending on its severity. They may be advised to take frequent sips of water or sucking on finely crushed ice and keep hydrated. Chewing gum or lozenges with xylitol or artificial saliva or salivary substitutes can be prescribed. Anticholinergic sialogogues such as pilocarpine and cevimeline can be prescribed for better patient comfort and helps in chewing, swallowing, eating, and speaking. Patients with TMJ problems and tenderness of the muscles of mastication should also be referred to oral medicine specialist. Depending on TMJ involvement or the muscles of mastication or both the management of these patients varies. Usually, conservative management should be started advising the patient not to eat hard, chewy food, and to cut their food into small pieces and eat. The patient should be advised to avoid any activity that would require opening their mouth wide. Warm or cold compression can be applied on the areas where pain is present due to the TMJ pain or myalgia. Analgesics may be given to relieve the pain. However, if the patient has pain in other joints, the patient should be referred to a rheumatologist for management. The rheumatologist may prescribe non-steroidal anti-inflammatory drugs (NSAIDs) or a short course of oral steroids such as prednisolone, for flare ups and ongoing inflammation of the joints, like painful swelling of the joints. Immunosuppressants that are used for cases of persistent inflammatory arthritis such as hydroxychloroquine or methotrexate are given to prevent flare-up of joint disease. These medications may act on the TMJ and the muscles of mastication to relieve pain. Therefore, the oral medicine specialist and rheumatologist may need to work closely with regards to the management of joint problems in SS patients. Patients should be referred to an ophthalmologist for their dry eyes and other medical specialists as SS may affect extraglandular tissues. As oral hygiene needs to be maintained in SS patients, they should be reviewed every 4 months for dental caries and periodontal status by the general dental practitioners.

Salient features of SS	
Clinical features	Primary SS: Xerostomia (dry mouth) and keratoconjunctivitis sicca (dry eyes). Secondary SS: Xerostomia (dry mouth) and keratoconjunctivitis sicca (dry eyes) with other systemic autoimmune or connective tissue disease such as rheumatoid arthritis (RA), scleroderma or systemic lupus erythematosus (SLE).
Radiographic features	Sialography: Snowstorm appearance or cherry blossom appearance.
Histopathological features	Minor salivary gland tissues show periductal lymphocytic clusters (>50 lymphocytes) adjacent to normal minor salivary gland acini which is referred to as focal lymphocytic sialadenitis. The focus score is measured by counting the number of lymphocytic aggregates per 4 mm^2. If the focus score is ≥1 then it is considered that the patient has SS. Acinar destruction can also be seen in some areas of the minor salivary gland.
Criteria for diagnosis	1. Anti-SSA/Ro antibody positivity = 3. 2. Focal lymphocytic sialadenitis with a focus score of ≥1 foci/4 mm^2 = 3. 3. Abnormal ocular staining score of ≥5 (or van Bijsterveld score of ≥4) = 1. 4. Schirmer test result of ≤5 mm/5 min = 1. 5. Unstimulated salivary flow rate of ≤0.1 mL/min = 1. Individuals with signs and/or symptoms suggestive of SS with a total score of ≥4 for the above items meet the criteria for primary SS.
Treatment	Oral hygiene education and instructions. Extraction of teeth that cannot be restored. Non-surgical prophylactic treatment. Cervical caries restored with fluoride-releasing glass-ionomer cements. Prosthetic replacement of extracted tooth. Referral to oral medicine specialist for management of dry mouth and TMJ pain and/or myalgia of muscles of mastication. Referral to ophthalmologist for management of dry eyes. Referral to rheumatologist for management of joint pain.

Self-Assessment Questions

1. State the difference between primary and secondary SS.
2. List the investigations required to diagnose SS.
3. State the diagnostic criteria for primary SS.
4. Describe the histopathological features seen in the lip biopsy of the minor salivary gland in patients with SS.
5. Discuss the management plan for SS.

57

- **Diagnostic Algorithm**

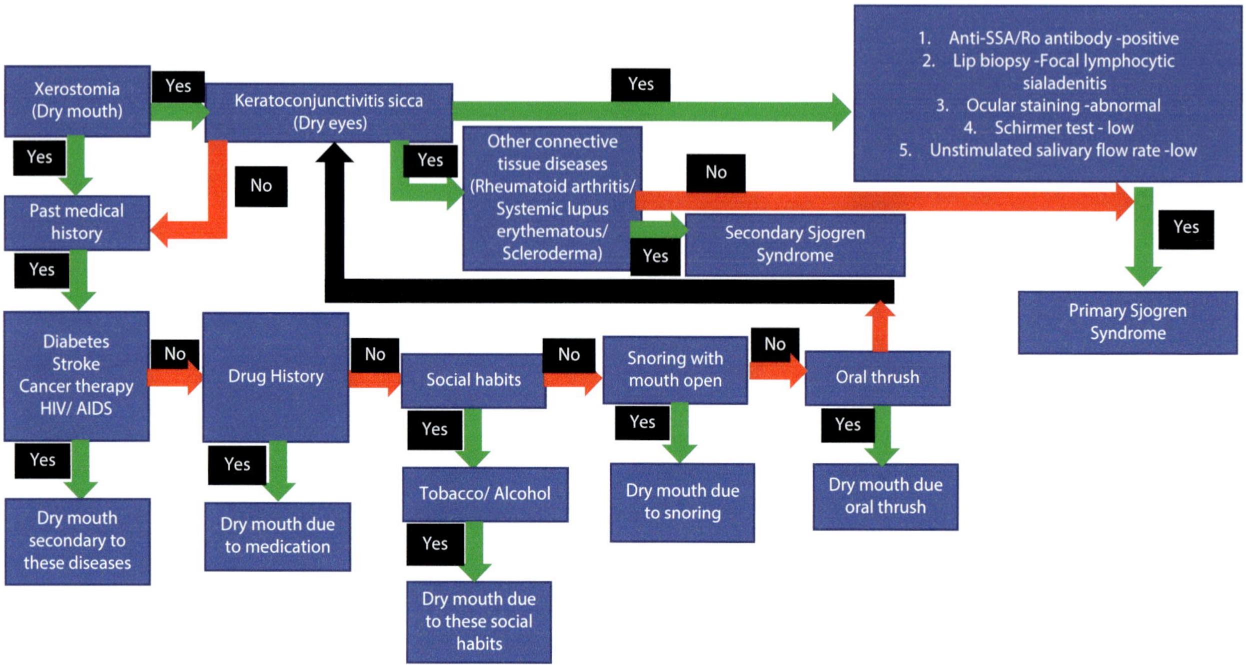

Summary

The clinical feature of primary SS is xerostomia (dry mouth) and keratoconjunctivitis sicca (dry eyes), whereas those of secondary SS are dry mouth and dry eyes with other systemic autoimmune or connective tissue disease. Sialography shows snowstorm appearance or cherry blossom appearance. The diagnostic criteria used is the 2016 American College of Rheumatology/European League Against Rheumatism classification criteria for Primary SS with labial biopsy playing an important role. Histopathology of minor salivary gland tissues shows periductal lymphocytic clusters (>50 lymphocytes) adjacent to normal minor salivary gland acini which is referred to as focal lymphocytic sialadenitis. The focus score is measured by counting the number of lymphocytic aggregates per 4 mm^2. If the focus score is ≥ 1 then it is considered that the patient has SS. Treatment of these patients involves oral hygiene education and instructions, extraction of teeth that cannot be restored, non-surgical prophylactic treatment, restoration of cervical caries with fluoride-releasing glass-ionomer cements and prosthetic replacement of extracted tooth by general dental practitioners. Effective management of patients with SS requires referral to oral medicine specialist for management of dry mouth and TMJ pain and/or myalgia of muscles of mastication as well as, referrals to ophthalmologist and rheumatologist for management of dry eyes to joint pain, respectively.

Suggested Reading

Cha S. Sjögren's syndrome and oral health disease characteristics and management of oral manifestations. 1st ed. Cham: Springer; 2021.

Glick M, Greenberg MS, Lockhart PB, Challacombe SJ. Burket's oral medicine. 13th ed. Wiley-Blackwell; 2021.

Sivapathasundharam B. Shafer's textbook of oral pathology. 9th ed. Elsevier Health Sciences; 2020.

Warnakulasuriya S, Tilakaratne WM. Oral medicine & pathology. A guide to diagnosis and management. 1st ed. Jaypee; 2014.

Swelling over the Right Cheek: Pleomorphic Adenoma

Zuraiza Mohamad Zaini and Nur Fauziani Zainul Abidin

Contents

W. M Tilakaratne, T. G. Kallarakkal (eds.), *Clinicopathological Correlation of Oral Diseases*,
https://doi.org/10.1007/978-3-031-24408-7_58

Learning Goals

1. Devise the correct way of compiling the history with appropriate questions.
2. Develop a differential diagnosis after history taking.
3. Deduce appropriate procedures in clinical examination.
4. Formulate a differential diagnosis combining findings in the history and clinical examination.
5. Justify the relevant investigations required to arrive at the diagnosis.
6. Comprehend the importance of clinicopathological correlation in arriving at the correct diagnosis.
7. Outline the management plan.
8. Recognize the importance of a diagnostic algorithm in arriving at a diagnosis.

58.1 Main Complaint

A 44-year-old man complains of swelling over his right cheek since 3 years.

58.2 History of Complaint

Question: How and when did you notice the swelling?

The swelling started as a small lump 3 years ago. It has been slowly growing until it reached present size.

58.3 Additional Information

Question: Is there any pain associated with the swelling or pain when you move your jaw to eat and talk?

The swelling does not cause pain, and I have no pain during eating or talking.

Question: Have you noticed any variation in the size of the swelling? Is the lesion persistent or appear in an episodic manner?

The swelling is persistent. It does not vary in size.

Question: Did you notice any redness on the skin overlying the swelling?

I have not noticed any redness on the skin overlying the swelling.

Question: Does your mouth feel dry? Do you need to frequently sip water especially while eating due to dryness since the onset of the swelling?

I did notice slight dryness but not to the extent that I need frequent sips of water during eating. I do not feel any discomfort while eating.

Question: Do you have any discharge from the inner side of the right cheek?

I did not notice any discharge inside the mouth.

Question: Did you seek any medical advice or treatment for this problem before?

I did not seek any medical advice or treatment as the swelling is painless and did not affect my daily activities and functions.

Question: Are you on follow-up or taking medications for any medical problems that you are having?

I have hypertension which was diagnosed 8 years ago and I am currently on perindopril 8 mg and amlodipine 10 mg. I was recently prescribed atorvastatin 10 mg for dyslipidaemia.

Question: Do you experience any weight loss or loss of appetite?

My body weight has been between 65 and 72 kg since the last 20 years. I have not noticed any significant weight loss recently. My appetite is normal.

Question: Do you smoke, drink alcohol or chew betel/areca nut?

I am not a smoker and drink alcohol occasionally, mainly during social functions. I do not chew betel/areca nuts.

Question: Do you have any difficulty in breathing or have been coughing before or after the swelling appeared?

I have no difficulty breathing. I have not had any episodes of coughing after the swelling appeared.

Question: Did you notice any sudden increase in size of the swelling?

I have never noticed any sudden increase in the size of the swelling. It has been growing slowly over the years.

58.4 With the Findings from the History, What is Your Differential Diagnosis?

1. Benign salivary gland neoplasms such as Pleomorphic adenoma or Warthin tumour.
2. Non-neoplastic salivary gland diseases such as sialadenitis.
3. Immune-mediated syndromes such as Sjogren syndrome or sarcoidosis.

58.5 How Do You Justify Your Differential Diagnosis After History Taking?

1. The absence of symptoms and progressive growth since the onset 3 years ago suggests a tumour of benign nature. Benign salivary gland neoplasms typically present as an asymptomatic, slow growing mass. A vast majority of salivary gland tumours occur in the parotid gland. Pleomorphic adenoma is the most common salivary gland neoplasm. About 80% of benign salivary gland neoplasms occurring in the parotid gland are pleomorphic adenomas followed by Warthin tumour. However, there are several malignant salivary gland neoplasms with an indolent clinical behaviour that has predilection for parotid gland, one of which is acinic cell carcinoma. Apart from benign neoplasms, few non-neoplastic lesions almost exclusively occur within the parotid gland. These include nodular oncocytic hyperplasia.
2. Sialadenitis is the most common non-neoplastic cause of parotid gland swelling. Sialadenitis is the inflammation of the gland, which is caused by stasis of salivary secretions that leads to retrograde seeding of bacteria from the oral cavity. Acute sialadenitis is usually due to bacterial or viral infections and usually presents with rapid onset, pain and swelling. Fever may be present. Chronic sialadenitis manifests as a recurrent or persistent swelling of the salivary gland without erythema of the overlying skin and is usually due to obstruction from calculus, strictures, scarring, foreign bodies or extrinsic compression by a tumour. Physical examination to confirm the diagnosis should include visual inspection of glands to observe erythema of overlying skin, palpation of the gland to note for tenderness, massaging of the gland to express salivary discharge from the duct orifice and identify if there is suppurative discharge.
3. Immune-mediated parotid swellings such as sarcoidosis and Sjogren syndrome need to be considered in this case as it is the common cause of chronic parotid gland swelling. The definitive diagnosis is cumulatively based on the patient's medical history, clinical examination, and presence of key diagnostic features of a particular syndrome. Sarcoidosis is characterized by non-caseating granulomas involving multiple organs, particularly lung, lymph nodes, skin, and glands. Patients with sarcoidosis often present with unexplained cough, shortness of breath and constitutional symptoms that are absent in this case. Sjogren syndrome is an autoimmune chronic inflammatory disorder characterized by dry mouth and dry eyes. The patient did not complain about these symptoms during history taking.

58.6 Findings of Examination

Extraorally, there is a firm swelling over the right preauricular region extending to the angle of the mandible measuring about 3 × 2 cm (◘ Fig. 58.1). The overlying

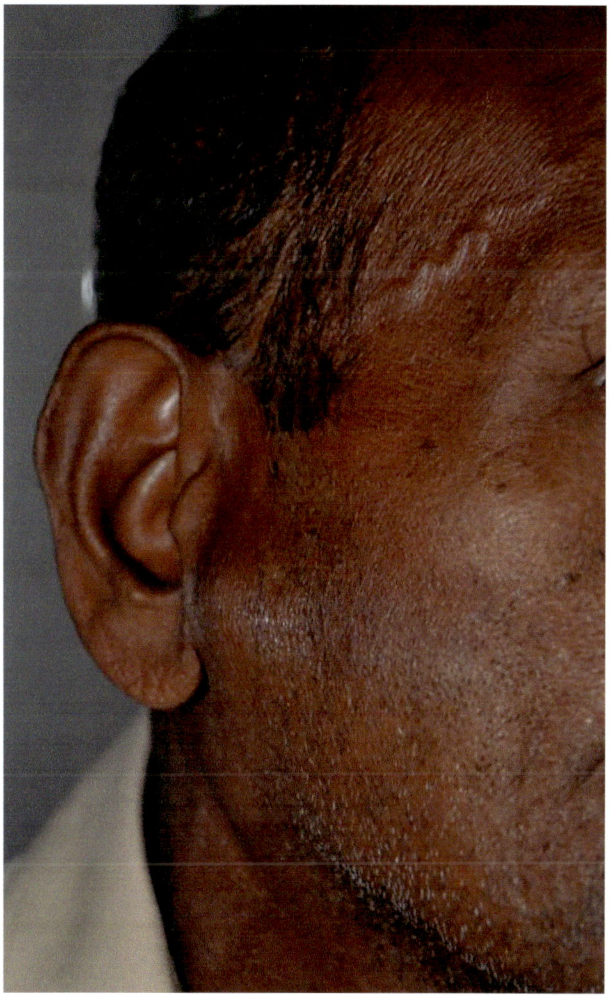

◘ **Fig. 58.1** A swelling over right preauricular region extending to the angle of mandible measuring about 3 × 2 cm (Courtesy Dr. Nadeena Jayasuriya)

skin is normal in colour with no signs of inflammation. The swelling is well demarcated, firm in consistency, mobile and non-tender to palpation. He has no lymphadenopathy and his mouth opening is not restricted, with a maximum mouth opening of 41 mm. He is partially dentate and wearing an acrylic partial denture. There is no mucosal lesion or swelling on the corresponding mucosal site intra-orally. All remaining teeth are free from caries. His mucosa is moist with salivary pooling in the floor of mouth. There is also no obstruction within the right Stensen duct as saliva flow from the right parotid gland is observed upon milking the right parotid gland area around the swelling. Facial and trigeminal nerve examination revealed intact nerve function with no paralysis or paraesthesia.

58.7 What is Your Provisional Clinical Diagnosis?

Benign salivary gland neoplasm (most likely a pleomorphic adenoma or Warthin tumour).

58.8 What is the Justification for Your Provisional Clinical Diagnosis?

Clinically the swelling presents as a painless, slow growing, single mobile and nodular firm mass that is not associated with pain, discharge, and change in skin colour or impeding jaw movement. In addition, he does not have facial nerve palsy which is a feature of possible malignancy involving the parotid gland. The patient also does not have systemic symptoms that would suggest parotid gland swelling due to sarcoidosis or Sjogren syndrome. Furthermore, the salivary gland swelling in those diseases would be more diffuse rather than a well demarcated, nodular mass. Thus, it is likely to be a benign tumour arising from the parotid gland. The most common benign tumour involving the parotid gland is a pleomorphic adenoma. Warthin tumour is the second most common benign salivary gland neoplasm in the parotid gland and occurs predominantly in men. Although these two tumours are the most likely differential diagnoses, the possibility of other rare benign salivary gland tumours cannot be excluded.

58.9 How Would You Investigate This Patient?

1. Ultrasound to assess presence of duct obstruction or inflammation.
2. Computed tomography (CT) scan to detect small calculi that may not be seen on ultrasound, duct dilatation, acute or chronic sialadenitis or cellulitis.
3. Magnetic Resonance Imaging (MRI) to further assess tumour mass whether solid or cystic and presence of malignant features such as extracapsular spread and nerve involvement.
4. Ultrasound guided Fine Needle Aspiration Cytology (FNAC) provides preoperative diagnosis of mass as a primary salivary gland neoplasm.

Patient was sent for radiographic examinations with the findings given in the table below.

Investigations	Findings
1. Ultrasound	A well-defined hypoechoic lesion in the superficial lobe of right parotid gland. There is no calcification or cystic changes in the lesion.
2. CT scan	Right parotid gland with sharply marginated homogenous round mass, hyperdense to the surrounding tissue with no necrosis, calcification or infiltration of the adjacent structure.
3. MRI	MRI through the right parotid demonstrates a sharply circumscribed solid mass in the superficial aspect of the gland. The lesion is isotense to the muscle on T1 and markedly hypertense on T2, reflecting the myxoid component of the tumour. A rim of decreased signal intensity in the T2 weighted image represents the surrounding capsule.

Ultrasound guided FNAC was performed for this patient and the cytological features are as follows.

The smear shows a unique fibrillary stroma consisting of a mixture of myoepithelial cells, ductal cells and extracellular matrix. The cells do not show cytological atypia. Myoepithelial cells are usually the predominant cell type with a variable cytomorphology, including round, polygonal, plasmacytoid and spindle cells (◘ Fig. 58.2). The extracellular matrix shows characteristic feathery/fibrillary borders and bright magenta colour on Giemsa stain and grey-green colour on Papanicolaou stain.

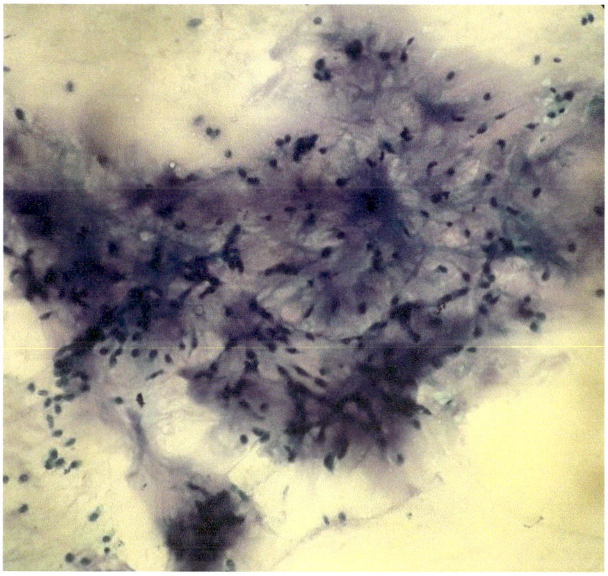

◘ **Fig. 58.2** The smear stained with Papanicolaou stain shows fibrillary stroma consisting of a mixture of myoepithelial cells, ductal cells and extracellular matrix

58.10 What is the Most Likely Diagnosis Based on Cytological Findings?

Pleomorphic adenoma

58.11 How Would You Manage This Patient?

Wide excision of lesion via superficial parotidectomy under general anaesthesia.

58.12 The Specimen was sent for Histopathological Examination. What are the Features That Confirm the Diagnosis?

Histopathology revealed an encapsulated salivary gland tumour (◘ Fig. 58.3a) composed of epithelial and myoepithelial cells arranged in sheets, cords and occasional bilayered ductal structures containing eosinophilic material within the lumen (◘ Fig. 58.3b, c). The myoepithelial cells are predominantly epithelioid, and some are spindle and stellate in shape. Plasmacytoid cells are scarce. The stroma is fibro-myxoid and shows chondroid changes in areas (◘ Fig. 58.3d). Surrounding salivary acini lobules, adipocytes and ductal ectasia are also evident.

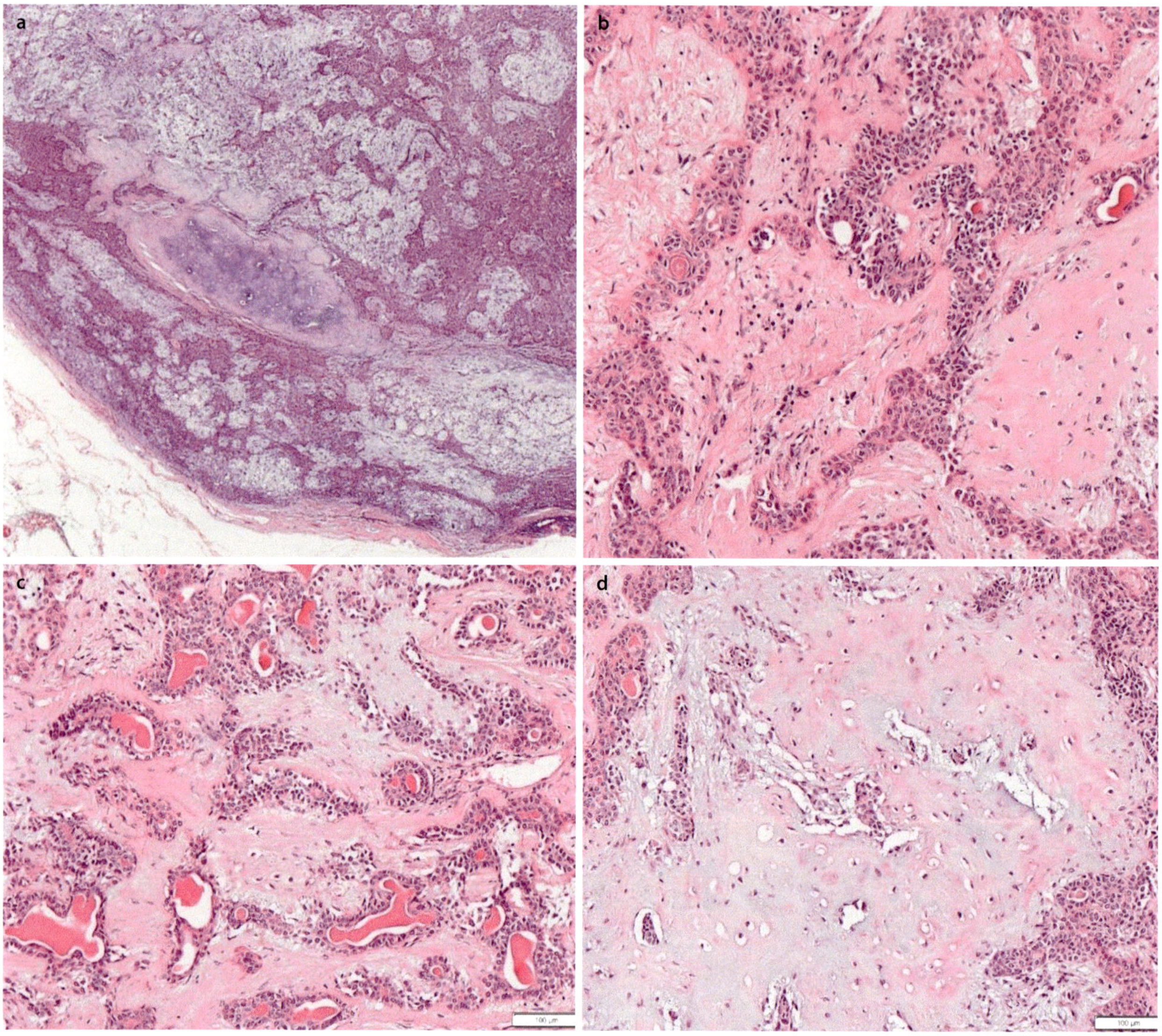

Fig. 58.3 Encapsulated tumour **a** with epithelial and myoepithelial cells arranged in sheets, cords **b** and occasional bilayered ductal structures containing eosinophilic material within the lumen **c**. The stroma shows chondroid changes in areas **d**

58.13 What is Your Definitive Diagnosis Based on the Histopathological Findings?

Pleomorphic adenoma

58.14 Pleomorphic Adenoma

Pleomorphic adenoma (PA), also known as benign mixed tumour, is a tumour with both epithelial and myoepithelial cell proliferation in a myxochondroid stroma. It is the most common salivary gland neoplasm in children and adults, accounting for more than 60% of all salivary gland neoplasms. It comprises about 75% of major salivary gland neoplasm with parotid being the most common affected gland and approximately 40% of minor salivary gland neoplasms. PA can occur in patients of any age but most common in the third and sixth decade of life. The female to male ratio is 2:1. Being a benign neoplasm, PA presents clinically as a slow growing, painless mass. PA can grow to an enormous size if left untreated. Paraesthesia due to facial nerve compression may be associated with tumour of a significant size as well as in PA with malignant transformation.

Macroscopically, PA is well circumscribed with light tan to grey cut surface. Recurrent PA is generally multinodular, and areas of haemorrhage or infarction can be present in cases with prior fine needle aspiration. The key histopathologic features of PA are its diverse cytomorphological and architectural patterns. It is usually well circumscribed but in minor glands or those that are rich in stroma, the encapsulation may be absent. In such lesions, direct interface between the tumour and adjacent normal glands or connective tissue is seen. Its bosselated periphery may resemble tumour invasion into and beyond the capsule hence be mistaken as a malignant lesion. The myoepithelial component of PA often predominates the lesion, presenting with a wide range of cytomorphology including plasmacytoid, spindled, basaloid and stellate cells. These myoepithelial cells can be abluminal, individual and scattered, or in nests, solid sheets or trabeculae. The epithelial cells in PA form variably sized ductal or cystic structures or are arranged in sheets or strands. The ductal structure in PA is typically bilayered with luminal, cuboidal to low-columnar epithelial cells and abluminal spindled or stellate cells that typically stream or 'melt-away' into the adjacent stroma. The stromal element of PA is characteristic and can range from loose myxoid to dense and hyalinized collagen. Chondromyxoid change is common while foci of osteoid, chondroid and adipose-like changes can be present. PA with frequent mitosis and mild to moderate pleomorphism may be regarded as atypical but if definite malignant features that include marked nuclear pleomorphism, tumour necrosis and atypical mitosis are seen, diagnosis of carcinoma ex pleomorphic adenoma is favoured. When the malignant cytological features are confined within the tumour, or in the absence of capsular invasion, the diagnosis of intra-capsular carcinoma ex PA is given.

PA mimics a handful of both benign and malignant salivary gland neoplasms due to its diverse histopathologic features, thus, the diagnosis of PA is difficult in a small biopsy. The diagnosis of myoepithelioma should be considered when a neoplasm contains predominantly myoepithelial cells and the ductal component is absent. PA in minor salivary glands can be misdiagnosed as polymorphous adenocarcinoma (PAC) as both present with poor tumour circumscription, pale myxoid background stroma and numerous growth patterns. The latter, however, is a tumour of single cell population, consisting of uniform oval cells. Bi-layered ductal structures with clear outer cells may resemble epithelial–myoepithelial carcinoma (EMC) but the stromal elements as seen in PA are absent in EMC. In addition, capsule may not be complete in a majority of minor salivary gland PA.

The diverse morphologic features seen in histologic sections are reflected in cytological preparations of PA. In most cases, presence of bland epithelial cells with mucoid to myxoid stroma, that appears fibrillar and bright magenta in Diff-Quik stain, mixed with spindled and plasmacytoid cells is diagnostic.

More than 70% of PA is characterized by recurrent chromosomal rearrangements of the Pleomorphic adenoma gene 1 (PLAG1) and High mobility group AT-hook 2 (HMGA2) genes. This genetic feature is retained in carcinoma ex PA. Immunohistochemistry carries little diagnostic value in PA as the diagnosis is established mainly on its morphologic features. However, in small biopsies, nuclear positivity for PLAG1 and cytoplasmic expression of glial fibrillary acid protein (GFAP) by the tumour cells is useful, as in the context of its mimics, these staining patterns are almost specific for PA. Cytokeratin is strongly positive in the epithelial component in PA but variably positive or weakly positive in the myoepithelial cells. The myoepithelial cells of variable morphology will stain for cytokeratin 14, α-smooth muscle actin (α-SMA) or calponin.

Complete tumour resection is curative and decreases the risk for recurrence. Incomplete tumour excision, tumour rupture and spillage due to lack of encapsulation increase the risk for tumour recurrence. Tumours with predominant myxoid stroma (Fig. 58.4) may lead to higher recurrence as myxoid material can spill into surrounding tissue during surgery. Reports showed that 26.9% of ruptured tumours and 80% of cases with spill-

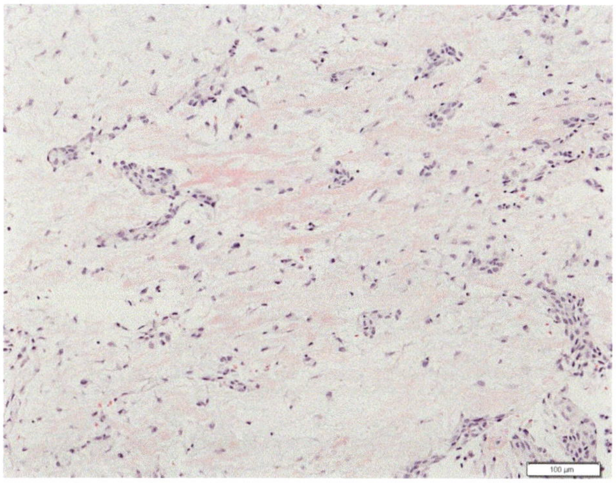

Fig. 58.4 Pleomorphic adenoma with predominant myxoid stroma

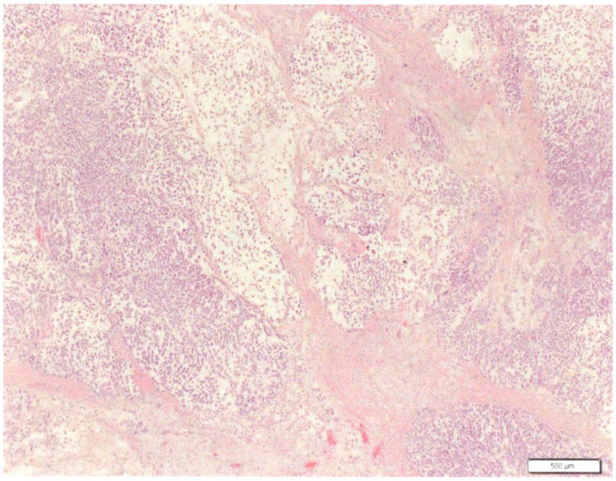

Fig. 58.5 The cellular and mesenchymal components of recurrent pleomorphic adenoma present in multiple nodules

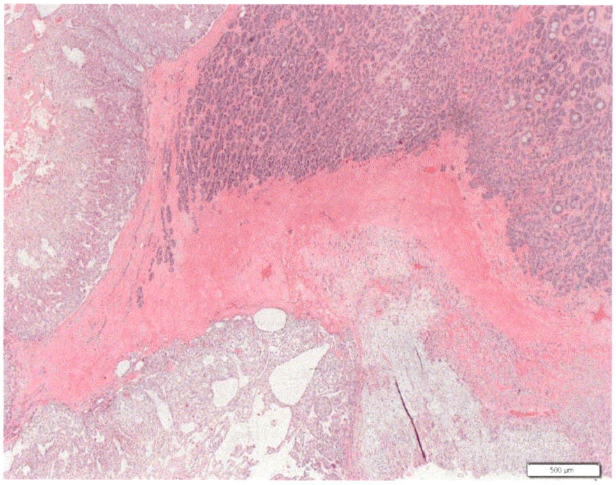

Fig. 58.6 Carcinoma ex pleomorphic adenoma with the malignant component consisting of adenoid cystic carcinoma (upper right) and clear cell predominant myoepithelial carcinoma (upper left). An area with epithelial and myoepithelial cells within myxoid stroma shows the evidence of existing PA (bottom)

age recurred. Recurrent PAs are often multinodular, comprising numerous individual and coalescing islands of varying sizes and shaped with smooth outlines (Fig. 58.5). Recurrent tumour is associated with increased risk of postoperative facial nerve paralysis and malignant transformation. Progression to carcinoma, known as carcinoma ex pleomorphic adenoma (ca ex PA), occurs in about 6% of PAs and on average, 12% of ca ex PAs develop in the setting of recurrent PA. The risk factors for malignant transformation include untreated long-standing tumour, multiple recurrences, old age, male gender, tumour in the deep parotid lobe and large tumours. Observation of rapid enlargement of the mass or pain can help to early diagnosis. The histopathological features of Ca ex PA include both benign and malignant components. The latter can be of any type of salivary gland carcinoma and may be extensive (Fig. 58.6).

Self-Assessment Questions

1. List the clinical features of pleomorphic adenoma (PA).
2. Describe the histopathological features of PA.
3. Describe the cytopathological features of PA.
4. List the common salivary gland diseases affecting the parotid gland
5. Outline the management of PA.
6. State the risks of incomplete resection of PA.

Suggested Reading

Andreasen S, Therkildsen MH, Bjørndal K, Homøe P. Pleomorphic adenoma of the parotid gland 1985–2010: a Danish nationwide study of incidence, recurrence rate, and malignant transformation. Head Neck. 2016;38(Suppl 1):E1364–9. https://doi.org/10.1002/hed.24228.

El-Naggar AK, Chan JKC, Grandis JR, Takata T, Slootweg PJ. WHO classification of head and neck tumours, vol. 9. 4th ed. IARC Publications.

Hernandez-Prera JC, Skálová A, Franchi A, et al. Pleomorphic adenoma: the great mimicker of malignancy. Histopathology. 2021;79(3):279–90. https://doi.org/10.1111/his.14322.

Khurram SA, Barrett AW, Speight PM. Diagnostic difficulties in lesions of the minor salivary glands. Diagn Histopathol. 2017;23(6):250–9. ISSN 1756-2317

Lewis AG, Tong T, Maghami E. Diagnosis and management of malignant salivary gland tumors of the parotid gland. Otolaryngol Clin N Am. 2016;49(2):343–80.

Thompson LDR, Bishop JA. Head and neck pathology, Foundation in diagnostic pathology. 3rd ed. Elsevier.

Thompson LDR, Wenig BM. Diagnostic pathology: head and neck. 2nd ed. Elsevier.

Swelling in the Floor of the Mouth: Adenoid Cystic Carcinoma

Kathreena Kadir, Yet Ching Goh, and Chuey Chuan Tan

Contents

W. M Tilakaratne, T. G. Kallarakkal (eds.), *Clinicopathological Correlation of Oral Diseases*,
https://doi.org/10.1007/978-3-031-24408-7_59

Learning Goals

1. Devise the correct way of compiling the history with appropriate questions.
2. Develop a differential diagnosis after history taking.
3. Deduce appropriate procedures in clinical examination.
4. Formulate a differential diagnosis combining findings in the history and clinical examination.
5. Justify the relevant investigations required to arrive at the diagnosis.
6. Comprehend the importance of clinicopathological correlation in arriving at the correct diagnosis.
7. Outline the management plan.
8. Recognize the importance of a diagnostic algorithm in arriving at a diagnosis.

59.1 Main Complaint

A 42-year-old gentleman presented to the Oral and Maxillofacial Surgery (OMFS) clinic with a swelling in the floor of the mouth.

59.2 History of Complaint

Question: How long have you been noticing the swelling?

I have been noticing the swelling since 4 months and it has been slowly increasing in size.

Question: Is this the first time you have experienced a swelling in this region?

I have not experienced any swelling in this region previously.

59.3 Additional Complaints

Question: Do you experience any other symptoms besides the swelling?

I experience intermittent pain which radiates along the left lower jaw region. My tongue has become more sensitive on the left side to hot and cold since the swelling was noticed.

Question: Is the pain felt during eating?

The pain is spontaneous and is not associated with eating.

Question: Does the swelling increase in size during meal time?

There is no significant change in the size of the swelling during mealtime.

Question: Did it change your meal habits? Have you been losing weight?

I have a normal appetite and I have been eating well. I have not lost weight.

Question: Do you recall any foul-smelling discharge coming from the swelling site?

I cannot recall any discharge in relation to the swelling.

Question: Did you notice any lumps elsewhere on other parts of your body?

I think there is a lump growing in my neck just beneath the jaw.

59.4 Past Medical/Dental and Social History

Question: Are you suffering from any other medical problems like heart disease, high blood pressure, diabetes, bleeding disorder, or respiratory diseases? If yes, what kind of medications have you been taking until now?

I have hypertension and has been taking amlodipine 10 mg for the past 10 years. I am under regular follow up with the physician and my blood pressure is well controlled with medication.

Question: Have you undergone any dental treatment?

I have undergone scaling, several restorations and extraction previously. I did not have any post-treatment complications. My last dental visit was 6 months ago for a restoration of my front tooth.

Question: Are you married and having children? What do you do for a living?

I am not married and currently staying alone. I work as an executive in an advertising company.

Question: Are you a smoker?

I smoke about ten cigarettes daily.

Question: Do you take alcohol?

I drink alcohol occasionally during social functions.

59.5 With the Findings from the History, What Is Your Differential Diagnosis?

1. Malignant salivary gland tumour or any other malignant soft tissue tumour.
2. Benign salivary gland tumour or any other benign soft tissue tumour.
3. Cystic lesion, such as dermoid/epidermoid cyst.

59.6 How Do You Justify Your Differential Diagnosis After History Taking?

Floor of the mouth is anatomically close to submandibular and sublingual salivary glands. There could be neoplastic changes involving either gland. A salivary gland neoplasm could be either benign or malignant. However, the occurrence of it being malignant is higher when involving the submandibular and sublingual gland or minor salivary glands in the floor of the mouth compared to the parotid gland. In this case, the tendency for the lump being a malignant tumour is supported by the patient's history of having intermittent pain over the same side of his jaw and altered sensation on the tongue. In addition, a history of short duration may also suggest it to be a malignancy. He also mentioned having another lump on his neck suggesting a possible metastatic deposit. Furthermore, he does have risk habits commonly associated with malignancy such as the use of tobacco and alcohol consumption. Therefore, the findings of the history are more in favour of a malignant lesion. Although, dermoid and epidermoid cysts occur usually at this site, other associated features such as intermittent pain, short duration, and paraesthesia do not support them to be the possible diagnosis. Benign tumours of soft tissue origin, such as lipoma, neurilemmoma, or leiomyoma, may occur in the floor of the mouth but may be an unlikely diagnosis in this case due to the presence of obvious clinical features suggestive of malignancy.

59

59.7 Findings of Clinical Examination

There is an indurated nodular growth measuring 2 × 1 cm in the anterior aspect of the floor of the mouth towards the left side (Fig. 59.1). Upon palpation, the growth appears fixed to the underlying structures. The overlying mucosa is normal in colour. There is no apparent saliva discharging from the left Warthon duct.

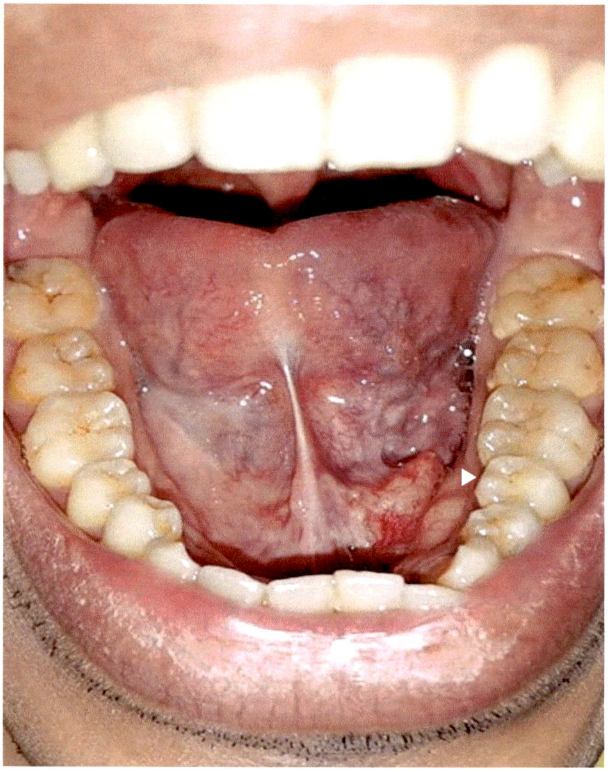

Fig. 59.1 A nodular growth with prominent telangiectasia is seen in the anterior aspect of the floor of the mouth

59.8 What Other Relevant Features Are Evident?

A solitary left submandibular lymph node is enlarged. The node is firm and tender on palpation. A solitary submental lymph node is also enlarged and tender on palpation. The nodes are not fixed to the underlying tissues or overlying mucosa. Clinical examination reveals paraesthesia of the left side of the tongue. There is no limitation of tongue movements.

59.9 What Is Your Clinical Differential Diagnosis?

1. Malignant tumour highly suggestive of salivary gland origin.
2. Any other soft tissue malignancy.

59.10 How Would You Exclude Other Conditions and Justify the Inclusion of the Disease That You Have Mentioned in the Differential Diagnosis to Arrive at a Working Diagnosis?

In this particular case, the suspicion of a malignant tumour is very high due to the obvious clinical findings such as the appearance of an indurated nodular growth in the floor of the mouth. Furthermore, the patient's claim that his left tongue had altered sensation since the swelling was noticed, is a strong indication of neural involvement. Hence, any benign lesion or tumour in the floor of the mouth can be excluded from the clinical differential diagnosis. In addition, majority of salivary tumours in the sublingual area are malignant. Absence of ulceration and an intact normal mucosa close to the appearance of the normal mucosa would enable us to rule out a clinical diagnosis of squamous cell carcinoma as this tumour commonly appears as an indurated ulcer with rolled border or a cauliflower-like growth when present in the floor of the mouth.

59.11 What Is the Most Likely Diagnosis?

Malignant salivary gland tumour (Mucoepidermoid carcinoma, Adenoid cystic carcinoma or Polymorphous adenocarcinoma is most likely as they are the most common intra oral salivary gland malignancies). However, the possibility of other salivary gland malignancies and soft tissue tumours cannot be excluded completely.

59.11.1 Mucoepidermoid Carcinoma

Mucoepidermoid carcinoma (MEC) is the most common malignancy arising from minor salivary glands. It occurs mostly in the third to fifth decade of life with a slight female predilection. The possible risk factors include exposure to radiation and chemotherapy in childhood. The clinical presentation of MEC is highly variable depending on the tumour site and size. It may present as slow growing lesion associated with pain, trismus, and dysphagia depending on the site. It can also present as a bluish and fluctuant cyst-like growth resembling a mucocele or a vascular lesion. Occasionally, it invades the underlying bone causing bone resorption.

59.11.2 Adenoid Cystic Carcinoma

Adenoid cystic carcinoma is an aggressive malignant salivary gland tumour which accounts for less than 10% of all salivary gland tumours. It commonly affects middle-aged adults without gender and ethnic predilection. Adenoid cystic carcinoma occurs in the minor salivary glands, major salivary glands, and in glands of upper aerodigestive tract. It presents clinically as a firm lump and is associated with paraesthesia, pain, or sometimes ulceration. Therefore, adenoid cystic carcinoma should be considered very highly in the working diagnosis.

59.11.3 Polymorphous Adenocarcinoma

Polymorphous adenocarcinoma (PAC) is a common minor salivary gland tumour which mostly occurs on the palate, buccal mucosa and upper lip although it can occur anywhere in the oral cavity. PAC can occur over a wide age range from the third to seventh decades of life with a female predilection. It is a slow growing but locally invasive tumour. Its clinical characteristics are similar to other benign and malignant salivary gland tumours making it difficult to diagnose clinically.

59.12 How Would You Investigate This Patient?

- Fine needle aspiration biopsy (FNAB)
- Incisional biopsy for histopathological examination (HPE)
- Radiographic investigations

59.13 How Would You Perform FNAB and What Are the Important Considerations?

There are several options available to biopsy a lesion involving salivary glands. In a situation where there is a palpable swelling, FNAB should be performed either using intra-oral or extra-oral approach depending on

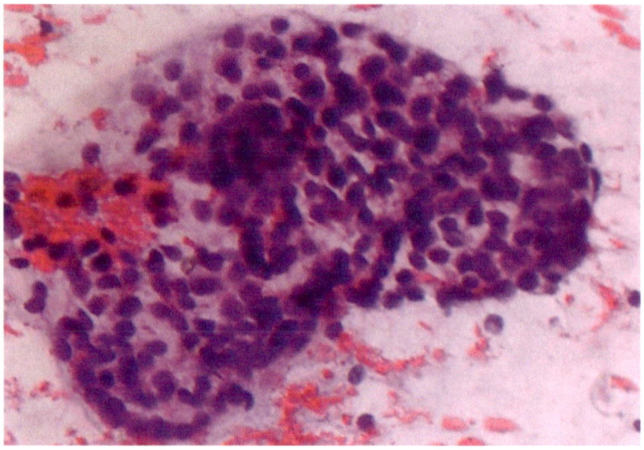

Fig. 59.2 Hematoxylin and Eosin (H&E) stained smear shows cells with scant cytoplasm and hyperchromatic angular nuclei (Courtesy: Dr. Cherine Sosai)

where the swelling is more apparent. It is a non-invasive and easy to perform procedure under local anaesthesia. The important thing to consider when performing FNAB is to ensure that adequate material is harvested for cytological evaluation.

The cytology report confirms the diagnosis of adenoid cystic carcinoma.

59

59.14 What Cytopathological Features Would You Expect to See in This Lesion?

The smear shows aggregates of small-sized, round to ovoid cells with angular nuclei in a background of purplish hyaline spheres of mucopolysaccharide material. The hyaline spheres are stained purplish pink with Giemsa stain and pale green or light orange with Papanicolaou stain. The neoplastic cells exhibit scant cytoplasm, indistinct cytoplasmic borders, and nuclei with evenly distributed chromatin (Fig. 59.2).

An incisional biopsy is not necessary if the definitive diagnosis can be confirmed with the FANB. However, incisional biopsy is mandatory when the definitive diagnosis is doubtful or in deciding whether the tumour is benign or malignant.

59.15 What Would Be the Best Imaging Modality to Investigate This Lesion?

Any lesions or tumours involving the salivary gland would be best viewed using MR imaging. However, since this lesion is a malignancy, it is necessary to extend the imaging to the neck and rest of the body in order to rule out any possibility of regional or distant metastasis. The best imaging for tumour staging purposes would be contrast enhanced CT scan or Pet scan from the level of the head down to the pelvic region.

The patient underwent a CT and MRI prior to formulating his treatment plan. The MRI (Fig. 59.3a) was carried out to assess the extension of the tumour in the primary and loco-regional areas, while CT scans (Fig. 59.3b) were performed to rule out any possibilities of distant metastases. Both images confirmed an ill-defined extensive heterogeneously enhancing area at the left anterior and lateral floor of the mouth consistent with a malignant lesion. The lesion crossed the midline anteriorly to extend into the sublingual spaces bilaterally (left > right), submandibular spaces (left > right), and left side of the tongue. There was enlargement of the left submandibular gland measuring 2.2 cm (AP) × 2.5 cm (W) × 3.3 cm (H). Cervical lymph nodes of less than a centimetre were also noted bilaterally.

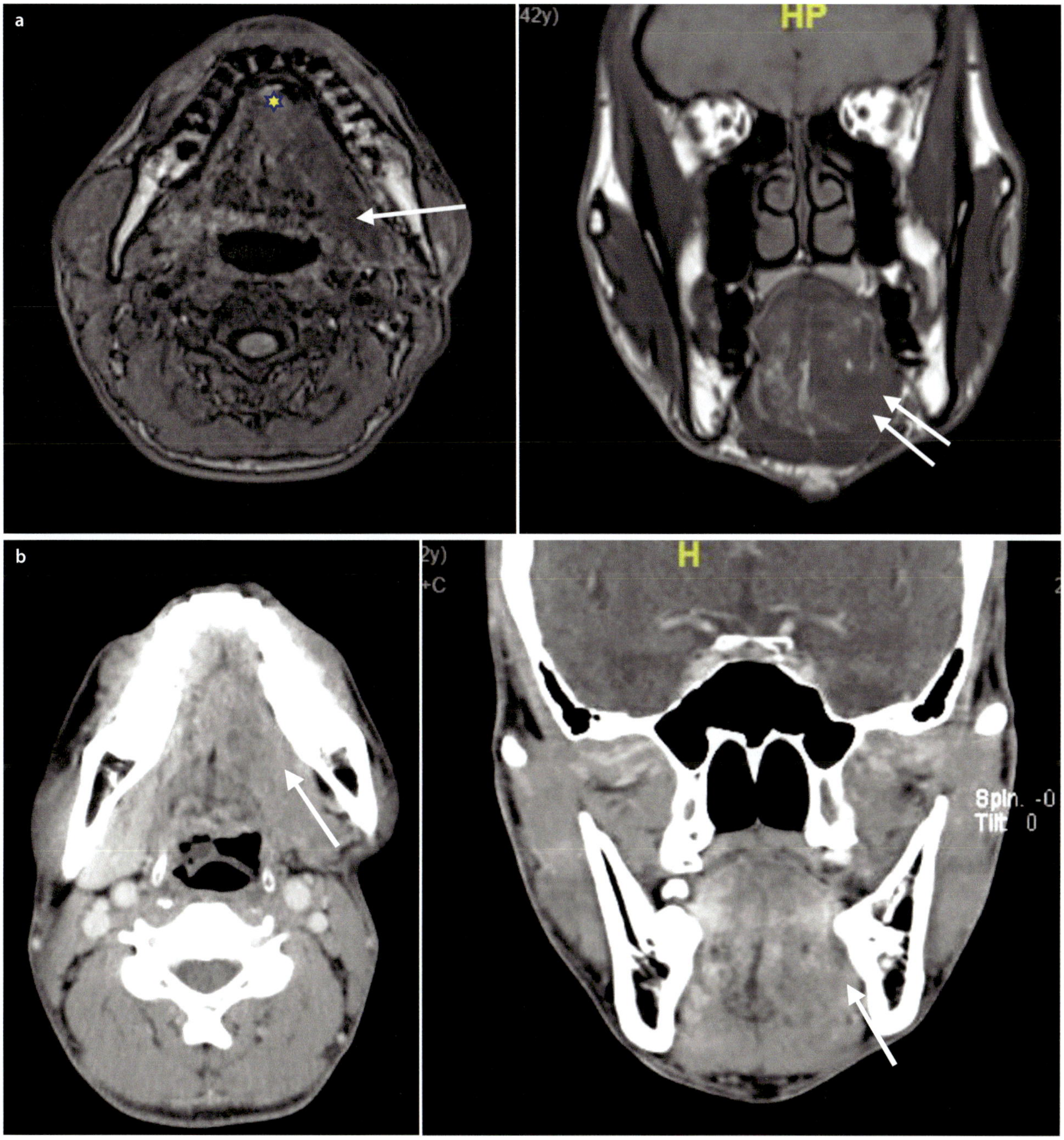

Fig. 59.3 (**a**) MRI axial view (L) and coronal view (R) show tumour extension involving left floor of the mouth (white arrow). The lesion crossed the midline anteriorly to extend into the sublingual spaces bilaterally (left > right), submandibular spaces (left > right), and left side of the tongue (double white arrow). (**b**) CT axial view (L) and coronal view (R). There was enlargement of the left submandibular gland measuring 2.2 cm (AP) × 2.5 cm (W) × 3.3 cm (H) (white arrow). Cervical lymph nodes of less than a centimetre were also noted bilaterally

59.16 How Would You Treat This Patient?

Surgery is the mainstay of treatment for adenoid cystic carcinoma. The amount of surgical defect and complications following resection of the involved salivary gland with wide free margins usually depends on the location of the tumour. The present case occurred in the floor of the mouth in relation to sublingual gland. Based on the imaging, the tumour is large and extends beyond the mylohyoid muscles and occupies both the sublingual and submandibular spaces bilaterally. Since tumour removal was done clearing the entire content of the floor of the mouth as well as two thirds of the tongue, an appropriate reconstruction option needs to be applied to ensure that post-operative form and function are well maintained. Surgical access to the tumour is via pull-through method as clearance to the regional cervical lymph nodes were also indicated bilaterally. In such a case, a bulky soft tissue flap would be most suitable to reconstruct the floor of the mouth and create neo tongue with sufficient bulk to achieve good palato-glossal contact during the swallowing process. Nevertheless, using a composite bone and soft tissue flap to reconstruct the surgical defect is another option whenever there is tumour involvement of the adjacent mandibular bone.

59.17 What Are the Histopathological Features That You Would Expect to See in the Excised Specimen?

Histopathological examination shows histologically polymorphous but cytologically rather isomorphous tumour cells arranged in islands, strands, and nests of variable sizes within a fibromyxoid stroma (◘ Fig. 59.4).

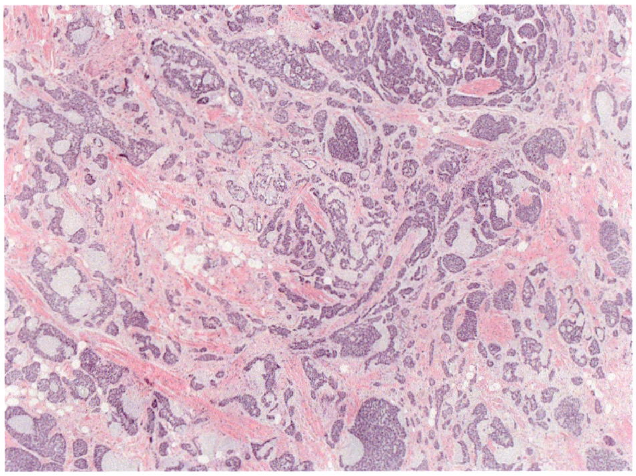

◘ **Fig. 59.4** Photomicrograph shows tumour cells arranged in islands, strands, and nests of variable sizes within a fibromyxoid stroma

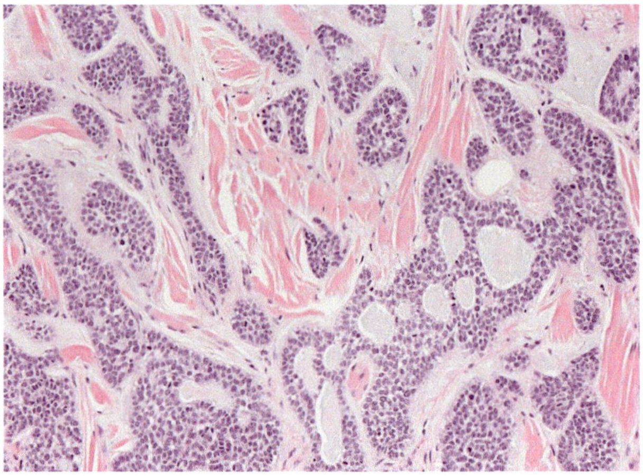

◘ **Fig. 59.5** Photomicrograph shows tumour cells in a cribriform pattern of arrangement with punched-out spaces filled with basophilic material. Nuclei are hyperchromatic and angular in shape

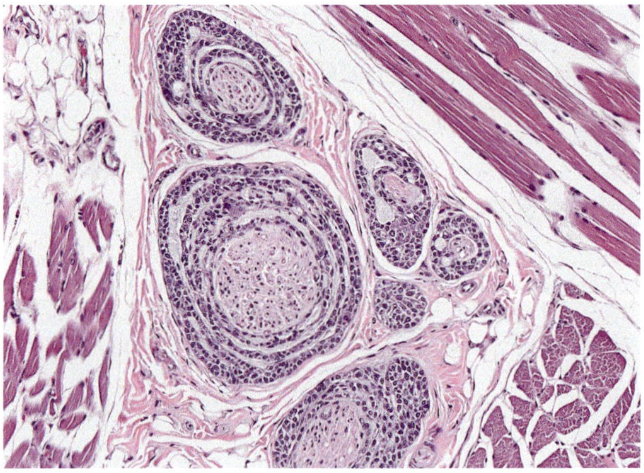

◘ **Fig. 59.6** Perineural invasion involving nerve bundles of variable size. Bands of tumour cells encircle the nerves of variable sizes

The tumour cells exhibit hyperchromatic angular nuclei with scant cytoplasm. Cribriform pattern is predominant with punched-out cyst-like spaces containing basophilic substances (◘ Fig. 59.5). The tumour demonstrates pronounced perineural invasion involving variable sized nerve bundles (◘ Fig. 59.6). Mitotic figures are inconspicuous in this cribriform pattern predominant tumour.

59.18 Follow Up and Prognosis

Adenoid cystic carcinoma has a varying prognosis depending on the histological subtype. It tends to grow into and along the nerves of the face referred to as perineural invasion. Regional lymphatic spread and even distant metastasis take place after many years. The prognosis of ACC often depends on its histological grading upon diagnosis whereby those with more solid components end up with poorer prognosis. Although having a higher histopathological grading often indicates unfavourable prognosis, the treatment of choice most often would not differ between an early and late stage. As ACC behaves aggressively with a high tendency for perineural spread, adjuvant radiotherapy following radical resection is warranted for most cases. Five-year survival rate is usually good (60–90%) at early stage; however, long-term survival is poor with involvement of distant sites.

In terms of follow up, it is advised to review every 3–6 months within or beyond 5 years after treatment. A thorough head and neck clinical examination is mandatory. MRI, CT, and/or PET-CT is indicated if there is any suspicion of loco-regional recurrence or distant metastasis.

59.19 Adenoid Cystic Carcinoma

ACC is a rare form of adenocarcinoma that begins in glandular tissues with highest prevalence in patients in their sixth decades of life. It occurs frequently in the major and minor salivary glands of the head and neck. The age of patients affected with major salivary gland tumours is documented to be younger than those with minor salivary gland tumours. ACC can also occur in the breast, uterus, skin, or other locations in the body.

Clinically, ACC often manifests as a swelling and may have pain and/or numbness as accompanying symptoms. The signs and symptoms of ACC vary according to the location of the tumour. Those affecting the larynx and trachea or vocal cords may cause respiratory symptoms or changes in speech, respectively, while those affecting the lacrimal gland may cause bulging of the eye or changes in vision. When it occurs in the parotid gland, facial nerve palsy is a pathognomonic clinical feature in most patients. ACC often spreads along the nerves and sometimes through the bloodstream. Only a small fraction of cases spread along the lymphatics. The exact aetiological factors for ACC are still unknown, and there is no evidence of hereditary basis for occurrence.

Investigations

- Imaging features help to distinguish between low- and high-grade adenoid cystic carcinomas. Low-grade tumours tend to be well defined, in contradistinction to high-grade tumours, which appear infiltrative. However, both subtypes are usually homogeneously enhancing after contrast administration. Typically, an ACC would demonstrate significant characteristic features in MRI. They often appear hypo to isointense in T1 window, while it tends to be slightly hyperintense in T2 window which increases significantly with higher grades of tumour. When viewed together with contrast medium such as Gadolinium (Gd), the tumour would appear as a homogenous enhancement. The same modality would be able to capture perineural involvement by the tumour especially if it involves cranial nerve VII.
- Histopathological features: The neoplastic cells feature scant cytoplasm and small hyperchromatic and angular nuclei arranged in variable patterns, such as solid, cribriform, and tubular forms. The tumour cells are composed of both epithelial and myoepithelial elements. ACC often shows prominent perineural invasion histopathologically. The tumour is divided into three histopathological types. Cribriform pattern is the most frequent and solid form is the least frequently encountered pattern. The third type is defined as tubular pattern. The cribriform pattern has a Swiss cheese-like appearance exhibiting islands of neoplastic cells containing pseudocystic structures. The tubular pattern is composed of bilayered epithelium with conspicuous luminal spaces. The tumour cells are characteristically hyperchromatic with angular nuclei. Sheets or lobular aggregates of tumour cells form the solid pattern of adenoid cystic carcinoma. Marked pleomorphism and high-grade features can be seen in solid pattern compared to cribriform and tubular patterns (◘ Fig. 59.7). Inevitably, the amount of solid pattern in the tumour content would relatively indicate a poor prognosis.

In the past, the prognosis of ACC was graded depending on the growth pattern. The tumours with at least 70% of the tumour volume exhibiting a solid growth pattern were considered to have poor prognosis. It is believed that the T status and nodal involvement are better prognosticators than growth pattern.

Adenoid cystic carcinoma is a slow growing and rare tumour. Even though the tumour has high incidence for local recurrences and distant metastasis, it is often successfully removed via surgical resection with or without adjuvant radiotherapy. Since this tumour

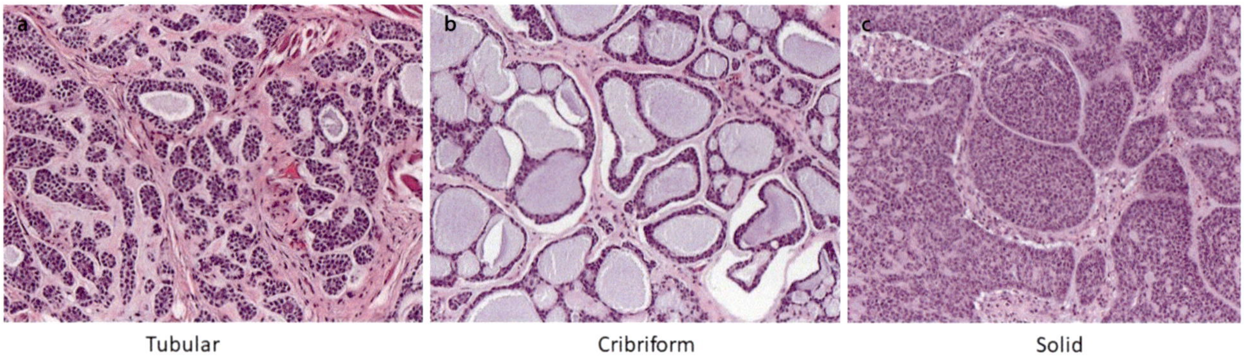

Fig. 59.7 Different histopathological variants of ACC (**a**) tubular. (**b**) cribriform. (**c**) solid

has the tendency to spread via neural invasion, it is difficult to determine the clinical margin of the tumour intraoperatively. Hence, a concurrent radiation therapy following surgery is often indicated for most patients especially when there is evidence of involved margins, perineural invasion, and regional metastasis. The disease is most often regarded as a locoregional disease, but when there is relapse, it often occurs at distant sites with late recurrence. Tumour size (T3 or T4), presence of lymphovascular invasion, and positive/close margins are independent risk factors for distant metastasis. Meanwhile, loco-regional recurrence is affected independently by T stage, presence of lymphovascular invasion, and nodal status. Besides tumour staging, the location of the tumour especially if it originates from the floor of the mouth, sinonasal tract, and hard palate are adverse predictors for survival. Complexity of the surgical anatomy inevitably complicates the treatment planning. ACC originating from certain sites are usually symptomless and lead to delay in patient seeking for help. Further, tumours occurring in the mobile tongue may increase the risk of nodal involvement while late-stage ACC of the hard palate and maxillary sinus may involve the base of the skull and cranial nerves. Among all salivary gland tumours, those occurring in the submandibular and sublingual glands have poorer prognosis. Other than the site of occurrence, age has also been recognized as a predictive factor in disease survival. Older patients tend to have a poor prognosis compared to younger patients.

Salient features of adenoid cystic carcinoma	
Clinical	• Often presents as a swelling which may be ulcerated. • May manifest paraesthesia or pain. • Muscle weakness may be encountered if motor nerves are involved. • Macroscopically, the tumour is usually non- encapsulated and fixed to adjacent tissue. • Facial nerve palsy is common in parotid tumours.
Imaging	• Infiltrative margin is indicative of high-grade tumour.
Histopathology	• Manifests as tubular, cribriform or solid types. • Tumour cells show scanty cytoplasm with small angular and hyperchromatic nuclei. • Perineural invasion is an unequivocal feature in adenoid cystic carcinoma.
Treatment	• Treatment of choice is radical excision, with or without postoperative radiotherapy/chemotherapy.

59.20 Diagnostic Algorithm

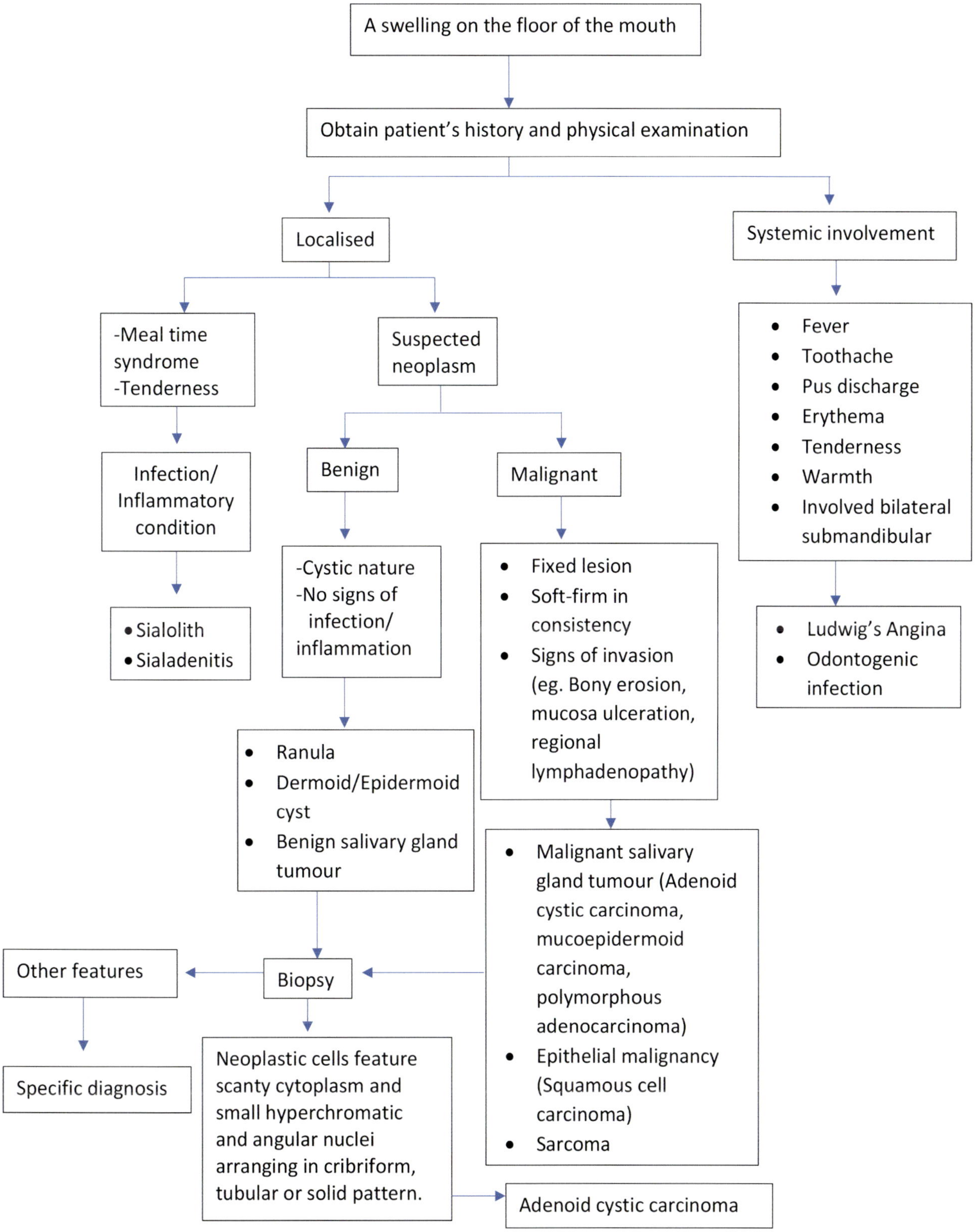

Self-Assessment Questions

1. List the pathognomonic clinical features of ACC.
2. State the important conditions that need to be included in the differential diagnosis for swellings in the floor of the mouth.
3. Describe the histopathological features of ACC.
4. Outline the management plan according to the stage of the disease.
5. Describe the grading criteria for ACC.

Suggested Reading

Amit M, Na'Ara S, Trejo-Leider L, Ramer N, Burstein D, Yue M, et al. Defining the surgical margins of adenoid cystic carcinoma and their impact on outcome: an international collaborative study. Head Neck. 2017;39:1008–14.

Chundru NS, Amudala R, Thankappan P, Nagaraju CD. Adenoid cystic carcinoma of palate: a case report and review of literature. Dent Res J. 2013;10(2):274–8. https://doi.org/10.4103/1735-3327.113372.

Ellis GL, Auclair PL. Tumours of the salivary glands. AFIP Atlas of Tumour Pathology; 2008.

El-Naggar AK. Tumours of salivary glands. WHO classification of tumours of the head and neck. 4th ed. Lyon: IARC Press; 2017.

Godge P, Sahrma S, Yadav M. Adenoid cystic carcinoma of parotid gland. Contemp Clin Dent. 2012;3:223–6.

Ouyang DQ, Liang LZ, Zheng GS, et al. Risk factors and prognosis for salivary gland adenoid cystic carcinoma in southern China: a 25-year retrospective study. Medicine. 2017;96:e5964.

van Weert S, van der Waal I, Witte BI, René Leemans C, Bloemena E. Histopathological grading of adenoid cystic carcinoma of the head and neck: analysis of currently used grading systems and proposal for a simplified grading scheme. Oral Oncol. 2015;51(1):71–6.

59

A Painless Swelling on the Left Cheek: Warthin Tumour

Kathreena Kadir, Yet Ching Goh, and Chuey Chuan Tan

Contents

W. M Tilakaratne, T. G. Kallarakkal (eds.), *Clinicopathological Correlation of Oral Diseases*,
https://doi.org/10.1007/978-3-031-24408-7_60

60.1 Main Complaint

A 65-year-old man presented to the Oral and Maxillofacial Surgery (OMFS) clinic with a complaint of a large lump over the angle of his left lower jaw.

60.2 History of Complaint

❓ Question: How long have you noticed the lump?

✅ I noted the lump about 2 years ago.

❓ Question: What is the nature of the lump?

✅ It started off as a small swelling beneath my left ear. The swelling is persistent and is gradually increasing in size.

❓ Question: Is the swelling painful? Were there any episodes of fever concurrent with the swelling?

✅ It is painless and I have never experienced any fever prior to it.

❓ Question: Do you feel any salty or foul taste in the mouth?

✅ No, I don't feel so.

❓ Question: Did you seek for any medical advice prior to the visit?

✅ No, I didn't. Most of my family and friends had noticed it too and they did advise me to seek medical attention.

❓ Question: Are you finding it difficult to open your mouth wide with the present swelling?

✅ I have no such difficulty.

❓ Question: How is your meal habits? Are you experiencing any pain while eating? Does your mouth feel dry?

✅ I cannot recall any difficulty or changes in my meal habits since the swelling appeared. I do not experience any pain or dryness in the mouth while eating.

❓ Question: Have you noticed any facial weakness over the same side of the face such as asymmetrical smile, inability to puff cheeks, or raise your eyebrow?

✅ I did not notice any facial weaknesses.

❓ Question: Do you experience any numbness over you left ear lobe?

✅ I don't experience any numbness.

❓ Question: Did you notice any lumps elsewhere on your body?

✅ I can feel another lump over the angle of my right jaw.

60.3 Past Medical/Dental and Social History

❓ Question: Are you currently being treated for any medical problems or taking any medications prescribed by your physician?

✅ I do not suffer from any medical condition and I do not take any prescribed medication.

❓ Question: Have you been admitted to the hospital before or undergone any surgical procedure?

✅ I was admitted to the hospital 30 years ago to remove my appendix. The whole experience was uneventful.

❓ Question: Do you have any known allergies towards any types of drugs or foods?

✅ I am unaware of any such allergies.

❓ Question: Do you see your dentist regularly?

✅ I don't see my dentist on a regular basis.

❓ Question: Are you married and have children? What do you do for a living?

✅ I am married and I have three children. I run my own business in the city.

❓ Question: Are you a smoker?

✅ I smoke half a pack of cigarettes per day since my teenage years and I still do so.

❓ Question: Do you take alcohol?

✅ I do enjoy social drinking with my friends over the weekends or over some special occasions.

Question: Do you have any specific chewing habits?

I do not have any chewing habits.

60.4 With the Findings from the History, What Is Your Differential Diagnosis?

1. Benign salivary gland tumour (SGT) (Pleomorphic Adenoma, Warthin Tumour).
2. Malignant SGT (Mucoepidermoid Carcinoma, Adenoid cystic Carcinoma, Acinic Cell Carcinoma).
3. Non-neoplastic salivary gland disease (SGD) (Sialadenosis, Sialadenitis).

60.5 How Do You Justify Your Differential Diagnosis After History Taking?

The patient gives a history of a painless slow growing lump over his left angle of the mandible. Swellings over this region are usually associated with the parotid gland owing to the typical location of the parotid salivary gland. The parotid gland is located anteriorly to the auricular meatus and over the posterior border of the ramus of the mandible. Hence, any associated lesion or common disease in the parotid gland should be considered.

60

Benign SGTs such as pleomorphic adenoma is included in the differential diagnosis as it is the most common benign salivary gland neoplasm. Approximately, 53–77% of these tumours occur in the parotid gland. Warthin tumour is included in the differential diagnosis as it is the second most common type of salivary gland neoplasm occurring in the parotid gland. Furthermore, his chronic history of cigarette smoking would have been associated with Warthin tumour. Apart from that, he also mentioned of a similar swelling occurring on the right side of the jaw. This could be a feature of Warthin tumour whereby 5–17% of these tumours have been reported to occur bilaterally. Most of these bilateral tumours do not occur synchronously but are metachronous.

Mucoepidermoid carcinoma, adenoid cystic carcinoma, and acinic cell carcinoma are the three most common malignant neoplasms occurring in the salivary glands. The parotid gland is, however, less commonly involved, when compared to the submandibular gland or other minor salivary glands. Even though the patient did not complain of any neuromotor or sensory disturbances over the ipsilateral facial region, the diagnosis of malignancy cannot be totally ruled out until further investigations are made.

Other non-neoplastic SGDs such as sialadenosis is listed in the differential diagnosis as it is a term referred to any swelling of the parotid gland with unknown cause. A history of excessive alcohol usage has been associated with this condition. Sialadenitis, sialolithiasis, and all other lesion associated with inflammation of the parotid gland could easily be ruled out since the patient is not experiencing any pain, dryness, or difficulty during eating and functioning. There was no history of any systemic involvement suggestive of diseases such as Sjogren syndrome.

60.6 Findings of Examination

Extra-orally the lump is located at the tail of the left parotid gland with a well-demarcated boundary measuring 3.5 × 4 cm in greatest dimension (Fig. 60.1). The lesion is firm in consistency and is not fixed to the overlying skin. The skin is of normal colour and temperature. Left facial nerve examination appears to be normal with no reported paraesthesia over the left ear lobe. The right side of the face appears to have another smaller swelling with almost similar features. Further examination of the neck did not reveal any cervical lymphadenopathy.

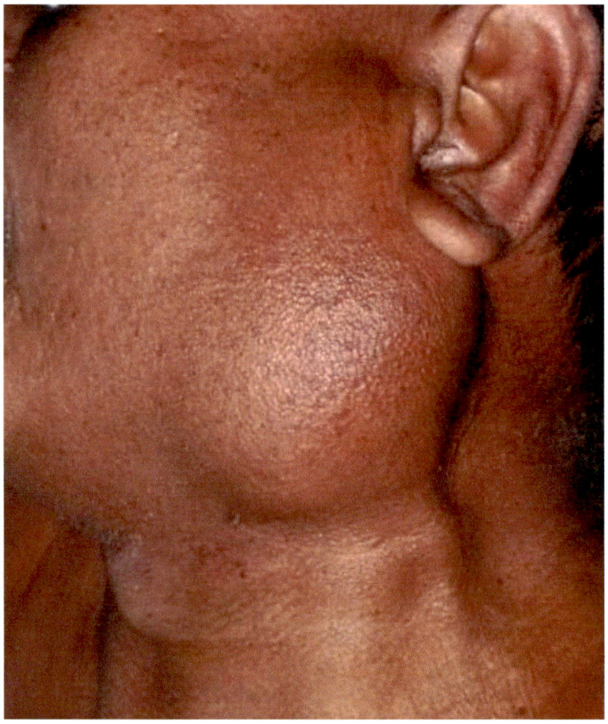

Fig. 60.1 A well-demarcated lump noted at the tail of the left parotid gland measuring 3.5 × 4 cm in greatest dimension (Courtesy: Dr. Nadeena Jayasuriya)

60.7 What Is Your Clinical Differential Diagnosis?

1. Pleomorphic Adenoma (PA)
2. Warthin Tumour (WT)

60.8 How Would You Justify the Inclusion of the Diseases That You Have Mentioned in the Differential Diagnosis to Exclude Other Conditions?

Pleomorphic Adenoma and Warthin tumour are listed on top of the differential diagnoses since these two are the common types of neoplasms that occur in the parotid gland.

60.8.1 Pleomorphic Adenoma

Pleomorphic adenoma is the commonest salivary gland tumour in both adults and children. It commonly occurs in the fourth–sixth decade of life with a female predilection. Majority of major gland PAs occur in parotid glands, followed by the submandibular and sublingual glands. Approximately, 70% of parotid swelling are PAs. Intraoral pleomorphic adenoma usually presents on the palate, buccal mucosa or lips. The typical presentation of a pleomorphic adenoma is a slowly growing and mobile, painless swelling without skin or mucosal ulceration. Therefore, PA is a highly possible differential diagnosis.

60.8.2 Warthin Tumour

Warthin Tumour is the second commonest salivary gland neoplasm affecting the parotid gland after pleomorphic adenoma. It appears as painless slow growing parotid mass that usually affects older men. Clinically, the tumour is located at the parotid tail and may occur bilaterally with a strong predilection in chronic smokers. WT is a likely differential diagnosis according to the findings of the history and clinical examination.

Other types of benign SGTs such as oncocytomas, myoepitheliomas, monomorphic adenomas, and basal cell adenomas are worth to be mentioned but are relatively rare benign tumours of the parotid gland. Meanwhile, all other non-neoplastic diseases of the salivary glands can be excluded since the clinical features of the lump are suggestive of a tumour rather than a non-neoplastic disease. It has a clear boundary and appeared firm in consistency with a history of long-standing nature SGDs of inflammatory origin are usually accompanied by symptoms such as pain and increase in the size of the swelling particularly at mealtimes. A malignant SGT is also a possibility. However, important clinical findings such as the absence of neuromotor and sensory disturbances as well as tumour not being fixed to the underlying structures or overlying skin excludes all other potential malignant salivary gland neoplasms. Furthermore, 80% of all parotid masses are benign. Nevertheless, the final definitive diagnosis could only be determined after proper investigations are carried out.

60.9 How Would You Investigate the Patient?

- Fine needle aspiration cytology (FNAC)
- Radiographic investigations

60.10 What Is the Reason to Perform an FNAC Without Performing an Incisional Biopsy?

Performing an open biopsy in the parotid gland carries a significant morbidity due to the location of facial nerve within the gland. Therefore, FNAC is the best option as a definitive diagnosis can be obtained for most salivary tumours. The important point to consider when performing FNAC is to ensure adequate cells are harvested for cytological evaluation and the procedure is performed as atraumatic as possible to avoid injury to the facial nerve within the gland.

60.11 The Cytology Report Confirms the Previous Clinical Diagnosis of Warthin Tumour. What Are the Cytological Features?

The smears prepared from the aspirate show fragments of oncocytic epithelium exhibiting moderate to abundant eosinophilic cytoplasm and uniform centrally placed nuclei within a proteinaceous background (◘ Fig. 60.2). The epithelial clusters are surrounded by numerous lymphocytes. The epithelial cells are cytologically bland and do not demonstrate cytological atypia. The lymphoid component comprises predominantly of small lymphocytes and shows fewer large cells as part of the germinal centres. Occasional, pseudopapillary arrangements consisting of double oncocytic cell layers surrounding lymphoid aggregates are also present.

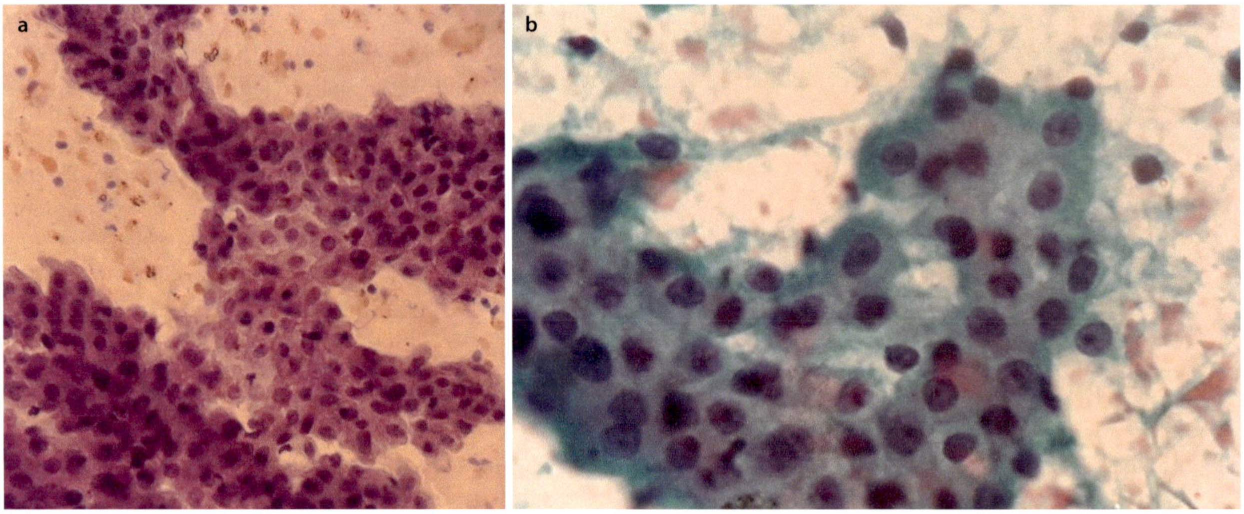

Fig. 60.2 (**a**) Giemsa staining showing oncocytic epithelium exhibiting moderate to abundant eosinophilic cytoplasm and uniform centrally placed nuclei. (**b**) Papanicolaou stain showing cells with clear cytoplasmic borders (right) (Courtesy: Dr. Cherine Sosai)

60.12 What Would Be the Best Imaging Modality to Investigate This Lesion?

One may first decide which type of imaging is available within the facility. Magnetic resonance imaging (MRI) would be the best choice of modality to view any lesions or tumour involving the salivary gland compared to both computed tomography scan (CT scan) and ultrasonography. When viewed using CT scan or MRI, the tumour has a significant proportion of cystic change.

- Ultrasound

  Warthin tumour usually appears as a round or ovoid hypoechoic mass, with well-defined margins and multiple irregular, small, sponge-like anechoic areas. Larger tumours (>5 cm) tend to be more cystic compared to smaller tumours. They are often hypervascular.

- CT scan

  Warthin tumour appears as a well-defined heterogeneous solid or cystic lesion within the superficial lobe of the tail of the parotid. It is moderately enhanced but with no calcification noted within. Presence of mural nodules is strongly suggestive of Warthin tumour (Fig. 60.3)

- MRI

  Signal characteristics according to different relaxation times

  - **T1:** Low-to-intermediate signal and isointensity when compared to adjacent muscle. Warthin tumours with microscopic cysts containing cholesterol components or proteinaceous fluid will display a focal high-signal intensity.
  - **T2:** Heterogeneous and variable signal intensity.
  - **T1 C+ (Gd):** Cystic components do not take up contrast while solid parts usually enhance.

60

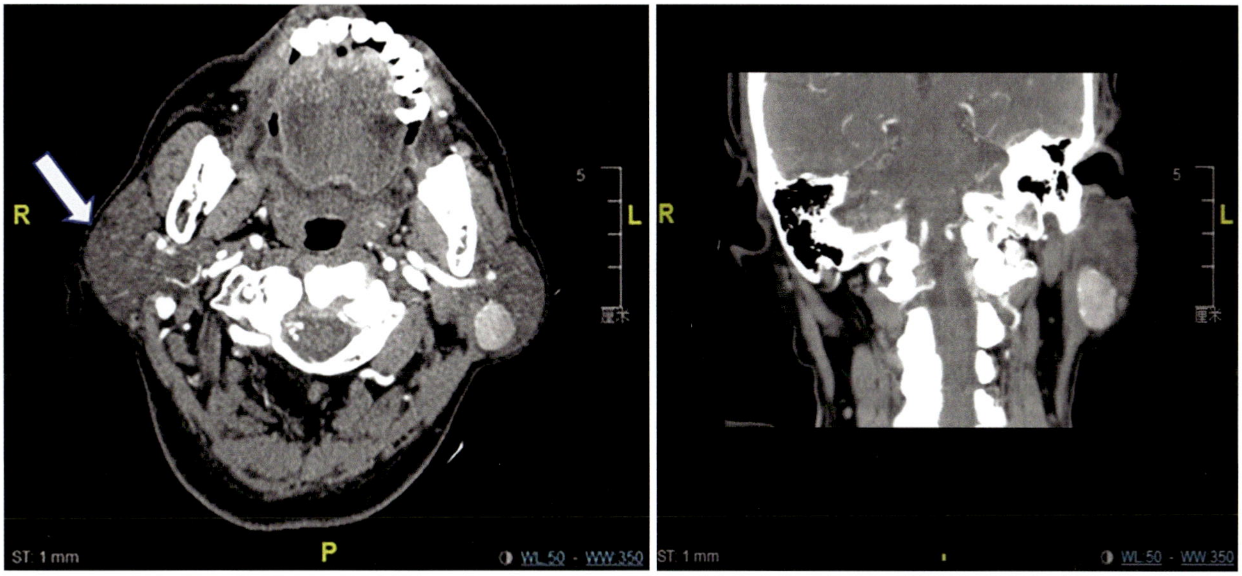

Fig. 60.3 Computed tomography shows well-defined heterogeneous solid to cystic lesion within the left parotid gland. It is moderately enhanced but with no calcification noted within. The right parotid gland is also enlarged (white arrow)

60.13 How Would You Treat This Patient?

Warthin tumour is a slow growing benign lesion with a very low risk of malignant transformation. Most often, when the size is relatively small and asymptomatic, the tumour would go unnoticed. When indicated for removal, most surgeons prefer to either do an excision of the tumour alone or a complete superficial parotidectomy with preservation of the facial nerve. Recent knowledge of functional MRI allows for sufficient diagnostic value for Warthin tumour. Hence, some surgeons may proceed to undertake surgical removal of the tumour even without performing any biopsy prior to the surgery.

60.14 What Are the Common Complications with Surgery to the Parotid Gland?

Surgery to the parotid gland may lead to several complications, which may be detrimental. These complications can be divided into early and late complications due to the complexity of all the vital structures that lie within the gland, especially the facial nerve. Among the most common early complications post-parotidectomy is injury to any of the facial nerve branches that may cause either temporary facial nerve paresis or complete facial palsy especially with total parotidectomy. The most common nerve branch to be involved is the marginal mandibular branch. However, if facial paresis causes incomplete closure of the eye due to injury to the superior trunk, the patient must be advised to use ophthalmic moisture drops frequently during the day and an ophthalmic ointment and eye protection at night. Regular follow-up with an ophthalmologist is mandatory. Other less common early complications following surgery to the parotid glands are hypoesthesia of greater auricular nerve, amputation neuroma, facial depression which causes cosmetic concern, haemorrhage or haematoma, skin flap necrosis, infection, trismus, and parotid fistula.

Other common complications that may appear later but pose a great concern to patient is gustatory sweating or Frey syndrome. Frey syndrome occurs due to the aberrant regeneration of sectioned parasympathetic secretomotor fibres of the auriculotemporal nerve with inappropriate innervation of the cutaneous facial sweat glands that are normally innervated by sympathetic cholinergic fibres. As a consequence, Frey syndrome is a disorder characterized by unilateral sweating and flushing of the facial skin in the area of the parotid gland occurring during meals that becomes evident usually 1–12 months after surgery. To avoid this, prophylactic measures are done intraoperatively including the use of the superficial musculoaponeurotic system (SMAS) as a flap or the superficial temporal artery fascial flap. These techniques aim to create a physical barrier between the divided fibres of the auriculotemporal nerve and the sweat glands in the facial skin. Recently, the use of botulinum toxin injection has been reported as the gold standard in treating Frey syndrome.

The best means of reducing all these complications after parotid surgery is a clear understanding of the anatomy and good surgical technique. It is mandatory for the surgeon to discuss clearly with the patient and explain the goals, rationale, and risk of the operation at pre-operative level when getting consent for the surgery. Furthermore, patient has to be informed about the cosmetic sequelae of the resection if total parotidectomy is the only option of getting clearance of the disease. This is usually the case when treating malignant salivary gland tumours.

60.15 What Histopathological Features Would You Expect to See in the Excision Specimen?

Histopathologically, the tumour is characterized by a well-circumscribed lesion containing cystic spaces with papillary-projections lined by bilayered epithelium and supported by prominent lymphoid stroma (◘ Fig. 60.4). Well-formed germinal centres are observed. The epithelium component features tall columnar luminal cells with palisaded nuclei and basal columnar cells (◘ Fig. 60.5). Mucous cells, squamous metaplasia, and ciliation can be found within the luminal layer. The lumen contains eosinophilic coagulum.

60

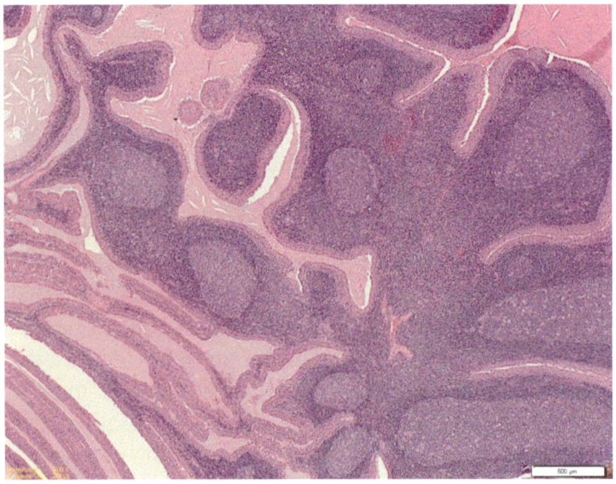

◘ **Fig. 60.4** Cystic spaces containing papillary proliferations of epithelial components supported by prominent lymphoid stroma with well-formed germinal centres

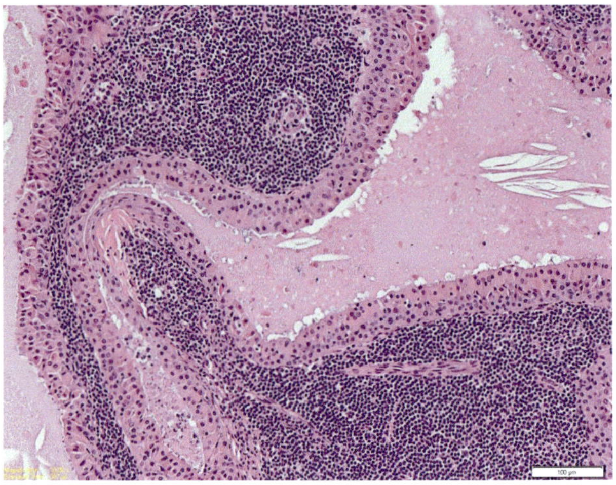

◘ **Fig. 60.5** The epithelium shows a bilayered configuration with luminal columnar cells and outer cuboidal cells

60.16 Follow-Up and Prognosis

Once the tumour is removed, the incidence of recurrence is very rare or less than 5%.

60.17 Warthin Tumour

Warthin tumour also known as papillary cystadenoma lymphomatosum is a benign neoplasm which occurs predominantly in the parotid gland and represents approximately 15% of all parotid tumours. It is the second most common benign salivary gland neoplasm in the parotid gland following pleomorphic adenoma. Fewer than 10% of cases occur outside this gland. Furthermore, bilateral occurrence is described in 5–15% of cases and multifocality in 6–20% of cases.

Warthin tumour most often occurs in older adults between sixth and seventh decades of life with a male predilection. Warthin tumour is associated with cigarette smoking which most often explains why this particular tumour could present bilaterally though not synchronously but metachronously. It usually appears as a firm or fluctuant mass located at the angle of the mandible or in the tail of the parotid gland.

The pathogenesis of these tumours is traditionally hypothesized as arising from heterotopic salivary gland tissue found within parotid lymph nodes. The predilection for parotid salivary gland supports the proposal that Warthin tumour is a neoplasm that develops from heterotopic salivary ducts within intraparotid or paraparotid lymphoid tissue. Unlike other salivary glands, parotid salivary glands normally contain lymphoid tissue in the form of small intraglandular lymph nodes or small unorganized aggregates of lymphoid cells. Others have also suggested that it may develop from a proliferation of salivary gland ductal epithelium that is associated with secondary formation of lymphoid tissue.

Warthin tumour is histopathologically characterized by cystic spaces lined by bilayered oncocytic epithelium showing papillary proliferations and supported by dense lymphoid tissue. Warthin tumour usually has a thin capsule and is sharply demarcated from the surrounding parenchyma. The bilayered epithelium consists of luminal tall columnar cells and outer basaloid appearing cuboidal cells. The tall columnar cells display palisading ovoid nuclei and finely granular eosinophilic cytoplasm. The luminal surface of the cells may demonstrate apocrine-like secretions in the form of small protuberances and cilia. As for the outer cuboidal cells, they are smaller cells with fusiform nuclei and more haphazardly arranged than the luminal cells. The epithelium forms papilla that projects into the luminal spaces. The supporting fibrovascular connective tissue is often obscured by dense lymphoid element principally of mature, small uniform lymphocytes. In most cases, well-formed germinal centres are present.

Warthin tumour has been subclassified into typical, stroma-poor, stroma-rich, and metaplastic forms according to the proportion of the epithelial and lymphoid components. Microscopic changes such as squamous metaplasia, mucous metaplasia, oncocytosis, necrosis, fibrosis, and inflammation are sometimes observed.

Surgical removal of the tumour via local resection with minimal surrounding tissue is the most preferred treatment modality among surgeons. Some may opt for a more aggressive approach such as superficial parotidectomy to avoid violating the tumour capsule especially in cases where pre-operative diagnosis is not ascertained. Others may even choose for a more conservative method if the lesion is small due to fear of causing facial nerve dysfunction or Frey syndrome post-operatively. Most often, if removed completely, the incidence of recurrence is really low. However, many reports suggest that these tumours are multicentric in nature. Hence, it is difficult to determine on long-term follow-up if there is a true recurrence or a secondary tumour.

Salient features of Warthin tumour	
Clinical	A firm to fluctuant well-defined mass located at the tail of parotid near the angle of mandible. The tumour is unique as it may present bilaterally and is highly associated with cigarette smoking.
Radiology	Best viewed using MRI under T1 window. A typical tumour would exhibit low to intermediate signal with cyst containing cholesterol components containing focal high signal.
Histopathology	A well-demarcated lesion containing cystic spaces with papillary projections-lined by bilayered epithelium and supported by prominent lymphoid stroma.
Treatment	Local resection with minimal surrounding tissue and preservation of the facial nerve would be the treatment of choice.
This is a benign neoplasm of the salivary gland with very low risk of malignant transformation. Incidence of recurrence is almost rare if removed completely.	

60.18 Diagnostic Algorithm

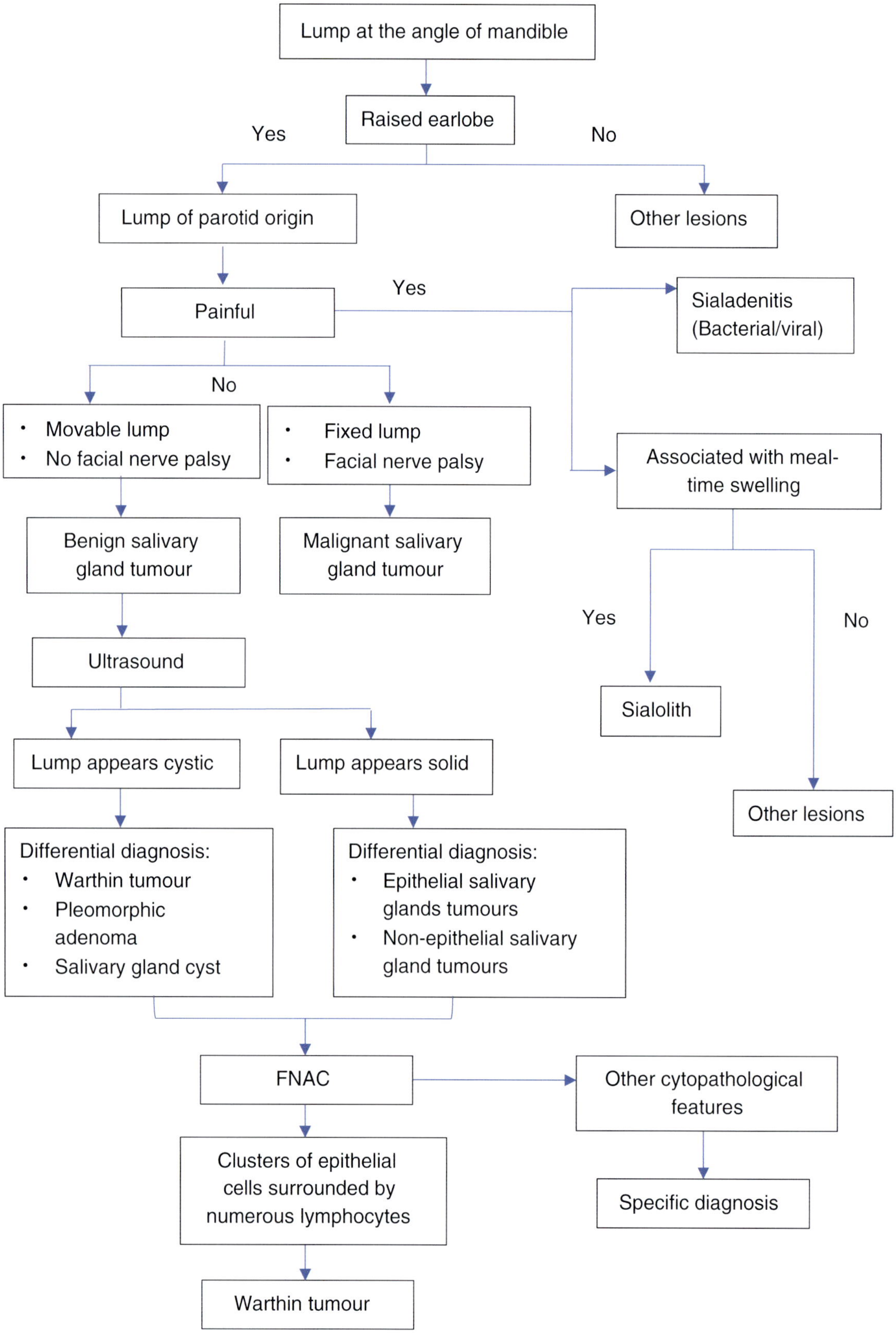

Self-Assessment Questions

1. State the typical clinical characteristics of Warthin tumour.
2. Discuss the etiopathogenesis of Warthin tumour.
3. Discuss the differential diagnosis for parotid gland swellings.
4. Describe the histopathological features of Warthin tumour.
5. Discuss the treatment of Warthin tumour.

Suggested Reading

Chulam TC, Noronha Francisco AL, Goncalves Filho J, Pinto Alves CA, Kowalski LP. Warthin's tumour of the parotid gland: our experience. Acta Otorhinolaryngol Ital. 2013;33(6):393–7.

Ellis GL, Auclair PL. Tumors of the salivary glands. AFIP atlas of tumor pathology, vol. 9. 4th ed. Silver Spring, MD: ARP Press; 2008. p. 85–100.

El-Naggar AK, Takata T, Slootweg PJ, editors. Tumours of salivary glands. In: WHO classification of tumours of the head and neck. 4th ed. Lyon: IARC Press; 2017.

Kim J, Kim EK, Park CS, Choi YS, Kim YH, Choi EC. Characteristic sonographic findings of Warthin's tumor in the parotid gland. J Clin Ultrasound. 2004;32(2):78–81. https://doi.org/10.1002/jcu.10230.

Kuzenko YV, Romanuk AM, Dyachenko OO, Hudymenko O. Pathogenesis of Warthin's tumours. Interv Med Appl Sci. 2016;8(2):41–8.

Marchese-Ragona R, De Filippis C, Marioni G, Staffieri A. Treatment of complications of parotid gland surgery. Acta Otorhinolaryngol Ital. 2005;25(3):174–8.

Pinkston JA, Cole P. Cigarette smoking and Warthin's tumour. Am J Epidemiol. 1996;144(2):183–7.

Intermittent Pain and Swelling in the Floor of the Mouth: Sialolithiasis

Ajith Manjula Attygalla

Contents

W. M Tilakaratne, T. G. Kallarakkal (eds.), *Clinicopathological Correlation of Oral Diseases*,
https://doi.org/10.1007/978-3-031-24408-7_61

Learning Goals

1. Devise the correct way of compiling the history with appropriate questions
2. Develop a differential diagnosis after history taking
3. Deduce appropriate procedures in clinical examination
4. Formulate a differential diagnosis combining findings in the history and clinical examination
5. Justify the relevant investigations required to arrive at the diagnosis
6. Comprehend the importance of clinicopathological correlation in arriving at the correct diagnosis
7. Outline the management plan
8. Recognise the importance of a diagnostic algorithm in arriving at a diagnosis

61.1 Main Complaint

A 57-year-old female presented with a complaint of intermittent pain and swelling of the left floor of the mouth.

61.2 History of Complaint

Question: How long have you been having this problem and can you explain the nature of it?

I noticed it about 8 months ago. There was on and off pain and swelling under the tongue. The pain gradually worsened from time to time and sometimes there was a foul taste. The occurrence of the episodes became more frequent later

61.3 Additional Complaints

Question: Can you tell about any features associated with the pain and swelling you experienced?

I could feel a kind of lump under the tongue. It comes up especially during mealtimes. There was much discomfort with swelling and pain in relation to that area which often lasted few hours.

Question: Do you have any other medical problems such as diabetes, eating disorders, congestive heart failure, hepatic failure, renal failure, any neoplastic disease, radiotherapy, or immunocompromised conditions?

No. I do not have anything as such.

Question: Have you undergone any surgery recently?

I haven't undergone any surgery.

Question: Have you experienced recent fever, diarrhoea or mumps, dry mouth or dry eyes or any recent urinary tract infections with difficulty in passing urine or severe intermittent abdominal colicky pain?

I cannot remember anything as such but felt only a painful on and off lump under the tongue.

61.4 With the Findings from the History, What is Your Differential Diagnosis?

1. Recurrent sialadenitis of the left submandibular gland
2. Submandibular sialolithiasis
3. Salivary duct stricture
4. Tumour of the left submandibular salivary gland
5. Submandibular lymphadenopathy
6. Angioneurotic oedema
7. Dermoid/epidermoid cyst
8. Parasitic infection

61.5 How do You Justify Your Differential Diagnosis after History Taking?

1. Recurrent sialadenitis of the left submandibular gland

   She had intermittent swelling in the left floor of the mouth with discomfort during mealtimes for few months. The patient has experienced foul taste on and off as well. According to the site and the nature of the complaint, there is a high degree of suspicion of a submandibular salivary gland infection.
2. Submandibular sialolithiasis

   Presence of features in the history of salivary gland involvement and discomfort under the tongue together with the fact that highest incidence of sialolith formation in the submandibular gland suggests the possibility of submandibular sialolithiasis.
3. Salivary duct stricture

   Salivary duct strictures are the second most frequent cause of obstructions in the salivary glands, representing 5–10% of all obstructions of the submandibular gland. Painful swelling of the submandibular glands during eating as seen in this patient is a characteristic clinical manifestation in patients with salivary duct strictures.

4. Tumour of the left submandibular salivary gland

   The findings from the history and complaint are not characteristic of a neoplastic disease. Further, obstructive and infective features are frequent in the submandibular salivary gland while submandibular salivary gland neoplasms are not uncommon. Therefore, this is an unlikely differential diagnosis.

5. Submandibular lymphadenopathy

   Submandibular lymphadenopathy is anatomically related to the site of the complaint and is one of the commonest swellings of the submandibular region.

6. Angioneurotic oedema

   Recurrent nature of the swelling is consistent with angioneurotic oedema.

7. Dermoid/epidermoid cyst

   These cysts occur most often in patients in their second or third decade of life. Clinically, the lesion presents as a slow-growing asymptomatic mass, usually located in the midline.

8. Parasitic infection

   A rare possibility of parasitic infection such as filariasis in the endemic areas as well as conditions such as hydatid cyst may occur in the submandibular salivary gland.

61.6 Findings of Examination

There is no visible swelling in the submandibular region extra orally. Intra orally the submandibular salivary gland orifice is slightly inflamed (Fig. 61.1). Bimanual palpation of the floor of the mouth reveals a firm mass in the posterior aspect of the left floor of the mouth and a separate mobile hard lump in the anterior floor of the mouth of the size of 12 × 5 mm. Milking of the submandibular gland results in slight purulent discharge. There are no enlarged submandibular lymph nodes evident. Her oral hygiene is satisfactory without any signs of acute infections of pulpal or periodontal origin.

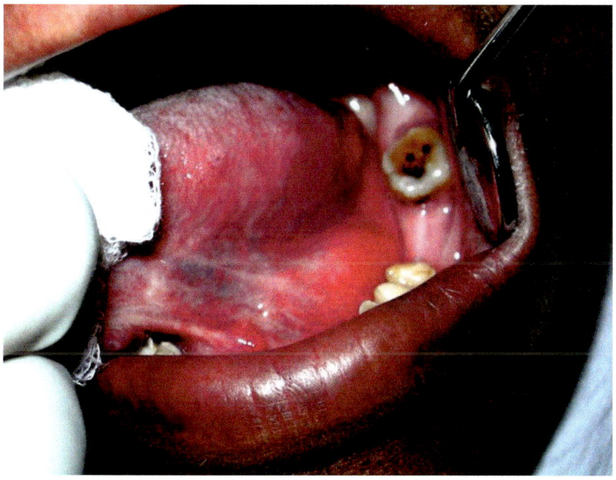

Fig. 61.1 Intra oral photograph of the left side floor of the mouth. Swelling of the left floor of the mouth is evident with inflamed left submandibular salivary duct

61.7 What is Your Clinical Differential Diagnosis?

1. Submandibular sialolithiasis

61.8 How would You Justify Your Clinical Diagnosis?

The presence of obstructive features such as intermittent pain and swelling especially during mealtimes highly suggests that it could be a sialolith obstructing the submandibular salivary duct. This is supported by the examination findings of a firm lump under the tongue which is bimanually palpable and a separate mobile non-tender, smaller hard mass more anteriorly.

61.9 What are the Investigations that should be Carried Out in Logical Sequence?

1. Full blood count
2. ESR/CRP
3. Lower standard occlusal radiograph
4. Ultrasound (US) scan of the floor of the mouth
5. Sialography (if not acutely infected, it has more therapeutic significance than diagnostic value)
6. If the above investigations are negative but the patient continues to have symptoms, an MRI/CT should be performed
7. FNAC

61.10 What are the Findings of Investigations?

Both the full blood count (FBC) and the ESR were within the normal range.

Lower posterior oblique occlusal radiograph revealed a well-defined radiopaque mass in relation to the left floor of the mouth (Fig. 61.2) in favour of a submandibular salivary calculus.

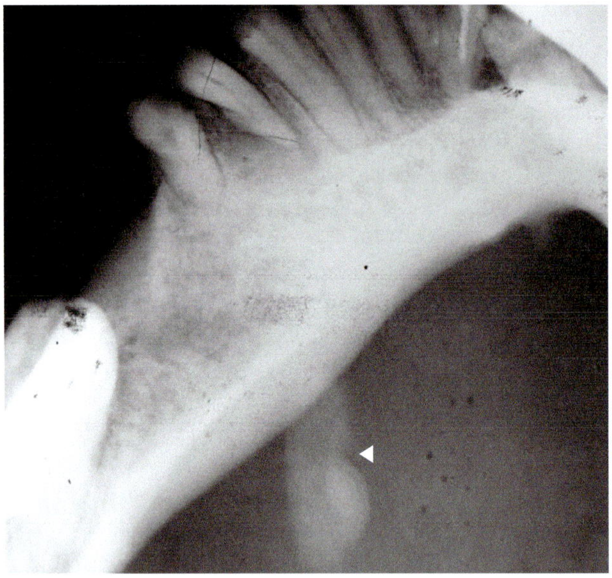

Fig. 61.2 Posterior lower oblique occlusal radiograph revealing a well-defined radiopaque mass in relation to the left floor of the mouth

61.11 What is the Definitive Diagnosis?

A salivary calculus in the left submandibular salivary gland duct with minimal gland destruction.

This diagnosis was arrived as there was clear evidence of intermittent pain and swelling specially during mealtimes and an enlarged left submandibular gland which is bimanually palpable with no hard masses felt in the gland itself but a separate hard mobile mass in the anterior floor of the mouth in relation to the left submandibular duct. The consistency of the gland was uniformly firm with minimal expression of pus when milking out indicating minimal gland destruction due to the chronic infection (Chronic sialadenitis). This suggested that the gland was functional and can be left behind following removal of the calculus. FBC and CRP values were within the normal range indicating minimal infection of the gland. Left posterior oblique occlusal radiograph revealed a well-defined radiopaque mass in the anterior floor of the mouth with confirmation of the presence of a calculus. US Scan/CT and MRI and FNAC were not carried out in the present case.

61.12 How would You Manage This Patient?

The presence of a hard lump anteriorly separated from the more posterior larger diffuse bimanually palpable mass helped to arrive at a tentative diagnosis of a submandibular sialolith in the duct. This was supported by the presence of a radiopaque mass in the lower occlusal radiograph. Although there was minimal discharge, the inflamed duct orifice indicated a chronic low-grade infection of the left submandibular salivary gland.

There was no evidence of acute spreading infection with fever. The patient had no immunocompromising conditions or any other predisposing medical issues. The patient was not acutely ill and she could take oral feeds as well. Therefore, there was no need of in-ward treatment but could be managed as an outpatient initially. She was asked to have adequate hydration and massaging of the gland. Surgical extirpation of the salivary calculus was planned under local anaesthesia. The patient was informed regarding the diagnosis and informed consent was taken for surgical removal of the calculus under local anaesthesia as it was located anteriorly in the floor of the mouth anterior to the second lower molar tooth. The patient was explained about the possibility of lingual paraesthesia and anaesthesia.

Following local anaesthesia injection into the floor of the mouth, a stay suture was placed behind the calculus in the region of the posterior aspect of the left side submandibular duct to prevent the calculus displacing into the gland with manipulation. With a no. 15 scalpel, a 1.0 cm incision was made parallel to the submandibular duct in the region of the calculus on the mucosa only. The incision was deepened bluntly with the surgical scissors and area of the duct enlarged with the calculus was approached. Following confirmation with palpation, an incision was made over the calculus on the duct exposing the calculus (Fig. 61.3). Adequate exposure was gained with blunt dissection and the calculus was expressed out of the duct (Fig. 61.4). The surgical area and the duct were irrigated thoroughly with saline and checked on haemostasis. The wound was left open without suturing to prevent the risk of duct obstruction with fibrosis.

The patient was advised to have adequate hydration and to use sialogogue such as vitamin C to be sucked three times a day and to gently massage and milk out the gland. Oral antibiotics and analgesics along with a

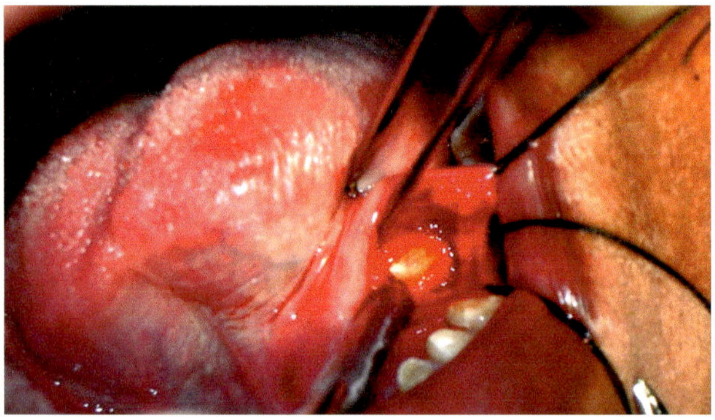

Fig. 61.3 Intra oral view showing exposure of the calculus within the duct with an incision in the floor of the mouth made parallel to the lingual nerve

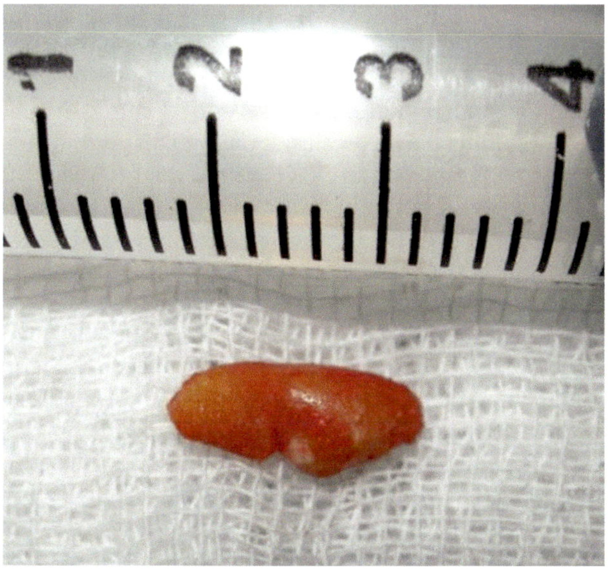

Fig. 61.4 Excised salivary calculus

mouth wash were prescribed and the patient was advised to maintain good oral hygiene.

The patient was reviewed 1 week later and there was good healing without any signs of infection or obstruction. The patient was advised to have good hydration and continue with sialogogue for a while together with massaging of the gland to prevent a recurrence.

61.13 Sialolithiasis

Sialolithiasis is a condition affecting the salivary glands with formation of calcified mass/masses within the excretory duct or within the gland itself. Sialolithiasis primarily affects the submandibular salivary gland (84–94%) followed by the parotid gland (4–10%). Sialolithiasis constitutes of one-third of all salivary gland disorders. These calcified masses or calculi lead to obstruction of the salivary flow resulting in stagnation of saliva with secondary infection of the salivary gland termed as sialadenitis.

Sialolith formation may occur due to irregularities, inflammation or local irritants in the ductal system. As a result of infection or rarely chemicals become crystallised and block the ducts. Calcifications around the degenerative substances liberated by saliva could also lead to calculi formation. Therefore, causes of salivary stone formation could be summarised as mechanical, inflammatory, chemical and neurohumoral.

Multiple internal microcalculi within salivary gland secretory granules act as nidus to form larger calculi. External material from the oral cavity such as bacteria or food debris enter the distal duct to contribute for sialolith formation. Elevated position of the duct orifice with antigravity flow, long course of the duct with bends, more viscous nature of saliva and higher alkalinity of the submandibular saliva may contribute to the increased incidence of sialoliths in the submandibular salivary gland. These patients are also more susceptible for nephrolithiasis.

Differential diagnoses of well-defined radio-opacities in the floor of the mouth region include sialolithiasis, phleboliths, calcification of lymph nodes, dystrophic calcification leading to calcification of muscles and myositis ossificans, tonsilloliths, calcified arterial atheromas and elongated styloid process.

A patient with sialolithiasis may present with a history of recurrent swelling of the gland region specifically aggravated during meal times. Males are more affected than females and the age range varies from 30 to 60 years. Secondary infection is common with possible spread of infection. There may be predisposing factors including underlying medical conditions such as diabetes. Any general condition which contributes for dehydration may predispose to salivary stasis and calculi formation. In a certain percentage of patients, there may be concurrent renal stone formation. If the cause has not been treated early, there will be irreversible destruction in the gland leading to chronic infection and atrophy of the gland. Foul taste and smell could be features when there is acute pyogenic infection secondary to sialolithiasis. Patients may give a history of dry eyes and dry mouth in case of systemic conditions such as Sjogren syndrome. Drug history for anticholinergic medications, antidepressants, antihistamines is important in the case of sialolithiasis. Other relevant points that should be asked in the history include recent fever, mumps, hyposalivation with ageing, chemotherapy and radiotherapy.

The commonest site for sialolithiasis is the submandibular gland with an incidence of 84–94% followed by the parotid gland 4–10%. There may be a visible swelling of the corresponding area extra orally (a submandibular swelling or a preauricular swelling) and a bony hard lump in the gland area or the duct upon palpation. The duct orifice may be inflamed and milking out of the gland may express pus from the duct if acutely infected. Bimanually palpable mass in the floor of the mouth may indicate an enlarged submandibular salivary gland in contrast with an enlarged submandibular lymph node which could be mainly palpated against the medial border of the mandible extra orally. A discrete mass in the submandibular region or the floor of the mouth may indicate a salivary tumour which may give a similar clinical picture as a sialolith. Absence of pus in the case of viral infections is a contrasting feature to acute bacterial infections with abscess formation.

61.14 Differential Diagnosis of Sialolithiasis

- Sialadenitis
- Salivary gland tumour
- Submandibular lymphadenopathy

Sialadenitis or inflammation of the salivary glands is a common inflammatory condition affecting mainly major salivary glands, namely the parotid and the submandibular glands especially with sialoliths. It may present as an acute or chronic condition. During the pre-antibiotic era, sialadenitis was a much-feared life-threatening post-operative complication. When the gland is surgically removed, it shows characteristic histopathological features. The gland maintains its lobular architecture with significant acinar atrophy and associated fibrosis (◘ Fig. 61.5a). In addition, a diffuse mixed inflammatory cell infiltrate is also present. Acute sialadenitis is characterised by the presence of numerous neutrophils (◘ Fig. 61.5b).

Investigations for patients with a swelling in the floor of the mouth should include full blood count (FBC) and serum C-reactive protein (CRP) to assess possible infection and its nature and severity. Plain radiography including lower occlusal radiograph and dental panoramic tomograph (DPT) are essential to diagnose sialolithiasis. Ultrasound scan (USS) helps to assess for neoplastic disease, presence of calculi and gland destruction. Computerised tomography (CT) and magnetic resonance imaging (MRI) detect the number and location of salivary gland calculi within the glandular structure. Normal sialography and CT or MRI sialography may be therapeutic and diagnostic in certain cases with calculi and gland destruction. Scintigraphy is useful for assessment of gland destruction. Sialoendoscopy is a minimally invasive technique for the effective treatment of obstructive salivary gland disorders and other salivary gland conditions. The patient should also be investigated for any other coexisting general medical conditions.

61

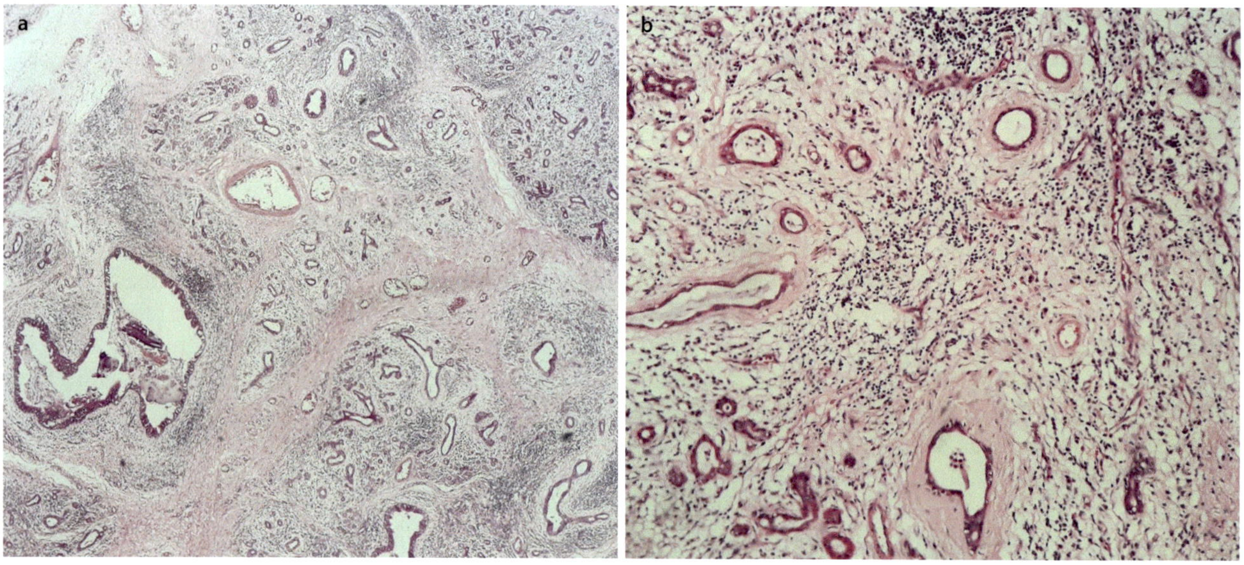

◘ **Fig. 61.5** (**a**) Atrophic salivary gland with a calculus within the dilated duct. (**b**) A patchy chronic inflammatory cell infiltrate and marked periductal fibrosis

Symptomatic treatment should be initiated especially in case of secondary infections. It is necessary to consider about hydration and nutrition. Care should be taken to prevent spread of infection that may be a threat to the airway and progress to involve the fascial spaces. A decision should be made regarding inpatient or outpatient management depending on whether the treatment necessitates the administration of intravenous (IV) antibiotics and IV fluids. In addition, patients who undergo surgical removal of the sialolith together with the involved gland and those with underlying medical conditions will need to be warded in the hospital.

Patients who do not require inpatient treatment should be managed with oral antibiotics, oral hydration together with sialogogue, massaging and removal of calculus under anaesthesia, if it is in an accessible place such as within the duct. Latest techniques for the management of sialoliths include sialoendoscopy-assisted sialolithectomy, basket retrieval, lithotripsy and balloon inflation of the duct.

Lithotripsy techniques may involve either intracorporeal or extracorporeal techniques. In intracorporeal lithotripsy, the fragmentation and removal of the salivary calculus will be performed within the salivary duct endoscopically whereas in extracorporeal lithotripsy, the sialolith will be fragmented using Extracorporeal Shock Wave Lithotripsy (ESWL) externally as an alternative to surgery preserving the gland. Following are some examples for intracorporeal techniques:

(a) Mechanical fragmentation
(b) Intracorporeal laser lithotripsy
(c) Pneumatic lithotripsy

The complications in the management of sialoliths include (a) inability to remove the stone or an associated fragment, (b) post-operative infection, (c) changes in peripheral nerve functions, (d) intra ductal adhesion formation, (e) sub-glossal scar formation, (f) sialocele formation and (g) ranula formation.

Salient features of sialolithiasis	
Clinical	• Mostly asymptomatic • Mealtime syndrome—recurrent painful swelling during mealtimes • Recurrent infection of the gland • Visible or palpable mass in the gland region • Inflammation of the duct orifice • Reduced or absent salivary flow
Histopathological	• Significant acinar atrophy and associated fibrosis with preservation of the lobular structure • Presence of neutrophil infiltration in acute sialadenitis
Treatment	• Symptomatic treatment with hydration and pain relief • Emergency surgical management and IV antibiotics ~~if~~ in case of spreading cellulitis • Management of any underlying medical conditions, e.g. Diabetes • Definitive management with surgical removal of the calculus/gland excision or other conservative methods such as intracorporeal or extracorporeal lithotripsy

61.15 Diagnostic Algorithm for Salivary Calculi

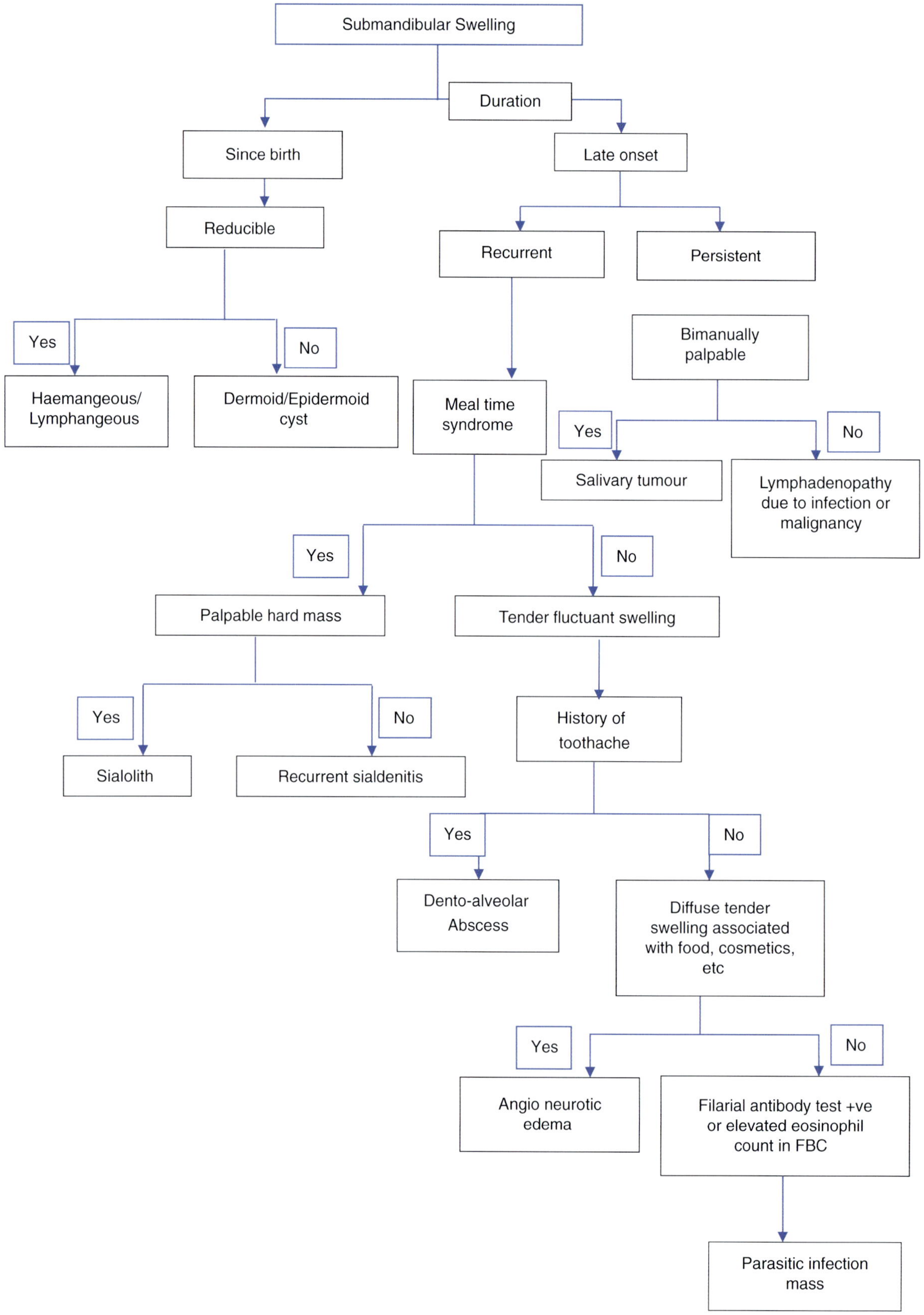

Self-Assessment Questions

1. List the symptoms suggestive of a patient presenting with a salivary calculus.
2. Explain the technique for examining a submandibular swelling to exclude a sialolith.
3. Outline the imaging modalities available and their advantages in assessing a salivary calculus.
4. Discuss the factors that determine the treatment method of a salivary calculus.
5. List the treatment options available for a salivary calculus.

Suggested Reading

Andretta M, Tregnaghi A, Prosenikliev V, Staffieri A. Current opinions in sialolithiasis diagnosis and treatment. Acta Otorhinolaryngol Ital. 2005;25(3):145–9.

Carlson ER. Diagnosis and management of salivary gland infections. Oral MaxillofacSurg Clin North Am [Internet]. 2009;21(3):293–312. https://doi.org/10.1016/j.coms.2009.04.004.

Hammett JT, Walker C. Sialolithiasis [internet]. StatPearls; 2020. p. 363–4. http://www.ncbi.nlm.nih.gov/pubmed/31751035.

Harrison JD. Causes, natural history, and incidence of salivary stones and obstructions. Otolaryngol Clin N Am. 2009;42(6):927–47.

Stelmach R, Pawłowski M, Klimek L, Janas A. Biochemical structure, symptoms, location and treatment of sialoliths. J Dent Sci [Internet]. 2016;11(3):299–303. https://doi.org/10.1016/j.jds.2016.02.007.

Turner MD. Sialoendoscopy and salivary gland sparing surgery. Oral MaxillofacSurg Clin North Am [Internet]. 2009;21(3):323–9. https://doi.org/10.1016/j.coms.2009.05.003.

Warnkulsooriya S, Tillakaratne WM. Oral medicine and pathology. p. 222–58.

A Lump on the Palate: Mucoepidermoid Carcinoma

Chuey Chuan Tan, Yet Ching Goh, and Kathreena Kadir

Contents

W. M Tilakaratne, T. G. Kallarakkal (eds.), *Clinicopathological Correlation of Oral Diseases*,
https://doi.org/10.1007/978-3-031-24408-7_62

Learning Goals

1. Devise the correct way of compiling the history with appropriate questions
2. Develop a differential diagnosis after history taking
3. Deduce appropriate procedures in clinical examination
4. Formulate a differential diagnosis combining findings in the history and clinical examination
5. Justify the relevant investigations required to arrive at the diagnosis
6. Comprehend the importance of clinicopathological correlation in arriving at the correct diagnosis
7. Outline the management plan
8. Recognize the importance of a diagnostic algorithm in arriving at a diagnosis

62.1 Main Complaint

A 25-year-old female was referred to the Oral and Maxillofacial Surgery (OMFS) clinic with an ulcerated lump on the palate.

62.2 History of Complaint

Question: How long have you been having this lump?

I have been noticing the lump on the palate for the past 6 months. It is persistent and has been growing progressively in size. However, I have noticed that the lesion has been rapidly increasing in size recently.

Question: Did you notice an ulcer on the lump? Was it there before?

I noted the ulcer on the lump; however, the ulcer just appeared around a week ago.

Question: Did you experience any toothache or pain in the jaw prior to the development of the lump?

I did not have any toothache or jaw pain prior to the development of the lump.

Question: Did you have any fever when you noted this lump?

I had an episode of fever few months ago and was given a course of antibiotics for 1 week. My family physician had advised me to consult a dentist following the course of medication as he suspected the swelling was of a dental origin. However, I forgot to get an appointment with the dentist as I wasn't having any discomfort. I only went to see a dentist when an ulcer appeared on the lump and the attending dentist referred me to the OMFS clinic.

Question: Did you experience any trauma to the facial region (i.e. a fall or get involved in any fight) prior to the swelling?

I do not have any history of trauma to the facial region.

Question: How is your current dietary habit? Have you been noticing any changes?

Ever since the ulcer appeared, I have lesser appetite and have been slowly losing weight.

Question: Did you notice any foul-smelling yellowish discharge coming from the lump before?

I don't recall any such changes.

Question: Does your nose bleed easily ever since you noticed this lump on the palate?

I do not recall any spontaneous nasal bleeding.

62.3 Past Medical, Dental and Social History

Question: Are you currently being treated for any medical problems or taking any medications prescribed by your physician?

I don't have any medical conditions and not taking any medication.

Question: Have you been admitted to the hospital before or undergone any surgical procedure?

I have not been hospitalized or undergone a surgical procedure before.

Question: Do you have any known allergies towards any types of drugs or foods?

I don't have any such allergies.

Question: Do you see your dentist regularly?

I see my dentist twice a year for dental scaling. During my last dental visit, the dentist referred me to the OMFS clinic after noticing the lump and the ulcer.

Question: Are you married and have children? What do you do for a living?

I am married and have a daughter. I teach arts for primary school children.

Question: Do you smoke or take any tobacco products?

I don't have any such habits.

Question: Do you take alcohol?

I enjoy social drinking with my friends over the weekends or over some special occasions.

Question: Do you have any specific chewing habits?

I don't have any betel quid chewing habits.

Question: Does anyone in your family have had the same condition as yours before?

No one in my family have had a similar condition before.

62.4 With the Findings from the History, What Is Your Differential Diagnosis?

1. Malignant salivary gland tumour (SGT) (Mucoepidermoid Carcinoma, Adenoid Cystic Carcinoma, or Polymorphous Adenocarcinoma)
2. Benign SGT (Pleomorphic Adenoma)
3. Odontogenic cysts or infection
4. Other soft tissue tumours such as vascular or a neural tumour

62.5 How Do You Justify Your Differential Diagnosis After History Taking?

1. A firm soft tissue swelling over the palate for a duration of 6 months would include either a benign or malignant salivary gland neoplasm like pleomorphic adenoma, mucoepidermoid carcinoma, adenoid cystic carcinoma and polymorphous adenocarcinoma. However, the posterior palatal location of an ulcerated swelling is more compatible with a malignant salivary gland neoplasm. It is supported by the fact that the swelling is persistent and rapidly increasing in size.
2. A benign salivary gland neoplasm would be the second differential diagnosis for a palatal lump such as pleomorphic adenoma as it is the most common benign salivary gland tumour. It represents 45–75% of all salivary gland tumours. Nevertheless, the occurrence in minor salivary glands is only less than 10%.
3. A lump on the palate may resemble an odontogenic cyst such as a radicular cyst or a dental abscess. A brief episode of fever may indicate an odontogenic infection or an infected odontogenic cyst. However, they are listed last in the differential diagnosis as the patient gave a negative history for any toothache prior to the swelling or foul discharge from the lump.
4. A firm soft tissue lump on the palate should include a vascular or soft tissue tumour such as a haemangioma or a leiomyoma in the differential diagnosis. However, leiomyoma is common in individuals over 30 years old and affects males more than females. Haemangioma is unlikely in this case as it is usually congenital in nature. The lesion is compressible with well-circumscribed or sometimes diffuse appearance. A negative history of bleeding from the ulcerated mucosa over the lump excludes the likeliness of haemangioma as the diagnosis. A traumatic neuroma can be excluded as patient denied any history of a traumatic injury.

62.6 Findings of Examination

The patient is well nourished and looks otherwise healthy without any apparent distress. There is no facial asymmetry or swelling. She has an exophytic growth over the right posterior lateral part of hard palate measuring about 2.0 × 1.5 cm in size (Fig. 62.1). There is an ulcer measuring about 1.0 cm at the centre of the

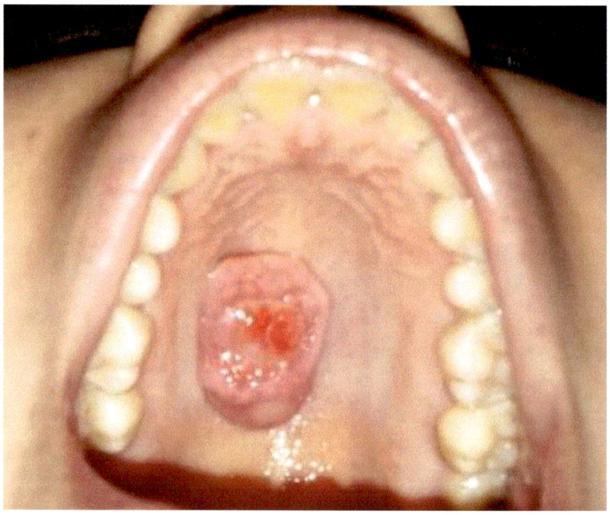

Fig. 62.1 An exophytic growth over the right palate with surface ulceration

lump. The growth is pinkish with slight bluish colour at the posterior inferior region with well-defined margins. Upon palpation, the growth is firm in consistency, non-tender, non-pulsatile and is not warm. The dentition is in good condition.

62.7 What Other Relevant Features Would You Look for with the Findings You Have So Far?

A malignant tumour has a high tendency for regional and distant metastasis. Hence, it is crucial to examine the neck in order to rule out any cervical lymphadenopathy. In this case, the patient did not present with any enlarged cervical lymph nodes.

62.8 What Is Your Clinical Differential Diagnosis?

1. Mucoepidermoid Carcinoma
2. Adenoid Cystic Carcinoma
3. Polymorphous Adenocarcinoma
4. Pleomorphic Adenoma

62.9 How Would You Exclude Other Conditions and Justify the Inclusion of the Diseases that You Have Mentioned in the Differential Diagnosis to Arrive at a Working Diagnosis?

62.9.1 Mucoepidermoid Carcinoma (MEC)

Mucoepidermoid carcinoma is the most common malignant neoplasm of salivary glands. It usually arises from parotid glands with minor salivary glands being the next common site. It is the commonest minor salivary gland malignancy. Majority of palatal mucoepidermoid carcinomas appear as painless firm swellings mimicking a mucocele or a vascular lesion. Uncommonly, it can present with pain, numbness, bleeding or paraesthesia of surrounding mucosa. The growth of the lesion can cause erosion of the underlying palatal bone. Low-grade MEC is known to display a wide variety of clinical appearances. The possibility of this lesion being a MEC is high considering the site, surface characteristics such as bluish area towards one area and surface ulceration. Further, a relatively short duration of the lesion also suggests that it may be a malignancy.

62.9.2 Adenoid Cystic Carcinoma

Adenoid cystic carcinoma is a rare tumour accounting for <1% of all head and neck tumours and about <10% of salivary gland tumours. It is frequently found in those in fifth to sixth decades of life without gender predilection. It commonly affects major salivary glands like parotid and submandibular glands and minor salivary glands over the palate, floor of mouth, lip and tongue. The clinical presentation of adenoid cystic carcinoma will be more aggressive in nature. However, it is difficult to exclude the possibility of adenoid cystic carcinoma with certainty in this case.

62.9.3 Polymorphous Adenocarcinoma

Polymorphous adenocarcinoma is usually found in the minor salivary glands especially on the palate, buccal mucosa and lips even though it can be found at any another site in the oral cavity. It is the second most common malignant tumour of minor salivary glands after mucoepidermoid carcinoma. It occurs over a wide age range with a female predilection particularly in the fourth to fifth decades of life. Its clinical behaviour is similar to other minor salivary gland tumours. It is normally described as a slow growing painless mass with intact overlying mucosa and size ranging from 1 to 4 cm. This tumour can infiltrate the underlying bony tissue. Nevertheless, the existing evidences are inadequate to rule out the diagnosis of polymorphous adenocarcinoma in this case.

62.9.4 Pleomorphic Adenoma

Pleomorphic adenoma is the commonest salivary gland tumour in the head and neck region in both adults and children. It commonly affects individuals in their fourth to sixth decades of life with a female predilection. Majority of the pleomorphic adenomas arise from parotid glands (50–70%), followed by submandibular/sublingual glands (40–60%) and minor salivary glands (10%). Intra-oral pleomorphic adenomas usually present on the palate, buccal mucosa or lips. On the palate, it occurs over the posterior-lateral region unlike midline swellings such as torus palatinus, which usually is located at the centre of the hard palate. The typical presentation of pleomorphic adenoma is a slow progressively enlarging, painless mass/swelling that rarely causes skin or mucosal ulceration. However, features such as recent ulceration and rapid growth as seen in this case are unlikely for pleomorphic adenoma.

62.10 What Is the Most Likely Diagnosis?

Mucoepidermoid carcinoma, however the possibility of other salivary gland malignancies cannot be excluded completely.

62.11 How Would You Investigate This Patient?

- Biopsy for histopathological examination (HPE)
- Radiographic investigation once HPE results are known

62.12 How Would You Biopsy the Lesion? What Are the Important Considerations?

There are several options available to biopsy lesions involving salivary glands. In a situation where there is no apparent ulceration/lesion whereby the tumour appears as a nodular swelling, we can opt to perform fine needle aspiration cytology (FNAC). For major salivary glands, the FNAC could be carried out either from an intra-oral or extra-oral approach depending on which area the swelling is more apparent. However, in this case, presence of ulcer over the lump mandates for an incisional biopsy. An incisional biopsy is helpful to grade the degree of malignancy which is difficult to achieve with an FNAC. An important consideration when performing the biopsy is that the specimen should be taken from the lesion proper with a margin of adjacent normal palatal mucosa.

62.13 Biopsy Report Confirms the Previous Clinical Diagnosis of Mucoepidermoid Carcinoma. What Are the Histopathological Features that Will Help in the Diagnosis?

Histopathological evaluation shows an unencapsulated and infiltrative tumour (◘ Fig. 62.2) with predominant mucous-producing cells and less frequent intermediate cells and epidermoid cells with prominent cystic areas and occasional solid growth pattern (◘ Fig. 62.3). Eosinophilic coagulum is seen within the cystic spaces (◘ Fig. 62.4). The solid area is mainly arranged into lobules, separated by fibrous/hyalinized stroma. Mitoses or areas of necrosis are not evident. A diagnosis low-grade mucoepidermoid carcinoma is considered in view of the predominance of mucous cells, cystic areas and inconspicuous cellular atypia.

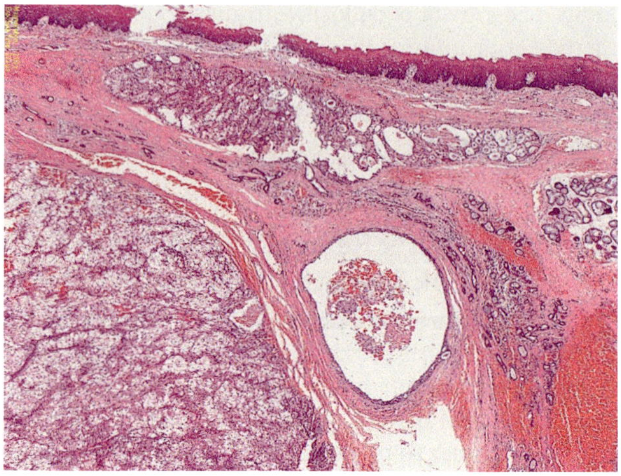

◘ **Fig. 62.2** Histopathological examination shows an infiltrative and unencapsulated tumour

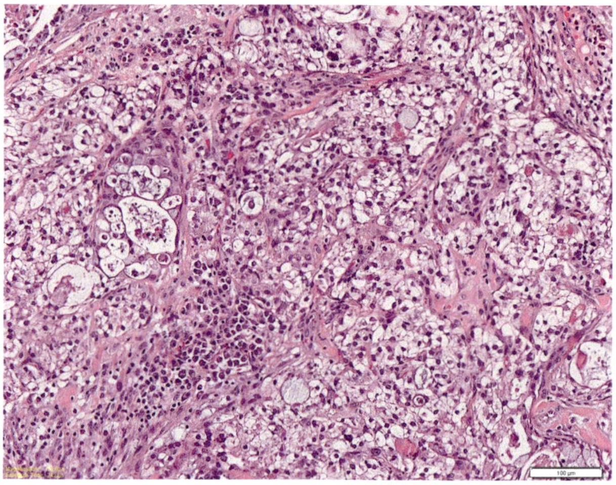

◘ **Fig. 62.3** The tumour is mucous cell-rich, admixed with lesser proportions of intermediate and epidermoid cells arranged into sheets

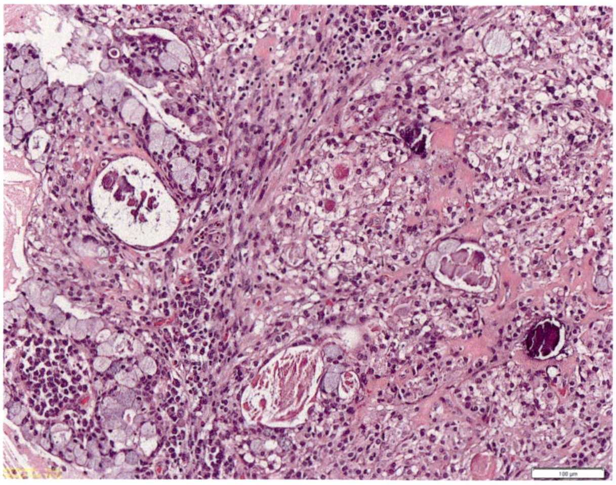

◘ **Fig. 62.4** Multiple cystic spaces containing eosinophilic coagulum

62.14 What Would Be the Best Imaging Modality to Investigate This Lesion?

Magnetic resonance (MR) imaging would be the best choice of modality to view any lesions or tumour involving the salivary gland compared to both computerized tomography (CT) scans and ultrasonography. However, when the lesion involves a nearby bony structure such as the palate, a CT is best to rule out any bone erosion/infiltration of the lesion.

62.15 How Would You Manage This Patient?

MEC is a malignant salivary gland tumour. Hence, surgery is still the best treatment of choice. Prior to surgery, a baseline blood investigation is carried out in order to rule out any underlying medical illness. A CT with contrast media is helpful in identifying local extension and distant metastasis. Wide local excision with tumour-free margins of 1 cm and local palatal flap reconstruction was performed for this case (◘ Fig. 62.5a, b). Prophylactic neck dissection was not performed as this was a stage I tumour and histologically a low-grade MEC. Histopathological examination of the surgical specimen confirmed the diagnosis of low-grade MEC with free margin of more than 5 mm. This patient is on her periodical follow-up in the clinic (◘ Fig. 62.6).

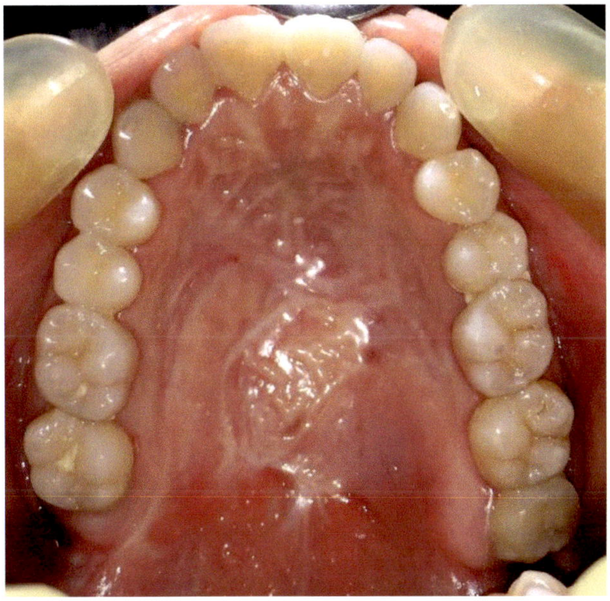

◘ **Fig. 62.6** 6 months post-operative appearance of the palatal defect, well-healed with no signs of recurrence

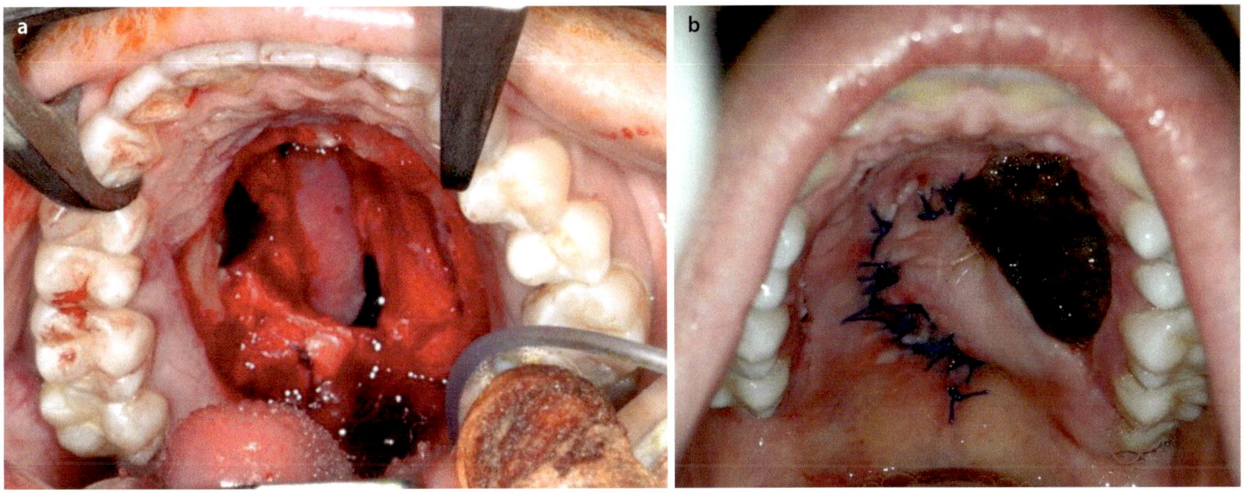

◘ **Fig. 62.5** (**a**) Wide surgical excision of MEC over the palate with 1 cm free margin. (**b**) Post-excision defect over the palate reconstructed with a palatal flap

62.16 Mucoepidermoid Carcinoma

Masson and Berger in 1924 were the first to describe MEC as mucoepidermoid tumour. Subsequently, it was popularized by Steward et al. in 1945 who introduced it as a different entity of salivary gland tumours. Mucoepidermoid carcinoma (MEC) accounts for about 10% of all salivary gland tumours. However, it represents almost 30% of all malignant tumours of salivary glands. MEC not only involves the major salivary glands (60%), but it also occurs in minor salivary glands (35%) and other locations (5%). MEC has a predilection for parotid glands, minor salivary glands in the buccal mucosa followed by palate, maxillary antrum, tongue, gingiva and floor of the mouth. Rarely, it arises in an intraosseous location in both maxilla and mandible. It occurs at any age but most frequently during the third to fifth decades of life with a slight female predominance. The aetiology of MEC of salivary glands remains unknown and neither oncogenic viruses nor chemical carcinogens are found to be associated with MEC. Nevertheless, the pre-exposure to ionizing radiation can be a contributing factor for the occurrence of MEC. An increased relative risk of 9.3 has been reported for atomic bomb survivors exposed to ionizing radiation in Hiroshima and Nagasaki to develop MEC. The occurrence of MEC was proportionate to the exposing doses of radiation. MEC has been reported in patients who received ionizing radiotherapy to head and neck region for other neoplastic conditions.

Genomic analysis has identified that t (11;19) translocation of CRTC1-MAML2 is the protein involved in tumourigenesis for about 40–60% of MEC cases. The CRTC1-related CREB-Regulated Transcription Coactivator 1 binding protein plays an important role in initialization of MEC. CRTC1 is also known as mucoepidermoid carcinoma translocated 1 gene. It causes disruption of the cell-cycle by expressing the CRTC1 protein in the morphogenesis phase of SMG epithelia, missing in differentiation phase and emerges again in MEC. The mutation of somatic TP53 and POU6F2 genes is also believed to be involved in the pathogenesis of MEC.

Low- and intermediate-grade MECs may appear as slow-growing rubbery/soft masses, whilst high-grade MEC generally presents as a rapidly expanding mass. Majority of the cases present as asymptomatic swellings and only minority experience pain sensation. MEC in parotid or submandibular glands generally presents as a solitary mass localized to preauricular or submandibular region with fixation of the mass either to skin or underlying deep tissue. Occasionally, partial or complete facial nerve palsy with skin ulceration is reported in high-grade MEC. MECs arising from minor salivary glands shows a wide variation in presentation. It is often mistaken as a benign tumour or inflammatory condition. MEC can appear as bluish fluctuant/firm, smooth surface swelling mimicking a mucocele. Other symptoms like dysphagia, dysphonia, paraesthesia, ulceration and bleeding have been reported depending on the location of the MEC. Cervical lymph node involvement related to metastasis in MEC is about 29%. It commonly occurs in MEC of submandibular glands and recurrent high-grade parotid tumours compared to tumours of minor salivary gland origin.

The morphologic features in the FNA smears of MEC show variable cellularity. In low-grade tumours, fragments of epidermoid cells, mucous cells in a background of mucinophages, mucin and nuclear debris can be seen (Fig. 62.7a, b). High-grade tumours are more cellular, with poorly cohesive clusters and singly scattered squamous cells with moderate to abundant eosino-

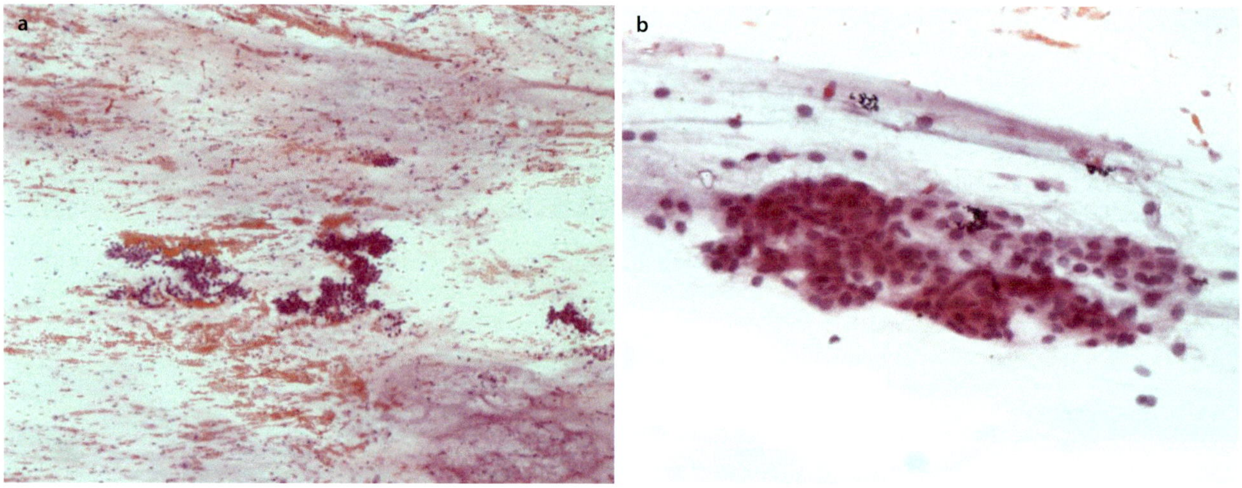

Fig. 62.7 (a) Clusters of epithelial cells in abundant background mucin Pap stain 10×. (b) Epidermoid cells and mucin-producing cells in streams of mucin. Pap stain 40×

philic cytoplasm, pleomorphic hyperchromatic nuclei and mitosis.

The histopathological features of MEC show an unencapsulated tumour containing varying proportions of epidermoid, intermediate and mucous-secreting cells. Mucous cells are predominant in low-grade tumours whilst epidermoid cells/squamoid cells predominate in high-grade tumours. Intermediate cells and clear cells are also present in varying proportions. The amount of cystic areas, number of mitosis, anaplasia, vascular/neural invasion and presence of necrosis are important features in grading the tumours into low-, intermediate- and high-grade. ◻ Table 62.1 shows the histopathological features of different grades of MEC.

All these three classifications use similar parameters. Nevertheless, the AFIP system tend to 'down-grade' the intermediate group of MEC into low-grade while the Brandwein system upgrades the staging of intermediate-grade MEC. These differences might affect the therapeutic choices and prognostic outcomes of the tumour.

Immunohistochemical stains are helpful in the diagnosis of MEC in some cases where it mimics the appearance of other tumours. MEC usually shows positive reactivity for Cytokeratin 5/6/7/8/14/18/19, EMA, carcinoembryonic antigen (CEA) and p63. CK7 shows higher reactivity in luminal cells and intermediate cells. p63 staining often shows strong staining in the epidermoid cell component. p63 staining is used to differentiate MEC from acinic cell carcinoma, unusual mucous retention cyst and papillary cystadenomas of salivary glands. The high expression of PCNA and other proliferative markers are associated with poorer prognosis.

The diagnosis of MEC is a challenge as majority of these cases are asymptomatic. More than two-thirds of MEC cases are diagnosed when disease has progressed to advanced stages. It has been shown that 55.9% of the cases are in stage III due to local-regional dissemination at the time of diagnosis. Staging affects the survival rate and treatment outcomes. The clinical staging of MEC is shown in ◻ Table 62.2.

◻ Table 62.1 Histopathological features of different grades of MEC (Adapted from Seethala 2009)

Modified healey (qualitative)	AFIP (point based)	Brandwein (point based)
Low-grade • Macrocysts, microcysts, transition with excretory ducts • Differentiated mucin-producing epidermoid cells, often in a 1:1 ratio; minimal to moderate intermediate cell population • Daughter cyst proliferation from large cysts • Minimal to absent pleomorphism, rare mitoses • Broad-front, often circumscribed invasion • Pools of extravasated mucin with stromal reaction	• Intracystic component <20% = 2 pts • Neural invasion present = 2 pts • Necrosis present = 3 pts	• Intracystic component <25% = 2 pts • Tumour invades in small nests and islands = 2 pts • Pronounced nuclear atypia = 3 pts
Intermediate-grade • No macrocysts, few microcysts, solid nests of cells • Large duct not conspicuous • Slight to moderate pleomorphism, few mitoses, prominent nuclei and nucleoli • Invasive quality, usually well- defined and uncircumscribed • Chronic inflammation at periphery, fibrosis separates nests of cells and groups of nests	• Mitosis (4 or more per 10 HPF) = 3 pts • Anaplasia = 4 pts	• Lymphatic and/or vascular invasion = 3 pts • Bony invasion = 3 pts • >4 mitoses per 10 HPF = 3 pts
High-grade • No macrocysts, predominantly solid but may be nearly all glandular • Cell constituents range from poorly differentiated to recognizable epidermoid and intermediate to ductal type adenocarcinoma • Considerable pleomorphism, easily found mitoses • Unquestionable soft tissue, perineural and intravascular invasion • Chronic inflammation less prominent, desmoplasia of stroma may outline invasive cluster		• Perineural spread = 3 pts • Necrosis = 3 pts
	Low-grade = 0–4 pts Intermediate-grade = 5–6 pts High-grade = 7–14 pts	Low-grade = 0 pts Intermediate-grade = 2–3 pts High-grade = 4 or more pts

Table 62.2 Staging of salivary tumours according to AJCC 8th, 2018

Tumour (T)	• T1: Tumour 2 cm or smaller in greatest dimension without extraparenchymal extension • T2: Tumour larger than 2 cm but not larger than 4 cm in greatest dimension without extraparenchymal extension • T3: Tumour larger than 4 cm and/or tumour having extraparenchymal extension • T4a: Moderately advanced. Tumour invades skin, mandible, ear canal and/or facial nerve • T4b: Very advanced disease. Tumour invades skull base and/or pterygoid plates and/or encases carotid artery
Lymph node (N)	• N0: No regional lymph node metastasis • N1: Metastasis in a single ipsilateral lymph node, 3 cm or smaller in greatest dimension and ENE (−) • N2a: Metastasis in a single ipsilateral node larger than 3 cm but not larger than 6 cm in greatest dimension and ENE (−) • N2b: Metastases in multiple ipsilateral lymph nodes, none larger than 6 cm in greatest dimension and ENE (−) • N2c: Metastases in bilateral or contralateral lymph nodes, none larger than 6 cm in greatest dimension and ENE (−) • N3a: Metastasis in a lymph node larger than 6 cm in greatest dimension and ENE (−) • N3b: Metastasis in any node(s) with clinically overt ENE (+)
Metastasis (M)	• M0: No distant metastasis • M1: Distant metastasis • M2: Distant metastasis, microscopically confirmed
Overall stage	• I—T1N0 • II—T2 N0 • III—T3 N0–1, or T1–3 N1 • IVA—T4a N0–2, or T1-4a N2 • IVB—T4b N0–3, or T1-4b N3 • IVC—M1

Metastases of MEC to regional lymph nodes or distant site occur in about 15–35% of cases. Primary tumour location and histological grading are two key factors affecting the risk of metastases to cervical lymph nodes. It has been revealed that lymph node metastases are more common in males, high-grade tumours and lesions originating from submandibular glands and parotid glands rather than minor salivary glands. MEC of submandibular glands always behave aggressively and local resection with tumour-free margins is difficult to achieve due to surrounding vital structures.

Surgery remains the standard treatment modality in managing MEC. Wide surgical excision with 1 cm margin is recommended to prevent recurrence. Prophylactic neck dissection is proposed for high histological grade, clinically T3/T4 tumours or proximity of tumour to regional lymph nodes. Adjuvant therapy like chemoradiotherapy is recommended for patients with high-grade tumours, positive tumour margins and extra-nodal extension. The possible surgical complications include risk of failure on regional reconstruction of post-radical excisional defect, facial nerve palsy, Frey's syndrome, wound infection and others.

The survival rate of MEC depends mainly on the disease stage, histopathological grading and the site of involvement. The reported 5-year survival rate for low-grade MEC can be as high as 90–100% excluding the submandibular gland. The 5-year disease-free survival rate for high-grade and low-grade MEC is 22.5% and 97.0% respectively. In general, low- to intermediate-grade of MEC is associated with a better prognosis compared to high-grade tumours. The palatal MEC may metastasize to skull base and respiratory tract while advanced stage MEC can involve the brain, liver, lung and bones. The late recurrence and metastasis in malignant salivary gland tumour are a well-known fact, thus patients are required to be on long-term follow-up after treatment.

62.17 Diagnostic Algorithm

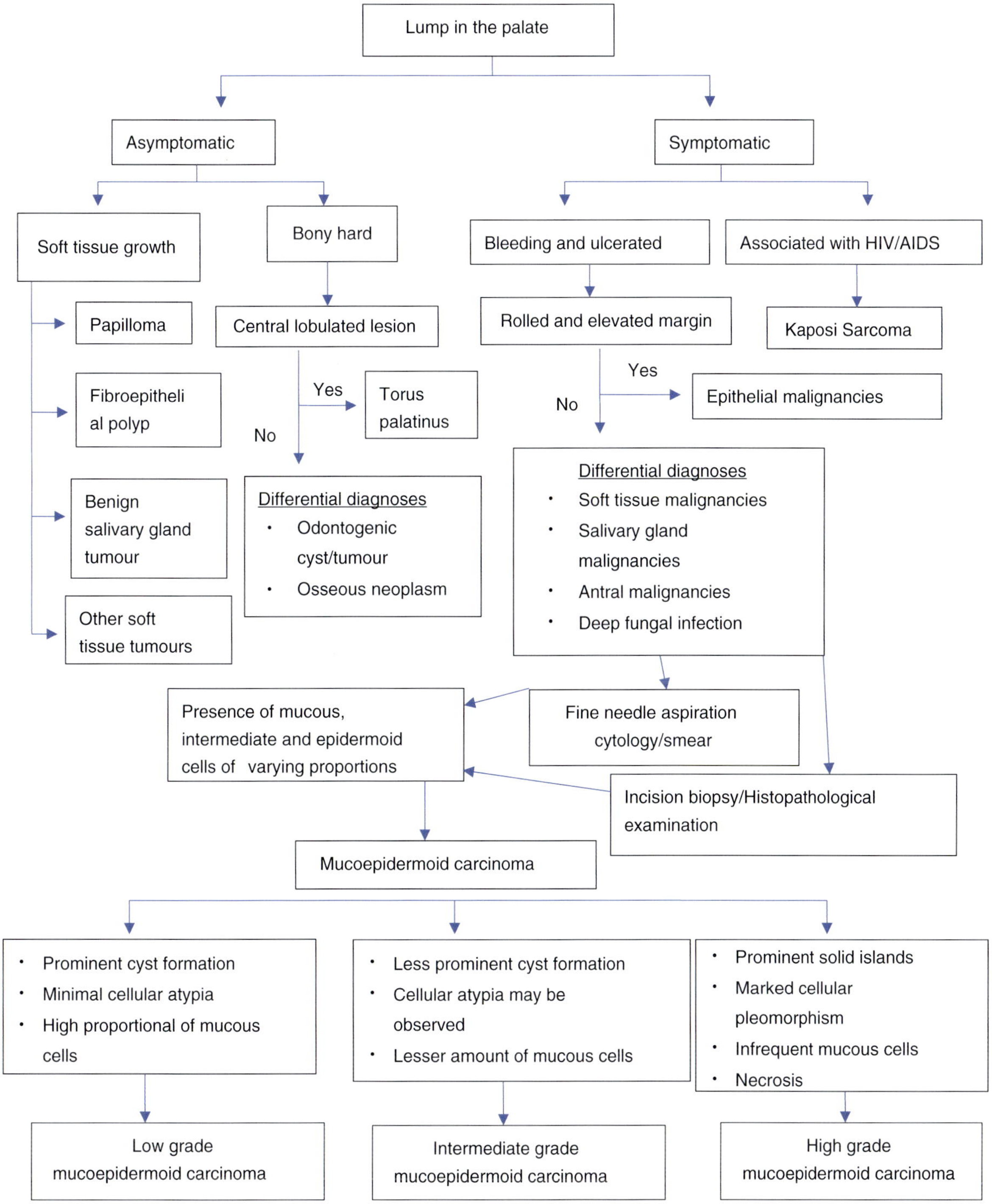

Self-Assessment Questions

1. List the pathognomonic clinical features of MEC.
2. State the important conditions that need to be included in the differential diagnosis for MEC.
3. Describe the histopathological features of MEC.
4. Outline the grading of MEC.
5. Outline the management plan according to the stage of the disease.

Summary

Diagnostic dilemma of a lump on the palate could be solved with proper history taking and investigations. Mucoepidermoid carcinoma should be considered in the differential diagnosis of a palatal lump for early diagnosis and optimal care.

Suggested Reading

Amin MB, Edge SB, Greene FL, et al., editors. AJCC cancer staging manual. 8th ed. New York: Springer; 2017.

Brandwein MS, Ivanov K, Wallace DI, Hille JJ, Wang B, Fahmy A, Bodian C, Urken ML, Gnepp DR, Huvos A, Lumerman H. Mucoepidermoid carcinoma: a clinicopathologic study of 80 patients with special reference to histological grading. Am J Surg Pathol. 2001;25(7):835–45.

Chou C, Zhu G, Luo M, Xue G. Carcinoma of the minor salivary glands: results of surgery and combined therapy. J Oral Maxillofac Surg. 1996;54:448–53. https://doi.org/10.1016/S0278-2391(96)90119-6.

Cornog JL. Surgical and clinical pathology of salivary gland tumours. In: Rankow RM, Polayes IM, editors. Diseases of the salivary glands; 1976. p. 99–142.

Gao M, Hao Y, Huang MX, Ma DQ, Chen Y, Luo HY, et al. Salivary gland tumours in a northern Chinese population: a 50-year retrospective study of 7190 cases. Int J Oral Maxillofac Surg. 2017;46:343–9. https://doi.org/10.1016/j.ijom.2016.09.021.

Land CE, Saku T, Hayashi Y, Takahara O, Matsuura H, Tokuoka S, Tokunaga M, Mabuchi K. Incidence of salivary gland tumours among atomic bomb survivors, 1950–1987. Evaluation of radiation-related risk. Radiat Res. 1996;146(1):28–36.

Lanzel E, Robinson RA, Zimmerman MB, Pourian A, Hellstein JW. The use of immunohistochemistry in detection of perineural invasion in mucoepidermoid carcinoma. Oral Surg Oral Med Oral Pathol Oral Radiol. 2016;121:636–42. https://doi.org/10.1016/j.oooo.2016.01.026.

Luna MA. Salivary mucoepidermoid carcinoma: revisited. Adv Anat Pathol. 2006;13(6):293–307. https://doi.org/10.1097/01.pap.0000213058.74509.d3.

Martínez-Madrigal F, Pineda-Daboin K, Casiraghi O, Luna MA. Salivary gland tumours of the mandible. Ann Diagn Pathol. 2000;4(6):347–53.

Peraza A, Gomez R, Beltran J, Amarista FJ. Mucoepidermoid carcinoma. An update and review of the literature. J Stomatol Oral Maxillofac Surg. 2020; https://doi.org/10.1016/j.jormas.2020.06.003.

Seethala RR. An update on grading of salivary gland carcinomas. Head Neck Pathol. 2009;3(1):69–77.

Spiro RH, Huvos AG, Berk R, et al. Mucoepidermoid carcinoma of salivary gland origin. A clinicopathologic study of 367 cases. Am J Surg. 1978;136:461–8.

Stewart FW, Foote FW, Becker WF. Muco-epidermoid tumours of salivary glands. Ann Surg. 1945;122(5):820.

Whatley WS, Thompson JW, Rao B. Salivary gland tumours in survivors of childhood cancer. Otolaryngol Head Neck Surg. 2006;134(3):385–8.

Zhu S, Schuerch C, Hunt J. Review and updates of immunohistochemistry in selected salivary gland and head and neck tumours. Arch Pathol Lab Med. 2015;139(1):55–66.

Orofacial Syndromes

Contents

Multiple Asymptomatic Cysts in the Jaws: Naevoid Basal Cell Carcinoma Syndrome

Nadeena S. S. Jayasuriya and Wanninayake M Tilakaratne

Contents

W. M Tilakaratne, T. G. Kallarakkal (eds.), *Clinicopathological Correlation of Oral Diseases*,
https://doi.org/10.1007/978-3-031-24408-7_63

Learning Goals

1. Devise the correct way of compiling the history with appropriate questions
2. Develop a differential diagnosis after history taking
3. Deduce appropriate procedures in clinical examination
4. Formulate a differential diagnosis combining findings in the history and clinical examination
5. Justify the relevant investigations required to arrive at the diagnosis
6. Comprehend the importance of clinicopathological correlation in arriving at the correct diagnosis
7. Outline the management plan
8. Recognise the importance of a diagnostic algorithm in arriving at a diagnosis

63.1 Main Complaint

A 32-year-old lady presented to the clinic complaining of a swelling and discomfort on her left posterior upper jaw.

63.2 History of Complaint

Question: When did you first notice this?

I felt the discomfort 5 months ago and the swelling was very insignificant.

63.3 Additional Complaints

Question: Have you had pain from that area?

I have never had any pain related to that area.

Question: Do you have pain in the teeth on that side when eating?

I don't have any pain in the teeth on that side during eating.

Question: Have you felt that your upper left teeth are loose or shaking?

I have not felt any abnormality in my teeth.

Question: Have you felt any discharge from that area?

I have had no symptoms to suggest a discharge from the area.

Question: Have you felt any unusual taste in the mouth?

I have not felt any unusual taste in the mouth.

Question: Do you feel that your left side nostril is blocked?

I don't feel that my left nostril is blocked.

Question: Have you experienced bleeding from your nose or heaviness on that side of the face?

I have had no such symptoms before.

Question: Do you feel a numbness over your left side cheek?

I have a normal sensation over the skin on my left cheek.

Question: Do you feel that you can open your mouth normally?

I can open my mouth normally.

Question: Do you have any other swellings in your jaws?

Apart from the swelling on the left side, I don't have any other problems in my mouth or jaws. I have a small lump on my left upper eyelid. It is slowly enlarging and is not painful.

Question: Did you have any previous illnesses or surgeries?

I had a small lump removed from my hand 5 years ago. But I don't have any biopsy report for the same.

Question: Do you have any family history of such diseases?

My father had undergone multiple surgeries in his jaws and on the skin. I don't know the diagnosis of my father's illness. My father passed away 2 years ago due to a cardiovascular complication.

63.4 With the Findings from the History, What Is Your Differential Diagnosis?

1. Odontogenic cyst; Dentigerous cyst, odontogenic keratocyst with Gorlin-goltz syndrome (GGS)
2. Benign odontogenic tumour
3. Fibrous dysplasia or other fibro-osseous lesion affecting the left side maxillary bone
4. Neoplasm of the left side maxillary antrum

63.5 How Do You Justify Your Differential Diagnosis After History Taking?

The patient has no significant symptoms. She has no dental problems and no pain and signs of inflammation to suggest an odontogenic infection.

The most common reason for the patient's complaint would be an odontogenic cyst or an odontogenic tumour. As these lesions can grow into the maxillary antrum, cysts and tumours may not show a significant bony swelling. They are slow growing and can be asymptomatic in the early stages. A dentigerous cyst related to an impacted left upper third molar or an odontogenic keratocyst (OKC) are most likely differential diagnoses. The patient mentioned about a soft tissue lump that was removed from her arm and also currently has a similar lesion on her left upper eyelid. In addition, she also gives a family history of jaw and skin surgeries for her father. Considering these facts, GGS should be suspected.

Odontogenic tumours may cause some symptoms and should be included in the differential diagnosis. Tumours can grow into the maxillary sinus and the swelling may not be significant as in this patient. However, mobility of teeth and pain are frequently associated symptoms with odontogenic tumours though it can also be seen in cysts.

63

Monostotic fibrous dysplasia (MFD) affects the maxillary bone and can appear as an asymptomatic bony swelling. MFD usually occurs at a much younger age and affects the maxillary bone and other adjacent bones appearing as a facial swelling. Even though it affects young individuals, it may only be diagnosed in the second or third decades of life. The possibility of other fibro-osseous lesions such as ossifying fibroma and cemento-osseous dysplasias should also be considered.

Bony swellings (buccal and palatal) can appear due to neoplastic lesions of the maxillary antrum. Maxillary swelling, mobility of teeth and symptoms of sinus obstruction and nerve involvement would be expected from such lesions. These are absent in this patient making it an unlikely differential diagnosis.

63.6 Findings of Clinical Examination

The patient's mouth opening is normal. She has a very slight swelling on her upper posterior alveolar region on the left side. The area is non-tender and bony hard in consistency. The adjacent teeth have no signs of decay, mobility or any other pathology. There is no significant palatal swelling associated with the lesion. All her third molar teeth are absent clinically.

63.7 What Other Relevant Features Would You Look for with the Findings You Have So Far?

The patient is an otherwise healthy woman with a normal BMI. Her face shows frontal bossing with a mild increase in her inter-canthal distance. A well-circumscribed non-tender soft tissue lump measuring 0.5 cm in diameter is seen on her mid left upper eyelid (▢ Fig. 63.1). On her right and left hands, numerous palmar pits are noted (▢ Fig. 63.2).

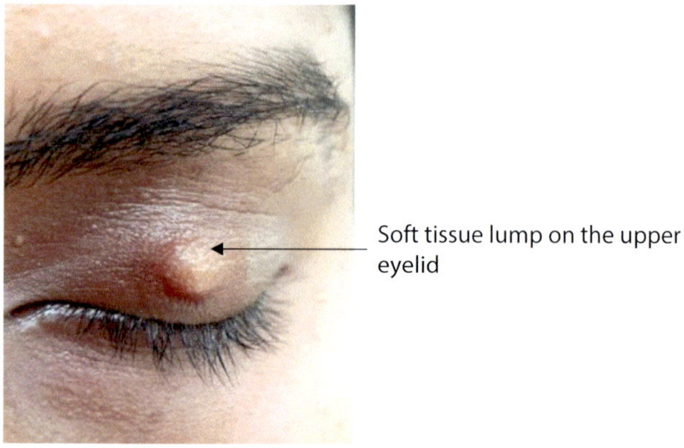

▢ **Fig. 63.1** A well-defined soft tissue lesion was found on the left side upper eyelid

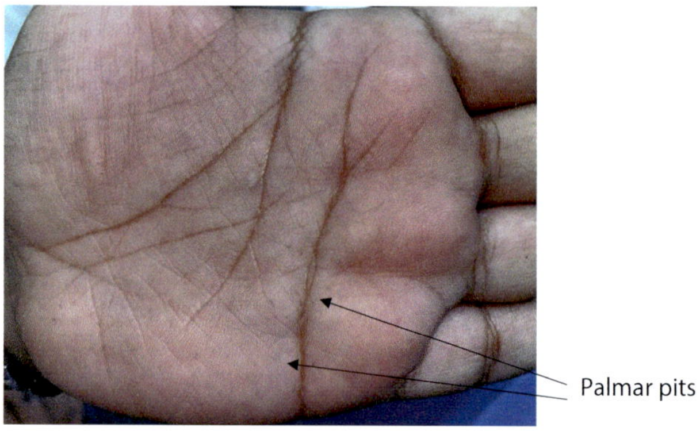

▢ **Fig. 63.2** Numerous palmar pits are seen on the palms of the patient

On general examination, two black-coloured naevi (less than 0.5–1 cm diameter) are noted on her chest region.

63.8 What Is Your Clinical Differential Diagnosis?

1. Odontogenic cyst (OKC with GGS)
2. Odontogenic tumour
3. Antral-pathology such as a tumour

63.9 How Would You Exclude Other Conditions and Justify the Inclusion of the Diseases That You Have Mentioned in the Differential Diagnosis to Arrive at a Working Diagnosis?

63.9.1 Odontogenic Cyst with Possible Gorlin-Goltz Syndrome (GGS)

Considering the fact that an obvious swelling is not noted, an odontogenic cyst extending into the maxillary sinus is very likely. The absence of a non-vital tooth, excludes a radicular cyst. As the upper third molar tooth is not seen erupted, a dentigerous cyst cannot be excluded. An odontogenic keratocyst (OKC) is also a possibility.

The family history of possible jaw and skin lesions, facial appearance (frontal bossing and increased intercanthal distance), the presence of neavi, palmar pits and the soft tissue lesion on her upper eyelid should lead to the suspicion of GGS. Therefore, an OKC would be a possible diagnosis with a suspicion of multiple asymptomatic cysts in other locations.

63.9.2 Odontogenic Tumours

Lack of bony expansion excludes odontogenic tumours such as an ameloblastoma. However, extension of the lesion into the sinus cavity is possible. Therefore, further radiographic investigations are necessary to narrow down the differential diagnoses. An early ameloblastoma extending to the maxillary sinus may also be considered in the differential diagnosis.

63.9.3 Pathology of the Maxillary Sinus

A neoplasm extending from the left maxillary antrum can be a rare possibility. The lack of obstruction in the left nostril, absence of a significant bony swelling, lack of mobility of teeth in this region and absence of any numbness over the face makes an antral pathology unlikely.

63.10 What Is the Most Likely Diagnosis?

Odontogenic keratocyst (OKC) with GGS.

63.11 How Would You Investigate This Patient?

1. Dental panoramic tomograph (DPT) / Cone Beam CT scan to exclude multiple cysts
2. Postero-anterior skull radiograph- to visualise calcifications of the falx cerebri
3. Anterio-posterior chest radiograph to identify any deformities of the ribs or clavicle
4. Excisional biopsy of the pigmented neavi on the chest
5. Biopsy of the cystic lesion/s
6. Antero-posterior and lateral radiographs of the cervical spine

63.12 What Findings Would You Expect from the Above Investigations?

The DPT and the CBCT scans show multiple cystic lesions in the posterior bilateral mandibular rami and in the posterior left side maxilla. Well-defined radiolucent lesions with a cortical border are seen involving the unerupted upper left third molar tooth (▪ Fig. 63.3). The lesions in the mandibular rami are multilocular in nature.

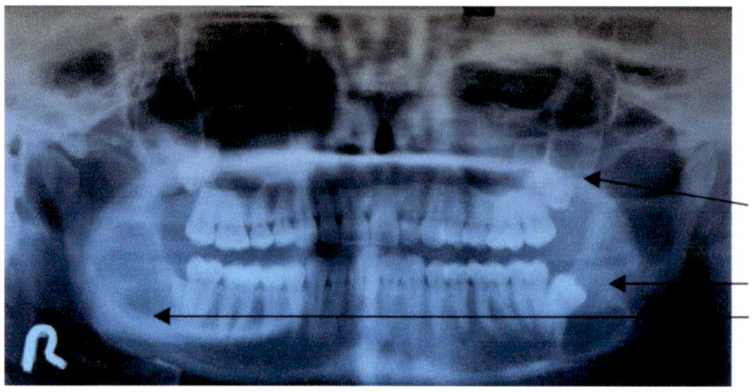

Fig. 63.3 DPT showing multiple cystic lesions in bilateral mandibular body and ramus. In addition, a cystic lesion is seen in the left posterior maxillary region

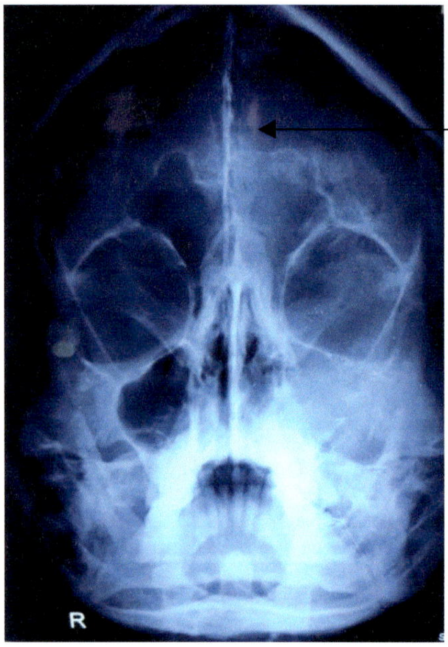

Fig. 63.4 Occipitomental view shows calcified falx cerebri

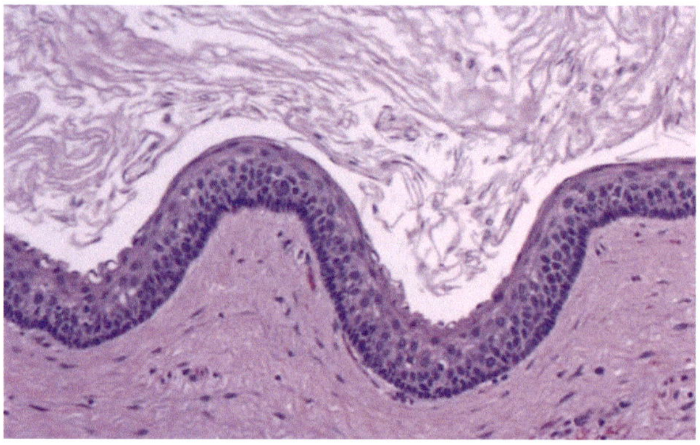

Fig. 63.5 Odontogenic Keratocyst; The hematoxylin and eosin (H&E) stained section shows thin uniform parakeratinised stratified squamous epithelium with uninflamed cyst wall. The cyst lumen contains keratin

Postero-anterior skull radiograph shows a radio-opaque line on the mid skull region which denotes the calcification of the falx cerebri (Fig. 63.4).

The chest radiographs showed no anomalies of ribs and clavicles.

Histopathology of the right maxillary cyst confirmed the diagnosis of an OKC.

Histopathology of the pigmented lesions confirmed the diagnosis of early basal cell naevi.

63.13 What Are the Histopathological Features of the Biopsy from the Cystic Lesion?

The fibrous cyst wall is lined by parakeratinised stratified squamous epithelium showing a corrugated surface. Marked palisading of the basal cell is evident. The cyst wall is uninflamed and contains daughter cysts in some areas. The lumen contains keratin material. These histopathological features confirm the diagnosis of an OKC (Fig. 63.5).

63.14 How Would You Confirm the Diagnosis of GGS?

GGS is diagnosed based on the presence of two major or one major and two minor criteria (Table 63.1). This patient has multiple odontogenic cysts, a strong family history and calcification of the falx cerebri and palmar pits which are all major criteria. She has two basal cell naevi detected on her chest. She has an unusual fibrous growth on her upper eyelid and also a mild degree of frontal bossing, which are minor criteria. Combination of these features confirm the diagnosis of GGS.

Table 63.1 Diagnostic criteria of GGS by Evans et al. (1993)

Major criteria	Minor criteria
• Multiple basal cell carcinomas or one occurring under the age of 20 years or more than ten basal cell naevi	Congenital skeletal anomalies Bifid (Fig. 63.6), fused, or markedly splayed ribs
• Histologically proven OKCs of the jaws	Increased occipital-frontal circumference with frontal bossing
• Palmar or plantar pits (Fig. 63.7) (three or more)	Cardiac or ovarian fibromas
• Calcifications of the falx cerebri under the age of 20 years	Medulloblastomas
• First-degree relative with naevoid basal cell carcinoma syndrome	Lymphomesenteric cysts
	Other congenital anomalies such as cCleft lip and palate and ocular anomalies

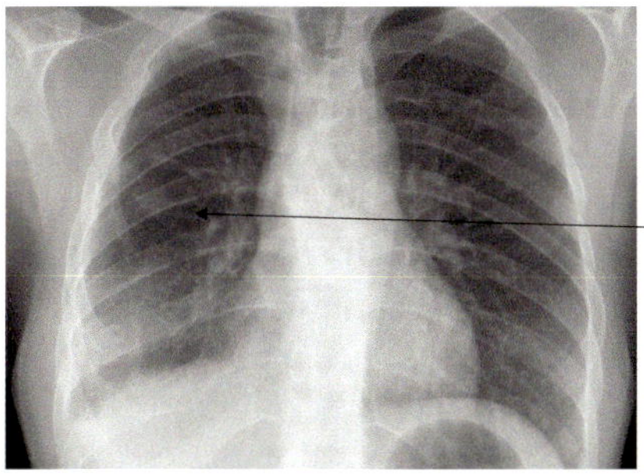

Fig. 63.6 The antero-posterior chest radiograph shows the occasional bifid ribs on the right side on a patient diagnosed with GGS (Courtesy of Dr. Ankita Chugh, Additional Professor, OMFS, Department of Dentistry, AIIMS Jodhpur, India)

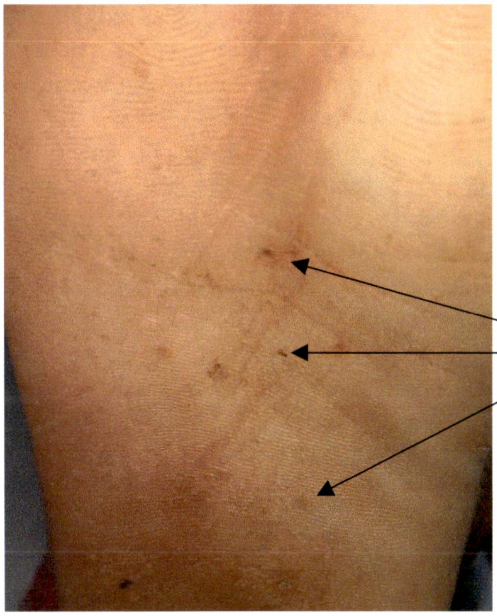

Fig. 63.7 Plantar pits seen on the sole of the foot in a patient with GGS (Courtesy of Dr. Ankita Chugh, Additional Professor, OMFS, Department of Dentistry, AIIMS Jodhpur, India)

63.15 What Other Additional Investigations Would You Perform?

Genetic testing for Human PTCH 1 gene is confirmatory of the inherited nature.

63.16 How Would You Manage This Patient?

The multiple OKCs should be enucleated with mechanical curettage and application of Carnoy's solution/liquid nitrogen to eliminate the potential residual cells of the cyst lining. Use of Carnoy's solution is a controversial issue in the recent past. Technique of dredging can also be used in larger OKCs which helps as a conservative treatment. Regular follow-up with routine radiographs is advised over a long time.

The basal cell naevi should be surgically excised as prophylaxis or kept under close observation. Patient should be followed up long term to identify any new basal cell naevi or their malignant transformation.

Other anomalies such as the fibroepithelial lesion of the upper eyelid should be surgically removed as a cosmetic treatment. The patient should be referred to a cardiologist and a gynaecologist to exclude possible cardiac and ovarian pathologies. A dermatology follow-up is essential in early diagnosis of neavi and to identify possible malignant transformation. The patient should also be referred for genetic counselling to avoid possible familial transmission.

63.17 Gorlin-Goltz Syndrome (GGS)

Multiple odontogenic keratocysts (OKC) can occur in patients with GGS, Elher-Danlos syndrome, Noonan syndrome and oro-facial digital syndrome. Apart from GGS, occurrence of multiple OKCs in other syndromes is very rare. GGS is a syndrome associated with multiple odontogenic keratocysts, basal cell carcinomas' skeletal and dental anomalies. It is also known as Naevoid Basal Cell Carcinoma Syndrome (NBCCS) or Basal Cell Naevi Syndrome (BCNS). It was first described by Robert Gorlin and William Goltz in 1958. GGS is an uncommon autosomal dominant disease with a variable inheritance and a high genetic expression. The incidence in the general population is estimated to be one in 50,000–150,000. The genetic mutation occurs in the human patch gene (PTCH 1) located on chromosome 9q in these patients. GGS usually presents at a younger age (10–30 years) and more common in females.

63

The skeletal anomalies in GGS include bifid ribs, frontal bossing and increased inter-canthal distance (hypertelorism) (Fig. 63.8). Calcification of the falx cerebri is also seen. Basal cell naevi which occur with GGS have a higher tendency to transform to basal cell carcinomas, thus it was named BCNS. The diagnosis of GGS is made when either two major or one major and two minor criteria (Table 63.1) are fulfilled.

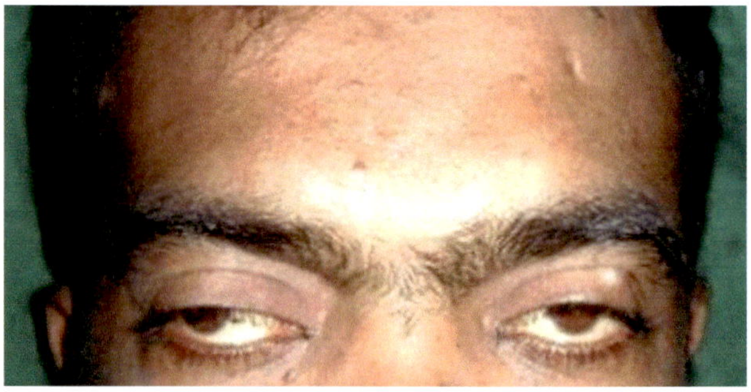

Fig. 63.8 Hypertelorism and frontal bossing seen in a man with GGS, increased inter-canthal distance due to increased interorbital distance is also observed (Courtesy of Dr. Padma Pandeshwar, Bangalore)

The OKCs that occur in GGS are said to be different from the OKCs that occur in isolation. OKCs in GGS has a higher affinity to occur in the mandible (69%) than in the maxilla (31%). In the mandible, OKCs occur mostly in the ramus region and in the maxilla it may occur in the anterior maxilla or at the maxillary tuberosity.

OKCs associated with GGS are usually diagnosed as an incidental finding. They cause minimum bony expansion as they grow along the intramedullary bone space. In some patients, symptoms such as swelling, discharges and numbness of the lower lip may occur as the cysts become larger. The treatment of OKCs at an early stage may be conservative to preserve the developing dentition. Simple enucleation and curettage (mechanical or chemical), dredging techniques cause healing or reduction in the size of lesions with less morbidity. OKCs associated with GGS are more locally aggressive and have a higher tendency for recurrence (12–62%). Lesions that do not respond to conservative treatment may require en-bloc resection and reconstruction.

The management of a patient diagnosed with GGS should focus on a holistic approach. A team of specialists should be involved in the management of each area of concern (Table 63.2).

Table 63.2 Management of GGS

Disease manifestation	Clinical presentation	Investigations	Management
Multiple OKCs	Multiple swellings in bilateral maxillae and mandible. In the early stage of the disease, they are asymptomatic and maybe an incidental finding in the DPT.	Dental panoramic tomogram Cone Beam CT scan	Surgical excision with topical methods to eliminate the potential residual cyst lining cells. Methods include – Photodynamic treatment – Carnoy's solution – Cryotherapy Recurrent OKCs may require more aggressive surgical excision.
Basal cell naevi	Pigmented lesions that appear as birthmarks.	Biopsy and histopathology	Prophylactic removal or close observation. Excision with a margin for BCC.
Skeletal anomalies	Frontal bossing, some degree of hypertelorism is seen with anomalies of the ribs and clavicle.	Skull radiographs Chest radiographs and CT scan of the chest	No treatment unless for cosmetic reasons.
Ocular manifestations	Ocular changes such as colobomas to cataracts, cysts, nystagmus.	Ophthalmological investigations	Referral to an ophthalmologist.
Skin manifestations	Skin pits (palmar pits) can occur in the palms and soles. Epidermal cysts and skin fibromas (Fig. 63.9) can occur in any part of the body.	Excision biopsy and histopathological examination	Surgical removal
Other	Calcification of the falx cerebri and medulloblastoma	Occipitomental view radiograph CT scan of the skull MRI brain	In case of intracranial medulloblastomas, neurological referral is recommended.

Salient features of Gorlin-Goltz syndrome	
Clinical/radiographical features	Family history, multiple OKCs, basal cell naevi and skin manifestations such as fibromas and epidermoid cysts, palmar plantar pits, calcification of falx cerebri and skeletal abnormalities.
Treatment	OKCs should be surgically treated and followed up for recurrences. The naevi should be removed and observed regularly for malignant transformation. Skin lesions maybe surgically removed as they can be aesthetically unpleasing.

GGS is important due to the multiple odontogenic cysts that can cause recurrences. Suspicion of this syndrome helps to diagnose these cysts at an early stage. The basal cell naevi that have a chance of malignant transformation are of a significant risk and need close follow up by a dermatologist. Genetic counselling is important for affected patients.

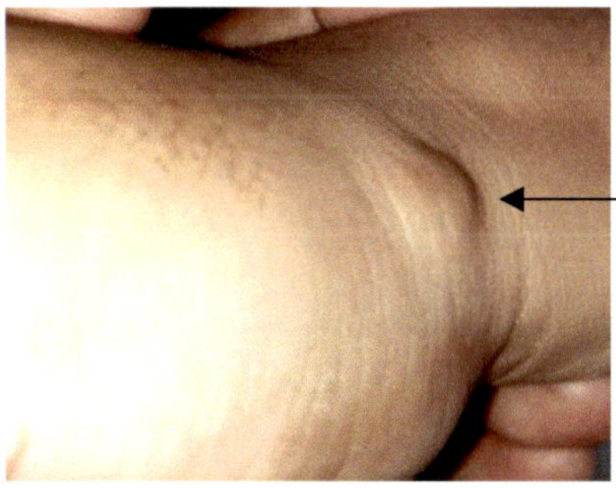

Fig. 63.9 A soft tissue lump noted in the arm of a patient suspected of GGS

63.18 Diagnostic Algorithm

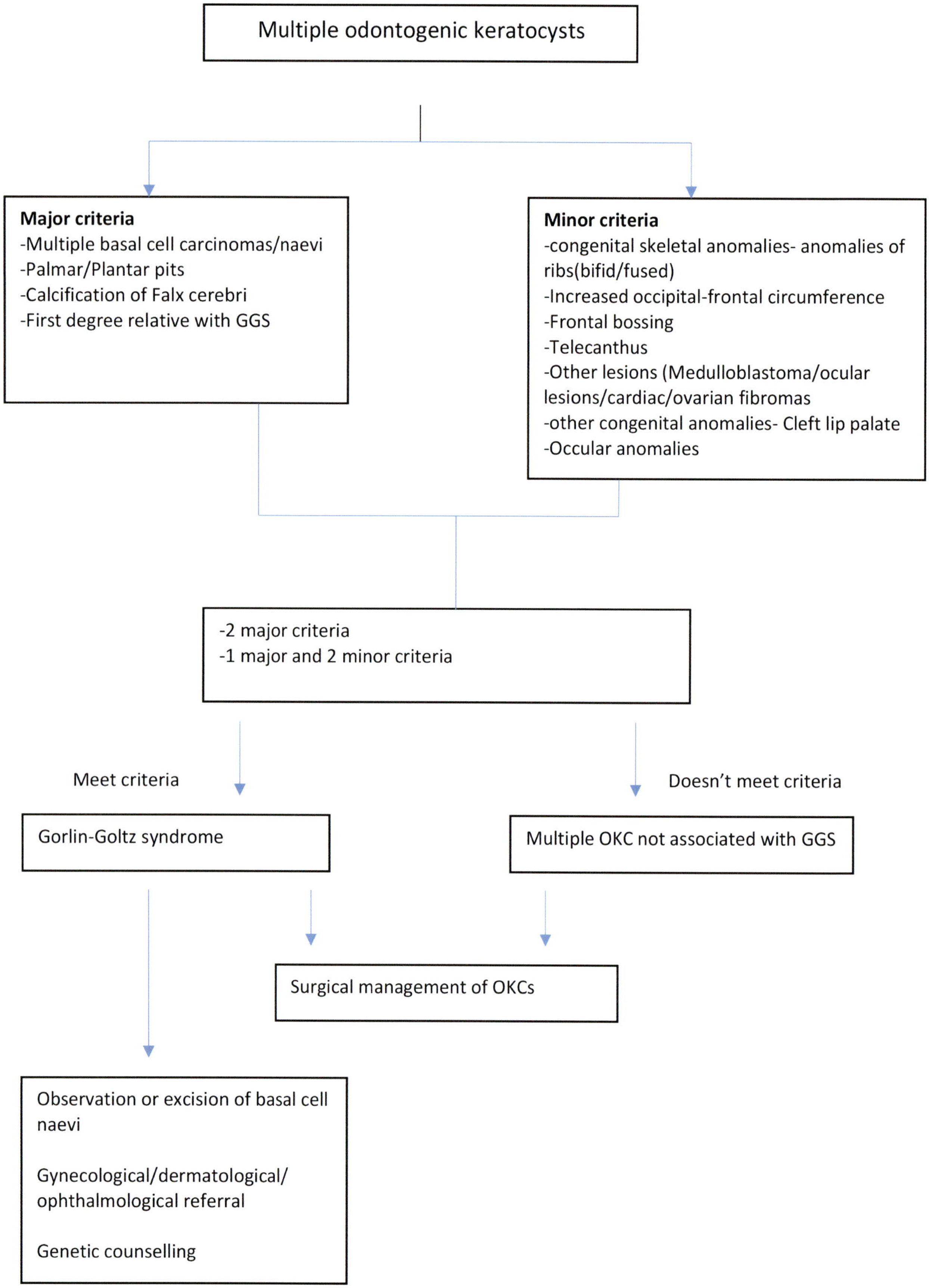

Self-Assessment Questions

1. Explain the classical clinical triad of GGS.
2. List the major and minor criteria used in the diagnosis of GGS.
3. List other syndromes that can give rise to multiple OKCs.
4. Describe the histopathological features of OKC.
5. Explain the clinical significance of OKCs found in GGS.
6. Discuss the management of GGS.

Suggested Reading

Dixit S, Acharya S, Dixit PB. Multiple odontogenic keratocysts associated with Gorlin-Goltz syndrome. Kathmandu Univ Med J. 2009;7(4):414–8.

Eleuch A, Ayachi S, Ayed MB, Tritar S, Mziou Z, Moatemri R, et al. Gorlin-goltz syndrome: a case series of 12 patients. Int J Oral Maxillofac Surg. 2019;48:90.

Evans DG, Ladusans EJ, Rimmer S, Burnell LD, Thakker N, Farndon PA. Complications of the naevoid basal cell carcinoma syndrome: results of a population based study. J Med Genet. 1993;30(6):460.

Hasan A, Akintola D, Hasan A, Akintola D. An update of Gorlin-Goltz syndrome. Prim Dent J. 2018;7(3):38–41.

Joshi PS, Deshmukh V, Golgire S. Gorlin-Goltz syndrome. Dent Res J. 2012;9(1):100–6.

Main B, Felstead A, Hughes C, Thomas S. A guide to skin cancer of the face for the dental team [internet]. Dent Update. 2014;41(2):111–8. https://pubmed.ncbi.nlm.nih.gov/24783879/

A Hard Lump at the Back of the Lower Jaw: Gardner Syndrome

Nadeena S. S. Jayasuriya and Wanninayake M Tilakaratne

Contents

W. M Tilakaratne, T. G. Kallarakkal (eds.), *Clinicopathological Correlation of Oral Diseases*,
https://doi.org/10.1007/978-3-031-24408-7_64

Learning Goals

1. Devise the correct way of compiling the history with appropriate questions
2. Develop a differential diagnosis after history taking
3. Deduce appropriate procedures in clinical examination
4. Formulate a differential diagnosis combining findings in the history and clinical examination
5. Justify the relevant investigations required to arrive at the diagnosis
6. Comprehend the importance of clinicopathological correlation in arriving at the correct diagnosis
7. Outline the management plan
8. Recognize the importance of a diagnostic algorithm in arriving at a diagnosis

64.1 Main Complaint

A 28-year-old female patient, complaining of a bony lump on her right lower jaw presented to the clinic.

64.2 History of Complaint

Question: When did you first notice the lump?

The bony swelling appeared around 5 years back and has been enlarging slowly. It has not been associated with pain. At present, it has grown to a size that is very obvious.

Question: What is your concern now?

I am worried now as it changes my appearance to some extent. Other than that I have no functional issues such as restriction of mouth opening.

64.3 Additional Complaints

Question: Have you had any pain or infections related to any of the lower jaw teeth?

I have not experienced dental pain or related infections in the past.

Question: Do you have missing teeth, mobile teeth or any discharge from your mouth on the right side mouth?

I have no such issues involving right side of the lower jaw.

Question: Do you have similar swellings in any other areas on the body?

I have a similar bony hard swelling on upper left forehead, but it is small in size to be obliviously noticed.

Question: Do you have any other soft or hard lumps on your body?

I underwent a minor procedure to remove a cyst from my left arm 1 year ago.

Question: Have you had any problems in the stomach or when passing stools?

I have no history of abdominal pain, constipation, diarrhoea or bleeding from the rectum.

Question: Have you lost weight recently? Do you feel lethargic, have palpitations and pain in your legs?

I have no history of an unusual loss of weight and I don't have any of those symptoms.

Question: Are you suffering from any other medical problems such as heart disease, high blood pressure, diabetes, bleeding disorder, respiratory diseases? If yes, what kind of medications, have you been taking until now?

I have not been diagnosed with any medical condition till now.

Question: Have you undergone any surgery?

I underwent surgery to remve a cystic lesion from my left arm under local anaesthesia which was diagnosed as an epidermoid cyst.

Question: Have you undergone any dental treatment?

✔ I had an extra tooth removed from my upper anterior jaw few years ago.

? Question: Do you have any family members with such lumps or cysts on the body?

✔ My elder sister and father had similar bony lumps in the lower jaw and in the skull. My father's brother and his two sons also had such bony lumps on the face.

? Question: Has anyone in your family been diagnosed with disease conditions related to the stomach?

✔ My father died 3 years ago due to cancer of the bowel.

64.4 Findings of Clinical Examination

She has a very obvious facial asymmetry with a swelling on her lower jaw on the right side (Fig. 64.1). A bony hard swelling is present at her lower border of the mandibular angle on the right side. It is well-demarcated, oval in shape and measures 3 × 2 cm in dimensions. The lesion is not warm and not attached to the overlying skin. The overlying skin is normal. There is no cervical lymphadenopathy. She has good oral hygiene. Intraoral examination reveals no obvious anomaly.

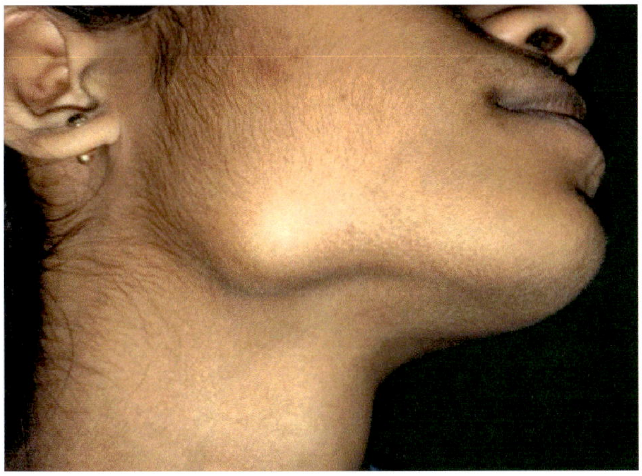

Fig. 64.1 A prominent bony swelling is present on the right side at the lower border of the mandibular angle

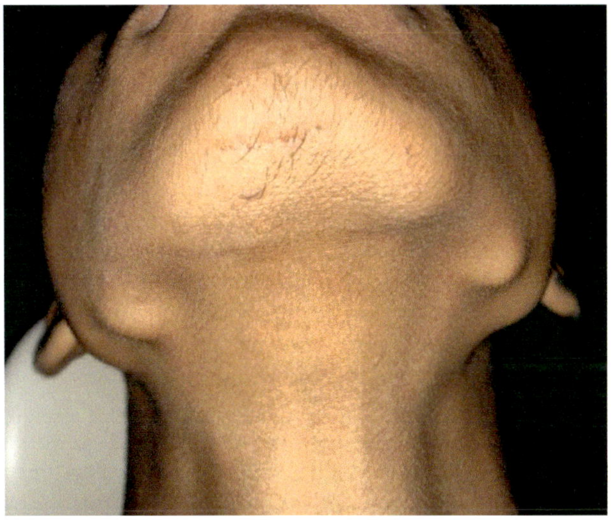

Fig. 64.2 Patient's sister: two bony prominences were noted bilaterally at the lower borders of the mandible

64.5 What Other Relevant Features Would You Look for with the Findings You Have So Far?

A thorough examination for bony prominences and soft tissue lesions/cysts is important. In this patient, apart from the additional bony prominence on the forehead, no other obvious lesions were found. The medical records of the father revealed a carcinoma of the large intestine. Her sister was asked to attend the clinic and similar bony lesions were confirmed. Her sister had bilateral bony prominences along the lower border of the mandible (Fig. 64.2). She had no other bony or soft tissue lesions. Her mother had no detectable lesions.

64.6 With The Findings From The History And Clinical Examination, What is Your Differential Diagnosis?

1. Gardner syndrome (GS)
2. Odontogenic tumour or an Odontogenic cyst
3. Prominent antegonial notch
4. Fibrous dysplasia
5. Osteoma

64.7 How Do You Justify Your Differential Diagnosis?

She has a progressively enlarging bony prominence in her mandible and a smaller prominence on her forehead. Such multiple bony prominences are seen in GS. Odontogenic tumours such as ameloblastoma may occur at the angle of the mandible, but a prominent intraoral swelling (bucco-lingual expansion) with involvement of teeth was not seen. Odontogenic cysts and tumours cause buccal expansion of the mandibular cortical bone. However, odontogenic keratocyst expands more antero-posterioly than bucco-lingually. Fibrous dysplasia is a differential diagnosis, but the presentation would be more of a diffuse swelling rather than a well-defined swelling as seen in this patient. A prominent antegonial notch is seen as bilateral bony prominences in people with a high angled mandible. It is unlikely in this patient as she has the lesion only on her right side of the mandible. An isolated osteoma of the mandible is a possibility. However, strong family history of multiple bony lumps in family members is more supportive of GS.

The patient gave a history of an epidermoid cyst which was removed from her arm. The incidence of epidermoid cysts accompanied by bony swellings are supportive for the diagnosis of GS.

The multiple bony lesions, cystic lesions in her arm, presence of bony lesions in her sister and father and the history of intestinal cancer in her father are strongly suggestive that the patient is having GS.

64.8 What Is the Most Likely Clinical Diagnosis?

Gardner syndrome

Gardner syndrome typically presents with multiple osteomas and with positive family history of similar lesions. In addition, earlier occurrence of a soft tissue cyst, supernumerary teeth and multiple polyps on colonoscopy together with positive family history for colon cancer are confirmatory of GS.

64.9 How Would You Investigate This Patient?

1. Maxillofacial Radiography
2. Endoscopy for the intestinal polyps or tumours
3. Genetic study to confirm GS and the risk of malignant change
4. Genetic studies of family members

64.10 What Are the Investigation Indings?

Dental-panoramic tompograph (DPT), occipitomental view radiographs and cone beam computerized tomography (CBCT) are adequate for diagnosis. A 3 × 2 cm well-defined homogeneously radioopaque mass is noted at the lower border of the mandible on the right side (■ Fig. 64.3). A radiopaque lesion of 1 cm diameter is noted at the left frontal bone. In addition, multiple supernumerary teeth are present in the anterior region of the mandible (■ Fig. 64.4). No other dental or bony lesions are noted. Osteomas in GS commonly occur in

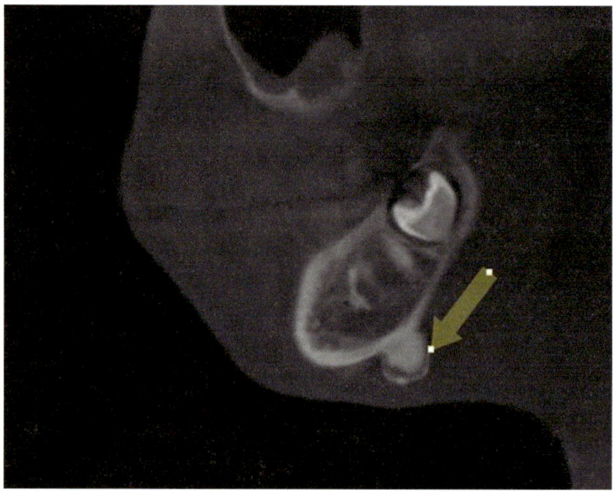

■ Fig. 64.3 CBCT shows an osteoma in the mandible

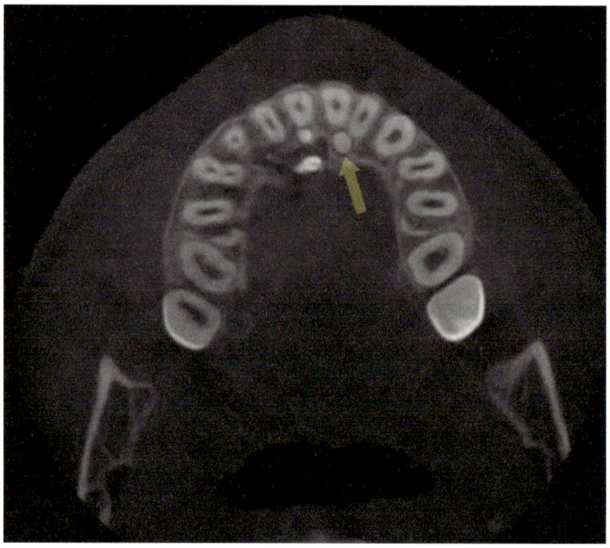

■ Fig. 64.4 CBCT shows multiple supernumerary teeth in the anterior mandible

64

the mandible. Less commonly, they may involve the other maxillofacial bones including paranasal sinuses and long bones. Radiological evaluation of the whole skeleton may reveal other lesions, though it is not usually performed unless symptomatic.

Colonoscopy was performed by a gastrointestinal surgeon and the report confirmed a large number of mucosal polyps throughout the colon. No malignant change was noted but the need for regular reviews was emphasized.

64.11 What Is the Importance of Investigating Intestinal Symptoms in a Suspected Patient with GS?

Gardner syndrome may present with bony and dental deformities as the initial presentation. As GS has a higher chance of intestinal polyps that have a risk for malignant transformation, early diagnosis and regular follow-up will reduce the morbidity and mortality.

64.12 How Do You Confirm the Diagnosis of GS?

GS is typically a triad of multiple osteomas, colonic (large intestine) polyps, epidermoid or sebaceous cysts and mesenchymal tumours of the skin. The presence of the above features confirms the clinical diagnosis of the syndrome. Multiple supernumerary teeth are also present in a majority of patients. Though, the osteomas and skin lesions are easily detectable, colonic and rectal polyps are not unless symptomatic. Symptomatic polyps would give rise to abdominal pain, bleeding from the rectum resulting in anaemia. The polyps can be diagnosed with colonoscopy.

Mutations of the APC tumour suppressor gene are linked with the formation of multiple colonic and rectal polyps and their malignant transformation. Therefore, detection of the APC gene mutation is confirmative of the diagnosis of GS. Genetic testing should be performed on all family members at risk.

64.13 What Is Your Definitive Diagnosis?

Gardner syndrome

64.14 How Would You Manage This Patient?

The main complaint of the patient was the aesthetical concern due to the large bony swelling. She had few unerupted supernumerary teeth in the anterior maxilla, palatal to the incisors. Skin lesions or intestinal symptoms were not noted. The bony prominence of the mandible can be surgically removed to obtain the contour of the mandible accessing through an intraoral incision. The unerupted supernumerary teeth can be surgically removed under local anaesthesia.

The most important aspect of her management is the diagnosis of colonic or rectal polyps and possible malignant change. Referral to a gastrointestinal surgeon for colonoscopy and further management is a must. In addition, genetic profiling of her family members would be beneficial. The importance of investigating for intestinal polyposis should be emphasized to her sister and relatives.

64.15 What Histopathological Features Would You Expect to See in the Excised Lesion?

The hematoxylin and eosin (H&E) stained sections show an encapsulated tumour composed of normal trabeculae of woven and lamellar bone. The bulk of the lesion is composed of cortical type lamellar bone (◘ Fig. 64.5). A fibrocellular stroma of varying density

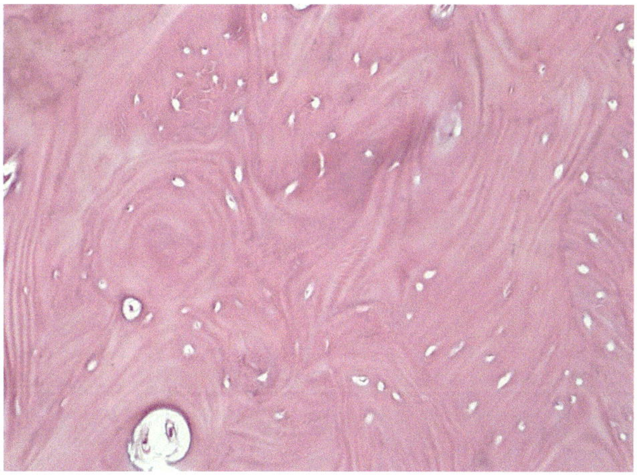

◘ **Fig. 64.5** Compact osteoma: H&E section shows mature lamellar bone containing Haversian canals and osteocytes within bone

in between bony trabeculae may be present in some cases. Osteoblastic riming around bony islands is not conspicuous. There is no cytological atypia either in the osteoblasts or in stromal cells.

64.16 Gardner Syndrome (GS)

Gardner syndrome is a multi-organ disease inherited as an autosomal dominant trait. It has a characteristic clinical triad of multiple osteomas, mesenchymal skin lesions and intestinal (colon and rectum) polyposis. GS and familial adenomatosis coli (FAC) are believed to be variants of the same disorder with a mutation of the adenomatous polyposis coli (APC) tumour suppressor gene located at the chromosome 5q21-q22. GS was first described by Gardner in 1950s as a syndrome associated with extra-colonic features. GS may affect both genders and present at any age from 2 years to 70 years. Usually the symptoms arise after the age of 20 years and colorectal polyps are said to be rare before the age of 10 years.

Gastrointestinal manifestations may occur as adenomatous polyps in the stomach, small intestines and in the colon and peri-ampular carcinomas. The polyposis mainly affects the colon. The risk of malignant transformation is close to 100% with late diagnosis of the syndrome. Patients may present with abdominal pain, vomiting and rectal bleeding.

The osseous lesions predominantly occur in the skull, mandible and the maxilla. Osteomas can even occur in the long bones, but the mandible is most commonly affected. Osseous lesions commonly precede colonic polyps. Therefore, these patients may present initially to a dentist. Presence of more than three osteomas is an indication to screen a patient for GS. Apart from endosteal or exosteal osteomas, various dental anomalies have been described in patients with GS. Patients with GS, have a higher incidence of supernumerary teeth, compound odontomas and impacted permanent teeth compared to the normal population. In addition, missing teeth, hypercementosis, fused or unusually long roots and dentigerous cysts are found in these patients. Epidermoid or sebaceous cysts are the most common skin manifestations (66%) while fibromas, neurofibromas, lipomas and leiomyomas are less common. In some patients, pigmented skin lesions may also be found. Apart from the classical clinical triad, GS can involve multiple organs. They include, retinal hypertrophy, papillary thyroid cancer, benign intracranial neoplasms, hepatomas, hepatoblastomas, biliary and adrenal neoplasms.

The diagnosis of GS is based on eliciting the clinical triad with primary emphasis on the colorectal polyposis by colonoscopy. Genetic confirmation can be through demonstrating the mutation of the APC gene in the patient as well as in relatives.

Treatment of patients with GS depends on the clinical presentation and the stage of the disease with regard to the colorectal polyps. The bony lesions and the skin lesions can be surgically removed for cosmetic reasons as they give minimal symptoms. Dento-alveolar anomalies can be managed according to the clinical presentation. The most important part of the management includes regular follow-up of the gastrointestinal system and the thyroid glands for pathology. The number of intestinal polyps and the risk of malignant transformation are key factors to be taken into account when surgery is considered. Due to the autosomal dominant nature of transmission, genetic screening is recommended for the family members at risk.

Management of Gardner syndrome

Disease manifestation	Clinical presentation	Investigations	Management
Osseous lesions	Osteomas of the facial bones and the skull. Mandibular lower border is most commonly involved. Long bones can also be affected.	Maxillofacial radiographs – DPT – OM view – Cone beam/CT scans	Treat only if aesthetically or functionally a problem.
Skin lesions	Epidermoid cysts Sebaceous cysts Pigmented lesions	Ultra sound scan	Epidermoid and sebaceous cysts can be surgically removed.
Intestinal manifestations	Abdominal pain, vomiting and rectal bleeding	Colonoscopy/proctoscopy incisional biopsy when needed and genetic screening for detection of APC gene mutation.	Regular screening Surgical excision and reconstruction if malignancy is suspected or there is a high risk for malignant transformation

Disease manifestation	Clinical presentation	Investigations	Management
Dental anomalies	Multiple supernumerary teeth, odontomas, missing teeth, or impacted teeth	Dental panoramic tomogram (DPT) Cone beam CT scan	Surgical removal of supernumerary teeth/odontomas/impacted teeth Replacement of missing teeth
Involvement of other organs	Papillary adenocarcinoma of the thyroid gland	Magnetic resonance imaging (MRI)/CT scan, US scan	Thyroidectomy if carcinoma is detected

Salient features of Gardner syndrome	
Clinical	Multiple osteomas occurring in the facial bones predominantly involving the mandible. Abdominal pain, vomiting and rectal bleeding due to intestinal polyps that can transform to malignancy. Multiple epidermoid and sebaceous cysts. In some cases, multiple supernumerary teeth may be present.
Treatment	The osteomas and cysts of the skin are surgically removed mainly for aesthetic reasons. Abdominal polyps should be investigated for malignant transformation and surgically removed if necessary. Thyroid gland should be investigated and treated if malignant changes are observed.
GS can initially present only with multiple osteomas in the facial skeleton. Such patients should be suspected of GS and investigated for intestinal polyposis that can transform to malignancies. Investigations to detect the APC gene mutation and family screening are important.	

64.17 Management Algorithm of GS

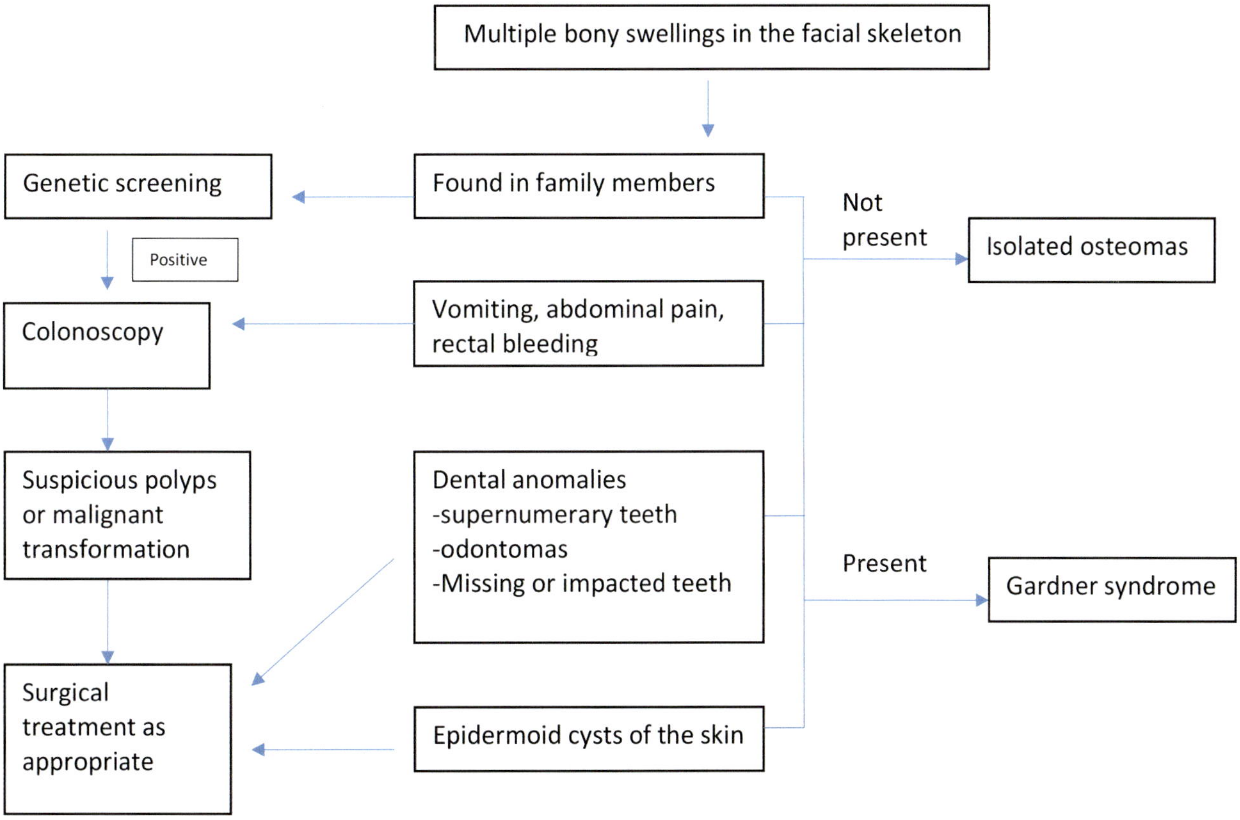

Self-Assessment Questions

1. List the clinical triad in diagnosing GS.
2. State the oncogene that is mutated in GS.
3. State the pattern of genetic transmission in GS.
4. List the possible oro-facial manifestations of GS.
5. Discuss the management plan of GS.
6. Outline the importance of early diagnosis in GS.
7. Describe the role of the dentist in the management of GS.

Suggested Reading

Fotiadis C, Tsekouras D, Antonakis P, Sfiniadakis J, Genetzakis M, Zografos G. Gardner's syndrome: a case report and review of the literature. World J Gastroenterol. 2005;11(34):5408–11.

Halling F, Merten HA, Lepsien G, Honig JF. Clinical and radiological findings in Gardner's syndrome: a case report and follow-up study [internet]. Dentomaxillofac Radiol. 1992;21(2):93–8.

Jones EL, Cornell WP. Gardner's syndrome: review of the literature and report on a family. Arch Surg. 1966;92(2):287–300.

Leppard B, Bussey HJR. Epidermoid cysts, polyposis coli and Gardner's syndrome. Br J Surg. 1975;62(5):387–93.

Nandakumar G, Morgan JA, Silverberg D, Steinhagen RM. Familial polyposis coli: clinical manifestations, evaluation, management and treatment. Mt Sinai J Med N Y. 2004;71(6):384–91.

Naylor EW, Lebenthal E. Gardner's syndrome. Dig Dis Sci. 1980;25(12):945–59.

Panjwani S, Bagewadi A, Keluskar V, Arora S. Gardner's syndrome. J Clin Imaging Sci [Internet]. 2011;1.

Perniciaro C. Gardner's syndrome. Dermatol Clin. 1995;13(1): 51–6.

Takeuchi T, Takenoshita Y, Kubo K, Iida M. Natural course of jaw lesions in patients with familial adenomatosis coli (Gardner's syndrome). Int J Oral Maxillofac Surg. 1993;22(4):226–30.

Thomas KE, Watne AL, Johnson JG, Roth E, Zimmermann B. Natural history of Gardner's syndrome. Am J Surg. 1968;115(2):18–26.

Forensic Odontology

Contents

Burning Sensation of the Tongue: Burning Mouth Syndrome

Zuraiza Mohamad Zaini and Nur Fauziani Zainul Abidin

Contents

W. M Tilakaratne, T. G. Kallarakkal (eds.), *Clinicopathological Correlation of Oral Diseases*,
https://doi.org/10.1007/978-3-031-24408-7_65

Learning Goals

1. Devise the correct way of compiling the history with appropriate questions
2. Develop a differential diagnosis after history taking
3. Deduce appropriate procedures in clinical examination
4. Formulate a differential diagnosis combining findings in the history and clinical examination
5. Justify the relevant investigations required to arrive at the diagnosis
6. Comprehend the importance of clinicopathological correlation in arriving at the correct diagnosis
7. Outline the management plan
8. Recognize the importance of a diagnostic algorithm in arriving at a diagnosis

65.1 Main Complaint

A 65-year-old lady presents with burning sensation and discomfort in the tongue for the past 6 months.

65.2 History of Complaint

Question: What is the nature of burning sensation?

I have been having a constant burning sensation throughout the day. It starts early in the morning and mainly affects the tongue but sometimes I feel that the whole mouth is sore. My tongue feels sticky when I wake up which is relieved by taking a sip of water.

Question: Does the burning sensation affect your sleep?

It does not disturb my sleep.

Question: Are there any factors that aggravate the discomfort?

I tend to avoid spicy and salty food as it worsens the symptoms. I feel that the burning sensation becomes intolerable sometimes when I talk.

65.3 Additional Information

Question: Does the burning sensation and discomfort radiate to other sites for example to the face or throat?

I do not feel it radiating elsewhere.

Question: Have you noticed any changes in the mouth other than the burning sensation?

I have not noticed any changes or lesions inside the mouth.

Question Do you feel any dryness in the mouth or eyes?

I do not have such a feeling.

Question: How do you rate the severity of the symptom on a scale from 0 to 10?

I rate the burning sensation at 10 when it becomes severe at times but most of the time it is around 8.

Question: Did you seek any medical advice or treatment for this problem before?

I consulted a neurologist for the pain on the tongue and had an MRI taken but there were no abnormalities detected. A laryngoscopy was performed by an Ear, Nose and Throat (ENT) specialist who prescribed me with Difflam™ mouthwash. However, I felt that the mouthwash causes heartburn and increases the dryness in my mouth.

Question: Are you on follow-up or taking medications for any medical problems that you are having?

I have been on multiple medications for many years. I was diagnosed with hypertension 10 years ago and I take carvedilol for hypertension and atorvastatin for cholesterol. I reached menopause 9 years ago and has been on paroxetine. My ENT specialist recently prescribed pantoprazole for gastritis. I am also taking medication for vertigo. However, I do not have diabetes and my routine blood investigations that included the HbA1c test showed normal reading.

Question: Can you relate the appearance of your symptoms with any new medication that you have taken?

I cannot relate that as I have been on the same medication throughout.

Question: Have you had any surgery in the past?

Yes. I had right lobe thyroidectomy 15 years ago and at present I am not on any follow-up or taking medications for my thyroid problem.

Question: Do you have any allergies?

I am not aware of any.

Question: Do you get tired easily when you work?

I can carry out my routine work without any problem.

Question: When was your last dental visit?

I had scaling done a year ago without any complications.

Question: How do you maintain your oral hygiene?

I brush my teeth twice a day using herbal toothpaste and soft bristle toothbrush.

Question: Do you tend to thrust your tongue towards the roof of the mouth or the teeth?

I do not have any such habits.

Question: Do you or any family members notice that you grind the teeth when asleep?

I live alone and I am not aware of having any teeth grinding habit at night.

Question: Do you have habits such as betel chewing or smoking?

I do not practise such habits.

Question: Do you drink alcohol?

I do not consume alcohol.

Question: Are you a vegetarian or on a specific diet?

I am a vegetarian. In order to have a balanced diet, I eat protein-rich food like tofu and nuts as a substitute for meat. I also drink milk.

65.4 With the Findings from the History, What is Your Differential Diagnosis?

1. Burning mouth secondary to underlying systemic illness or medications.
2. Oral burning/discomfort due to oral lesions such as oral lichen planus, erythema migrans or oral candidiasis.
3. Burning mouth secondary to mucosal dryness due to illness/disease involving salivary glands such as Sjogren syndrome
4. Burning mouth syndrome

How do you justify your differential diagnosis after history taking?

1. Burning mouth could possibly be a manifestation of underlying systemic illness, hormonal dysfunction, or nutritional deficiency. Elements of the patient's history that support the diagnosis are thyroidectomy, antihypertensive medication and certain diet restriction (plant-based diet) leading to anaemia.
2. There are many oral mucosal diseases and infections that may cause burning sensation in the mouth. However, oral lichen planus, oral candidiasis, oral blistering disorders or erythema migrans are unlikely as she has not notice any changes in the oral mucosa.
3. Burning mouth can also be an indirect manifestation of diseases affecting salivary glands that cause diminished salivary flow. Sjogren syndrome is an autoimmune disease characterized by destruction of glandular structure by lymphocytic infiltrate. Patients with Sjogren syndrome complain of dry mouth and eyes. Burning mouth in this setting can be due to the discomfort imposed by dry mucosa or Candidal infection that is common in patients with dry mouth. The patient however did not report any dry mouth or eyes.
4. Burning mouth syndrome is an idiopathic condition that is present in the absence of any organic disease. It is a diagnosis by exclusion and an extensive diagnostic workout is essential before such a diagnosis could be made.

65.5 Findings of Examination

Her face is symmetrical and there is no lymphadenopathy or cranial nerve dysfunction. Intraorally, her mouth appears dry with frothy saliva and shiny oral mucosa (Fig. 65.1a, b, and c). The tongue appears fissured (Fig. 65.1d). There are no other oral mucosal lesions detected elsewhere including the floor of the mouth, buccal and labial mucosa, sulcus/ vestibules, gingiva, hard and soft palate. She is partially dentate but does not wear a denture. Her oral hygiene is good.

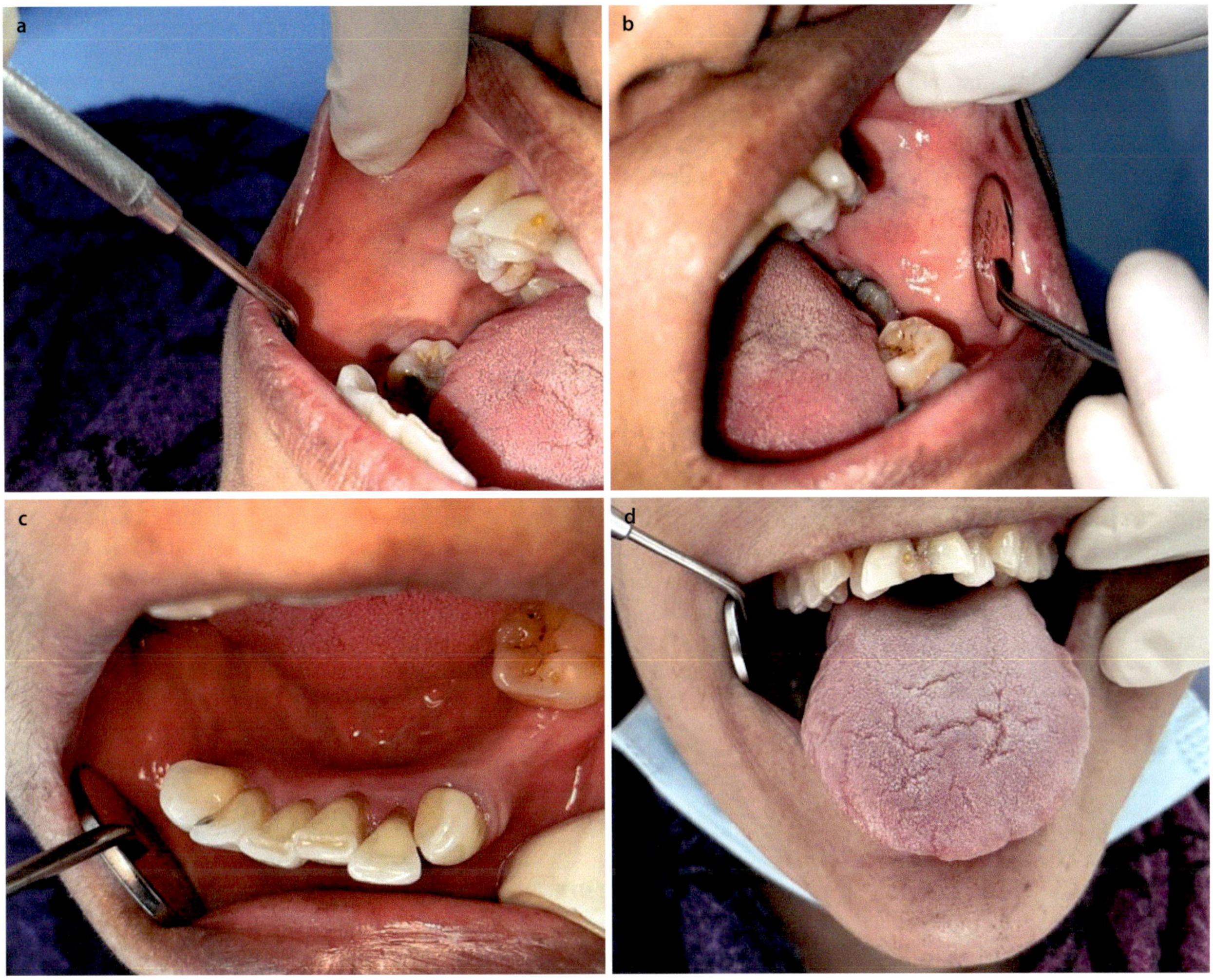

Fig. 65.1 (**a** & **b**) Shiny right and left buccal mucosa, (**c**) lack of saliva pooling in the floor of the mouth and (**d**) the tongue is well-papillated with prominent fissures

65.6 What is Your Provisional Clinical Diagnosis?

Burning mouth syndrome (BMS)

65.7 How Would You Exclude Other Conditions and Justify the Inclusion of the Disease That You Have Mentioned as the Diagnosis?

65.7.1 Oral Mucosal Lesions/Diseases

Oral lichen planus (OLP), oral lichenoid reaction (OLR), chronic ulcerative stomatitis, vesiculobullous disease such as mucous membrane pemphigoid and pemphigus vulgaris, benign migratory glossitis and recurrent aphthous ulcers are often associated with burning or discomfort in the mouth. The symptoms of burning and pain occur most often with erosive and atrophic types of OLP and OLR and are typically aggravated by spicy food, citrus fruits and alcohol. The presence of interlacing white striae is pathognomonic for OLP and OLR. Vesiculobullous diseases affecting oral mucosa also cause burning sensation and intense pain following rupture of bullae leading to formation of diffuse/multiple mucosal erosions. Benign migratory glossitis is a benign oral inflammatory condition characterised by loss of epithelium, particularly of the filiform papillae on the dorsum of the tongue. Burning sensation occurs in areas of depapillation which may be exacerbated by spicy food and alcohol. These oral mucosal diseases are diagnosed in correlation with distinct clinical findings. The patient did not have oral mucosal lesions that are characteristic of the mentioned diseases. Hence none of these can be considered in the differential diagnosis. In patients with BMS, the oral mucosa appears normal.

65.7.2 Oral Candidiasis

Oral burning sensation can also be a presentation of infections in the oral cavity. Candida albicans is the most common causal agent of burning mouth and needs to be ruled out first. It is frequently found in elderly patients, those who are immunodeficient either due to prolonged use of antibiotics, immunosuppressant medication, antiretroviral drugs, corticosteroids or having conditions causing dysfunction of the immune response such as diabetes. Oral candidiasis is also common among denture wearers (denture stomatitis) as well as in those with hyposalivation. Typically, oral candidiasis is associated with a pseudomembranous plaque, erythema or atrophy or hyperplastic mucosa. All forms of candidiasis can be excluded in this case as the patient did not have any such oral manifestations. BMS patients often report diminished or decreased pain during eating whilst patients with oral candidiasis commonly feel increased pain during eating even when the atrophic change is minimal, and the mucosa is almost normal in appearance.

65.7.3 Local Trauma

Oral burning sensation or discomfort could be caused by injury to the oral mucosa resulting from mechanical, chemical or thermal trauma. Such injuries could arise from parafunctional habits such as cheek biting and cheek sucking habit, sharp edges of the teeth or dental prosthesis, hot food or drink, ill-fitting dentures, inappropriate use of medication or iatrogenic damage during dental treatment. The cause of trauma that possibly underlies the patient's complaint of oral burning sensation could be identified from history. The patient may not be aware of the oral lesions and burning sensation may be the chief complaint. A thorough intra-oral examination would reveal clinical evidence of local trauma and the associated oral mucosal changes such as erythema, erosion, ulcerations or keratosis. Absence of mucosal lesions or history of trauma with concurrent complaint of burning mouth would highly suggest BMS as the clinical diagnosis.

65.7.4 Hyposalivation

Patients with an oral burning sensation often have concomitant dry mouth. Dry mouth can either be an objective finding of hyposalivation (through salivary flow test) or a subjective feeling of dryness termed xerostomia. Hyposalivation can be idiopathic or secondary to certain medications, radiation therapy or autoimmune disease. There are many medications that are known to cause reduction in salivary flow, the most common being anticholinergic agents, antihistamines, anti-retroviral drugs, tricyclic antidepressants, serotonin uptake inhibitors and diuretics. Radiotherapy following head and neck cancer could cause irreversible acinar destruction depending on the radiation dose (>40 Gy). Sjogren syndrome is an autoimmune disorder characterized by progressive immune-mediated impairment of exocrine glands which include salivary glands. Abnormal immunological features particularly elevated rheumatoid factor (RF) and antinuclear antibody (ANA) are clues to diagnosis. Dry mouth and dry eyes are the two common clinical manifestations of Sjogren syndrome with some of the patients also presenting with salivary gland swelling, particularly the parotid gland. Patients with Sjogren syndrome have increased risk of candidal infection due to diminished salivary flow and that may cause oral burning sensation.

65.7.5 Endocrine-Related Disorders

Oral burning sensation has been attributed secondary to diabetes, poor glycaemic control and peripheral neuropathy. Dry mouth in diabetic patients is usually a result of polyuria and dehydration. There is a correlation between dry mouth and increased haemoglobin A1c (HbA1c) levels and better glycaemic control reduces symptoms of oral burning sensation. Increased salivary glucose, hyposalivation and decreased neutrophil activity in diabetic patients promote candidal infection causing burning mouth. As burning mouth has a high incidence in post-menopausal women, a decrease in oestrogen levels has been suggested as a cause for burning symptoms. However, hormone replacement therapy has showed insignificant improvement in these patients. There is a also a substantial proportion of BMS patients having abnormal taste perception who showed a variety of thyroid abnormalities such as euthyroidism, hypothyroidism and echographic abnormality. There is a neuronal connection between taste and oral pain, in which stimulation of the gustatory system decreases/inhibits oral pain. Thyroid hormones on the other hand are involved in the maturation and specialization of taste buds. Therefore, reduction in taste (diminished stimulation of gustatory system) following thyroid hormone dysfunction will consequently intensify normal trigeminal sensation that can manifest as burning sensation. The patient's history and clinical findings are not supportive of any endocrine problem.

65.7.6 Nutritional Deficiency

Patients with oral burning sensation were shown to have significant deficiencies of some major nutrients including riboflavin (Vitamin B2), thiamine (vitamin B1), niacin (vitamin B3), pyridoxine (Vitamin B6), folic acid (Vitamin B9), cobalamin (vitamin B12), iron and zinc. These major nutrients are all essential to the normal functioning of oral epithelial cells and are involved in proliferation and repair of oral epithelial cells. Thus, deficiency in riboflavin, niacin, pyridoxine, folic acid, vitamin B12, iron and zinc as well as the subsequent low Hb levels (due to iron and/or vitamin B12 deficiency) may result in atrophy of oral mucosa. The alteration may be so subtle that it cannot be recognized by clinical visual examination. In such situations, spicy molecules in the saliva could easily diffuse through the atrophic epithelium and irritate the free sensory nerve endings, and in turn induce burning sensation. Atrophic glossitis characterized by partial or complete loss of filiform papillae on the dorsal surface of the tongue is the most common oral manifestation of nutritional deficiency and can be easily detected clinically. The patient does not show any clinical features to support nutritional deficiency.

65.7.7 Medications

There are several medications known to cause oral burning sensation. Thus, in the absence of oral lesions or underlying systemic illnesses that cause hyposalivation, medications taken by patients for other comorbidities may be the reason for oral burning sensation. Anti-hypertensive drugs are most often associated with burning mouth particularly those that act upon the angiotensin-renin system. Anti-retroviral drugs (efavirenz), antibiotics (cephalosporins, chloramphenicol, penicillin), antidepressants (fluoxetine, sertraline and venlafaxine) and antianxiety drugs can also cause burning mouth. These medications may also cause hyposalivation resulting in oral burning sensation. The pain-inducing mechanism in the absence of hyposalivation is not well known. About a quarter of the cases were seen to be dose-dependent phenomena and no relationship was found between the duration of treatment and appearance of the symptoms.

65.8 How Would You Investigate This Patient?

1. Swab from the site of complaint to exclude oral candidiasis
2. Blood investigation:
   (a) Diagnostic screening for nutritional deficiency and anaemia such as iron studies, vitamin B12 and folate.
   (b) HbA1C for diabetes mellitus, thyroid-stimulating hormone (TSH) for thyroid function, autoantibody tests such as RF (rheumatoid factor), ANA (antinuclear antibody), ENA (extractable nuclear antigen to rule out anti-Ro and anti-La) to rule out autoimmune diseases such as Sjogren syndrome, ESR (erythrocyte sedimentation rate) for inflammatory diseases and oestradiol for hormonal imbalance.
3. Salivary flow rate to exclude hyposalivation
4. Skin patch test for allergic contact dermatitis
5. Psychological assessment using questionnaires on anxiety, depression, post-traumatic stress disorder and neuropathic pain
6. Evaluation of trigeminal nerve (chorda tympani) with chemo-gustometry or electro-gustometry taste test and mechanical sensory tests such as light tactile, two-point discrimination test, and pinprick to assess for taste alteration and somatosensory change such as allodynia and hyperalgesia

The patient's blood investigations, salivary flow rate and skin patch test showed normal findings and negative somatosensory change.

65.9 What is Your Definitive Diagnosis Based on the Clinical and Laboratory Results/Findings?

Burning mouth syndrome

65.10 How Would You Manage This Patient?

Management of this patient is centred upon symptomatic relief and psychological support. The patient needs to be informed that there is no cure for her condition, but the aim of therapy is to reduce pain and to improve comfort over time. Keeping the mouth moist using commercial oral rinses to improve dryness and lubrication will reduce oral discomfort. This can also be achieved by taking frequent sips of water. Any food, drink or substances which trigger or worsen the burning sensation should be avoided. The use of oral hygiene products without sodium lauryl sulphate may help ease the symptoms. Psychological support includes exploring and addressing issues that may contribute to the pain as well as identify and change negative thoughts about the condition and help the patient to adopt positive ways of coping with the pain.

65.11 Burning Mouth Syndrome

Burning mouth syndrome (BMS) is a type of chronic pain characterized by burning or dysaesthetic sensation of the oral mucosa. Epidemiologic data on BMS are limited and reports from previous population-based studies provide a wide range of prevalence, varying from 0.7 to 18%. BMS is most common among middle-aged and elderly women and high preponderance is observed in post-menopausal women.

The aetiopathogenesis of BMS is not fully understood, but both psychogenic factors and peripheral and central neuropathies appear to be involved. While observational studies suggest an association between anxiety and depression and BMS, it is unclear whether psychogenic factors are primary or secondary to a particular case of BMS. This is because, like other chronic neuropathic pain conditions, BMS can trigger psychological symptoms or itself be a somatic feature of a psychological disorder. Apart from psychogenic factors, several neuronal dysfunctions have been linked to BMS. Objective testing methods such as quantitative sensory testing (QST), electrogustatometry, trigeminal neurography, neurotransmitter–positron emission tomography, indicate that BMS, in most cases, is a chronic neuropathic pain condition. QST utilizing argon laser stimulators revealed a high pain threshold to heat and low pain threshold/sensory threshold ratio on tongue mucosa of BMS patients. Through Doppler flowmetry, the intra-oral mucosa of BMS patients was shown to have increased vasoreactivity following dry ice stimulation, which is consistent with the sensory phenomenon of decreased pain tolerance. Small diameter nerve fibres loss has also been suggested as one of the possible causes of BMS. Neuroanatomical studies showed that there is a decreased number in small diameter nerve fibres in the tongue mucosa of BMS patients and coherently, immunohistochemical studies showed up-regulation of transient receptor potential subfamily member V1 (TRPV1) ion channel, P2X3 receptors and nerve growth factor (NGF). Up-regulation of these factors has been linked to hypersensitivity and neuropathic pain symptoms in various experimental models and human pain conditions. Thus, they may be related to the burning sensation in patients with BMS. In addition, studies utilizing positron emission tomography (PET) demonstrated a decline in endogenous dopamine levels in BMS patients suggesting deficiencies in central pain modulation.

65

Pain in BMS is usually bilateral and rarely unilateral. Patients often complain of pain that fluctuates in intensity, spontaneous in nature and difficult to be described. The oral burning sensation in BMS is poorly localized but patients may have clinical manifestations at a specific site, most commonly at the tip of the tongue. Burning sensation can also be felt on the labial mucosa, buccal mucosa, palate, gingiva or generalized to the entire oral cavity. Subjective xerostomia, dysaesthesia and altered taste are experienced by two-thirds of patients with BMS. Night-time awakening due to pain is not common in BMS but some patients do have a concomitant sleep disorder. Salient features of BMS are summarized in ▶ Box 65.1.

Box 65.1 Burning Mouth Syndrome: Salient Features

1. Burning sensation in the oral cavity that is often poorly localized but felt superficially.
2. Recurring daily for more than 2h per day for more than 3 months (ICOP 2020).
3. Normal oral mucosa and local or systemic diseases have been excluded through thorough investigations.

The diagnosis of BMS should follow a set of strict criteria and is not merely based on complaints of oral mucosal pain in the absence of oral mucosal lesions. According to the International Classification of Orofacial Pain (ICOP 2020), BMS is an oral pain fulfilling the following criteria: (1) recurring daily for more than 2 h per day for more than 3 months, (2) pain of burning quality and felt in superficial oral mucosa, (3) oral mucosa is of normal appearance, (4) local and systemic causes have been excluded (◘ Tables 65.1 and 65.2). Diagnosis of proba-

◘ Table 65.1 Local factors that may cause oral burning sensation

Local factors	
Oral lesion/disease	Immune-mediated conditions: • Oral lichen planus, vesiculobullous lesions, erythema migrans, atrophic glossitis Infection: • Oral candidiasis
Trauma	Mechanical • Ill-fitting dentures, sharp restorations, or teeth Chemical • Medications such as aspirin, dental irrigation solution such as sodium hypochlorite Thermal • Hot food or beverage
Hyposalivation	Consequence of salivary gland hypofunction/destruction: • Radiotherapy, Sjogren syndrome, salivary gland disease Medication side effects: • Antihistamines, antidepressants, diuretics
Contact allergy	Dental material: • Monomer, nickel sulphate, mercury, cobalt, zinc Food additives and colouring Oral care products

■ **Table 65.2** Systemic factors that may cause oral burning sensation

Systemic factors	
Nutritional deficiencies	Decreased levels of vitamin B1, B2, B3, B6, B9 and B12, iron and zinc
Medications	Angiotensin-converting enzyme inhibitors, anticoagulants, antipsychotics, antiretrovirals and benzodiazepines
Autoimmune disease	Sjogren syndrome, systemic lupus erythematosus
Endocrine disorder	Diabetes mellitus, hypothyroidism, hormonal disorders (adrenal cortisol/gonadal steroids)
Gastrointestinal disease	Gastroesophageal reflux disease, inflammatory bowel disease hindering vitamin B absorption
Peripheral/central neuropathy	Diabetic neuropathy, peripheral neuropathies associated with connective tissue disease
Psychological	Depression, anxiety, post-traumatic stress, eating disorder such as bulimia

ble burning mouth syndrome is considered in a patient who has a burning mouth that confirms to the above characteristics but is of less than 3 months duration. An extensive clinical and laboratory investigation is essential to exclude any possible contributable organic disease in diagnosing BMS (■ Fig. 65.2).

65.11.1 Management

To date, there is no standard treatment for BMS as the treatment is often empirical and mostly based on expert opinion and experience. The mechanisms of many treatments used in BMS are unclear and not well described. As both neuropathological changes and psychological co-morbidities are involved in BMS, it is anticipated that BMS may respond to those treatments offered for other neuropathic and psychological conditions, such as antidepressants, anticonvulsants, dietary/nutritional supplements and topical anaesthetic or analgesic agents. However, the level of evidence on the interventions used in the treatment of BMS currently is low in quality. Essentially, patients need to be informed that BMS is a complex disorder for which there is no cure, treatment is

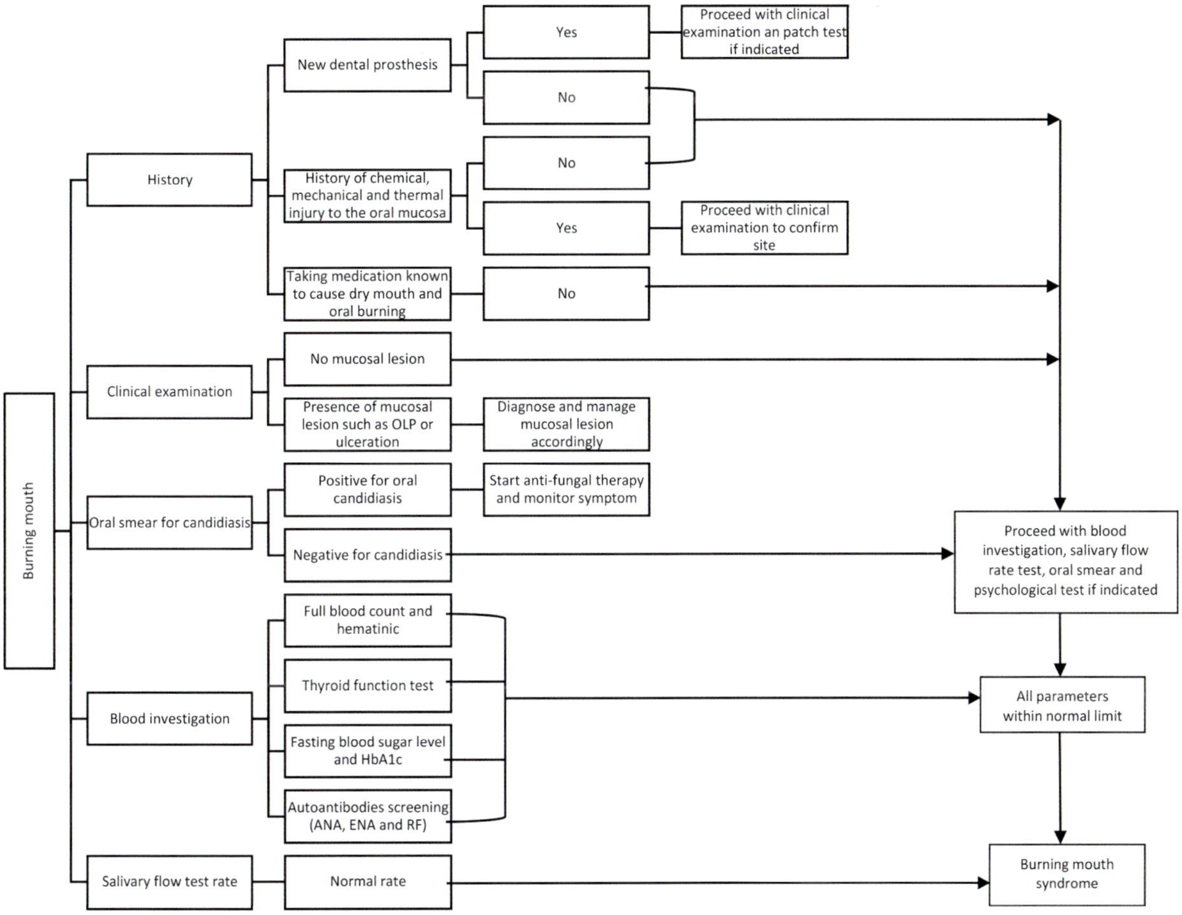

■ **Fig. 65.2** Diagnostic algorithm for burning mouth syndrome

purely aim for symptomatic relief and that the therapeutic outcomes vary with individuals.

65.11.2 Topical

Capsaicin, benzodiazepines such as clonazepam, benzydamine hydrochloride and topical anaesthetics are the common topical agents used in the management of BMS. Combination of topical anaesthetics and benzydamine hydrochloride provides a transient analgesic effect while capsaicin therapy aims to desensitize peripheral nerves. Clonazepam is an agonist to gamma-amino butyric acid (GABA) receptors that cause mild inhibition of the central nervous system and is widely used as an anxiolytic. When applied topically to the oral mucosa, clonazepam is thought to decrease the excitability of peripheral sensory nerve fibres and central sedative, anxiolytic and analgesic effects are achieved when it is taken systemically.

65.11.3 Systemic

Systemic interventions include alpha-lipoic acid (ALA), anticonvulsants and tricyclic antidepressants (TCA). ALA is a potent antioxidant that has a neuroprotective effect and has been used to treat diabetic neuropathies. ALA is shown to be beneficial in the treatment of BMS, either alone or in combination with anticonvulsants or with cognitive behaviour therapy. Amitriptyline is the commonly used TCA in managing BMS. It has a complex pharmacodynamics and functions by inhibiting multiple CNS receptors. This lack of specificity may in part be the reason for it to be clinically effective in managing BMS at low dose.

65.11.4 Others

Recently, electromagnetic radiation by low-level laser and transcranial magnetic stimulation has been used as a non-invasive analgesic intervention for chronic pain, and its application in BMS is being explored. Cognitive behavioural therapy and group psychotherapy are other non-pharmacological approaches aiming to enable self-controlled pain intensity through individual understanding and perception of symptoms and emotional distress.

? Self-Assessment Questions

1. List the causes of oral burning sensation.
2. State the salient features of BMS.
3. State the important conditions that need to be included in the differential diagnosis of BMS.
4. Outline the management plan of BMS.

Suggested Reading

Femiano F, Lanza A, Buonaiuto C, Gombos F, Nunziata M, Cuccurullo L, Cirillo N. Burning mouth syndrome and burning mouth in hypothyroidism: proposal for a diagnostic and therapeutic protocol. Oral Surg Oral Med Oral Pathol Oral Radiol Endod. 2008;105(1):e22–7. https://doi.org/10.1016/j.tripleo.2007.07.030.

ICOP. International Classification of Orofacial Pain, 1st edition (ICOP). Cephalalgia. 2020;40(2):129–221. https://doi.org/10.1177/0333102419893823.

Patton LL, Siegel MA, Benoliel R, De Laat A. Management of burning mouth syndrome: systematic review and management recommendations. Oral Surg Oral Med Oral Pathol Oral Radiol Endod. 2007;103:S39.e1–S39.e13. https://doi.org/10.1016/j.tripleo.2006.11.009.

Tan HL, Renton T. Burning mouth syndrome: an update. Cephalalgia Rep. 2020; https://doi.org/10.1177/2515816320970143.

Teruel A, Patel S. Burning mouth syndrome: a review of etiology, diagnosis, and management. Gen Dent. 2019;67(2):24–9.

Forensic Age Estimation: Forensic Odontology

Rabi'ah Al-Adawiyah Rahmat and Phrabhakaran Nambiar

Contents

W. M Tilakaratne, T. G. Kallarakkal (eds.), *Clinicopathological Correlation of Oral Diseases*,
https://doi.org/10.1007/978-3-031-24408-7_66

Learning Goals
1. To learn the importance of the dentition for forensic age estimation
2. To improve the understanding of the different timing and sequence of the developing teeth and also their degenerative and chemical changes
3. To appreciate different methods of age estimations for infants, juveniles and adults
4. To understand the influence of sex and ethnicity in age estimation procedures

66.1 Main Complaint

Two male siblings who had no identification documents were referred by the Department of Social Welfare to a forensic odontologist for age estimation.

66.2 History of Complaint

Question: Why were the siblings referred for age estimation?

A woman who claimed to be an acquaintance of the late mother of the two siblings wanted to obtain legal guardianship of them. She claimed that the siblings were 16 years old (Mr X) and 10 years old (Mr Y). The woman wanted to institute the adoption process of the siblings. The siblings were considered stateless and placed under the care of the Department of Social Welfare. To provide identification documents, the siblings were then referred for dental age estimation. This is a standard operating procedure recognised by legal authorities to verify their age and issue a legal identification document.

66.3 Past Dental and Medical History

Question: Did the siblings have any dental or medical condition that could affect their dental development?

The siblings did not have any known dental or medical condition and they appeared to be physically normal and healthy.

66.4 Family History

Question: What is the ethnicity of the siblings?

Both siblings are Malay. Their father is a Malaysian and their late mother was an Indonesian.

66.5 Social History

Question: Did the siblings receive formal education?

Both of them did not attend school because they lacked identification documents.

66.6 Examination

Question: How would you assess the dental age of the siblings?

Dental age estimation (DAE) is a method of estimating age of a person whose formal birth registration document is absent or the chronological age (CA) is not known. The dental age is calculated by using an established method based on a population-specific dataset.

66.7 What is the Protocol of Conducting Dental Age Estimation?

The dental age estimation protocol is as the following (Fig. 66.1):
1. To receive a referral letter from an authorised body such as the Court, Department of Social Welfare or a medical department
2. To obtain personal information comprising date of birth (if known), race, sex, parents/guardian information, socio-economic status and background on his/her formal education
3. To conduct a thorough history taking, including history of complaint, past dental and medical history, family history and social history
4. To perform an oro-facial examination that includes assessment of oral or facial abnormality and dental charting
5. To take an appropriate maxillofacial radiograph/image (dental panoramic image or CBCT scan) to assess dental development
6. To calculate the dental age using maturity scores/formulae/dental development atlases for age estimation
7. To prepare a report stating the estimated age for submission to legal authorities

66

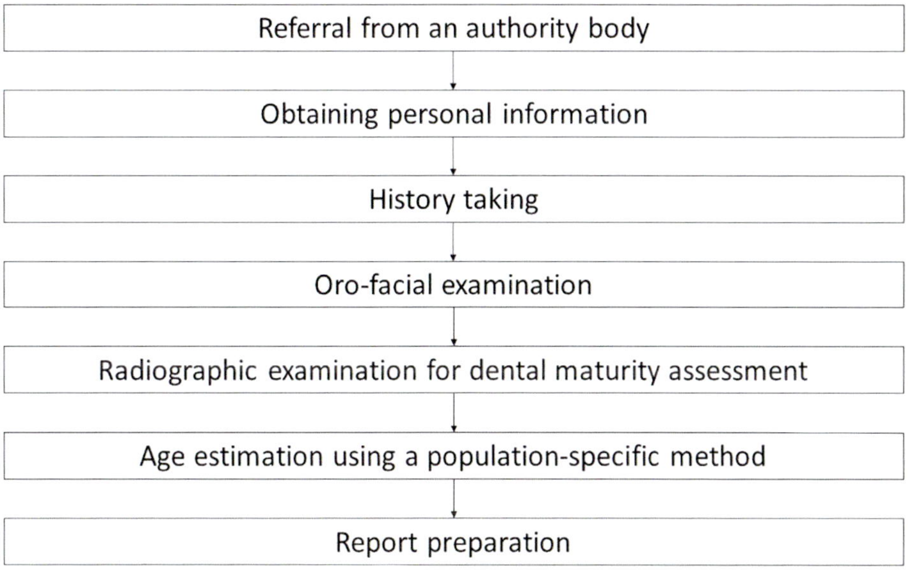

Fig. 66.1 Sequence of dental age estimation procedure upon referral from an authorised body

66.8 Why is Obtaining Personal Information of a Person Important?

Unverified age, sex and race/ethnicity are crucial information prior to determining dental age. Unverified age is merely a reference to compare the resultant estimated dental age. Sometimes the age claimed by the undocumented person is not true. Sex and ethnicity are factors influencing the growth, maturity and eruption of dentition. This explains developmental variations between male and female, and also racial origin.

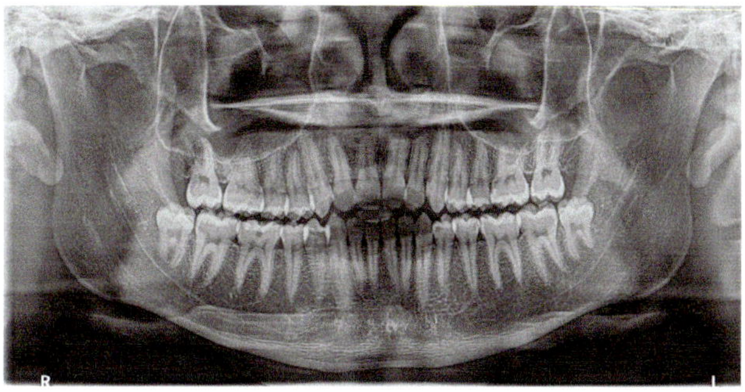

Fig. 66.2 Dental panoramic tomograph of Mr. X who claimed to be 16 years old

66.9 What is the Type of Radiograph Taken for Dental Age Estimation?

Dental panoramic image/tomograph (DPT) is the most frequently used radiograph for dental age estimation. DPT provides a two-dimensional overview of the complete dentition, enabling the evaluation of all developing and erupting teeth. In this case, DPT of both siblings were taken for radiographic assessment of their dental maturation status (Figs. 66.2 and 66.3).

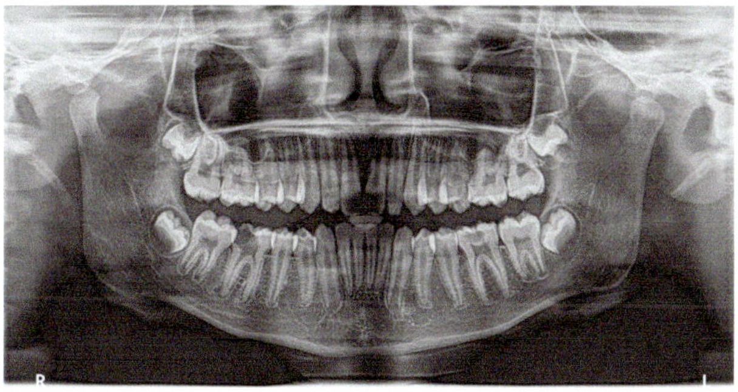

Fig. 66.3 Dental panoramic tomograph of Mr. Y who claimed to be 10 years old

66.10 Radiographic Findings

The development of dentition was assessed using the Demirjian's staging system. The system has often been adopted in numerous population-specific age estimation methods to define the tooth mineralization stages and assigns them according to pre-determined scores. The dental age estimation was performed based on the development of the permanent teeth on the left side of the mandible, tooth numbers 31–37 according to FDI nomenclature. Tooth formation was divided into eight stages (Table 66.1).

66.10.1 *Mr X*

On DPT examination (Fig. 66.2), a permanent type of dentition was observed. All teeth were present except for maxillary right and left third molars. Based on the Demirjian's staging system, the radiographic findings were as follows:

1. The permanent mandibular left incisors, canine, premolars, first and second molars were fully erupted in the oral cavity. All teeth developments corresponded to stage H.
2. The apical roots of the left third mandibular molar are open and the root canal walls were parallel. This morphological development corresponded to stage G.

66.10.2 *Mr Y*

On DPT examination (Fig. 66.3), a permanent dentition was observed. All permanent teeth had emerged into the oral cavity except third molars. Based on the Demirjian's staging system, the radiographic findings were as follows:

1. The roots of left incisors, first premolar and first molar were completely formed. All teeth developments corresponded to stage H.
2. The root apices of the left second premolar and second molar are open, and the root canal walls were

Table 66.1 Description of the developmental stages of the permanent dentition according to Demirjian's system

Stage	Description
A	In both uniradicular and multiradicular teeth, a beginning of calcification is seen at the superior level of the crypt in the form of an inverted cones or cones. There is no fusion of these calcified points.
B	Fusion of the calcified points forms one or several cusps which unite to give a regularly outlined occlusal surface.
C	(a) Enamel formation is complete at the occlusal surface. (b) The beginning of a dentinal deposit is seen. (c) The outlie of the pulp chamber has a curved shape at the occlusal border.
D	(a) The crown formation is completed down to the cementoenamel junction. (b) The superior border of the pulp chamber in the uniradicular teeth has a definite curved form, being concave towards the cervical region. The projection of the pulp horns if present, gives an outline shaped like an umbrella top. In molars, the pulp chamber has a trapezoidal form. (c) Beginning of root formation is seen in the form of a spicule.
E	Uniradicular teeth: (a) The walls of the pulp chamber now form straight lines, whose continuity is broken by the presence of the pulp horn, which is larger than in the previous stage. (b) The root length is less than the crown height. Molars: (a) Initial formation of the radicular bifurcation is seen in the form of either a calcified point or a semi-lunar shape. (b) The root length is still less than the crown height.
F	Uniradicular teeth: (a) The walls of the pulp chamber now form a more or less isosceles triangle. The apex ends in a funnel shape. (b) The root length is equal to or greater than the crown height. Molars: (a) The calcified region of the bifurcation has developed further down from its semilunar stage to give the roots a more definite and distinct outline with funnel-shaped endings. (b) The root length is equal to or greater than the crown height.
G	The walls of the root canal are now parallel, and its apical end is still partially open (distal root in molar).
H	(a) The apical end of the root canal is completely closed (distal root in molar). (b) The periodontal membrane has a uniform width around the root and apex.

parallel. This morphological development corresponded to stage G.
3. The root of the mandibular left canine is open, and the root canal walls were diverged. This tooth development corresponded to stage F.
4. The left mandibular third molar is still forming, with a completed crown formation and no evidence of root formation. This morphological development corresponded to stage D.

66.10.3 Analysis

66.10.3.1 *Mr X*

Mr. X's dental age was estimated using the following methods:

1. Age estimation employing a sex-specific age prediction model for Malay children based on Demirjian's seven-tooth method demonstrated that his age is more than 16 years old.
2. The calculated age based on Mincer's method for White male population was 18.3 years with a standard deviation of 1.93.
3. Based on the lower third molar development data in Northeast Malaysian population, the mean of his estimated dental age for males was 19.03 years with a standard deviation of 2.03.

66.10.3.2 *Mr Y*

Mr. Y's dental age was estimated using a sex-specific age prediction model for Malay children and adolescent. This model was developed using the Demirjian's seven-tooth scoring method. The mean of his estimated dental age is 13.3 years.

66.10.4 Results

66.10.4.1 *Mr X*

After considering the developmental stages of Mr. X's permanent dentition, his estimated age is 18 years and 4 months. However, he might be between 17 and 20 years due to the biological variability of human growth.

66.10.4.2 *Mr Y*

After considering the developmental stages of Mr. Y's dentition, his estimated age is 13 years and 4 months. However, there is a possibility of a minor deviation (approximately 6 months) of the estimated age due to the biological variability of human growth.

66.10.5 Conclusion

Initially, these siblings claimed that their age was 2–3 years younger than the estimated age. This case has shown that dental age estimation is crucial and reliable in verifying a person's chronological age.

66.11 Forensic Age Estimation

Age estimation has an important role in various disciplines, mainly forensic odontology, anthropology, archaeology, palaeontology, paediatric dentistry and orthodontic. From forensic perspective, age estimation is important for verifying identity in both the living and the dead. Dental age is the most reliable and comparable biological age to that of chronological age. This is because teeth demonstrate low variability in relation to chronological age in comparison to other skeletal structures. This is possible due to predictable timing of tooth formation and maturation. Dental formation and eruption are less likely affected by nutrition, hygiene, medical condition and economic status. But subsequently racial and familial factors might dictate, in addition to possible hormonal and environmental factors. In addition, dental mineralisation can be subjected to periodic disturbances such as birth, diseases and drug intake. These changes in some instances, may be retrospectively linked to a specific time or event during an individual's life.

Historically, dental age estimation for legal purposes was first proposed in 1837, which was before birth registration became compulsory in England. The Factory Acts concerning the employment of child labour in a factory stated that the minimum legal age to work was 9 years old and children between 9 and 13 years old were only allowed to work not more than 9 h a day. At the time, the only way to prove the age of a child was based on strength and appearance of a child at least 9 years of age. This rendered the children vulnerable to exploitation by factory owners and parents. To address this issue, Saunders had suggested the use of teeth for age verification in factory working children to replace the age estimation using their height. When the mummy of the Pharaoh, King Tutankhamun of ancient Egypt was found in 1922, the age was estimated then as around 18–22 years as the autopsy revealed three partially erupted third molars. This evidently proved that developing teeth were used for age estimation during previous times.

After the completion of eruption, structural changes that occur in the teeth may be considered as degenerative changes. Here technology advancements became useful in age estimations. In 2008, Jeong et al., reported that three Korean mummies had their ages determined using 3D-reconstructed CT images based on dental attrition observed. The estimated dental ages of the mummies were 51.01, 64.45 and 23.57 years. Recession of the periodontal ligament, secondary dentine deposition, cementum apposition, root resorption and root transparency (translucency) are other structural changes that can be evaluated to estimate dental age in adults. Even changes in the chemical composition of teeth have been utilised for age estimation.

Dental age estimation is widely accepted in many countries and employed in medicolegal situations. These include:

- Human identification process
- Absence of birth certificate or other official proof of age
- Criminal and civil responsibility—A person's age determines the sentence that will be imposed, especially in cases of confirming juvenile versus adult status. In addition, some countries have lawful corporal punishment by caning as a sentence for serious crimes. However, caning is spared for males above 50 years.
- Abuse of child labour
- Consent for medical treatment
- Amnesia

Dental age of humans can be classified in two phases:

1. Childhood up to 18 years of age: This is the phase during which teeth are developing continuously in the jaw.
2. Adulthood: This phase starts after the completion of tooth development based on degenerative age-dependent changes.

66.11.1 Dental Age Estimation of Infants, Children and Adolescents

66

The application of progressive dental developmental changes is the most accurate technique for estimating the ages of infants, children and adolescents. Dental developmental data are usually established based on formative or developmental changes and are good age predicators of age from birth until about early twenties. The sequence of tooth maturation and eruption follows a specific chronological order. Starting with deciduous dentition, the mineralisation commences at 16th week of intrauterine life (IUL) and around 30th week, IUL cusp tips of all deciduous teeth (A, B, C, D and E) can be observed on radiographic images. Following that, the permanent mandibular first molar starts to mineralise and the mesiobuccal cusp tip can be evident radiographic images just before birth.

66.11.1.1 Histological Assessment

The shift from an intrauterine life to extrauterine life is marked by neonatal line, an accentuated hypomineralised incremental line in enamel and dentine of a developing tooth. Its presence indicates live birth and a separate existence. This is especially important in the forensic identification case of a dead foetus. Generally, a foetus is considered as viable by 28 weeks of gestation and could have been born alive. Thus, any incidence whereby a foetus is found dead should raise suspicion. Neonatal lines can be used as a reference to estimate the survival period of an infant in perinatal period. One limitation of estimating age through neonatal lines is that at least a couple of days of survival of the newborn baby is necessary for the maturation of neonatal lines to be identified. However, it must be noted that the absence of the neonatal line is not always an indicator of still birth.

Age after birth of an infant can be estimated by measuring the amount of dentine laid down after the neonatal line. Coronal dentine is deposited at a rate of 4 μm per day, both during the intrauterine period and for some time after birth. Similarly, the rate of enamel formation in deciduous enamel is 2.5–4.5 μm per day. Daily incremental depositions of enamel are seen across enamel rods as cross striations. Counting these cross striations from neonatal line can be used as an additional method to estimate the age of a newborn.

66.11.1.2 Atlas of Tooth Development

Schematic diagrams illustrating the different stages of tooth development and eruption have been established. A specific diagram is chosen and used as a standard when assessing teeth on a radiographic image for age estimation. Comparing dental status on a radiograph with a concordant stage in an atlas is simple and quick, but the stage usually shows the mean age and age interval. One of the earliest dental development charts was developed by Schour and Massler. It presented 22 stages of tooth development ranging from the fifth month of IUL to 35 years of age. Alqahtani et al. published a holistic London atlas of human tooth development and eruption to estimate age of individuals between 28 weeks IUL and 23 years. The atlas was developed according to the median tooth stage and eruption level.

66.11.1.3 Radiographic Assessment

Various age estimation methods based on radiographic investigation are available and often differentiated by the number of tooth formation stages and population-specific data. Appropriate training and experience are important when performing age estimation and distinguishing between dental developmental stages on a radiograph. Moorrees was the earliest to propose dental maturation staging. In his model, 14 dental stages were produced, from initial cusp formation to apical closure for ten permanent teeth including maxillary incisors and all eight mandibular teeth. Mean ages of teeth in Moorrees' stages of tooth formation and resorption of deciduous teeth are tabulated with a guidance when performing age estimation. The data were developed separately for males and females.

The most famous dental age estimation that applied radiographic method is Demirjian's eight stages tooth development model. The eight stages (stage A–H) consist of the crown and root calcification till the apex closure was customised according to the tooth types that are incisor, canine, premolar and molar. Score is assigned to each stage of seven permanent teeth of left mandibular region (31, 32, 33, 34, 35, 36 and 37). The total score then correlates with the value in the sex-based tooth maturity scoring table to obtain an estimated dental age. Demirjian's tooth staging chart is versatile as it has been adopted to various population data for age estimations around the world.

Thirty decades later, Chaillet and Demirjian improvised dental maturity standards for southern French children using the Demirjian's method. In this method, the alphabetical eight-stage system was converted to numerical system with additional two initial stages to become ten-stage tooth developmental model (0–9). The initial stages are, Stage 0 is when there is no evidence of tooth development and Stage 1 is when the bony crypt is without any dental germ inside. Moreover, a dental maturity score of third molar was included because it is the only tooth that is developing for predicting age past 16 years.

66.11.1.4 Measuring the Apical Foramen of Developing Teeth

During tooth development, the root tapers and becomes conical and blunt at the apex. This has led to the development of an age estimation method based on the measurement of the open apices of developing seven left mandibular teeth using dental panoramic images of European children aged between 4 and 16 years old. The method proved to be effective and was successfully applied on various populations around the world. It provides a better accuracy in comparison to Demirjian's method.

Nevertheless, dental panoramic image is two-dimensional, unequal magnification causing distortion of anatomical structures and inability to assess sectional details. To overcome the limitations of dental panoramic image, a new dental age estimation method based on cone-beam computed tomography (CBCT)-scanned data was introduced. In this method, three-dimensional (3D) surface area analysis of the developing maxillary canine root apices of Malaysian children was performed using Mimics and 3-matics software. The results showed an excellent correlation of the surface area with chronological age. Subsequently, the same technique was used to assess two-rooted mandibular third molars to ascertain juvenile versus adult status.

66.11.1.5 Third Molar Development

Third molar development is the final developing permanent tooth after all 28 permanent teeth have completely developed. It is a reliable tooth for estimating chronological age in adolescence between 14 and 25 years old. Mincer investigated the accuracy of estimating chronological age based on radiographical assessment of third molar development. Modified Demirjian's eight stages of crown and root formation was used to score third molar development. The results showed that third molars of stage A, B, C or D are most likely indicate a person's age to be less than 18 years, while third molars with stage H are a suggestive marker that a person is at least 18 years of age.

66.11.2 Dental Age Estimation of Adults

Six multi-factorial age-determinant parameters for adults are secondary dentin formation, periodontal recession, attrition, apical translucency, cementum apposition and external root resorption. Various age estimation methods have been developed based on these parameters using histological examination, radiographic assessment and chemical analysis.

66.11.2.1 Secondary Dentin Formation

Secondary dentin formation is one of the reliable methods to estimate age as it forms throughout life once root formation is completed. Kvaal's method described the measurement of secondary dentin formation using periapical radiographs. An age predicting formula was produced based on six different teeth and various

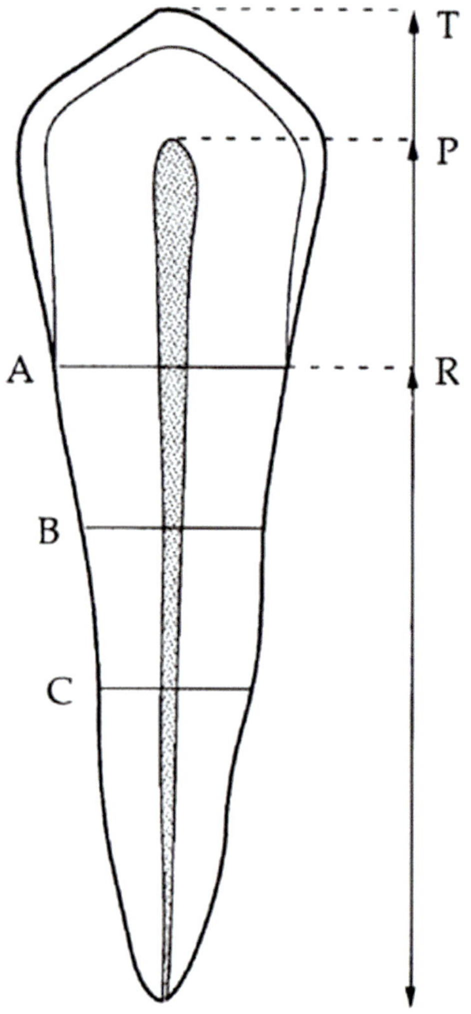

Fig. 66.4 The measurements made on the radiograph of a tooth. *T:* maximum tooth length, *R:* root length on the mesial surface, *P:* maximum pulp length, *A:* root and pulp width at cementoenamel junction (CEJ), *B:* root and pulp width midway between measurement levels A and C, *C:* root and pulp width midway between apex and CEJ

measurement ratios of teeth and pulp cavity (Fig. 66.4). Statistical analysis showed strong correlation between all the measured ratios and chronological age, except for tooth/root length ratio.

At present, age estimation methods based on secondary dentin formation have been developed using CBCT data of a population. CBCT scans can provide volumetric value of a whole tooth and its tooth part (Fig. 66.5). In this method, volume ratio of a tooth was used to form an age prediction regression mode. Two types of tooth volume ratio that can be used are:

1. Pulp cavity/tooth ratio
2. Pulp chamber/crown ratio

The volumetric analysis of the pulp chamber/crown ratio gives a higher accuracy of the estimated age compared to pulp cavity/tooth ratio. The advantage of using this method is that a single permanent tooth is sufficient to estimate the age of an adult, with permanent central incisors being the most reliable tooth. However, any multi-rooted tooth can also be used for the analysis.

66.11.2.2 Attrition

Attrition is the loss of tooth structure on the occlusal/incisal surface that is caused by constant contact with the opposing teeth. It is a tooth wearing process associated with ageing. At 30 years of age, attrition is usually limited to enamel. At 40 years of age, the process begins to involve dentine and it occurs deep into dentine when a person reaches 50 years old. At 60 years of age, the whole of the occlusal surface may be missing and at 70 years the tooth crown itself is steadily lost. However, the degree of attrition is subjected to dietary intake and personal habits. For instance, attrition may be accelerated in a person who regularly chew raw and hard food or has a night grinding.

66.11.2.3 Root Transparency

Root transparency forms gradually with ageing when dentinal tubules become sclerosed with hydroxyapatite mineral, decreasing the amount of light refracted through the tubules. Root dentin translucency initiates in the apical portion of the root and increases in the coronal direction. The length of the root and the translucent zone can be measured through microscopic analysis of ground sections of a tooth. However, the clinical application of this method is not suitable for the living individuals. This is because the procedure requires the tooth to be removed, sectioned and polished before measurement.

66.11.2.4 Cementum Annulations

Tooth is held in alveolar socket by fibres that are attached onto the cementum covering the root. The cementum increases in thickness, particularly towards the apex. It was found that the thickness of the cementum was nearly three times thicker at the age of 76 years as it was at 11 years. Cementum is deposited on the root surface in layers as dense bundles of collagen that are subsequently mineralised by hydroxyapatite crystals. These layers are known as cementum annulations which can be observed microscopically as alternating light and dark bands, each layer corresponding to approximately one year of life. Thus, counting cementum annulation is useful for age estimation. However, this method is an invasive procedure as it requires tooth extraction and histological examination of tooth sections.

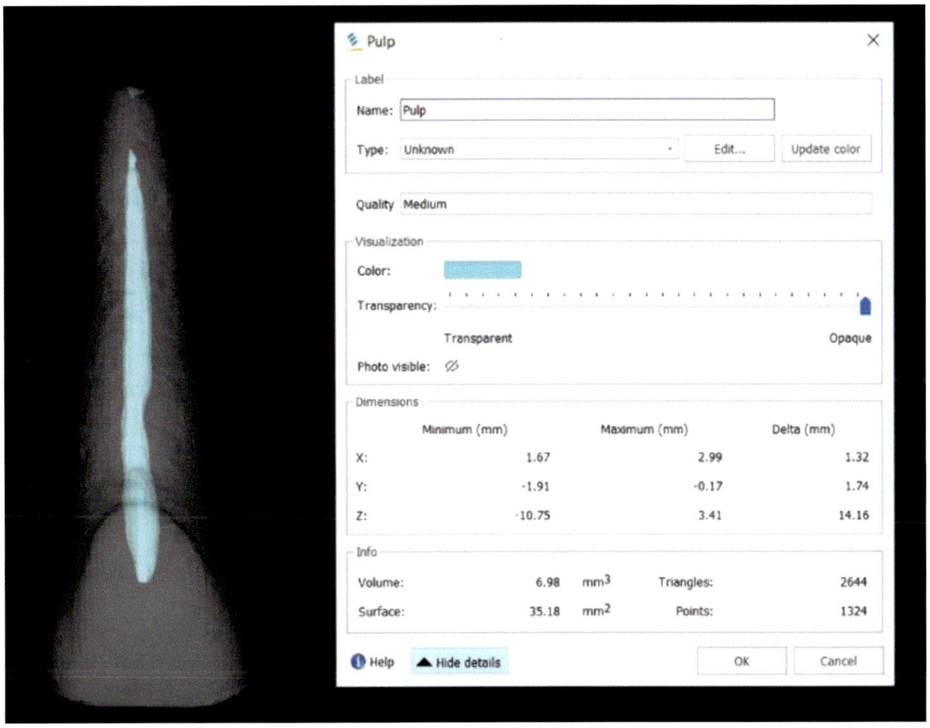

Fig. 66.5 A 3D-model of a tooth and its volume generated from CBCT-scanned data that can be used for age estimation

66.11.2.5 Aspartic Acid Racemisation

Aspartic acid is a type of amino acid that has been shown to undergo racemisation in all dental hard tissues. Racemisation is a process whereby L-isomer of the amino acid converts to D-isomer towards equilibrium and occurs continuously throughout life. Thus, age can be estimated by quantifying the relative amounts of the L- and D-isomer of aspartic acid in the enamel or dentin of a tooth. The quantification of aspartic acid can be performed using amino acid analyser or a high-performance liquid chromatography. This chemical analysis is suitable to be used to estimate age of an individual at death.

66.11.2.6 DNA Methylation

DNA methylation-based age estimation method has been increasingly used in forensic science. DNA methylation is a type of epigenetic modification in which gene expression in DNA is altered. It affects the chemical base of DNA resulting in an addition of methyl group to 5′ carbon of DNA nucleotides. DNA methylation patterns of CpG dinucleotides in the human genome have been shown to be correlated with age. Dentin has demonstrated a high potential for age estimation using DNA methylation in archaeological samples or forensic biological evidence, especially when blood and soft tissues are absent.

66.11.3 Conclusion

Dental age estimation contributes profoundly to forensic investigations of civil and criminal cases. When conducting an age estimation, it is wise to deploy more than one method that are most appropriate for a person. Sex and ethnicity should be taken into consideration. Moreover, dental age estimation is a preferred biological profiling method for it is widely accepted, rapid and least invasive. Hence, a rigorous improvement for dental age estimation is needed to ensure its continuous validity, reliability and acceptance by the legal enforcement authorities.

Self-Assessment Questions

1. Why is dental age estimation a reliable method to predict chronological age of a person?
2. What are the available dental age estimation methods for children and adolescents?
3. List six degenerative changes that can be used for age estimation in adults.
4. Describe the sequence and timing of emergence of deciduous and permanent dentition.
5. How reliable is it to use the developing third molar for determining juvenile versus adult status of a person?

Suggested Reading

AlQahtani SJ, Hector MP, Liversidge HM. Brief communication: the London atlas of human tooth development and eruption. Am J Phys Anthropol. 2010;142(3):481–90.

Asif MK, Nambiar P, Mani SA, Ibrahim NB, Khan IM, Sukumaran P. Dental age estimation employing CBCT scans enhanced with Mimics software: comparison of two different approaches using pulp/tooth volumetric analysis. J Forensic Legal Med. 2018;54:53–61.

Chaillet N, Demirjian A. Dental maturity in South France: a comparison between Demirjian's method and polynomial functions. J Forensic Sci. 2004;49(5):JFS2004037-8.

Demirjian A, Goldstein H, Tanner JM. A new system of dental age assessment. Hum Biol. 1973:211–27.

Gustafson G. Age determinations on teeth. J Am Dent Assoc. 1950;41(1):45–54.

Mincer HH, Harris EF, Berryman HE. The ABFO study of third molar development and its use as an estimator of chronological age. J Forensic Sci. 1993;38(2):379–90.

Rötzscher K, editor. Forensic and legal dentistry. Switzerland: Springer; 2014.

Schour I, Massler M. Development of human dentition chart. 2nd ed. Chicago: American Dental Association; 1944.

Senn DR, Stimson PG, editors. Forensic dentistry. CRC Press; 2010.

Supplementary Information

W. M Tilakaratne, T. G. Kallarakkal (eds.), *Clinicopathological Correlation of Oral Diseases*,
https://doi.org/10.1007/978-3-031-24408-7

Index

D

E

F

G

H

I

J

K

L

M

N

O

P

R

S

T

U

V

W

X

Z

GPSR Compliance

The European Union's (EU) General Product Safety Regulation (GPSR) is a set of rules that requires consumer products to be safe and our obligations to ensure this.

If you have any concerns about our products, you can contact us on ProductSafety@springernature.com

In case Publisher is established outside the EU, the EU authorized representative is:

Springer Nature Customer Service Center GmbH
Europaplatz 3
69115 Heidelberg, Germany

Batch number: 08328717

Printed by Printforce, the Netherlands